IMAGING IN
OTOLARYNGOLOGY

GURGEL | HARNSBERGER

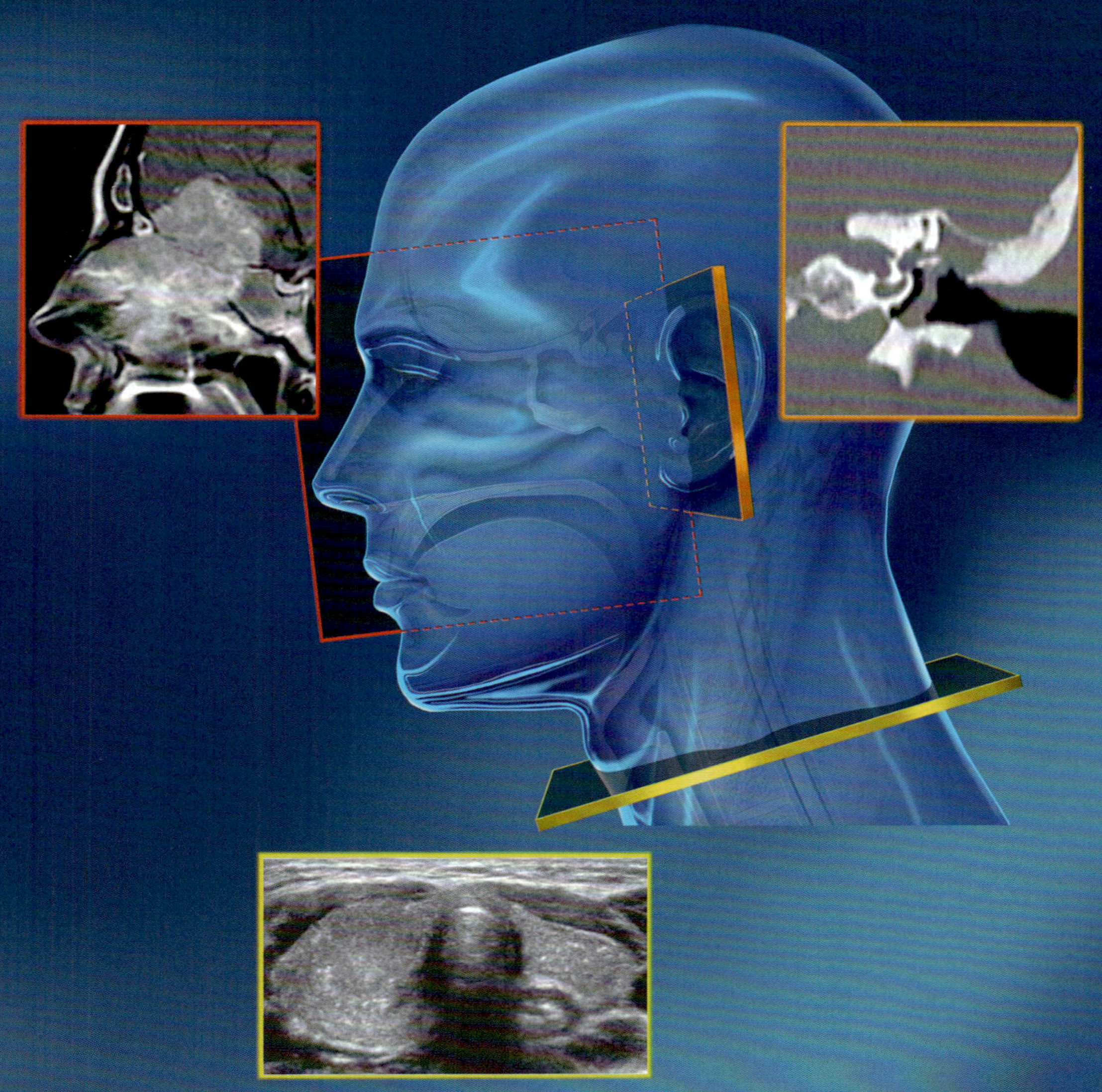

ELSEVIER

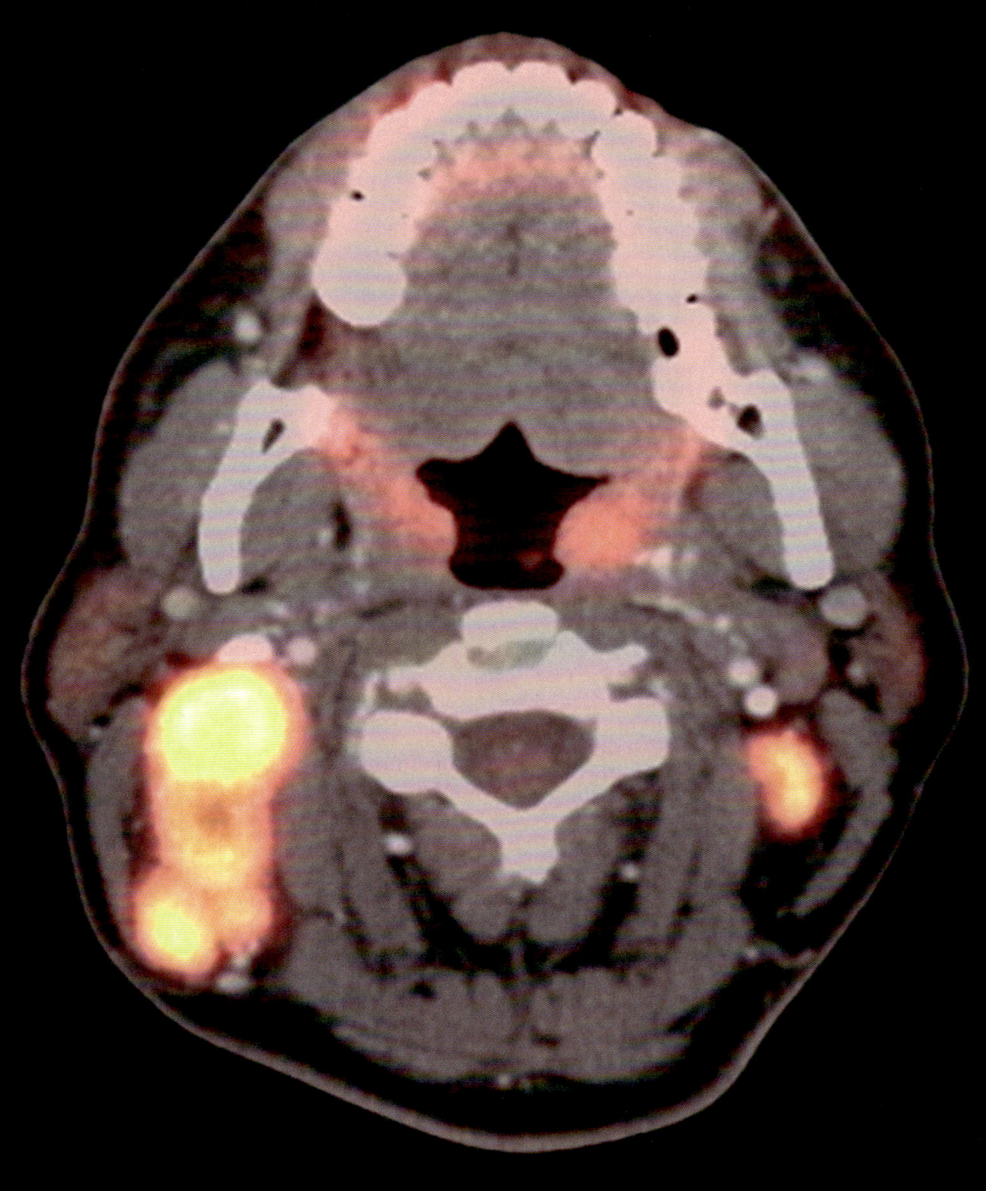

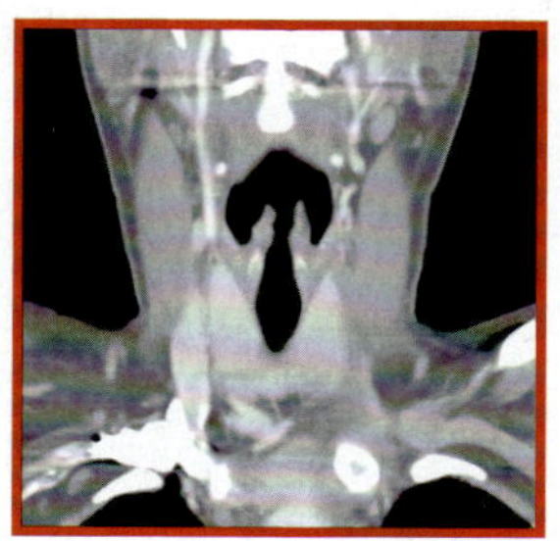

IMAGING IN OTOLARYNGOLOGY

Richard K. Gurgel, MD
Associate Professor Otolaryngology – Head and Neck Surgery
University of Utah School of Medicine
Salt Lake City, Utah

H. Ric Harnsberger, MD
R.C. Willey Chair in Neuroradiology
Professor of Radiology and Otolaryngology
University of Utah School of Medicine
Salt Lake City, Utah

ELSEVIER

1600 John F. Kennedy Blvd.
Ste 1800
Philadelphia, PA 19103-2899

IMAGING IN OTOLARYNGOLOGY, FIRST EDITION

ISBN: 978-0-323-54508-2

Notices

Knowledge and best practice in this field are constantly changing. As new research and experience broaden our understanding, changes in research methods, professional practices, or medical treatment may become necessary.

Practitioners and researchers must always rely on their own experience and knowledge in evaluating and using any information, methods, compounds, or experiments described herein. In using such information or methods they should be mindful of their own safety and the safety of others, including parties for whom they have a professional responsibility.

With respect to any drug or pharmaceutical products identified, readers are advised to check the most current information provided (i) on procedures featured or (ii) by the manufacturer of each product to be administered, to verify the recommended dose or formula, the method and duration of administration, and contraindications. It is the responsibility of practitioners, relying on their own experience and knowledge of their patients, to make diagnoses, to determine dosages and the best treatment for each individual patient, and to take all appropriate safety precautions.

To the fullest extent of the law, neither the Publisher nor the authors, contributors, or editors, assume any liability for any injury and/or damage to persons or property as a matter of products liability, negligence or otherwise, or from any use or operation of any methods, products, instructions, or ideas contained in the material herein.

Publisher Cataloging-in-Publication Data

Names: Gurgel, Richard K. | Harnsberger, H. Ric.
Title: Imaging in otolaryngology / [edited by] Richard K. Gurgel and H. Ric Harnsberger.
Description: First edition. | Salt Lake City, UT : Elsevier, Inc., [2018] | Includes bibliographical references and index.
Identifiers: ISBN 978-0-323-54508-2
Subjects: LCSH: Otolaryngology--Handbooks, manuals, etc. | Ear--Diseases--Handbooks, manuals, etc. | Throat--Diseases--Handbooks, manuals, etc. | Magnetic resonance imaging--Diagnostic use--Handbooks, manuals, etc. | MESH: Otolaryngology--Atlases. | Ear Diseases--diagnostic imaging--Atlases. | Magnetic Resonance Spectroscopy--Atlases.
Classification: LCC RF56.I434 2018 | NLM WV 39 | DDC 617.51--dc23

International Standard Book Number: 978-0-323-54508-2

Cover Designer: Tom M. Olson, BA

Printed in Canada by Friesens, Altona, Manitoba, Canada

Last digit is the print number: 9 8 7 6 5 4 3 2 1

Dedications

I would like to dedicate this book to my wife, Kristie, and five daughters, Anna, Kennedy, Taylor, Elizabeth, and Heidi, who represent my greatest support and will be my most important legacy. I would also like to dedicate this work to my dad, Klaus, the consummate academician.

RKG

This last book is dedicated to my wife and much better half, Janet. You keep my world hopping, vital, and happy! Also to Dave, Dan & Dylan, Danielle, and grandson Roen. You all are the living branches of our Harnsberger family tree.

HRH

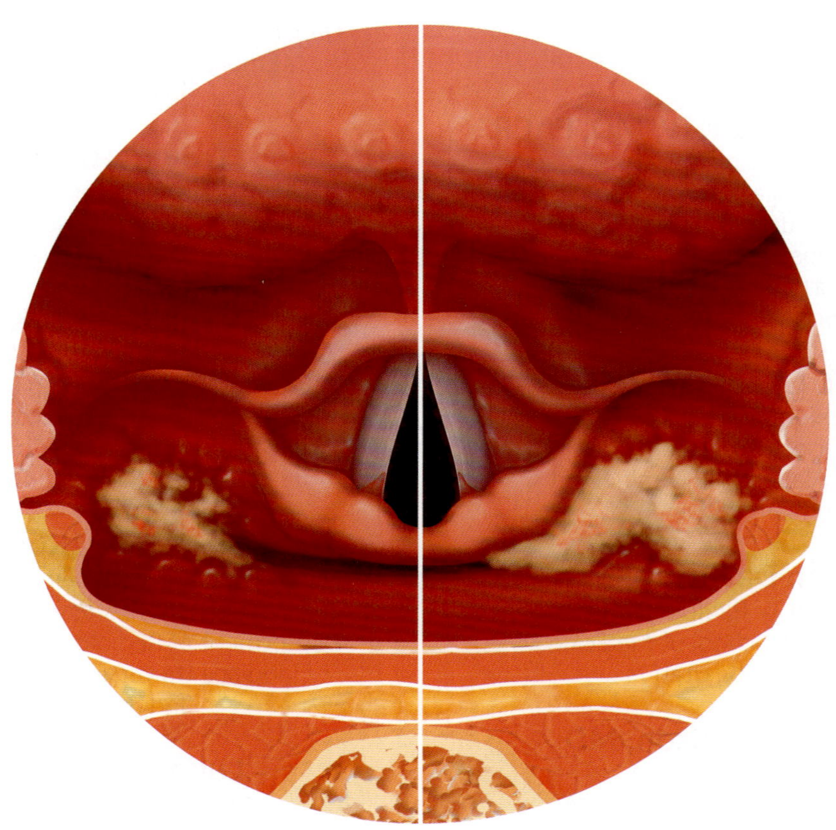

Contributing Authors

Atul Mallik, MD, PhD
Visiting Instructor Neuroradiology Fellow
Radiology and Imaging Sciences
University of Utah
Salt Lake City, Utah

Additional Contributors

Yoshimi Anzai, MD, MPH
Professor of Radiology
Associate Chief Medical Quality Officer
University of Utah
Salt Lake City, Utah

Barton F. Branstetter, IV, MD, FACR
Associate Professor of Radiology, Otolaryngology, and Biomedical Informatics
University of Pittsburgh School of Medicine
Director of Head and Neck Imaging
University of Pittsburgh Medical Center
Pittsburgh, Pennsylvania

Philip R. Chapman, MD
Section Chief, Neuroradiology
Associate Professor
University of Alabama at Birmingham
Birmingham, Alabama

H. Christian Davidson, MD
Professor of Radiology
University of Utah School of Medicine
Salt Lake City, Utah

Bronwyn E. Hamilton, MD
Professor of Radiology
Director of Head & Neck Radiology
Oregon Health & Science University
Portland, Oregon

Patricia A. Hudgins, MD, FACR
Professor of Radiology and Otolaryngology
Director of Head & Neck Radiology
Department of Radiology and Imaging Sciences
Emory University School of Medicine
Atlanta, Georgia

Troy A. Hutchins, MD
Assistant Professor of Radiology
University of Utah School of Medicine
Salt Lake City, Utah

Bernadette L. Koch, MD
Associate Director of Radiology
Cincinnati Children's Hospital Medical Center
Professor of Clinical Radiology and Pediatrics
University of Cincinnati College of Medicine
Cincinnati, Ohio

Nicholas A. Koontz, MD
Dean D. T. Maglinte Scholar in Radiology Education
Assistant Professor of Radiology
Department of Radiology and Imaging Sciences
Indiana University School of Medicine
Indianapolis, Indiana

Luke N. Ledbetter, MD
Assistant Professor of Radiology
Division of Neuroradiology
University of Kansas Medical Center
Kansas City, Kansas

Daniel E. Meltzer, MD
Associate Clinical Professor of Radiology
Icahn School of Medicine at Mount Sinai
New York, New York

A. Carlson Merrow, Jr., MD, FAAP
Corning Benton Chair for Radiology Education
Cincinnati Children's Hospital Medical Center
Associate Professor of Clinical Radiology
University of Cincinnati College of Medicine
Cincinnati, Ohio

Kristine M. Mosier, DMD, PhD
Associate Professor of Radiology
Chief, Head and Neck Radiology
Indiana University School of Medicine
Department of Radiology & Imaging Sciences
Indianapolis, Indiana

C. Douglas Phillips, MD, FACR
Professor of Radiology
Director of Head and Neck Imaging
Weill Cornell Medicine
NewYork-Presbyterian Hospital
New York, New York

Caroline D. Robson, MBChB
Operations Vice Chair, Radiology
Chief, Neuroradiology & Head and Neck Imaging
Boston Children's Hospital
Associate Professor of Radiology
Harvard Medical School
Boston, Massachusetts

Karen L. Salzman, MD
Professor of Radiology
Chief of Neuroradiology
Leslie W. Davis Endowed Chair in Neuroradiology
University of Utah School of Medicine
Salt Lake City, Utah

Hilda E. Stambuk, MD
Attending Radiologist
Clinical Head of Head and Neck Imaging
Memorial Sloan-Kettering Cancer Center
Professor of Clinical Radiology
Weill Cornell Medicine
New York, New York

Richard H. Wiggins, III, MD, CIIP, FSIIM
Director of Head and Neck Imaging
Director of Imaging Informatics
Professor, Departments of Radiology,
Otolaryngology, Head and Neck Surgery, and
BioMedical Informatics
University of Utah Health Sciences Center
Salt Lake City, Utah

Blair A. Winegar, MD
Assistant Professor of Medical Imaging
Division of Neuroradiology
University of Arizona College of Medicine
Banner - University Medical Center
Tucson, Arizona

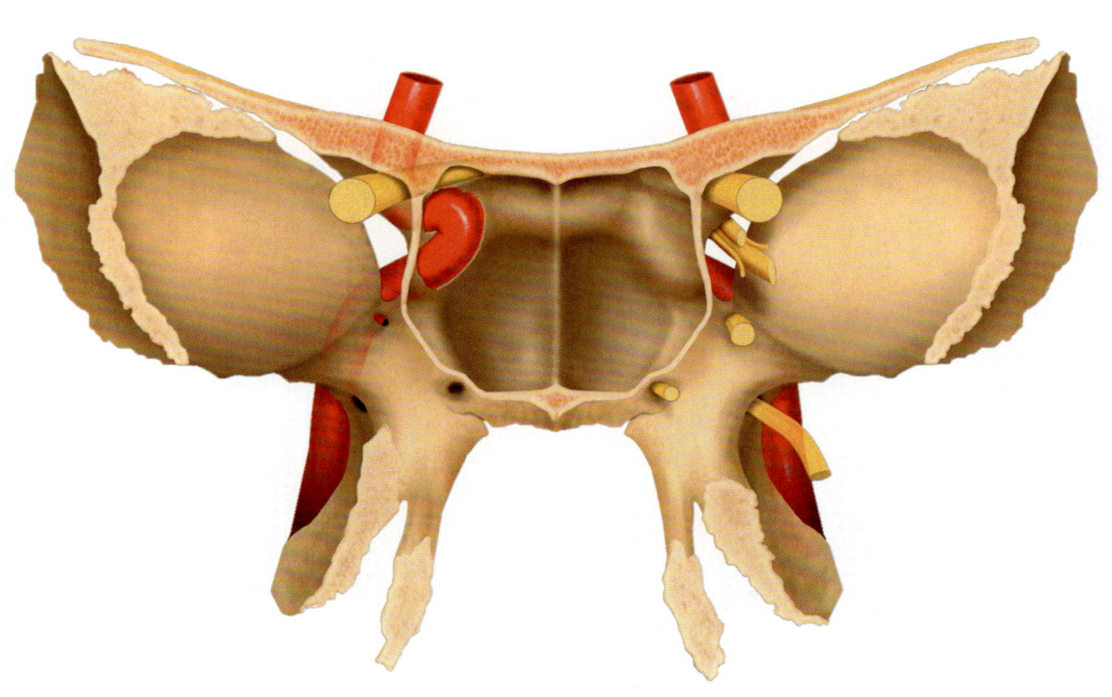

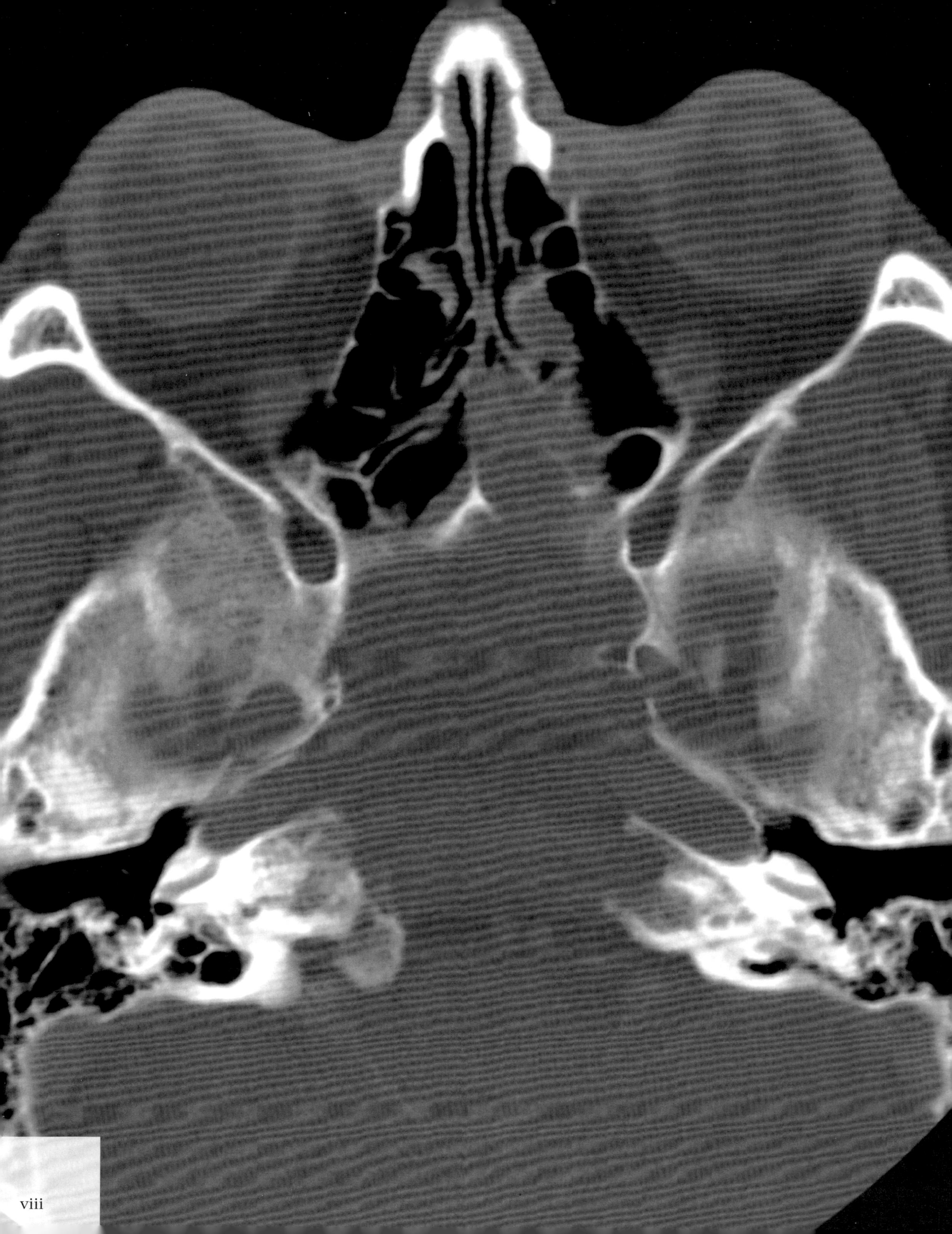

Preface

Imaging plays a critical role in otolaryngology. Appropriate management of patients with disorders of the ear, nose, and throat requires a thorough understanding of the complexity of head and neck anatomy. One of the foundational principles of surgery is knowing how a disease affects a patient's anatomy, and how a patient's anatomy affects the disease. Imaging helps clinicians gain the necessary understanding of this process.

Multiple imaging modalities are employed in otolaryngology. Computed tomography (CT) is widely used to evaluate the structures of the temporal bone and skull base, sinonasal cavity, and soft tissues of the neck, including tumor staging. Magnetic resonance (MR) imaging provides exquisite detail of the cerebellopontine angle and brain, tumor anatomy, and other soft tissue pathology, especially when multiple different MR sequences are utilized. Ultrasound is often the imaging modality of choice for thyroid disease. Functional imaging, such as positron emission tomography (PET) imaging, can be used for staging and surveillance of patients with head and neck malignancies. Angiography is utilized for vascular lesions or highly vascular neoplasms in the head and neck. Understanding which modality will yield the most useful information for any given patient is essential for the discerning clinician.

This book grew from the collegial relationship of the two senior authors, Drs. Harnsberger and Gurgel, a relationship that developed over years of weekly radiology conferences and discussing individual patients. It is our hope that a similar relationship between clinicians and radiologists is replicated in the readers' home institutions. Each specialty can inform the other, and being able to communicate openly about interesting clinical and radiographic findings enhances patient care.

This book will provide clinicians with a fund of knowledge that is directly applicable to their practice. In addition to the four key images printed for each condition, there is a rich online repository of digital images, both histological and clinical, that exhibit variations in disease presentation and severity. These are all accessible via the mobile application so the clinician can have easy access virtually anywhere.

We hope that you find this resource useful as you further develop your clinical acumen in reading and interpreting imaging studies.

Enjoy!

Richard K. Gurgel, MD
Associate Professor Otolaryngology – Head and Neck Surgery
University of Utah School of Medicine
Salt Lake City, Utah

H. Ric Harnsberger, MD
R.C. Willey Chair in Neuroradiology
Professor of Radiology and Otolaryngology
University of Utah School of Medicine
Salt Lake City, Utah

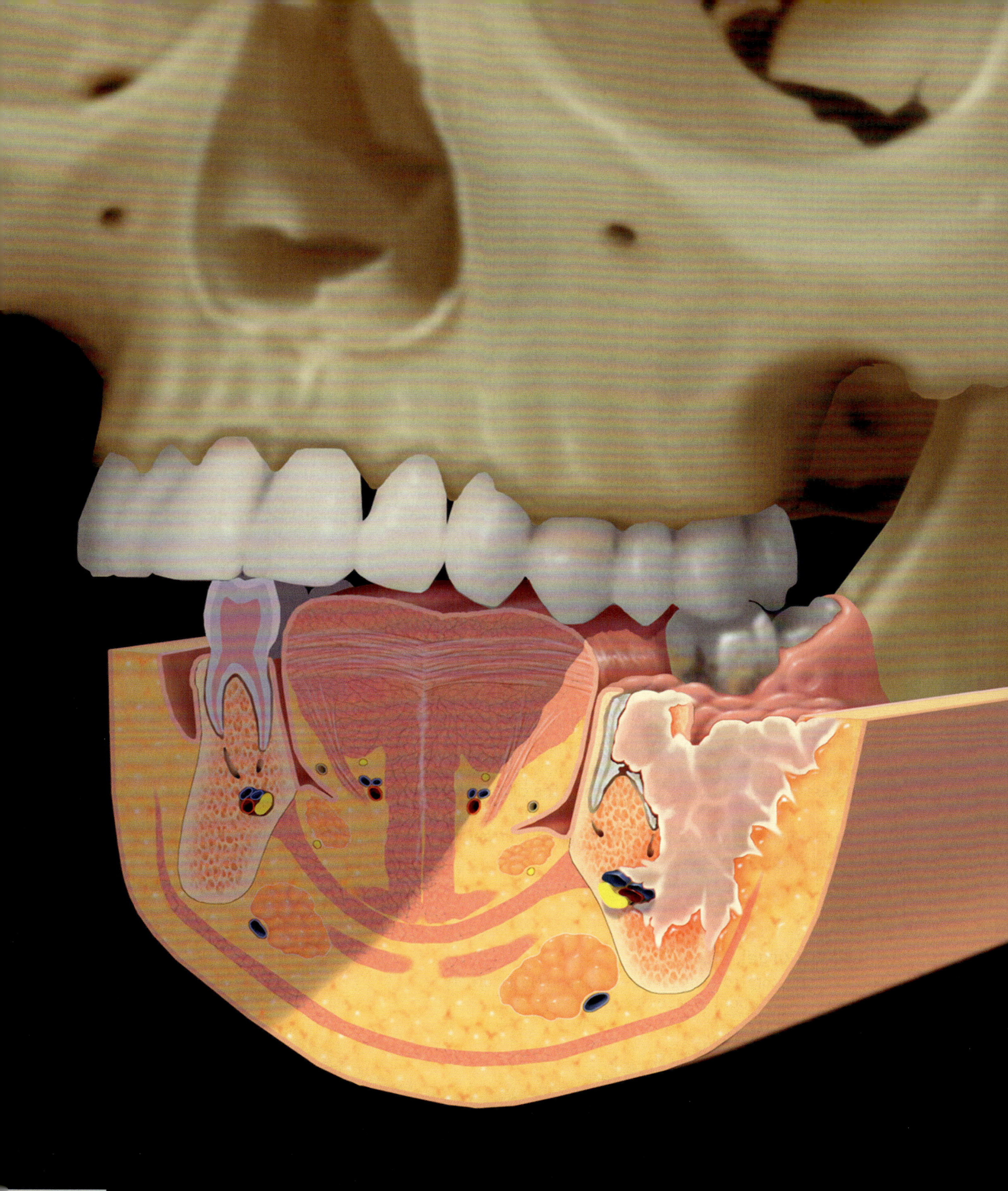

Acknowledgments

Lead Editor

Nina I. Bennett, BA

Text Editors

Arthur G. Gelsinger, MA
Rebecca L. Bluth, BA
Terry W. Ferrell, MS
Lisa A. Gervais, BS
Matt W. Hoecherl, BS
Megg Morin, BA

Image Editors

Jeffrey J. Marmorstone, BS
Lisa A. M. Steadman, BS

Illustrations

Richard Coombs, MS
Lane R. Bennion, MS
Laura C. Wissler, MA

Art Direction and Design

Tom M. Olson, BA
Laura C. Wissler, MA

Production Coordinators

Angela M. G. Terry, BA
Emily C. Fassett, BA

ELSEVIER

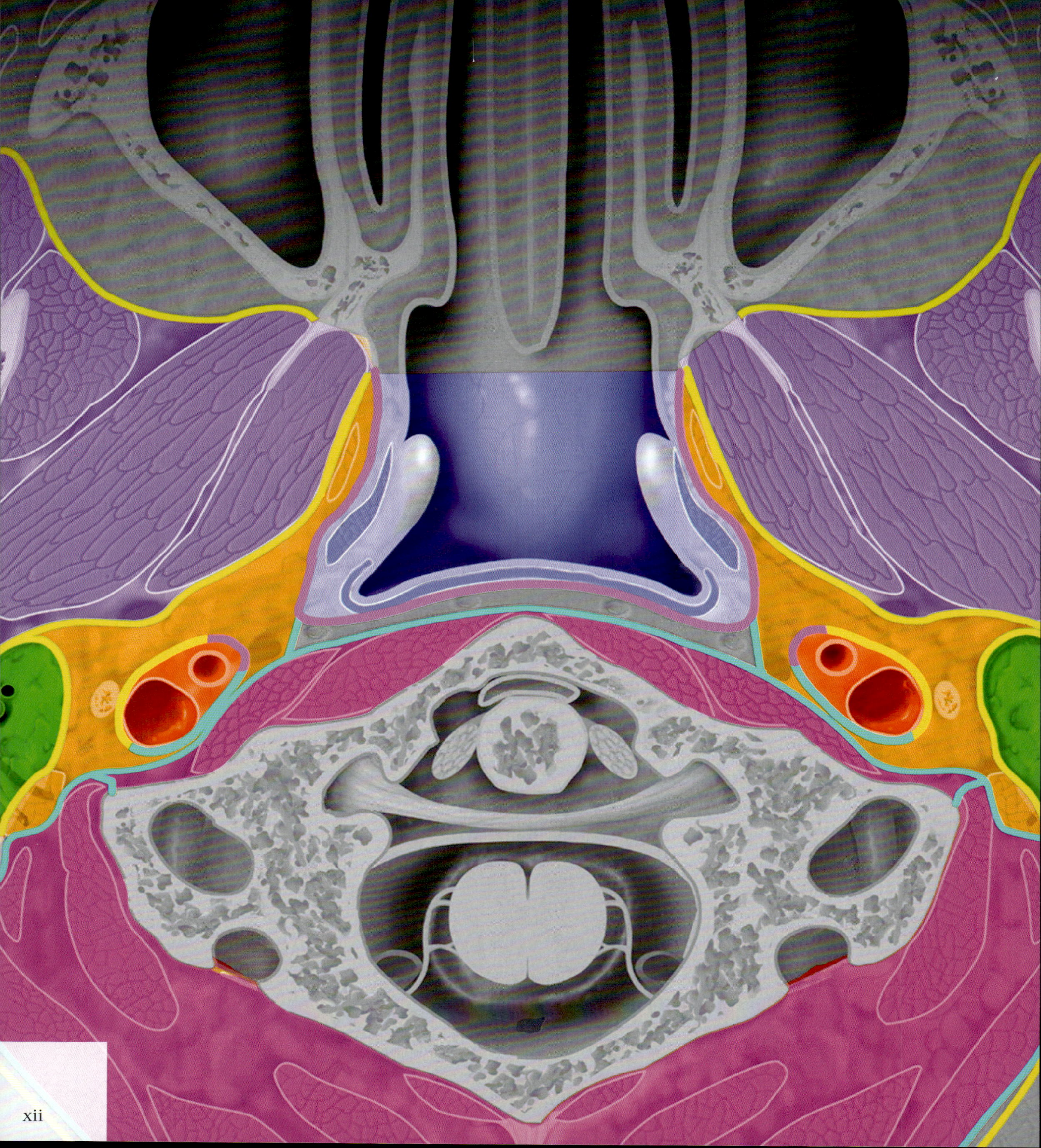

Sections

TABLE OF CONTENTS

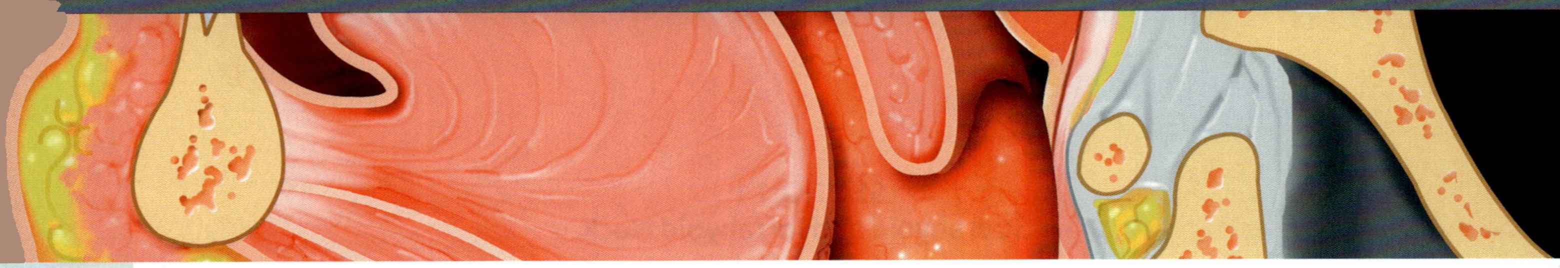

TABLE OF CONTENTS

TABLE OF CONTENTS

TABLE OF CONTENTS

TABLE OF CONTENTS

TABLE OF CONTENTS

TABLE OF CONTENTS

TABLE OF CONTENTS

TABLE OF CONTENTS

TABLE OF CONTENTS

TEMPORAL BONE, NO SPECIFIC ANATOMIC LOCATION

CPA-IAC

CONGENITAL LESIONS

INFECTIOUS AND INFLAMMATORY LESIONS

BENIGN AND MALIGNANT TUMORS

VASCULAR LESIONS

RADIOLOGY ABBREVIATION INDEX

11C: carbon-11

123-FP-CIT: [123I]N-ω-co-fluoropropyl-2β-carbomethoxy-3β-(4-iodophenyl)nortropane)

15O: oxygen-15

99mTC: technetium-99m

A

ACCa: adenoid cystic carcinoma

ADC: apparent diffusion coefficient

AP: anteroposterior

ASL: arterial spin labeling

ASVD: atrioventricular septal defect

B

BMT: benign mixed tumor

C

CBF: cerebral blood flow

CBV: cerebral blood volume

CECT: contrast-enhanced computed tomography

Cho: choline

CISS: constructive interference in steady state

CPA: cerebellopontine angle

Cr: chromium

CT: computed tomography

CTA: computed tomography angiography

CTP: computed tomography perfusion

CTV: computed tomography venography

D

DaT: dopamine transporter

DCE: dynamic contrast-enhanced (MR)

DSA: digital subtraction angiography

DSC: dynamic susceptibility contrast-enhanced (MRI)

DST: dural sinus thrombosis

DTI: diffusion tensor imaging (MRI)

DWI: diffusion-weighted imaging

DWI MR: diffusion-weighted imaging using MR

E

EAC: external auditory canal

ECD: Tc N,N'-l,2-ethylenediylbis-L-cysteine diethyl ester

ENog: electroneuromyography

EMG: electromyography

F

F-18 FDG: F-18 fluorodeoxyglucose

FESS: functional endoscopic sinus surgery

FIESTA: fast imaging employing steady-state acquisition

FISP: fast imaging with steady-state precession

FLAIR: fluid-attenuated inversion recovery

fMRI: functional magnetic resonance imaging

FSE T2: T2 fast-spin echo imaging

FS-PGR: focal segmental pulse-generated runoff

G

Glx: glutamic acid

GRE: gradient echo

H

HMPAO: hexamethylpropyleneamine oxime

HU: Hounsfield unit

I

I&D: incision and drainage

IAC: Internal auditory canal

ICA: internal carotid artery

IVJ: internal jugular vein

K

kPS: endothelial transfer coefficient

L

Lac: lactate

M

MDCT: multidetector computed tomography

MIP: maximum intensity projection

MP-RAGE: magnetization-prepared rapid acquisition gradient echo

MR: magnetic resonance

MR T1: magnetic resonance T1

MRA: magnetic resonance angiography

MRP: magnetic resonance perfusion

MRS: magnetic resonance spectroscopy

MRV: magnetic resonance venography

MTT: mean transit time

N

NAA: N-acetylaspartate

NASCET: North American Symptomatic Carotid Endarterectomy Trial

NCS: nerve conduction study

NCV: nerve conduction velocity

NECT: nonenhanced computed tomography

P

PACS: picture archiving and communications system

PC: phase contrast

pCT: positron computed tomography

PD: pulsed Doppler (wave)

PET: positron emission tomography

PE (tubes): pressure equalizer

PiB: Pittsburgh compound B

pMR: proton magnetic resonance

PORP: partial ossicular replacement prosthesis

PPS: parapharyngeal space

PVT: portal vein thrombosis

PWI: perfusion-weighted (MR) imaging

R

RF: radiofrequency

S

SCC: semicircular canal

SCCa: squamous cell carcinoma

SNHL: sensorineural hearing loss

SPACE: sampling perfection with application-optimized contrast with different flip-angle evolutions

SPECT: single photon emission computed tomography

SPGR: spoiled gradient echo

SRT: stereotactic radiotherapy

SSP: section sensitivity profile

STIR: short tau inversion recovery

STIR MR: short tau inversion recovery MR

SWI: susceptibility weighted imaging

T

T1: spin lattice or longitudinal relaxation time (MR scan)

T1 C+: T1 contrast enhanced

T1 C+ FS: T1 contrast enhanced with fat suppression

T1WI: T1-weighted imaging

T2: spin-spin or transverse relaxation time

T2*: T2 star, observed or effective T2

T2* GRE: gradient echo T2 star

T2* SWI: T2 star susceptibility weighted imaging

T2WI: T2-weighted imaging

T2WI FS MR: T2-weighted magnetic resonance imaging with fat suppression

TE: echo time

TEF: tracheoesophageal fistula

TM: tympanic membrane

TOF: time of flight

TORP: total ossicular replacement prosthesis

tPA: tissue plasminogen activator

TR: recovery time

TTP: time to peak

X

XRT: radiation therapy

IMAGING IN OTOLARYNGOLOGY

GURGEL | HARNSBERGER

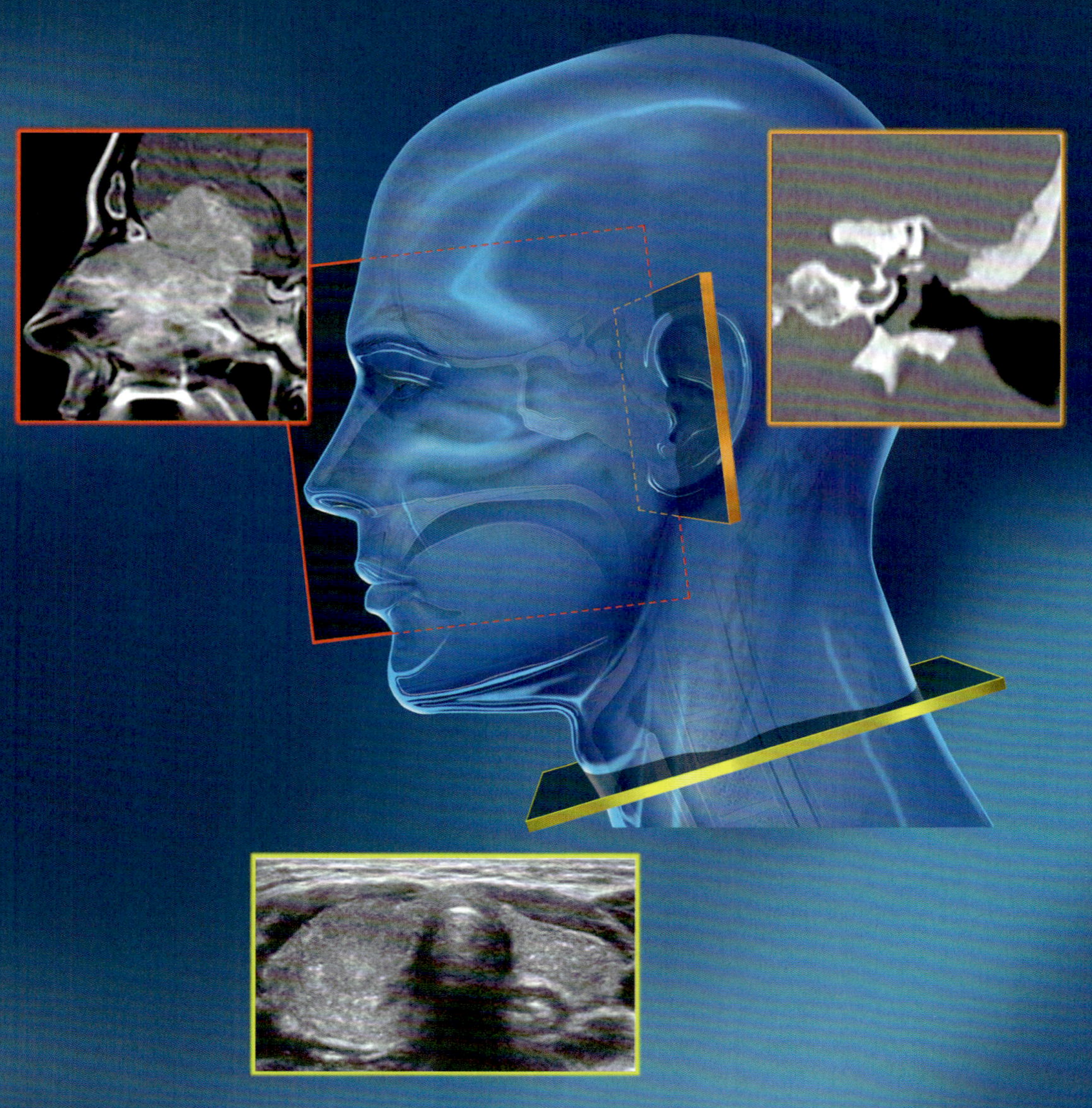

ELSEVIER

Introduction

Rapid advancement of medical imaging in the last few decades has significantly enhanced the role of imaging in medicine. Imaging plays an integral role in the evaluation of many of the diseases confronted by the otolaryngologist. It is performed for diagnosis, staging of tumors, assessing efficacy of therapy, follow-up, and guidance for procedures.

Imaging in the head and neck, like no other area of the human body, differs considerably based on the specific anatomic area of interest. In fact, unique imaging protocols have been designed for at least 9 specific areas of the head and neck. These include from superior to inferior the cerebellopontine angle-internal auditory canal (CPA-IAC), skull base, temporal bone, orbit, sinus and nose, suprahyoid neck, infrahyoid neck, pharynx, and larynx. Clinical history and physical findings in combination with high-resolution imaging available today create the possibility of a highly specific clinical-radiologic diagnosis. Computed tomography (CT) and magnetic resonance (MR) form the backbone of the imaging work-up of patients with diseases of the head and neck.

Imaging Modalities

In the past, radiography ("plain films" and "tomography") played a significant, but not very effective, role in imaging of the head and neck. With the emergence of advanced imaging, the role of radiography has virtually disappeared. Currently, CT, MR, and PET/CT are the most commonly performed imaging modalities for diseases of the head and neck. Modern multidetector, multiplanar CT now creates exquisite anatomical detail allowing the diagnosis of very small lesions, such as temporal bone otosclerosis, not thought possible even a decade ago. MR techniques, such as multiplanar thin-section enhanced, fat-saturated T1, allow the imager to identify subtle findings, such as perineural tumor spread along extracranial portions of cranial nerves. The use of a variety of MR sequences (T1, T2, FLAIR, GRE, enhanced T1 fat-saturated) permit the imager to differentiate tissue types, such as normal muscle from tumor. Other unique MR sequences can suggest specific diagnoses, such as the case of diffusion weighted imaging (DWI) MR sequence being highly specific for the diagnosis of epidermoid.

Likewise, fluorodeoxyglucose positron emission tomography (FDG-PET)/CT imaging has a distinct role in the imaging of patients with squamous cell carcinoma (SCCa) staging and follow-up. Metabolically active primary tumor and malignant nodes mapped against an underlying contrast-enhanced CT can help differentiate normal tonsillar tissue and reactive nodes from invasive SCCa primary and metastatic nodes. Ultrasound and color Doppler are useful in evaluating the head and neck vasculature. Ultrasound is also used to evaluate neck masses and localize them for fine-needle aspiration.

CT

CT technology relies on the same physical principles as x-rays. The differential absorption of the x-ray beam by different tissues produces varied levels of density in the image (see Table 1), which on CT scans are measured in **Hounsfield units** (HU). This can be displayed in cross-sectional format or in multiple planes. Multidetector CT has enlarged the capability of CT with faster scans, greater spatial resolution, and multiplanar reformations.

Nonenhanced CT (NECT)

The role for NECT in head and neck imaging is small. A ductal stone, lesion chondroid (cartilaginous) or osteoid (bony) matrix, or radiopaque foreign body can be seen in the presence of contrast in the vessels of the neck. As a rule, contrast-enhanced CT (CECT) is done in all soft tissue neck imaging examinations if renal function and allergy history allow.

CECT

CECT is the workhorse in imaging the soft tissues of the extracranial head and neck. CECT is often preferred to MR because the images are acquired rapidly (fractions of seconds), whereas MR sequences require the patient to remain still for 3-5 minutes at a time (see Table 2). This is especially true in the infrahyoid neck area where movement artifact degrades MR images considerably.

CECT is routinely used as a starting exam in most patients who need imaging of the head and neck to evaluate a deep tissue clinical question. Staging and follow-up of pharyngeal and laryngeal SCCa, abscess search, and suspected mass evaluation are but a few of the uses of CECT.

Thin-Section Bone CT

Temporal bone, skull base, and sinonasal CT evaluations begin with unenhanced, multiplanar, thin-section, and bone algorithm CT. Slice thickness varies by area (temporal bone: 0.6 mm; skull base: 1-2 mm; sinuses: 2-3 mm). If soft tissue questions remain after the CT is completed in these 3 areas, enhanced fat-saturated T1 MR is used to analyze tissue type and extent instead of repeating the CT with contrast at a later date.

CT Angiogram (CTA)

For many, CTA remains the study of choice for all emergent and nonemergent vascular conditions, such as carotid atherosclerotic stenosis, dissection, and pseudoaneurysm. It can also be used in the setting of a suspected dural arteriovenous fistula and carotid cavernous fistula. Other uses of CTA include assessing the integrity of the internal carotid artery when it is involved by dural tumors, such as meningioma or invasive neck SCCa. When significant neck trauma suggests the possibility of arterial injury, CTA is ideal to answer this clinical question. CTA is fast and less prone to artifact than MR angiography (MRA). A combined CTA of the head and neck, from the aortic arch to the cranial vertex, can be obtained with as little as 70 ml of IV contrast in < 15 seconds.

CT Venogram (CTV)

CTV is similar to CTA except for an added delay for optimal visualization of the venous system. It is a fast, reliable modality to exclude dural sinus thrombosis in an emergent setting. It is particularly helpful in the search for venous sinus thrombosis in the posterior fossa and skull base.

MR

The primary origin of the MR signal used to generate clinical images comes from hydrogen nuclei. Hydrogen nuclei consist of a single proton that is constantly spinning. A radio frequency pulse (RF pulse) emitted from the scanner results in some of the hydrogen protons being "knocked" out of alignment with the static magnetic field. As the energy from the RF pulse is dissipated, the hydrogen protons will return to alignment with the static magnetic field. The MR signal is derived from the hydrogen protons as they move back into alignment with the magnetic field. The MR signal is then broken down and spatially located to produce images.

The movement of the neck, which occurs during swallowing, coughing, sneezing, scratching, and breathing, often degrades the diagnostic quality of MR images of the neck. Enhanced fat-saturated MR is preferred over CECT in the suprahyoid neck where movement is less frequent and in the oral cavity when dental amalgam artifact obscures the CT image. MR is also a powerful imaging tool for mass lesions in the CPA-IAC, orbit, skull base, and sinonasal areas.

T1 and T2 are the fundamental parameters of MR and determine the contrast between tissues. MR sequences that emphasize tissue differences in T1 relaxation are called **T1 weighted**, and those that emphasize T2 relaxation are called **T2 weighted**. Tissues with short T1 relaxation time, such as fat, melanin, and protein, produce high signal on T1-weighted sequences and appear "bright," whereas fluid is relatively dark. Fluid has a long T2 relaxation time and appears bright on T2-weighted sequences.

Spin-echo and gradient-echo are 2 basic sequences in MR. All other sequences are variations of one of these sequences and are used to better characterize specific tissue types.

Fluid-attenuation inversion recovery (FLAIR) sequence eliminates fluid signal, which thus appears dark. It is useful for highlighting cisternal lesions. "Bright" CSF sulcal signal on FLAIR may suggest leptomeningeal disease with replacement of normal CSF by pus (meningitis), blood (subarachnoid hemorrhage), or tumor cells (leptomeningeal carcinomatosis).

Short-tau inversion recovery (STIR) sequence is used to eliminate signal from fat. In the head and neck area, STIR often displays fluid-containing lesions (cysts, abscess) as conspicuous high-signal (bright) lesions. It is also used in diagnosing fat-containing lesions like lipoma and dermoid cyst.

Diffusion-weighted imaging (DWI) shows the molecular motion or diffusion of water protons within tissue. DWI generates diffusion and apparent diffusion coefficient (ADC) maps. ADC is a measure of the magnitude of diffusion. True restricted diffusion will be bright on diffusion and dark on ADC maps. Restricted diffusion can be seen in processes like pyogenic abscess, highly cellular tumor, and epidermoid cyst. Generally, the ADC value of malignant tissue is < the ADC value of benign tumors.

Gradient-echo sequence (GRE) is sensitive to small amounts of blood breakdown products as well as calcium and metallic deposits, fat, and air. In lesions with blood products (lymphatic malformation, cholesterol granuloma, paraganglioma) or calcifications (osteosarcoma, chondrosarcoma, meningioma), the focal areas of blood will be low signal and bloom on GRE sequences.

MRA

Time-of-flight (TOF) imaging is most commonly used for MRA. Signal in intracranial arteries is related to flow phenomenon, and thus no IV gadolinium is needed. TOF MRA can be performed by both 2D and 3D techniques.

Contrast-enhanced MRA is often used to evaluate the neck vasculature. Contrast-enhanced intracranial MRA is useful in patients with stents &/or coils.

MR Venogram (MRV)

MRV can be performed with 2D/3D TOF techniques, which do not need administration of IV gadolinium. Contrast-enhanced MRV is, however, more robust and is less susceptible to artifacts compared with the TOF techniques.

PET/CT

PET/CT is the best imaging modality for staging, monitoring, and surveillance of advanced head and neck SCCa. It is superior to PET, CECT, or MR imaging alone. It is also superior for identifying 2nd primary tumors.

A basic understanding of the core workings of PET is essential. Fluorodeoxyglucose (FDG) is transported into a cell in the same manner as normal glucose. There, it becomes trapped and accumulates in cells with high glucose metabolism. Fused PET/CT offers the imager combined anatomic and physiologic information. It distinguishes extensive physiologic FDG uptake in the head and neck from true pathologic uptake. **Standardized uptake value** (SUV) provides a quantified measure of FDG uptake.

The clinical utility of PET/CT for SCCa of the head and neck depends on the size of primary tumor. This technique is most useful for evaluating for nodal and distant metastases with locally **advanced T3 or T4 tumors** or those with known nodal metastases. It also supplies specific information about the presence of **2nd primary tumors** in the body. In the clinical setting of malignant metastatic nodes without a clinically identified primary tumor ("**unknown primary**"), PET/CT at times will locate the hidden primary tumor.

Pitfalls of PET/CT are multiple. False-positive uptake from normal physiology, inflammation, and posttreatment changes must be guarded against. False-negative uptake from cystic lesions (necrotic primary or nodal metastases), small tumors, and non-FDG-avid tumors may be encountered. Reading head and neck PET/CT scans requires intimate knowledge of head and neck anatomy and tumor behavior for correct interpretation to be rendered.

Ultrasound and Doppler

Grayscale is used to for extracranial atherosclerotic disease and plaque morphology. Color Doppler detects turbulent blood flow. Doppler spectral analysis measures blood flow velocity, which correlates with the degree of vascular stenosis. Ultrasound is also used to evaluate neck masses (especially in children) and localize them for fine-needle aspiration.

Digital Subtraction Angiography (DSA)

DSA is still considered the "gold standard" in vascular imaging. However, DSA is an invasive procedure associated with risk of complication, with 1% overall incidence of neurologic deficit and 0.5% incidence of persistent deficit. CTA and CTV have made the use of DSA for diagnosis extremely limited. Instead, DSA is used to confirm the diagnosis of arteriovenous fistula while at the same time completing endovascular treatment. It is additionally used for preoperative embolization of vascular tumors, such as paraganglioma and meningioma.

Selected References

1. Dickerson E et al: Advanced imaging techniques of the skull base. Radiol Clin North Am. 55(1):189-200, 2017
2. Corrales CE et al: Imaging innovations in temporal bone disorders. Otolaryngol Clin North Am. 48(2):263-80, 2015
3. Srinivasan A et al: Biologic imaging of head and neck cancer: the present and the future. AJNR Am J Neuroradiol. 33(4):586-94, 2012
4. Fortnum H et al: The role of magnetic resonance imaging in the identification of suspected acoustic neuroma: a systematic review of clinical and cost effectiveness and natural history. Health Technol Assess. 13(18):iii-iv, ix-xi, 1-154, 2009

Table 1: CT Hounsfield Units

Tissue Type	Hounsfield Unit Range
Air	-1000
Fat	-130 to -70
Water/cerebrospinal fluid	0-30
Muscle	40-60
Hemorrhage	70-80
Calcification	80-100
Bone	+400

Table 2: Comparison of CT & MR in Head & Neck Imaging

CT	MR
Few contraindications	Multiple contraindications (implantable devices)
Fast, less motion sensitive	Slower, extremely motion sensitive
Radiation exposure	No radiation exposure
Very good for acute hemorrhage	Excellent for different phases of hemorrhage
Poor soft tissue contrast	Excellent soft tissue contrast
Nephrotoxic contrast	Nephrogenic systemic fibrosis (rare)
Higher incidence of contrast reaction	Lower incidence of contrast reaction
Need contrast for CTA	Noncontrast MRA (flow related)

Table 3: MR Signal Characteristic of Different Tissues

Tissue Type	T1	T2
Dense bone	Low (dark) signal	Low (dark) signal
Fat	High (bright) signal	Loses signal compared with T1
Water	Low (dark) signal	High (bright) signal
Hemorrhage	Variable (hemoglobin breakdown stage dependent)	Variable (hemoglobin breakdown stage dependent)
Muscle	Intermediate signal	Intermediate signal

Table 4: Summary of Preferred Imaging Studies in Head & Neck

Area of Imaging	Preferred 1st Imaging Study
Cerebellopontine angle-internal auditory canal	MR: T1 C+ fat saturated with thin-section T2 (FIESTA, CISS, etc.) for surgical planning
Temporal bone	Bone CT: 0.6-mm thick axial & coronal planes If lesion extends regionally, add MR: 2- to 3-mm thick T1 C+ fat saturated axial & coronal; include DWI
Skull base	Both MR (T1 C+ FS axial & coronal) & CT (bone only, no contrast) for complete lesion analysis
Orbit	MR: T1 C+ fat-saturated; add bone CT for bone changes, calcifications as needed
Sinus & nose	Sinusitis: Bone CT, multiplanar; in invasive fungal sinusitis need T1 C+ fat saturated axial & coronal Tumor: MR, T1 C+ fat saturated axial & coronal; add unenhanced bone CT for surgical planning PRN
Suprahyoid neck	CECT: Base of skull to clavicles; soft tissue & bone algorithms If lesion involves skull base, add enhanced MR for perineural tumor, dural, & vascular invasion
Infrahyoid neck	CECT: Skull base to clavicles; extend to carina if left vagal neuropathy, parathyroid adenoma (PTA) at issue; ultrasound 1st for PTA, then Sestamibi scan, then CECT if anatomic localization needed
Pharynx in staging of squamous cell carcinoma (SCCa)	CECT: Base of skull (BOS) to clavicles; soft tissue & bone algorithms PET/CT controversial: Best for staging, monitoring, & surveillance of **advanced stage SCCa** Add enhanced MR for perineural tumor, dural, vascular invasion or cartilage invasion
Larynx	CECT: BOS to clavicles, quiet respiration; 2nd pass angled along hyoid bone plane with breath holding Add MR if cartilage invasion question on CECT to confirm CT impression

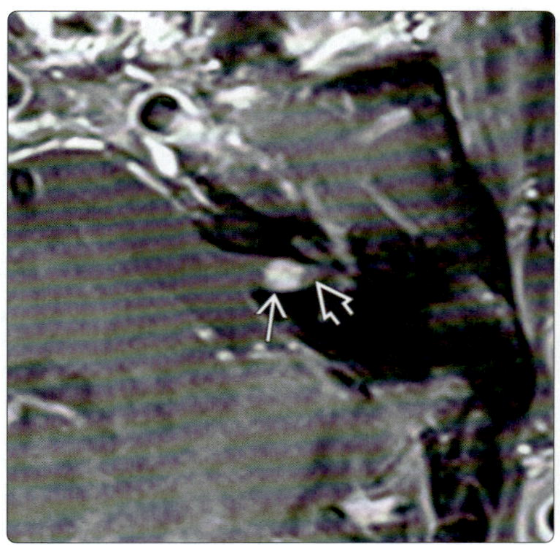

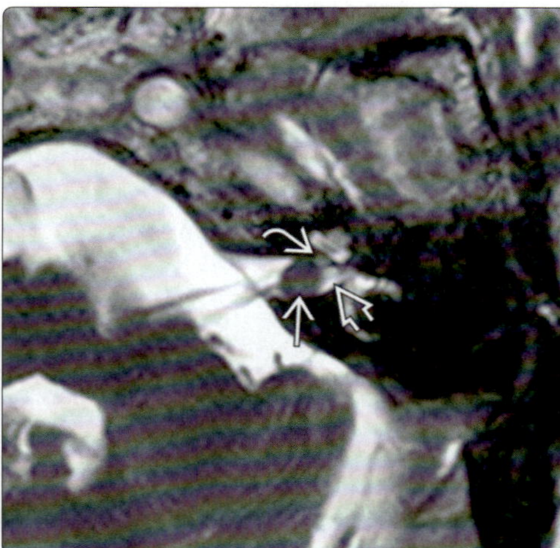

(Left) *Axial T1WI C+ FS MR of the CPA-IAC in a patient with left sensorineural hearing loss shows a small enhancing vestibular schwannoma (VS) ➡ within the IAC with a 3-mm fundal CSF cap ➡ lateral to the tumor. Enhanced T1 FS MR is the gold standard of imaging for CPA-IAC pathology.* **(Right)** *Axial CISS MR in the same patient shows a VS defect ➡ in the high-signal CSF of the IAC. Surgical information like fundal CSF cap size ➡ & the relationship to the cochlear nerve canal ➡ are more readily seen with T2 or T2-like CISS MR sequences.*

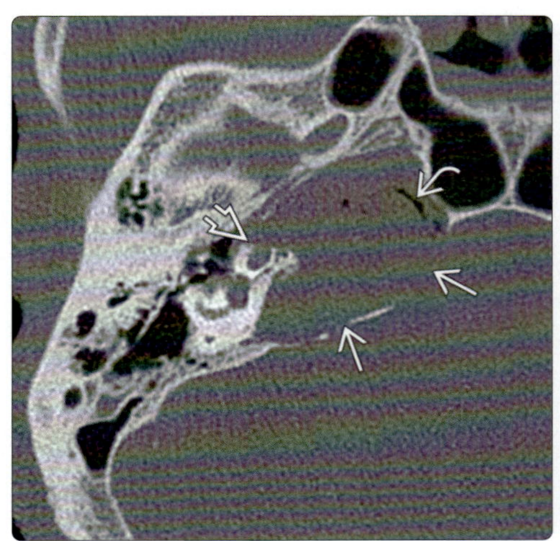

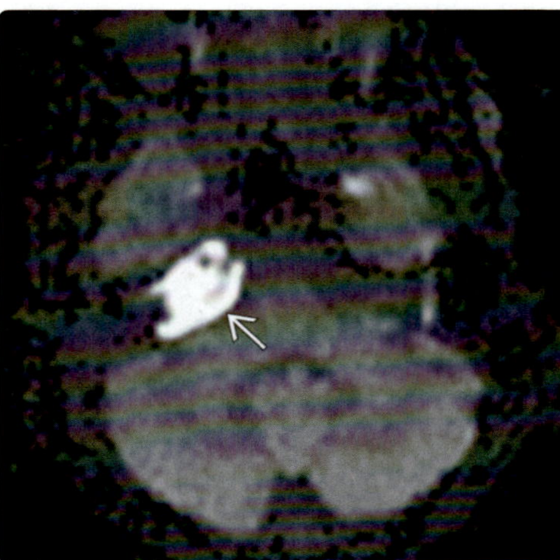

(Left) *Axial bone CT in a patient with a "dead" right ear shows an ovoid petrous apex mass ➡ with intramural air ➡ & cochlear destruction ➡. Cholesteatoma, cholesterol granuloma, and chondrosarcoma are in the differential diagnosis.* **(Right)** *Axial diffusion-weighted MR in same patient shows hyperintense restricted diffusion ➡ diagnostic of cholesteatoma. When CT shows a lesion spreading into adjacent structures, contrast-enhanced MR with special sequences, such as MRA, MRV, and DWI, is recommended.*

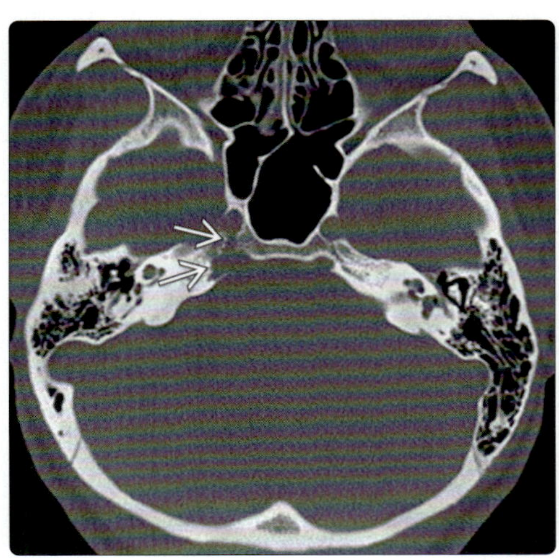

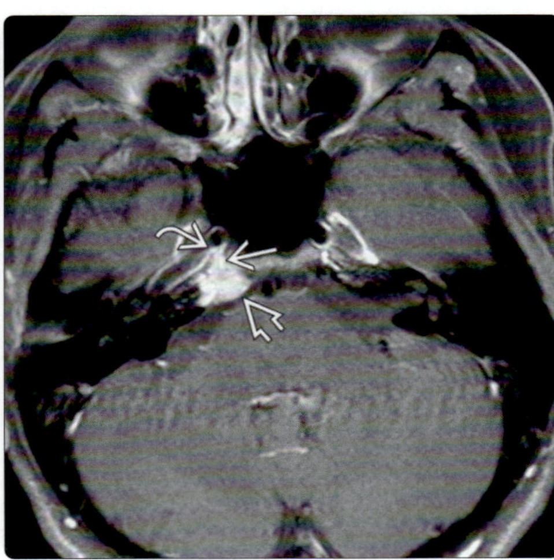

(Left) *Axial 1-mm thick skull base CT in a patient with right cranial nerve VI palsy shows an erosive bone lesion in the right petrooccipital fissure ➡ suspicious for small chondrosarcoma.* **(Right)** *Axial T1WI C+ FS MR in the same patient reveals enhancing tissue within the right petrooccipital fissure ➡, enlarging the fissure posteriorly and pushing into the prepontine cistern ➡. There is involvement of the petrous ICA wall ➡. MR shows true soft tissue extent of tumor, while bone CT shows associated bony changes.*

(Left) *Axial T1 FS MR in patient with proptosis & decreased right eye vision reveals globular configuration of avidly enhancing optic nerve sheath meningioma (ONSM) ➡ eccentrically surrounding orbital segment of right optic nerve. Note the tumor spares optic nerve immediately posterior to globe ➡, a common pattern.* **(Right)** *Axial orbital CECT shows another enhancing ONSM ➡ with punctate & linear calcification surrounding left optic nerve complex extending through orbital apex. Note adjacent hyperostosis ➡.*

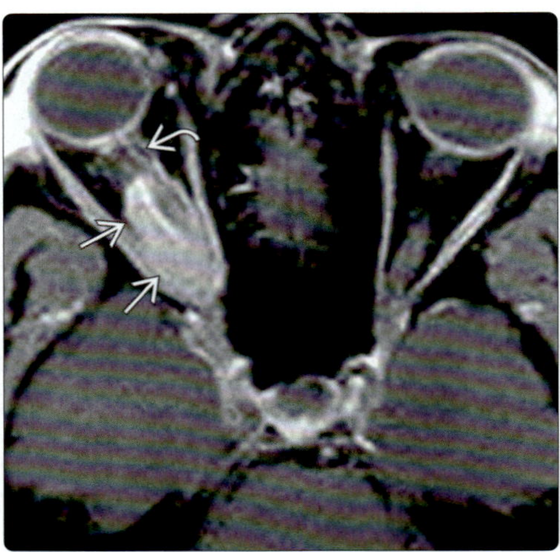

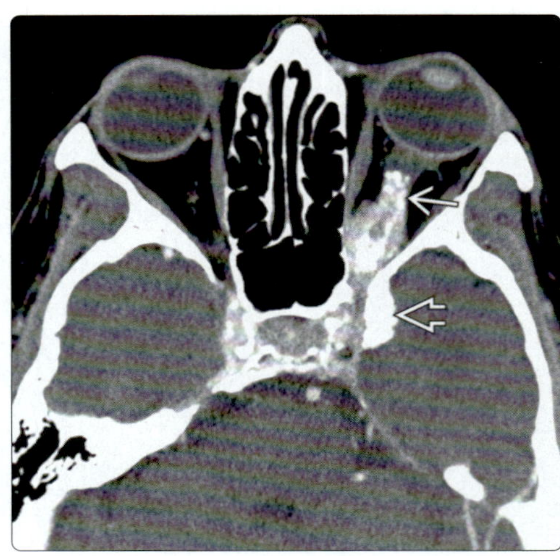

(Left) *Axial sinonasal bone CT in a immunocompromised patient with clinical suspicion of invasive fungal sinusitis shows left nose and maxillary sinus disease with loss of medial sinus wall ➡ and trabecular bone ➡. Note premaxillary soft tissue swelling ➡.* **(Right)** *Axial T1 C+ FS MR in the same patient shows acute invasive fungal sinusitis in premaxillary soft tissues ➡, retromaxillary fat pad ➡, and masticator space ➡. Bone CT alone is not adequate for evaluation of invasive sinonasal infection or tumor.*

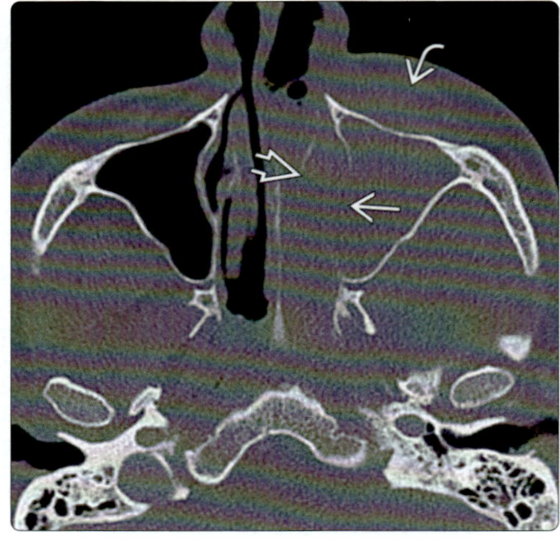

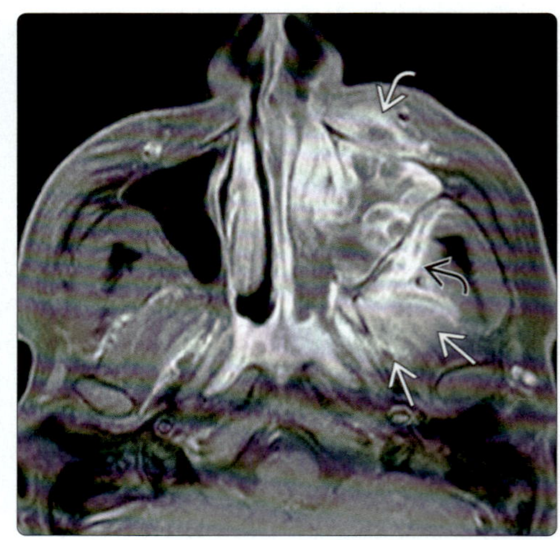

(Left) *Axial CECT of the suprahyoid neck shows a carotid body paraganglioma ➡ with avid, uniform enhancement. Note that the tumor sits in the notch between the ICA ➡ & ECA ➡. This location is diagnostic of paraganglioma.* **(Right)** *Axial T1WI MR reveals a carotid body paraganglioma in the left carotid space ➡, between 2 flow voids representing the ICA ➡ and ECA ➡. Small internal foci of signal void ("pepper") represent vascular flow of feeding vessels ➡. This characteristic finding is only present on MR, not on CT.*

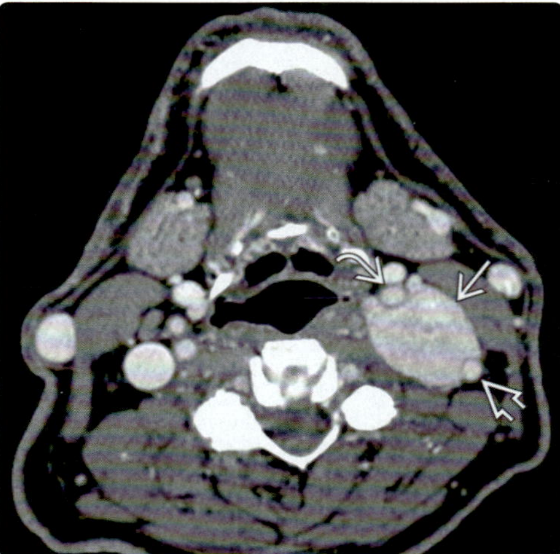

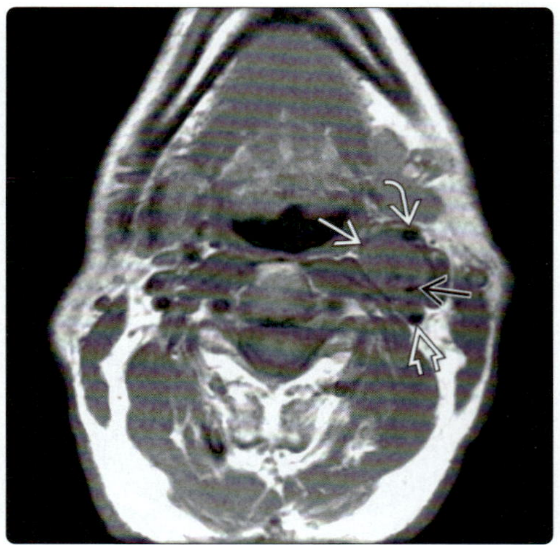

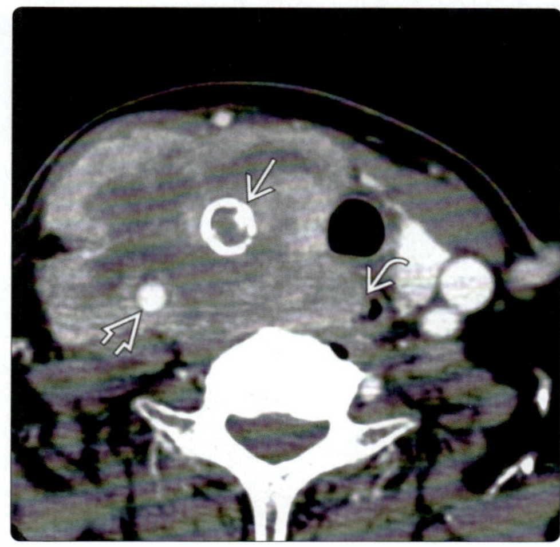

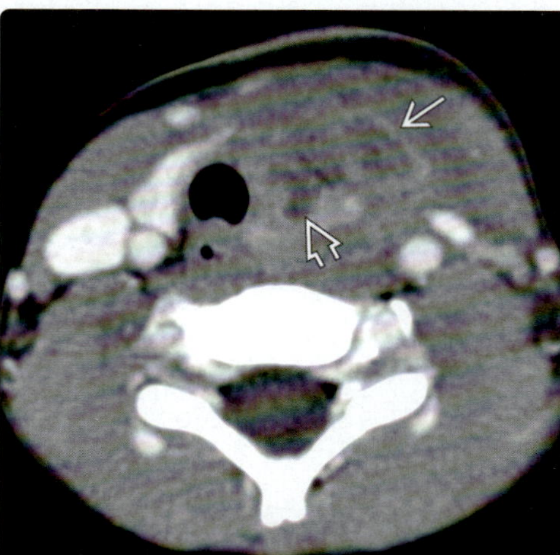

(Left) *Axial CECT reveals a large, invasive anaplastic thyroid carcinoma with dense, focal calcification →, right common carotid artery encasement →, & lateral wall of esophagus invasion →. CECT is the best 1st exam for infrahyoid neck masses as it is less affected by motion than MR.* **(Right)** *Axial CECT in a child with acute neck infection shows a phlegmonous mass → in the left neck involving the left thyroid lobe →. Fourth branchial arch anomaly connects the pyriform sinus to left thyroid lobe. CECT is the best 1st exam in this setting.*

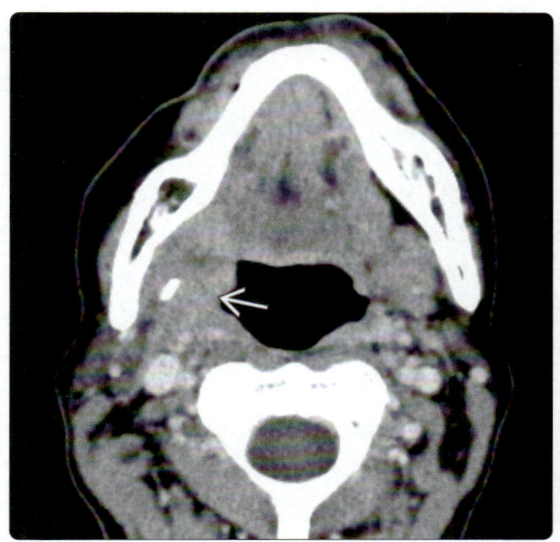

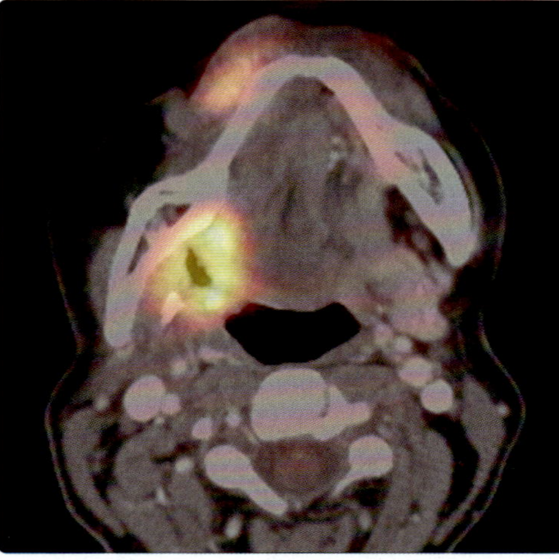

(Left) *Four months following combined surgery, radiation, and chemotherapy for right inferior palatine tonsil SCCa, this patient's axial CECT shows fullness in the right lateral pharyngeal wall →.* **(Right)** *Axial PET/CT in the same patient reveals hypermetabolic tissue in the area of anatomic distortion seen on CECT only, diagnostic of recurrent SCCa. PET/CT provides both anatomic and physiologic information in advanced stage SCCa of the head and neck.*

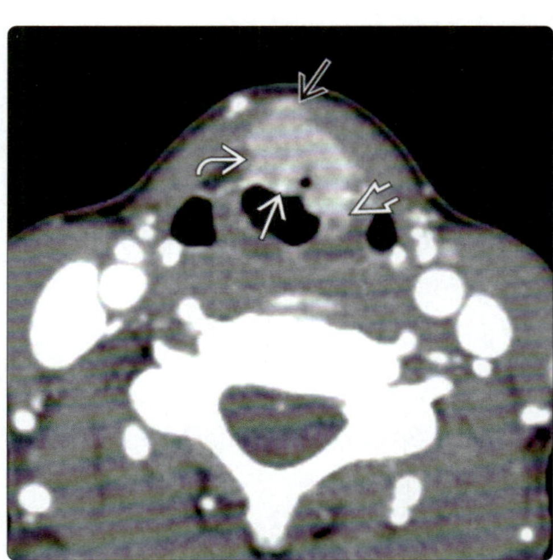

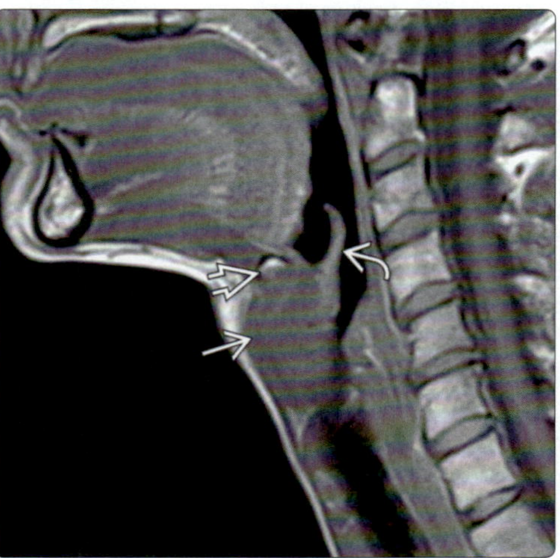

(Left) *Axial CECT in a patient with epiglottic SCCa shows involvement of the inferior epiglottis → and left aryepiglottic fold →. Tumor involves preepiglottic fat → and bulges through the thyroid cartilage notch →. CECT is the best 1st exam for the larynx due to movement issues.* **(Right)** *Sagittal T1WI MR shows supraglottic SCCa in preepiglottic space fat → that spares the suprahyoid epiglottis →. Note the hyoid is invaded →. MR is used in imaging the larynx after CECT if specific issues like cartilage invasion are present.*

SECTION 1

Suprahyoid and Infrahyoid Neck

Imaging Approaches & Indications

Neither CT nor MR is a perfect modality for imaging the extracranial H&N. MR is most useful in the suprahyoid neck (SHN) because it is less affected by oral cavity dental amalgam artifact. The SHN tissue is less affected by motion compared with the infrahyoid neck (IHN); therefore, the MR image quality is not degraded by movement seen in the IHN. Axial and coronal T1 fat-saturated enhanced MR is superior to CECT in defining soft tissue extent of tumor, perineural tumor spread, and dural/intracranial spread. When MR is combined with CT of the facial bones and skull base, a clinician can obtain precise mapping of SHN lesions.

CECT is the modality of choice when IHN and mediastinum are imaged. Swallowing, coughing, and breathing makes this area a "moving target" for the imager. MR image quality is often degraded as a result. Multislice CT with multiplanar reformations now permits exquisite images of the IHN unaffected by movement.

High-resolution ultrasound also has a role. Superficial lesions, thyroid disease, pediatric neck lesions, and nodal evaluation with biopsy are often best done by ultrasonography.

Many indications exist for imaging the extracranial H&N. Exploratory imaging, tumor staging, and abscess search comprise 3 common reasons imaging is ordered in this area. Exploratory imaging, an imaging search for any lesion that may be causing the patient's symptoms, is best completed with CECT from skull base to the clavicles.

Squamous cell carcinoma (SCCa) staging is best started with CECT, as both the primary tumor and nodes must be imaged, requiring imaging from the skull base to clavicles. MR imaging times and susceptibility to motion artifact make it a less desirable exam in this setting. Instead, MR is best used when specific delineation of exact tumor extent, perineural spread, or intracranial invasion is needed.

When the type and cause of H&N infection are sought, CECT is the best exam. CECT can readily differentiate inflammation from abscess. CT can also identify salivary gland ductal calculi, odontogenic infections, mandible osteomyelitis, and intratonsillar abscess as causes of infection.

Imaging Anatomy

In discussing the extracranial H&N soft tissues, a few definitions are needed. The **SHN** is defined as deep facial spaces **above the hyoid bone**, including parapharyngeal space (PPS), pharyngeal mucosal space (PMS), masticator space (MS), parotid space (PS), carotid space (CS), retropharyngeal space (RPS), danger space (DS), and perivertebral (PVS) space. The **IHN** soft tissue spaces are predominantly **below the hyoid bone** with some continuing inferiorly into the mediastinum or superiorly into the SHN, including the visceral space (VS), posterior cervical space (PCS), CS, RPS, and PVS.

Important **SHN** space **anatomic relationships** include their interactions with the skull base, oral cavity, and infrahyoid neck. When one thinks about the SHN spaces and their relationships with the skull base, perhaps the most important consideration is to examine each space alone to see what critical structures (cranial nerves, arteries, veins) are at the point of contact between the space and the skull base. Space by space, the **skull base interactions** above and IHN extension below are apparent.

- **PPS** has bland triangular skull base abutment without critical foramen involved; it empties inferiorly into submandibular space (SMS)
- **PMS** touches posterior basisphenoid and anterior basiocciput, including **foramen lacerum**; PMS includes nasopharyngeal, oropharyngeal, and hypopharyngeal mucosal surfaces
- **MS** superior skull base interaction includes zygomatic arch, condylar fossa, skull base, including **foramen ovale (CNV3)**, and **foramen spinosum** (middle meningeal artery); MS ends at inferior surface of body of mandible
- **PS** abuts floor of external auditory canal, mastoid tip, including **stylomastoid foramen (CNVII)**; parotid tail extends inferiorly into posterior SMS
- **CS** meets **jugular foramen (CNIX-XI)** floor, hypoglossal canal (CNXII), and petrous internal carotid artery canal; CS can be followed inferiorly to aortic arch; also called poststyloid parapharyngeal space
- **RPS** contacts skull base along lower clivus without involvement of critical structures; it continues inferiorly to empty into DS at T3 level
- **PVS** touches low clivus, encircles occipital condyles and foramen magnum; PVS continues inferiorly to level into thorax

In addition to skull base interactions, the relationships of the SHN spaces to the fat-filled PPSs are key to analyzing SHN masses. The PPSs are a pair of fat-filled spaces in the lateral SHN surrounded by the PMS, MS, PS, CS, and RPS. When a mass enlarges in one of these spaces, it displaces the PPS fat. Larger masses define their space of origin based on this displacement pattern.

- Medial PMS mass displaces PPS laterally
- More anterior MS mass displaces PPS posteriorly
- Lateral PS mass displaces PPS medially
- Posterolateral CS mass displaces styloid process and PPS anteriorly
- More posteromedial lateral RPS nodal mass displaces PPS anterolaterally

The **IHN** space **anatomic relationships** are defined by their superior and inferior projections. The VS has **no** SHN component, instead projecting only inferiorly into the superior mediastinum. The PCS extends superiorly to the mastoid tip and ends inferiorly at the clavicle. It is predominantly an IHN space, however. The CS begins at the floor of jugular foramen and carotid canal and extends inferiorly to the aortic arch. The RPS begins at the ventral clivus superiorly and traverses SHN-IHN to T3 level. The DS is immediately posterior to the RPS but continues beyond T3 level into mediastinum. For imaging purposes, RPS and DS can be considered a single entity. The PVS can be defined from skull base above to clavicle below. The PVS is divided by fascial slip into prevertebral and paraspinal components.

Understanding the **deep cervical fasciae (DCF)** of the neck can be challenging. However, it is these fasciae that define the very spaces we use to subdivide neck diseases and construct space-specific DDx lists. It is imperative that a clear understanding of these fasciae be grasped by any clinician caring for patients with disease in this area.

Many nomenclatures have been used to describe the neck fascia. The following is a practical distillate meant to simplify

Common Benign and Malignant Tumors in Spaces of Neck

Pharyngeal mucosal space	Warthin tumor	**Posterior cervical space**
Pharyngeal SCCa	**Carotid space**	Pharyngeal SCCa nodal metastasis (VA-VB)
Tonsillar NHL	Glomus vagale paraganglioma	NHL nodal disease
Masticator space	Carotid body paraganglioma	Differentiated thyroid carcinoma nodes
Sarcoma	Schwannoma of CNIX-XII	**Visceral space**
Perineural CNV3 SCCa	**Retropharyngeal space**	Differentiated thyroid carcinoma
Parotid space	SCCa nodal metastasis	Anaplastic thyroid carcinoma
Mucoepidermoid carcinoma	NHL nodal disease	Thyroid NHL
Adenoid cystic carcinoma	**Perivertebral space**	Cervical esophageal carcinoma
Malignant nodal metastases	Vertebral body systemic metastasis	Parathyroid adenoma
Benign mixed tumor	Brachial plexus schwannoma	

SCCa = squamous cell carcinoma; NHL = non-Hodgkin lymphoma.

this challenging subject. There are 3main DCF in the neck. The same names are used in the SHN and IHN. The superficial layer (**SL-DCF**), the middle layer (**ML-DCF**), and deep layer of DCF (**DL-DCF**) are the 3 important fascia in the neck.

In the SHN, the **SL-DCF** circumscribes **MS** and **PS** and contributes to the carotid sheath. In the IHN, it "invests" neck by surrounding the infrahyoid strap, sternocleidomastoid, and trapezius muscles, which are derived from the same embryologic origin. It also contributes to the carotid sheath of the CS in the IHN.

The **ML-DCF** in the SHN defines the deep margin of the PMS. It contributes to carotid sheath in both the SHN and IHN. In the IHN, it also circumscribes the VS.

In both the SHN and IHN, the **DL-DCF** surrounds **PVS**. A slip of DL-DCF dives medially to the transverse process, dividing PVS into prevertebral and paraspinal components. Another slip of DL-DCF, the alar fascia, provides the lateral wall to RPS and DS, as well as the posterior wall to RPS, separating RPS from DS. DL-DCF contributes to carotid sheath, like the SL and ML-DCF.

The internal structures of the spaces of the neck are for the most part responsible for the diseases there. Let us begin by defining the **critical contents of the SHN spaces.**

- **PPS** contains fat with rare minor salivary glands
- **PMS** contains mucosa, lymphatic ring, and minor salivary glands; in nasopharyngeal mucosal space, opening of eustachian tube, torus tubarius, adenoids, superior constrictor, and levator palatini muscles can be seen; oropharyngeal mucosal space contains anterior and posterior tonsillar pillars, palatine, and lingual tonsils
- **MS** includes posterior mandibular body and ramus, TMJ, CNV3, masseter, medial and lateral pterygoid and temporalis muscles, and pterygoid venous plexus
- **PS** contains parotid, extracranial CNVII, nodes, retromandibular vein, and external carotid artery
- **CS** contains CNIX-XII, internal jugular vein, and internal carotid artery
- **RPS** has fat and medial and lateral RPS nodes inside
- Prevertebral **PVS** contains vertebral body, veins and arteries, and prevertebral muscles (longus colli and capitis); in paraspinal PVS resides posterior elements of vertebra and paraspinal muscles

The **critical contents** of **IHN spaces** are defined next.

- **VS** contains thyroid and parathyroid glands, trachea, esophagus, recurrent laryngeal nerves, and pretracheal and paratracheal nodes
- **PCS** has fat, CNXI, and level V nodes inside
- **CS** houses common carotid artery, internal jugular vein, and CNX
- **IHN RPS** has **no** nodes and contains only fat
- Prevertebral **PVS** has brachial plexus and phrenic nerve, vertebral body, veins, arteries, and prevertebral and scalene muscles within; paraspinal PVS contains only posterior vertebra elements and paraspinal muscles

Approaches to Imaging Issues in SHN and IHN

It is crucial that the clinician has a method of analysis when a mass is found in the neck. In the SHN, mass evaluation methodology begins with defining mass **space of origin** (PMS, MS, PS, CS, lateral RPS). When small, this is simple, as the mass is seen within the confines of one space. In larger masses, ask, "How does the mass displace the PPS?" Next, utilize a **space-specific DDx** list. Match the imaging findings to the diagnoses within this list to narrow your differential.

With IHN masses, a similar evaluation methodology can be employed. First, determine what space the mass originates in (VS, CS, PCS). Then, review space-specific DDx list. Match radiologic findings of your case to this DDx list. The clinical findings will guide a clinician's differential.

Lesions of posterior midline spaces (RPS and PVS) of the neck need different image evaluation. When a lesion is defined here, 1st ask, "How does mass displace prevertebral muscles (PVM)?" In the case of an **RPS mass**, PVMs are flattened posteriorly or invaded from anterior to posterior. Contrast this imaging appearance to that of the **PVS mass** in which the PVMs are lifted anteriorly or invaded from posterior to anterior. Since most PVS lesions arise from vertebral body, vertebral body destruction and epidural disease will be linked. The DL-DCF "forces" PVS disease into the epidural space.

Selected References

1. Harnsberger HR et al: Differential diagnosis of head and neck lesions based on their space of origin. 1. the suprahyoid part of the neck. AJR Am J Roentgenol. 157(1):147-54, 1991
2. Smoker WR et al: Differential diagnosis of head and neck lesions based on their space of origin. 2. the infrahyoid portion of the neck. AJR Am J Roentgenol. 157(1):155-9, 1991

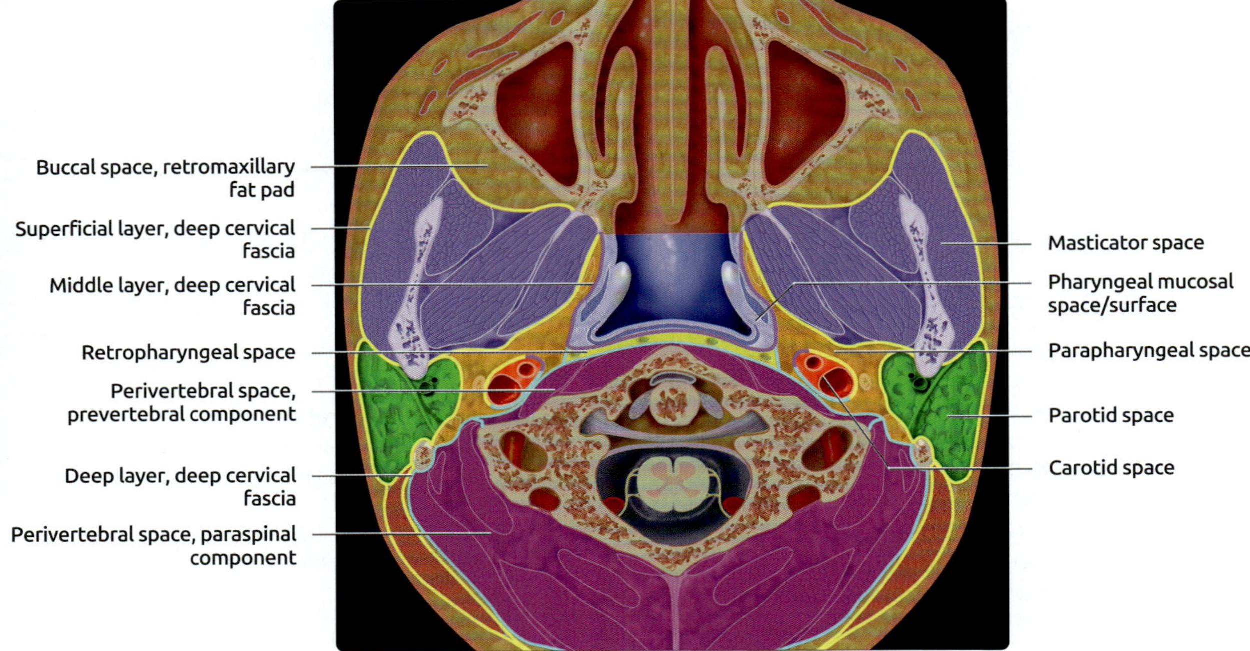

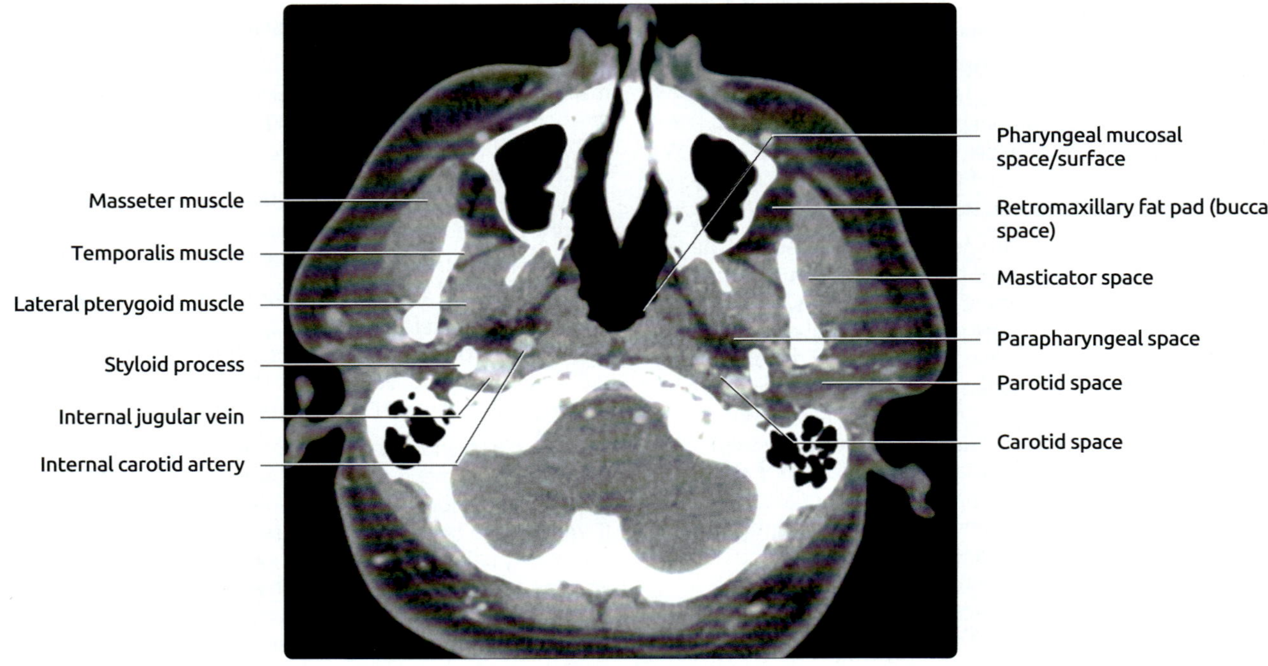

(Top) *Axial graphic depicts the spaces of the suprahyoid neck. Surrounding the paired fat-filled parapharyngeal spaces (PPS) are the 4 critical paired spaces of this region, the pharyngeal mucosal (PMS), masticator (MS), parotid (PS), and carotid spaces (CS). Retropharyngeal (RPS) and perivertebral spaces (PVS) are the midline nonpaired spaces. A PMS mass pushes the PPS laterally, an MS mass pushes the PPS posteriorly, a PS mass pushes the PPS medially, and a CS mass pushes the PPS anteriorly. Lateral RPS mass pushes PPS anteriorly without lifting styloid process. The superficial (yellow line), middle (pink line), and deep (turquoise line) layers of deep cervical fascia outline the spaces.* **(Bottom)** *Axial CECT at the level of the nasopharyngeal suprahyoid neck shows the 4 key spaces surrounding the PPS: The PMS, MS, PS, and CS. Notice the retropharyngeal fat stripe is not seen in the high nasopharynx between the prevertebral muscles and the pharyngeal mucosal surface.*

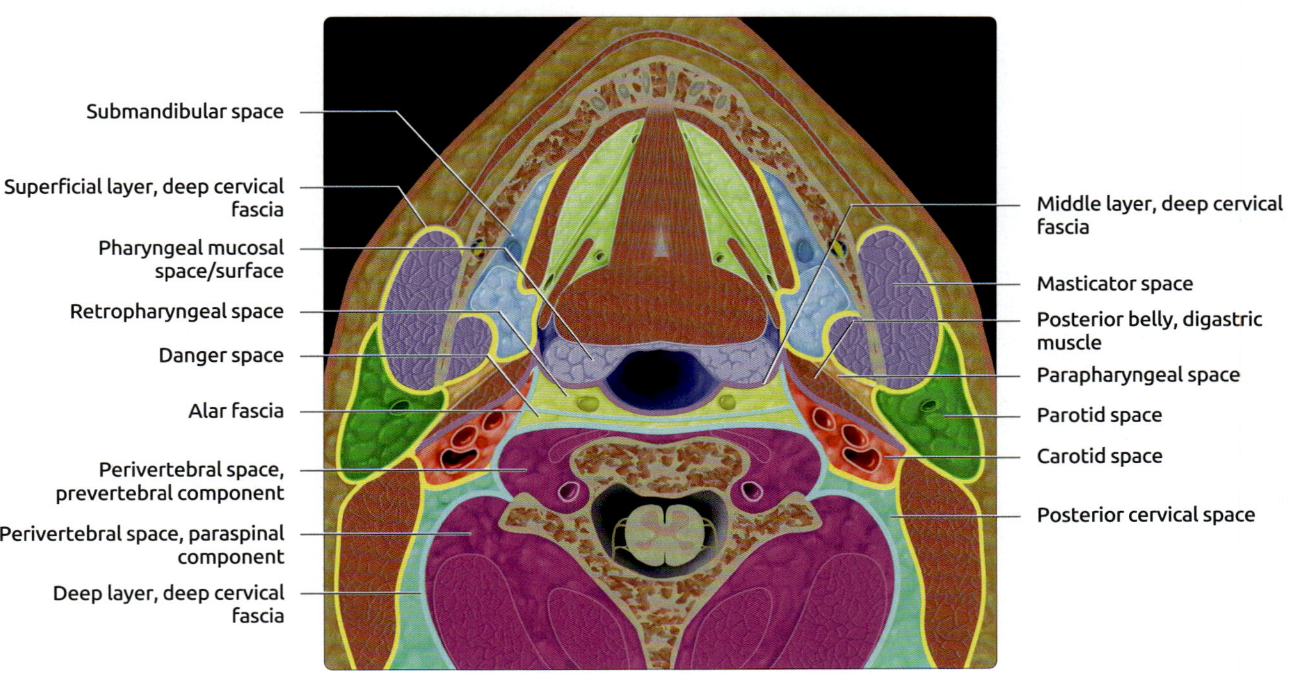

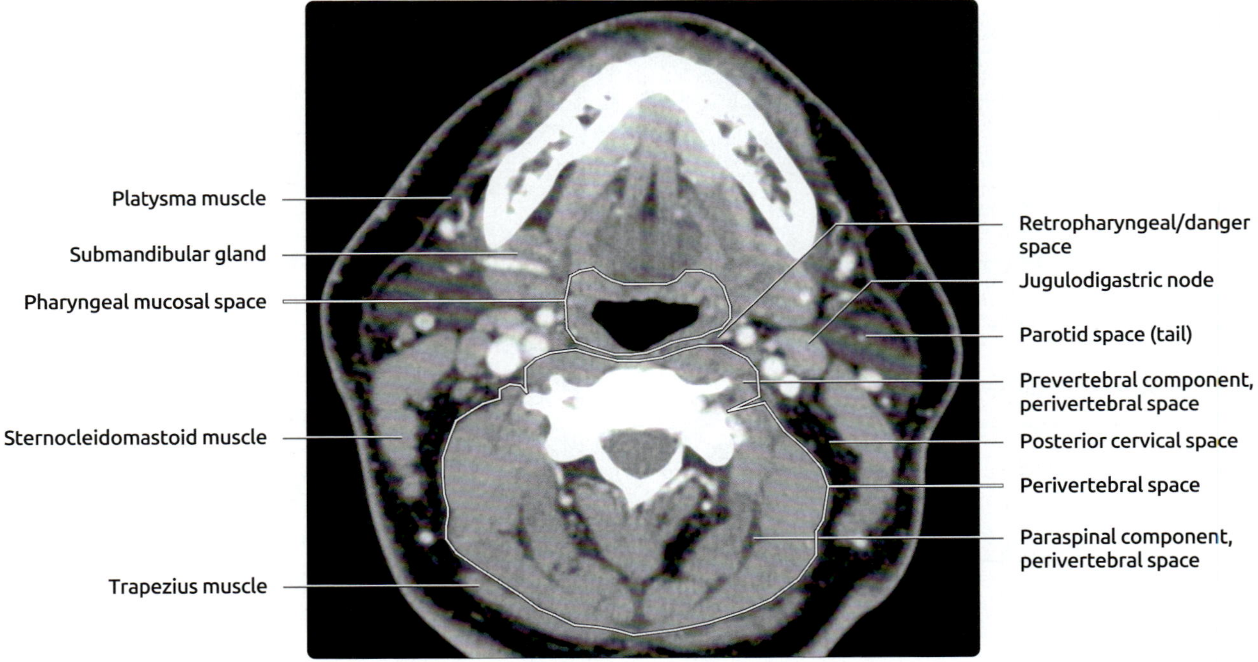

(Top) *Axial graphic shows the suprahyoid neck spaces at the level of the oropharynx. The superficial (yellow line), middle (pink line), and deep (turquoise line) layers of deep cervical fascia outline the suprahyoid neck spaces. Notice the lateral borders of the RPS and danger spaces are called the alar fascia, which represents a slip of the deep layer of deep cervical fascia. The CS has a tricolored fascial representation for the carotid sheath. This is because all 3 layers of deep cervical fascia contribute to the carotid sheath.* **(Bottom)** *In this image, through the low oropharynx, the PMS and the PVS have been outlined. The space between them is the RPS. The alar fascia that makes up the lateral borders of the RPS is not shown.*

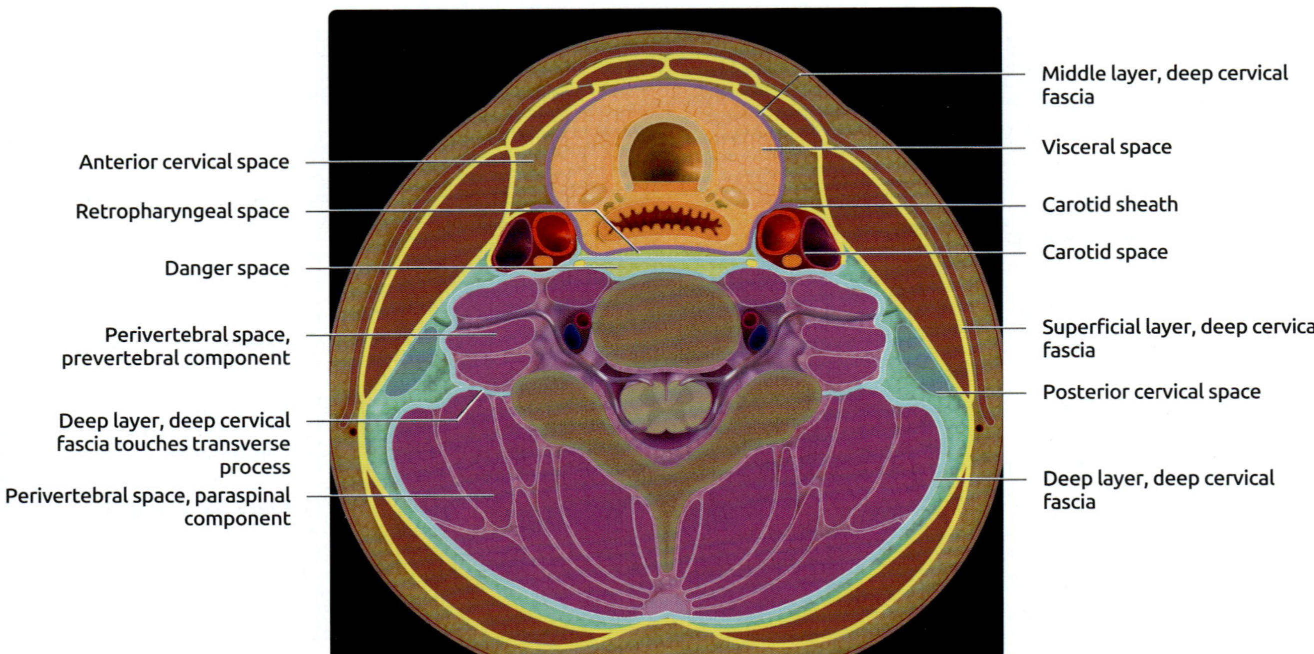

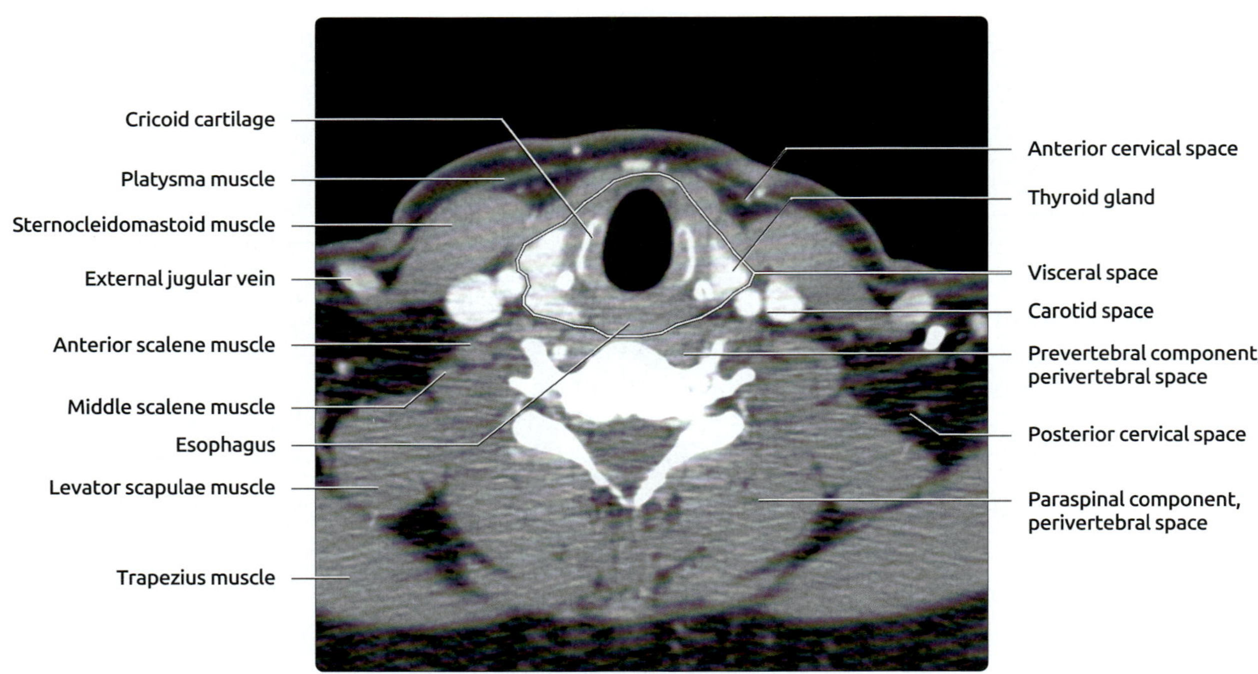

(Top) *Axial graphic depicts the fascia and spaces of the infrahyoid neck. The 3 layers of deep cervical fascia are present in the suprahyoid and infrahyoid neck. The carotid sheath is made up of all 3 layers of deep cervical fascia (tricolor line around CS). Notice the deep layer (turquoise line) completely circles the PVS, diving in laterally to divide it into prevertebral and paraspinal components. The middle layer (pink line) circumscribes the visceral space, while the superficial layer (yellow line) "invests" the neck deep tissues.* **(Bottom)** *In this axial CECT, the middle layer of deep cervical fascia is drawn to delineate the margins of the visceral space. The visceral space contains the high-density thyroid gland, the upper cervical esophagus, and the cricoid cartilage. The CS are lateral to the visceral space, while the RPS and PVS are posterior.*

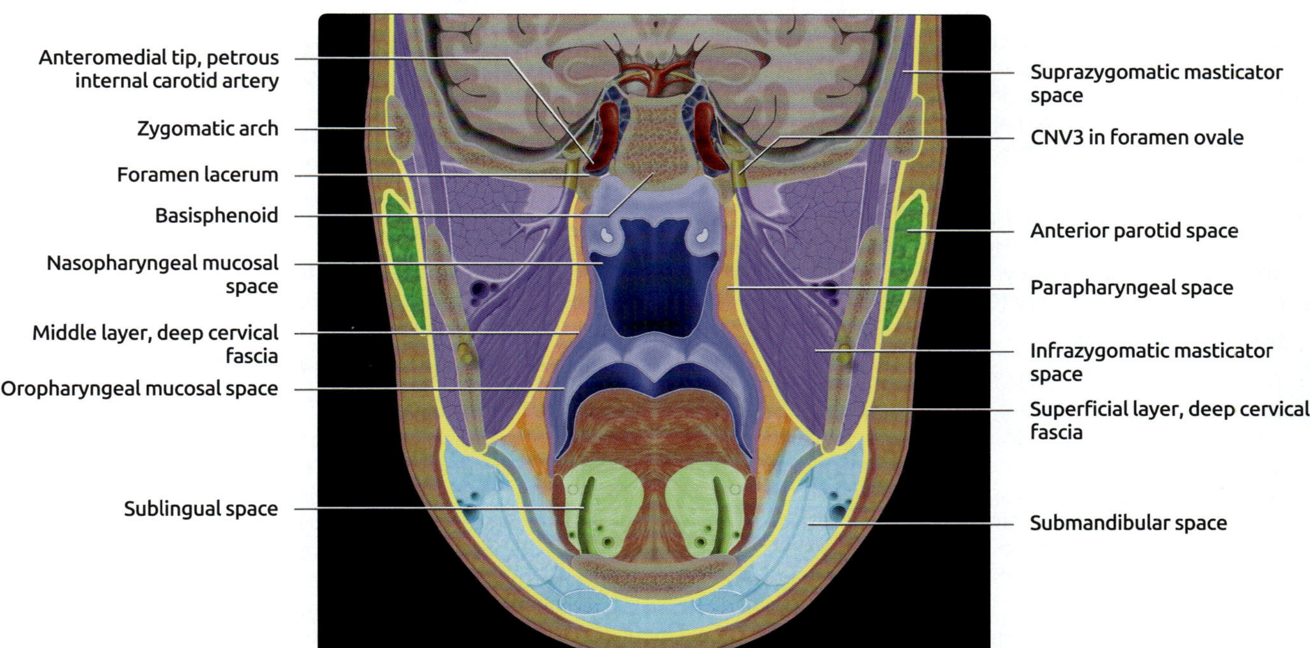

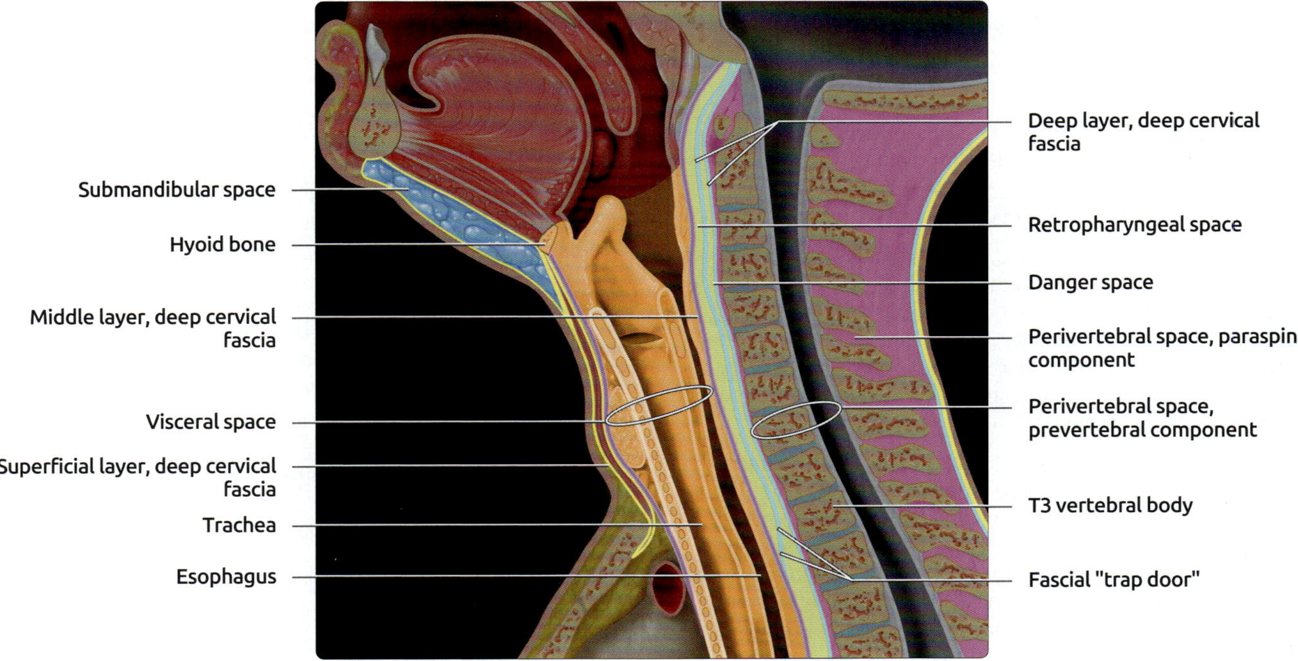

(Top) *Coronal graphic shows suprahyoid neck spaces as they interact with the skull base. The MS has the largest area of abutment with the skull base, including CNV3. The PMS abuts the basisphenoid and foramen lacerum. The foramen lacerum is the cartilage-covered floor of the anteromedial petrous internal carotid artery canal.* **(Bottom)** *Sagittal graphic depicts longitudinal spatial relationships of the infrahyoid neck. Anteriorly, the visceral space is seen surrounded by middle layer of deep cervical fascia (pink line). Just anterior to the vertebral column, the RPS and danger space run inferiorly toward the mediastinum. Notice the fascial "trap door" found at the approximate level of T3 vertebral body that serves as a conduit from the RPS to the danger space. RPS infection or tumor may access the mediastinum via this route of spread.*

Summary Thoughts: Parapharyngeal Space

The 4 key spaces of the suprahyoid neck (SHN) surround the parapharyngeal space (PPS), which is the fat-filled lateral SHN space. When large lesions of the SHN become hard to localize to a space of origin, the direction of the PPS displacement may be used in combination with the space where most of the tumor is located to make a determination as to where the lesion originated. Once a space of origin is assigned, the space-specific differential diagnosis can be applied to narrow the diagnostic possibilities.

The PPS has been described in terms of prestyloid and poststyloid compartments. Here we will define the **PPS** as the **prestyloid component only**. The poststyloid component will be called the **carotid space (CS)**.

Imaging Anatomy

The PPSs are paired, fat-filled spaces in the lateral SHN around which most of the important spaces are located. These surrounding important spaces are the pharyngeal mucosal space (PMS), masticator space (MS), parotid space (PS), CS, and the lateral retropharyngeal space (RPS). The PPS contents are limited; therefore, few lesions actually occur in this space. Diseases (tumor and infection) of the PPS usually arise in adjacent spaces (PMS, MS, PS, CS), spreading secondarily into the PPS.

The importance of the fat-filled PPS is its conspicuity on CT and MR. Even when large lesions are present in the SHN it is still usually possible to find the PPS. Identifying the direction of displacement of the PPS by a mass lesion from a surrounding space can be a **key finding** in determining its **space of origin**. The PPS displacement direction defines the space of the primary lesion.

- **PMS** (pharyngeal surface) mass lesion pushes PPS **laterally**
- **MS** mass lesion pushes PPS **posteriorly**
- **PS** mass lesion pushes PPS **medially**
- **CS** mass lesion pushes PPS **anteriorly**
- **Lateral RPS** mass (nodal) pushes PPS **anterolaterally**

The PPS is a crescent-shaped, fat-filled space in a craniocaudal dimension extending from the skull base superiorly to the superior cornu of the hyoid bone inferiorly. As paired fatty tubes separating other SHN spaces from one another, the PPS functions as an elevator shaft through which infection and tumor from these adjacent spaces may travel from the skull base to the hyoid bone.

The PPS has multiple important **anatomic relationships** with surrounding spaces. As there is no fascia separating the inferior PPS from the submandibular space (SMS), open communication between the PPS and posterior SMS exists. Superiorly, the PPS interacts with the skull base in the **"bland" triangular area** on the inferior surface of the petrous apex. No exiting skull base foramina are found in this area of attachment. In the axial plane the PMS is medial, the MS anterior, the PS lateral, the CS posterior, and the lateral RPS posteromedial to the PPS.

PPS **internal structures** are few. There is no mucosa, muscle, bone, nodes, or major salivary gland tissue within the PPS boundaries. The PPS principal content is **fat**. **Minor salivary glands** can be found there but are ectopic and rare. Although most of the **pterygoid venous plexus** is in the deep portion of the MS, a part of the plexus spills into the PPS.

The **fascia** surrounding the PPS is complex. Different layers of the deep cervical fascia combine to circumscribe the PPS. The medial fascial margin of PPS is made up of the middle layer of the deep cervical fascia as it curves around the lateral margin of the PMS. The lateral fascial margin of the PPS is comprised of the medial slip of the superficial layer of deep cervical fascia along the deep border of the MS and PS. The posterior fascial margin of the PPS is formed by the deep layer of the deep cervical fascia on the anterolateral margin of the RPS and the anterior part of the carotid sheath (made up of components of all 3 layers of deep cervical fascia).

Clinical Implications

Since the PPS empties inferiorly into the SMS, PPS infection or malignancy spread inferiorly from the upper SHN to present as an angle of mandible mass.

Approaches to Imaging Issues of Parapharyngeal Space

When you discover a lesion in the PPS on CT or MR, answer the following question 1st: "Is this lesion really primary to the PPS?" This question needs to be answered because there are so few things that occur initially in the PPS. In fact, the vast majority of lesions of the PPS arise in adjacent spaces and spread from there into the PPS. To conclude that a lesion is primary to the PPS, it must be completely surrounded by PPS fat. In most cases where a lesion is thought to be primary to the PPS, careful observation will find a connection to one of the surrounding spaces.

Lesions that are primary to the PPS itself include atypical 2nd branchial cleft cyst, benign mixed tumor (BMT), and lipoma. All are rare. Far more common lesions can be seen spreading into the PPS, such as intratonsillar abscess becoming peritonsillar and squamous cell carcinoma of the nasopharynx and oropharyngeal palatine tonsil. When a large parotid deep lobe BMT pedunculates into the PPS, it may at 1st glance appear to be primary to the PPS. Careful inspection will reveal a connection to the deep lobe of the parotid in the vast majority of cases. This is particularly true of parotid deep lobe BMT.

Differential Diagnosis

DDx of PPS lesion includes

- Congenital: Atypical 2nd branchial cleft cyst, lymphatic malformation, venous malformation
- Congenital/Inflammatory: Large diving ranula spreading from SMS into PPS
- Infection: Spreading from PMS, MS, PS or RPS; most commonly peritonsillar abscess from palatine tonsil (PMS) involving PPS
- Benign tumor: Lipoma, BMT from minor salivary gland rest in PPS
- Malignant tumor: Spreading from PMS, MS, PS or RPS into PPS; most often squamous cell carcinoma spreading from naso-, hypo- or oropharynx (PMS) into PPS

Selected References

1. Gamss C et al: Imaging evaluation of the suprahyoid neck. Radiol Clin North Am. 53(1):133-44, 2015
2. Mendelsohn AH et al: Parapharyngeal space pleomorphic adenoma: a 30-year review. Laryngoscope. 119(11):2170-4, 2009
3. Piccin O et al: Branchial cyst of the parapharyngeal space: report of a case and surgical approach considerations. Oral Maxillofac Surg. 12(4):215-7, 2008
4. Monobe H et al: Peritonsillar abscess with parapharyngeal and retropharyngeal involvement: incidence and intraoral approach. Acta Otolaryngol Suppl. (559):91-4, 2007

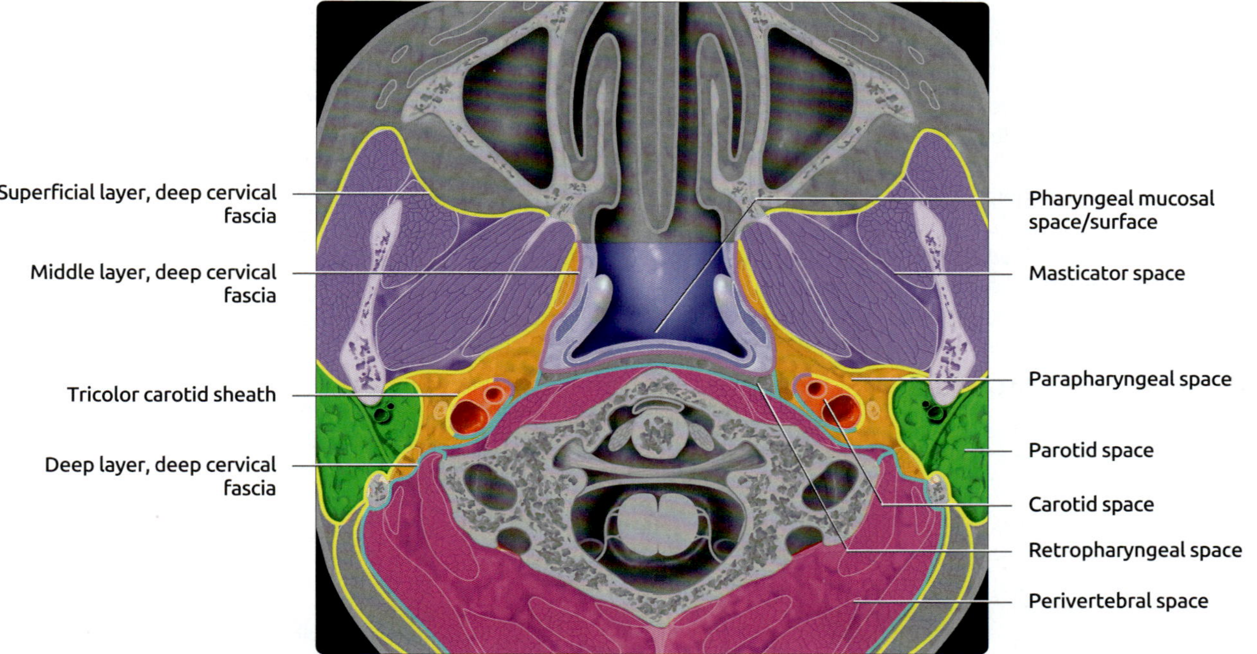

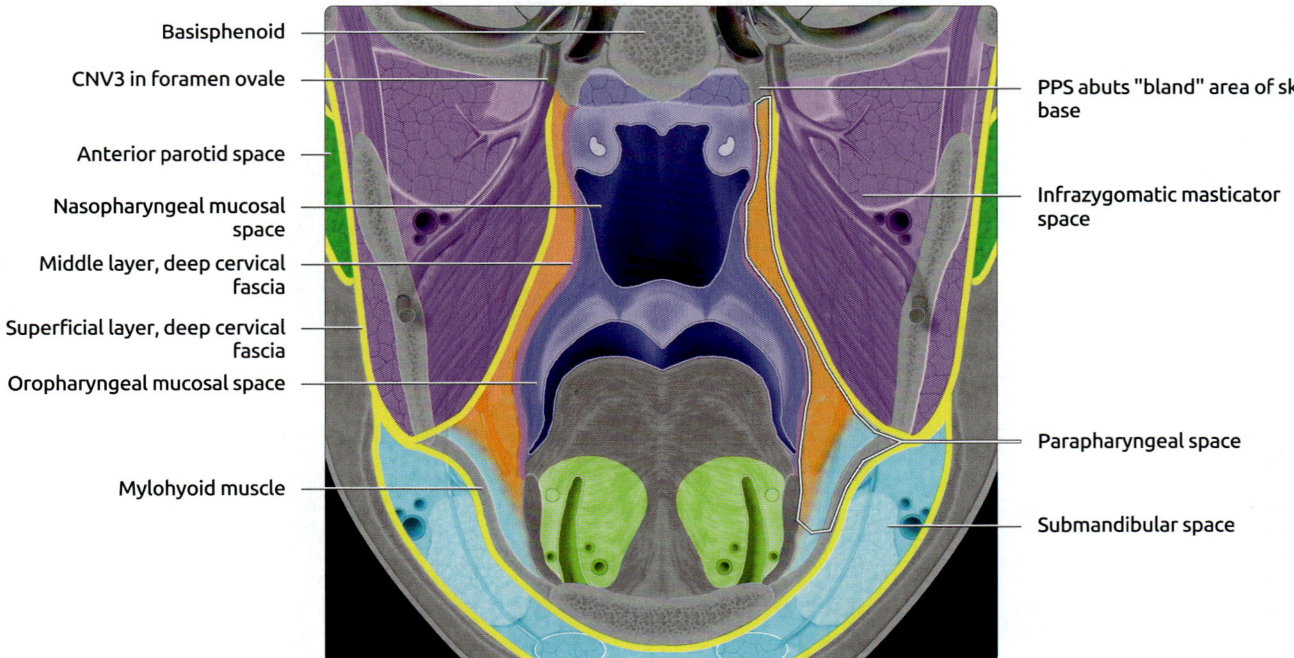

(Top) *Axial graphic of the normal parapharyngeal space at the level of the nasopharynx demonstrates the complex fascial margins and the fat-only contents. Mass lesions originating in the surrounding pharyngeal mucosal, masticator, parotid, and carotid spaces can extend into the parapharyngeal space. The resulting displacement pattern of the parapharyngeal space may be helpful in defining the space of origin of a mass in the suprahyoid neck.* **(Bottom)** *Coronal graphic shows suprahyoid neck spaces as they interact with the skull base superiorly and submandibular space inferiorly. The parapharyngeal space interacts with no critical structures as it abuts the skull base. Inferiorly it empties into the posterior submandibular space along the posterior margin of the mylohyoid muscle. As a consequence of this anatomic arrangement, it is possible for an infection or a malignant tumor that breaks into the parapharyngeal space to present inferiorly as an angle of a mandible mass.*

Parapharyngeal Space Benign Mixed Tumor

KEY FACTS

TERMINOLOGY

- Parapharyngeal space benign mixed tumor (PPS-BMT): BMT is primarily in PPS, not extension of deep lobe parotid BMT into PPS

IMAGING

- Rounded, well-defined ovoid lesion within PPS fat
  - Distinct from parotid deep lobe
- CECT findings
  - Heterogeneous, moderately enhancing PPS mass
- MR findings
  - Fat plane between deep lobe parotid & PPS-BMT
  - T1 C+ MR: Uniform enhancement when small
    - Heterogeneous enhancement when large
  - T2 MR: Marked T2 hyperintensity similar to CSF

TOP DIFFERENTIAL DIAGNOSES

- BMT of parotid deep lobe
- Pterygoid venous plexus asymmetry
- Neurogenic tumor in PPS

PATHOLOGY

- Rare lesion; much more common than parotid deep lobe BMT
- Benign tumor arising in aberrant salivary gland rests in PPS
- Solid but often heterogeneous with hemorrhage, cystic degeneration, or necrosis
- Occasional ossific or calcific degeneration

CLINICAL ISSUES

- Most asymptomatic, or minimally so, because of deep location and slow growth
- Small lesion usually incidental imaging finding
- Surgery: Typically cervical-parotid approach, occasionally with mandibulotomy
  - Resection without violation of tumor capsule is critical to prevent recurrence, often multifocal
  - ± total parotidectomy with facial nerve preservation

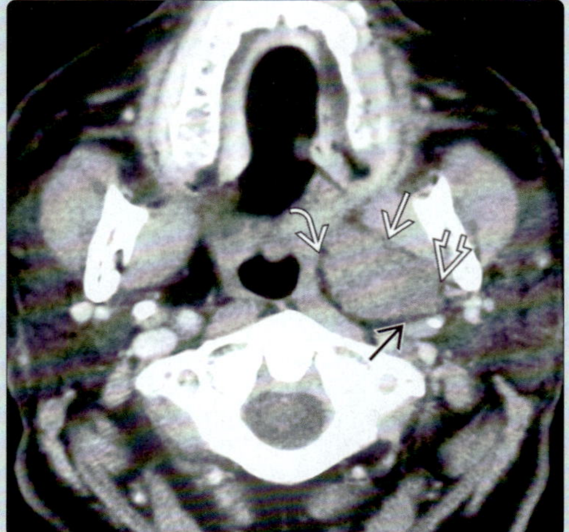

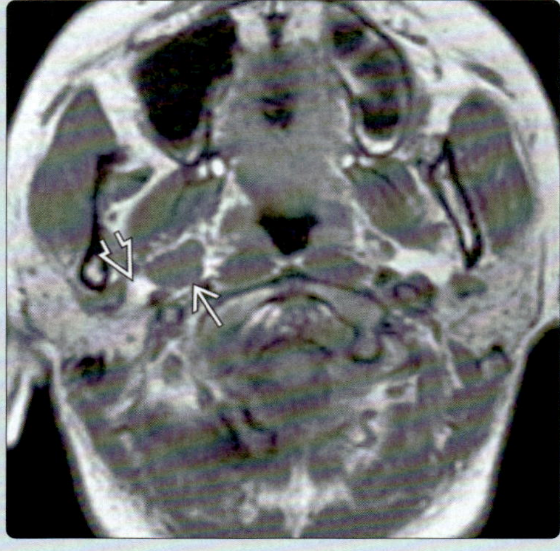

(Left) *Axial CECT demonstrates a well-defined, benign mixed tumor (BMT) ➡ within the left parapharyngeal space. The lesion is completely surrounded by parapharyngeal space (PPS) fat separating it from pharyngeal mucosal space medially ➡, parotid deep lobe laterally ➡, and carotid space posteriorly ➡.* **(Right)** *Axial T1WI MR reveals a well-defined PPS BMT within the right deep face ➡, completely surrounded by parapharyngeal fat. Note the mass is separated from the deep parotid by PPS fat ➡.*

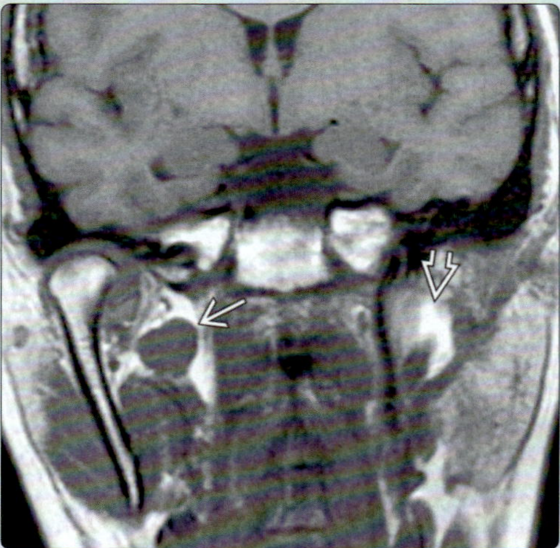

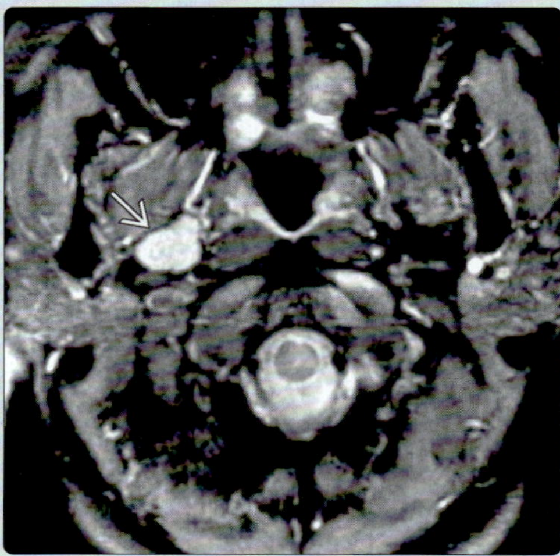

(Left) *Coronal T1WI MR shows a well-defined BMT ➡ to be surrounded by high-signal parapharyngeal fat. The mass is too small to have mass effect on adjacent tissues and was incidentally found on brain MR. There is normal PPS fat ➡ on the left.* **(Right)** *Axial T2WI FS MR shows homogeneous hyperintensity of a slightly lobulated PPS BMT ➡. Hyperintensity similar to CSF is typically seen with BMTs, although postcontrast images confirm it to be a solid mass (not shown).*

TERMINOLOGY

Abbreviations

- Parapharyngeal space, benign mixed tumor (PPS-BMT)

Synonyms

- Pleomorphic adenoma of PPS

Definitions

- Benign tumor arising from **aberrant minor salivary gland rests** in PPS
- Surgeons often describe lesions as "parapharyngeal," whether arising in PPS proper, parotid deep lobe, pharyngeal mucosal space or masticator space

IMAGING

General Features

- Best diagnostic clue
  - Rounded, well-defined ovoid lesion within PPS fat
    - Distinct from parotid deep lobe
- Location
  - Within parapharyngeal fat of suprahyoid neck
- Size
  - Variable: 1-8 cm
  - Large lesion often indistinguishable from parotid deep lobe tumor
- Morphology
  - Well-defined, rounded lesion when small
  - Often lobulates with increasing size

Imaging Recommendations

- Best imaging tool
  - Readily detected on CT or MR
  - MR allows better characterization & improved delineation from adjacent structures
    - Parotid deep lobe, internal carotid artery
- Protocol advice
  - T1 MR best to delineate parotid deep lobe

CT Findings

- CECT
  - Heterogeneous, moderately enhancing PPS mass
  - Surrounded by PPS fat

MR Findings

- T1WI
  - Fat plane seen between deep parotid & PPS-BMT
- T2WI FS
  - **Marked hyperintensity** similar to CSF
- T1WI C+ FS
  - Small lesions uniformly enhance
  - Heterogeneous enhancement especially when large

DIFFERENTIAL DIAGNOSIS

Benign Mixed Tumor of Parotid Deep Lobe

- Identical appearance but **within** parotid deep lobe

Pterygoid Venous Plexus Asymmetry

- Tubular enhancing structures in PPS or medial masticator space

Neurogenic Tumor in Parapharyngeal Space

- Well-defined, oval mass
- Intermediate T2, homogeneous CE if small

2nd Branchial Cleft Cyst

- Type IV branchial cleft cyst lies within PPS
- Cystic mass abutting lateral pharyngeal wall

PATHOLOGY

General Features

- Etiology
  - Benign tumor arising in **aberrant salivary gland rests**

Gross Pathologic & Surgical Features

- Solid but often heterogeneous with hemorrhage, cystic degeneration, or necrosis
- Occasional ossific or calcific degeneration

Microscopic Features

- As name implies, morphologically diverse
  - Epithelial and myoepithelial cells, mesenchymal or stromal elements

CLINICAL ISSUES

Presentation

- Most common signs/symptoms
  - Most asymptomatic because of deep location and slow growth
    - Small lesion usually **incidental imaging finding**
    - Large lesion may be found at dental/oral exam
  - Large mass often has minimal symptoms
    - Painless oral swelling or dysphagia

Demographics

- Age
  - Adults; peak in 5th decade
- Gender
  - Slight female predominance

Natural History & Prognosis

- Slow growing; may be asymptomatic even when large
- Uncommonly degenerates to malignant mixed tumor (carcinoma ex pleomorphic adenoma)

Treatment

- Resection for definitive pathological diagnosis or if large and symptomatic
- Operative cell spillage may result in multifocal recurrence

DIAGNOSTIC CHECKLIST

Image Interpretation Pearls

- Primary PPS lesions are rare
  - Should be entirely surrounded by fat
- Look for fat at posterolateral margin to distinguish PPS-BMT from parotid deep lobe BMT

SELECTED REFERENCES

1. Pelaz AC et al: Simultaneous pleomorphic adenomas of the hard palate and parapharyngeal space. J Craniofac Surg. 20(4):1298-9, 2009
2. Zhi K et al: Management of parapharyngeal-space tumors. J Oral Maxillofac Surg. 67(6):1239-44, 2009

Summary Thoughts: Pharyngeal Mucosal Space

Clinically, the upper aerodigestive track is often divided into the naso-, oro-, and hypopharyngeal subsites. Each of these subsites is unified, however, with mucosa that is subject to shared pathology. The pharyngeal mucosal space (PMS) is a key suprahyoid neck (SHN) space that represents the pharyngeal surface. The PMS has on its non-airway surface the **middle layer of deep cervical fascia** (ML-DCF). Important PMS contents include the mucosal surface of the pharynx, pharyngeal lymphatic ring (adenoidal, palatine, and lingual tonsils), and submucosal minor salivary glands.

An enlarging PMS mass of the palatine tonsil or nasopharyngeal lateral pharyngeal recess displaces the parapharyngeal space (PPS) fat laterally. Disruption of the mucosal and submucosal landmarks also occurs in PMS masses.

Important PMS malignancies include **squamous cell carcinoma** (SCCa) arising from the mucosal surface, **non-Hodgkin lymphoma** (NHL) from the pharyngeal lymphatic ring, and **minor salivary gland carcinoma** from the normal submucosal minor salivary glands. Of these, SCCa is by far the most frequent. Staging of SCCa primary and nodal disease is one of the most common reasons for imaging studies in the head and neck.

The PMS is not a true space as it is not enclosed on all sides by fascia. It is an imaging construct to overcome the problems encountered in describing a lesion of the pharynx as nasopharyngeal, oropharyngeal, and hypopharyngeal. These terms, although universally applied to lesions of the pharyngeal surface, do not address the deep tissue component of an invasive PMS mass. Describing a lesion as primary to the PMS with extension into the adjacent SHN spaces clearly delineates lesion extent in a radiologic report.

Imaging Techniques & Indications

Both CECT and enhanced MR can be used to image the PMS. If tonsillar or peritonsillar abscess is the major clinical concern, CECT of the soft tissues with bone CT of the mandible is a better choice. For tumor staging of pharyngeal SCCa neoplasms, enhanced fat-saturated multiplanar MR is the better exam. MR is usually less affected by dental amalgam artifact than CT and visualizes perineural and perivascular tumor spread more readily. In larger tumors of the oropharynx and nasopharynx already imaged with MR, the addition of noncontrast bone CT provides information regarding bone invasion, particularly of the skull base with staging implications, that may be difficult to derive from MR imaging.

Imaging Anatomy

The **anatomic relationships** of the PMS and surrounding deep tissue anatomy are extremely important because both PMS malignancy and infection readily spread into these adjacent areas. Directly posterior to the PMS is the retropharyngeal space (RPS). The PPS is lateral to the PMS.

Superiorly, the **PMS** abuts the **skull base** along the roof and posterosuperior portion of the nasopharynx. This broad abutment with the skull base includes the posterior basisphenoid (sphenoid sinus floor) and the anterior basiocciput (anterior clival margin). The **foramen lacerum** (cartilaginous floor of the anteromedial petrous internal carotid artery canal) is a key area of abutment of the PMS with the skull base. Nasopharyngeal carcinoma (NPCa) accesses the intracranial compartment via the **perivascular spread** along the internal carotid artery beginning at the foramen lacerum or **perineural spread** along V3.

The PMS extends from the roof of the nasopharynx above to the hypopharynx below as a continuous mucosal sheet. This mucosal space/surface is subdivided into **nasopharyngeal**, **oropharyngeal**, and **hypopharyngeal** components.

The PMS is a space with fascia on each deep margin but no superficial fascia. With no fascia on the surface of the PMS, it is not a true fascia-enclosed space. In fact it represents a conceptual construct to complete the spatial map of the SHN. The term "pharyngeal mucosal surface" functions just as well as PMS.

The **ML-DCF** defines the deep margin of the PMS. Just below the skull base, the ML-DCF encircles the lateral and posterior margins of the pharyngobasilar fascia (dense aponeurosis connecting the superior constrictor muscle to the skull base). In the more inferior nasopharynx and oropharynx, the ML-DCF resides on the deep margin of the superior and middle constrictor muscles.

Important **PMS internal structures** include the mucosa, lymphatic ring (of Waldeyer), and minor salivary glands. The pharyngeal lymphatic ring is divided into 3 components: The nasopharyngeal **adenoids** and the oropharyngeal **palatine** (faucial) and **lingual tonsils** (base of tongue). The lymphatic tissue normally declines in volume with age. Minor salivary glands are found in the submucosa throughout the oral cavity, pharynx, larynx, and trachea. Their highest concentration is found in the oral cavity and at the hard-soft palate junction.

The nasopharyngeal mucosal space also contains the superior constrictor muscle and the **pharyngobasilar fascia**. Along the posterosuperior margin of the pharyngobasilar fascia, there is a notch referred to as the **sinus of Morgagni**. The levator palatini muscle and the distal eustachian tube (torus tubarius) project into the PMS through this notch. NCPa may escape the PMS through this notch.

Approaches to Imaging Issues of Pharyngeal Mucosal Space

The answer to the question, **"What imaging findings define a PMS mass?"** depends on the area of the PMS where the mass originates. The most common PMS mass arises in the lateral pharyngeal recess of the nasopharynx or in the palatine tonsil of the oropharynx. As such, it is medial to the PPS, displacing the PPS fat laterally as it enlarges. A PMS mass of the lingual tonsil projects into the posterior sublingual space of the tongue as it enlarges. The rare posterior nasopharyngeal or oropharyngeal wall mass pushes posteriorly into the RPS as it grows. No matter where in the PMS a mass grows, disruption of the mucosal and submucosal architecture occurs. In addition, the growing airway side of the mass projects out into the adjacent PMS airway.

Traditionally, the pharynx is divided into the nasopharynx, oropharynx, and hypopharynx as a method to describe where on this continuous sheet of mucosa a SCCa is found. This **surface of the pharynx** is referred to here as the **PMS**. To unify these 2 terminologies, it is possible to refer to the nasopharyngeal, oropharyngeal, or hypopharyngeal mucosal space. It is not helpful to merely refer to a tumor as either of the oropharynx or found in the oropharyngeal mucosal space. The clinician must also understand what other deep facial spaces are involved by a PMS tumor. For treatment planning,

Differential Diagnosis of Pharyngeal Mucosal Space

Pseudolesions	**Malignant tumor**
Asymmetric lateral pharyngeal recess	Nasopharyngeal carcinoma
Fluid in lateral pharyngeal recess	Oropharyngeal squamous cell carcinoma (SCCa)
Asymmetric tonsillar tissue	Palatine tonsil SCCa
Inflammatory lesions	Lingual tonsil SCCa
Mucosal inflammation (pharyngitis, post radiation)	Non-Hodgkin lymphoma
Tonsillar lymphoid hyperplasia	Minor salivary gland carcinoma
Retention cyst	Rhabdomyosarcoma
Postinflammatory dystrophic calcifications	Extraosseous chordoma
Tonsillar inflammation (tonsillitis)	**Miscellaneous**
Infectious lesions	Tornwaldt cyst
Tonsillar/peritonsillar abscess	Patulous lateral pharyngeal recess + palate atrophy
Benign tumor	In proximal vagal neuropathy
Benign mixed tumor, minor salivary gland	

this requires reviewing the other deep facial spaces, including the PPS, masticator space (MS), parotid space (PS), carotid space (CS), RPS, and perivertebral space.

When a PMS lesion is identified on imaging, there are a limited number of common diseases to consider. If the patient is imaged to evaluate for possible infection, 3 lesions may be identified. **Tonsillar lymphoid hyperplasia** is commonly found in children and young adults, resulting from multiple bouts of tonsillar inflammation. **Tonsillar inflammation** is suggested when enhancing, enlarged tonsil(s) possess "stripes." **Tonsillar abscess** is diagnosed when focal rim-enhancing pus collections are seen. A **peritonsillar abscess** has ruptured from the tonsil into the adjacent PPS, RPS, or MS.

If the PMS lesion lacks a clinical infectious context but has invasive imaging features, a limited group of **malignant tumors** must be considered. SCCa is by far the most common malignancy of the PMS with NHL, next in frequency followed by minor salivary gland carcinoma. These neoplasms arise from the normal structures found within the PMS.

- Mucosal epithelium → SCCa
- Pharyngeal lymphatic ring → **NHL**
- Minor salivary glands → **minor salivary gland carcinoma**
- Notochordal remnant → extraosseous chordoma
- Constrictor and levator palatini muscles → rhabdomyosarcoma

The most common **interpretation pitfall** associated with the PMS occurs when large adenoidal tonsillar tissue is misinterpreted as tumor. Recurrent tonsillar inflammation in the young may lead to disturbingly prominent, often asymmetric tonsillar hyperplasia on CT or MR imaging. If the prominent lymphatic tissue in the PMS has no invasive deep margins, demonstrates no inflammatory septa, and is found in a patient less than 20 years of age, lymphoid hyperplasia is the most likely explanation.

A 2nd common interpretation pitfall occurs when the lateral pharyngeal recess is asymmetric either because of retained secretions, retention cysts, or unevenly distributed adenoidal tissue. Suggesting NPCa in this setting creates great patient and physician consternation. Suggesting normal asymmetry and recommending clinical inspection usually suffice to clear the nasopharynx of significant pathology.

Clinical Implications

Remember that a lesion of the PMS can often be directly visualized. Lesions of the lateral pharyngeal recess of the nasopharynx may be the exception to this rule. In the case of SCCa, the appearance of the mucosal lesion is often diagnostic. Knowing what the physical examination of the pharynx shows at the time imaging is reviewed allows for a richly detailed and highly relevant interpretation.

When staging a **SCCa of the pharyngeal surface** with CT or MR, the clinician should focus on both the **primary tumor (T) and nodal (N) stage**. The 2010 American Joint Committee on Cancer (AJCC) staging manual defining the T and N stages of each of the subsites of the pharynx is an important reference for the clinician doing this type of work. Familiarity with the routes of spread of SCCa of the PMS by primary site and subsite also permits the clinician to thoroughly utilize the associated imaging.

NPCa, because of its proximity to the skull base, spreads early into the intracranial compartment. The ML-DCF and the pharyngobasilar fascia direct NPCa growth superiorly where it will invade directly into the upper clivus, floor of the sphenoid sinuses, and the foramen lacerum. When the tumor invades through the foramen lacerum, it accesses the anteromedial internal carotid artery. **Perivascular spread** takes it into the cavernous sinus from there. The proximity of the nasopharyngeal CS to lateral pharyngeal recess NPCa makes early invasion of the internal carotid artery and cranial nerves IX-XII likely.

Selected References

1. Gamss C et al: Imaging evaluation of the suprahyoid neck. Radiol Clin North Am. 53(1):133-44, 2015
2. Parker GD et al: The pharyngeal mucosal space. Semin Ultrasound CT MR. 11(6):460-75, 1990

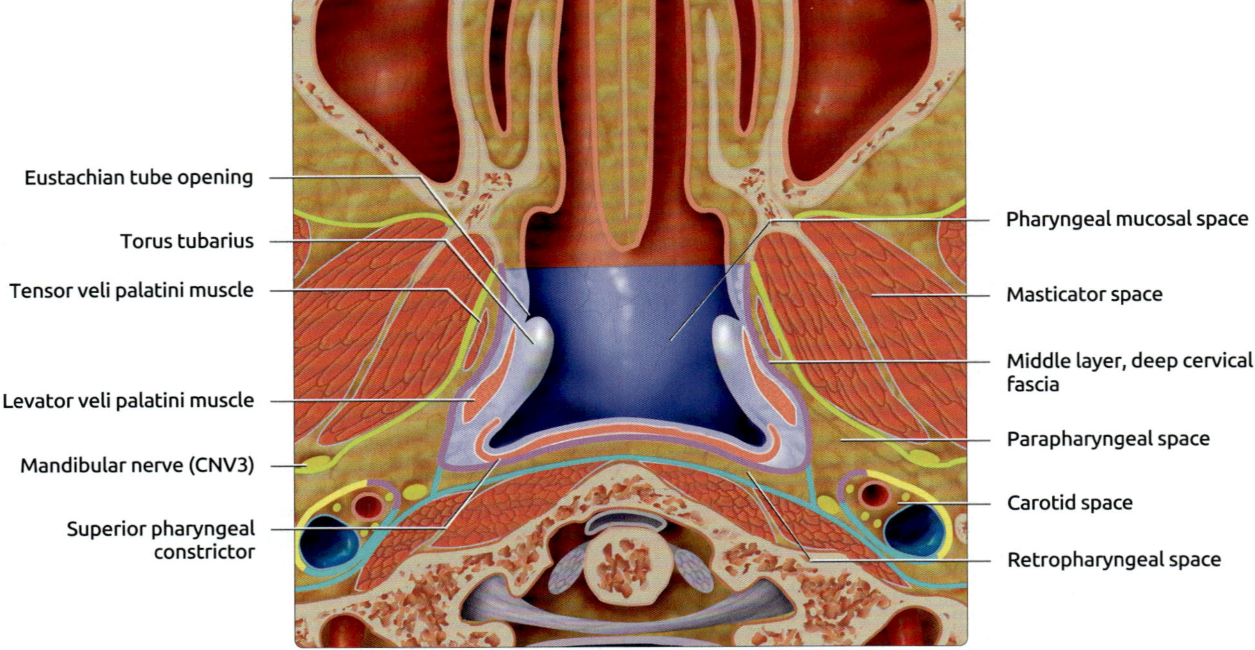

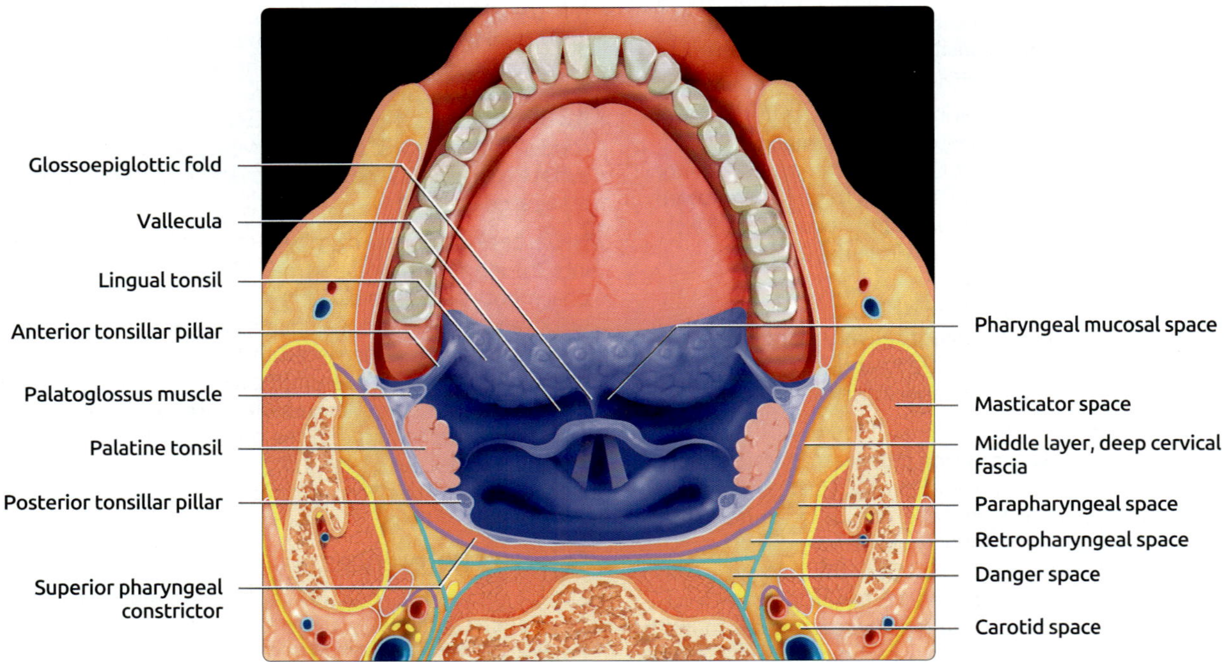

(Top) *Axial graphic of the nasopharyngeal mucosal space (in blue) shows that the superior pharyngeal constrictor, levator veli palatini muscles, and the cartilaginous eustachian tube ending (torus tubarius) are within the space. The levator veli palatini and eustachian tube access the pharyngeal mucosal space (PMS) via the sinus of Morgagni in the upper margin of the pharyngobasilar fascia. The middle layer of deep cervical fascia provides a deep margin to the space. The retropharyngeal space is behind and the parapharyngeal space is lateral to the PMS.* **(Bottom)** *Axial graphic of the oropharyngeal mucosal space (in blue) viewed from above reveals that the superior pharyngeal constrictor and the tonsillar pillars along with the palatine and lingual tonsils are all occupants of this space. The middle layer of deep cervical fascia provides a deep margin to the space. The retropharyngeal space is behind and the parapharyngeal space is lateral to the PMS.*

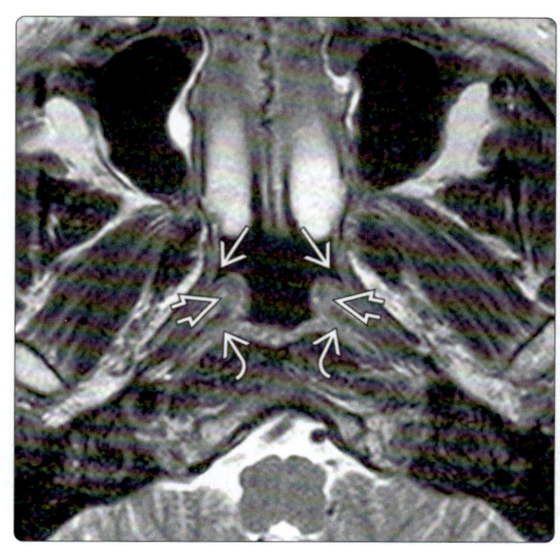

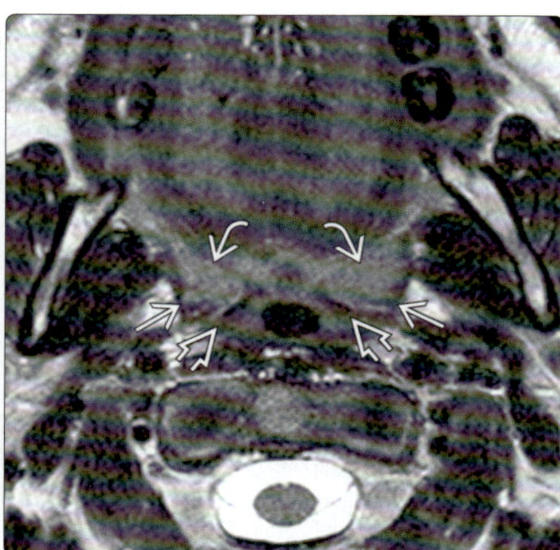

(Left) *Axial T2WI MR shows the PMS at the level of the nasopharynx. Notice the opening to the eustachian tube* ➡ *and torus tubarius* ➡*. The lateral pharyngeal recess is collapsed* ➡ *with the 2 mucosal surfaces touching each other.* **(Right)** *Axial T2WI MR through the mid oropharynx reveals the palatine tonsil* ➡ *as the main occupant of the PMS. The superior constrictor muscle* ➡ *and the palatopharyngeus muscles* ➡ *are visible.*

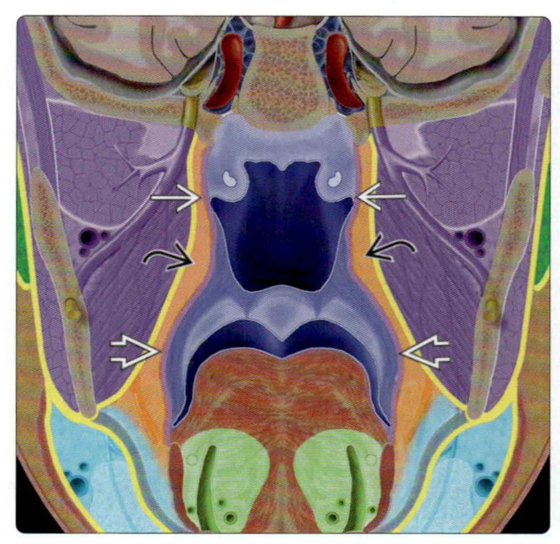

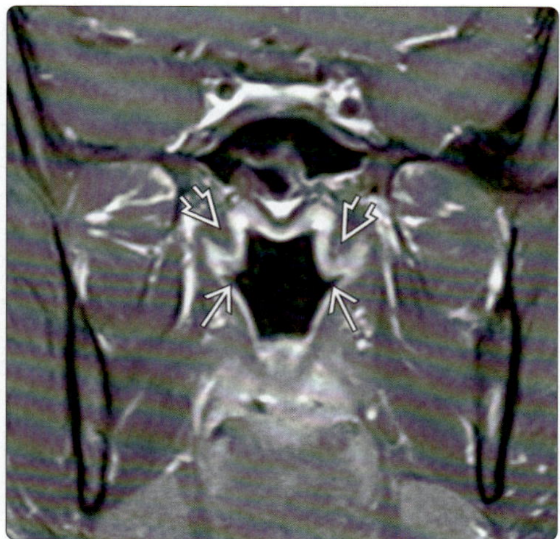

(Left) *Coronal graphic shows the nasopharyngeal and oropharyngeal mucosal spaces. Note the middle layer of deep cervical fascia defining the lateral margin of the nasopharyngeal PMS* ➡ *and the oropharyngeal PMS* ➡*. The parapharyngeal spaces are paired fatty spaces* ➡ *lateral to the PMS.* **(Right)** *Coronal C+ FS T1WI MR reveals the normal enhancing sheet of mucosa. Notice the torus tubarius (cartilaginous eustachian tube)* ➡ *& lateral pharyngeal recesses* ➡*.*

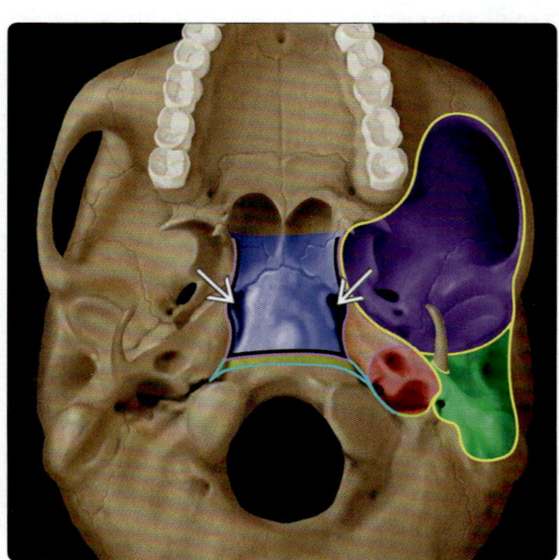

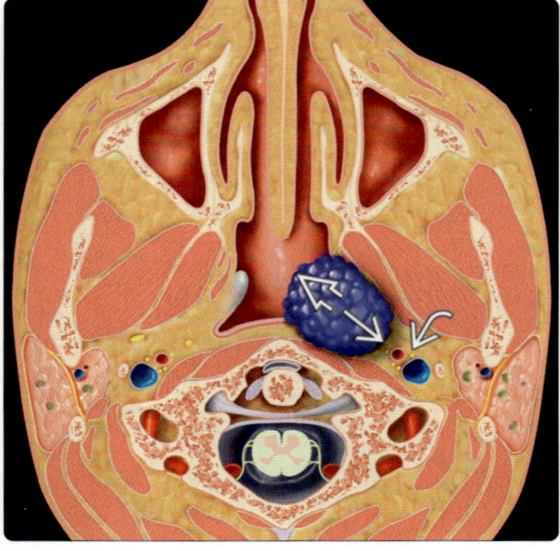

(Left) *Skull base graphic viewed from below highlights an area of PMS abutment (blue). Note the posterior basisphenoid & clival basiocciput are both involved. Bilateral foramina lacerum* ➡ *are within the abutment area.* **(Right)** *Axial graphic through the nasopharynx depicts a generic PMS mass. The lesion projects into the nasopharyngeal airway* ➡ *as well as pushes from medial to lateral on the adjacent parapharyngeal space* ➡*. Notice the close proximity of the nasopharyngeal carotid space* ➡ *with CNIX-XII.*

KEY FACTS

TERMINOLOGY

- Definition: Benign **developmental midline cyst** in pharyngeal mucosal space (PMS) covered by mucosa anteriorly & bounded by longus muscles posteriorly

IMAGING

- General features: Ovoid, cystic mass in midline nasopharyngeal mucosal space
- CT findings
  - Midline, nasopharyngeal well-circumscribed cyst
  - If enhanced CT, no cyst enhancement present
- MR findings
  - T1: Intermediate to high signal depending on cyst fluid protein concentration
  - T2: Homogeneously high signal with no deep extension into surrounding structures
    - Low signal if contains highly proteinaceous fluid
  - T1 C+: May have minimal enhancement of cyst wall

TOP DIFFERENTIAL DIAGNOSES

- Retention cyst in PMS
- Adenoidal hyperplasia
- Benign mixed tumor in PMS
- Nasopharyngeal carcinoma

PATHOLOGY

- **Notochordal remnant** where embryologic notochord & endoderm of primitive pharynx come into contact
- Histology: Cyst lined by **respiratory epithelium**

CLINICAL ISSUES

- Usually asymptomatic and incidental
  - Seen on **5%** of routine brain MR
  - If large, seen on CECT of brain
- Most common lesion of nasopharyngeal mucosal space occurring in 4% at autopsy
- Rarely, chronically infected large cyst (> 2 cm) causes periodic halitosis and unpleasant taste in mouth

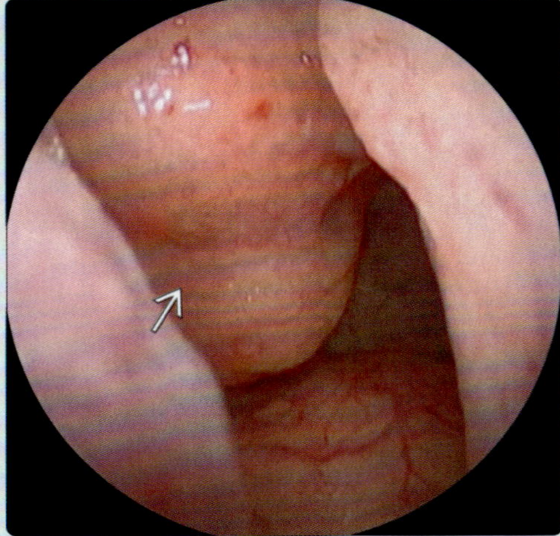

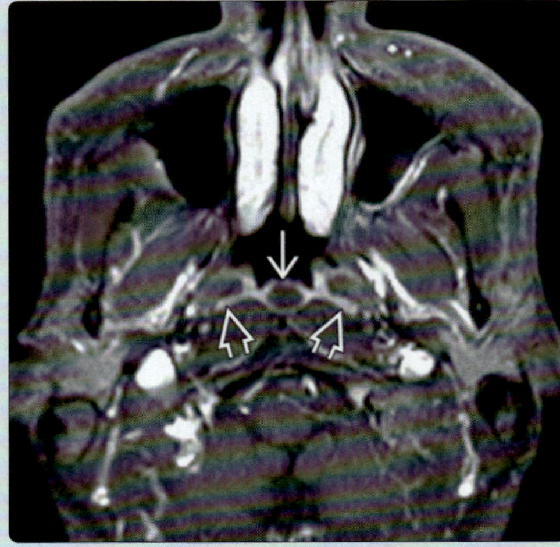

(Left) *Endoscopic view of a Tornwaldt cyst ➡ shows that it appears as a submucosal mass in the right nasopharynx obscuring the eustachian tube opening. Notice the overlying mucosa is normal. (DP: H&N, 2e.)* **(Right)** *Axial T1 enhanced fat-saturated MR demonstrates a classic small, submucosal, nonenhancing Tornwaldt cyst ➡ in the midline nasopharynx. The mucosal surface enhances ➡ and is seen as a thin white line.*

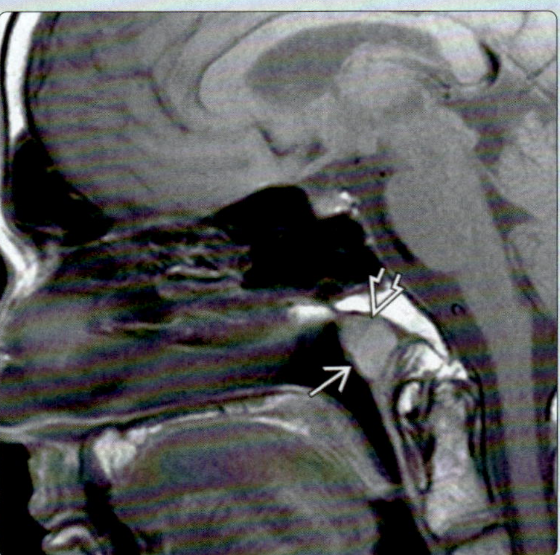

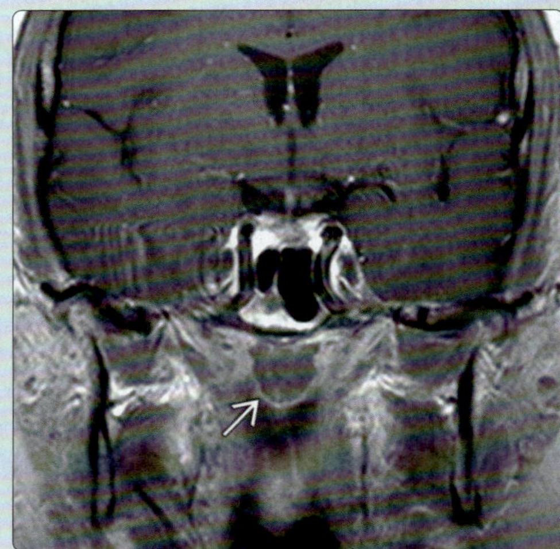

(Left) *Sagittal T1 nonenhanced MR shows a patient with a medium-sized Tornwaldt cyst ➡. The cyst is slightly hyperintense, presumably due to increased protein content. Subtle internal septation ➡ is present.* **(Right)** *Coronal T1 enhanced fat-saturated MR through the pituitary gland in the same patient reveals the midline nonenhancing Tornwaldt cyst ➡ within the otherwise enhancing nasopharyngeal mucosal space.*

KEY FACTS

TERMINOLOGY

- Abbreviations: Retention cyst (RC) of pharyngeal mucosal space (PMS)
- Synonyms: Postinflammatory cyst, tonsillar cyst
- Definition: Benign, asymptomatic PMS cyst

IMAGING

- RC of PMS in nasopharynx (adenoids) or oropharynx (palatine or lingual tonsil)
  - If in adenoids, often **pear-shaped** as it extends into lateral pharyngeal recess
- CECT imaging findings
  - Size: Usually < 1-cm low-density (cystic) mass
  - If in tonsils, **ovoid or round**, well circumscribed
  - No cyst wall enhancement
- MR imaging findings
  - T1 MR: May be hyperintense if proteinaceous
  - T2 MR: Homogeneously hyperintense mucosal cyst
  - T1 C+ MR: No significant enhancement in wall

TOP DIFFERENTIAL DIAGNOSES

- Thyroglossal duct cyst at foramen cecum: Midline tongue base
- Tornwaldt cyst: Midline nasopharynx PMS
- Tonsillar abscess: Wall enhances; > 1 cm
- Vallecular cyst: Tongue base of infant

CLINICAL ISSUES

- Typical presentation: Incidental finding on CT or MR
  - Lesion found on routine brain MR, cervical spine MR, CECT of head and neck
  - May be confused with tonsillar abscess but RC is small with no wall enhancement
  - In general should be considered benign, "leave alone" lesion requiring no treatment
- Rare presentation
  - Lateral pharyngeal recess RC can rarely obstruct eustachian tube with middle ear-mastoid effusion
  - If clearly symptomatic, surgical resection merited

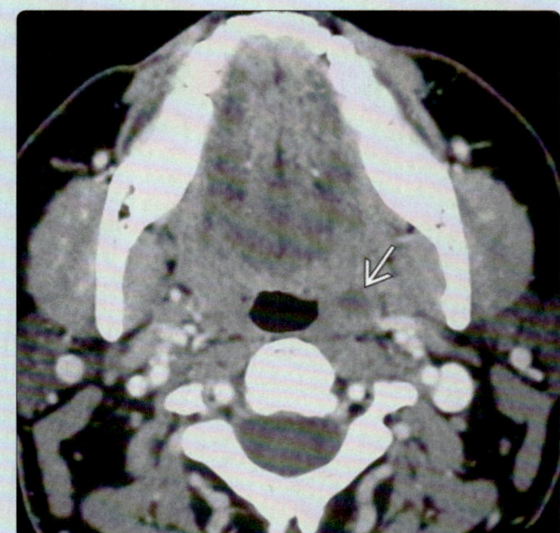

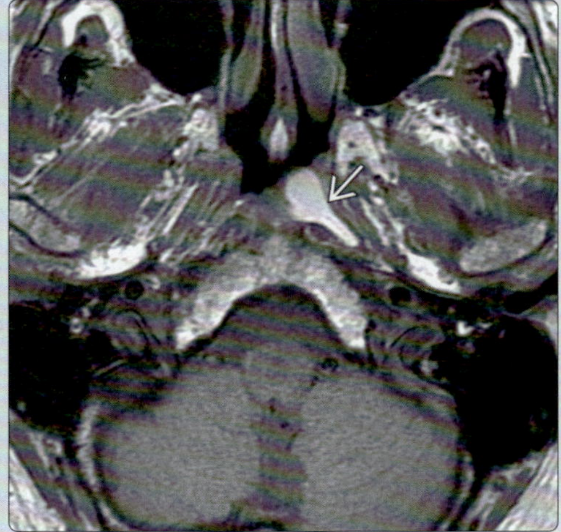

(Left) *Axial CECT in a patient with a cervical neck mass reveals a typical incidental left palatine tonsil retention cyst (RC) ➡. These cysts are postinflammatory retention cysts and are considered "leave alone" lesions.* **(Right)** *Axial T1WI MR in the same patient shows the characteristic high-signal pear-shaped RC ➡ in the lateral pharyngeal recess. The high-signal fluid within the cyst suggests the cyst contents are either hemorrhagic or proteinaceous.*

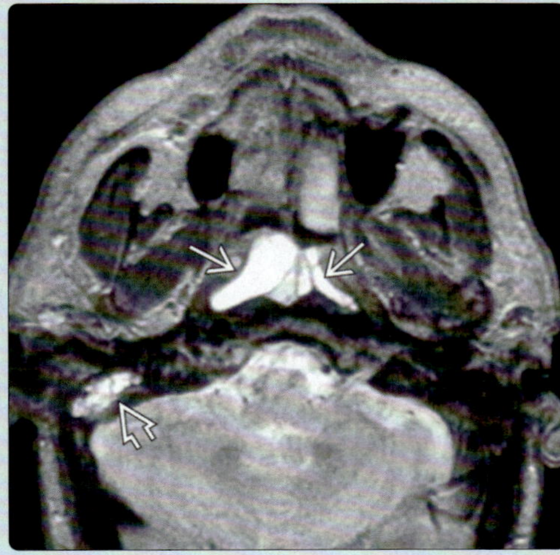

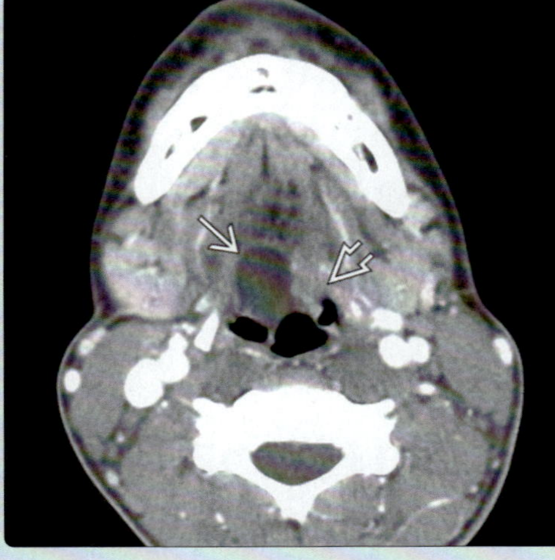

(Left) *Axial T2WI MR shows bilateral nasopharyngeal RCs ➡, larger on the right. Note that the small left RC is septated. Effusion present in the right mastoid ➡ is secondary to eustachian tube obstruction.* **(Right)** *Axial CECT at the base of the tongue in an adult reveals a right low lingual tonsil RC ➡. The left vallecula is partially filled with enhancing lingual tonsillar tissue ➡. A foramen cecum thyroglossal duct cyst would be more midline and not fill the vallecula. This lesion is different from the congenital vallecular cyst of a newborn.*

KEY FACTS

TERMINOLOGY

- Synonym: Tonsillitis/tonsillopharyngitis
- Definition: Acute, nonsuppurative tonsillar inflammation

IMAGING

- Bilateral > unilateral tonsillar enlargement with variable density and enhancement
- CECT used to distinguish acute tonsillitis from tonsillar/peritonsillar abscess (TA/PTA)
  - Well-formed capsule and homogeneous internal hypodensity in TA/PTA
- CECT **nonsuppurative tonsillar inflammation** (tonsillitis)
  - **Striated pattern** of internal enhancement (tiger stripe sign) relatively specific for tonsillar inflammation
  - Lower density area(s) may be present as transitions to TA
- Reactive adenopathy common

TOP DIFFERENTIAL DIAGNOSES

- Tonsillar/peritonsillar abscess
- Tonsillar hyperplasia (hypertrophy)
- Palatine tonsil squamous cell carcinoma

PATHOLOGY

- Most commonly secondary to respiratory virus
- 30% bacterial: Group A β-hemolytic strep most common
- Less commonly, Epstein-Barr virus mononucleosis

CLINICAL ISSUES

- Predominantly affects children and young adults
- Presentation: Fever, sore throat, tender nodes
- For diagnosis: Rapid strep test and monospot
- Treatment options
  - Tonsillar inflammation: ± antibiotics, clinical observation
  - TA/PTA: I&D with antibiotics, ± steroids and inpatient admission for airway compromise

DIAGNOSTIC CHECKLIST

- CECT: Striated pattern of internal enhancement + absence of well-defined capsule help rule out TA/PTA

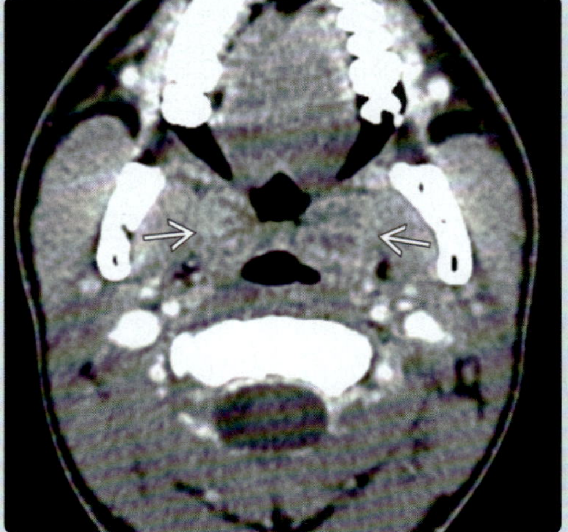

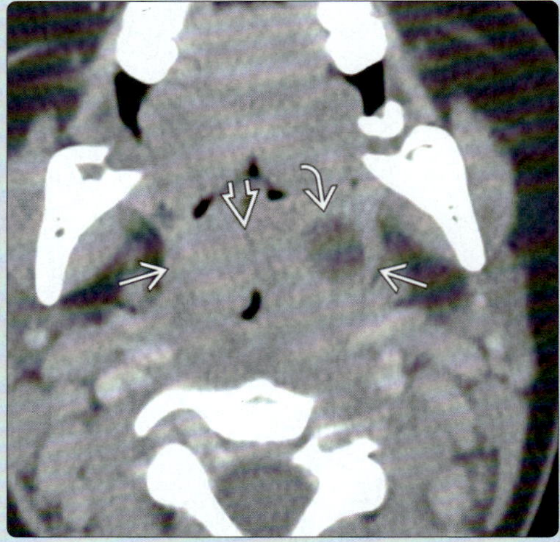

(Left) *Axial CECT in a child with fever and sore throat shows the typical striated ➡ appearance of the bilaterally enlarged palatine tonsils consistent with tonsillar inflammation (nonsuppurative tonsillitis).* **(Right)** *Axial CECT in a child with a fever and sore throat shows that both palatine tonsils ➡ are enlarged and are "kissing" in the midline ➡. There is also a low-attenuation focus within the left tonsil ➡ without a well-defined capsule, which did not yield pus at aspiration, consistent with nonsuppurative tonsillitis.*

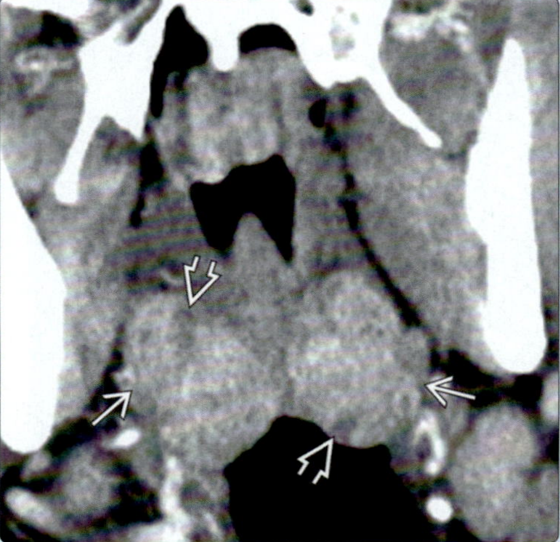

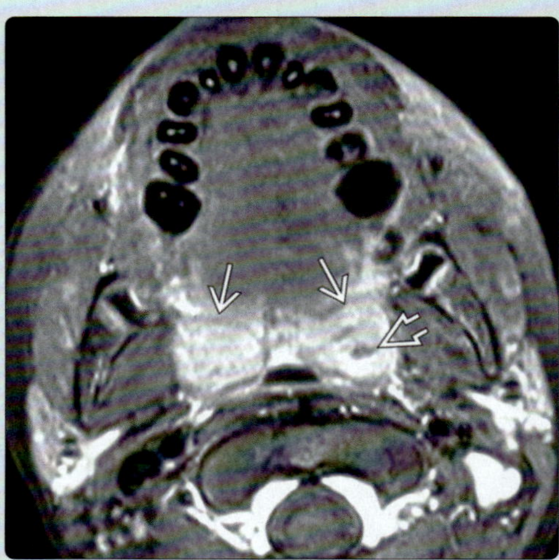

(Left) *Coronal CECT in an 11 year old with a sore throat and fever demonstrates diffuse, bilateral enlargement of the palatine tonsils ➡, both with small areas of heterogeneity ➡, consistent with edema, without frank abscess. CECT diagnosis was nonsuppurative tonsillar inflammation.* **(Right)** *Axial T1WI C+ FS MR shows bilateral tonsillar enlargement ➡ and pronounced enhancement typical of tonsillar inflammation. Small internal areas of low signal ➡ are compatible with intratonsillar edema.*

Tonsillar/Peritonsillar Abscess

KEY FACTS

TERMINOLOGY

- Definitions
  - Tonsillar abscess (TA): Palatine tonsil suppurates with abscess forming within tonsil
  - Peritonsillar abscess (PTA): Infection spreads to adjacent parapharyngeal (PPS) ± masticator (MS) ± submandibular (SMS) spaces

IMAGING

- CECT
  - TA: Swollen tonsil with central low-density & peripheral enhancing rim
  - PTA: Focal low-density pus in adjacent PPS ± MS ± SMS
  - Reactive bulky bilateral cervical adenopathy common
  - Must differentiate tonsillar inflammation from TA
    - TA may be treated with surgery
  - If indicated, CECT is recommended modality for TA or PTA
    - If PTA suspected, CECT

TOP DIFFERENTIAL DIAGNOSES

- Tonsillar hyperplasia (hypertrophy): Tonsils do not enhance or show low-density center (TA)
- Tonsillar inflammation (tonsillitis): Acute onset; unilateral or bilateral tonsil enlargement with enhancement but without low-density center (TA)
- Tonsillar retention cyst: Focal cyst with no inflammation
- Oropharyngeal neoplasia: Will usually not present with acute inflammation, swelling, and pain

CLINICAL ISSUES

- Presentation: Fever, sore throat, dysphagia, tender cervical nodes, uvular deviation, and trismus
  - Usually occurs in child or young adult
- Treatment options
  - Tonsillitis: Antibiotics & clinical observation
  - TA: Initially intravenous antibiotics alone
  - TA or PTA: I&D & antibiotics
    - Steroids; airway management for airway compromise

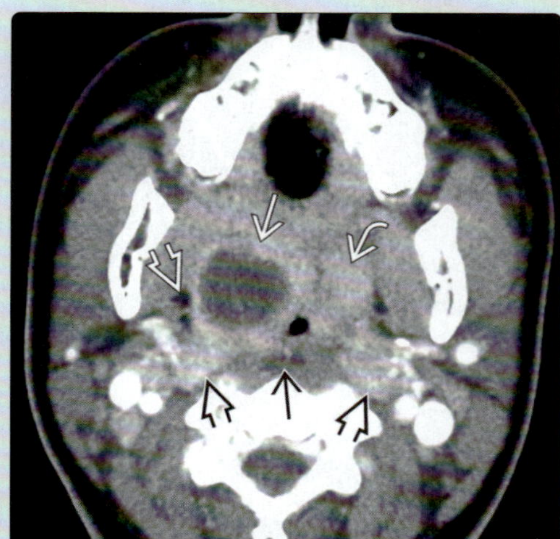

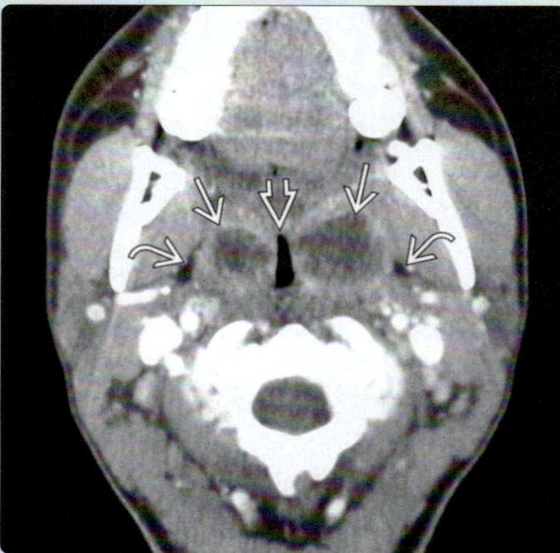

(Left) *Axial CECT shows a large, low-density tonsillar abscess. No extension through the capsule into the parapharyngeal space (PPS) is present. The left tonsil is prominent and enhancing, but no abscess is seen. Note effusion in the retropharyngeal space and reactive retropharyngeal nodes.* **(Right)** *Axial CECT reveals bilateral tonsillar abscesses, the left larger than the right. Note the mass effect on both PPSs but no extra- or peritoneal abscess. The airway is narrowed with a slit-like appearance.*

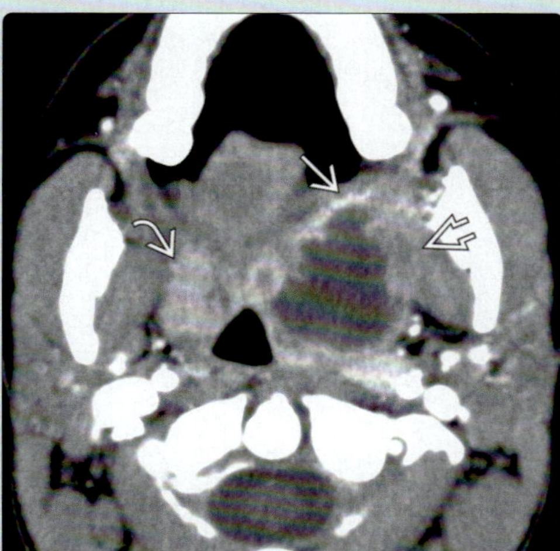

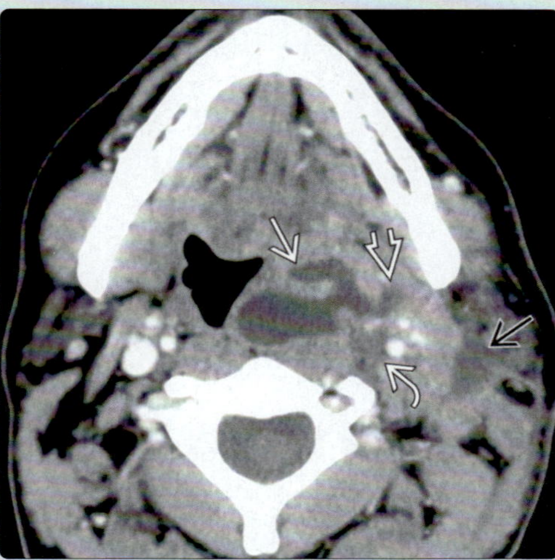

(Left) *Axial CECT demonstrates left tonsillar and peritonsillar abscess with extension through the capsule into the posterior buccal space and medial pterygoid muscle of the masticator space. Note enhancement in the inflamed right tonsil without abscess formation.* **(Right)** *Axial CECT reveals a complicated large left tonsillar abscess. Infection has ruptured posteriorly into the carotid space, anterolaterally into the upper submandibular space, and laterally into the inferior parotid space.*

Minor Salivary Gland Malignancy of Pharyngeal Mucosal Space

KEY FACTS

TERMINOLOGY

- Abbreviations: Minor salivary gland malignancy (MSGM) of pharyngeal mucosal space (PMS)
- Rare malignancy arising from minor salivary glands in pharyngeal surface
- Most common pathology: Adenoid cystic carcinoma (ACCa) > mucoepidermoid carcinoma > adenocarcinoma

IMAGING

- Locations: Oral cavity (**hard palate**) > > oropharynx (**soft palate**, base of tongue) > > nasal cavity/sinus
- CECT findings
  - Enhancing, infiltrating mass centered in PMS
  - Bone CT shows hard palate, skull base, mandible invasion
- MR findings
  - Submucosal mass usually **high T2 signal intensity**
  - T1 helpful to detect mandible or maxilla invasion, **perineural tumor**
  - T1 C+ fat saturation helps define perineural spread

TOP DIFFERENTIAL DIAGNOSES

- PMS squamous cell carcinoma
  - Naso- or oropharyngeal (palatine or lingual tonsil)
- PMS non-Hodgkin lymphoma
- PMS benign mixed tumor

CLINICAL ISSUES

- ACCa has high affinity for pulmonary metastasis
- Presentation: Painful submucosal pharyngeal surface mass
  - ACCa may present with pain & V2, V3 neuropathy
  - Imaging critical to evaluate perineural spread
- Image-guided biopsy usually needed if mass not palpable
- Management issues
  - Wide local excision via transoral (robotic) or transcervical approach, depending on location and T stage
  - Elective neck dissection (ND) controversial but is often used for high-grade MSGM; therapeutic ND when positive for nodal disease
  - Adjuvant XRT often utilized

(Left) *Axial CECT in patient with left pharyngeal mucosal space (PMS) adenoid cystic carcinoma shows a mildly enhancing invasive mass in the left nasopharynx ➡ involving the skull base ⇨ and deeper soft tissues ➡.* **(Right)** *Axial CECT in the same patient reveals the left PMS adenoid cystic carcinoma ➡ invading the prevertebral soft tissues ➡ and distorting the anatomy of the lateral pharyngeal wall ➡.*

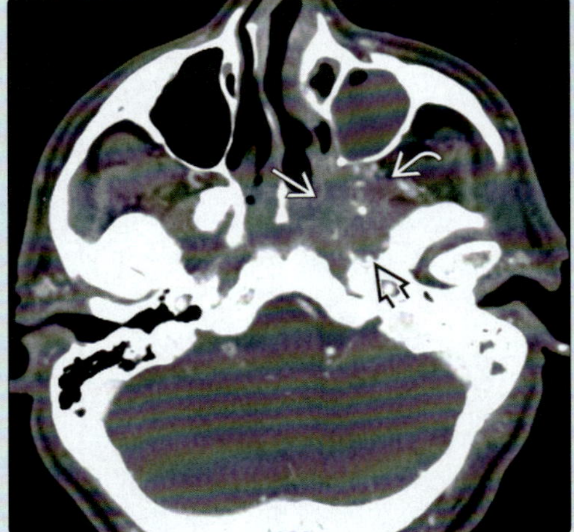

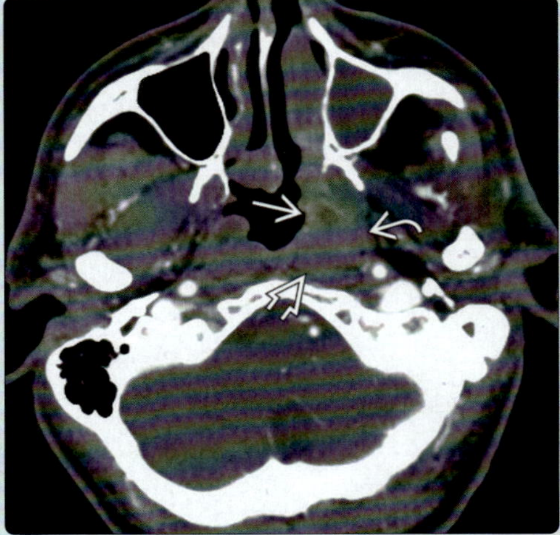

(Left) *Axial STIR MR in a patient with a left palatine tonsil adenoid cystic carcinoma ➡ reveals a heterogeneous invasive mass with both areas of high-signal and linear low-signal strands ➡ (most likely secondary to fibrous bands within the tumor).* **(Right)** *Axial enhanced fat-saturated MR in the same patient with a heterogeneously enhancing adenoid cystic carcinoma of the oropharyngeal mucosal space ➡ shows the early invasion of the left posterior tongue base ➡.*

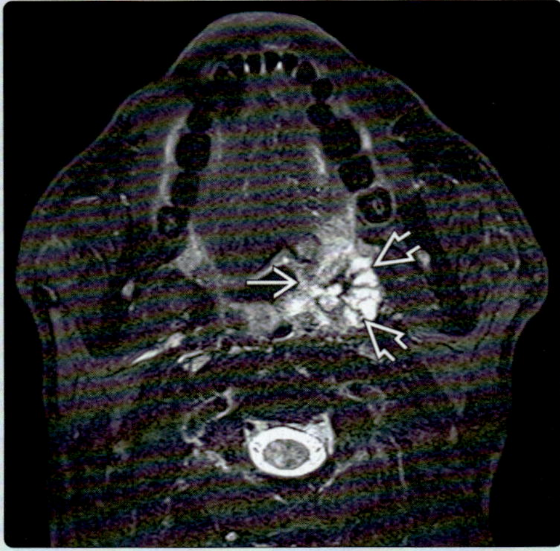

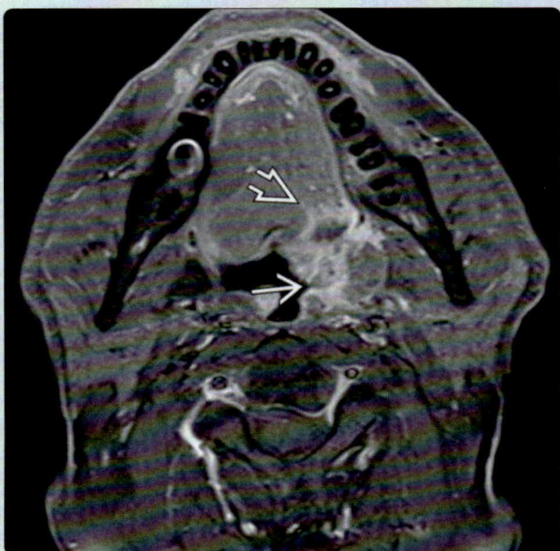

KEY FACTS

TERMINOLOGY

- Non-Hodgkin lymphoma (NHL) of pharyngeal mucosal space (PMS)
- 3 subsites of Waldeyer lymphatic ring: Nasopharyngeal adenoids, palatine & lingual tonsils

IMAGING

- CECT findings
  - **Minimally enhancing** bulky mass filling PMS airway; often without deep extension
  - Associated NHL nodal disease present **50%** of time
- MR findings
  - T2: Varies in signal intensity depending on cellularity
    - Often lower than squamous cell carcinoma (SCCa)
  - DWI: Restricted because of high cellularity

TOP DIFFERENTIAL DIAGNOSES

- Tonsillar lymphoid hyperplasia
- Nasopharyngeal, palatine or lingual tonsil SCCa
- PMS minor salivary gland malignancy
- Infectious lymphoid hyperplasia, especially mononucleosis

PATHOLOGY

- Multiple subtypes, usually B- or T-cell categories
- **Overall survival rate** for H&N PMS NHL is **60%**
- 35% of extranodal NHL in H&N occurs in PMS

CLINICAL ISSUES

- ↑ incidence in AIDS, Sjögren syndrome, Hashimoto thyroiditis, IgG4 disease, transplants
- Clinical presentation
  - Nasopharyngeal NHL: Nasal obstruction, otitis media
  - Palatine or lingual tonsil NHL: Sore throat, otalgia, mass
  - B systemic symptoms: Fever, sweats, weight loss
- Treatment approaches
  - Based on clinical stage/aggressive vs. indolent subtypes
    - Chemoradiotherapy (aggressive NHL)
    - "Watch and wait" (indolent types) in elderly

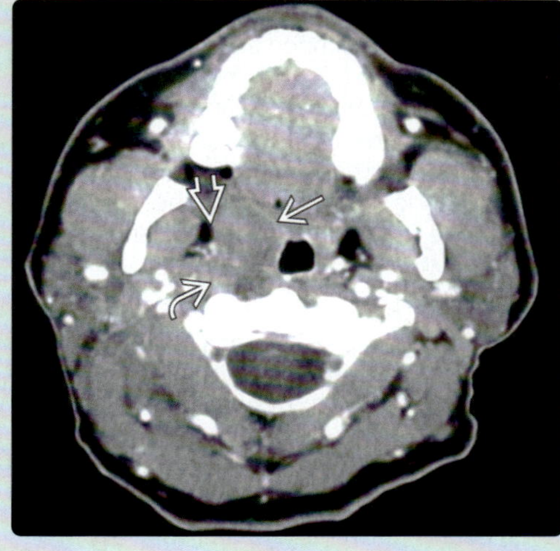

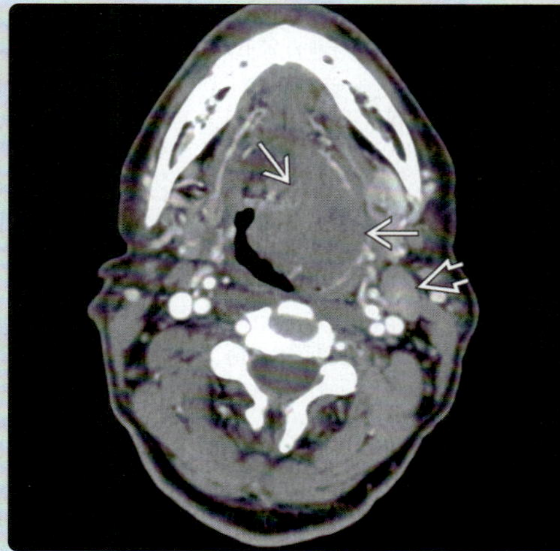

(Left) *Axial CECT shows a large, low-density mass ➡ in the right tonsil. The smooth interface between parapharyngeal fat ➡ implies no extension through the lateral capsule. Note fullness in right prevertebral muscles ➡, suggesting the mass has invaded through the posterior tonsillar capsule.* **(Right)** *Large, exophytic, minimally enhancing NHL ➡ arises in left lingual lymphoid tissue, with near-complete airway obstruction. Note the level IIA node ➡ with no central necrosis, a common finding in nodal lymphoma.*

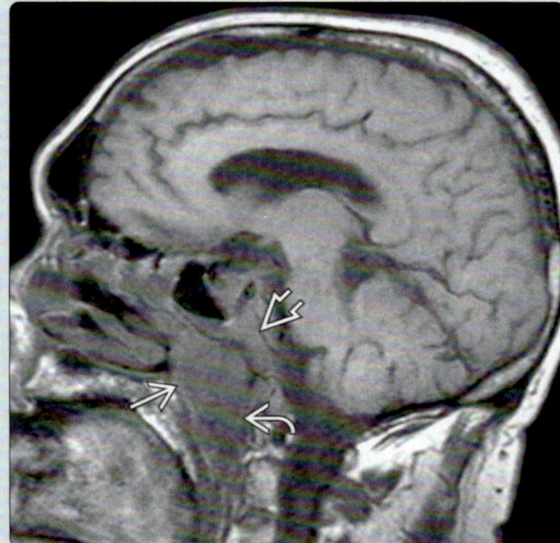

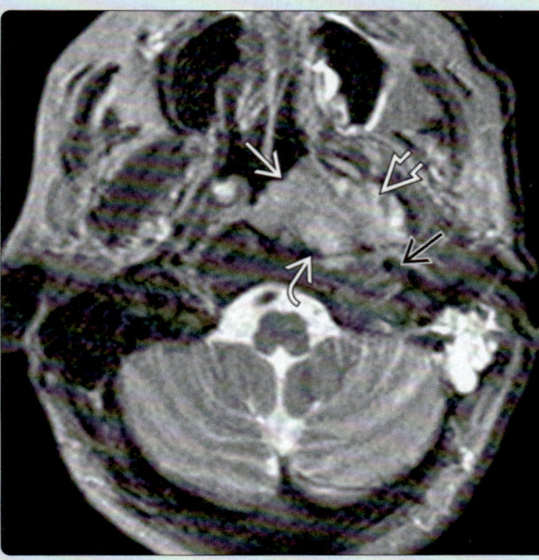

(Left) *Sagittal T1WI MR shows a bulky nasopharyngeal mass ➡ extending to the oropharyngeal level ➡. Abnormal signal intensity in the clivus ➡ implies central skull base invasion.* **(Right)** *Axial T2WI FS MR in the same patient reveals the mass ➡ is relatively low signal intensity, with invasion of prevertebral muscles ➡, parapharyngeal ➡, and carotid ➡ spaces. Note mastoid effusion secondary to tumor invasion of the eustachian tube orifice. Nasopharyngeal carcinoma could exactly mimic this imaging appearance.*

Summary Thoughts: Masticator Space

The 3 most frequently encountered abnormalities in the masticator space (MS) are infection, infection, and infection. Odontogenic infection should always cross the clinician's mind 1st when evaluating abnormalities in this space.

When evaluating tumors of the MS, the presence of **perineural CNV3 tumor spread** is of critical importance because it is easily overlooked but can have a dramatic effect on treatment and prognosis.

The MS includes the posterior body and ramus of the mandible, the 4 muscles of mastication (masseter, temporalis, medial pterygoid, lateral pterygoid), and the mandibular branch of the trigeminal nerve (CNV3). It has greater extension in the craniocaudal dimension than commonly recognized, as it reaches from the bottom of the mandible nearly to the vertex of the skull.

The MS is divided at the level of the zygomatic arch into the suprazygomatic MS (**temporal fossa**) and the infrazygomatic MS (**infratemporal fossa**).

Imaging Techniques & Indications

Because **odontogenic infection** is by far the **most likely pathology** to affect the MS, CECT is the preferred imaging modality. The tooth of origin can be best identified with bone CT. This is important because the infection will recur until the offending tooth is treated. To be sure that a worrisome tooth is the true site of origin, look for mandibular cortical erosions that communicate between the apical tooth abscess and the soft tissue MS abscess. Contrast is needed to determine how far the infection has spread into soft tissues. Contrast also helps differentiate cellulitis and phlegmon from surgically drainable abscess.

Either CECT or enhanced MR cover the entire length of **CNV3** in the MS, in the jaw, and up to the skull base to assess for perineural tumor spread (**PNT**). Ideally, imaging should include the lateral pons, Meckel cave, foramen ovale, the mandibular foramen (where the inferior alveolar nerve enters the mandible), the entire inferior alveolar canal, and the mental foramen.

Imaging Anatomy

The MS is the largest suprahyoid neck space. In the superior direction its suprazygomatic component extends along the parietal skull almost to the vertex, enclosing the temporalis muscle. There is a broad abutment of the MS to the skull base. Within this area of contact with the skull base is the **foramen ovale (CNV3)** and the **foramen spinosum** (middle meningeal artery). Inferiorly, the MS terminates at the inferior margin of the posterior body of the mandible.

MS regional anatomic relationships are important as both tumor and infection of the MS tend to spread into adjacent spaces. The buccal space is found anteriorly, including the retromaxillary fat pad. The parotid space is posterolateral, while the parapharyngeal space is posteromedial to the MS. The relationship between the MS & PPS is important because the PPS fat will be displaced posteromedially by an enlarging MS mass. Medial to the MS is the pharyngeal mucosal space. The subcutaneous fat of the cheek is seen lateral to the MS.

The **superficial layer** of the **deep cervical fascia** divides around the inferior margin of the mandible. This split fascia encases the mandible and the muscles of mastication. The medial slip of the fascia runs along the deep surface of the pterygoid muscles to insert on the undersurface of the skull base just **medial** to **foramen ovale**. The medial slip is also known as the medial pterygoid fascia. The lateral slip covers the superficial surface of the masseter muscle and attaches to the zygomatic arch, where the masseter muscle originates. This lateral fascia continues over the temporalis muscle to the top of the suprazygomatic MS. There is no fascia separating the suprazygomatic and infrazygomatic portions of the MS. In fact, there are no horizontal fascia anywhere in the MS, facilitating craniocaudal spread of disease.

Most of the MS is filled by the **4 muscles of mastication**. The masseter muscle originates at the zygomatic arch and inserts on the inferior mandibular body. The temporalis muscle takes its origin from a semicircular area of bone splayed across the parietal skull. Inferiorly, the temporalis inserts on the coronoid process of the mandible. The medial pterygoid arises from the medial pterygoid plate and inserts on the lingual surface of the mandibular angle and ramus. The lateral pterygoid muscle originates from the lateral pterygoid plate and greater wing of sphenoid and inserts on the pterygoid fovea under the mandibular condyle. The lateral pterygoid is unique among the muscles of mastication because it serves to open the jaw instead of close it.

The mandibular division of the **CNV3** emerges into the MS from the middle cranial fossa via the **foramen ovale**. CNV3 gives off a masticator branch (motor innervation to the muscles of mastication), a mylohyoid branch (motor innervation to the mylohyoid and anterior digastric muscles), and an auriculotemporal branch (sensory innervation to the skin overlying the parotid gland). The nerve continues as the inferior alveolar nerve, entering the mandible via the **mandibular foramen** on the lingual surface of the mandibular ramus.

The remaining contents of the MS are the inferior alveolar artery and veins (which accompany the inferior alveolar nerve into the mandibular foramen), the **pterygoid venous plexus** (which lies amongst the fibers of the pterygoid muscles), and the ramus and posterior body of the mandible. The posterior teeth are considered part of the oral cavity, not the MS. Remember the TMJ is within the superior aspect of the infrazygomatic MS. Tumefactive TMJ lesions must be considered in the differential diagnosis of an MS mass.

Approaches to Imaging Issues of Masticator Space

The answer to the question, "What imaging findings define a MS mass?" depends on what part of the MS is primarily involved. If the lesion is in the infrazygomatic MS, the muscles of mastication, ramus, and posterior body of the mandible are involved. If a larger mass is present, the parapharyngeal fat is displaced posteromedially. If the lesion begins in the suprazygomatic MS, it is within or immediately adjacent to the temporalis muscle in the temporal fossa.

The MS is one of the suprahyoid neck spaces that is connected to the intracranial compartment via a major cranial nerve branch, CNV3. As a result, all MS masses should be assessed for possible **PNT** along CNV3 into the middle cranial fossa. Squamous cell carcinoma from the chin skin, alveolar ridge, and retromolar trigone may demonstrate PNT spreading through the foramen ovale into the Meckel cave and beyond. Alternatively, a parotid space malignancy may travel along the

Differential Diagnosis of Masticator Space

Pseudolesions	Malignant tumor, primary
Asymmetric pterygoid venous plexus	Chondrosarcoma
Asymmetric accessory parotid lobe	Osteosarcoma
Motor denervation CNV3 (acute or chronic)	Synovial sarcoma
Benign masticator muscle hypertrophy	Rhabdomyosarcoma
Infectious	Malignant schwannoma
Odontogenic abscess	Non-Hodgkin lymphoma (primary H&N)
Inflammatory	**Malignant tumor, metastatic**
Postradiation scarring	SCCa from retromolar trigone (direct invasion)
Vascular	SCCa from oral cavity (perineural spread along V3)
Venous or venolymphatic malformation	Intracranial tumor spread (glioblastoma, meningioma)
Benign tumor	SCCa from nasopharynx (direct spread)
Fibromatosis	Systemic hematogenous metastasis
Neurofibroma	Non-Hodgkin lymphoma (direct invasion from jaw primary)
Schwannoma (CNV3)	Non-Hodgkin lymphoma (systemic)
Infantile hemangioma	

SCCa = squamous cell carcinoma.

auriculotemporal nerve to CNV3 and then through the foramen ovale to the intracranial compartment.

When CNV3 is injured, the muscles that undergo denervation are the muscles of mastication, the tensor tympani and palatini, anterior belly of the digastric, and the mylohyoid. Remember that in acute-subacute denervation, the muscles often swell and enhance, whereas in more chronic denervation, the muscles lose volume and fatty infiltrate.

There are at least 4 **pseudolesions** that can mimic pathology in the MS. The most challenging of these is the **pterygoid venous plexus**. This structure has a wide range of size in normal individuals. It lies within and around the pterygoid muscles in the medial MS. Asymmetric pterygoid venous plexus can mimic an infiltrative mass or PNT involving the pterygoid muscles.

A 2nd pseudolesion of note is **denervation of the muscles of mastication**. In the acute phase of denervation, the affected muscles may be mistaken for tumor infiltration as they enlarge and enhance. The sparing of the muscle ligaments is an important clue to the diagnosis. In late denervation, muscular atrophy can be mistaken for a tumor (due to asymmetric muscle bulk) on the contralateral side.

Similarly, **benign masticator muscle hypertrophy** is a 3rd potential pseudolesion. This can mimic a mass lesion due to asymmetric enlargement of the muscles of mastication; however, normal muscle attenuation and signal, lack of enhancement, and preserved internal architecture (with normal striated appearance typical of muscle tissue) helps distinguish this pseudolesion from pathology.

Finally, **prominent or asymmetric accessory lobe of the parotid gland** can mimic a mass on clinical examination, especially when asymmetrically enlarged on 1 side. The accessory lobe typically has the same density or signal and enhancement pattern as the remainder of the parotid gland on CT or MR imaging.

Clinical Implications

A common clinical presentation of a MS mass is **trismus,** which is defined as the inability to open the mouth due to masticator muscle spasm, inflammation, or fibrosis. Patients with trismus are notoriously difficult to examine clinically. Intubation also becomes challenging if patients need surgery. Imaging plays an even more important role in assessment of these patients.

The most frequent primary neoplasm of the MS is **sarcoma**, either from the mandible or soft tissues. However, extension of **oral cavity squamous cell carcinoma** from the **mandibular alveolar ridge** is far more common than primary MS malignancy, so evidence of a mucosal origin should be sought.

The presence of PNT is critical to the prognosis and care of cancer patients. PNT may require additional surgery, chemotherapy, &/or radiation therapy. If PNT reaches the intracranial compartment, the tumor may be rendered unresectable. Remember that enhanced, fat-saturated MR is far more sensitive than CECT for PNT. As a result, MR should be recommended in patients who are at risk for PNT. One final caveat regarding PNT: Only a high degree of suspicion during image analysis will allow the radiologist to make the diagnosis of subtle PNT.

Tumefactive TMJ lesions must also be considered whenever there is a mass found in the peri-TMJ portion of the MS. Pigmented villonodular synovitis, calcium pyrophosphate dihydrate deposition disease, and synovial chondromatosis are the principal TMJ lesions that must be added to the list of tumor-like lesions in the MS.

Selected References

1. Gamss C et al: Imaging evaluation of the suprahyoid neck. Radiol Clin North Am. 53(1):133-44, 2015
2. Faye N et al: The masticator space: from anatomy to pathology. J Neuroradiol. 36(3):121-30, 2009
3. Wei Y et al: Masticator space: CT and MRI of secondary tumor spread. AJR Am J Roentgenol. 189(2):488-97, 2007
4. Curtin HD: Separation of the masticator space from the parapharyngeal space. Radiology. 163(1):195-204, 1987

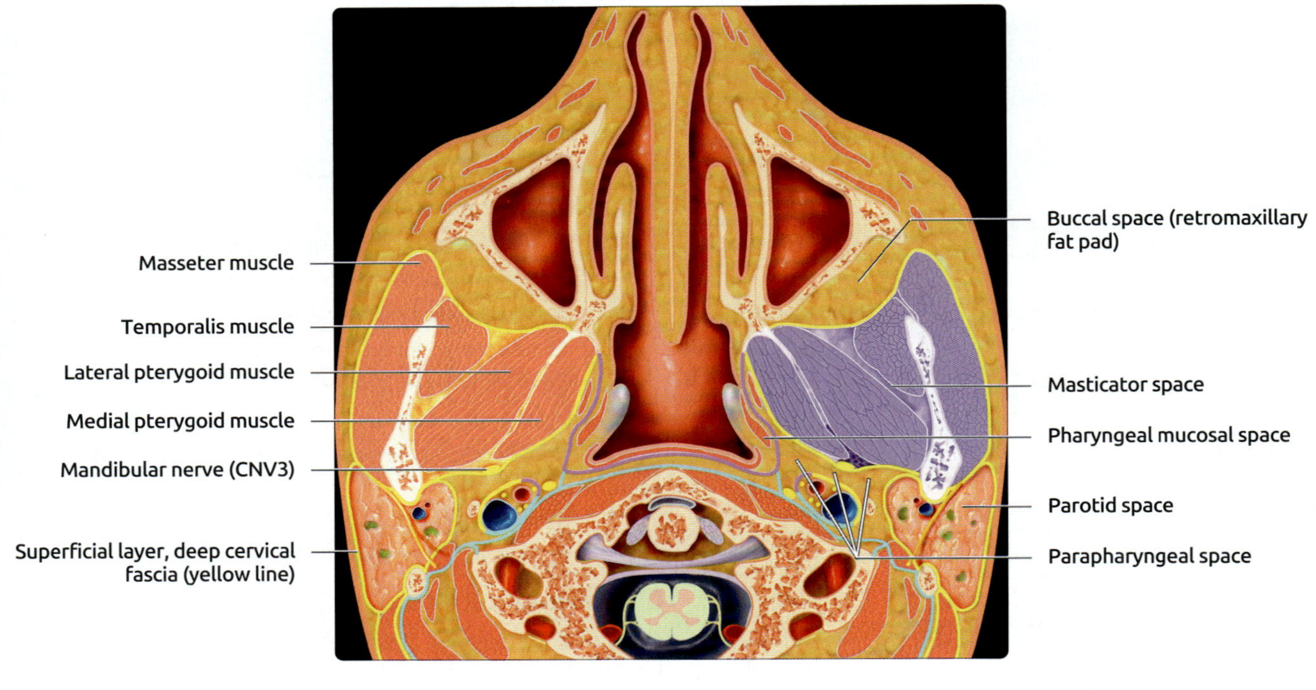

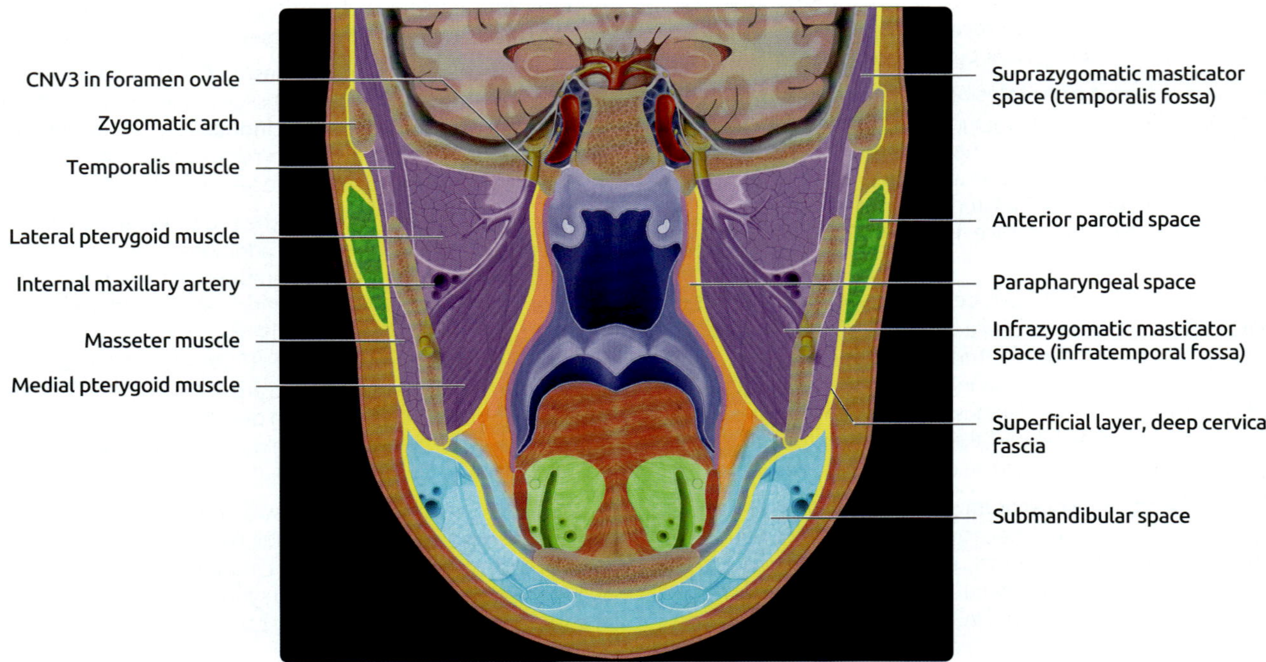

(Top) *Axial graphic shows the masticator space (MS) enclosed by the superficial layer (investing layer) of the deep cervical fascia (yellow line). The muscles of mastication from medial to lateral are the medial and lateral pterygoid, temporalis, and masseter muscles. Note the mandibular nerve (CNV3 main trunk) lies just posterior to the medial pterygoid muscle inside the superficial layer of deep cervical fascia. The buccal space is anterior, while the parapharyngeal and parotid space are posterior to the MS. The pharyngeal mucosal space is medial.* **(Bottom)** *Coronal graphic of the MS shows the suprazygomatic & infrazygomatic components. Note the medial slip of the superficial layer of the deep cervical fascia attaching to the skull base just medial to the foramen ovale, while the lateral slip continues over the zygomatic arch and up the parietal bone.*

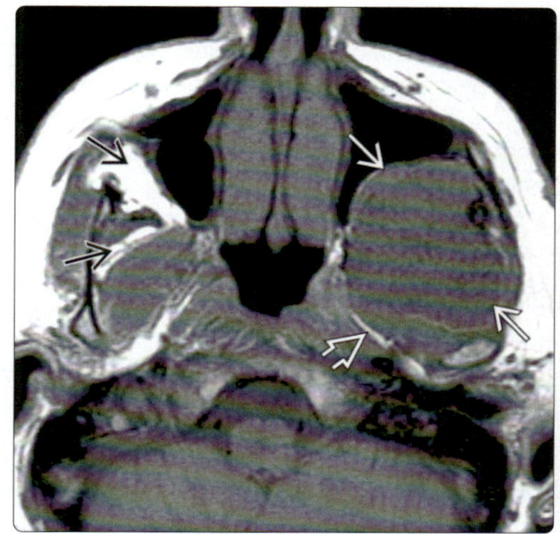

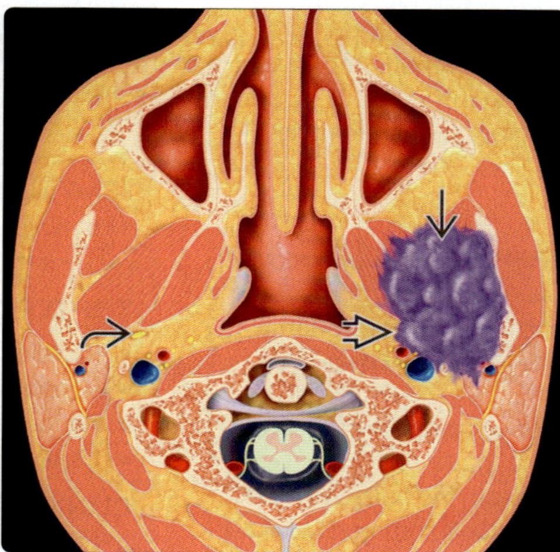

(Left) *Axial T1 MR shows a large MS mass . Parapharyngeal fat is displaced posteromedially. The muscles of mastication are invaded, and surrounding fat planes are replaced by tumor. Note preserved fat planes in the contralateral MS for comparison.* **(Right)** *Axial graphic shows a generic MS mass invading the parapharyngeal space from anterior to posterior. The CNV3 is engulfed by the tumor. Note the normal contralateral mandibular nerve for comparison.*

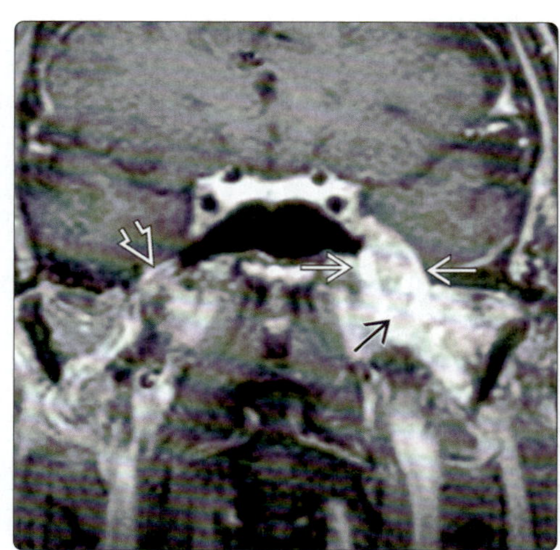

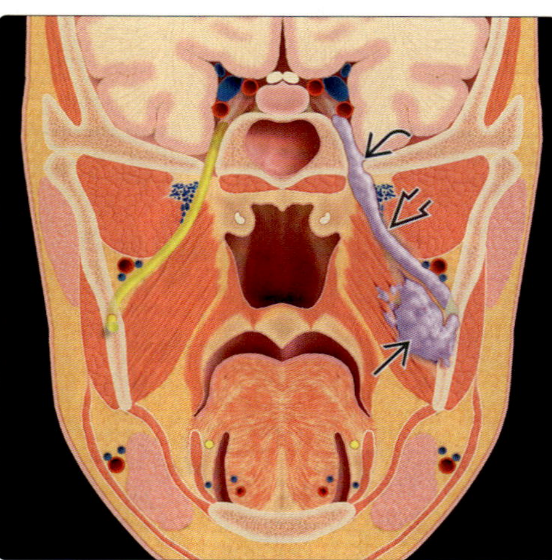

(Left) *Coronal T1 C+ FS MR shows a perineural tumor along CNV3, widening the foramen ovale as it extends intracranially. Compare the perineural tumor to the opposite normal size of the contralateral foramen , where normal perineural enhancement can be seen.* **(Right)** *Coronal graphic of the suprahyoid neck demonstrates a generic malignant tumor of the MS spreading in a perineural fashion along CNV3 . Notice the tumor traversing the foramen ovale into the intracranial compartment.*

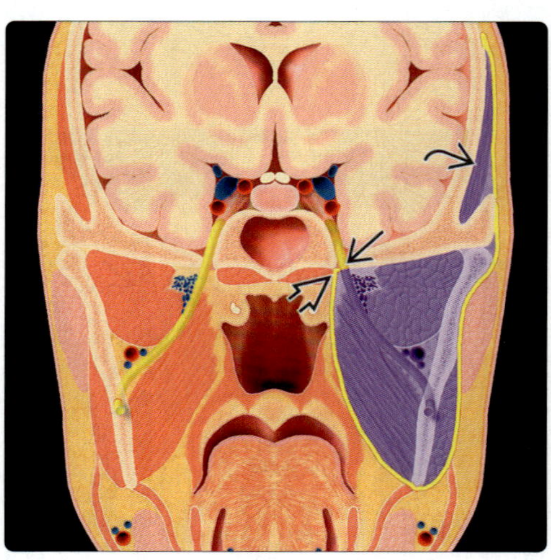

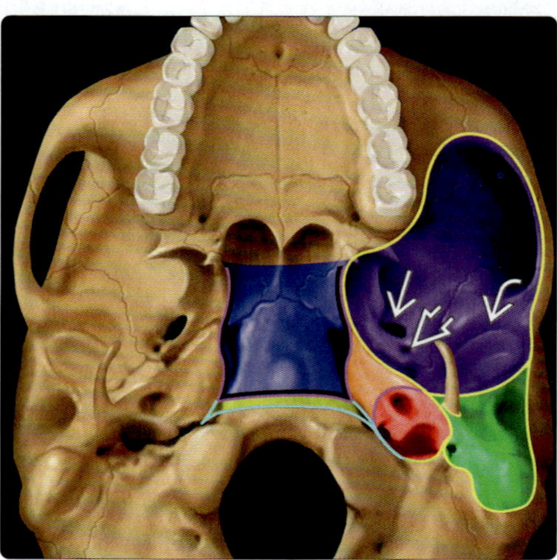

(Left) *Coronal graphic shows the craniocaudal extent of the MS. CNV3 passes through the foramen ovale near the medial attachment of the superficial layer of the deep cervical fascia . Note more superior suprazygomatic MS .* **(Right)** *Axial skull base graphic depicts the large area of abutment of the MS (purple). The yellow line around the outer MS margin represents the superficial layer of deep cervical fascia. Note the foramen ovale , spinosum , and TMJ within the MS skull base abutment.*

Pterygoid Venous Plexus Asymmetry

KEY FACTS

TERMINOLOGY

- Pterygoid venous plexus (PVP) asymmetry definition: Unilateral prominence of deep facial venous network draining cavernous sinus
  - Incidental finding at time of brain or neck imaging

IMAGING

- Relevant imaging anatomy
  - Cavernous sinus drains to PVP through foramina ovale, spinosum, & lacerum
  - PVP also connects with ophthalmic veins through inferior orbital fissure & anterior facial vein via deep facial branch
  - Receives tributaries from pterygopalatine maxillary artery
  - PVP drainage: Maxillary to retromandibular vein → IJV
  - PVP alternate drainage: Posterior & common facial veins → IJV
- CT or MR imaging
  - Tubular enhancing structures in medial masticator space ± parapharyngeal space
  - Identical enhancement in other neck veins
  - Caveat: May appear as "vascular mass" when asymmetry is prominent
    - PVP asymmetry knowledge prevents misdiagnosis
- MR imaging only
  - Flow signal may be seen in left > right PVP on 3T MRA images in normal patients

TOP DIFFERENTIAL DIAGNOSES

- Prominent internal maxillary arterial branches
- Venous vascular malformation
- Perineural V3 tumor of pterygopalatine fossa
- Carotid-cavernous fistula

CLINICAL ISSUES

- Must differentiate PVP asymmetry from CNV3 perineural tumor

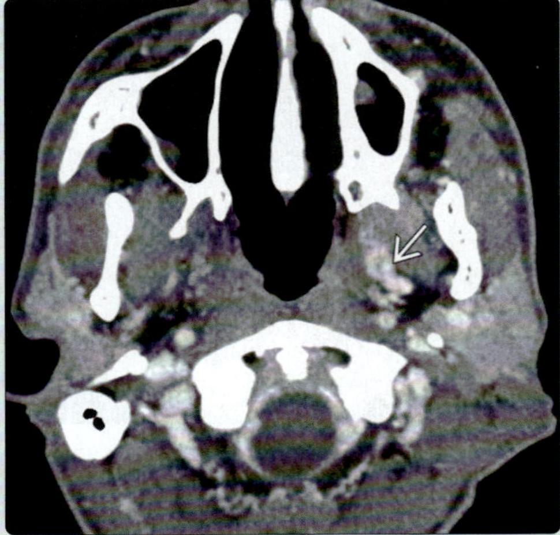

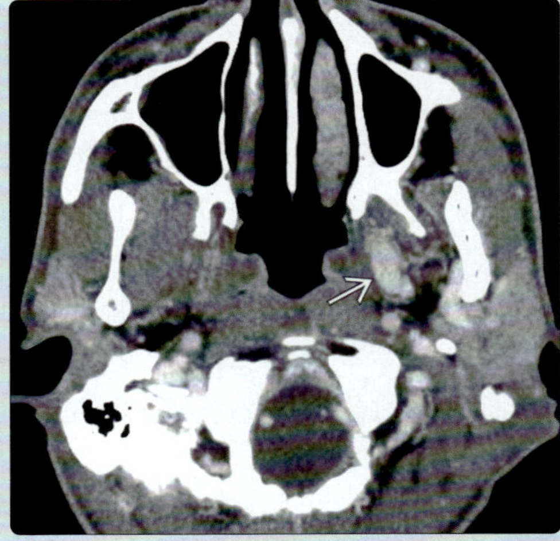

(Left) *Axial CECT shows curvilinear enhancement in the medial masticator and parapharyngeal spaces ➡ representing incidental enlarged asymmetric left PVP. Note enhancement is similar density compared to other veins.* **(Right)** *Axial CECT at a level just above the previous image shows a more mass-like appearance of incidental asymmetric enlarged pterygoid venous plexus ➡. Although this might raise concern for perineural tumor spread, enhancement does not parallel the expected course of CNV3.*

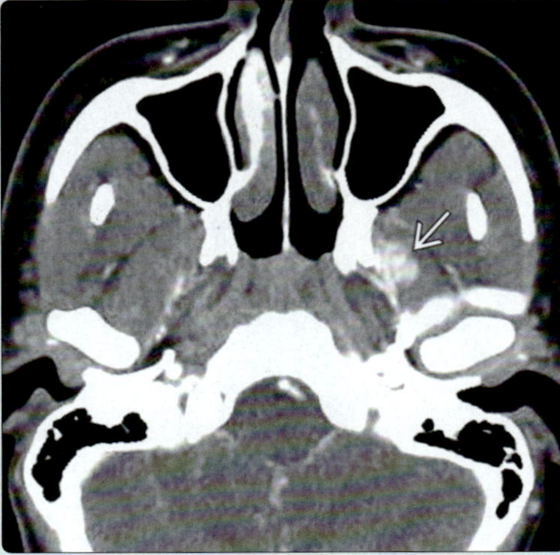

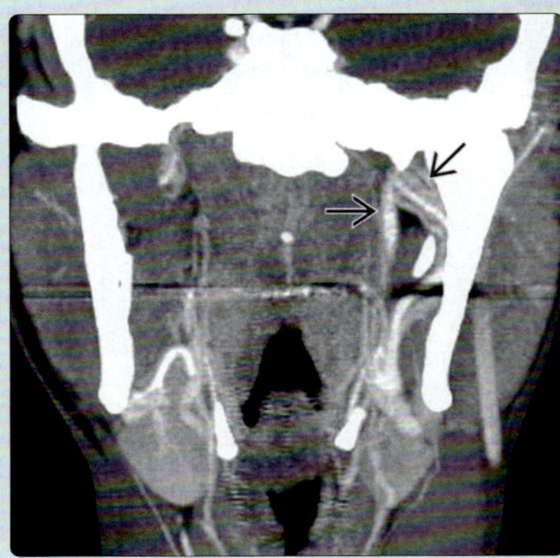

(Left) *Axial CECT shows mass-like enhancement in the medial masticator space ➡ representing incidental asymmetric enlargement of the left pterygoid venous plexus. Caveat: Do not mistake this normal variant for an "enhancing masticator space mass" or "vascular lesion."* **(Right)** *Coronal CECT reconstructed from the previous axial image better demonstrates the linear converging vascular structures ➡ representing incidental asymmetric enlargement of the left pterygoid venous plexus.*

Benign Masticator Muscle Hypertrophy

KEY FACTS

TERMINOLOGY

- Definition: Benign enlargement of muscles of mastication

IMAGING

- General features
  - Smooth, diffuse enlargement of masticator muscle(s)
    - Masseter, temporalis, medial, and lateral pterygoids
    - Masseter muscle most obviously affected
    - Masticator muscles enhance normally
  - 50% bilateral, usually asymmetric
- CT: Enlarged, normal-density masticator muscles
  - Cortical thickening affecting mandible & zygomatic arch
- MR: Enlarged, normal-intensity masticator muscles

TOP DIFFERENTIAL DIAGNOSES

- Masticator space abscess or neoplasm (sarcoma)
- Masticator space squamous cell carcinoma (SCCa)
  - SCCa enters masticator space directly (from retromolar trigone, palatine tonsil)
  - Skin of chin or mandibular alveolar ridge SCCa enters masticator space via perineural CNV3 route
- Parotid neoplasm

CLINICAL ISSUES

- Clinical causes
  - **Bruxism** (nocturnal teeth grinding)
  - Other: Habitual gum chewing, TMJ dysfunction, anabolic steroids, unilateral chewing
- Clinical presentation
  - Nontender lateral facial mass that enlarges with jaw clenching
    - Large masseter muscle most obvious clinical finding
  - Slowly progressive masticator muscle enlargement
- Treatment options
  - Surgery only for cosmetic reasons
  - Botulinum toxin A injection
  - Treat underlying cause

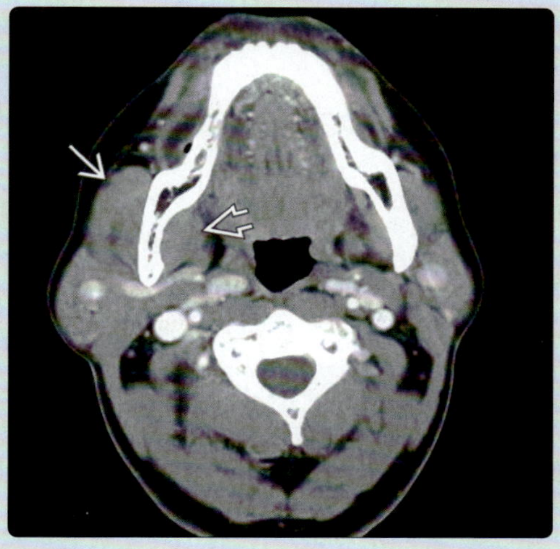

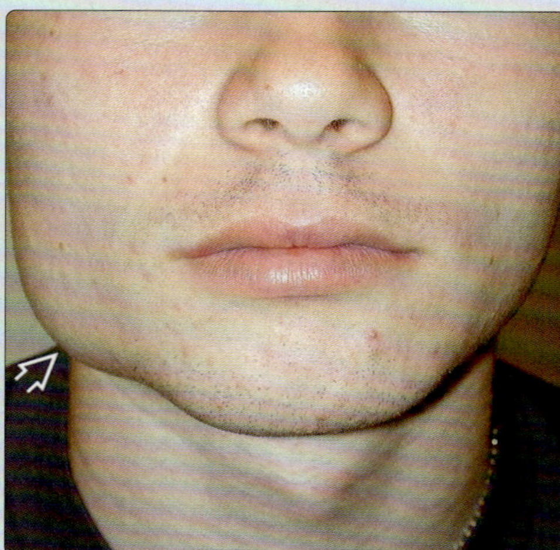

(Left) *Axial CECT demonstrates incidental unilateral asymmetric enlargement of the right masseter ➡ and medial pterygoid ➡ muscle. Enhancement and density of these muscles are equal to the opposite side. Patient was a nocturnal teeth grinder (bruxism).* **(Right)** *Clinical photograph demonstrates the clinical appearance of a patient with unilateral benign masticator muscle hypertrophy. Note the broad, smooth cheek bulge secondary to the enlarged masseter muscle ➡.*

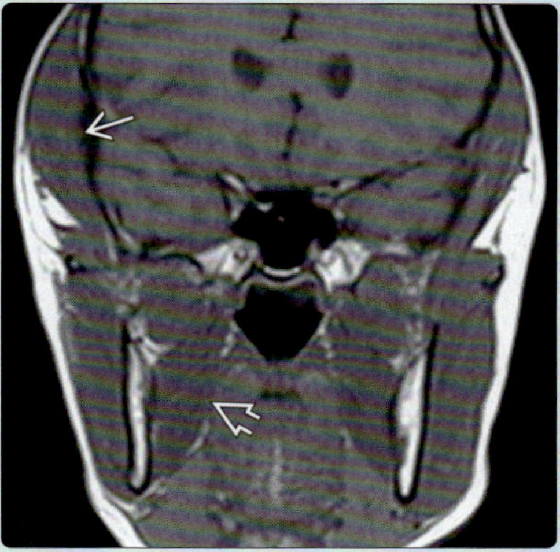

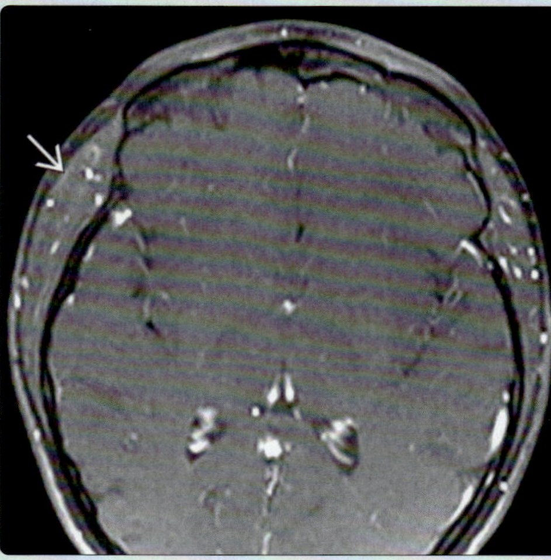

(Left) *Coronal T1 MR shows asymmetric enlargement of the right temporalis ➡ and medial pterygoid ➡ muscles in a young teenager complaining of the cosmetic deformity when wearing her hair pulled back in a ponytail. Any mixture of the muscles of mastication enlargement may be seen in benign masticator muscle hypertrophy.* **(Right)** *Axial T1 C+ FS MR in the same patient shows normal muscle signal intensity in the enlarged right temporalis without enhancement ➡.*

KEY FACTS

TERMINOLOGY

- Abbreviations: Trigeminal nerve (CNV)
- Mandibular nerve: 3rd division of CNV (CNV3) only division with motor function
- CNV3 denervation atrophy: Alteration in appearance of muscle groups from loss of innervation
    - **Acute** (< 1 month): Muscles slightly enlarged with edema; enhancement seen
    - **Subacute** (≤ 12-20 months): Fatty replacement and atrophy begins
    - **Chronic** (> 12-20 months): Fatty atrophic muscles with significant volume loss

IMAGING

- Involved muscles: Masticator space (muscles of mastication), nasopharynx (tensor veli palatini), and anterior belly digastric and mylohyoid muscles
- **Acute**: Increased T2 signal intensity with edema of muscles and abnormal contrast enhancement
- **Subacute**: T2 prolongation and abnormal contrast enhancement (diminishing) with early fatty replacement
- **Chronic**: Fatty infiltration of muscles with volume loss of muscles of mastication
- MR imaging tips
    - Fat saturation/STIR makes ↑ T2 signal more evident
    - Fat saturation on T1 C+ ↑ enhancement visibility

PATHOLOGY

- Malignant or benign tumors involving CNV3
- Surgical trauma 2nd most frequent cause

DIAGNOSTIC CHECKLIST

- 1st determine that CNV3 denervation present by analyzing muscles involved
- 2nd determine cause of CNV3 denervation
- Review history for obvious episodes of trauma or surgery
- If none, malignant tumor must be excluded
    - Search for CNV3 perineural tumor

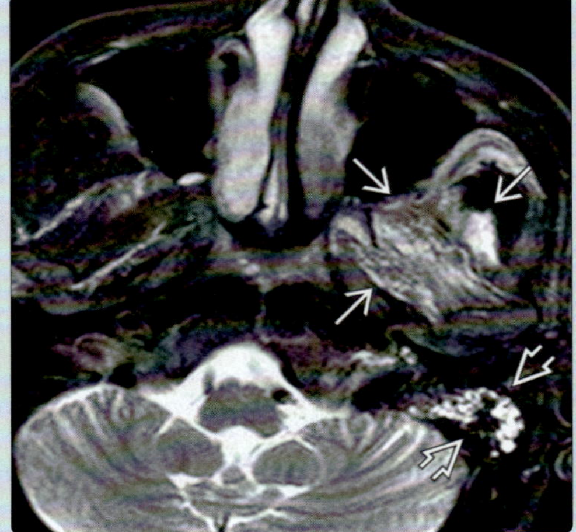

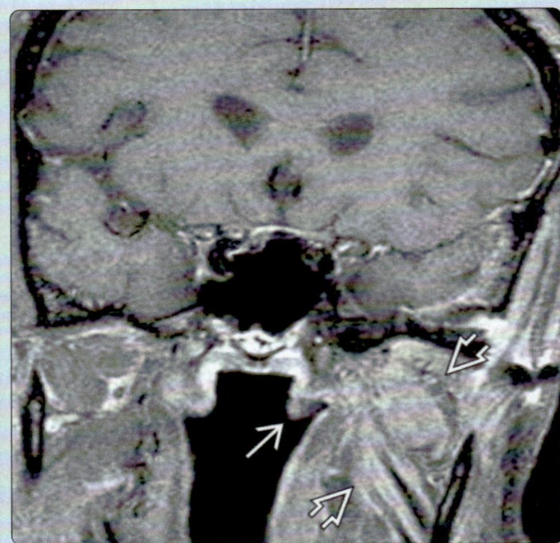

(Left) *Axial T2WI FS MR demonstrates increased signal in the pterygoid muscles and deep portion of temporalis muscle ➡. Mastoid opacification ➡ indicates eustachian tube obstruction due to tensor veli palatini dysfunction. This patient had meningioma in Meckel cave (not shown).* **(Right)** *Coronal T1WI C+ FS MR in the same patient shows mild pterygoid muscle enhancement ➡ as well as small size of left torus tubarius ➡ consistent with subacute denervation atrophy of CNV3.*

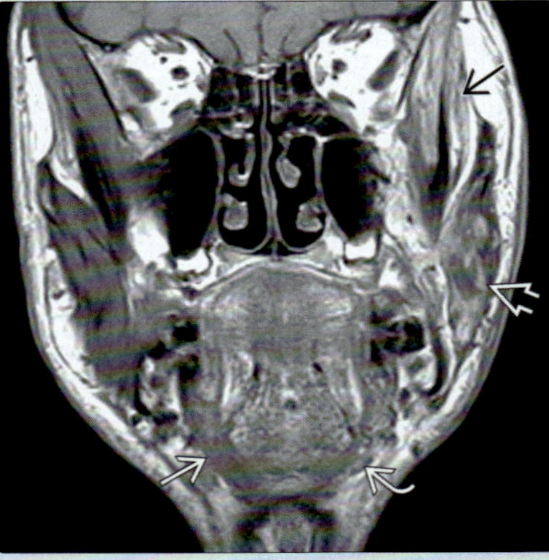

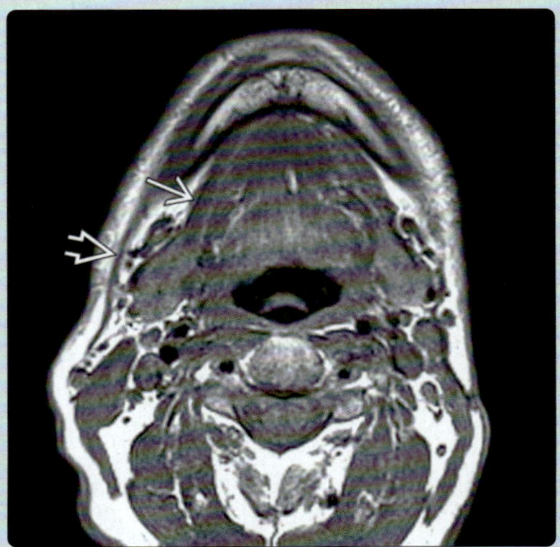

(Left) *Coronal T1WI MR reveals chronic fatty atrophy of the left temporalis ➡ and masseter ➡ muscle indicating chronic CNV3 injury. The left mylohyoid muscle ➡ is also small with fatty infiltration compared to the normal right mylohyoid muscle ➡.* **(Right)** *Axial T1WI MR in the same patient demonstrates the normal right mylohyoid muscle ➡ and platysma muscle ➡. Absence/marked atrophy on the left indicates that both CNV3 (mylohyoid) and CNVII (platysma) are chronically injured.*

KEY FACTS

TERMINOLOGY

- Definition: Abscess in masticator space (MS) from molar tooth infection or following dental procedure

IMAGING

- **CECT** preferred imaging modality in suspected infection
  - Soft tissue & bone algorithm CECT is best imaging approach in acutely infected patients with trismus
- CECT findings
  - **Focal fluid density** within muscles of mastication with thick **enhancing rim** = **MS abscess**
    - Adjacent muscles are swollen, enhancing without associated fluid = **myositis**
  - Bone CT: Tooth radiolucency or extraction socket ± gas
    - Periosteal elevation ± cortical erosion = **osteomyelitis**

TOP DIFFERENTIAL DIAGNOSES

- Cellulitis-phlegmon of MS
- Mandibular osteonecrosis
- TMJ degenerative disease
- Masticator muscle hypertrophy
- Sarcoma of MS

CLINICAL ISSUES

- Symptom: **Trismus**, fever, pain
  - Initial presentation may be confused clinically with TMJ disease (i.e., TMJ pain and trismus)
- Treatment options
  - Early MS abscess treated with involved molar extraction, ± I&D, + antibiotics
  - Late abscess treatment: Surgical drainage + IV antibiotics

DIAGNOSTIC CHECKLIST

- Questions for clinician and radiologist to address
  - What is potential source (specify offending tooth)
  - Is mandibular osteomyelitis present
  - Is MS only space with abscess (if others, name them)
  - Is suprazygomatic MS involved

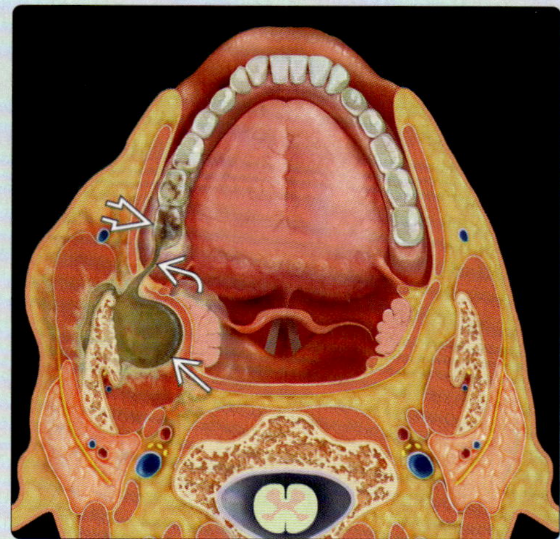

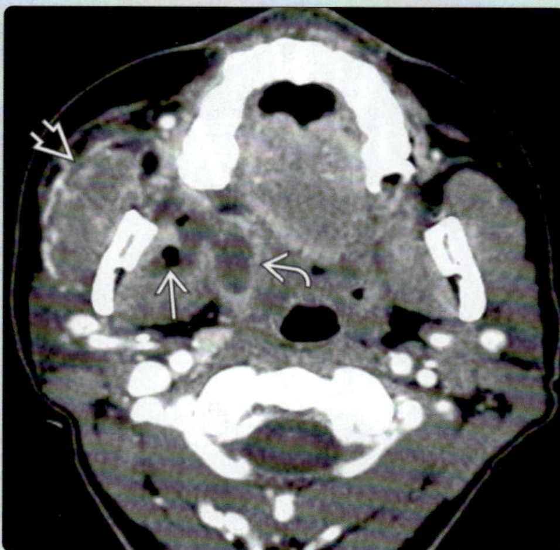

(Left) *Axial graphic depicts a masticator space (MS) abscess arising from an infected posterior mandibular molar tooth. Notice the fistula tract leading from the tooth to the abscess.* **(Right)** *Axial CECT in a 31 year old presenting with facial swelling, pain, and trismus demonstrates right medial MS abscess containing gas. There is inflammatory change in the lateral MS with edema and enlargement of the masseter muscle (myositis). Note medial extension into the deep right palatine tonsil.*

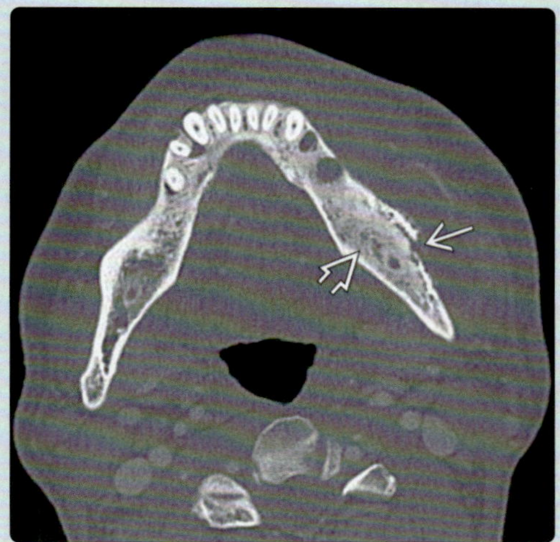

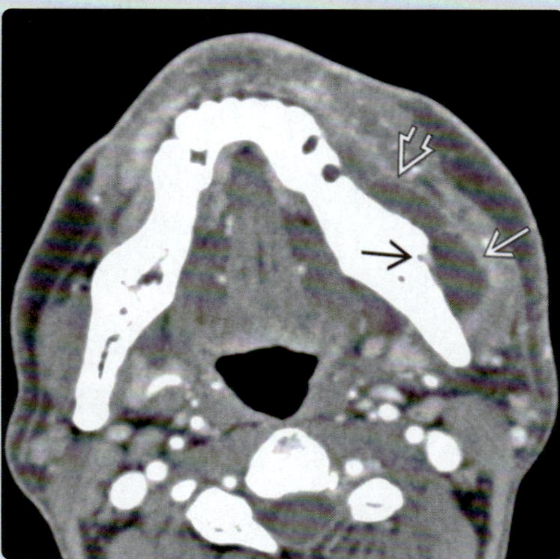

(Left) *Axial CECT in patient with mandibular osteomyelitis from an infected left molar tooth shows periosteal elevation and disruption. The underlying marrow space is sclerotic compared to the opposite normal right side.* **(Right)** *Axial CECT in same patient shows the mandibular cortical disruption connected to the lateral MS abscess. The abscess has ruptured anteriorly into the buccal space.*

Masticator Space CNV3 Schwannoma

KEY FACTS

TERMINOLOGY

- CNV3 schwannoma: Encapsulated tumor of Schwann cell origin, which displaces rather than infiltrates fascicles of CNV3 in masticator space

IMAGING

- General features: Well-circumscribed, fusiform, smoothly marginated soft tissue mass along course of CNV3
- Bone CT findings
  - **Smooth enlargement of bony foramen** involved
  - Foramen ovale most commonly enlarged
  - Mandibular foramen, inferior alveolar nerve canal, or mental foramen enlargement occurs with distal CNV3 schwannoma
- Enhanced MR findings
  - Homogeneous or heterogeneous enhancement
  - **Intramural cysts** are characteristic of schwannoma
  - Masticator muscle atrophy possible

TOP DIFFERENTIAL DIAGNOSES

- CNV3 neurofibroma
- Perineural tumor CNV3 in MS
- CNV3 malignant nerve sheath tumor
- Masticator space sarcoma

CLINICAL ISSUES

- Clinical presentation
  - Facial pain or numbness concentrated in jaw & chin
  - Rarely trigeminal neuralgia
- Treatment options
  - Surgical: Most definitive treatment option; open, external approaches vs. endoscopic resection
  - Radiotherapy: Stereotactic radiotherapy provides excellent tumor control rates
  - Observation: Reasonable option depending on tumor size, patient age, symptoms, and comorbidities

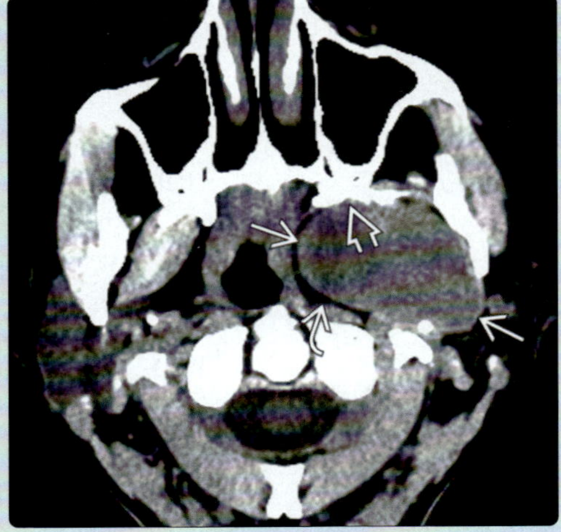
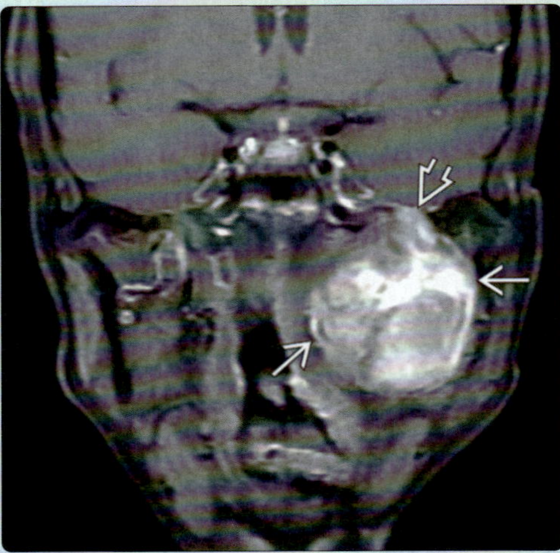

(Left) *Axial NECT in a patient with CNV3 schwannoma shows a circumscribed, heterogeneous, solid mass in the left masticator space ➡ with remodeling of the pterygoid plates ➡ suggesting a slow-growing lesion. Note the parapharyngeal fat ➡ is flattened from anterior to posterior.* **(Right)** *Coronal T1 C+ FS MR in the same patient demonstrates a heterogeneously enhancing masticator space schwannoma ➡ minimally projecting intracranially through an enlarged foramen ovale ➡.*

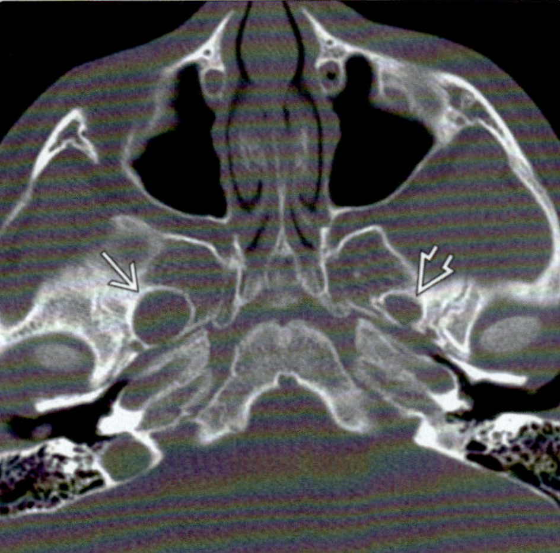
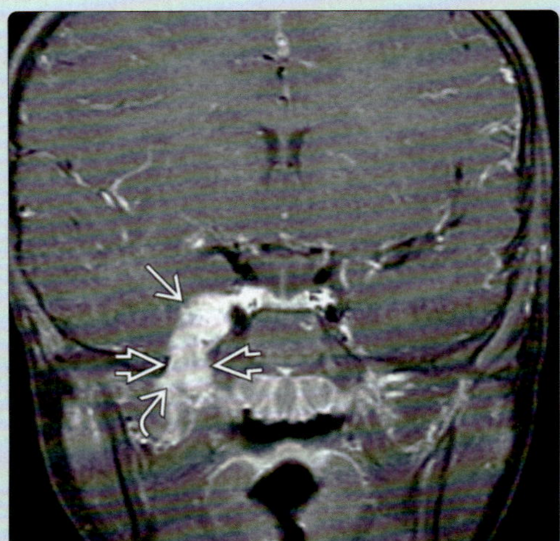

(Left) *Axial bone CT in a patient with known neurofibromatosis type 2 reveals a large right foramen ovale ➡. Note the normal left foramen ovale ➡. This foraminal enlargement with preservation of its cortical margin is characteristic of benign CNV3 schwannoma.* **(Right)** *Coronal T1 C+ FS MR in the same patient shows a tubular, enhancing CNV3 schwannoma coursing from the parasellar region ➡ through the enlarged foramen ovale ➡ into the nasopharyngeal masticator space ➡.*

KEY FACTS

TERMINOLOGY

- Perineural tumor (PNT) of masticator space (MS): Malignant spread along CNV3

IMAGING

- PNT occurs along all or part of V3 from mental foramen to lateral pons root entry zone of CNV
  - Nerve enlarged; may reach 1 cm in diameter
  - CNV3 may be normal size in early PNT
- Bone CT findings
  - **Enlarged** mandibular **inferior alveolar canal**, **mandibular foramen**, **foramen ovale**
- MR findings
  - Coronal T1 C+ best shows CNV3 PNT enhancement
  - Fat saturation ↑ conspicuity of PNT
- CECT less sensitive for PNT; MR recommended

TOP DIFFERENTIAL DIAGNOSES

- Normal pterygoid venous plexus asymmetry
- Normal vasa nervosa CNV3
- CNV3 schwannoma

PATHOLOGY

- Primary malignancies that may yield CNV3 PNT
  - Skin cancers of chin & jaw (SCCa, melanoma)
  - Oral cavity or pharynx primaries (SCCa, ACCa)
  - MS malignancy (sarcoma, non-Hodgkin lymphoma)
  - Parotid primary (spread via auriculotemporal nerve)

CLINICAL ISSUES

- Clinical presentation: **May be asymptomatic (40%)**
  - History of head and neck malignancy
  - Lower face paresthesias, numbness, pain
  - Masticator muscle denervation
- Treatment options
  - - intracranial extension, surgery with XRT or chemoXRT
  - + intracranial extension, XRT or chemoXRT, surgery not typically recommended

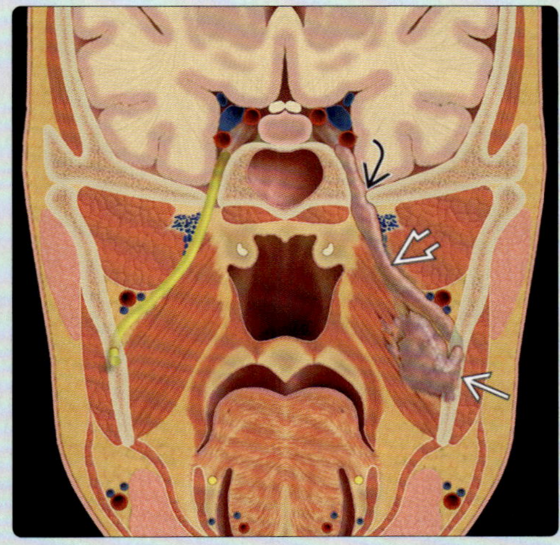

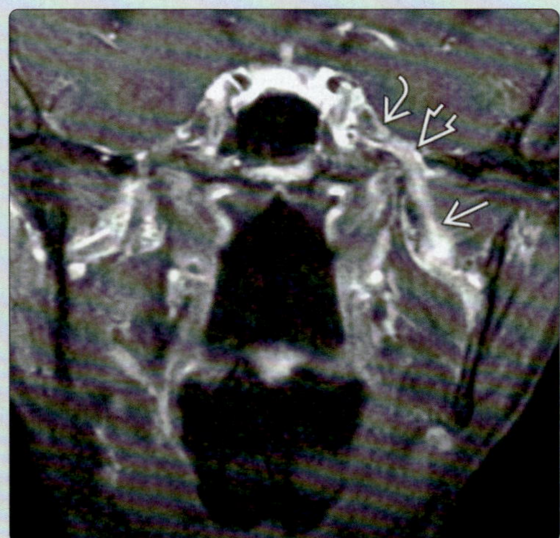

(Left) *Coronal graphic depicts a classic example of malignant masticator space tumor ➡ with perineural V3 spread ➡ through the foramen ovale ➡ into the intracranial compartment.* **(Right)** *Patient presents with a history of treated buccal space adenoid cystic carcinoma. New chin numbness creates concern for perineural CNV3 recurrence. Coronal T1WI C+ MR reveals perineural tumor involving CNV3 in nasopharyngeal masticator space ➡, passing through foramen ovale ➡, & beginning to invade Meckel cave ➡.*

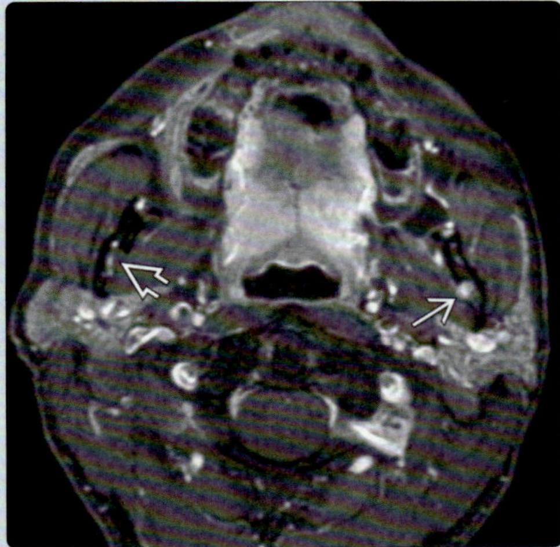

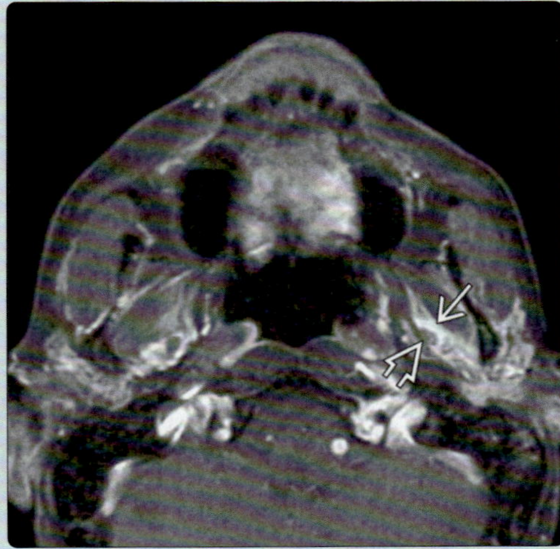

(Left) *Axial T1WI C+ FS MR in the same patient demonstrates the perineural tumor at the mandibular foramen ➡. Notice the minimal enhancement in the contralateral mandibular foramen ➡. Clearly if the clinician does not look for this specific finding, the observation of perineural tumor will not be made.* **(Right)** *Axial T1WI C+ FS MR in the same patient shows enhancing perineural tumor ➡ surrounding the CNV3 ➡ on its way to the foramen ovale.*

Masticator Space Chondrosarcoma

KEY FACTS

TERMINOLOGY

- Chondrosarcoma (CSa), masticator space (MS) definition: Malignant tumor of cartilage within MS

IMAGING

- General imaging findings & issues
  - Enhancing MS mass in or adjacent to mandible with variable Ca^{++} pattern
  - Molar region and ramus most frequent in mandible
  - May extend down from skull base or TMJ
  - CT shows characteristic Ca^{++} but MR better delineates extent of tumor
- Bone CT findings
  - **Radiolucent lesion ± areas of Ca^{++}**
  - Rings and crescents of calcium: Low-grade tumors
  - Amorphous or no Ca^{++}: High-grade tumors
  - When using CECT, view bone windows
- MR findings
  - Greater T1 C+ enhancement in high-grade CSa
  - T1 C+ heterogeneous, predominantly peripheral enhancement
  - Invasion of bone best delineated on T1 without contrast
  - **High signal typical on T2**
    - Extraosseous CSa tends to have intermediate signal
    - Flow voids may be present in extraosseous CSa

TOP DIFFERENTIAL DIAGNOSES

- TMJ synovial chondromatosis
- Mandibular ossifying fibroma
- Mandibular fibrous dysplasia
- Mandibular osteosarcoma

CLINICAL ISSUES

- Clinical presentation: Asymmetric mass, ± pain, paresthesia, trismus, and loose adjacent teeth if arising from mandible
- Treatment options
  - Complete surgical resection, ± reconstruction
  - Chemoradiation for residual or recurrent tumor

(Left) *Axial T1WI MR shows an intermediate-signal mass ➡ distending the masticator space and causing anterior bowing of the posterior wall of the left maxillary sinus ➡. A large focal Ca^{++} is seen as low signal intensity on all sequences ➡.* **(Right)** *Axial T2WI MR in the same patient shows the mass ➡ with characteristic pronounced T2 hyperintensity of chondroid tumors. Remember that all masticator space masses must be worked up until diagnosis is made so as to not miss sarcoma in this suprahyoid neck space.*

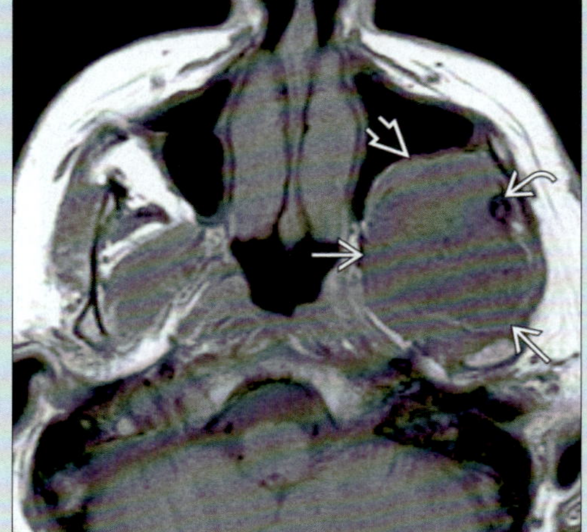

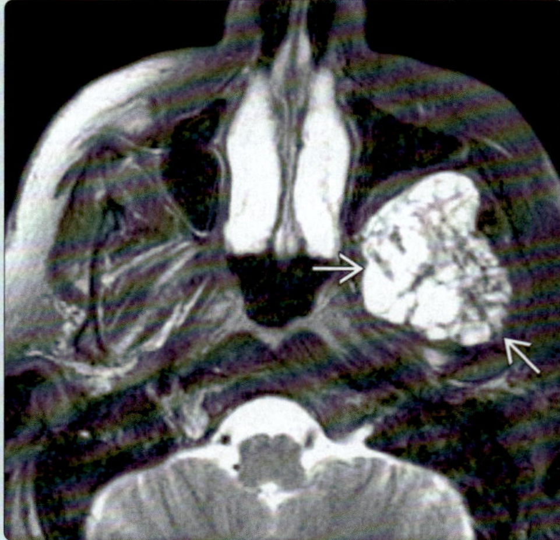

(Left) *Axial T1 C+ MR in the same patient shows the tumor ➡ is generally heterogeneous with intense enhancement with MR contrast.* **(Right)** *Axial CECT in bone window in the same patient shows a large mass with intrinsic Ca^{++} ➡, which are "fluffy," with rings and arcs. These are typical of chondroid Ca^{++}. Chondrosarcoma with visible chondroid Ca^{++} usually indicates low-grade tumor is present.*

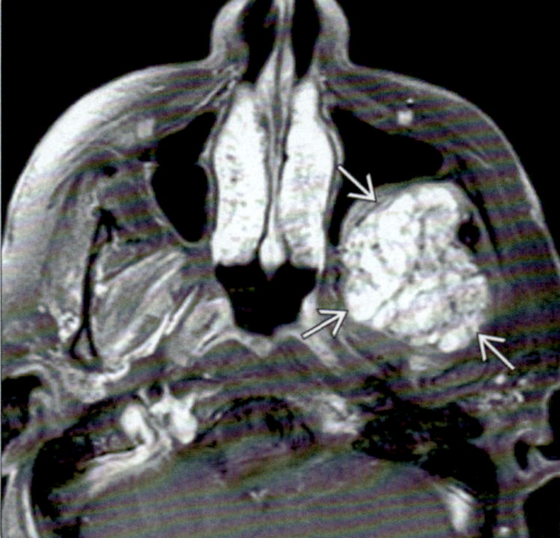

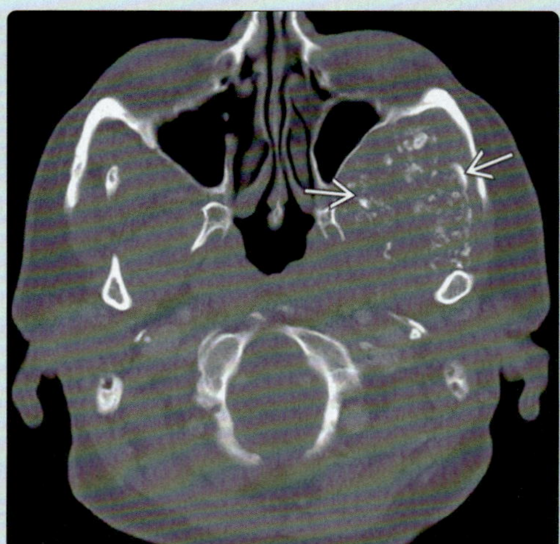

KEY FACTS

TERMINOLOGY

- Masticator space (MS) sarcoma: Malignant tumor of soft tissue origin (fat, muscle, nerve, joint, blood vessel, or deep skin tissues) in MS of suprahyoid neck

IMAGING

- Imaging recommendations: Bone CT and C+ MR
- General imaging findings
  - Aggressive, poorly marginated MS mass
  - ± bone destruction; ± invasion of adjacent fascial planes/spaces
- Bone CT: Allows assessment of tumor matrix ± bone destructive changes
  - **Invasive MS mass** with **bone destruction**
  - Any sarcoma may have bone production or Ca^{++}
- MR: Evaluation of soft tissues, possible mandibular invasion
  - Perineural tumor spread, commonly along CNV3
  - Skull base & intracranial invasion

TOP DIFFERENTIAL DIAGNOSES

- Masticator space abscess ± mandibular osteomyelitis
- Invasive SCCa: Palatine tonsil or retromolar trigone
- Mandible bony metastasis
- Masticator space venous malformation

PATHOLOGY

- Masticator space is most common site for sarcoma in suprahyoid neck spaces
- Many cell types in MS sarcoma group: Chondro-, rhabdo-, fibro-, osteo-, synovial, Ewing sarcomas

CLINICAL ISSUES

- Caveat: Absent known malignancy or infectious signs, MS mass should suggest sarcoma
- Symptoms: Enlarging mass cheek mass with ↑ pain
- Staging: T1 ≤ 5, T2 > 5 cm; A: Superficial; B: Deep
- Surgical excision is often primary modality with adjuvant chemoradiation, depending on histology

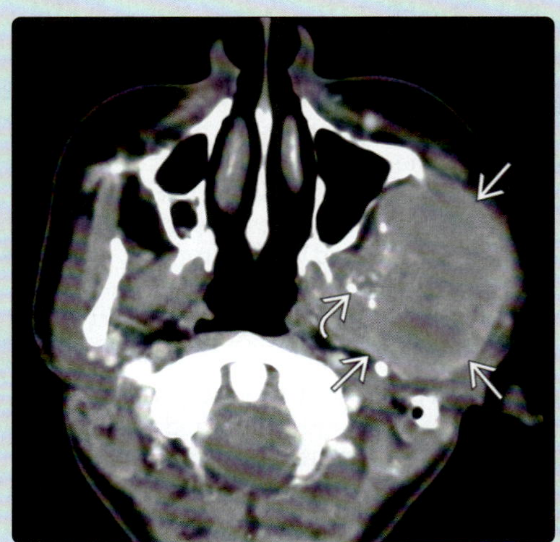

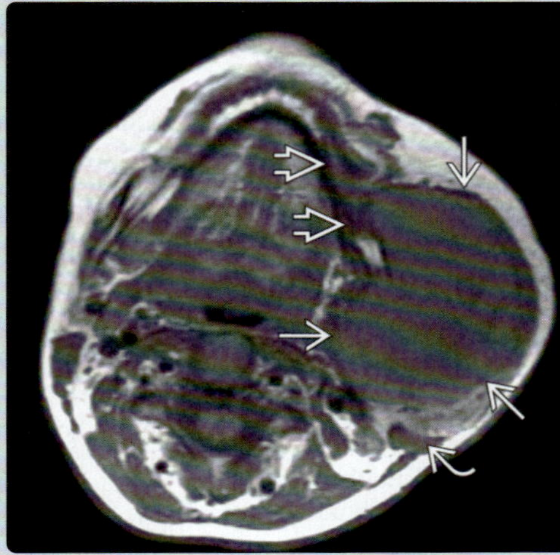

(Left) *Axial CECT shows a heterogeneous, necrotic masticator space (MS) mass ➡ with coarse Ca^{++} ➡. Mandibular destruction with invasion of the muscles of mastication is seen. Prior irradiation history suggests radiation-induced sarcoma. The pathology showed undifferentiated pleomorphic sarcoma.* **(Right)** *Axial T1WI MR in same patient shows the mass ➡ is isointense to the sternocleidomastoid muscle ➡. Loss of marrow fat within mandible ➡ suggests perineural spread on the inferior alveolar nerve.*

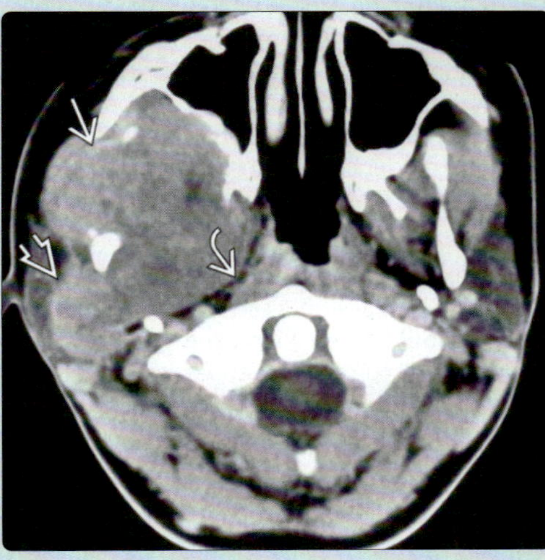

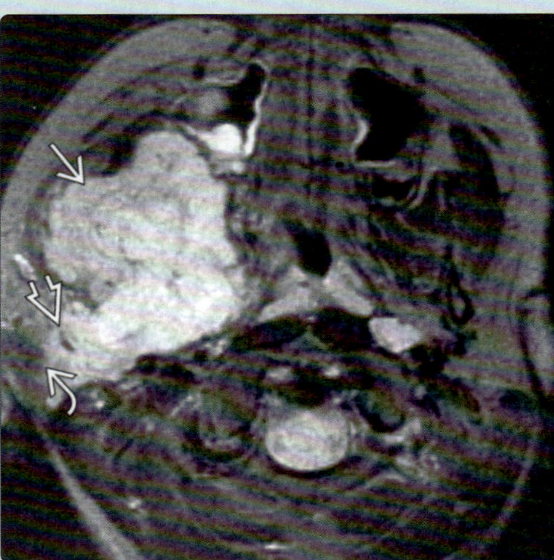

(Left) *Axial CECT in a 14-year-old patient with temporomandibular joint pain shows a large, invasive MS Ewing sarcoma ➡ invading the parotid space ➡ and destroying the mandible. Notice the lesion pushing the parapharyngeal space posteriorly ➡.* **(Right)** *Axial T2 MR in the same patient reveals an invasive hyperintense tumor ➡ destroying the mandible ➡ and invading the parotid gland ➡.*

Summary Thoughts: Parotid Space

The parotid space (PS) lies in the lateral suprahyoid neck in the cheek anterior to the external auditory canal (EAC). The main content of the PS is the parotid gland, but many other critical structures, such as the facial nerve (CNVII), external carotid branches, and intraparotid lymph nodes, also lie within the boundaries of this space.

The PS is traditionally divided into **superficial and deep compartments**. The true dividing line between these compartments is the CNVII, but the nerve is not visible on routine imaging, so an imaginary line between the stylomastoid foramen and the lateral margin of the retromandibular vein serves as a radiologic surrogate.

The deep PS compartment lies anterior to the styloid process and lateral to the parapharyngeal fat. The deep compartment was previously called the "**prestyloid parapharyngeal space**" to emphasize these anatomic relationships. Recalling the older name may help when determining the site of origin of a parapharyngeal mass; a mass arising anterior to the styloid process, displacing the parapharyngeal fat medially, is parotid in origin.

In the setting of a PS mass, the key findings are benign vs. aggressive margins, unifocal vs. multifocal, and homogeneity vs. heterogeneity. Potential involvement of CNVII must be carefully sought.

The main goal of imaging a parotid mass is not to provide a precise diagnosis (since this is often difficult). Instead, the **main goal is to guide the next step in the work-up**. For example, would a fine-needle aspiration be useful? Does the patient need an oncologic excision with neck dissection?

Key findings in PS inflammation include calculi, ductal dilatation, and the number of glands affected.

Imaging Techniques

Either CECT or MR can be used to evaluate diseases of the PS. The choice is often based on regional preferences.

In the setting of suspected inflammatory disease, CT is preferred because it can identify small calculi. Unenhanced CT images through the parotid before CECT are not generally useful as calcifications within the duct or parotid parenchyma can be seen on CECT. Enhanced CT images through the entire neck from the skull base to clavicles should be obtained. The patient's head should be positioned such that streak artifact from dental amalgam does not interfere with evaluation of the gland or the parotid duct (Stenson duct). Unfortunately, the punctum of the parotid duct lies alongside the 2nd maxillary molar, so dental amalgam often interferes with evaluation of the punctum. Open-mouthed images can avoid this pitfall.

MR is preferred in the setting of CNVII paralysis because it can better identify **perineural spread**. MR also allows sialography, in which heavily T2-weighted images emphasize the ductal system in settings like Sjögren syndrome.

Catheter sialography, once a mainstay of parotid radiology, has now become rare because of competition from MR sialography and sialoendoscopy.

Imaging Anatomy

The PS is a suprahyoid neck space only. PS anatomic relationships include the medial parapharyngeal space, anterior masticator space (MS), and posteromedial carotid space. The tail of the parotid projects into the posterior submandibular space below. Superiorly, the PS abuts the undersurface of the EAC and the mastoid tip.

The superficial layer of deep cervical fascia circumscribes the PS. This fascia surrounds the **superficial and deep lobes** of the parotid gland. The superficial lobe is about 2x as large as the deep lobe. There is an inconstant 3rd lobe, the **accessory lobe**, that lies superficial to the masseter muscle and occurs in 20% of patients.

The parotid duct emerges from the anterior PS and runs along the surface of masseter muscle. It then arches through the buccal space to pierce the buccinator muscle at the level of the maxillary 2nd molar. The normal duct is small and often not appreciable on cross-sectional imaging.

CNVII runs through the center of the PS. Although not usually visible radiographically, its course may be approximated by an imaginary line from the stylomastoid foramen to lateral aspect of the retromandibular vein. CNVII divides within the parotid, with 5 major branches arrayed in a sagittal plane. Superior to inferior, they are **temporal**, **zygomatic**, **buccal**, **marginal**, **and cervical branches**.

The external carotid artery is the medial and smaller of the 2 vessels seen just posterior to the mandibular ramus in the PS. The lateral and larger of the 2 vessels is the retromandibular vein.

Because the parotid gland undergoes late encapsulation during development, mature **lymph nodes are present within the parenchyma of the gland**. This differentiates the parotid gland from the other salivary glands and results in a longer differential diagnosis for parotid masses (including metastases, lymphoma, BLEL-HIV, and Warthin tumors). The intraparotid lymph nodes serve as 1st-order drainage for malignancies in the scalp, the EAC, and the deep face. Each gland contains ~ 20 nodes.

The parotid glands undergo progressive fatty degeneration throughout life. In childhood, the glands display radiodensity similar to that of underlying masseter muscle on CT. With age, the glands progressively decrease in density due to normal fatty degeneration. Occasionally, 1 parotid gland will undergo premature fatty degeneration.

Clinical Implications

80% of parotid masses are **benign**. Unfortunately, most parotid masses cannot be diagnosed by imaging findings alone. As a result, until biopsy or resection is performed, the exact diagnosis remains in question. Some benign lesions [benign mixed tumor (BMT)] in particular need to be surgically removed because they might degenerate into malignancy, for cosmetic reasons, or to relieve mass effect on surrounding structures.

BMT accounts for the majority of parotid masses. Although benign, it can undergo malignant degeneration. Consequently, **all BMTs should be surgically removed**. BMTs also have a high rate of local recurrence, so superficial or total parotidectomy is needed to avoid tumor "spillage."

Because a specific diagnosis is usually not possible radiographically, the goal of imaging is to **determine the next step in the diagnostic process and plan for surgery**.

- If discrete PS mass is seen, fine-needle aspiration or biopsy is most frequently employed; goal is not to

Parotid Space Overview

Congenital	Infectious-Inflammatory	Degenerative	Benign Tumor	Malignant Tumor, Primary	Neoplasm, Metastatic
Infantile hemangioma	Acute parotitis	Atrophy	Benign mixed tumor	Mucoepidermoid carcinoma	Skin cancer nodal metastasis
Venolymphatic malformation	Reactive adenopathy	Sialosis	Warthin tumor	Adenoid cystic carcinoma	NHL nodal metastasis
1st branchial cleft cyst	Chronic parotitis		Oncocytoma	Acinic cell carcinoma	Systemic nodal metastasis
	Benign lymphoepithelial lesions		Facial nerve schwannoma	Mammary analogue secretory carcinoma	
	Kimura disease		Lipoma	Adenocarcinoma	
	Kikuchi disease			Primary parotid non-Hodgkin lymphoma (NHL)	
				Salivary ductal carcinoma	
				Sebaceous carcinoma	

prevent surgery but to determine extent of surgery needed; malignancies often require wider excision ± neck dissection since surgical goal is to perform all procedures in single operative setting; palpable lesions can be needled without imaging guidance; sonographic guidance is most appropriate for superficial lobe lesions; CT guidance is most appropriate for deep lobe lesions

- If aggressive lesions present that clearly represent malignancy, resection and neck dissection may be performed even without definitive cytologic diagnosis; frozen section guidance is employed in such cases

Advanced imaging techniques, such as dynamic CT, dynamic MR, and quantitative ADC analysis, may increase diagnostic confidence in the probable diagnosis of a PS mass. However, they cannot provide a definitive diagnosis. As a result, the goal of imaging continues to be guidance of the next clinical step.

Facial nerve palsy in the setting of a PS mass suggests a malignant etiology. Imaging is aimed at determining if the deep PS lobe is affected, if a perineural tumor (PNT) is present, and if malignant adenopathy exists. MR is recommended in this setting as it is particularly sensitive to the presence of a PNT. In addition to PNT spread along the CNVII into the stylomastoid foramen, tumors may extend along the **auriculotemporal branch** of the trigeminal nerve. This PNT route runs through the parotid gland, around the posterior edge of the mandibular ramus, joining the main trunk of CNV3 in the masticator space below the foramen ovale.

Approaches to Imaging Issues of Parotid Space

The answer to the question, "What imaging findings define a PS mass?" is simple in a smaller intraparotid mass where the lesion is partially or completely surrounded by parotid tissue. It can be difficult to determine the space of origin for a larger, deep lobe PS mass, but in most cases **parapharyngeal space fat** is **displaced medially** with the MS pterygoid muscles pushed anteriorly. The stylomandibular tunnel is also often widened by a deep lobe mass.

When developing a differential diagnosis for parotid masses, the most important consideration is **multiplicity**. Solitary lesions should be distinguished from unilateral multifocal lesions and from bilateral lesions.

- **Multiple bilateral lesions** suggest unique differential diagnoses, including Sjögren syndrome, BLEL-HIV, Warthin tumor, NHL, and systemic metastases; for multifocal unilateral lesions, primary parotid lymphoma and regional metastases should be more strongly considered; BMT is not consideration in multifocal parotid masses
- Solitary intraparotid lesion is most often BMT; although Warthin tumor may be multifocal; most are actually solitary

Parotid mass margins can be used to suggest if a lesion is benign or malignant. Ill-defined, aggressive margins suggest a malignant lesion is present. A well-circumscribed lesion is usually benign. However, a **well-defined parotid mass should not be assumed to be benign** since a low-grade malignancy may have an imaging appearance identical to that of BMT.

Although there are no truly specific imaging findings to distinguish parotid masses, some diagnoses have characteristic features that may be helpful.

- **BMT** at times will have **hyperintense T2 signal** (> CSF); when present, which strongly suggests BMT
- **Warthin tumor** may appear as well-defined, cystic, rim-enhancing mass; unfortunately, PS carcinoma [especially mucoepidermoid carcinoma (MECa)] may have areas of cystic degeneration mimicking this appearance
- **PNT** spread is hallmark of malignancy; although adenoid cystic carcinoma is known for this tendency, lymphoma, MECa, and SCCa can spread this way

Always note the relationship of a PS mass to the CNVII plane. Designate the mass as superficial, deep, or in same plane as intraparotid CNVII. Superficial lobe masses are removed by superficial parotidectomy, while deep lobe masses require total parotidectomy. **Parotid tail masses** must be identified as intraparotid or their excision may injure CNVII. Remember that the platysma and sternocleidomastoid muscles are the superficial and deep borders of the parotid tail, respectively.

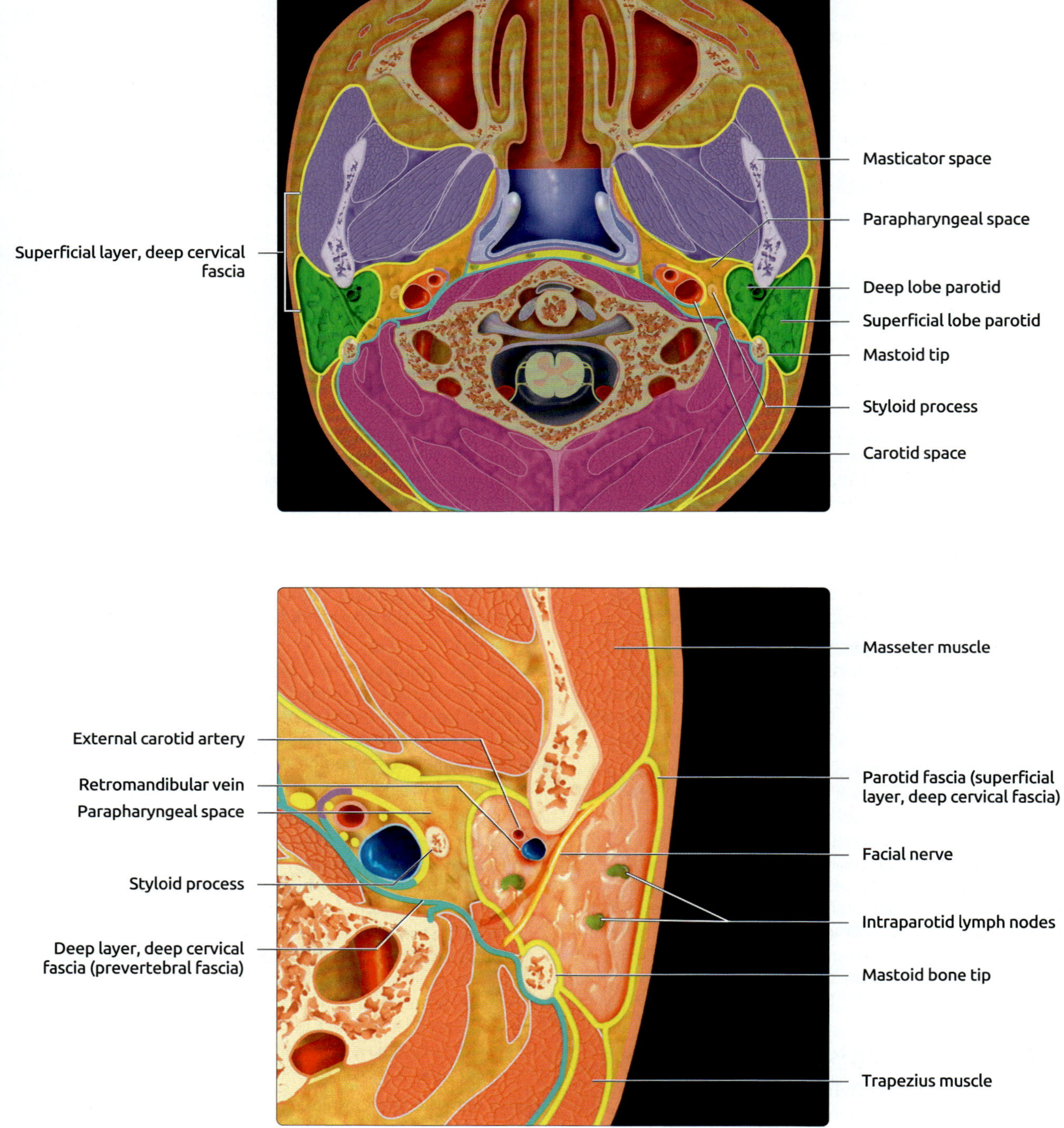

(Top) *Axial graphic of the suprahyoid neck soft tissues shows the relationships between the parotid space (green) and the surrounding spaces on the right. Notice the masticator space is anterior, while the parapharyngeal space is medial and the carotid space is posteromedial. On the left, the superficial layer of deep cervical fascia (yellow line) is seen to circumscribe both the masticator and parotid spaces.* **(Bottom)** *Axial graphic at the level of C1 vertebral body shows the contents of the parotid space. The intraparotid course of the facial nerve (not seen with imaging) extends from just medial to the mastoid tip to a position just lateral to the retromandibular vein. Within the superficial lobe (parotid superficial to the facial nerve), only parotid tissue and nodes are present. Within the deep lobe, notice the medial external carotid artery and retromandibular vein. The parapharyngeal space fat lies just medial to the deep lobe of the gland.*

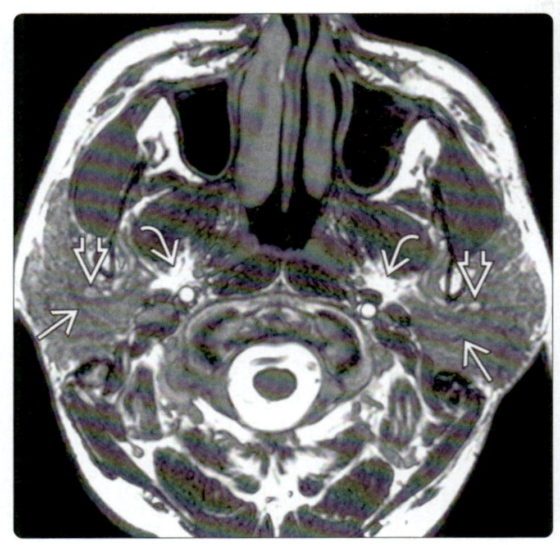

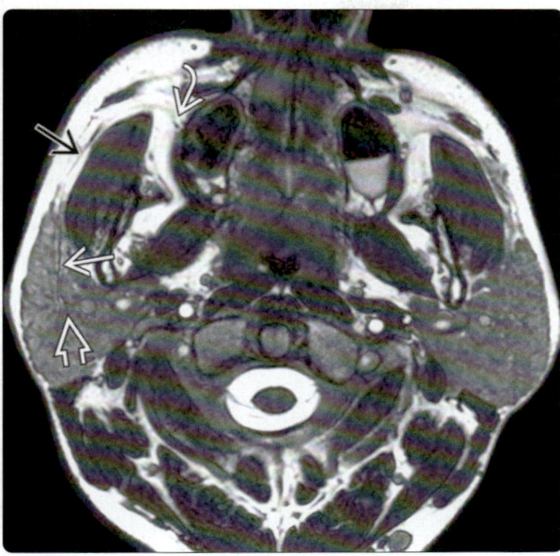

(Left) *Axial T2 high-resolution MR shows the intraparotid facial nerve ➡ dividing the parotid space into superficial and deep lobes. The retromandibular vein ➡ is visible just medial to the CNVII projected course. The parapharyngeal space fat ➡ is immediately medial to the deep lobe.* **(Right)** *Axial T2 high-resolution MR reveals the intraparotid duct ➡ and radicals ➡. The duct is seen superficial to the masseter muscle ⇒. It continues anteromedially to pierce the buccinator muscle ➡.*

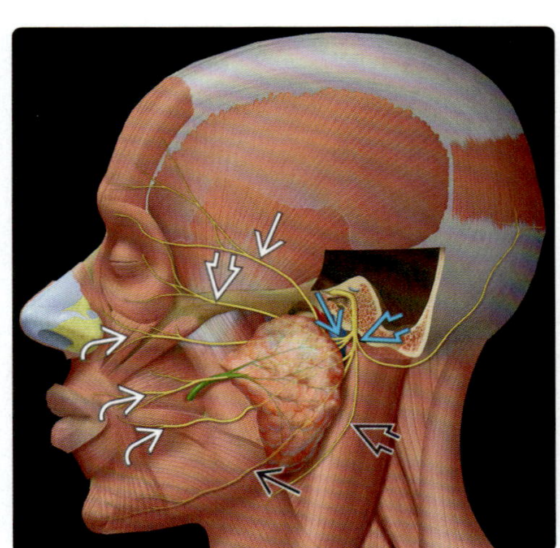

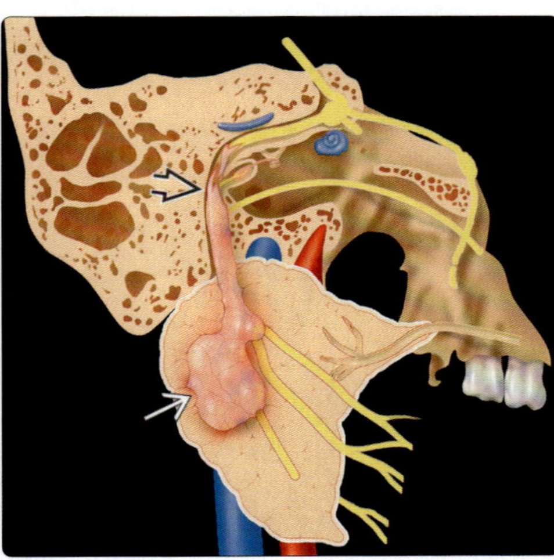

(Left) *Lateral view shows extracranial CNVII trunks & branches. After exiting stylomastoid foramen, CNVII divides into temporofacial ⇒ & cervicofacial ⇒ trunks. The temporofacial trunk divides into 2 branches: Temporal ➡ & ➡ zygomatic. Cervicofacial trunk divides into buccal ➡, marginal mandibular ⇒, cervical ⇒ & posterior auricular branches.* **(Right)** *Sagittal graphic of parotid malignancy ➡ shows perineural tumor spread along intraparotid CNVII along the mastoid segment to the posterior genu ⇒.*

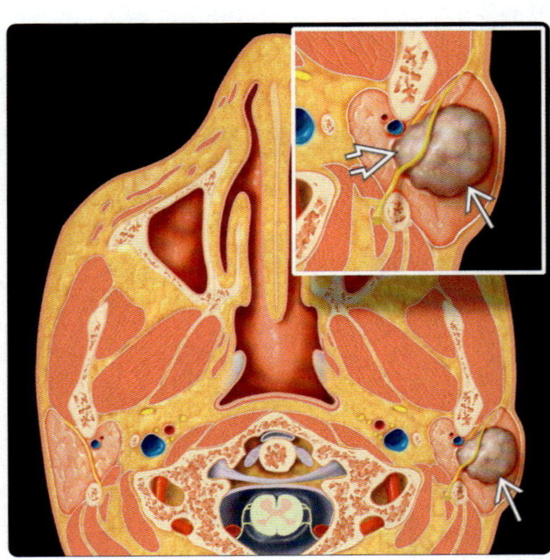

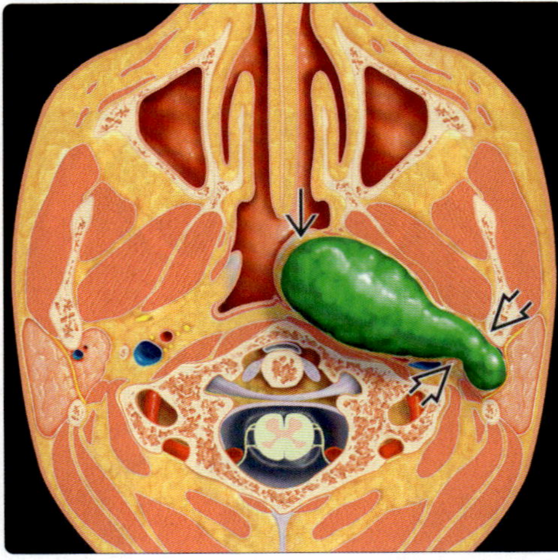

(Left) *Axial graphic of an intraparotid well-circumscribed tumor ➡ shows it is primarily in the superficial lobe but has a small component ➡ crossing facial nerve plane. If tumor needle biopsy revealed a benign mixed tumor diagnosis, it still may be possible to remove via superficial parotidectomy.* **(Right)** *Axial graphic of a deep lobe parotid mass shows medial displacement of parapharyngeal space fat ⇒. Note the widening of the stylomandibular tunnel ⇒. Total parotidectomy is necessary for removal.*

KEY FACTS

TERMINOLOGY

- Acute inflammation of parotid gland
  - Bacterial: Localized bacterial infection; ± abscess
  - Viral: Usually from systemic viral infection
  - Calculus-induced: Ductal obstruction by sialolith
  - Autoimmune: Acute episode of chronic disease

IMAGING

- Appearance: Enlargement of parotid gland with stranding of surrounding fat
- Bacterial parotitis
  - CECT and C+ MR shows enlarged, enhancing gland
  - Periparotid cellulitis/stranding common
  - Intra- or periparotid abscess may occur
- Parotitis with duct calculus
  - CECT shows large duct and intraluminal stone
- Viral parotitis
  - Clinical diagnosis; imaging rarely required
- Autoimmune parotitis
  - Diagnose with serum markers
  - Sialography for chronic complications
  - Usually involves entire gland but can be focal

TOP DIFFERENTIAL DIAGNOSES

- Sjögren syndrome
- Benign lymphoepithelial lesions of HIV

CLINICAL ISSUES

- Clinical presentation
  - Bacterial: Sudden onset of parotid pain and swelling
  - Viral: Prodromal symptoms of headaches, malaise, myalgia followed by parotid pain, earache, trismus
  - Calculus induced: Recurrent episodes of swollen, painful gland, usually related to eating
  - Autoimmune: Recurrent episodes of tender gland swelling, accompanied by dry mouth
- Treatment options: Antibiotics, sialogogues, hydration, warm compresses; plus I&D for abscess

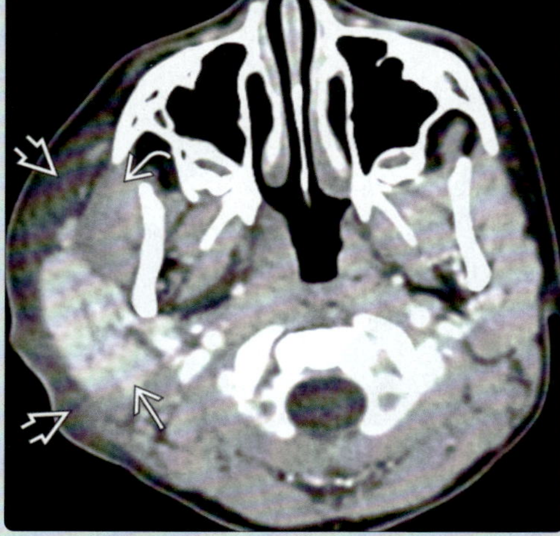

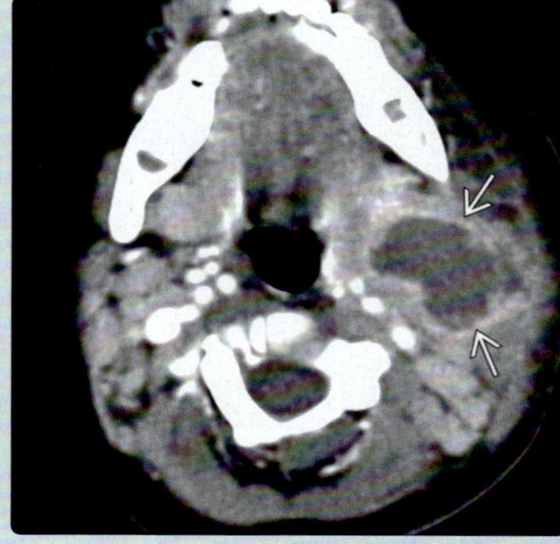

(Left) *Axial CECT in a child demonstrates diffuse enlargement and asymmetric enhancement of the right parotid gland ➡. There is associated facial cellulitis ➡ and masseter myositis ➡ that is typical of acute bacterial parotitis.* **(Right)** *Axial CECT shows a low-density collection ➡ replacing the left parotid gland. There is substantial surrounding fat stranding indicating an infectious source. These findings are diagnostic of intraparotid abscess complicating acute bacterial parotitis.*

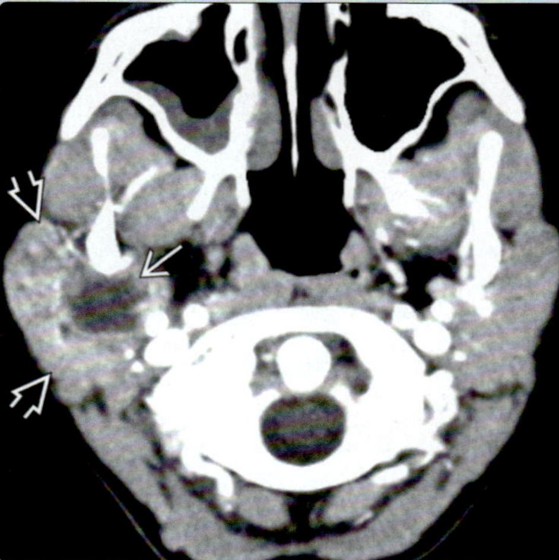

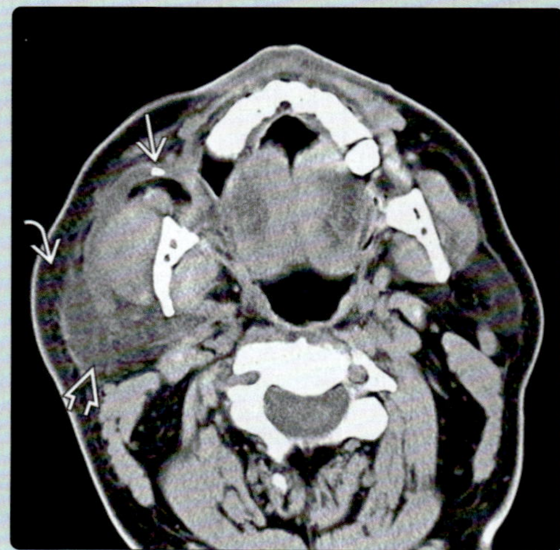

(Left) *Axial CECT shows a nonenhancing, irregular collection ➡ within the enlarged, asymmetrically enhancing right parotid gland ➡. Lack of rim enhancement suggests phlegmon rather than abscess; this is resolved with IV antibiotics.* **(Right)** *Axial NECT shows a stone in the right parotid duct ➡. The dilated parotid duct demonstrates graded attenuation due to the settling of pus. Note the enlarged, dense, inflamed parotid ➡ with stranding of subcutaneous fat ➡.*

KEY FACTS

TERMINOLOGY

- Definition: Chronic systemic **autoimmune exocrinopathy** that causes salivary & lacrimal gland tissue destruction
  - Primary Sjögren syndrome (SjS): Dry eyes & mouth; no collagen vascular disease (CVD)
  - Secondary SjS: Dry eyes & mouth with CVD; most commonly associated with **rheumatoid arthritis**

IMAGING

- Imaging appearance depends on SjS stage & presence or absence of lymphocyte aggregates within parotid
  - Earliest stage SjS: Parotids may appear normal
  - Intermediate-stage SjS: Miliary pattern of **small cysts** diffusely throughout both parotids
  - Late-stage SjS: Larger cystic (parenchymal destruction) & solid masses (lymphocyte aggregates) in both parotids
  - Dominant parotid mass + neck nodes, consider **lymphomatous transformation**
- CT: Punctate diffuse **calcifications** in both parotids
- Conventional or MR sialography
  - Alternating areas of ductal stenosis and dilatation (string of beads pattern)
  - Acinar spill into enlarged acini (apple tree pattern)
  - MR sialography is replacing conventional sialography

TOP DIFFERENTIAL DIAGNOSES

- Chronic infectious or obstructive parotitis
- Benign lymphoepithelial lesions of HIV
- Warthin tumor
- Parotid non-Hodgkin lymphoma (NHL) nodes

CLINICAL ISSUES

- Presentation: Tender bilateral parotid gland swelling
  - Striking **female** predominance (90-95%)
- Increased risk of malignancy (NHL) in primary SjS
- Treatment options
  - Sialogogues (drug/substance promoting saliva secretion)
  - Systematic treatment with immunomodulation

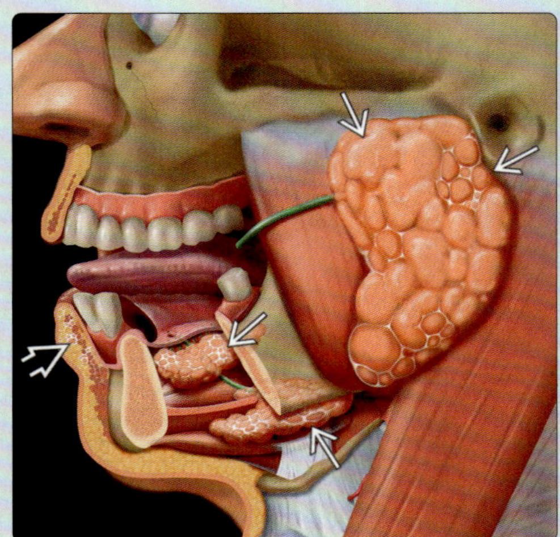

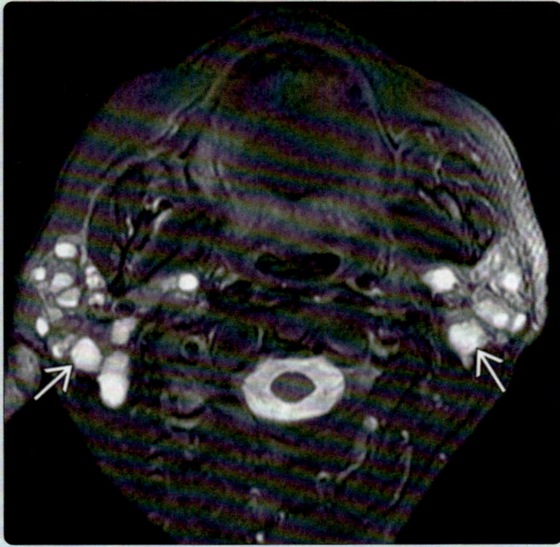

(Left) *Lateral graphic of face shows inflammatory-related enlargement of the major salivary glands ➡ (parotid, sublingual & submandibular) and minor glands of the lip ➡ in Sjögren syndrome. There is still preservation of the lobular architecture of the glands affected.* **(Right)** *Axial T2 FS MR shows high-signal masses ➡ within both parotid glands. These represent cystic dilatation of the intraglandular ducts in Sjögren syndrome, radiographically indistinguishable from lymphoepithelial lesions in HIV.*

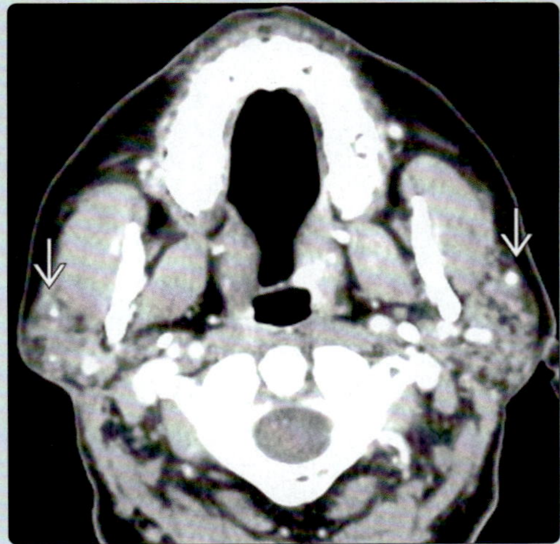

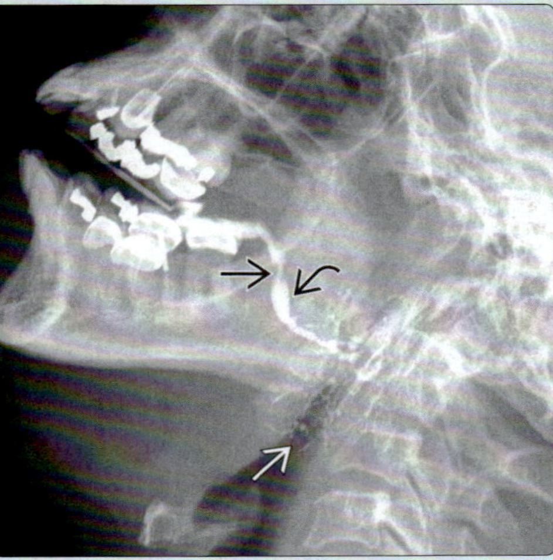

(Left) *Axial CECT shows multiple calcifications ➡ in parotid glands that have a multilobular configuration with fatty involution. Lobules of edematous glandular tissue with intervening fat & scattered calculi are characteristic of Sjögren syndrome.* **(Right)** *Lateral parotid sialogram shows stenosis ➡ & dilation ➡ in the Stensen duct (string of beads pattern). Intraglandular branches are truncated with cystic spaces (apple tree) ➡. Findings can be seen in any chronic sialadenitis but are classic for Sjögren syndrome.*

KEY FACTS

TERMINOLOGY

- 3-tiered classification
  - Persistent generalized parotid lymphadenopathy: **Solid** intraparotid lesions
  - Benign lymphoepithelial lesions (BLEL): **Mixed** solid and cystic lesions
  - Benign lymphoepithelial (BLE) cysts: **Cystic** lesions

IMAGING

- Enhanced CT or MR: Multiple bilateral, well-circumscribed cystic and solid masses within enlarged parotid glands
  - BLE cyst wall may be nodular (lymphoid follicles)
- Look for other CECT findings associated with HIV
  - **Reactive cervical adenopathy**
  - **Tonsillar hypertrophy**

TOP DIFFERENTIAL DIAGNOSES

- 1st branchial cleft cyst
- Parotid Sjögren syndrome
- Warthin tumor
- Non-Hodgkin lymphoma in parotid nodes

PATHOLOGY

- **Bilateral** parotid lesions: **60%**
- Florid follicular hyperplasia with attenuated to absent mantle lymphocytes with disruption of germinal centers
- Multinucleated giant cells in inter- and intrafollicular areas
- Ancillary test: **HIV p24 core antigen** immunoreactivity in germinal centers

CLINICAL ISSUES

- Clinical presentation
  - Bilateral painless enlargement of both parotid glands
    - BLEL may precede HIV seroconversion
    - **HIV testing** should be done on **any patient with BLEL**
- Historically, **5%** of HIV(+) patients develop BLEL
- Treatment options
  - HAART therapy treats BLEL manifestation of HIV

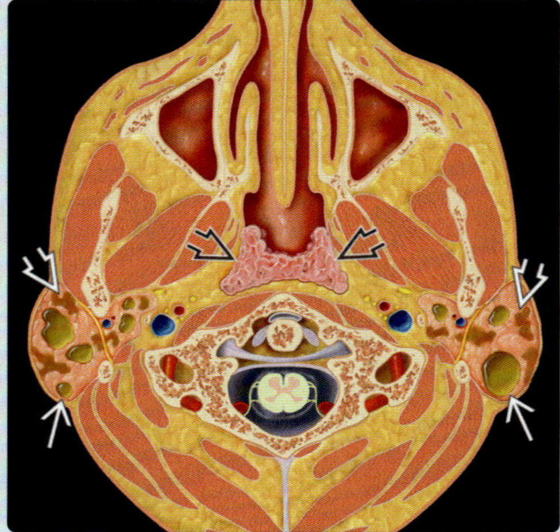

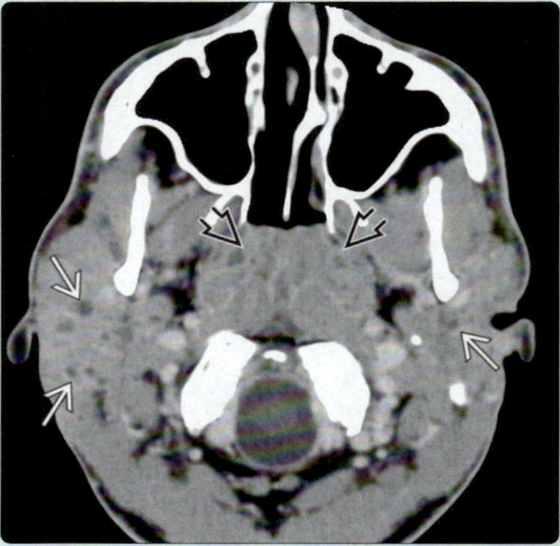

(Left) *Classic findings of benign lymphoepithelial lesions (BLEL) as bilateral intraparotid cysts ➡ are mixed with bilateral solid lymphoid aggregates ➡. Note associated adenoidal hypertrophy ➡ in the nasopharynx. Reactive adenopathy (not shown) is also a part of the imaging picture in BLEL-HIV.* **(Right)** *Axial CECT shows microcysts ➡ scattered throughout both hyperdense parotid glands in an HIV(+) patient, findings most consistent with BLE cysts. Note associated adenoidal hypertrophy ➡.*

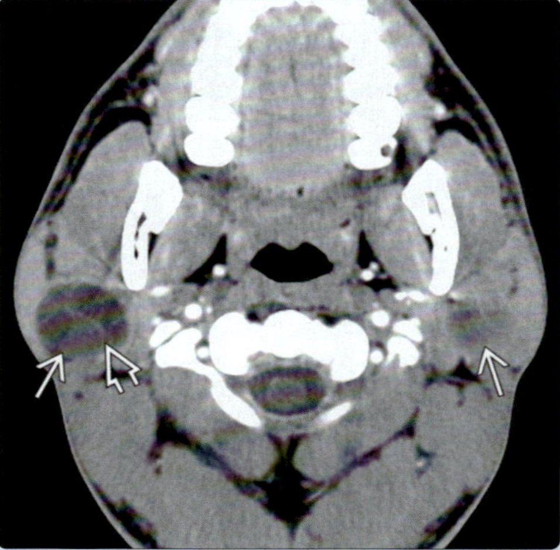

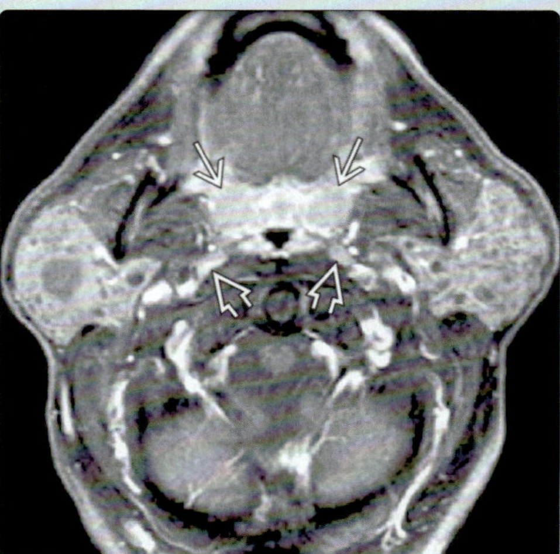

(Left) *Axial CECT in an HIV(+) patient shows larger loculated cystic lesions ➡ in both parotid glands. Septations can sometimes be seen within BLE cysts ➡.* **(Right)** *Axial T1WI C+ FS MR reveals bilateral cystic and solid intraparotid lesions of HIV. Palatine tonsils ➡ are hyperplastic bilaterally and associated with bilateral reactive lateral retropharyngeal nodes ➡.*

KEY FACTS

TERMINOLOGY

- Synonym: Pleomorphic adenoma

IMAGING

- Choice of imaging tool: CECT, MR, or US
  - CT or MR adequate to answer most imaging questions
    - MR best if specific signs (↑ T2 signal, ↑ ADC) present
  - Alternate approach: Use combination of US and FNAC
    - If US shows superficial lobe benign lesion and FNAC shows benign mixed tumor (BMT) cells, no further imaging needed
- CECT findings
  - Smooth, homogeneously enhancing, ovoid mass
  - **Pear-shaped** mass when in deep lobe
    - Larger lesions push parapharyngeal space medially
- MR findings
  - **Very high T2** signal **specific for BMT**
  - T1 C+ MR heterogeneous enhancement
  - ADC values higher than other parotid tumors

TOP DIFFERENTIAL DIAGNOSES

- Warthin tumor
- Metastatic nodes in parotid
- Adenoid cystic carcinoma
- Mucoepidermoid carcinoma

PATHOLOGY

- Tumor arising from distal portions of parotid ductal system
- Lobulated heterogeneous mass with **fibrous capsule**
- Interspersed **epithelial, myoepithelial, and stromal cellular components** needed to diagnose BMT

CLINICAL ISSUES

- Presentation: Painless, slow-growing cheek mass
- Rapid enlargement concerning for malignant degeneration
- Surgical issues
  - Complete removal **without violation of tumor capsule** is critical to prevent recurrence
  - Intraoperative monitoring may improve facial outcomes

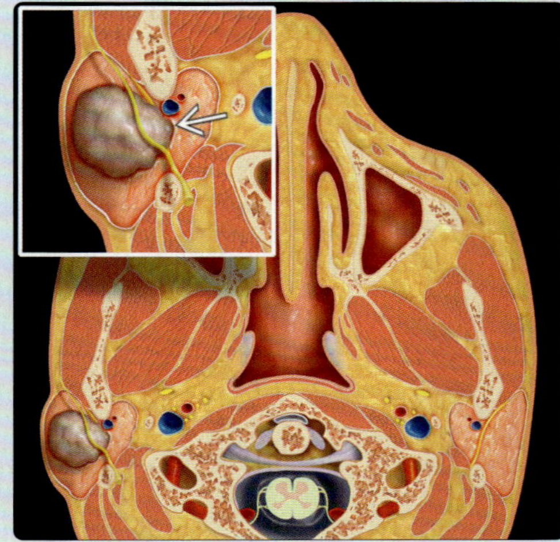

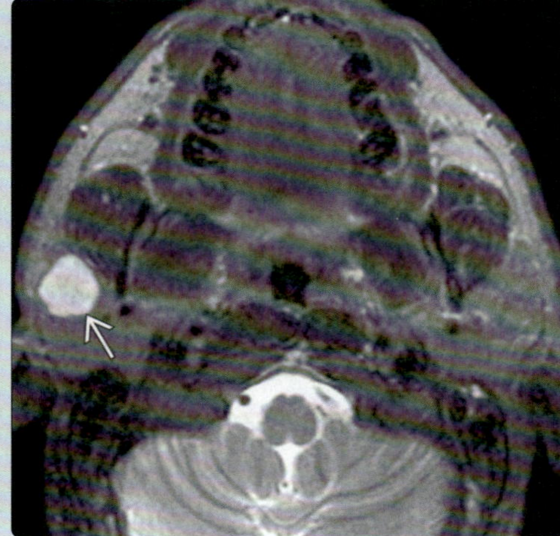

(Left) *Axial graphic depicts a small, predominantly superficial lobe, well-circumscribed benign mixed tumor (BMT). Notice in the insert the tongue of that tumor, which has insinuated itself between 2 facial nerve branches to involve the deep lobe* ➡. **(Right)** *Axial T2 FS MR reveals a sharply circumscribed, high-signal BMT* ➡ *in the superficial lobe of the parotid gland. This tumor likely abuts, if not crosses, the plane of the intraparotid facial nerve.*

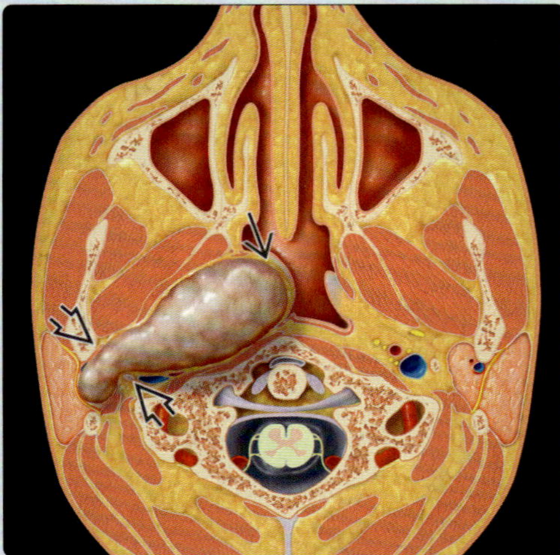

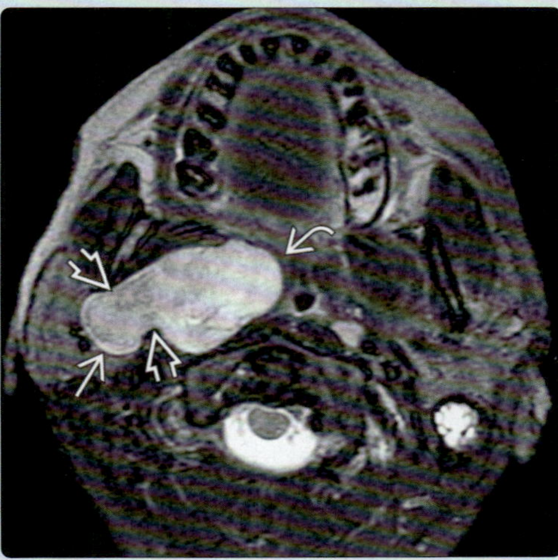

(Left) *Axial graphic reveals a pear-shaped BMT of the deep lobe of the parotid gland. Despite the size of this tumor, the parapharyngeal fat can still be seen* ➡ *as it is pushed superomedially. Note widened stylomandibular notch* ➡. **(Right)** *Axial T2 FS MR shows a pear-shaped high-signal mass extending from the deep lobe of the parotid gland* ➡, *through the enlarged stylomandibular notch* ➡, *displacing the parapharyngeal fat and palatine tonsil medially* ➡. *Large, deep lobe parotid tumors are almost always BMTs.*

Warthin Tumor

KEY FACTS

TERMINOLOGY

- Benign tumor arising from salivary-lymphoid tissue in intraparotid & periparotid nodes
  - a.k.a "papillary cystadenoma lymphomatosum"
- Most common mass to arise in **parotid tail**

IMAGING

- CECT or CEMR provides adequate presurgical information
- **20% multifocal**
  - May be **multiple lesions** in 1 gland or bilateral lesions
  - Multiplicity may be synchronous or metachronous
- Sharply marginated **parotid tail** mass
- **Parenchymal heterogeneity** is characteristic
- **Cystic** component in **30%** with thin, uniform walls
  - Difficult to differentiate radiographically from 1st branchial cleft cyst, infected lymph node, or other cystic mass
- Increased uptake of FDG
  - Incidental PET/CT finding
- Ultrasound highly suggestive
  - Well-defined hypoechoic mass or masses with multiple hypoechoic areas at lower pole of superficial parotid
  - Heterogeneous cystic & solid internal architecture
  - Multiseptated with debris

TOP DIFFERENTIAL DIAGNOSES

- Parotid benign mixed tumor (BMT)
- Benign lymphoepithelial lesions-HIV
- Parotid carcinoma
- Parotid metastatic nodal disease
- Parotid suppurative node

CLINICAL ISSUES

- Clinical presentation: Angle of mandible (tail of parotid) mass in **smokers,** typically **older patients**
  - **2nd** most frequent benign parotid tumor (BMT 1st)
- Treatment: Surgery with parotidectomy and facial nerve preservation

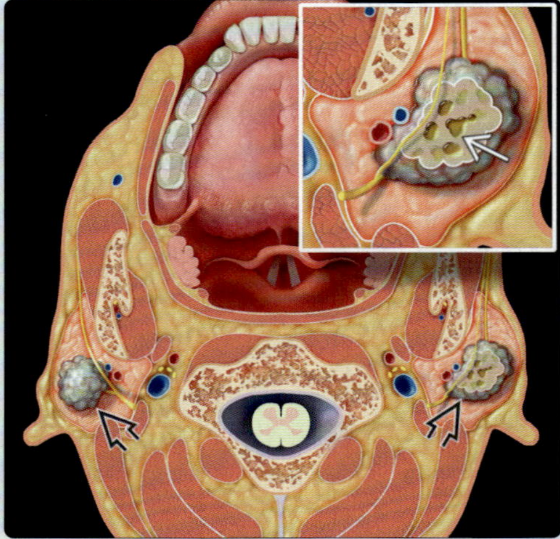

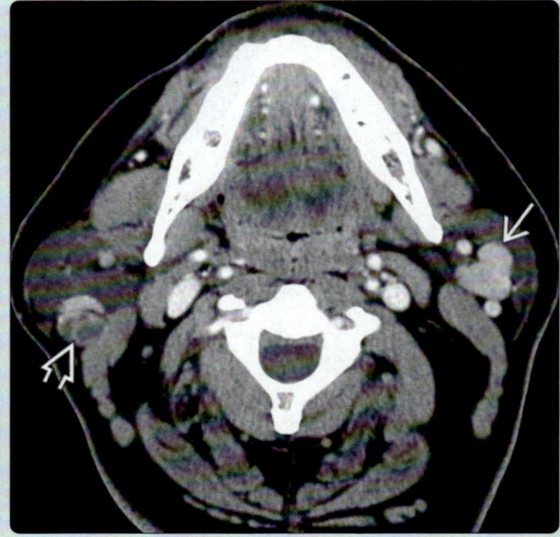

(Left) *Axial graphic depicts bilateral, mixed solid/cystic, parotid tail Warthin tumors ⇨. A larger left intraparotid tumor is cut in the insert to show characteristic parenchymal cystic changes ➡ seen in 30% of Warthin tumors.* **(Right)** *Axial CECT shows bilateral parotid masses. The left-sided lesion ➡ is lobular, well-circumscribed and homogeneously enhancing. The right-sided lesion ⇨ is heterogeneous with posterior margin cystic changes. Warthin tumors are 10-20% multifocal.*

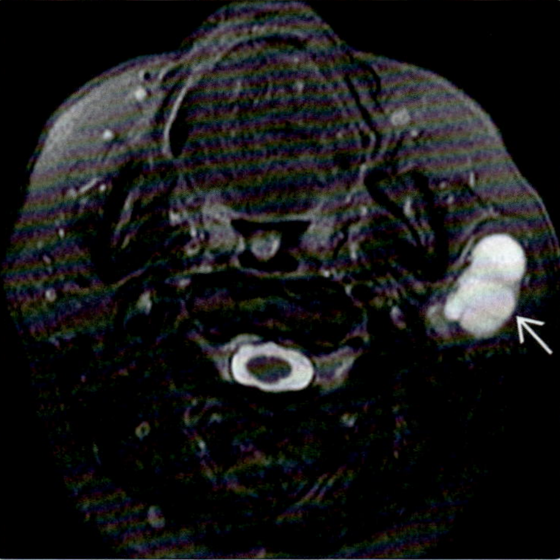

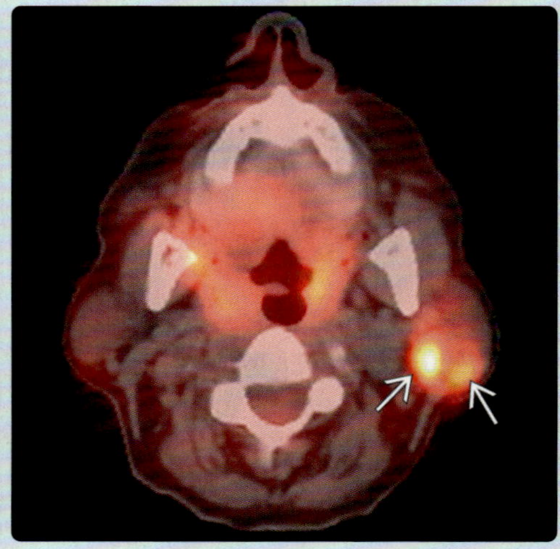

(Left) *Axial T2WI FS MR shows a high-intensity mass ➡ with thin septations in the superficial lobe of the parotid gland. On imaging, 30% of Warthin tumors appear cystic.* **(Right)** *Axial PET/CT done to stage a squamous cell carcinoma of the head and neck shows marked FDG uptake in 2 parotid masses ➡. Some benign glandular tumors, such as oncocytomas and Warthin tumors, are FDG avid but multifocality suggests a Warthin tumor. These lesions must be sampled to exclude metastatic disease.*

KEY FACTS

TERMINOLOGY

- Mucoepidermoid carcinoma (MECa): Malignant epithelial salivary gland neoplasm composed of epidermoid & mucus-secreting cells arising from ductal epithelium

IMAGING

- CECT & MR appearance based on histologic grade
  - **Low-grade**: Well-circumscribed, heterogeneous parotid space (PS) mass
  - **High-grade**: Invasive, ill-defined PS mass
    - Often has **nodal metastases**
- If lesion high grade, infiltrative, or near stylomastoid foramen, **perineural spread** along **CNVII** may occur
- MR findings
  - **Low T2** areas characteristic but not pathognomonic
  - T1 C+ shows heterogeneous tumor enhancement
  - MR useful for extent of lesion and facial nerve **perineural spread**
  - Enhanced images may "hide" lesion

TOP DIFFERENTIAL DIAGNOSES

- Benign: Benign mixed tumor, Warthin tumor
- Malignancy: Parotid adenoid cystic carcinoma, non-Hodgkin lymphoma, or metastasis

PATHOLOGY

- MECa is most common primary parotid malignancy
- Recurrence & survival rates depend on histologic grade
- Late local recurrence (after 5 years) possible

CLINICAL ISSUES

- Clinical presentation
  - Rock-hard cheek mass
  - ± pain, otalgia, facial nerve palsy (poor prognosis)
- Treatment options
  - Superficial or total parotidectomy depending on size
  - Elective neck dissection (ND) often indicated in N0 neck
  - Postoperative radiotherapy
    - Therapeutic ND recommended for N+ disease

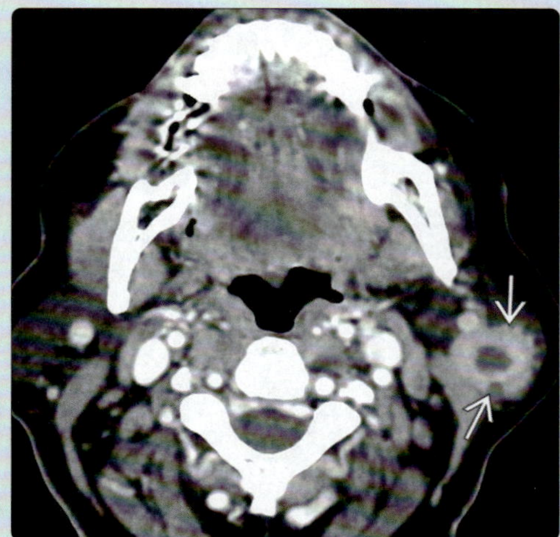

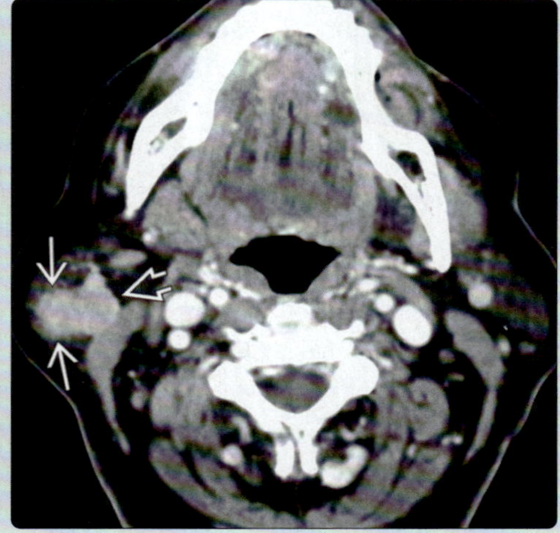

(Left) *Axial CECT reveals a well-defined mass ➡ in the superficial lobe of the parotid gland. It has a thick rind of peripheral enhancement and is centrally cystic or necrotic. This is a characteristic imaging appearance for a low-grade mucoepidermoid carcinoma (MECa).* **(Right)** *Axial CECT shows a mass in the parotid gland with ill-defined lateral borders ➡ and well-defined medial borders ➡. The tumor enhances uniformly. Although nonspecific, this is the expected appearance of an intermediate-grade MECa.*

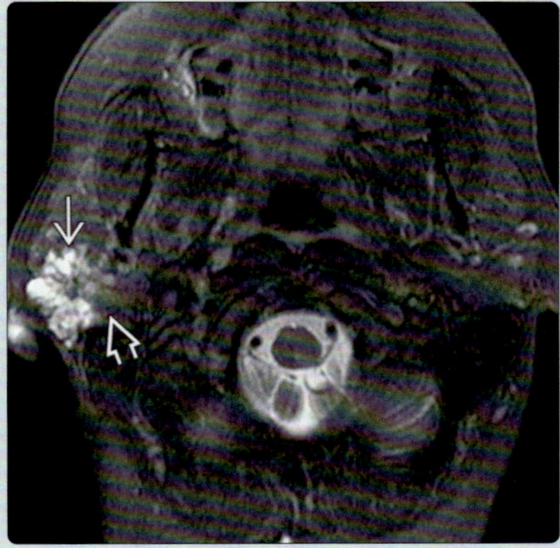

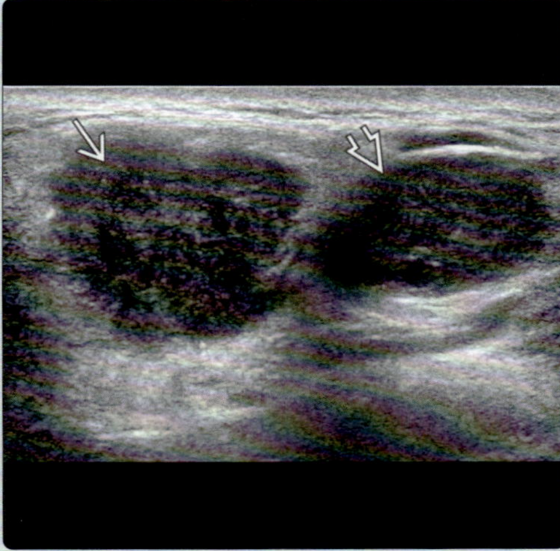

(Left) *Axial T2 FS MR shows an irregular mass in the parotid with mixed T2 signal. Laterally, there are high-signal cystic areas ➡, but medially there is a low-signal region ➡. Low T2 signal within the solid components of the tumor is characteristic of MECa.* **(Right)** *Longitudinal grayscale US shows a high-grade parotid MECa ➡. It is ill-defined, solid, hypoechoic, and heterogeneous with presence of metastasis in an associated level II lymph node ➡.*

Parotid Adenoid Cystic Carcinoma

KEY FACTS

TERMINOLOGY

- Parotid adenoid cystic carcinoma (ACCa): Malignant parotid gland neoplasm arising in peripheral parotid ducts

IMAGING

- **Low-grade ACCa**: Well-circumscribed, homogeneously enhancing parotid mass
- **High-grade ACCa**: Infiltrative, homogeneously enhancing parotid mass
- MR findings
  - Moderate T2 signal intensity
  - High-grade ACCa: Lower in T2 signal intensity
  - Look for **perineural tumor** CNVII or CNV3
- CT findings: Homogeneously enhancing parotid mass

TOP DIFFERENTIAL DIAGNOSES

- Parotid space benign mixed tumor
- Warthin tumor
- Parotid space mucoepidermoid carcinoma
- Intraparotid metastatic nodal disease

PATHOLOGY

- Tumor grading based on dominant histologic pattern
  - Tubular (grade 1); cribriform (grade 2); solid (grade 3)
- Greatest propensity of all H&N tumors to spread via perineural pathway
- Favorable short-term but poor long-term prognosis

CLINICAL ISSUES

- Clinical presentation
  - Adult tumor; peaks in 6th decade
  - Cheek mass ± pain & CNVII paralysis
  - Nodal metastasis very uncommon
- Treatment options
  - Treat with complete resection (parotidectomy)
  - Postoperative radiotherapy for all but lowest grade
- Prognosis: **Late recurrence** (up to 20 years) occurs, often with pulmonary metastasis

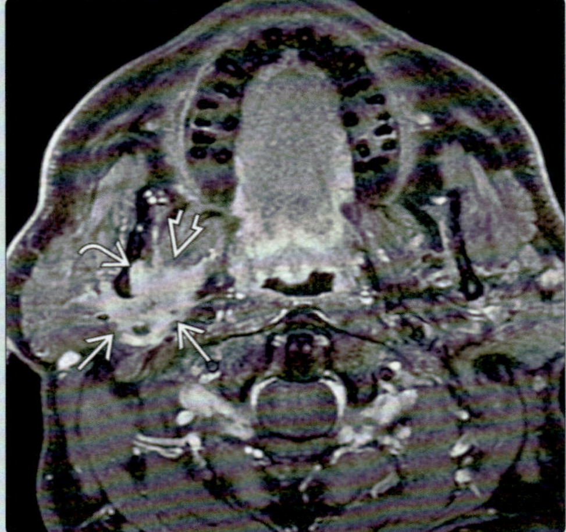

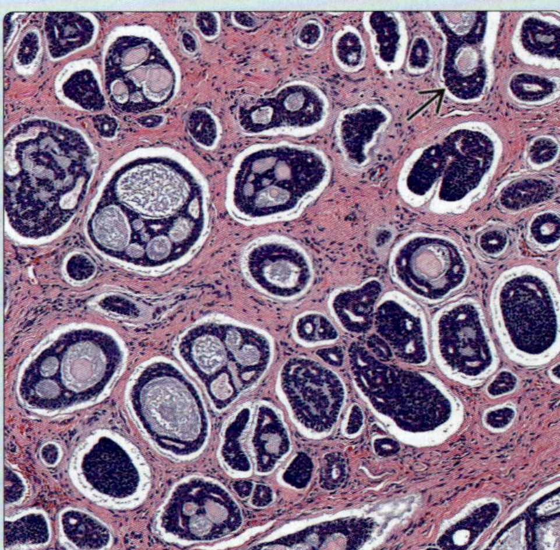

(Left) *Axial T1WI C+ FS MR shows an infiltrative, uniformly enhancing adenoid cystic carcinoma (ACCa) ➡ in the deep lobe of parotid gland. Tumor involves the masticator space ➡ & mandibular foramen ➡ (inferior alveolar nerve). Perineural spread is a clue that this is ACCa.* **(Right)** *Low-power H & E micrograph shows ACCa cribriform pattern (pierced by numerous small holes) or the so-called Swiss cheese pattern. This is the most common appearance of ACCa. The tumor cells are often described as creating C-shapes ➡.*

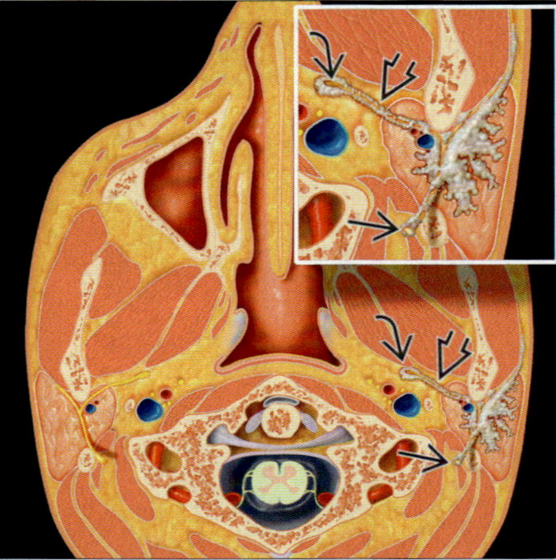

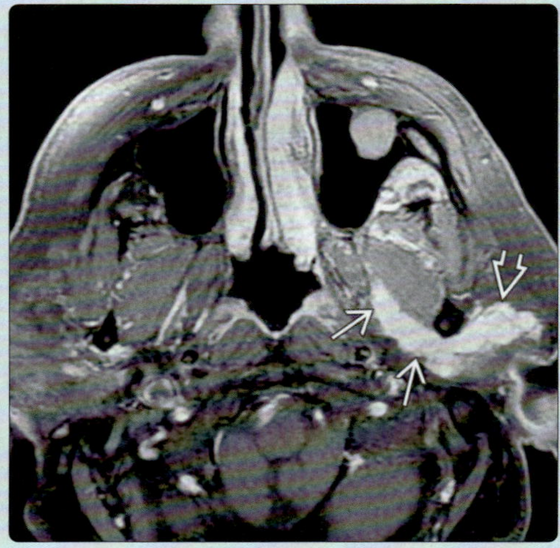

(Left) *Axial graphic depicts high-grade parotid ACCa spreading in a perineural fashion along the proximal facial nerve toward the stylomastoid foramen ➡ & via the auriculotemporal nerve ➡ to the mandibular branch (CNV3) of the trigeminal nerve ➡.* **(Right)** *Axial T1WI C+ FS MR shows marked thickening and enhancement of the auriculotemporal nerve ➡ from perineural spread of ACCa that originated in the superficial lobe of the parotid gland ➡.*

Parotid Non-Hodgkin Lymphoma

KEY FACTS

TERMINOLOGY

- 3 forms of parotid involvement with non-Hodgkin lymphoma (NHL)
    - **Nodal NHL: Primary nodal NHL**
    - **Nodal NHL: Systemic NHL** involving parotid nodes
    - **Primary parenchymal NHL**: Often mucosa-associated lymphoid tissue (MALT)

IMAGING

- CT or MR findings
    - Primary parotid NHL: Focal solid well-defined masses
    - Nodal parotid NHL + systemic NHL
        - Multiple parotid nodal masses + neck nodes
    - Primary parenchymal NHL: Infiltrating mass in parotid
    - Heterogeneous parotids with new parotid mass
        - Suspect NHL complicating Sjögren disease
- Ultrasound findings: Hypoechoic intraparotid mass(es)
    - Color Doppler shows hypervascular mass(es)
- PET/CT: Typically markedly FDG avid

TOP DIFFERENTIAL DIAGNOSES

- Benign lymphoepithelial lesions-HIV
- Parotid Sjögren syndrome
- Warthin tumor
- Parotid nodal metastatic disease

PATHOLOGY

- Overall 5-year survival = 72%
- Systemic NHL involves parotid in 1-8%
- Primary parotid NHL 4% of parotid malignancies

CLINICAL ISSUES

- Clinical presentation
    - Physical exam: Unilateral or bilateral cheek masses
        - Other neck masses/nodes: Consider systemic NHL
        - May have B-cell symptoms
    - History of Sjögren syndrome
    - FNA recommended for flow cytometry
- Treatment options: XRT and chemotherapy

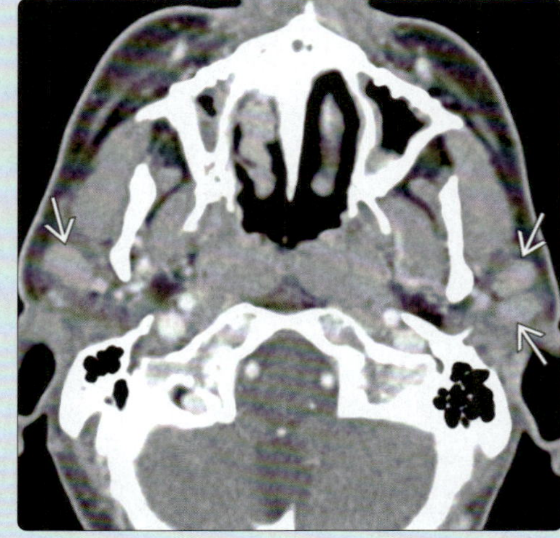

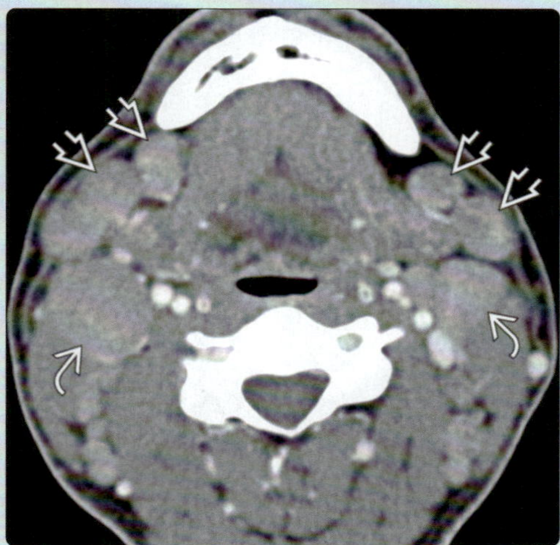

(Left) *Axial CECT shows multiple bilateral, well-defined, homogeneously enhancing masses ➡. Parotid gland nodules ≥ 1 cm deserve further evaluation to exclude multiple Warthin tumors, multiple metastatic nodes, or multiple lymphoma nodes. The remaining neck needs to be evaluated for nodes as a 1st step.* **(Right)** *Axial CECT in same patient shows extensive lymphadenopathy in upper neck, including level IB ➡ & IIA & B ➡ nodes. This case shows parotid node involvement with systemic lymphoma.*

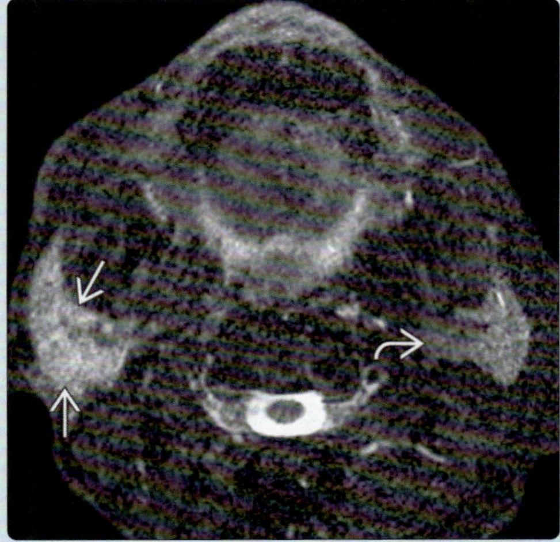

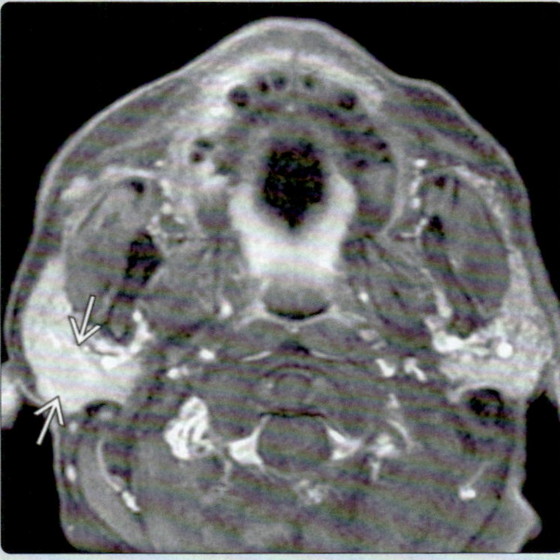

(Left) *Axial T2WI FS MR in a patient presenting with fullness of the right cheek demonstrates subtle enlargement & diffuse hyperintensity of right parotid gland ➡ as compared to the left side ➡. The prior CECT study was normal.* **(Right)** *Axial T1 C+ FS MR in the same patient reveals diffuse enhancement of right parotid with a more conspicuous ill-defined but homogeneous lesion ➡ in superficial lobe. FNA revealed mucosa-associated lymphoid tissue-type primary parotid lymphoma.*

Metastatic Disease of Parotid Nodes

KEY FACTS

TERMINOLOGY

- **Lymphangitic** or **hematogeneous** tumor spread to intraglandular parotid lymph nodes
- Parotid and periparotid nodes = **1st-order nodal station for skin** squamous cell carcinoma (SCCa) and melanoma from scalp, auricle, and face ("forgotten nodal station")

IMAGING

- CT or MR: Nodes usually well defined
  - Appear infiltrative if extranodal spread
  - Nodes may be homogeneous or heterogeneous with central necrosis
- PET/CT: Most sensitive for small node identification
- MR most sensitive for extranodal spread and perineural tumor spread on CNVII

TOP DIFFERENTIAL DIAGNOSES

- Benign parotid lymphoepithelial lesions
- Parotid Sjögren disease
- Warthin tumor
- Parotid non-Hodgkin lymphoma

PATHOLOGY

- **Skin cancers** of face, external ear, and scalp account for 75% of primary tumors
- **Metastatic SCCa is 2nd most common parotid malignancy**
- Systemic metastases to parotid nodes rare

CLINICAL ISSUES

- Clinical presentation: History of cutaneous malignancy, firm mass, ± pain, ± facial nerve weakness
- Treatment options: Surgical excision with parotidectomy and ipsilateral, selective neck dissection, depending on extent of metastasis
  - Important to find and treat primary site
  - Adjuvant XRT often indicated
- Prognosis depends on presence of extracapsular spread (8% vs. 79% local recurrence)

(Left) *Axial CECT shows multiple enhancing masses ➡ of varying size within the left parotid gland. This patient has squamous cell carcinoma of the face, and these nodes represent 1st-order lymphatic drainage.* **(Right)** *Axial T1WI C+ FS MR shows an ill-defined mass ➡ replacing the left parotid gland. The primary tumor, postauricular skin squamous cell carcinoma, is partially visible ➡. The ill-defined margins of the intraparotid metastasis indicate extracapsular spread is present.*

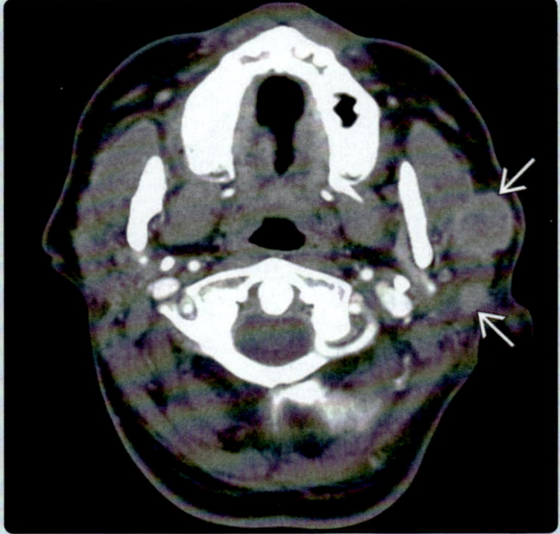

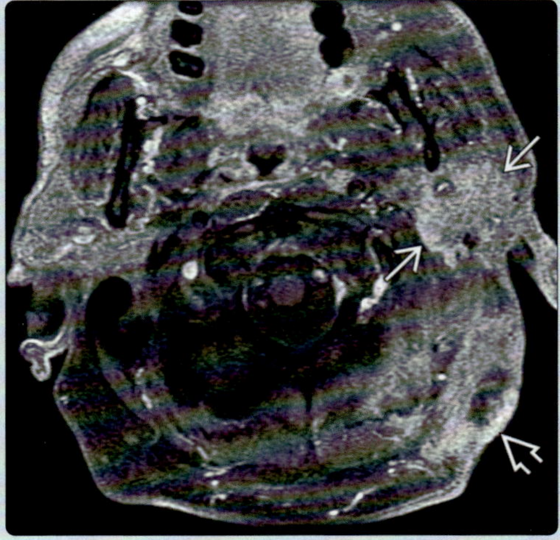

(Left) *Axial T1WI MR reveals numerous small masses ➡ in the left parotid gland. These regional metastases are clearly visible on unenhanced images because the parotid becomes fatty infiltrated with increasing age.* **(Right)** *Axial T2WI FS MR shows numerous masses ➡ in the left parotid gland with mildly increased T2 signal. Metastases may be more conspicuous on STIR images than on T2 images. These are a rare example of regional metastases from lymphoepithelial carcinoma of the base of tongue.*

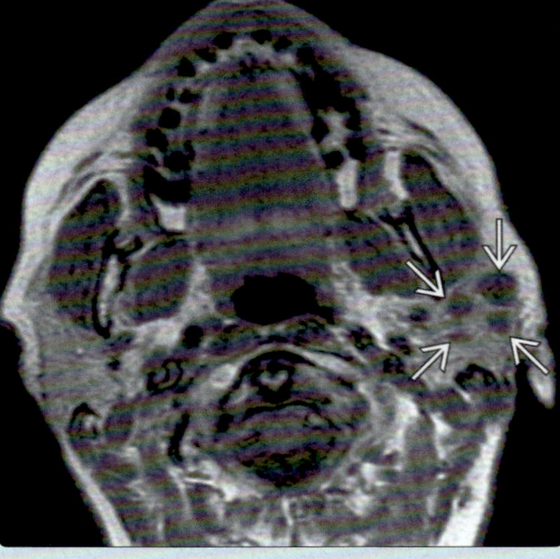

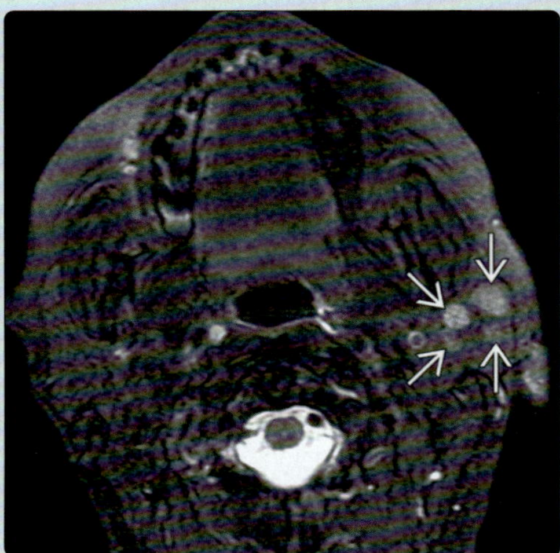

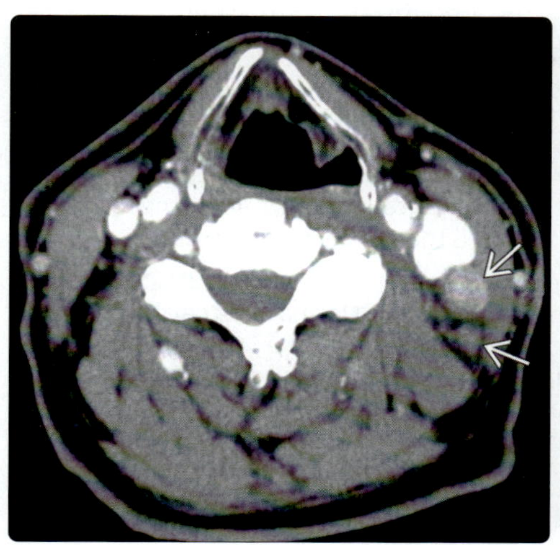

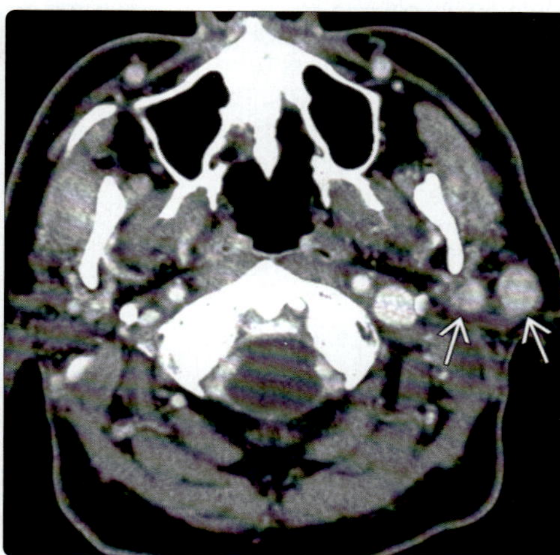

(Left) *Axial CECT in a patient with multiply treated ipsilateral forehead skin SCCa shows cervical neck metastatic nodal spread ➡ in addition to parotid nodal disease. This patient needs both parotidectomy and ipsilateral nodal dissection.* **(Right)** *Axial CECT in a patient with multiply treated ipsilateral forehead skin SCCa shows two intraparotid SCCa nodes ➡. Remember to look at the entire neck for other nodal metastases when nodes are seen in the parotid.*

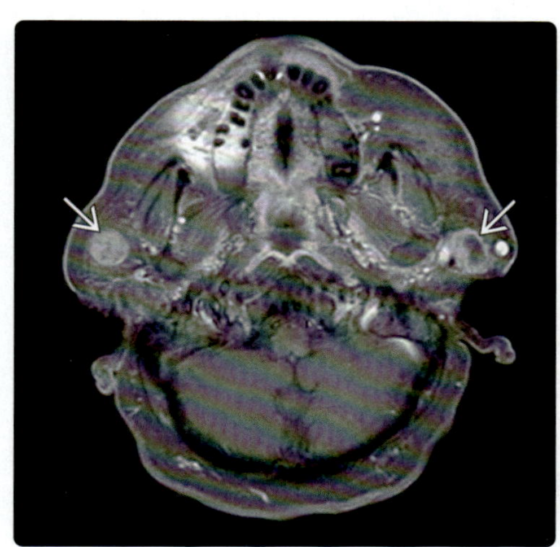

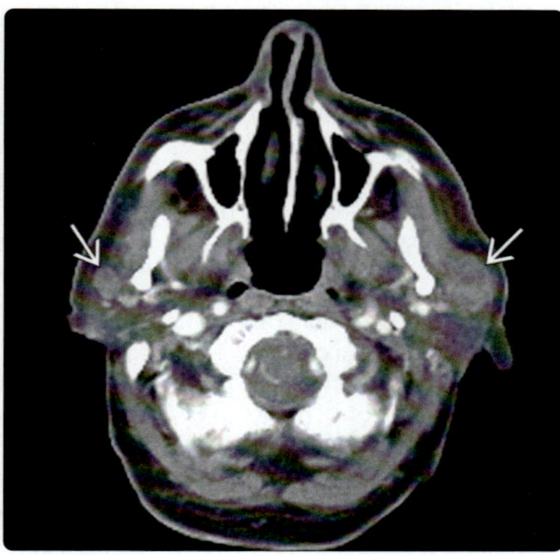

(Left) *Axial T1 fat-saturated enhanced MR in a patient with a multiply treated SCCa on the bridge of the nose shows bilateral parotid malignant nodes ➡. Forehead, nose and scalp SCCa often drain bilaterally.* **(Right)** *Axial CT in a patient with vertex scalp squamous cell carcinoma reveals bilateral parotid nodal metastases ➡. Any midline malignant tumor of the skin (scalp, nose, face) can spread bilaterally to both parotid glands.*

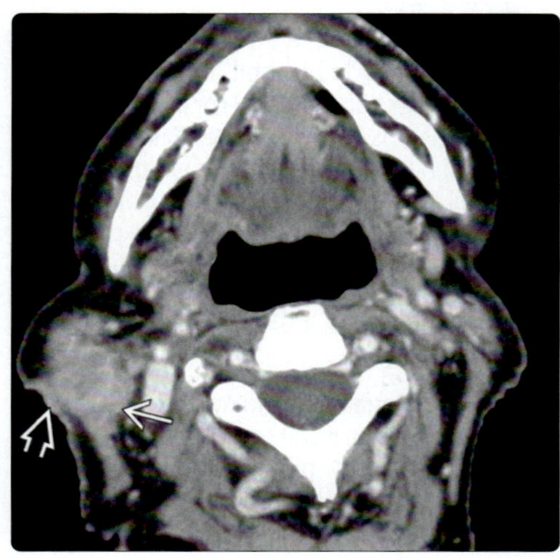

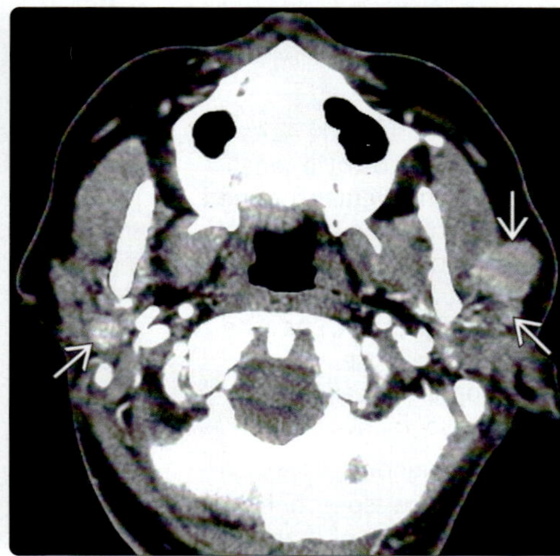

(Left) *Axial CECT shows parotid tail nodal conglomerate with extranodal markings from periauricular skin squamous cell carcinoma. Note the sternocleidomastoid invasion ➡ and skin thickening ➡, both imaging evidence of extranodal tumor.* **(Right)** *Axial CECT demonstrates numerous bilateral, well-defined, uniformly enhancing parotid masses ➡ in a patient with known breast cancer. These masses represent hematogeneous metastases.*

Summary Thoughts: Carotid Space

The carotid spaces (CSs) are paired tubular spaces that traverse the suprahyoid neck (SHN) and infrahyoid neck (IHN) just lateral to the retropharyngeal space (RPS). Another term for the CS is the retrostyloid parapharyngeal space (PPS). The CS is enveloped by the **carotid sheath**, which is made up of all **3 layers of deep cervical fascia**. The SHN CS contains the internal carotid artery (ICA), internal jugular vein (IJV), and cranial nerves (CN) IX-XII. The IHN CS has within it only the common carotid artery (CCA), IJV, and the vagus nerve (CNX) trunk.

A **SHN CS mass** displaces the anterior PPS fat anteriorly as it enlarges. Often the ICA is also displaced anteriorly by an enlarging SHN CS mass. An **IHN CS mass** engulfs the CCA or splays the carotid bifurcation (carotid body paraganglioma).

Important **CS tumors** include paraganglioma, schwannoma, neurofibroma, and sympathetic chain schwannoma. The internal jugular nodal chain is in close proximity to the superficial margin of the CS. As a result, when squamous cell carcinoma (SCCa) metastatic nodes undergo extranodal spread, they may involve the adjacent carotid artery and vagus nerve.

Imaging Techniques and Indications

CECT (+ CTA ± CTV) or MR (+ MRA ± MRV) easily identify most CS lesions. Certainly the CS mass lesions are readily seen using either technique. When using CT, CTA gives a multiplanar vascular-phase view of the intrinsic carotid diseases. CECT that allows contrast to penetrate into the soft tissues of the neck is better for delineation of CS mass lesions.

When using MR, remember to acquire T1 without contrast (to look for **high-velocity flow voids** imaging signature of paraganglioma). MRA & MRV may be helpful in defining a vascular CS lesion (ICA dissection, pseudoaneurysm, or IJV thrombosis).

Imaging Anatomy

The important **anatomic relationships** of the CS can be examined at the SHN and IHN level. At the SHN level the CS has the RPS medial, the perivertebral space (PVS) posterior, the deep lobe of the parotid space (PS) lateral, and the PPS anterior. At the IHN level, the CS is bounded by the visceral space (VS) & RPS medially, PVS posteriorly, anterior cervical space anteriorly, and posterior cervical space laterally.

The CS extends from the skull base to the aortic arch. At its superior skull base margin, the **ICA** enters the **carotid canal** just as the **IJV** emerges from the floor of the **jugular foramen** (JF). The sympathetic plexus leaves its position on the medial surface of the nasopharyngeal CS to ascend in the ICA adventitia as the carotid plexus along the ICA course through the temporal bone. At the CS inferior margin, the **CCAs** arise from the **aortic arch**, and the **IJVs** merge with the **brachiocephalic veins**. The CS has nasopharyngeal, oropharyngeal, cervical, and mediastinal segments.

The **carotid sheath** surrounds the CS throughout its passage through the soft tissues of the neck. A unique aspect of the carotid sheath is that it is made up of **all 3 layers of deep cervical** (superficial, middle, and deep) **fascia**. In the SHN, the carotid sheath is a considerably less substantial fascia than in the IHN. In the IHN, the sheath is a well-defined, tenacious fascia. This is fortunate as it is in the cervical neck that the CS suffers injury from trauma and spreading extranodal SCCa.

Important **CS internal structures** are best viewed from the perspective of what can be found in the SHN & IHN CS. The **SHN CS** contains the ICA & IJV along with the glossopharyngeal (**CNIX**), vagus (**CNX**), spinal accessory (**CNXI**), and hypoglossal (**CNXII**) CNs. Foci of normal neural crest derivative **glomus bodies** are found in the nodose ganglion of the vagus nerve approximately 2 cm below the floor of the JF of the skull base. They are also located in the JF above and the carotid bifurcation below. Along the medial border of the SHN CS is the **sympathetic plexus**.

All CNs but the vagus nerve have exited the SHN CS by the time it reaches the hyoid bone. **Normal internal structures** of the **IHN CS** include the vagus nerve, the CCA, and IJV. The **internal jugular nodal chain** is loosely wound into the external fascial layers along the surface of the CS. As such, this nodal chain is considered closely associated but **not** within the CS.

Approaches to Imaging Issues of Carotid Space

The answer to the question, **"What imaging findings define a CS mass?"** varies depending on the level of the lesion. If the lesion is in the **nasopharyngeal CS**, it displaces the PPS fat anteriorly and lifts the styloid process anterolaterally. At the level of the **oropharyngeal CS**, the PPS is again pushed anteriorly, but an important additional clue is the displacement of the posterior belly of the digastric muscle anterolaterally. At either the nasopharyngeal or oropharyngeal level, lesions in the posterior CS (vagal schwannoma, neurofibroma, paraganglioma) will bow the ICA anteriorly as they enlarge. A mass of the **infrahyoid CS** engulfs the CCA or splays the bifurcation (carotid body paraganglioma).

When a CS lesion is identified on imaging, matching its radiologic findings to common CS lesions is often very rewarding as many of the lesions have distinctive imaging findings. If the lesion is intrinsic to the carotid artery, ICA tortuosity, dissection, pseudoaneurysm, and thrombosis should all be considered. Intrinsic IJV lesions should suggest IJV asymmetry, thrombophlebitis, and thrombosis. Tumors within the space include paraganglioma (MR high-velocity flow voids), schwannoma (tubular lesions with intramural cysts), and neurofibroma (target appearance on MR; low density on CECT).

Nasopharyngeal CS tumors may "**dumbbell**" inferiorly from the **JF** above. A careful inspection of the JF for imaging signs of simultaneous involvement is in order. If the JF is abnormal, the main differential diagnoses of the CS mass are glomus jugulare paraganglioma, JF schwannoma (CNIX-XI), or JF meningioma. **Bone CT** imaging clues that may be helpful include permeative-destructive changes along the margin of the JF (glomus jugulare), smooth, expansile JF with sclerotic margins (schwannoma), and permeative-sclerotic or hyperostotic changes (meningioma).

MR clues to consider for a **JF mass** extending into nasopharyngeal CSs are plentiful. If the tumor has low-signal, high-velocity flow voids with vector of spread through the floor of the middle ear cavity, glomus jugulare is the 1st diagnostic consideration. A fusiform mass with intramural cystic change and a vector of spread that projects upward and medial toward the lateral medulla suggests schwannoma. JF meningioma lacks high-velocity signal voids and spreads centrifugally away from the JF.

Differential Diagnosis of Carotid Space Lesion

Pseudolesions	CCA or ICA aneurysm
Ectatic CCA or ICA	ICA pseudoaneurysm
Carotid bulb ectasia	Fibromuscular dysplasia
Asymmetric IJV	Takayasu arteritis
Congenital	**Benign tumor**
2nd branchial cleft cyst variant	Carotid body paraganglioma
Inflammation or infection	Glomus vagale paraganglioma
CS cellulitis	Glomus jugulare paraganglioma, inferior extension
CS abscess	CNIX-XII schwannoma
Acute idiopathic carotidynia	Sympathetic chain schwannoma
Vascular	CNIX-XII neurofibroma
IJV thrombophlebitis	Jugular foramen meningioma, inferior extension
IJV thrombosis	**Malignant tumor**
CCA or ICA atherosclerosis	SCCa primary tumor invasion, perifascial spread
CCA or ICA thrombosis	SCCa extranodal tumor invasion
ICA dissection	Extranodal NHL, internal jugular nodal chain

Above is an exhaustive list of all lesions that can be found in the carotid space. The table is organized by general pathology category. CCA = common carotid artery; ICA = internal carotid artery; IJV = internal jugular vein; SCCa = squamous cell carcinoma; NHL = non-Hodgkin lymphoma.

Vascular lesions in the CS arise within the IJV or carotid artery. IJV thrombophlebitis mimics a neck abscess clinically and is easily diagnosed because of the tubular luminal clot and surrounding soft tissue inflammatory changes. The more chronic IJV thrombosis clinically mimics a neck tumor, lacking the soft tissue inflammatory changes on imaging. Important carotid artery lesions include atherosclerosis, dissection with or without pseudoaneurysm, and fibromuscular dysplasia (FMD). This lesion group can be readily diagnosed with CTA with the exception of FMD, which may require angiography to diagnose.

Perhaps the most common image interpretation pitfall associated with CS lesions is the tendency to confuse SHN CS mass with lateral retropharyngeal nodal mass. **Lateral RPS mass** lesions displace the ICA-IJV in the CS posterolaterally whereas SHN CS mass lesions push the ICA anteriorly or anteromedially. As there are no nodes within the CS, if the imaging appearance suggests nodal disease, check to see if the ICA is pushed laterally. If so, you are looking at a lateral RPS lesion.

Clinical Implications

Lesions of the CS often present 1st with **hoarseness**. Endoscopy determines which vocal cord is paralyzed. **Left** vocal cord paralysis requires imaging from the posterior fossa to the aortopulmonic window, while **right** vocal cord paralysis only requires the scan to reach the clavicle inferiorly.

Proximal vagal neuropathy often includes other CN injury (CNIX, XI, or XII). Because the pharyngeal plexus branch of the vagus nerve is injured, the ipsilateral soft palate and superior constrictor muscles fasciculate in the acute phase and become patulous in the chronic phase of injury. In the chronic phase of proximal vagal neuropathy, imaging will show fatty infiltration of the ipsilateral soft palate and a patulous lateral pharynx due to constrictor muscle atrophy. Lesions causing proximal vagal neuropathy can be found involving the brainstem medulla, basal cistern, JF, or suprahyoid CS.

Distal vagal neuropathy is defined as isolated vagal neuropathy without the nasopharyngeal & oropharyngeal findings described above. In this setting, lesions are sought in the infrahyoid CS. Left-sided lesions may include diseases of the mediastinum, such as lung cancer. Right-sided lesions causing distal vagal neuropathy are usually clinically palpable at the time of imaging.

Postganglionic **Horner syndrome** presents loss of sympathetic tone and ptosis (droop of upper eyelid), miosis (decrease in pupil size), and anhydrosis (absence of sweat). The lesion causing Horner syndrome is sought along the segment of oculosympathetic pathway between the superior cervical ganglion and eye. Much of this pathway is found between the supraclavicular and nasopharyngeal CS. Remember the sympathetic chain passes with the ICA up the skull base carotid canal. The clinician must evaluate the cervical, oropharyngeal, and nasopharyngeal CS, the carotid canal in the skull base, cavernous sinus, & the orbit. In particular, ICA dissection must be excluded.

Selected References

1. Chong VF et al: The suprahyoid neck: normal and pathological anatomy. J Laryngol Otol. 113(6):501-8, 1999
2. Chong VF et al: Pictorial review: radiology of the carotid space. Clin Radiol. 51(11):762-8, 1996
3. Fruin ME et al: The carotid space of the infrahyoid neck. Semin Ultrasound CT MR. 12(3):224-40, 1991

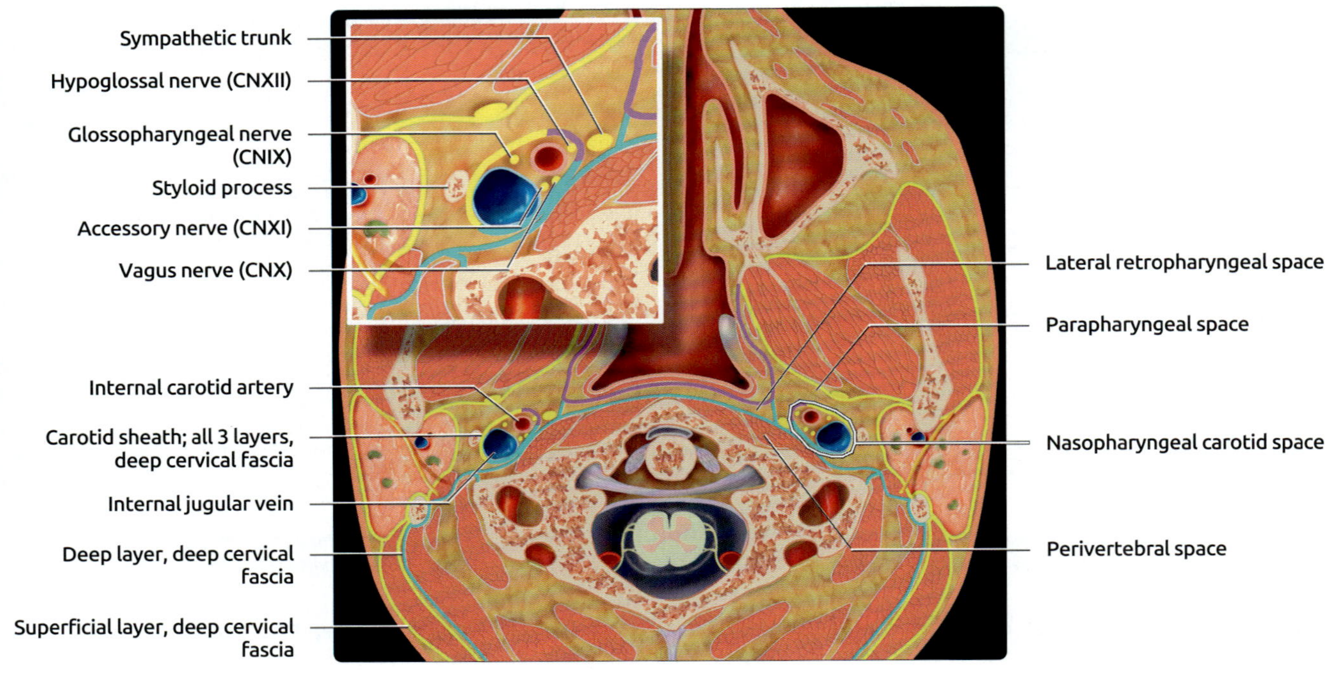

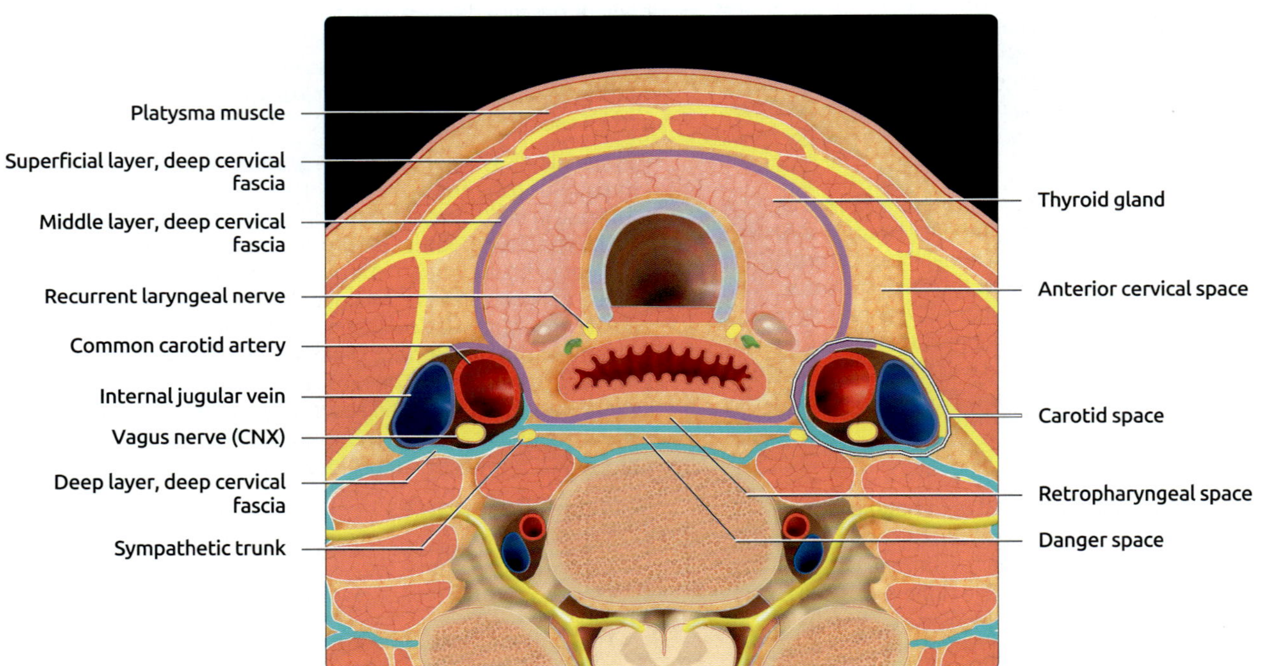

(Top) *Axial graphic of the suprahyoid neck (SHN) at the level of the C1 vertebral body with insert shows a magnified carotid space (CS). The suprahyoid CS contains CNIX-XII, the internal carotid artery (ICA), and the internal jugular vein (IJV). The carotid sheath is made up of components of all 3 layers of deep cervical fascia (tricolor line around CS). In the SHN, the carotid sheath is less substantial than in the infrahyoid neck (IHN). The sympathetic trunk runs just medial to the CS.* **(Bottom)** *Axial graphic shows the CS in the IHN. Note that the carotid sheath contains all 3 layers of the deep cervical fascia (tricolor line). In the IHN, the carotid sheath is tenacious throughout its length. The infrahyoid CS contains the common carotid artery (CCA), IJV, and only the vagus cranial nerve.*

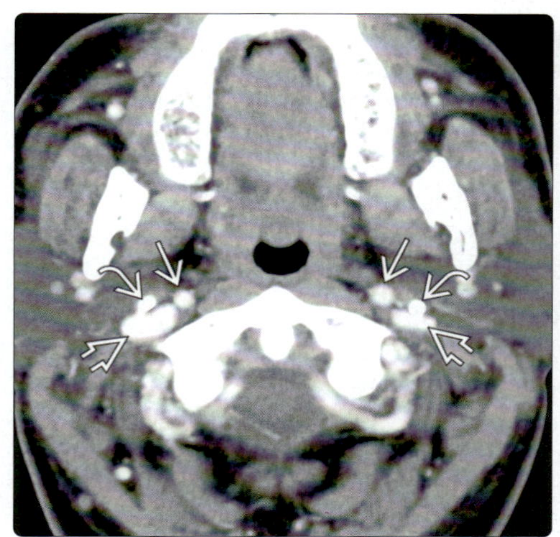

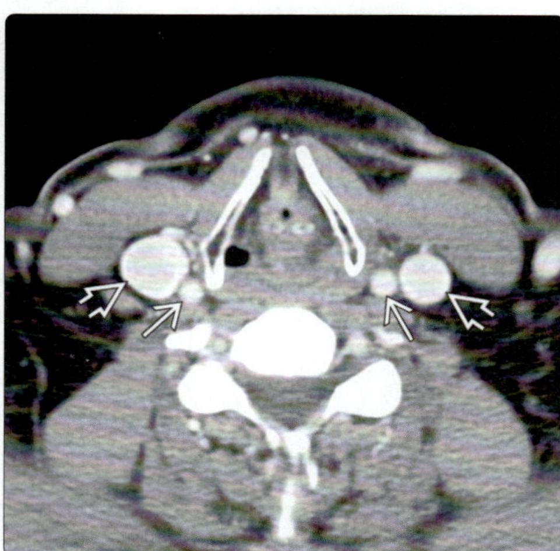

(Left) *Axial CECT at the level of C1 vertebral body shows the nasopharyngeal CS contains the ICA ➡, IJV ➡, and CNIX-XII (not visible). Note that the CS is posterior to the styloid process ➡.* **(Right)** *Axial CECT at the level of the glottic larynx shows that the infrahyoid CS contains the CCA ➡, IJV ➡, and vagus nerve (not visible). Notice that the carotid sheath is also not visible on imaging.*

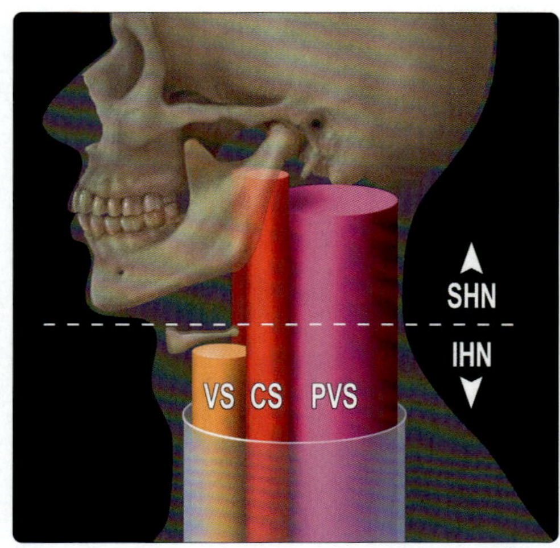

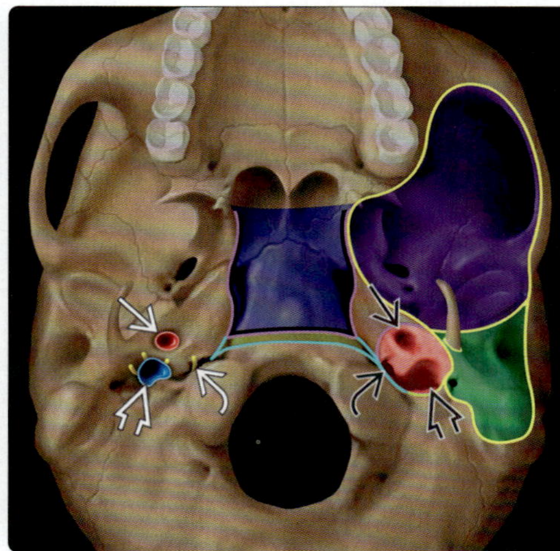

(Left) *Lateral graphic of the cervical neck shows the tubular CS extending from the skull base [carotid canal and jugular foramen (JF)] to the aortic arch.* **(Right)** *Axial graphic of the skull base viewed from below shows the CS abutting the skull base. The ICA ➡ enters the carotid canal ➡, while the IJV ➡ emerges from the JF ➡. CNIX-XI is exiting the JF. CNXII ➡ is more medial as it enters the CS from the hypoglossal canal ➡.*

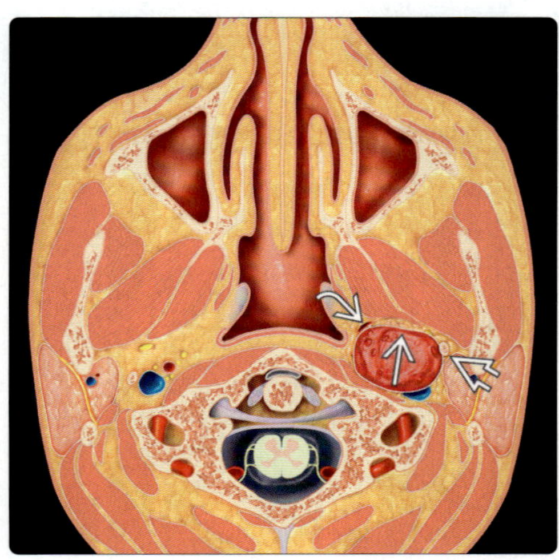

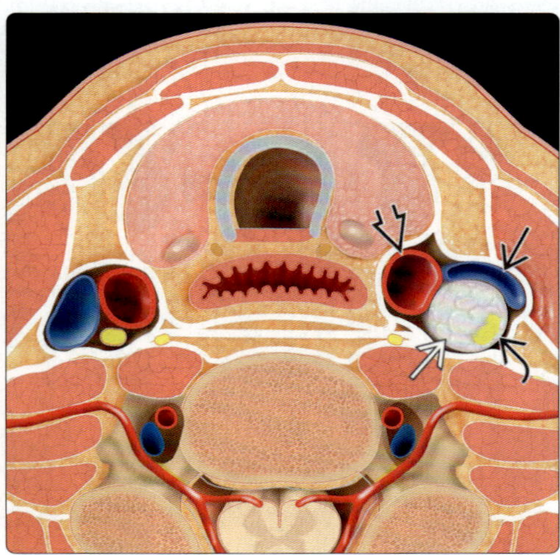

(Left) *Axial graphic reveals a generic nasopharyngeal CS mass. As the CS mass enlarges, it pushes the parapharyngeal space fat anteriorly ➡ as well as lifts the styloid process anterolaterally ➡. Often the ICA is also lifted anteriorly ➡ by a CS mass.* **(Right)** *Axial graphic of an infrahyoid CS mass ➡ shows that the CCA ➡ and the IJV ➡ are displaced anteriorly. Note the vagus nerve ➡ is visible in the posterolateral aspect of this vagal schwannoma.*

Tortuous Carotid Artery in Neck

KEY FACTS

TERMINOLOGY

- Synonyms: Retropharyngeal carotid, carotid transposition, kissing carotids, medialized carotid

IMAGING

- **CTA or MRA** easily establishes diagnosis
- CTA/CECT shows enhancing carotid artery (CA) in retropharyngeal space (RPS)
  - Round (axial) or tubular (coronal) vessel
  - Contiguous axial images reveal contiguous nature
- **Coronal reconstructions** best depict RPS CA

TOP DIFFERENTIAL DIAGNOSES

- CA pseudoaneurysm or dissection
- Carotid body paraganglioma

PATHOLOGY

- CA pushes medially from carotid space, bows ± violates **lateral slip of deep cervical fascia** to enter RPS

CLINICAL ISSUES

- Often incidental CT or MR finding
- Can be seen in 22q11 deletion syndrome
- If symptomatic, pulsatile retropharyngeal or retrotonsillar mass
  - Globus sensation
  - May potentiate obstructive sleep apnea
- Common pseudolesion of older population
- Correct imaging diagnosis prevents treatment

DIAGNOSTIC CHECKLIST

- Tortuous CA in differential diagnosis of prevertebral soft tissue widening on lateral plain film
  - Routine enhanced CT of neck easily makes diagnosis
- Clinician must recognize as **nonsurgical** lesion
- Key is recognizing **tubular nature** of ectatic CA
- **Must identify in patients undergoing pharyngeal surgery**

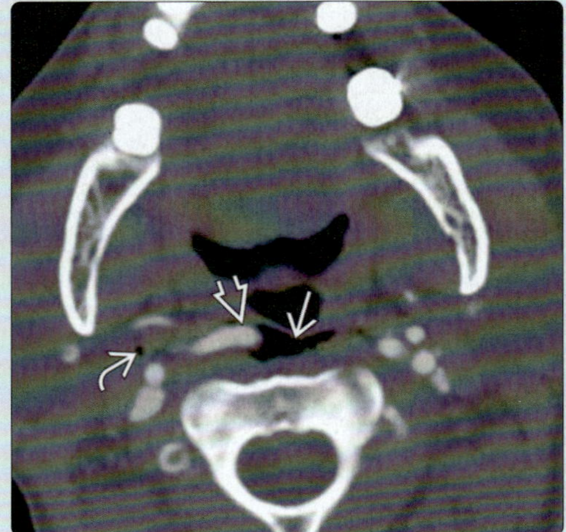

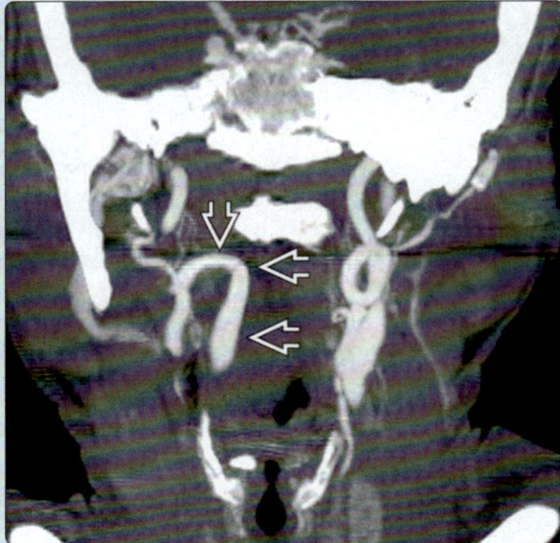

(Left) *Axial CT angiogram in a 62-year-old woman who suffered a stab wound to the right neck with a pharyngeal laceration demonstrates gas in the retropharyngeal ➡ and carotid spaces ➡. Medialized tortuous right internal carotid artery ➡ in the retropharyngeal space is incidentally seen.* **(Right)** *Coronal CT angiogram demonstrates the far medial course of the right internal carotid artery ➡ as it arches into the retropharyngeal space. Coronal images often best illustrate the serpiginous vascular nature of this variant.*

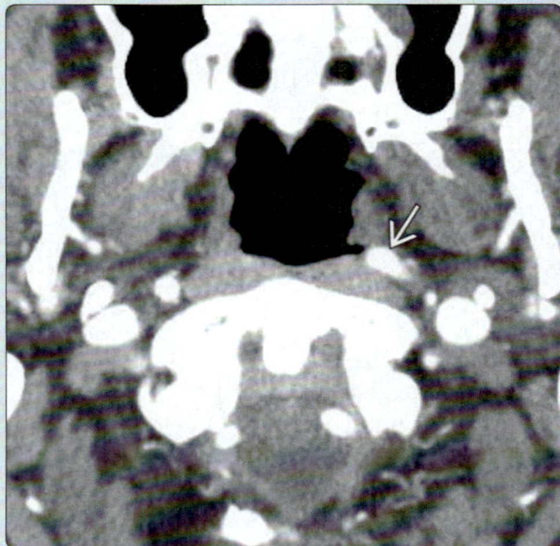

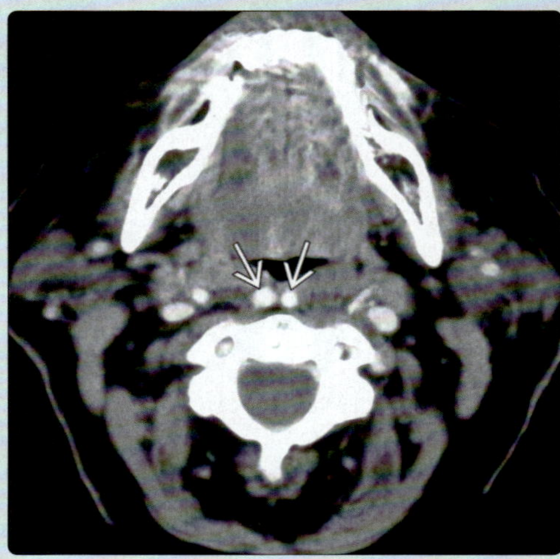

(Left) *Axial CECT demonstrates medial deviation of the left internal carotid artery ➡. Note its exposed position near the mucosal surface at the level of the nasopharynx. Reporting this variant is important to avoid iatrogenic injury if pharyngeal intervention is planned.* **(Right)** *Axial NECT demonstrates a classic example of "kissing" carotids as bilateral ectatic internal carotid arteries contacting in the midline ➡ retropharyngeal space.*

KEY FACTS

TERMINOLOGY

- Internal carotid artery dissection (ICAD): Tear in ICA wall allows blood to enter & delaminate wall layers

IMAGING

- Pathognomonic findings of dissection: **Intimal flap** or **double lumen** (seen in < 10%)
- Aneurysmal dilatation seen in 30%
  - Commonly in distal subcranial segment of ICA
  - Focal **pseudoaneurysm** unusual
- Flame-shaped ICA occlusion (acute phase)
- ICAD most commonly originates in ICA 2-3 cm above carotid bulb & variably involves distal ICA
  - Stops before petrous ICA
  - Long-segment irregularity of vessel
- CTA & MRA emerging as superior technologies to image intramural & extraluminal dissection components
  - CTA: Best shows **intimal flap**
  - T1 FS MR: Shows **hyperintense mural hematomas**

TOP DIFFERENTIAL DIAGNOSES

- Fibromuscular dysplasia
- Atheromatous plaque
- Traumatic ICA pseudoaneurysm
- Carotid artery fenestration
- Reversible cerebral vasoconstrictive syndrome

CLINICAL ISSUES

- Clinical presentation
  - Ipsilateral pain in face, jaw, head, or neck
  - Oculosympathetic palsy
    - Miosis & ptosis, partial Horner syndrome
  - Ischemic symptoms (cerebral or retinal TIA or stroke)
  - Neck bruit (40%) ± pulsatile tinnitus
  - Lower cranial nerve palsies (especially CNX)
- Treatment options: Preventing stroke is primary goal
  - Heparin followed by warfarin (3-6 months)
  - Antiplatelet meds: Aspirin, ticlopidine or clopidogrel

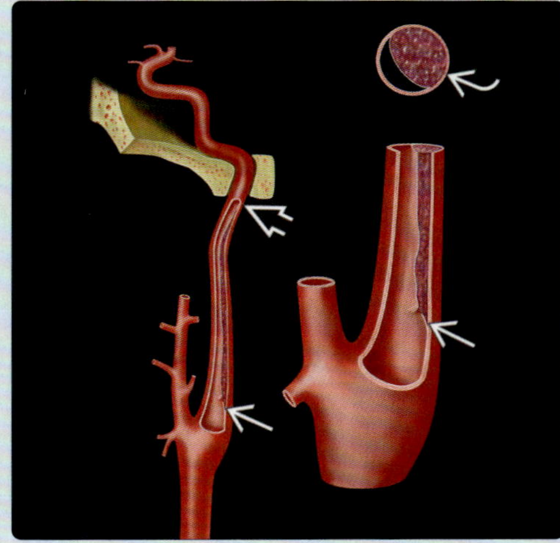

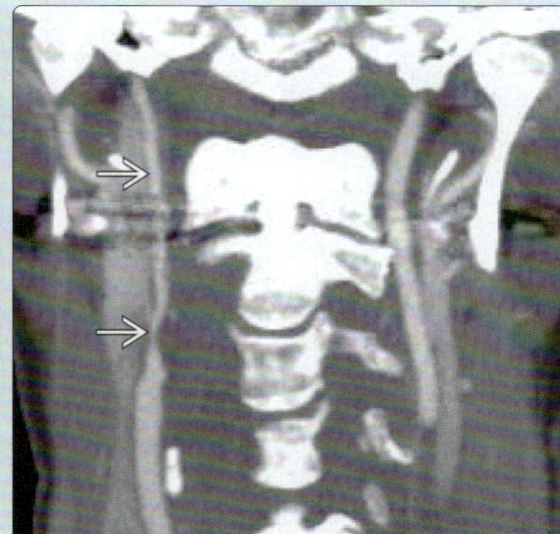

(Left) *Lateral graphic depicts typical internal carotid artery (ICA) dissection. Note that the dissection begins above bifurcation ➡ and ends just below the skull base ➡. Cross section of a subintimal hematoma ➡ is also shown.* **(Right)** *Coronal CTA multiplanar reconstruction demonstrates a long-segment irregular narrowing ➡ of the right ICA that is consistent with acute dissection.*

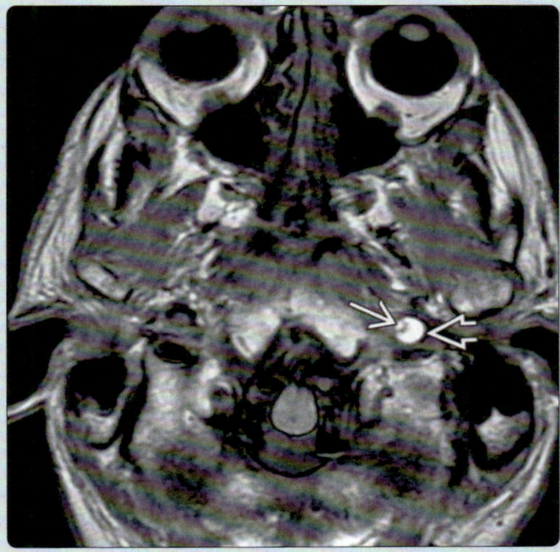

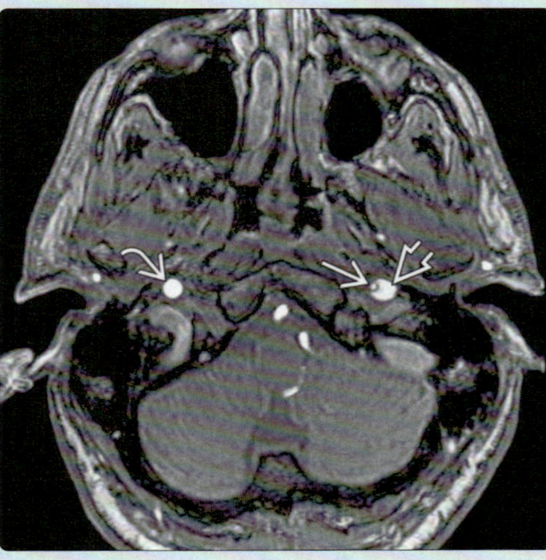

(Left) *Axial T1WI MR in an adult man who fell skiing 3 weeks prior to developing left temporal headache shows T1 shortening within the crescentic subacute clot ➡ in the false lumen of dissected left ICA. Note the high-signal thrombus ➡ within the true vessel lumen, which was occluded.* **(Right)** *Axial MRA source image in the same patient shows high-signal thrombus in the false lumen ➡ and thrombosed true lumen ➡. There is a signal difference of thrombosed vessel on the left compared to the patent right ICA ➡.*

Carotid Artery Pseudoaneurysm in Neck

KEY FACTS

TERMINOLOGY

- Abbreviation: Carotid artery pseudoaneurysm (CAPA)
- Synonyms: Carotid artery false aneurysm
- CAPA: Outpouching lacking part or all of carotid wall

IMAGING

- General findings
  - Internal carotid artery (ICA) lumen outpouching with extraluminal CAPA
  - Associated dissection often present
- CTA/CECT: **Focal increase in ICA wall-lumen diameter**
  - CECT & CTA show CAPA size, extent of intraluminal thrombus, & flow
- MR: Enlarged ICA with complex wall signal (stages of thrombosis with methemoglobin & hemosiderin)
  - Partly thrombosed CAPA may require enhanced MRA
- Conventional angiography
  - Gold standard for detection of CAPA ± ICA dissection

TOP DIFFERENTIAL DIAGNOSES

- Carotid bulb ectasia; tortuous or looping carotid artery in neck; carotid artery dissection in neck

PATHOLOGY

- Etiologies
  - **Post traumatic (with dissection or direct injury)**
  - Sporadic subadventitial ICA dissection
  - Atherosclerotic disease (frequently bilateral)
  - Iatrogenic: Radiation, carotid endarterectomy
  - Infection and congenital (ICA wall anomaly)

CLINICAL ISSUES

- Clinical: Pulsatile neck mass; TIA ± CVA
- Treatment options
  - Smaller CAPA + ICA dissection
    - Anticoagulation + observation ± aspirin
  - Larger CAPA: Endovascular stent graft
    - Surgical repair or vessel sacrifice as needed

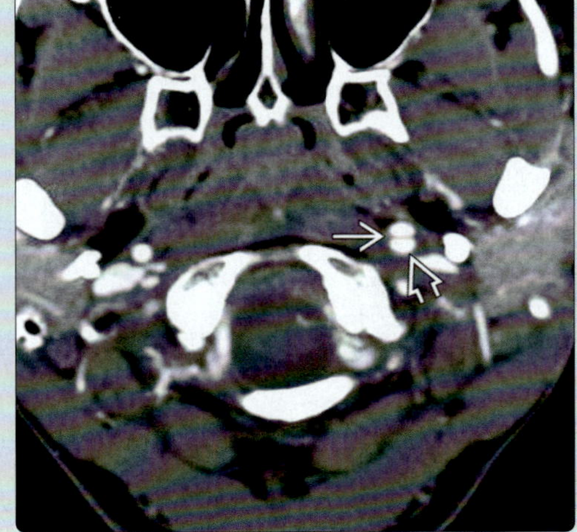

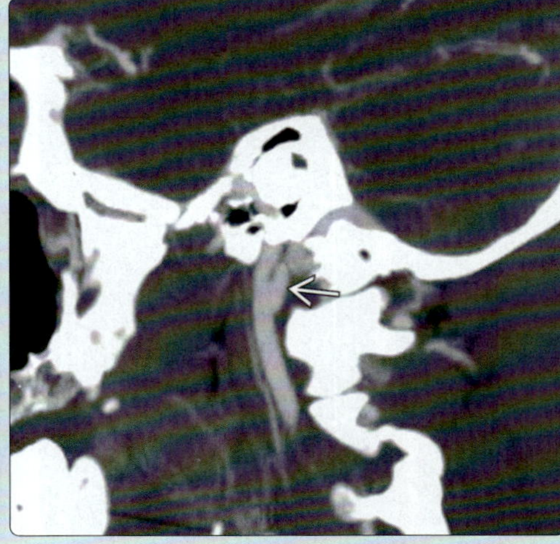

(Left) *Axial CTA in an adult man with cervical fractures following a motorcycle crash shows abnormality involving high cervical left internal carotid artery (ICA) with evidence of dissection with the intimal flap ➡ & focal outpouching along posterior wall of vessel (pseudoaneurysm)* ➡. **(Right)** *Sagittal CTA reformat in same patient clearly demonstrates pseudoaneurysm related to ICA dissection* ➡. *Note: Reformatted image allows clear morphologic characterization while axial image does not.*

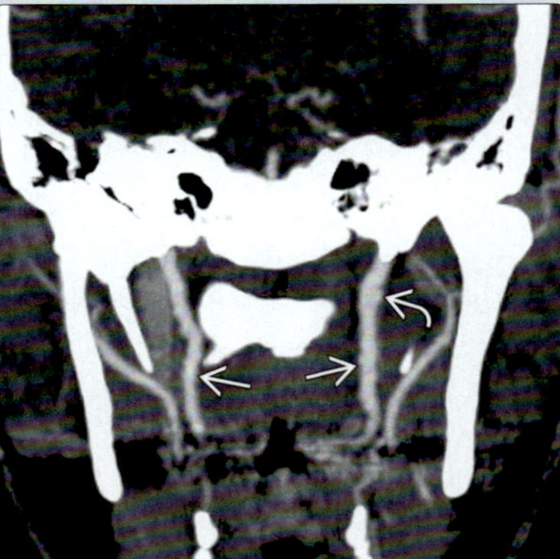

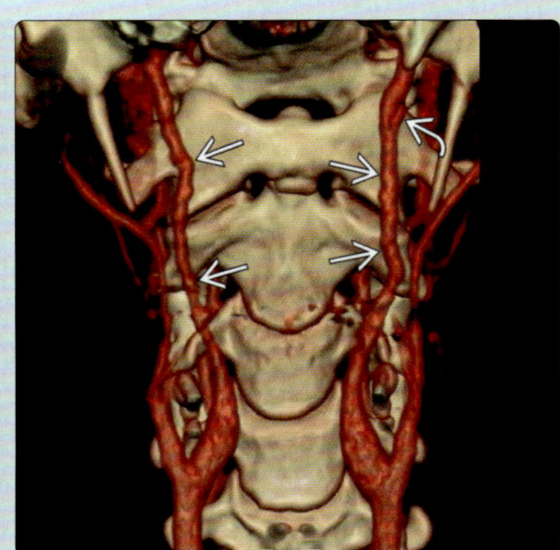

(Left) *Coronal CTA in a 44-year-old woman with fibromuscular dysplasia (FMD) shows diffuse irregularity of both ICAs* ➡*, consistent with FMD. There is a small focal dissection with the pseudoaneurysm involving the high cervical left ICA* ➡. **(Right)** *Coronal CTA volume-rendered image in the same patient more clearly demonstrates the left ICA pseudoaneurysm* ➡. *Diffuse vessel irregularity related to FMD is again seen* ➡.

KEY FACTS

TERMINOLOGY

- Fibromuscular dysplasia (FMD)
  - Arterial disease of unknown etiology
  - Overgrowth of smooth muscle, fibrous tissue
  - Affecting medium & large arteries

IMAGING

- Renal artery most common overall site (~ 75%)
- Cervicocranial FMD CTA/MRA findings
  - Vessel beading/irregularities: **String-of-beads appearance**
  - **Arterial stenosis** without mural Ca^{++} (compare to ASVD)
  - FMD associations: Dissection, pseudoaneurysm, intracranial aneurysms
- Digital subtraction angio: Gold standard; 3 appearances
  - **Type 1 (85%)**: Typical string-of-beads appearance; medial fibroplasia
  - **Type 2 (10%)**: Long tubular stenosis; intimal fibroplasia
  - **Type 3 (5%)**: Asymmetric outpouching along 1 side of artery; periadventitial or periarterial fibroplasia

TOP DIFFERENTIAL DIAGNOSES

- Atherosclerosis, nonatherosclerotic vasculopathies, standing waves on DSA, MRA motion artifact

PATHOLOGY

- 3 principal histopathologic varieties
  - **Medial fibroplasia**: Medial layer involvement (type 1)
  - **Intimal fibroplasia**: Intimal involvement (type 2)
  - **Perimedial fibroplasia**: Involvement of adventitia adjacent to media (type 3)
- Alternating zones of hyperplasia & weakening

CLINICAL ISSUES

- Presentation: TIA ± stroke
  - Hypertension 2° to renal artery stenosis
- Treatment: Antiplatelet ± anticoagulant therapy
  - Balloon angioplasty; covered stenting

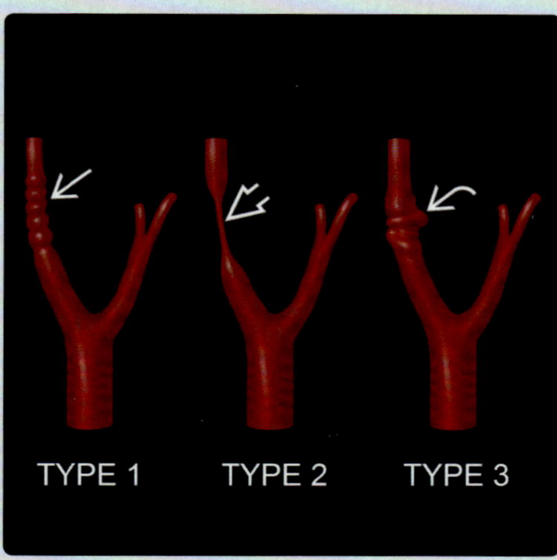

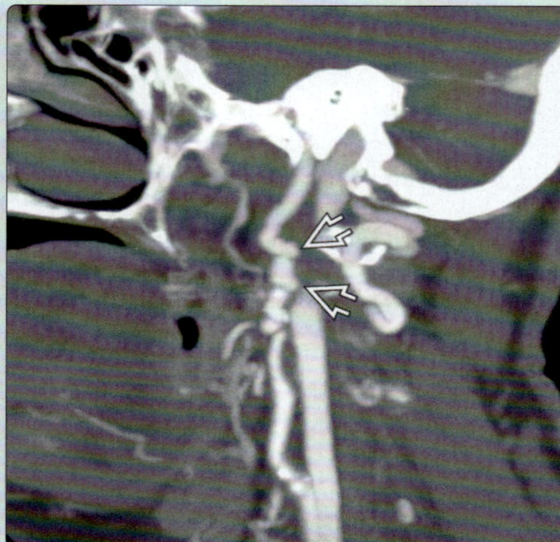

(Left) *Carotid bifurcation graphic shows the principal subtypes of fibromuscular dysplasia (FMD). Type 1 appears as alternating areas of constriction and dilatation ➡, type 2 as tubular stenosis ➡, and type 3 as focal corrugations ± a diverticulum ➡.* **(Right)** *Sagittal CTA reformation shows internal carotid artery (ICA) string-of-beads appearance. However, closer evaluation also shows focal outpouching ➡ along the course of both arteries, indicating that type 3 FMD is present.*

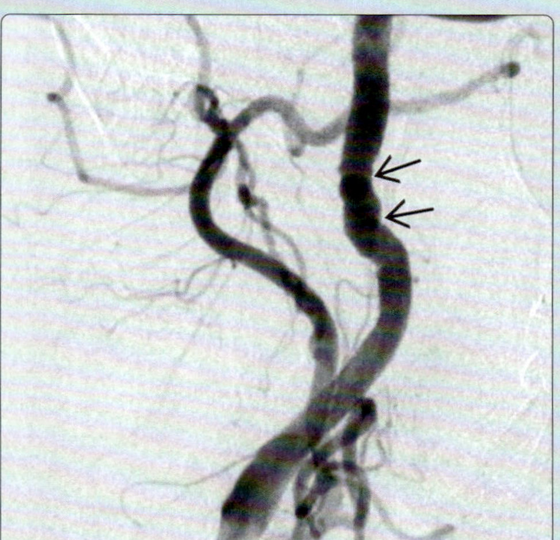

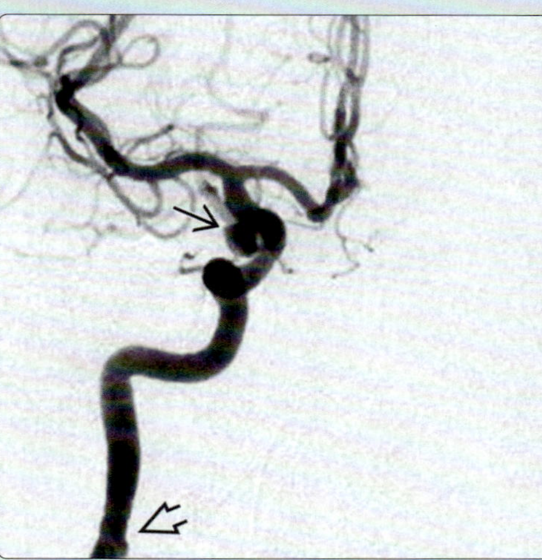

(Left) *Oblique right common carotid artery digital subtraction angiogram shows irregular outpouchings ➡ in the cervical ICA consistent with FMD.* **(Right)** *Anteroposterior right ICA digital subtraction angiogram in the same patient shows a 6-mm posterior communicating artery aneurysm ➡ that ruptured with resultant subarachnoid hemorrhage. Changes of FMD are again noted in the cervical ICA ➡.*

KEY FACTS

TERMINOLOGY

- Synonyms
  - Idiopathic or sclerosing (inflammatory) pseudotumor
  - Idiopathic carotiditis
  - Fay syndrome
- Controversial diagnosis: Syndrome vs. entity
- International Headache Society Classification Committee (IHSCC) criteria for diagnosis: Self-limited illness with ≥ 1 of following: Tenderness to palpation, swelling, ↑ pulsations over carotid
  - Imaging to exclude structural abnormality

IMAGING

- **Circumferential thickening of carotid wall**
  - Distal common carotid or carotid bifurcation area
  - Usually **no** luminal narrowing
- Contrast-enhanced MR better exam than CECT
  - **Markedly enhancing tissue only seen with MR**
  - CECT enhancement is poor
- Ultrasound: **Hypoechoic** soft tissue around distal common carotid artery and bifurcation

TOP DIFFERENTIAL DIAGNOSES

- Carotid artery dissection in neck
- Extracranial atherosclerosis
- Miscellaneous vasculitis

CLINICAL ISSUES

- Clinical presentation
  - Tenderness to palpation over carotid
  - Pulsatile neck mass, may be indurated
  - Typical symptomatic resolution in days to weeks
    - Repeat assessment after treatment to exclude other pathology
- Treatment options: Antiinflammatory medications
  - Migraine management if indicated
  - If early conservative management fails, histologic confirmation is important

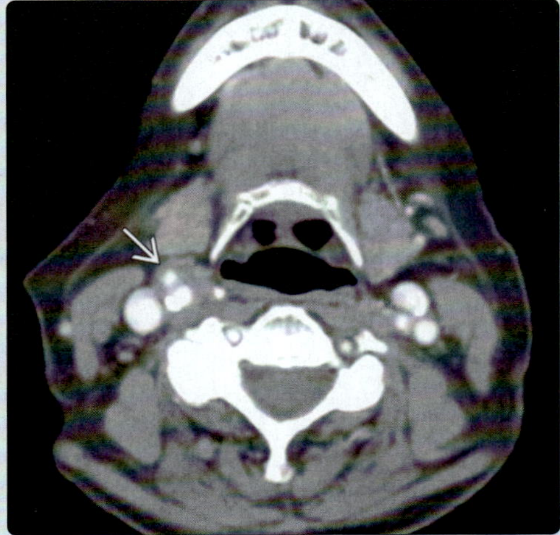

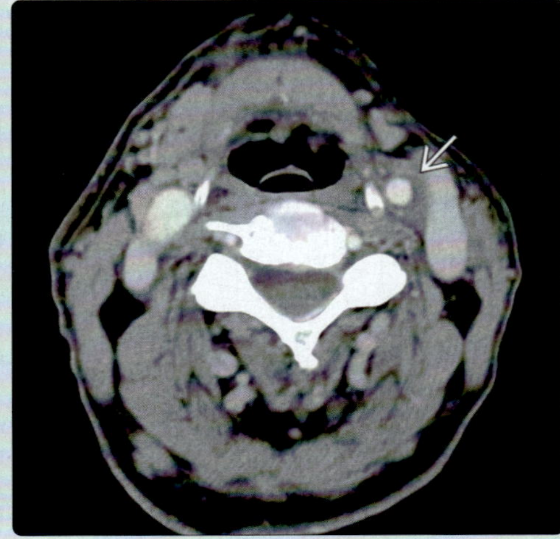

(Left) *Axial CECT of the neck reveals circumferential thickening of the common carotid wall ➡ at the carotid bifurcation. This patient was treated with steroids for presumptive diagnosis of carotidynia with symptoms resolving within 36 hours of treatment.* **(Right)** *Typical axial CECT of acute idiopathic carotidynia shows homogeneous soft tissue encasing the left distal common carotid artery ➡. There is no significant luminal narrowing.*

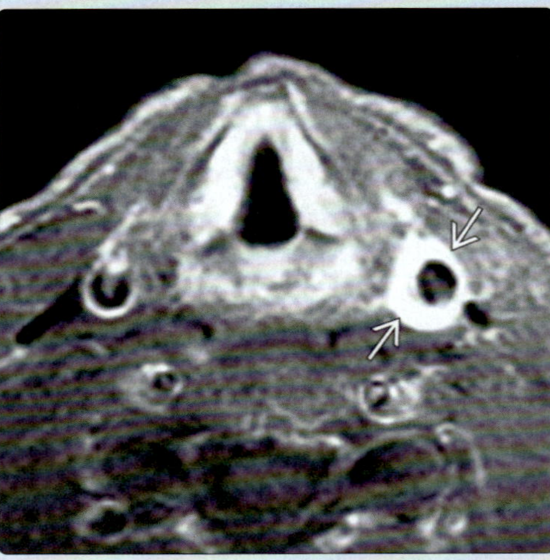

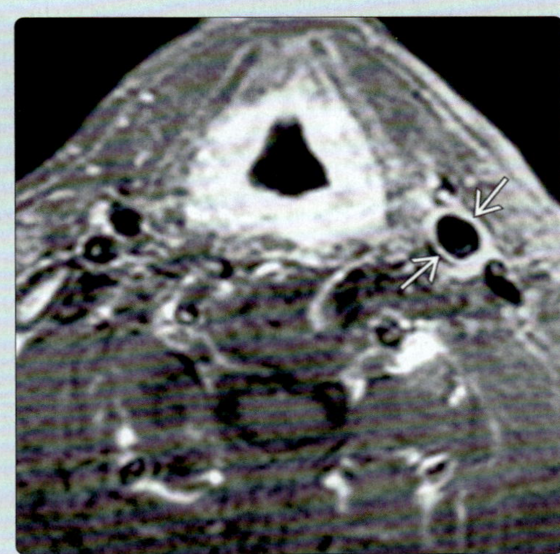

(Left) *Axial T1WI C+ FS MR in a patient with painful palpation in the left neck shows a thickened, intensely enhancing common carotid wall ➡ consistent with the diagnosis of carotidynia. Note the lack of luminal narrowing. (Courtesy G. W. Petermann, MD.)* **(Right)** *Axial T1 C+ FS MR in carotidynia post steroid therapy reveals mild residual wall thickening and enhancement involving the left common carotid wall ➡. (Courtesy G. W. Petermann, MD.)*

KEY FACTS

TERMINOLOGY

- Abbreviation: Jugular vein thrombosis (JVT)
- **JVT**: Chronic internal JV (IJV) thrombosis (> 10 days after acute event) in which clot persists within lumen after soft tissue inflammation is gone
- **JV thrombophlebitis**: Acute-subacute thrombosis of IJV with associated adjacent tissue inflammation

IMAGING

- CECT findings
  - Luminal clot (**filling defect**) in IJV with (thrombophlebitis) or without (thrombosis) associated soft tissue inflammatory changes
  - **Tubular** vascular lesion of cervical neck
- Ultrasound finding
  - **Noncompressible thrombus** and no flow

TOP DIFFERENTIAL DIAGNOSES

- Slow or turbulent flow in IJV (pseudothrombosis)
- Cervical neck abscess

PATHOLOGY

- JVT pathogenesis: 3 mechanisms for thrombosis
  - **Endothelial damage** from indwelling line or infection, altered blood flow, and hypercoagulable state
  - **Venous stasis** from neck IJV compression (nodes) or mediastinum (superior vena cava syndrome) incites JVT
  - Migratory IJV thrombophlebitis (Trousseau syndrome) associated with **malignancy** (pancreas, lung, and ovary)
- **Lemierre syndrome**: Pharyngeal infection causing septic IJV thrombosis from Fusobacterium necrophorum

CLINICAL ISSUES

- Clinical presentation
  - Acute-subacute: Swollen, tender neck mass with fever
  - Chronic: Woody neck mass may mimic tumor
- Treatment options
  - Aggressive intravenous antibiotics treat infection

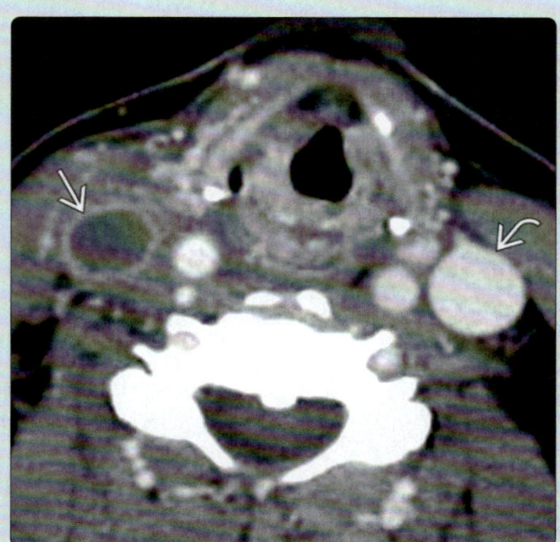

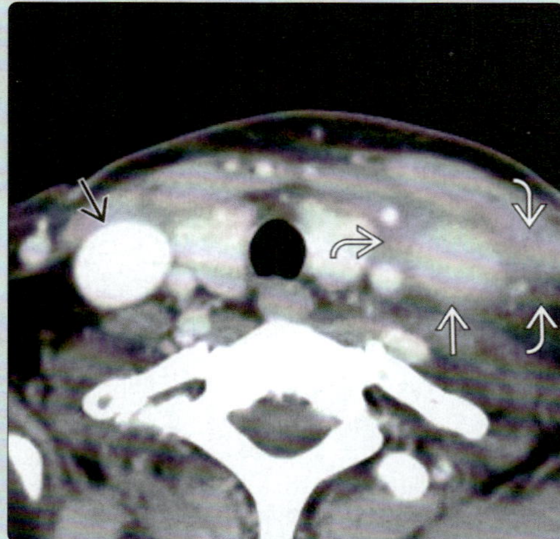

(Left) *Axial CECT in a 58-year-old woman with renal failure & a right internal jugular vein (IJV) hemodialysis catheter presented with right neck pain. Chronic right IJV thrombosis is seen ➡. Thin-wall enhancement of IJV venae vasorum and normal enhancement in patent left IJV ➡ are seen.* **(Right)** *Axial CECT in a 69-year-old woman with malignancy shows acute hyperdense thrombophlebitis involving the left IJV ➡. Note lower density compared with contrast-enhancing normal right IJV ➡ and surrounding tissue edema ➡.*

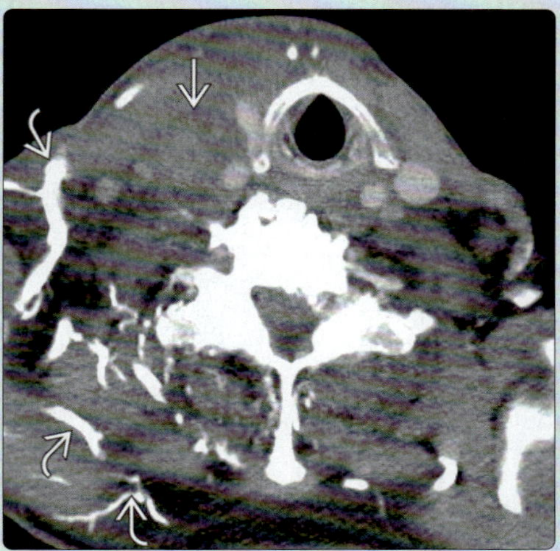

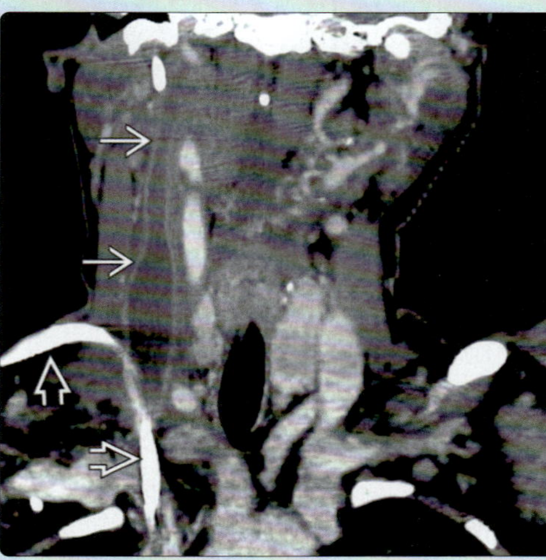

(Left) *Axial CECT shows low-density nonenhancing acute thrombophlebitis of the right IJV ➡. Note surrounding edema and extensive contrast reflux into small collateral veins ➡.* **(Right)** *Coronal CT reconstruction shows an IJV catheter ➡ and long-segment tubular thrombus within the right IJV ➡. Indwelling venous catheters in the cervical region predispose to jugular vein thrombosis*

Postpharyngitis Venous Thrombosis Lemierre Syndrome

KEY FACTS

TERMINOLOGY

- Lemierre syndrome or disease
- Postanginal sepsis or septicemia, necrobacillosis
- Opportunistic infection causing septic thrombophlebitis & metastatic infection

IMAGING

- CECT: Ipsilateral tonsillar fullness, edema; abscess atypical
  - Internal jugular vein ± tributary thrombophlebitis
  - Septic pulmonary emboli

TOP DIFFERENTIAL DIAGNOSES

- Jugular vein thrombosis, lung metastases

PATHOLOGY

- Usual agent is *Fusobacterium necrophorum*
  - Commensal anaerobic oral cavity bacillus
  - Many other agents possible, including *Staphylococcus aureus*
- Historical features
  - Common diagnosis in preantibiotic era
  - Reemergence due to antibiotic resistance
- **Preceding pharyngitis** in **90%** (less frequently after sinusitis, otitis, dental infection)
- **4-12% mortality** despite aggressive treatment

CLINICAL ISSUES

- Clinical presentation
  - Teenagers and young adults with pharyngitis
  - Atypical neck and face swelling
  - Classic imaging triad: Pharyngitis + neck vein thrombosis + cavitary pulmonary nodules
  - Imaging may suggest diagnosis before clinically evident
- Treatment options
  - Abscess drainage if present
  - IV antibiotics
    - Broad-spectrum antibiotics may **not** cover *F. necrophorum*

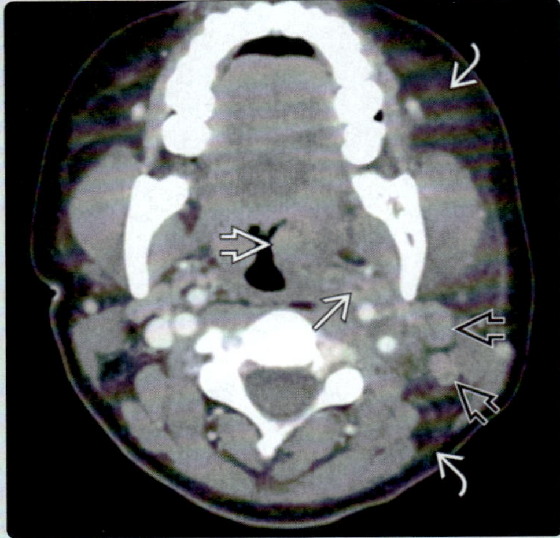

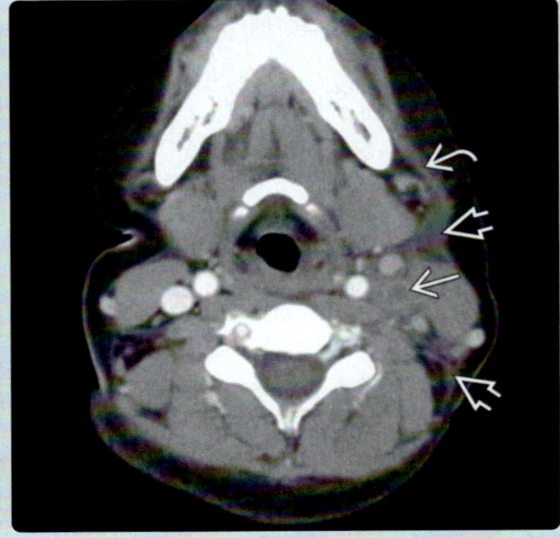

(Left) *Axial CECT shows tonsil edema ➡ and ipsilateral clot in venous tributaries ➡. Inflammatory changes of fat stranding ➡ and reactive lymph nodes ➡ are noted.* **(Right)** *Axial CECT shows nonopacification of the left internal jugular vein (IJV) consistent with thrombosis ➡. Acute inflammation is evidenced by stranding within regional fat pads ➡ and thickening of the platysma muscle ➡.*

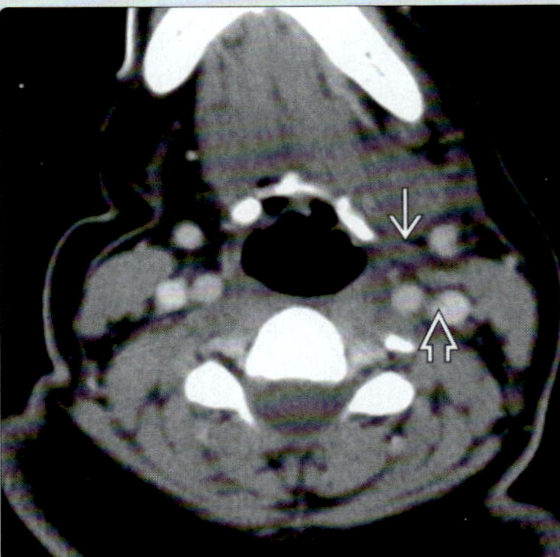

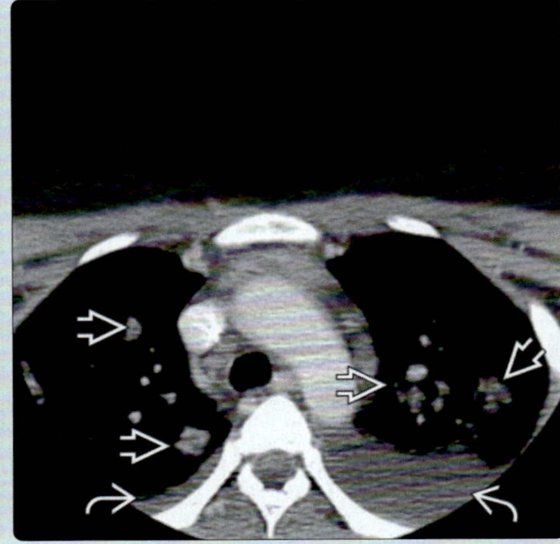

(Left) *Axial CECT shows an earlier, subtler case with few findings of neck inflammation. There is clot identified in the left facial vein ➡. Note that the IJV has suggestion of subtle, early intraluminal clot ➡.* **(Right)** *Axial CECT shows multiple pulmonary nodules ➡ due to septic emboli. There are bilateral pleural effusions ➡. Although the differential diagnosis may include metastatic disease, the clinical picture of sepsis establishes the correct diagnosis.*

KEY FACTS

TERMINOLOGY

- Synonyms: **Carotid body tumor**, glomus caroticum, chemodectoma, nonchromaffin paraganglioma

IMAGING

- General features: Vascular mass splaying external carotid artery and internal carotid artery at bifurcation (lyre sign on CTA, MRA, or angiography)
- CT and MR findings
  - Rapid dynamic enhancement on CT and MR
  - Serpentine or punctate vascular **flow voids** ("pepper") on MR, particularly in large lesions
- Ultrasound: Hypoechoic vascular mass on duplex US
- Angiography: Arteriovenous shunting, "early" veins

TOP DIFFERENTIAL DIAGNOSES

- Carotid space schwannoma or neurofibroma
- Carotid artery pseudoaneurysm or ectasia
- Glomus vagale paraganglioma

PATHOLOGY

- Multiple mutations (familial and sporadic) in *SDH* genes encoding for succinate dehydrogenase subunits
  - Paraganglioma syndromes
  - Multiple endocrine neoplasia syndromes
  - von Hippel-Lindau syndrome
- Staging: **Shamblin grouping** (types I, II, III, IIIb)
- Imaging surveillance with MR for familial disease

CLINICAL ISSUES

- Clinical presentation
  - Slow-growing, painless, pulsatile neck mass
  - Catecholamine-secreting carotid body paraganglioma; malignancy rare
    - Related to chronic hypoxia in some patients
- Treatment options: Surgery is treatment of choice
  - Preoperative embolization of larger lesions
  - Bilateral excision can cause baroreflex failure syndrome, unopposed sympathetic outflow

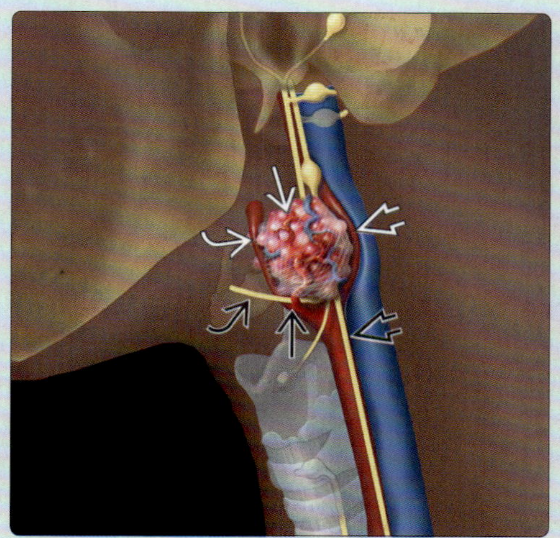

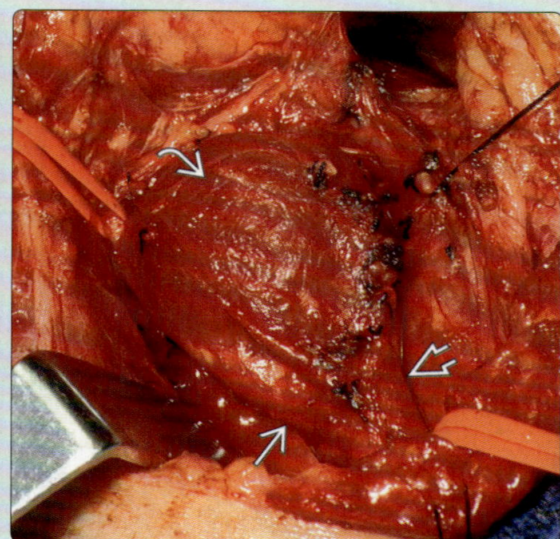

(Left) *Lateral graphic depicts a carotid body paraganglioma at the carotid bifurcation, splaying the internal carotid artery (ICA) and external carotid artery (ECA). The main arterial feeder is the ascending pharyngeal artery. The vagus and hypoglossal nerves are in close proximity.* **(Right)** *Intraoperative photograph shows splaying of the ICAs and ECAs as well as a large, richly vascularized carotid body paraganglioma set in the crotch of the carotid artery bifurcation.*

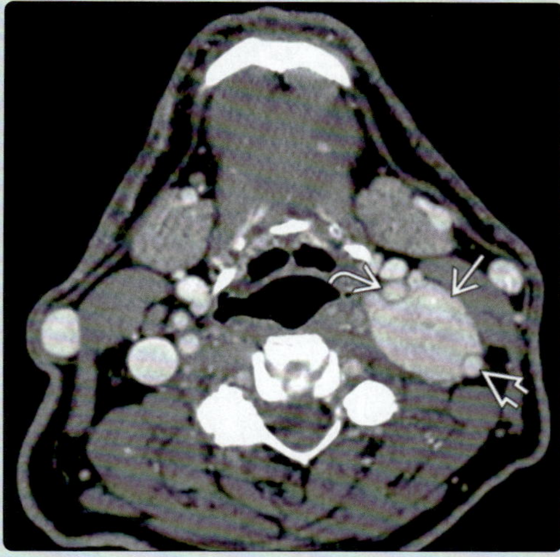

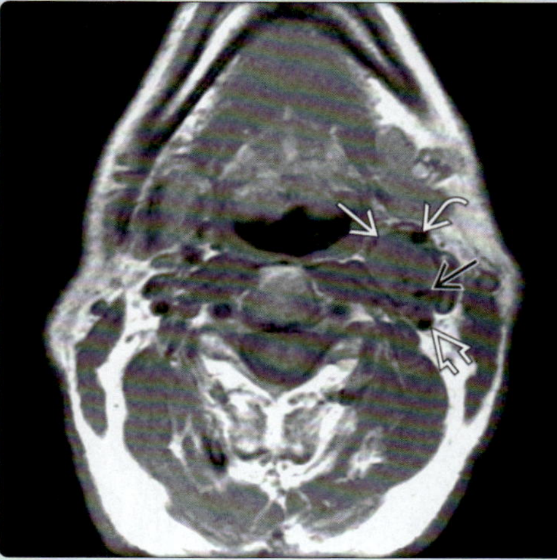

(Left) *Axial CECT shows a classic carotid body paraganglioma with avid, fairly uniform enhancement. Notice the clear definition of the tumor sitting in the notch between the ICA and ECA.* **(Right)** *Axial T1WI MR shows a rounded mass in the left carotid space located between 2 flow voids representing the ICA and ECA. Small internal foci of signal void ("pepper") represent the vascular flow of feeding vessels.*

KEY FACTS

TERMINOLOGY

- Glomus vagale paraganglioma (GVP)

IMAGING

- CT & MR (cross-sectional imaging) general imaging findings
  - Avidly enhancing GVP in nasopharyngeal carotid space centered ~ 2 cm below jugular foramen
    - Displaces carotid anteromedially
    - Displaces jugular vein posterolaterally
    - Displaces parapharyngeal fat anterolaterally
- MR only findings
  - Serpentine or punctate flow voids ("**pepper**")
  - Hyperintense on T2WI and STIR
- MR and CT appearances are diagnostic; modalities are complementary
  - CT useful to determine presence and extent of bone erosion at skull base
- When GVP is suspected, look for multiple lesions
- Imaging surveillance with MR in familial disease

TOP DIFFERENTIAL DIAGNOSES

- Carotid body paraganglioma
- Carotid space schwannoma
- Carotid space neurofibroma

PATHOLOGY

- Arises from glomus bodies in CNX nodose ganglion
- Multiple gene mutations (familial and sporadic)
  - Paraganglioma, multiple endocrine neoplasia type 2, & von Hippel Lindau syndromes

CLINICAL ISSUES

- Clinical presentation
  - Painless, pulsatile lateral cervical mass
  - Vagal neuropathy most common
  - CNIX, CNXI, & CNXII neuropathies (larger tumors)
- Treatment options
  - Surgery vs. observation (poor surgical candidates)
  - Stereotactic radiation effective to prevent growth

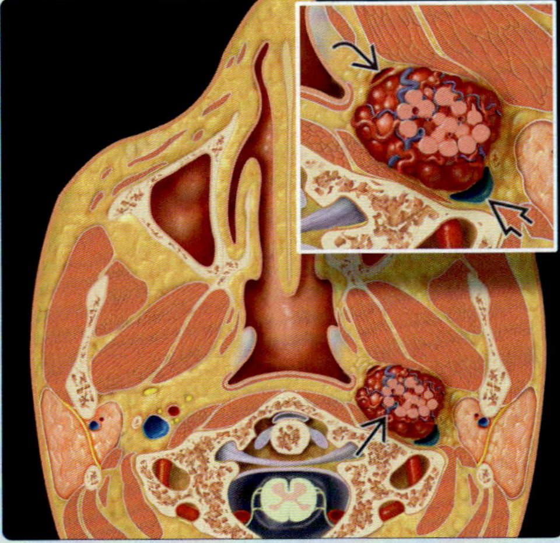

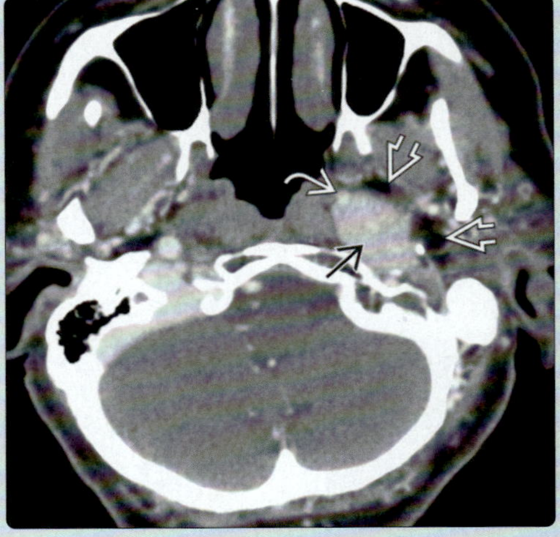

(Left) *Axial graphic depicts a glomus vagale paraganglioma ➡ located in the nasopharyngeal carotid space. The mass is interposed between and displacing the internal carotid artery (ICA) ➡ and jugular vein ➡ (inset).* **(Right)** *Axial CECT shows a large, ovoid, diffusely enhancing mass adjacent to the skull base ➡, centered high in the left carotid space medial to styloid process. Note displacement of the ICA ➡ anteromedially and parapharyngeal fat ➡ anterolaterally.*

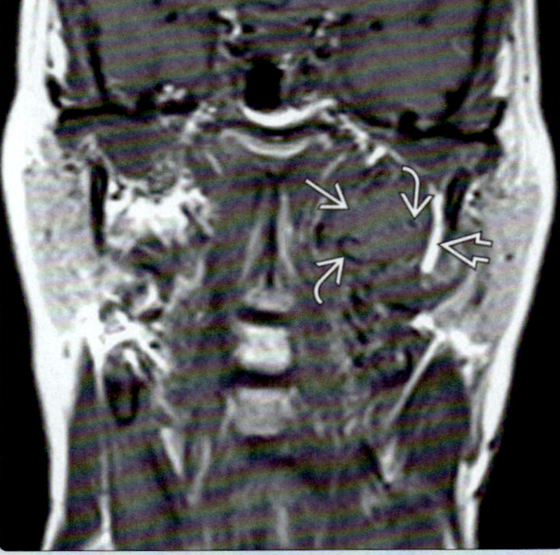

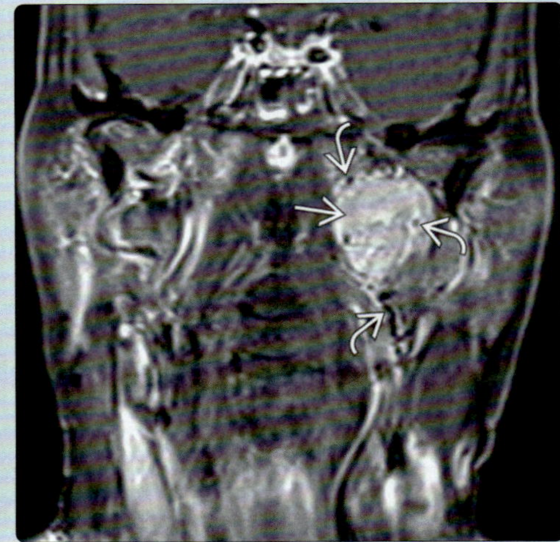

(Left) *Coronal T1 MR shows a solid, isointense mass high in the left carotid space ➡. Small internal punctate and serpentine flow voids ➡ indicate the vascular nature of this lesion. Note the lateral displacement of the parapharyngeal fat ➡ adjacent to the carotid space.* **(Right)** *Coronal T1 C+ FS MR in the same patient shows intense, homogeneous enhancement of the mass ➡, except for prominent vascular structures seen as focal flow voids ➡, despite the presence of intravascular contrast.*

Carotid Space Schwannoma

KEY FACTS

TERMINOLOGY

- **Benign tumor** of **Schwann cells** that wrap around cranial nerves in **carotid space** (CS)
- Nerve of origin: **CNIX-XII** possible; CNX (vagus nerve) most common

IMAGING

- Fusiform, enhancing CS mass
  - Larger schwannoma: Intramural cystic change
  - **MR: No high-velocity flow voids** characteristic
- Displacement pattern is characteristic
  - Nasopharyngeal CS schwannoma: Displaces PPS anteriorly & styloid process anterolaterally
  - Oropharyngeal CS schwannoma: Displaces PPS fat anteriorly & posterior belly of digastric laterally
  - Infrahyoid neck CS schwannoma: Displaces to contralateral neck, common carotid artery anteromedially, & posterior cervical space posterolaterally

TOP DIFFERENTIAL DIAGNOSES

- Carotid body paraganglioma
- Gomus vagale paraganglioma
- CS neurofibroma
- Vascular lesions (pseudoaneurysm or thrombosis)

PATHOLOGY

- Vagal schwannoma more common than other CN origins
- Antoni A & B cells characteristic on histology

CLINICAL ISSUES

- Typical presentation
  - Asymptomatic palpable mass
  - Symptoms often based on nerve of origin
  - Dysphagia, IJV occlusion, Horner syndrome, vocal cord paralysis may be seen
- Age range: 20-60 years (average: 45)
- **Suprahyoid** CS schwannoma > > infrahyoid
- Treatment: Surgery vs. SRT vs. observation

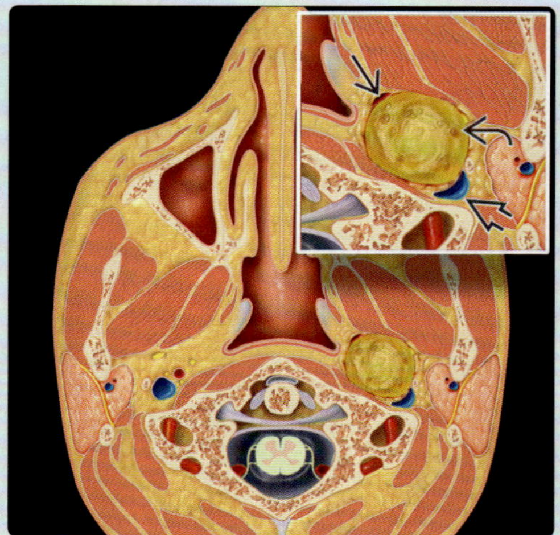

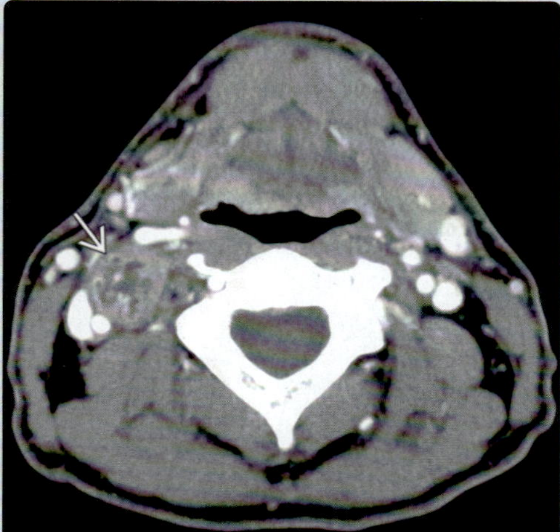

(Left) *Axial graphic depicts a nasopharyngeal carotid space (CS) schwannoma. The tumor is seen between the anteromedial internal carotid artery ⇒ and the posterolateral internal jugular vein ⇒. CS schwannomas are typically fusiform, enhancing masses and may contain cystic, nonenhancing areas ⇒.* **(Right)** *Axial CECT shows a right suprahyoid CS schwannoma ➡. Notice the mild enhancement and central intramural cystic change, both typical features of schwannoma of extracranial H&N.*

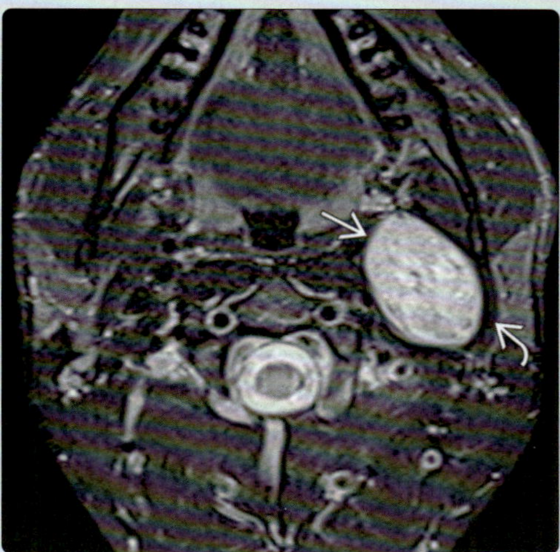

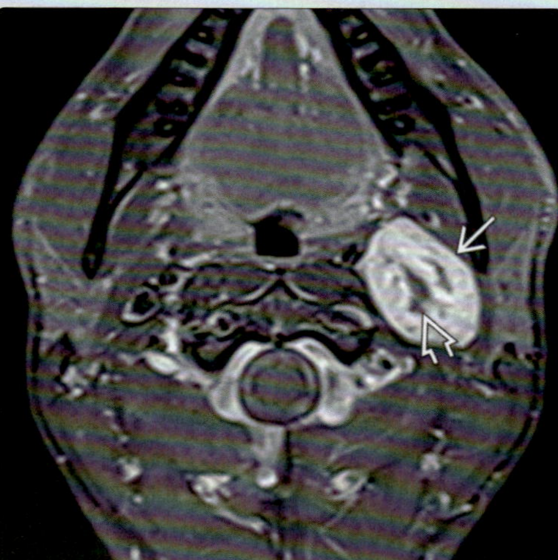

(Left) *Axial T2 FS MR shows a circumscribed, hyperintense CS mass ➡ with lateral displacement of the posterior belly of the digastric muscle ➡. The lack of flow voids help differentiate this schwannoma from a paraganglioma.* **(Right)** *Axial T1 C+ FS MR in the same patient reveals enhancement of the CS mass ➡ with regions of cystic change ➡ typical of a large schwannoma. CS schwannomas may arise from CNIX-XII or the cervical sympathetic chain, but most commonly arise from the vagus nerve (CNX).*

Sympathetic Schwannoma

KEY FACTS

TERMINOLOGY

- Sympathetic schwannoma: Benign, slow-growing tumor of Schwann cells investing cervical sympathetic chain

IMAGING

- Most common appearance
  - Fusiform enhancing carotid space (CS) mass that displaces both carotid artery & jugular vein anteriorly
- Tumor location
  - **Posterior** or posteromedial to CS vessels (sympathetic chain lies posterior or posteromedial in CS)
- CECT or enhanced MR findings
  - **Ovoid to fusiform** enhancing mass in posterior CS
  - Small lesion: Homogeneous enhancement
  - Large lesion: Intratumoral (intramural) nonenhancing **cysts** may be seen
- CECT often 1st exam for neck mass

TOP DIFFERENTIAL DIAGNOSES

- Carotid space schwannoma or neurofibroma
- Glomus vagale or carotid body paraganglioma
- Nodal SCCa in retropharyngeal space

PATHOLOGY

- Solitary, well-encapsulated tumor arising from peripheral nerve
- Arises from cervical sympathetic chain Schwann cell sheath
- Associated with neurofibromatosis type 2 (multiple schwannomas, meningiomas, & ependymomas)

CLINICAL ISSUES

- Presentation: Asymptomatic, palpable neck mass
  - **Horner syndrome** (miosis, ptosis, anhidrosis), headache
- Treatment options
  - Surgical excision is curative
    - Postoperative Horner syndrome is common

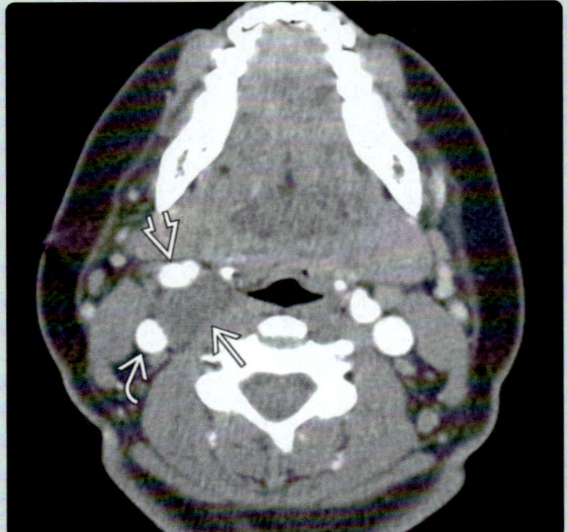

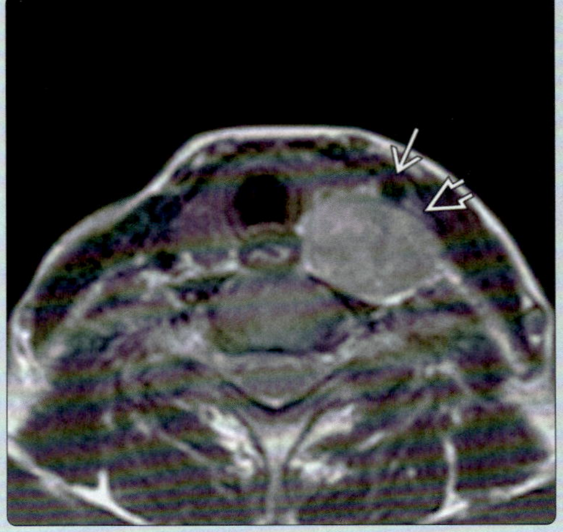

(Left) *Axial CECT shows an ovoid mass ➡ posteromedial within the carotid space (CS). Note the bifurcating carotid artery on the anterior surface ➡ with the jugular vein (JV) along the lateral surface of the mass ➡. Minimal enhancement is atypical of schwannoma.* **(Right)** *Axial T2WI MR reveals a heterogeneous, intermediate-signal, ovoid sympathetic schwannoma displacing the common carotid artery ➡ anteriorly. The internal JV is displaced with carotid artery ➡. Compression of JV may make it difficult to identify.*

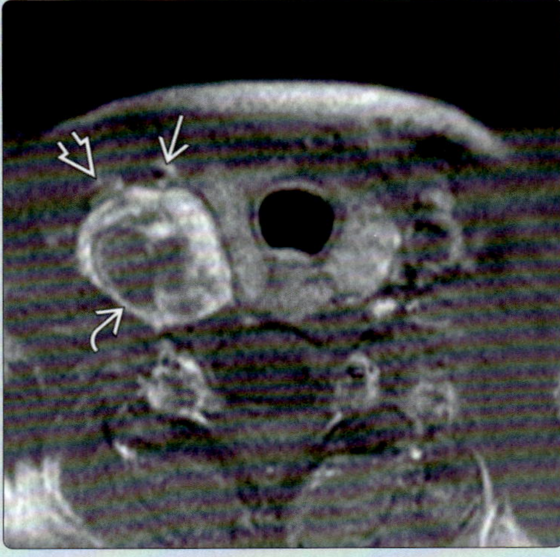

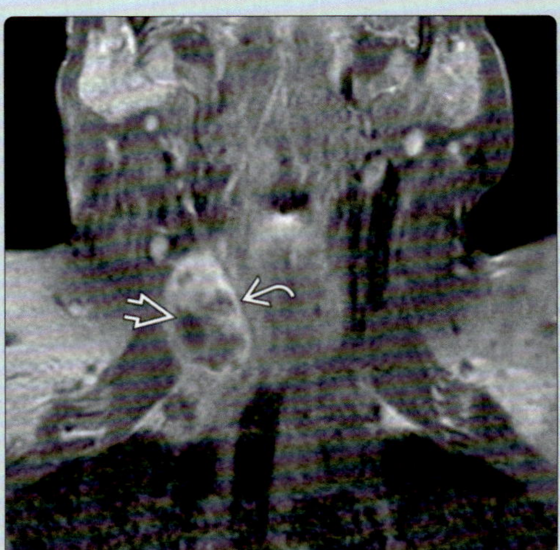

(Left) *Axial T1WI C+ FS MR reveals an ovoid mass in posterior infrahyoid CS ➡. The sympathetic schwannoma displaces both the internal JV ➡ and common carotid artery ➡ anteriorly. The simultaneous displacement of both CS vessels suggests the diagnosis of sympathetic schwannoma.* **(Right)** *Coronal T1WI C+ FS MR demonstrates a sympathetic schwannoma in the CS. The tumor is a heterogeneously enhancing mass ➡ posterior to the CS. Intramural cystic change ➡ is common in large schwannomas.*

KEY FACTS

TERMINOLOGY

- Benign nerve sheath tumor in carotid space, arising from vagus nerve, sympathetic chain, or hypoglossal nerve

IMAGING

- General features
  - Fusiform carotid space mass with patchy enhancement
  - Interposed between carotid artery and jugular vein
    - Displaces carotid anteromedially
    - Displaces jugular posterolaterally
  - Infrahyoid lesions typically posterior to vessels
    - Displaces carotid and jugular anterolaterally
- CT findings
  - Hypodense and poorly enhancing on CT
- MR findings
  - Hyperintense with target sign on STIR or T2WI MR
  - Homogeneous or patchy mild enhancement on MR

TOP DIFFERENTIAL DIAGNOSES

- Glomus vagale paraganglioma
- Carotid body paraganglioma
- Carotid space schwannoma

PATHOLOGY

- Benign spindle cell neoplasm; WHO grade 1 tumors

CLINICAL ISSUES

- Clinical presentation
  - Asymptomatic solitary or multiple neck masses
  - Lower cranial nerve palsies when large
  - Solitary neurofibroma (NF): Isolated soft tissue neck mass
  - Plexiform NF: Multinodular bag of worms appearance
  - 50% associated with neurofibromatosis type 1, 50% solitary
- Treatment options
  - Surgical removal of symptomatic isolated lesions
  - Excision much more difficult for plexiform lesions

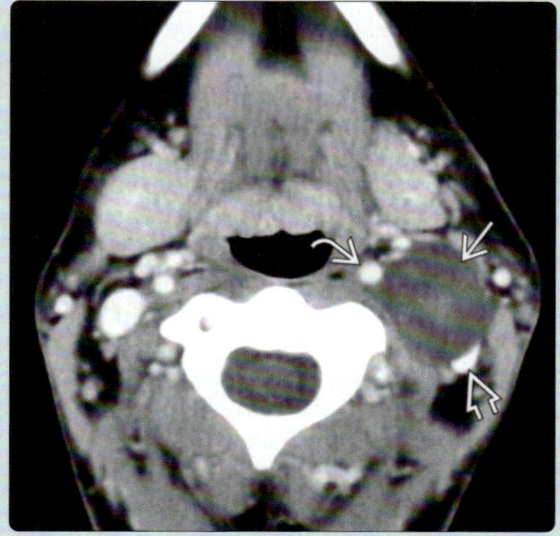

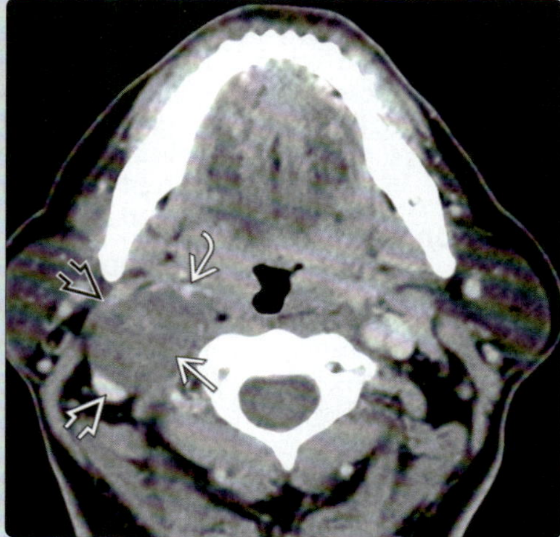

(Left) *Axial CECT demonstrates a low-density mass with faint internal enhancement ➡ located in the left carotid space. The internal carotid artery (ICA) ➡ is displaced anteromedially, while the internal jugular vein (IJV) ➡ is displaced posterolaterally.* **(Right)** *Axial CECT shows a carotid space neurofibroma ➡ with density similar to the cervical spinal cord and minimal enhancement. Note the ICA pushed anteromedially ➡, the IJV posterolaterally ➡, and the posterior belly digastric muscle laterally ➡.*

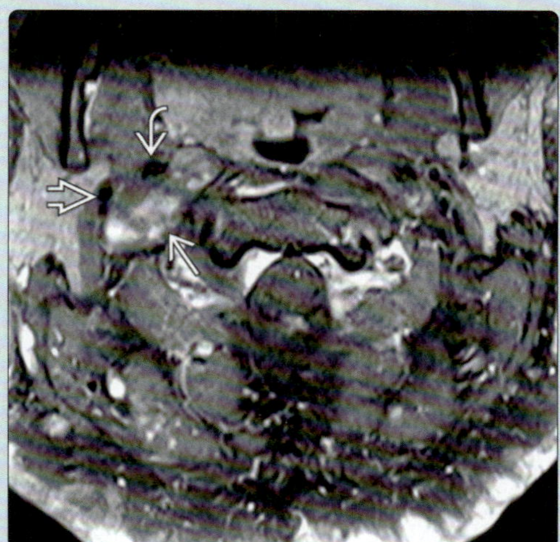

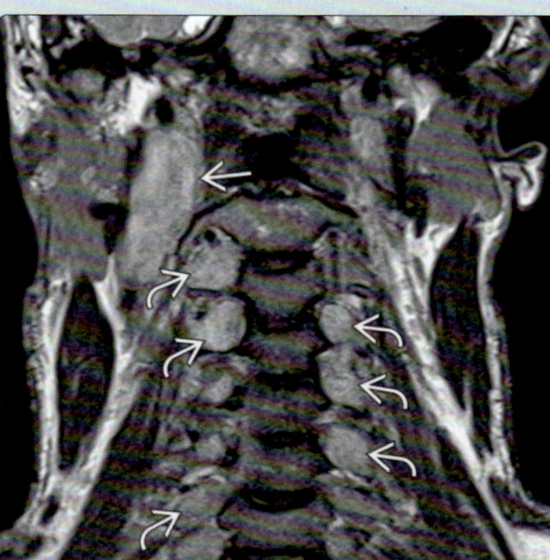

(Left) *Axial T1 C+ FS MR in a patient with neurofibromatosis type 1 (NF1) demonstrates an ovoid carotid space mass ➡ with patchy enhancement. The lesion displaces the ICA anteriorly ➡ and flattens and displaces the jugular vein anterolaterally ➡.* **(Right)** *Coronal T2 MR in the same patient demonstrates the typical elongated, oval contour and heterogeneous T2 hyperintensity of a vagal neurofibroma ➡. Stigmata of NF1 with multiple cervical nerve sheath tumors are evident ➡.*

Summary Thoughts: Retropharyngeal Space

The retropharyngeal space (RPS) spans the length of the neck from the skull base to the mediastinum. As its name indicates, it lies posterior to the pharynx. More inferiorly in the neck it lies posterior to the esophagus. It is located anterior to the cervical and upper thoracic spine and the prevertebral muscles. Anatomically, an additional fascia divides the RPS into 2 components: (1) an anterior true RPS and (2) a posterior danger space (DS). With imaging, it is rare to be able to delineate a lesion as residing in only 1 of these 2 spaces, so for most purposes the 2 are considered as 1 RPS.

The RPS contains only **medial** and **lateral** RPS **lymph nodes** and **fat**. This results in a very short differential diagnosis for pathology in this space, primarily a tumor or infection affecting the nodes. While this makes diagnosing easier, the RPS is actually an imaging and clinical "blind spot," with RPS nodes being inaccessible to direct observation or physical examination. Additionally, nonnecrotic nodes often appear isodense to prevertebral muscles on CECT and frequently lie far lateral in the RPS and medial to the internal carotid arteries. Therefore, it is critical that the clinician methodically searches the RPS for adenopathy on imaging, particularly in patients with head and neck (H&N) malignancies.

After nodal disease from tumor and infection, the next most common pathology is a frequently seen but poorly understood process known as **retropharyngeal edema**. While this process does not require treatment, it is a clue to other pathology in the H&N. Most importantly, it may pose a diagnostic challenge, as it mimics the appearance of retropharyngeal abscess, which often requires surgical intervention.

Imaging Approaches and Indications

The presence of fat in the RPS makes this space readily identifiable on CT (due to its low density) and MR (due to its intrinsic T1 and T2 hyperintensity). As CECT is the imaging technique of choice for evaluation of H&N infections, it is often the initial modality for detection of RPS pathology. Imaging of any RPS process must cover from the skull base to the mediastinum because of the potential for craniocaudal and mediastinal spread of disease. Intravenous contrast is important to determine enhancement characteristics of an RPS collection that suggests an abscess and for evaluation of nodal disease and nodal necrosis. It is also important for the evaluation of other neck structures, which may be responsible for RPS infection or edema. Review of the cervical spine for discitis-osteomyelitis as a potential infectious source is important during analysis of the neck CT or MR images.

MR allows excellent delineation of RPS contours but is less often used in evaluation of infection, except for discitis-osteomyelitis. MR is more sensitive than CT for detecting **retropharyngeal adenopathy**, which is important for the staging of many H&N tumors (particularly nasopharyngeal carcinoma).

Imaging Anatomy

The anterior margin of the RPS is delineated by the posterior pharyngeal wall and inferiorly by the posterior aspect of the esophagus. These structures are enveloped by a **middle layer of deep cervical fascia** (ML-DCF), also known as the buccopharyngeal and visceral fascia. The posterior margin of the RPS is defined by the **deep layer of deep cervical fascia** (DL-DCF), also called the prevertebral fascia.

Superiorly, the ML-DCF and DL-DCF insert on the central skull base, forming the superior boundary of the RPS. Inferiorly, the posterior fascial margin of the RPS (DL-DCF) blends with the anterior longitudinal ligament of the upper thoracic spine.

A 2nd component of the deep layer of deep cervical fascia, the **alar fascia**, separates the anterior **retropharyngeal space** from the posterior **danger space**. At approximately the T3 level, the alar fascia merges with the DL-DCF on the posterior aspect of the esophagus to form the inferior boundary of the true RPS. The danger space extends more inferiorly in the posterior mediastinum and typically reaches the diaphragm. It is not usually possible on imaging to delineate the RPS from the DS, so for all imaging purposes the RPS and DS are considered as 1 space. It is important, however, to remember the potential for posterior mediastinal extension of an RPS abscess.

The lateral margins of the RPS are defined by another piece of the alar fascia (alar for "wing-like"). This fascia separates the RPS contents from the more lateral carotid space and generally is less resistant to the spread of pathology. As a consequence, RPS edema frequently leaks out laterally to involve the carotid spaces. Similarly, RPS and DS often appear to communicate inferiorly despite the presence of the separating alar fascia.

Pseudolesions of the RPS include medial deviation of the carotid arteries and thyroid gland enlargement due to goiter. Both the carotid arteries and thyroid tissue may present in a near midline location in the RPS, which likely occurs from laxity or disruption of this lateral alar fascia. Medial deviation of the carotid arteries is important to report since iatrogenic injury can occur during transoral robotic surgery if this anatomic variant is not recognized.

Approaches to Imaging Issues of the Retropharyngeal Space

The answer to the question, "What imaging findings define an **RPS mass**?" varies slightly depending on the level in the neck. Throughout most of the neck, and particularly the infrahyoid neck, an RPS mass is clearly evident as a lesion posterior to the pharynx ± esophagus and anterior to the prevertebral muscles and spine. The pharynx and the esophagus may be deviated anteriorly, and there may by flattening of prevertebral muscles against the spine. These findings help to clarify an RPS location.

In the suprahyoid neck, and particularly just below the skull base, the RPS contains little fat and frequently appears to be more of a **potential space** with the prevertebral muscles and the pharynx closely opposed. Retropharyngeal nodes are located in the far lateral aspect of the RPS, immediately medial to the internal carotid arteries (ICAs). With a very thin RPS and prominent bellies of the prevertebral muscles, these RPS nodes appear to lie **lateral** to the prevertebral muscles. This is most evident in children, in whom large nonnecrotic RPS nodes, in association with prominent adenoidal tissue, are normal findings.

Nasopharyngeal or oropharyngeal infection, such as tonsillitis or pharyngitis, will result in reactive enlargement of these already prominent nodes in children. The presence of nonenhancing foci within RPS nodes in a child with infectious symptoms indicates **suppuration**. This is sometimes described as an intranodal abscess but does not typically require surgical intervention.

Differential Diagnosis of Retropharyngeal Space

Pseudolesion	Congenital	Inflammatory	Infectious	Vascular	Treatment Related	Benign Tumor	Malignant Tumor
Tortuous carotid artery	Venous malformation	Reactive or inflammatory RPS node (suprahyoid neck)	Cellulitis/ phlegmon from adjacent infection	Edema associated with IJV thrombosis	Edema from radiation	Lipoma	Direct invasion by SCCa
Thyroid enlargement (goiter or malignancy)	Lymphatic malformation	RPS edema from longus colli tendonitis	RPS abscess from adjacent infection	Edema from Kawasaki disease	Edema from neck dissection	Schwannoma	RPS nodal spread of systemic metastasis or NHL
	Ectopic parathyroid adenoma (infrahyoid)		Suppurative adenopathy (suprahyoid neck)		Edema, seroma or CSF leak from spine surgery	Neurofibroma	Primary or invasive sarcoma

IJV = internal jugular vein; NHL = non-Hodgkin lymphoma; RPS = retropharyngeal space; SCCa = squamous cell carcinoma.

In adults, normal RPS nodes are less frequently found and when seen are typically ≤ 5 mm. **Reactive enlargement** of RPS nodes may be found in adults with pharyngeal infection, although reactive nodal enlargement to 1 cm is unusual. RPS reactive adenopathy is distinctly less common in adults, which in part reflects the decreased frequency of pharyngeal infections in adults compared to children.

Enlarged RPS nodes in an adult > 8 mm are concerning for the possibility of **metastatic disease**. This is a 1st-order lymphatic drainage site for nasopharyngeal carcinoma, where unilateral or bilateral RPS metastases are designated as N1 disease. Other H&N tumors also drain to RPS nodes, either primarily or secondarily. Oropharyngeal squamous cell carcinoma (SCCa), sinonasal malignancies, middle ear malignancies, and thyroid carcinoma drain directly to RPS nodes. Other malignancies, such as posterior wall hypopharyngeal SCCa, invade the RPS and then drain through the lymphatic system to the RPS nodes. Non-Hodgkin lymphoma in the H&N frequently involves RPS nodes and may become particularly large without necrosis. Since RPS nodes are usually not detectable on clinical examination, it is important for clinicians to pay particular attention to this area. One effective method is carefully searching along the medial aspect of the suprahyoid ICA.

The differential diagnosis for a **well-defined, ovoid mass** in the suprahyoid RPS includes medial **carotid space (CS)** lesions that mimic RPS nodes by their location medial to the ICA. **Sympathetic chain schwannoma** typically lies medial to the ICA, and vagal paragangliomas may be posteromedial to the ICA. The absence of other adenopathy in the neck, or the clear demonstration of location in the CS, favors 1 of these 2 entities.

If an RPS abnormality is **diffuse** rather than a focal mass, the diagnostic approach is quite different and can be defined as collections or masses. **Collections** have fluid density (CT) or intensity (MR) and tend to enlarge the entire RPS into either a "bow-tie" or rectangular contour. Whenever a fluid-distended RPS is found, the 1st consideration is to exclude an **RPS abscess**, which is typically rim-enhancing rectangular distension of the RPS. More frequently evident in neck studies, however, is **RPS edema**, which is nonenhancing and tends to result in less marked RPS enlargement, with a lower volume rectangular contour. Once this diagnosis is suspected, the neck must be searched for an infectious source (typically of pharyngeal origin in children and spinal origin in adults), a vascular source (internal jugular vein thrombosis), inflammation (longus colli tendonitis), or evidence of recent treatment (spine or neck surgery, radiation).

Diffuse masses of the RPS may be lipomatous lesions, such as lipoma or liposarcoma, with fat density/signal on CT or MR imaging, other rare sarcomas, or congenital lesions, such as venous or lymphatic malformations, which share imaging characteristics with such lesions elsewhere in the H&N. These lesions are typically transspatial (in multiple contiguous spaces) involving adjacent H&N spaces, as are plexiform neurofibromas, which are characteristic of NF1.

Clinical Implications

Small lesions of the RPS are typically **not** evident on clinical examination. It is only when lesions become significantly enlarged that bulging of a posterior pharyngeal wall is seen. It cannot be emphasized enough that the clinician must consider the possibility of RPS metastatic nodal disease in **all H&N cancer patients** and must methodically search along the medial aspect of the cervical ICA. Nonnecrotic RPS nodes are more difficult to discern on CECT than MR, so vigilance is key.

Toxic patients with H&N infections, such as pharyngitis or tonsillitis, may be imaged to exclude the development of RPS abscess. This is a difficult clinical diagnosis because physical examination may not be fruitful. Thus, clinicians must rely largely on a high degree of clinical suspicion. The clinician must exclude RPS abscess, or, if one is found, must delineate the entire craniocaudal extent and specifically exclude mediastinal involvement. Large RPS abscesses may result in airway compromise, though it is rare that a patient presents with airway symptoms secondary to an RPS mass.

Selected References

1. Hoang JK et al: Multiplanar CT and MRI of collections in the retropharyngeal space: is it an abscess? AJR Am J Roentgenol. 196(4):W426-32, 2011
2. Chong VF et al: Radiology of the retropharyngeal space. Clin Radiol. 55(10):740-8, 2000
3. Davis WL et al: Retropharyngeal space: evaluation of normal anatomy and diseases with CT and MR imaging. Radiology. 174(1):59-64, 1990

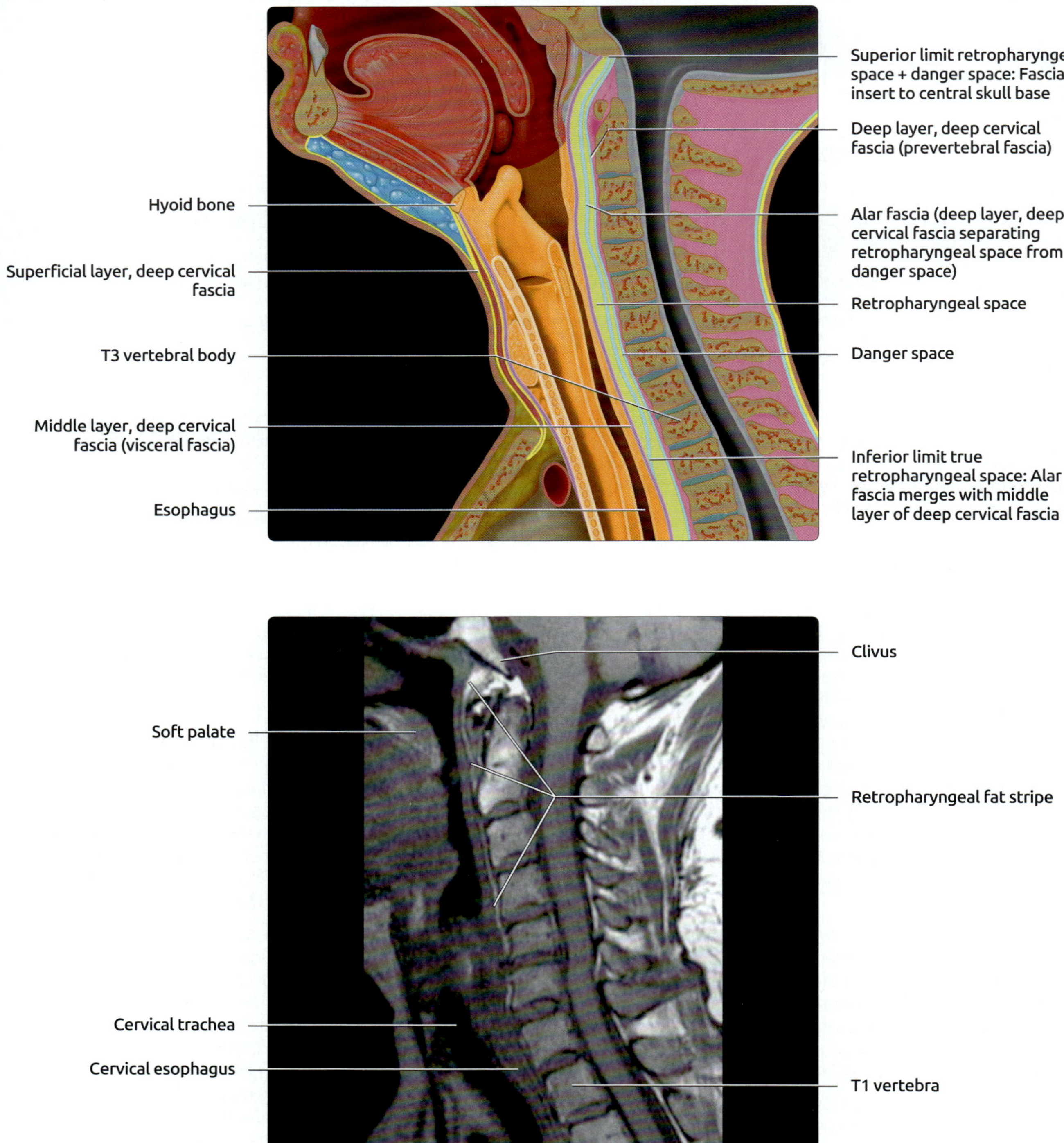

(Top) *Sagittal graphic shows the deep cervical fascia (DCF) layers, which determine and delineate the contours of the retropharyngeal space (RPS). The anterior contour of the RPS is defined by the middle layer, DCF (visceral fascia), which separates the RPS from the pharyngeal mucosal space of the suprahyoid neck and visceral space of the infrahyoid neck. The posterior contour is formed by the deep layer, DCF (prevertebral fascia). The alar fascia (also deep layer, DCF) anatomically defines an anterior true RPS and more posterior danger space, although this delineation is not typically evident at imaging. Inferiorly, the alar fascia blends with the middle layer, DCF at ~ T3, while superiorly the middle and deep layers of the DCF insert to the central skull base.* **(Bottom)** *Sagittal T1 MR shows thin, hyperintense signal corresponding to normal fat within the RPS. Contents include this thin fat stripe and the retropharyngeal lymph nodes in the lateral suprahyoid neck. It can be considered a potential space that is most visible when distended by disease.*

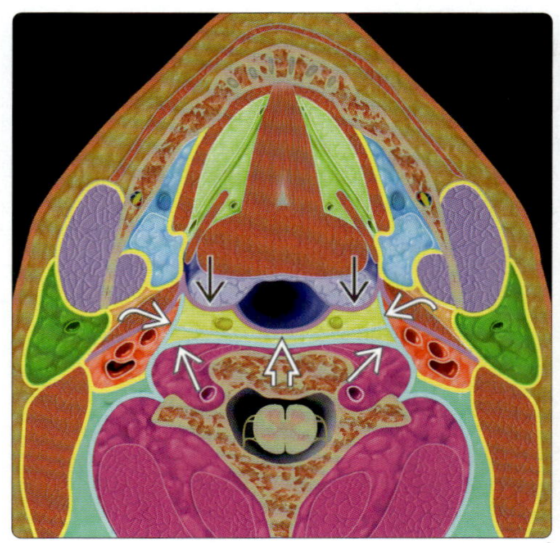

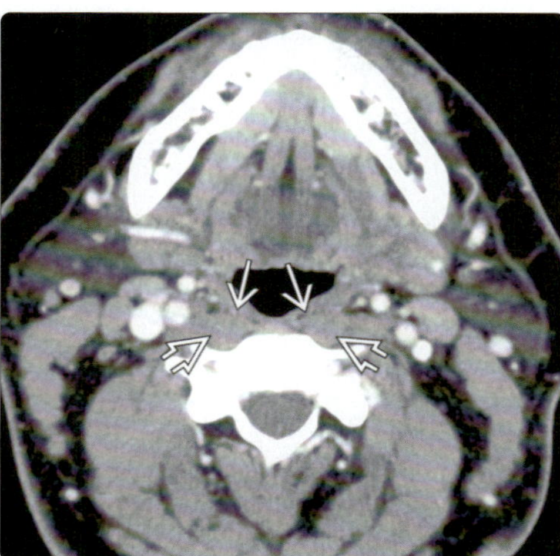

(Left) *Axial graphic at the level of oropharynx illustrates a predominantly fat-filled RPS. The anterior contour is delineated by middle layer of DCF and the posterior contour by deep layer DCF (prevertebral fascia) . Alar (wing-like) fascia forms the lateral margins and divides the RPS into anterior true RPS and posterior danger space.* **(Right)** *Axial CECT shows the typical appearance of RPS in a suprahyoid neck as a thin, low-density fat stripe anterior to prevertebral muscles .*

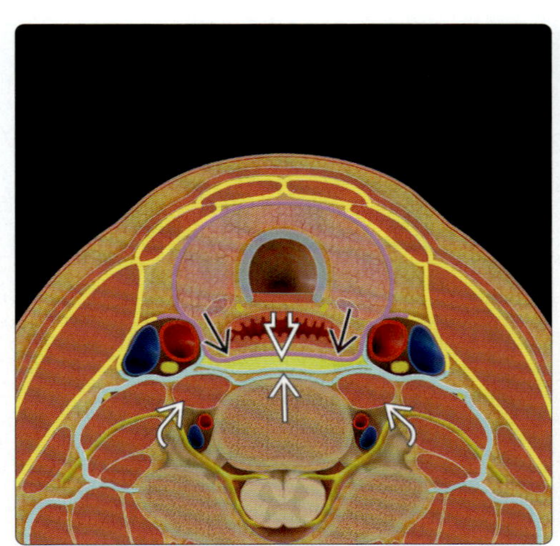

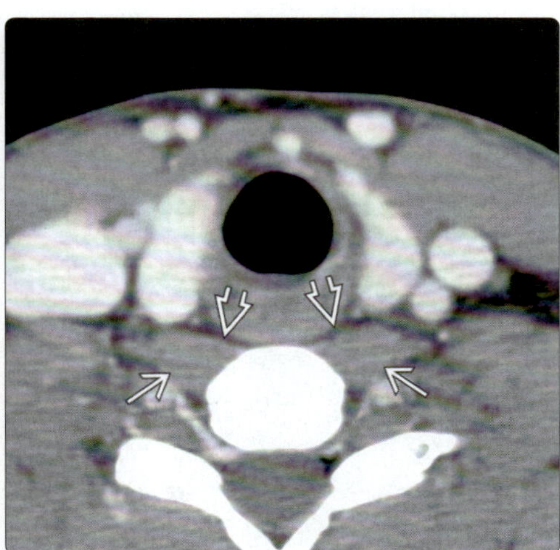

(Left) *Axial graphic at level of thyroid gland shows infrahyoid continuation of fat-filled RPS, again delineated anteriorly by the middle layer, DCF (visceral fascia) . Posterior danger space separates true RPS from prevertebral muscles and cervical vertebrae.* **(Right)** *Axial CECT shows RPS as a thin, low-density fat stripe anterior to perivertebral space and posterior to hypopharynx-esophagus junction . The prevertebral muscles are flattened posteriorly by RPS lesions, while the hypopharynx and esophagus are pushed anteriorly.*

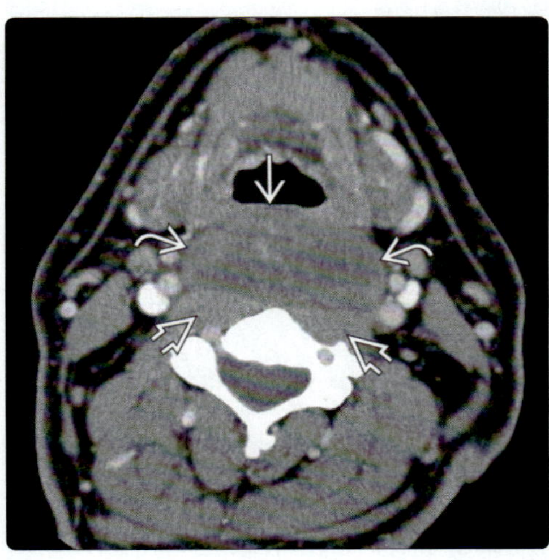

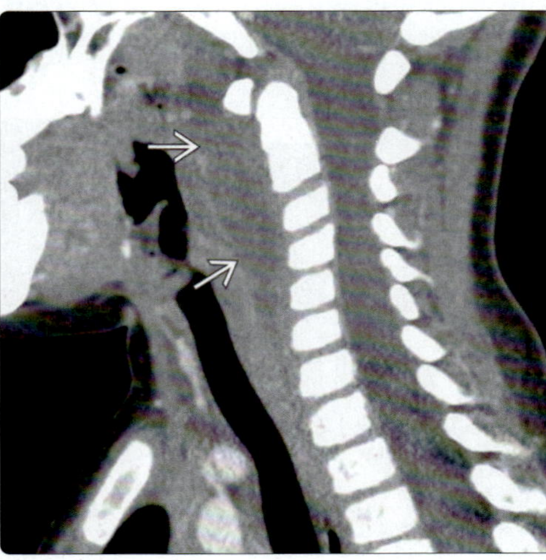

(Left) *Axial CECT shows a rare primary sarcoma of the RPS . Notice the comparatively lower density relative to the pharynx anteriorly and prevertebral muscles posteriorly that helps correctly localize this mass.* **(Right)** *Midline sagittal CECT MPR demonstrates an RPS abscess in a child. Infected & noninfected fluid collections are the most common source of RPS lesions. Infections are most often due to suppurative nodal disease in children and spread of spinal infection in adults.*

Reactive Adenopathy of Retropharyngeal Space

KEY FACTS

TERMINOLOGY

- Benign enlargement of nodes in response to antigen
- Lateral retropharyngeal space (RPS) nodes known as "nodes of Rouvière"

IMAGING

- General findings
  - RPS nodes found from skull base to hyoid bone
  - May be difficult to detect on CECT
    - CECT aids in detection of RPS nodes & intranodal suppurative change
  - Often elongate in craniocaudal direction
    - May appear round on axial CT
    - Oval on coronal or sagittal CT images
  - If large or associated with inflammatory change, may deform pharyngeal contour, narrowing airway
- CECT findings
  - Oval to round solid mildly enhancing mass medial to internal carotid artery
  - When enlarges, pushes anteriorly into medial parapharyngeal space
  - Pharyngeal tonsils enlarged (tonsillitis)

TOP DIFFERENTIAL DIAGNOSES

- Suppurative RPS node
- Squamous cell carcinoma (SCCa) RPS nodal metastasis
- Non-SCCa RPS nodal metastasis

PATHOLOGY

- Most often in response to infectious agent
- Reactive RPS nodes common in children because of oral exposure to antigens

CLINICAL ISSUES

- Clinical presentation
  - Sick child or young adult with pharyngitis
- Treatment: Treat pharyngitis as needed
- Caveat: RPS node(s) in patient > 35 years of age
  - Consider metastatic disease

(Left) *Axial CECT in a child with pharyngitis shows the difficulty in finding isodense retropharyngeal space (RPS) nodes on CT. Subtle mass effect is noted ➔ from the large right RPS node displacing ICA ➔. Low-density linear retropharyngeal edema ➔ delineates medial margin ➔ of reactive node.* **(Right)** *Axial T2 MR in a child shows prominent homogeneous RPS nodes ➔ and adenoid tissue ➔. Retropharyngeal nodes are much more evident on MR than CT; however, this is a normal finding in young children.*

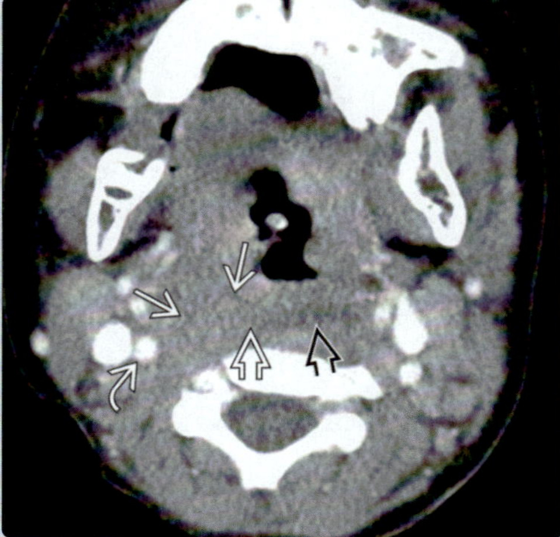

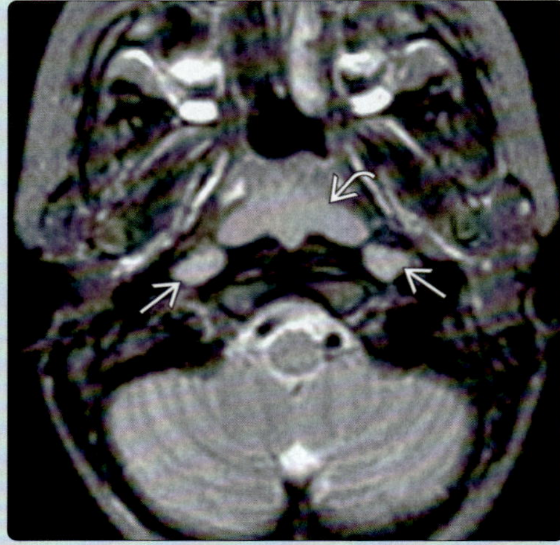

(Left) *Axial CECT in a teenage patient with pharyngitis shows large reactive left retropharyngeal node ➔ medial to the ICA ➔ and lateral to prevertebral muscle. Note bilaterally enlarged palatine tonsils ➔.* **(Right)** *Axial CECT in a young woman with clinical and radiographic evidence of tonsillitis reveals bilateral, mildly enhancing homogeneous nodes ➔ medial to the ICAs ➔. RPS reactive nodes are commonly seen on CT during episodes of tonsillitis.*

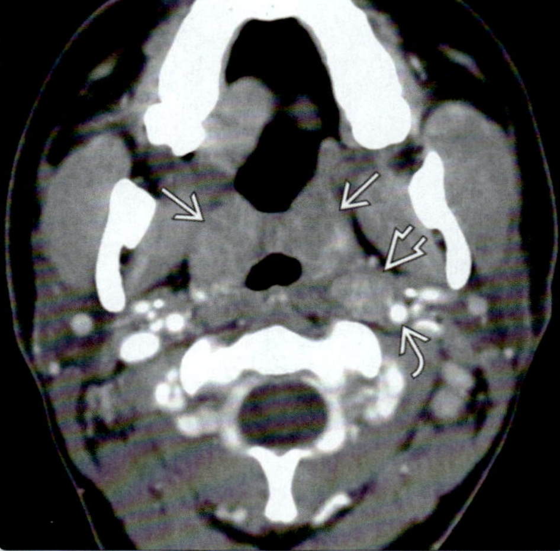

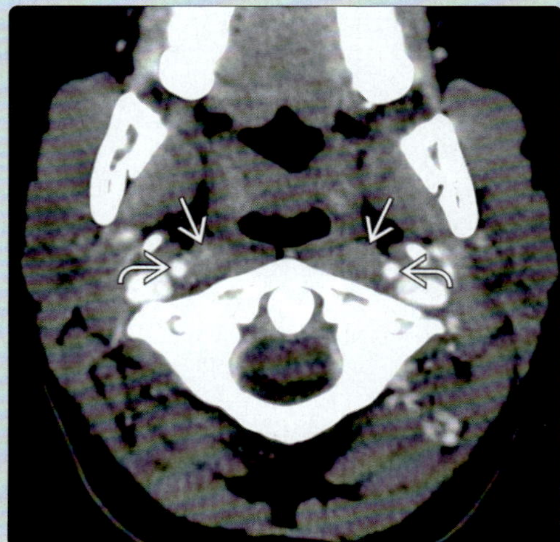

KEY FACTS

TERMINOLOGY

- Suppurative node = intranodal abscess
- Definition: Pus forms in retropharyngeal space (RPS) node draining H&N infection

IMAGING

- CECT is 1st-line tool for evaluation of H&N infection, best demonstrates suppuration
- CECT findings
  - Low density within enlarged RPS node
    - Primary location, medial to internal carotid artery
    - Node enlarges but does not cross midline
  - RPS cellulitis ± internal carotid narrowing (vasospasm more common in kids; usually self-limited)
  - Node may show peripheral enhancement
- MR: Restricted diffusion (high signal) in suppurative node

TOP DIFFERENTIAL DIAGNOSES

- RPS reactive adenopathy
- RPS abscess
- RPS nodal squamous cell carcinoma
- RPS edema

PATHOLOGY

- H&N infection seeds RPS nodes → node reacts → suppurates → ruptures → RPS abscess

CLINICAL ISSUES

- Clinical presentation
  - Child or young adult with sore throat, fever, neck pain
  - RPS suppurative nodes nonpalpable
  - RPS suppurative nodes can rapidly progress to abscess, sepsis, & airway compromise
- Treatment options
  - Oral antibiotics 1st, IV if nonresponsive
  - Surgical drainage if RPS abscess suspected
  - Airway management important; monitor for spread of infection to "danger space," mediastinitis

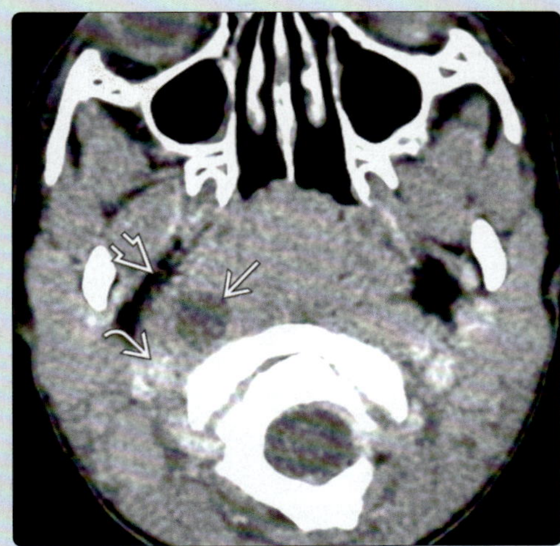

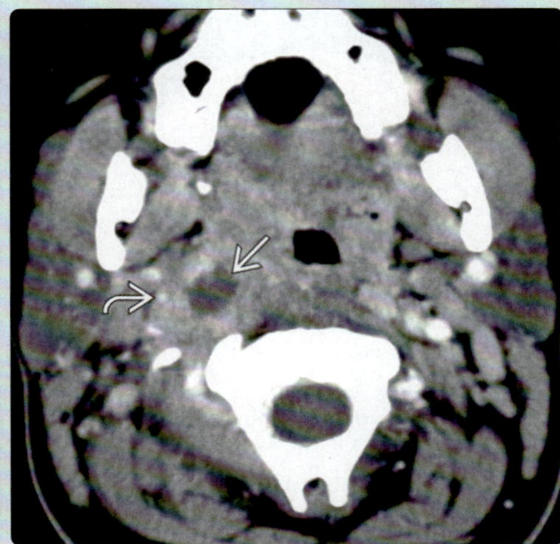

(Left) *Axial CECT in a young child demonstrates a well-defined, low-density lesion ➡ anteromedial to the right internal carotid artery (ICA) ➡. This represents pus within the right retropharyngeal lymph node and is associated with effacement of parapharyngeal fat ➡.* **(Right)** *Axial CECT in a young adult shows central low density within an enlarged lateral retropharyngeal space (RPS) node ➡. Extensive inflammatory change involves the right carotid sheath and is associated with narrowing of distal cervical ICA ➡.*

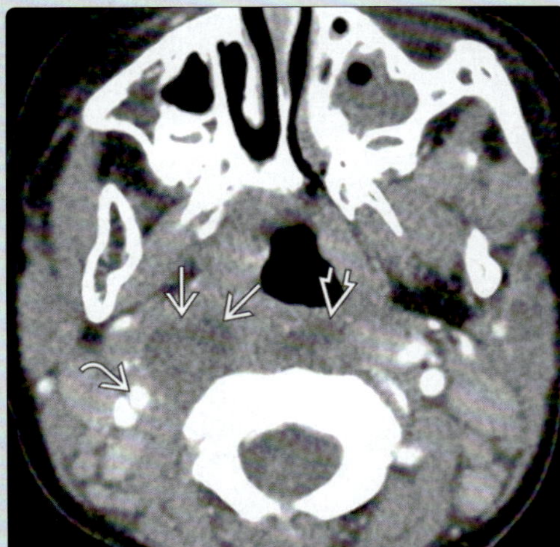

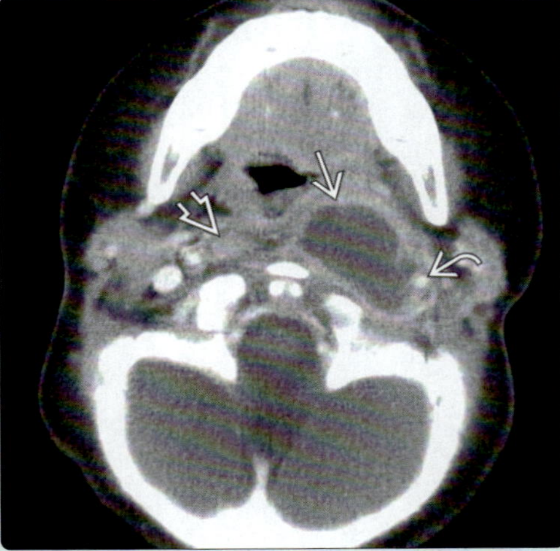

(Left) *Axial CECT reveals lateral displacement of the right ICA ➡ by a heterogeneous rounded mass ➡. The retropharyngeal node is enlarged, and low density indicates early suppurative change. Note RPS edema ➡, which may progress to abscess.* **(Right)** *Axial CECT shows a large suppurative node in the left RPS ➡. Rim-enhancing fluid partly surrounds the left ICA, which is narrowed due to spasm ➡. Although worrisome on imaging, ICA spasm is usually self-limited. Note reactive adenopathy in right RPS ➡.*

Retropharyngeal Space Abscess

KEY FACTS

TERMINOLOGY

- Retropharyngeal space (RPS) abscess definition: Extranodal purulent fluid collection in RPS

IMAGING

- Lateral plain radiograph: Wide prevertebral distance
- CECT findings
  - RPS distended by low-density collection
  - Convex anterior contour
  - **Enhancement of wall** suggests abscess
- CECT must cover skull base to carina to include full extent of RPS abscess; spread to "danger space" possible with mediastinitis
- MR can be helpful to determine extension to spine

TOP DIFFERENTIAL DIAGNOSES

- RPS edema or phlegmon
- RPS suppurative adenopathy
- Hypopharyngeal squamous cell carcinoma

PATHOLOGY

- Rupture of suppurative RPS node → RPS abscess
- Most commonly microorganisms: *Staphylococcus aureus*, *Haemophilus*, *Streptococcus*
- Other less common causes of RPS abscess
  - Ventral spread of discitis and prevertebral infection
  - Pharyngeal penetrating foreign body

CLINICAL ISSUES

- Clinical presentation
  - Septic patient: Fever, chills, elevated WBC and ESR
  - Stridor from narrowing of pharyngeal lumen
  - Most < 10 years old; can cause atlantoaxial subluxation due to inflammation (Grisel syndrome, rare)
  - Increasing incidence in adult population
- Treatment options
  - IV antibiotics, airway management, fluid resuscitation
  - Surgical intervention (incision & drainage) if drainable or complex abscess present

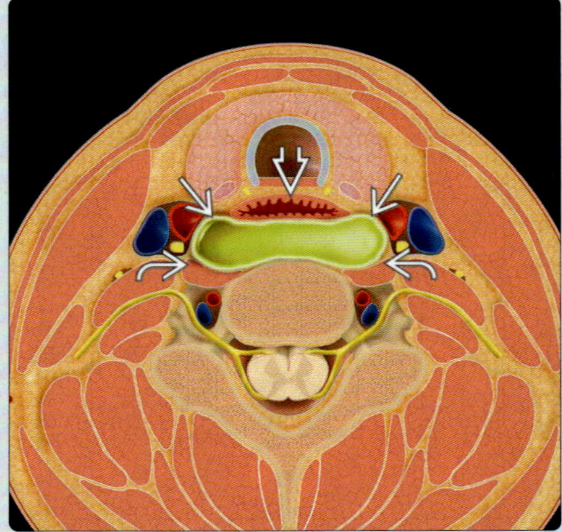

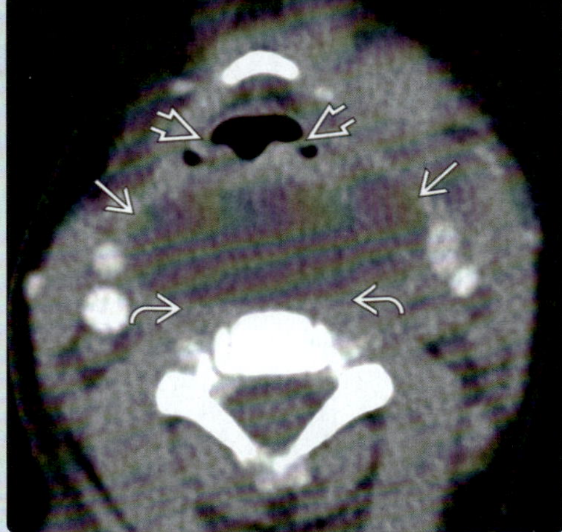

(Left) *Axial graphic illustrates the location and typical contour of a retropharyngeal space (RPS) abscess ➡ displacing the pharynx or cervical esophagus ➡ anteriorly and flattening the prevertebral muscles ➡.* **(Right)** *Axial CECT in a 10 month old with a 5-day history of febrile illness reveals a large, low-density ovoid collection distending the RPS ➡ with anterior displacement of the hypopharynx ➡ and flattening of the prevertebral muscles ➡.*

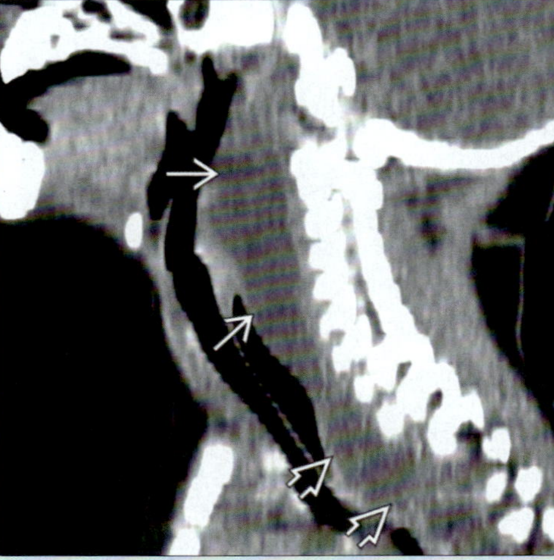

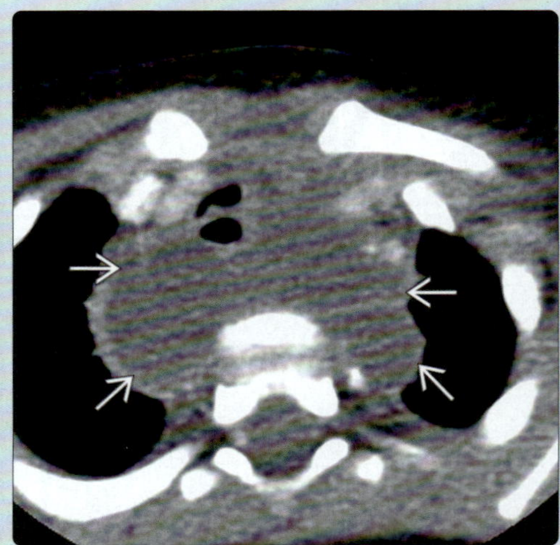

(Left) *Sagittal CECT in the same infant reveals an abscess ➡ displacing the pharynx and esophagus anteriorly and extending inferiorly into the danger space to involve the superior mediastinum ➡.* **(Right)** *Axial CECT reveals the inferior extent of methicillin-resistant Staphylococcus aureus abscess to the superior mediastinum ➡, which was drained following a transcervical approach to the abscess collection. There is no stridor or other signs of airway compromise, despite a displaced and narrowed airway.*

KEY FACTS

TERMINOLOGY

- Synonyms: Retropharyngeal space (RPS) effusion, benign retropharyngeal fluid
- Definition: Accumulation of sterile fluid within RPS

IMAGING

- General imaging features
  - Bland-appearing, small volume RPS fluid posterior to pharynx, anterior to prevertebral muscles
- CECT findings
  - Low-volume low-density RPS fluid
  - **No wall enhancement**
  - Usually no surrounding inflammatory change
- MR findings
  - Linear to lenticular ↓ T1 and ↑ T2 (**water signal**) in RPS

TOP DIFFERENTIAL DIAGNOSES

- RPS abscess or phlegmon
- Prominent normal retropharyngeal fat
- Posterior wall hypopharyngeal squamous cell carcinoma

PATHOLOGY

- Different inciting factors result in RPS transudate, cellulitis, or lymphatic fluid accumulation

CLINICAL ISSUES

- Self-limited or limited by course of causative process

DIAGNOSTIC CHECKLIST

- Key is to **differentiate from RPS abscess** 1st
  - Rim-enhancing collection distending RPS
  - Requires urgent management
- Then look for underlying cause; may be treatable
  - Venous occlusive disease
  - Recent chemotherapy or radiation therapy
  - Current infection: Pharynx, teeth, sinus
  - Longus colli tendinitis
  - Kawasaki disease

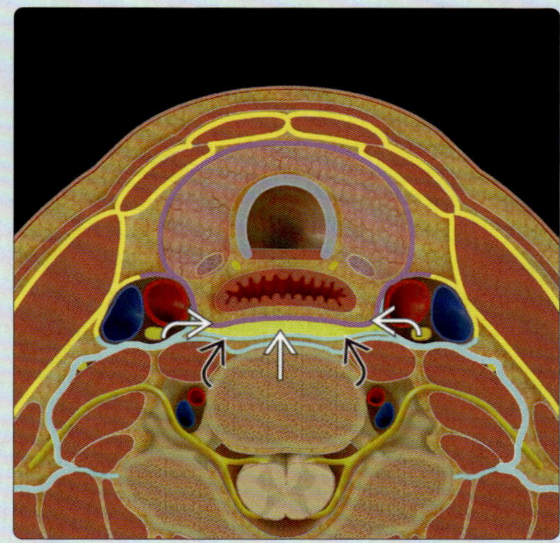

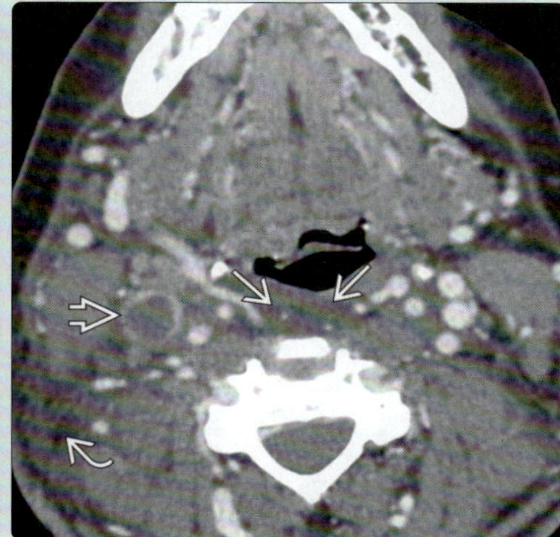

(Left) *Axial graphic illustrates retropharyngeal space (RPS) distension with edema ➡. Note fascial delineation of the RPS by a middle layer of deep cervical fascia (DCF) anteriorly ➡ and a deep layer of DCF posteriorly ➡.* **(Right)** *Axial CECT reveals RPS low-density fluid ➡ without peripheral enhancement due to right internal jugular vein (IJV) thrombosis ➡. Edematous changes are seen in the surrounding right carotid space and ipsilateral posterior cervical space deep fat ➡.*

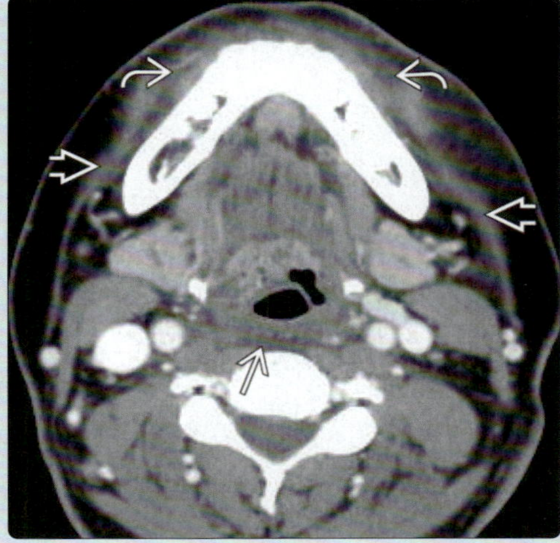

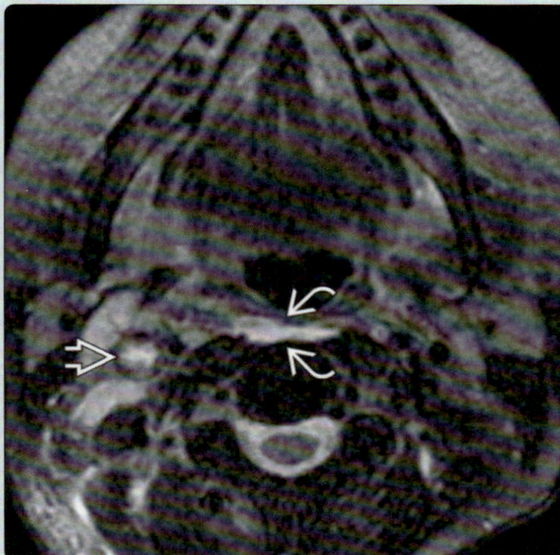

(Left) *Axial CECT shows bland RPS fluid without rim enhancement ➡. Note evidence of source: Cellulitis overlying the mandible ➡ and thickened platysma ➡ from nearby dental infection.* **(Right)** *Axial T2WI FS MR reveals RPS distension with thin, symmetric effusion ➡ of similar intensity to CSF. The source of the RPS fluid is due to right IJV thrombosis. Note the loss of IJV flow void with high signal intensity ➡.*

KEY FACTS

TERMINOLOGY

- Malignant retropharyngeal space (RPS) nodes: Squamous cell carcinoma (SCCa) RPS nodes from nasopharyngeal or posterior wall oro- or hypopharyngeal primary SCCa

IMAGING

- General CECT and MR imaging findings
  - Location SCCa nodes: Suprahyoid RPS only
    - Found just medial to ICA in lateral RPS
  - Oval to round, ± centrally necrotic mass > 0.8 cm
  - If extracapsular spread: Ill-defined margins ± stranding of surrounding fat
- CECT findings
  - Nodes difficult to identify on CT, especially if small
  - Nodal necrosis: Central low density with variably thick, irregular enhancing wall
- MR more sensitive to detect RPS nodes than CT
- PET has role in staging & follow-up of H&N SCCa
  - Cystic/necrotic nodes may be PET negative

TOP DIFFERENTIAL DIAGNOSES

- Suppurative RPS nodes
- Non-Hodgkin lymphoma RPS nodes
- Thyroid or systemic RPS nodal metastasis

PATHOLOGY

- RPS nodes = primary drainage for posterior nasal cavity, ethmoid & sphenoid sinus, palate, nasopharynx & posterior wall of oro- & hypopharynx

CLINICAL ISSUES

- Clinical presentation
  - Primary SCCa usually clinically apparent
  - RPS malignant adenopathy is often clinically occult
  - If large, bulging of posterolateral pharyngeal wall
- Treatment implications
  - For oro-/hypopharyngeal primary, chemotherapy & radiotherapy will often be treatment modality of choice
  - For posterior wall SCCa, surgical nodal dissection

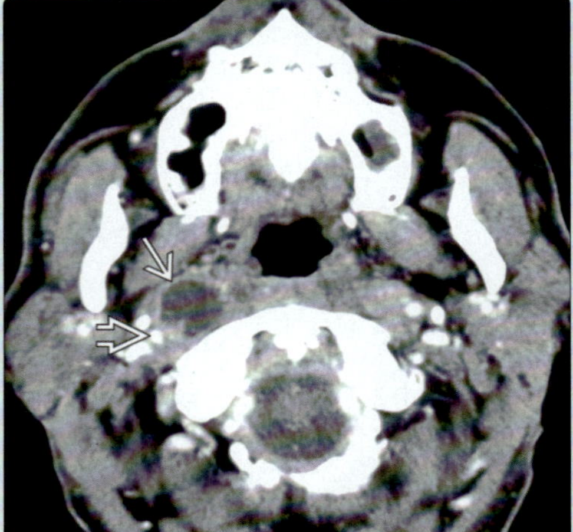

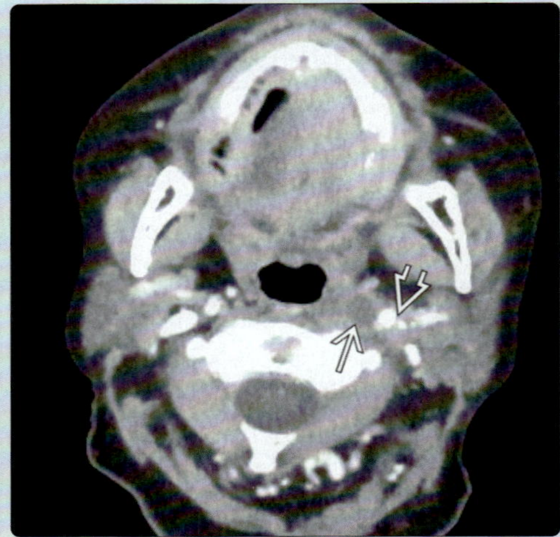

(Left) *Axial CECT through the nasopharynx shows a large, necrotic lateral retropharyngeal node ➡ just medial to the internal carotid artery (ICA) ➡. In an adult, squamous cell carcinoma (SCCa) from the pharynx is the most likely primary site for this suspected malignant retropharyngeal node.* **(Right)** *Axial CECT shows a cystic left retropharyngeal nodal metastasis ➡ in patient with posterior wall oropharyngeal SCCa. Note: Carotid space ➡ is laterally displaced by this lateral retropharyngeal space (RPS) SCCa nodal metastasis.*

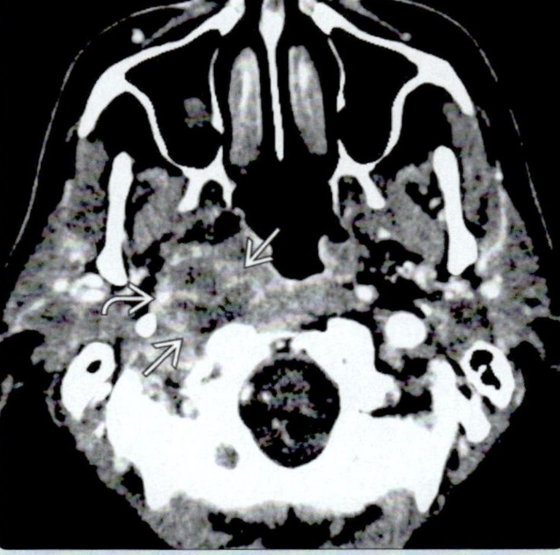

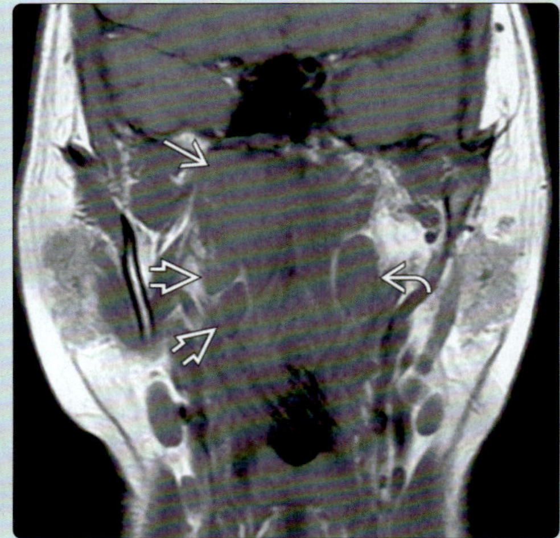

(Left) *Axial CECT in a 63-year-old man treated with surgery & radiation therapy 1 year prior for oropharyngeal SCCa shows a large, clinically silent recurrent RPS nodal mass with irregular rim enhancement ➡. Note its location medial to the narrowed and encased right ICA ➡.* **(Right)** *Coronal T1 MR in a patient with a mass in the upper pharynx ➡ shows a predominantly right-sided nasopharyngeal carcinoma with 2 right RPS ➡ nodes and 1 large left RPS node ➡.*

KEY FACTS

TERMINOLOGY

- Non-Hodgkin lymphoma (NHL) is lymphoreticular system malignancy
- Retropharyngeal space (RPS) from skull base to hyoid contains lateral & medial nodal groups
  - Lateral group = nodes of Rouvière
- H&N NHL has multiple forms
  - **Nodal**, nonnodal lymphatic, or extralymphatic

IMAGING

- CT or MR general findings
  - CT & MR cannot differentiate normal size, nonnecrotic NHL nodes from reactive nodes
  - Large, nonnecrotic nodes more likely NHL than SCCa
  - Oval-round, solid mass > **0.8 cm** (axial) in RPS
    - RPS nodes are medial to ICA above hyoid bone
    - Carotid space pushed laterally by RPS NHL node
  - **Typically associated with other neck adenopathy**
    - May have enlargement of Waldeyer ring
  - Necrosis ± extranodal spread suggest high-grade NHL
  - MR more sensitive than CT for detecting RPS nodes
- **Most NHL are FDG avid**; PET typically performed

TOP DIFFERENTIAL DIAGNOSES

- RPS reactive adenopathy
- RPS suppurative adenopathy
- RPS nodal SCCa or systemic metastasis

CLINICAL ISSUES

- Clinical presentation
  - Median age: 50-55 years
  - RPS nodes usually clinically occult
    - If large may see bulging of posterior pharyngeal wall
  - Other manifestations of NHL in H&N
    - Extranodal, lymphatic disease in Waldeyer ring
    - Extranodal, extralymphatic site involvement
- Treatment options depend on stage, cell type, patient age
  - Chemo, XRT, or combined modality therapy

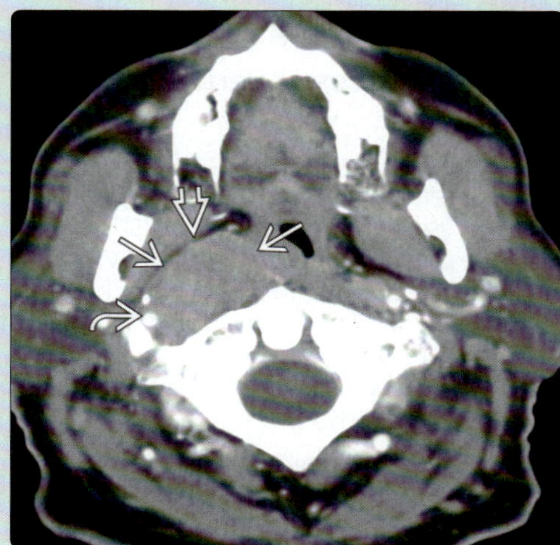

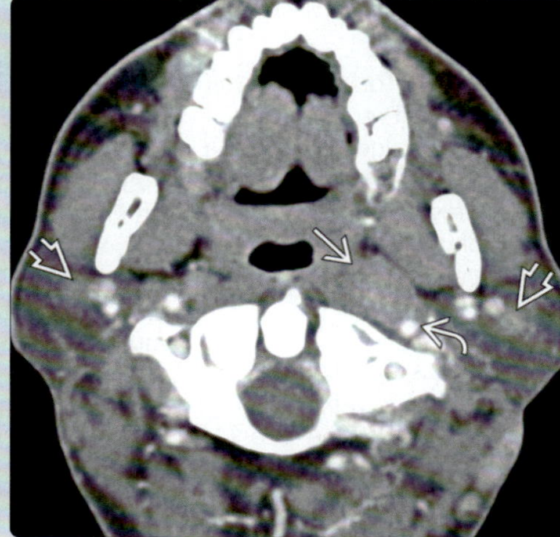

(Left) *Axial CECT in a patient with non-Hodgkin lymphoma (NHL) shows a large homogeneously enhancing mass ➡ medial to internal carotid artery ➡. Right retropharyngeal node displaces parapharyngeal fat ➡ anterolaterally and carotid space laterally.* **(Right)** *Axial CECT in a different patient shows a large, oval, homogeneous, nonnecrotic left retropharyngeal node ➡ displacing the left internal carotid ➡ posterolaterally. Mildly prominent parotid nodes are also noted ➡ in this patient with NHL.*

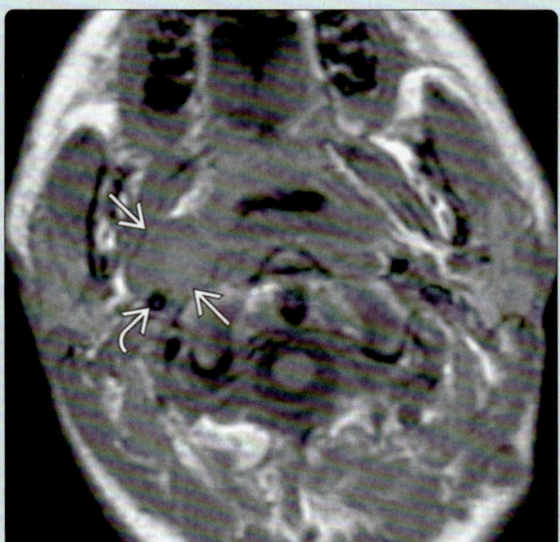

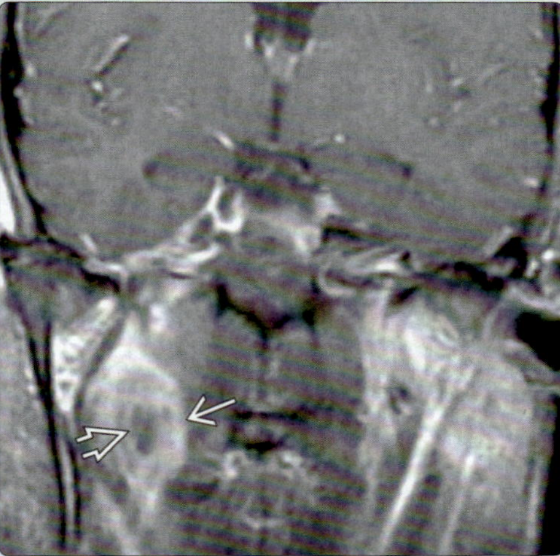

(Left) *Axial T1 MR reveals a soft tissue mass ➡ medial to the internal carotid artery ➡, representing abnormally enlarged lateral retropharyngeal node. Note that despite size this node does not deform the pharyngeal lumen enough to be clinically evident. This patient had history of aplastic anemia & bone marrow transplant.* **(Right)** *Coronal T1 C+ MR in same patient shows rim enhancement of the retropharyngeal node ➡ & central necrosis ➡. This patient was found to have posttransplant NHL.*

Summary Thoughts: Perivertebral Space

The perivertebral space (PVS) is a cylindrical space surrounding the vertebral column, extending from the skull base to the superior mediastinum. The **deep layer of the deep cervical fascia** (DL-DCF) completely encircles the PVS, which is subdivided into **prevertebral** (prevertebral-PVS) and **paraspinal** (paraspinal-PVS) portions or spaces.

A **prevertebral space mass** will displace the prevertebral muscles **anteriorly**, distinguishing it from a retropharyngeal space (RPS) mass, which pushes the muscles posteriorly. A **paraspinal space mass** bows the posterior cervical space (PCS) fat away from the posterior elements of the spine.

The DL-DCF serves as a tenacious barrier to the spread of malignancy or infection, and it will redirect extension of PVS disease to the **epidural space**.

The vast majority of PVS lesions originate in the **vertebral body** with **metastatic disease** and **infection** topping the list. Therefore, the vertebral body is usually diseased when a PVS lesion is found.

One imaging interpretation pitfall is mistaking a **hypertrophic levator scapulae muscle** for a mass. The hypertrophy is due to CNXI injury, usually from previous neck dissection. Ipsilateral atrophy of the trapezius and sternocleidomastoid (SCM) muscles help in making the correct diagnosis.

Imaging Techniques & Indications

Lateral cervical plain film provides a quick check for prevertebral soft tissue swelling and for cervical vertebral body integrity. **CECT** with soft tissue and bone algorithm, along with coronal & sagittal reformations, is the best exam to evaluate the **cervical soft tissues** and **bones**. Contrast-enhanced cervical spine **MR** is the exam of choice to evaluate for **epidural extension** of disease.

Imaging Anatomy

The name PVS nicely describes the anatomy. It is a cylindrical space that is quite literally around (or peri-) the vertebral column. This helpful naming system was not always the case as the entire region, including portions **beside** and **behind** the vertebrae, was historically called the **pre**vertebral space. Since it seemed counterintuitive to use **pre**vertebral to describe structures posterolateral to the vertebrae, the old terminology was upgraded to the new.

The PVS is bounded by the DL-DCF and extends from the skull base to the superior mediastinum T4 level. It consists of **2 major components**: The **prevertebral** and **paraspinal** portions or spaces. The attachments of the DL-DCF to the vertebral transverse processes mark the division, with the prevertebral-PVS lying anterior and the paraspinal-PVS lying posterior.

Important anatomic relationships can be examined as they relate to these 2 subdivisions. Directly in front of the **prevertebral space** throughout the extracranial head and neck are the retropharyngeal and danger spaces. Anterolateral are the paired carotid spaces, and lateral lie the anterior aspects of the PCSs. The **paraspinal space** lies deep to the PCSs and posterior to the cervical spine transverse processes.

The **DL-DCF** completely encircles the PVS. Its anterior portion (**anterior DL-DCF**) arches in front of the prevertebral muscles from 1 cervical spine transverse process to the opposite transverse process. The posterior portion (**posterior DL-DCF**) arches over the paraspinal muscles to attach to the nuchal ligament of the vertebral body spinous processes.

The **anterior DL-DCF** is often referred to as the "**carpet**" by surgeons because surgical approach reveals a smooth, carpet-like surface on which the pharynx slides up and down. The "carpet" is extremely tenacious and serves as a 2-way barrier to the spread of disease. Therefore, expanding **tumor or infection** of the prevertebral-PVS will be redirected by this tough fascia along the path of least resistance to the **epidural space**. Coming from the other direction, pharyngeal malignancy is usually blocked from accessing the PVS.

Only the **brachial plexus** roots pierce the tough DL-DCF. The C1-C5 roots exit the neural foramina, pass between the anterior & middle scalene muscles in the prevertebral-PVS, then out through an opening in the DL-DCF. From there, they traverse the PCS on their way to the axilla. This creates a bidirectional highway for perineural spread of malignancy.

A working knowledge of important **PVS internal structures** is key to understanding the pathology & pathology mimics (pseudolesions) found within. The prevertebral space contains the prevertebral muscles (longus colli and capitis), scalene muscles (anterior, middle, and posterior), brachial plexus roots, phrenic nerve (C3-C5), vertebral artery and vein, and vertebral body. The paraspinal space contains the paraspinal muscles and the posterior elements of the vertebrae.

Approaches to Imaging Issues of Perivertebral Space

When trying to define a lesion in the head and neck as in the PVS, one must 1st answer the question, "What **imaging findings** define a mass or lesion as **primary to the PVS**?" A lesion originates from the **prevertebral** aspect of the **PVS** if it is centered within the prevertebral muscles or vertebral body. Also, a mass that causes **anterior lifting** of the **prevertebral muscles** is arising from the prevertebral-PVS. In most cases, this feature clearly distinguishes a PVS mass from a RPS mass, which pushes the muscles posteriorly.

A mass is primary to the **paraspinal** aspect of the **PVS** if it is within the substance of the paraspinal musculature or if it bows the PCS fat away from the vertebral posterior elements.

When prevertebral space disease is noted, one should always check for **epidural extension**. Remember that infection or malignancy that breaks out of the vertebral body into the PVS will be blocked by the tough DL-DCF. As a result the path of least resistance is deep spread into the epidural space through the neural foramen, possibly leading to **spinal cord compression**.

A possible route of disease travel into or out of the PVS is along the **brachial plexus**. Extranodal tumor from the axilla (most frequently breast carcinoma) may access the PVS by retrograde perineural spread along the brachial plexus. Conversely, a PVS invasive malignancy may spread antegrade along this pathway to the axillary apex.

Once a lesion has been identified as originating in the PVS, the differential diagnosis unique to the PVS should be reviewed. Identifying characteristic imaging findings of common PVS lesions often yields a short list of possible diagnoses. By far, the **most common lesions** of the PVS originate in the **vertebral body**, with infection and metastatic disease at the

Perivertebral Space Lesion Differential Diagnosis

Pseudolesions	Vertebral body osteomyelitis, pyogenic
Levator scapulae hypertrophy	Vertebral body osteomyelitis, tuberculous
Cervical rib	**Benign tumor**
Large transverse process	Brachial plexus schwannoma
Degenerative	Brachial plexus neurofibroma
Anterior disc herniation	Vertebral body benign bony tumors
Hypertrophic facet joint	**Malignant tumor/metastatic tumor**
Vertebral body osteophyte	Vertebral body metastasis
Vascular	Epidural metastasis
Vertebral artery dissection	Chordoma
Vertebral artery aneurysm	Non-Hodgkin lymphoma
Vertebral artery pseudoaneurysm	Direct invasion, squamous cell carcinoma posterior pharyngeal wall
Inflammatory/infectious	Vertebral body primary malignant tumors
Longus colli tendonitis	

Above is an exhaustive list of lesions that can be found in the perivertebral space. The table is organized by general pathology category.

top of the list. Therefore, when a PVS lesion is identified, the vertebral body should be evaluated, as it is usually diseased.

Vertebral body osteomyelitis can be differentiated from other entities on the differential diagnosis list by noting destructive changes of adjacent vertebral endplates with increased T2 signal and enhancement of the intervertebral disc on MR. The disc space will be spared in metastatic disease or non-Hodgkin lymphoma, which are more likely to involve multiple bones than to be solitary. Epidural disease can be seen in either metastatic disease or non-Hodgkin lymphoma.

An inflammatory lesion that may be confusing to the radiologist is longus colli tendonitis. Neck pain that may be accompanied by fever may be imaged with CECT. Prevertebral soft tissue swelling secondary to RPS edema with focal prevertebral soft tissue calcification at the C1/2 level must not be confused with RPS abscess. The lesion is due to foreign body inflammatory reaction to deposited crystals of calcium hydroxyapatite, but its pathophysiology is not further understood.

Diagnosis of chordoma is suggested by a destructive mass centered at the sphenooccipital junction in the clivus or upper cervical vertebral body associated with a large, T2 hyperintense soft tissue mass, commonly with perivertebral & epidural extension. When epidural extension occurs in the neck, cord compression is an early & severe consequence.

Benign neurogenic PVS tumors include brachial plexus schwannoma & neurofibroma. Both appear as circumscribed, fusiform, enhancing masses situated between the anterior & middle scalene muscles.

PVS vascular lesions involve the vertebral arteries, including vertebral artery dissection, aneurysm, or pseudoaneurysm. While all can be usually diagnosed by CTA, axial fat-saturated T1 MR may help in cases of dissection, showing intramural hematoma as a hyperintense crescent.

With most PVS pseudolesions (cervical rib, large transverse process) and degenerative changes (anterior disc herniation, hypertrophic facet joint, and vertebral body osteophyte) there is little diagnostic dilemma on cross-sectional imaging.

Probably the biggest potential imaging pitfall when evaluating a PVS lesion is to mistake a hypertrophic LSM for an enhancing mass or recurrent tumor. This "pseudolesion" is secondary to spinal accessory nerve (CNXI) injury, usually from previous neck dissection. The levator scapulae hypertrophies to help lift the arm to compensate for the atrophy of the SCM and trapezius caused by spinal accessory neuropathy. On imaging, the LSM will be enlarged and may enhance. Look for small, fatty infiltrated ipsilateral trapezius and SCM muscles to confirm the diagnosis.

Clinical Implications

Clinical history provides important clues to differentiating PVS lesions. Fever, neck pain, and tenderness herald the onset of **vertebral body osteomyelitis** with possible progression to quadriparesis if there is epidural pus. Patients with **metastatic disease** usually have a known primary and those with **non-Hodgkin lymphoma** have known systemic disease when PVS disease is found. Both can present with neck pain, radiculopathy, or myelopathy.

Brachial plexus **schwannomas** may be seen sporadically or in the setting of neurofibromatosis type 2 (multiple schwannomas). **Neurofibromas** may also be sporadic but are most commonly found in the setting of neurofibromatosis type 1. Typically, both are painless, slow-growing masses.

Vertebral artery injuries can be from minor (chiropractic manipulation) or major trauma and may present with delayed **stroke**, possibly with a lateral medullary (Wallenberg) syndrome if the posterior inferior cerebellar artery is involved.

Longus colli tendonitis is associated with 2-7 days of neck pain and odynophagia. A history of previous surgical neck dissection can usually be elicited in patients with a **hypertrophic LSM**.

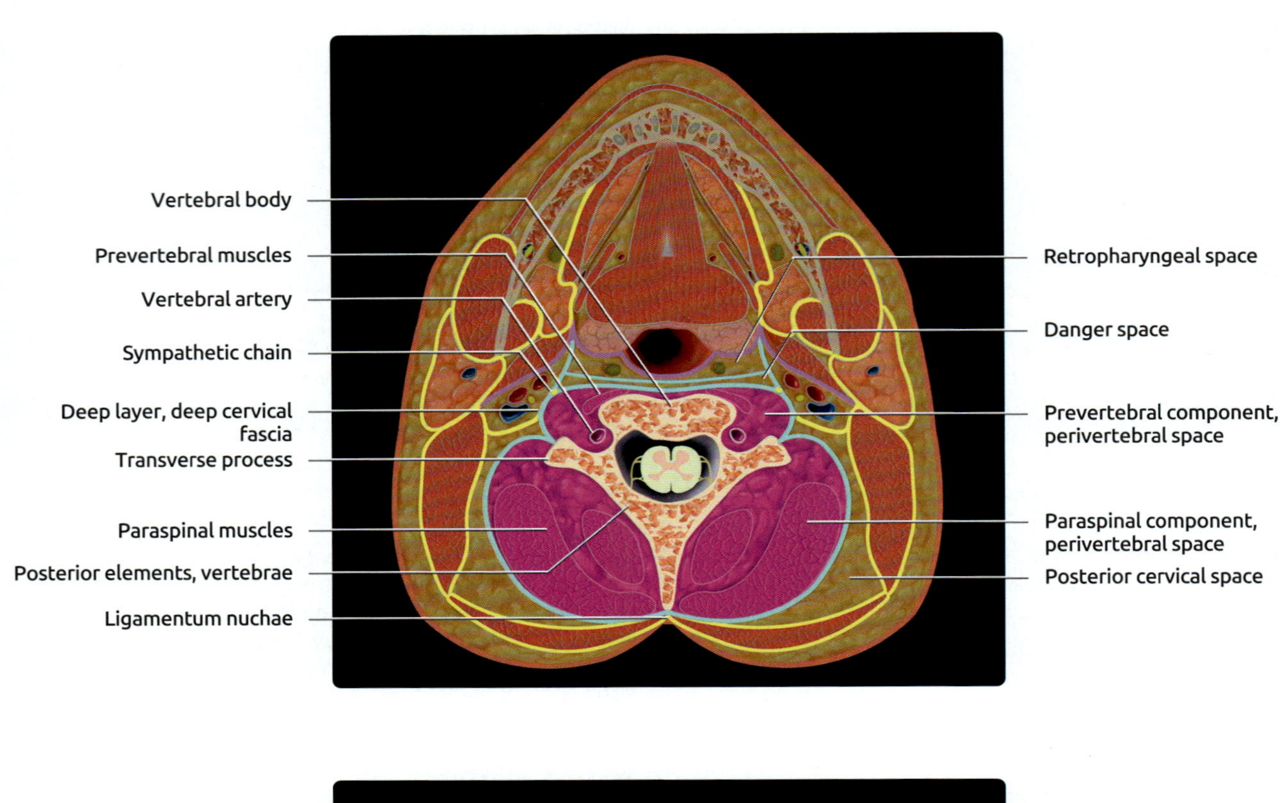

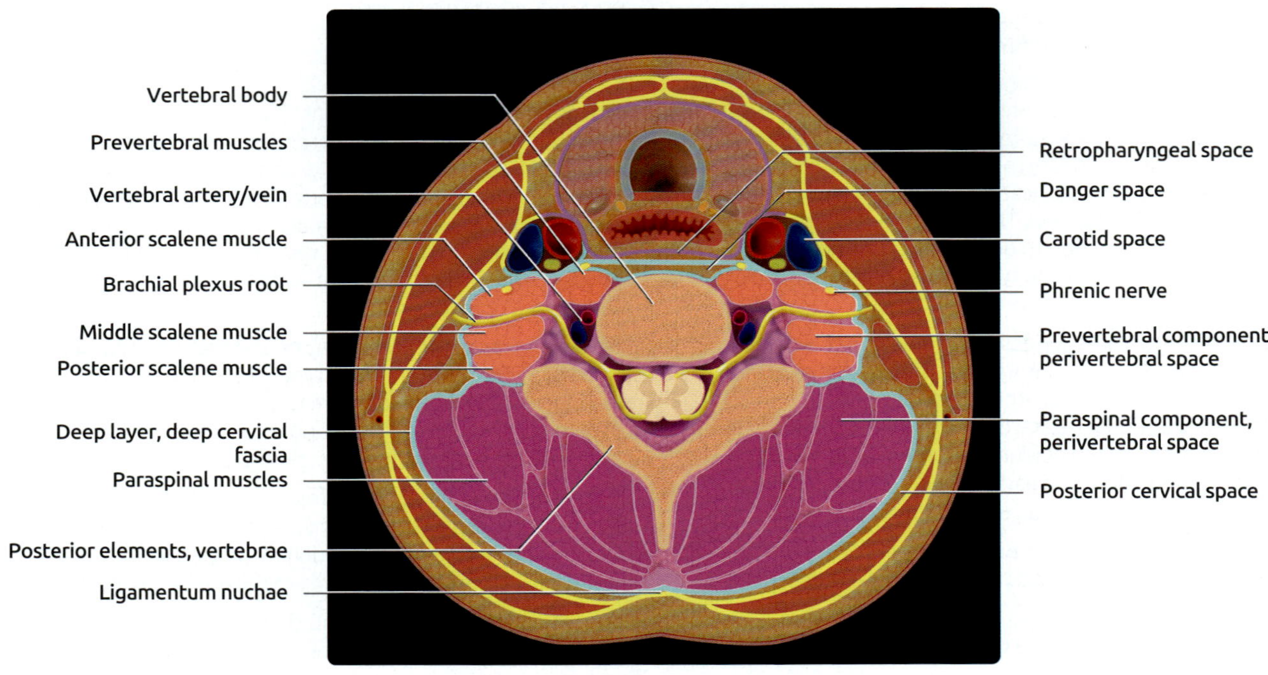

(Top) *Axial graphic through the level of the oropharynx shows prevertebral and paraspinal components of the perivertebral space (PVS) beneath the deep layer of deep cervical fascia (DL-DCF). Notice this fascia curves medially to touch the transverse processes of the vertebra, dividing the PVS into prevertebral and paraspinal components. The danger and retropharyngeal spaces are anterior to the PVS, while the posterior cervical space is lateral and posterior.* **(Bottom)** *Axial graphic through the thyroid bed shows prevertebral & paraspinal components of the PVS beneath the DL-DCF. The DL-DCF is a tenacious barrier to the spread of infection or malignancy, which will be redirected to the epidural space. The brachial plexus roots pass between the anterior and middle scalene muscles in the prevertebral-PVS and serve as a 2-way highway for perineural spread of malignancy between the PVS and axillary apex.*

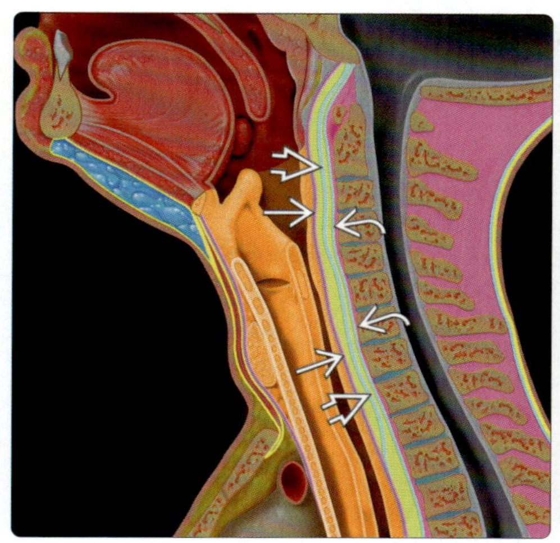

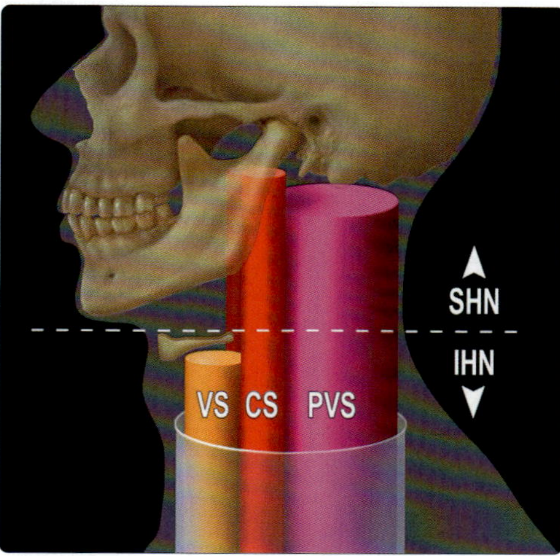

(Left) *Sagittal graphic depicts midline spacial relationships of the infrahyoid neck. Just anterior to the PVS (purple) are the danger space* ➡ *and retropharyngeal space* ➡*. The tenacious DL-DCF* ➡ *will usually redirect the spread of PVS disease to the epidural space.* **(Right)** *Lateral graphic of the extracranial head and neck shows the tubular PVS extending from the skull base to the mediastinum. DL-DCF completely encircles the PVS.*

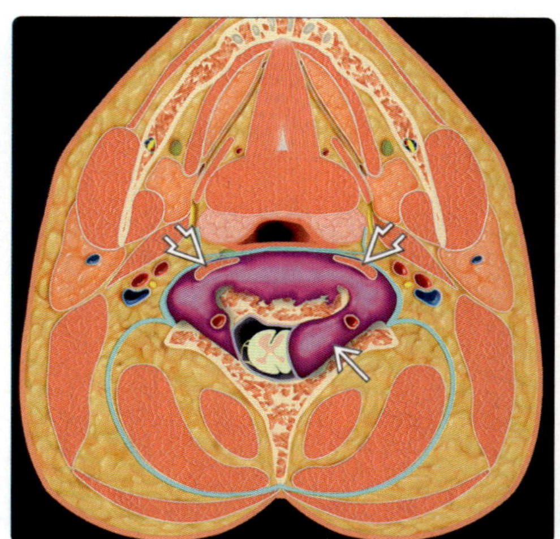

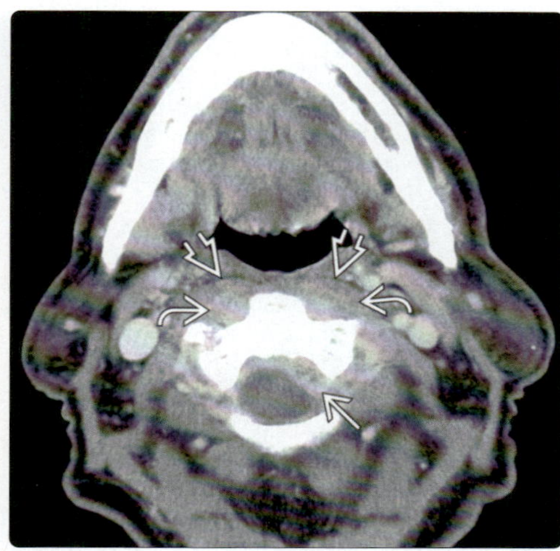

(Left) *Axial graphic at the suprahyoid neck oropharyngeal level shows a generic PVS mass that elevates prevertebral muscles* ➡ *& destroys vertebral body. Note DL-DCF (blue line) confines the mass and "forces" it into the epidural space* ➡*.* **(Right)** *Axial CECT at the same level reveals enhancing phlegmon-abscess in the prevertebral portion of the PVS* ➡*. Epidural abscess is seen on the left* ➡*. Note the anteriorly lifted prevertebral muscles* ➡*.*

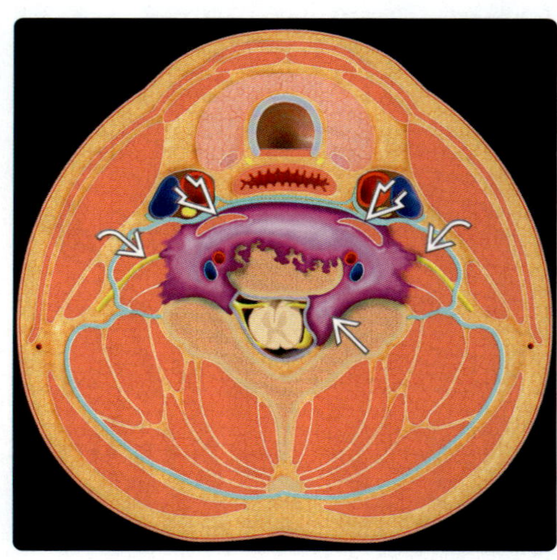

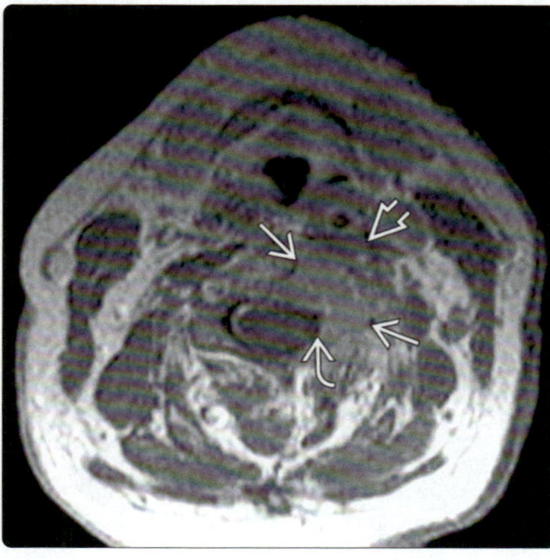

(Left) *Axial graphic at the thyroid level demonstrates a generic infrahyoid PVS mass arising from the vertebral body and elevating the prevertebral muscles* ➡*. Brachial plexus* ➡ *& vertebral arteries are engulfed, & epidural disease* ➡ *is present.* **(Right)** *Axial T1 MR shows an enhancing metastatic tumor involving the vertebral body and its posterior elements on the left* ➡ *with extensive epidural tumor visible* ➡*. Note the anteriorly displaced prevertebral muscle* ➡*.*

Acute Calcific Longus Colli Tendonitis

KEY FACTS

TERMINOLOGY

- Definition: Inflammatory condition due to **calcium hydroxyapatite deposition** in **longus colli tendon**
- Synonym: Longus colli tendonitis

IMAGING

- Process produces 3 distinct findings on CECT
  - **Calcifications** in prevertebral muscle tendons at C1-C2
  - Inflammation with swelling of prevertebral muscles
  - Retropharyngeal space (RPS) edema
    - **Calcification** at C1-C2 is pathognomonic
- Best imaging exam: CECT
  - Best identifies calcifications
- Caveat: Look for amorphous calcifications anterior to C1-C2 when unexplained RPS effusion identified
  - Do not mistake for RPS abscess
  - RPS edema is smoothly expansile, nonenhancing

TOP DIFFERENTIAL DIAGNOSES

- RPS effusion
- RPS abscess
- Prevertebral space infection

PATHOLOGY

- Deposition of **calcium hydroxyapatite crystals** with secondary inflammatory reaction
- Involves superior oblique fibers-tendon of longus colli that insert on C1 anterior tubercle

CLINICAL ISSUES

- Clinical presentation
  - Subacute neck pain, odynophagia, dysphagia
  - Low-grade fever possible
- Treatment options
  - Self-limiting condition; treat pain only
  - Analgesics & antiinflammatory medications

(Left) *Axial CECT (bone window) demonstrates pathognomonic focal central and left parasagittal amorphous calcification ➡ anteroinferior to the C1 arch within the prevertebral portion of the perivertebral space, corresponding to the longus colli tendon.* **(Right)** *Axial T1 C+ FS MR demonstrates focal low signal intensity representing calcification ➡, longus colli muscle enhancement ➡, and enhancing inflammatory change in the retropharyngeal space (RPS) ➡.*

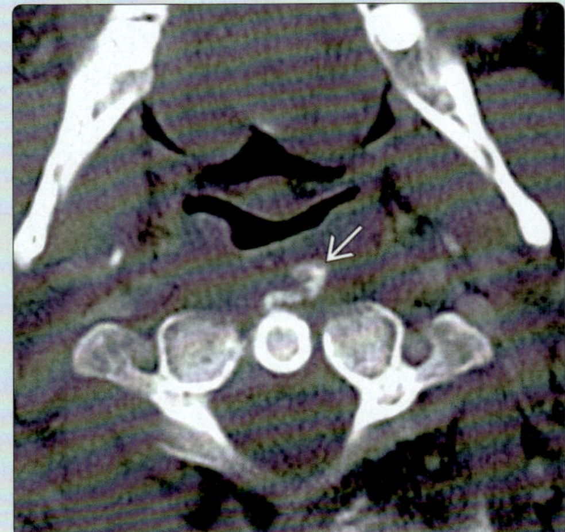

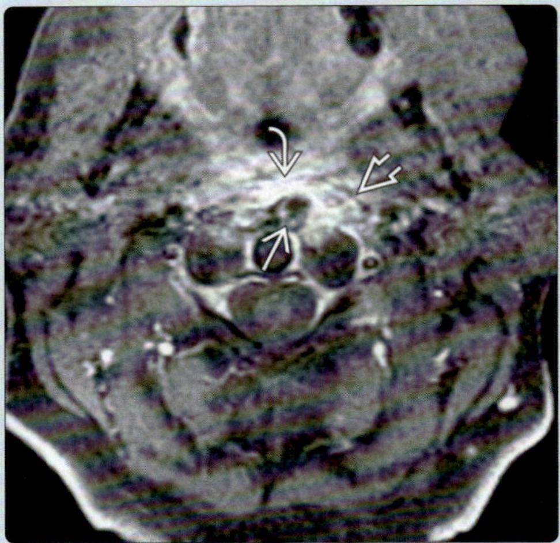

(Left) *Axial T2 MR reveals edema ➡ in the RPS associated with longus colli tendonitis. Fluid is anterior to the prevertebral muscles ➡ posteriorly and posterior to pharyngeal mucosal space. RPS effusion will not rim enhance.* **(Right)** *Sagittal T2 MR reveals marked focal hypointensity of calcification in longus colli muscle at mid C2 level ➡. Note hyperintense T2 signal of swollen prevertebral and retropharyngeal soft tissues ➡. There are no disc space changes that might reflect spondylodiscitis.*

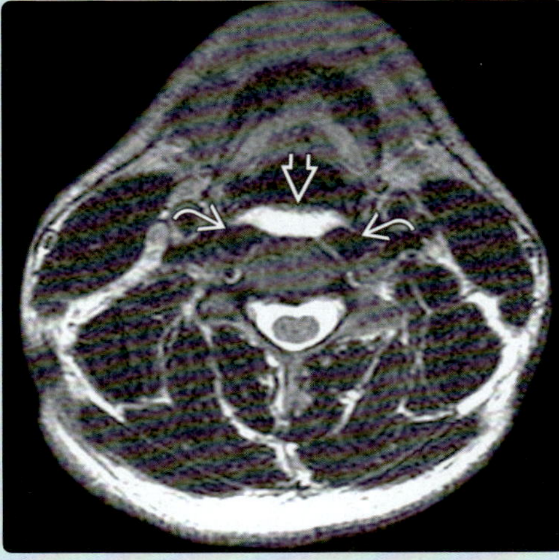

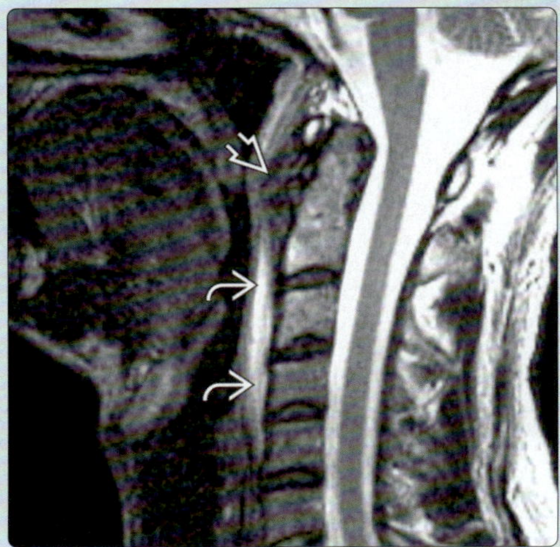

KEY FACTS

TERMINOLOGY

- Perivertebral space (PVS)
  - Prevertebral and paraspinal components (spaces)
- PVS infection: Deep neck infection centered on prevertebral muscles, disc space, vertebral body

IMAGING

- Plain film: Irregular end-plates, narrowed disc space, enlarged prevertebral soft tissues
- T1 C+ **MR best identifies epidural abscess**
- Enhanced CT and MR findings
  - Swollen, enhancing prevertebral soft tissues (phlegmon)
    - ± rim-enhancing fluid collection (abscess)
  - Enhancing epidural tissue (phlegmon)
    - Rim-enhancing epidural fluid (**epidural abscess**)
    - Cord inflammation or compression possible
  - Vertebral body end-plate erosions (CT)
  - Vertebral body marrow space enhancement (MR)

TOP DIFFERENTIAL DIAGNOSES

- Retropharyngeal space abscess
- Metastasis, lymphoma, chordoma

PATHOLOGY

- Most often due to spondylodiscitis
  - Uncommonly follows neck or spine surgery
  - Rarely direct seeding of PVS muscles
- **Spondylodiscitis** most often hematogenous infection
  - Primary pyogenic organism is *Staphylococcus aureus*
  - Worldwide, tuberculosis is most common cause

CLINICAL ISSUES

- Clinical presentation: Older patient (> 60 years) with neck pain, fever; neurologic deficits
- Treatment options
  - I&D of abscess
  - Long-term intravenous antibiotics
  - Dead bone debridement/fusion for collapse as needed

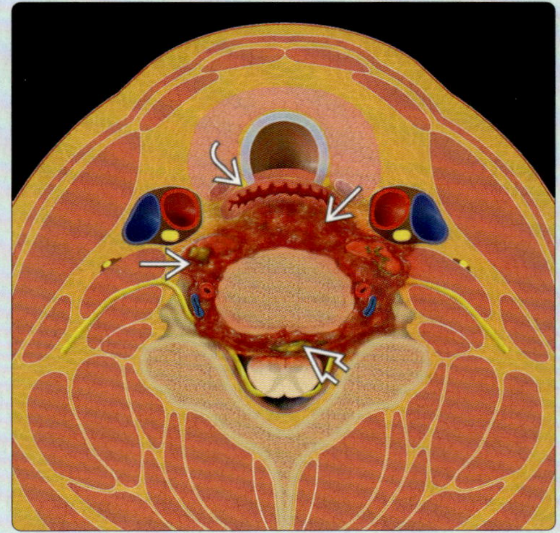

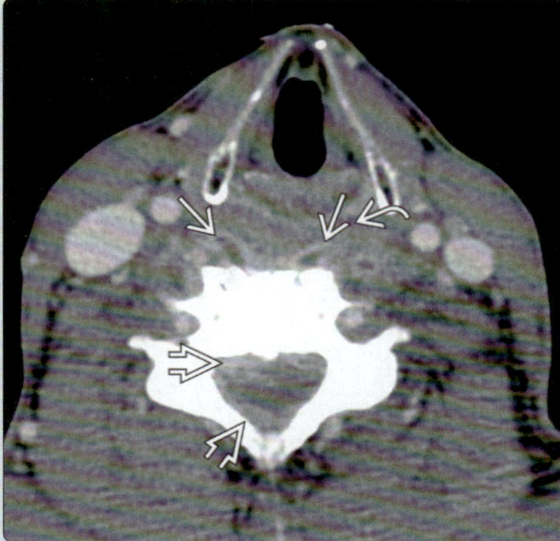

(Left) *Axial graphic depicts the typical findings of perivertebral space (PVS) infection. Phlegmonous soft tissue ➡ surrounds the vertebral body, displacing the esophagus ➡ anteriorly and producing epidural phlegmon/abscess posteriorly ➡.* **(Right)** *Axial CECT shows swollen, enhancing phlegmon in the prevertebral-PVS along with multifocal early abscesses ➡. Hypopharynx ➡ is displaced anteriorly. Careful evaluation of the spinal canal reveals densely enhancing tissue ➡ around cervical cord, indicating epidural phlegmon.*

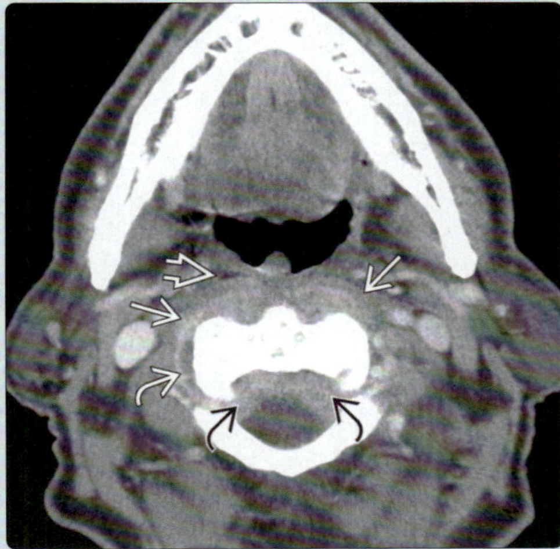

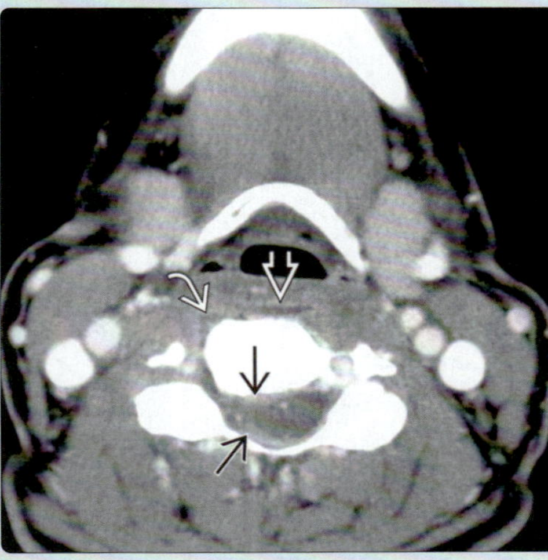

(Left) *Axial CECT at the C2 level shows a collar of heterogeneously enhancing tissue ➡ abutting vertebral body, directly posterior to the thin stripe of retropharyngeal fat ➡. Note the intraspinal epidural component ➡. A small area of early abscess is present ➡.* **(Right)** *Axial CECT reveals heterogeneously enlarged prevertebral tissues with a focal pool of rim-enhancing pus ➡. Inflamed tissues extend from epidural phlegmon ➡. A small retropharyngeal fluid collection is also noted ➡.*

KEY FACTS

TERMINOLOGY

- Vertebral artery (VA) dissection definition: Narrowing ± occlusion of VA secondary to intimal tear and subadventitial hematoma

IMAGING

- 2 typical forms of VA dissection
- **Stenoocclusive dissection**
  - Dissection to subintimal plane with vessel luminal narrowing or occlusion
- **Dissecting aneurysm**
  - Dissection into subadventitial plane with dilatation of outer wall
- Intramural hematoma is pathognomonic
  - Best seen as **bright crescent** on T1 FS MR
- CTA source images show contour changes of lumen
  - Suboccipital rind sign in V3 segment
- Conventional angiography is gold standard

TOP DIFFERENTIAL DIAGNOSES

- Extracranial atherosclerosis
- Fibromuscular dysplasia
- Miscellaneous vasculitis

PATHOLOGY

- **Traumatic** VA dissection
  - Direct or indirect arterial injury
- **Spontaneous** VA dissection
  - Many associations and predisposing factors

CLINICAL ISSUES

- Age: Majority < 45 years
- Symptoms: Head and neck pain, stroke symptoms (especially of posterior circulation)
- Treatment options
  - Stenoocclusive dissection → anticoagulation
  - Dissecting aneurysm → ligation or coil embolization
- Complete resolution of lumen abnormality in ~ 80%

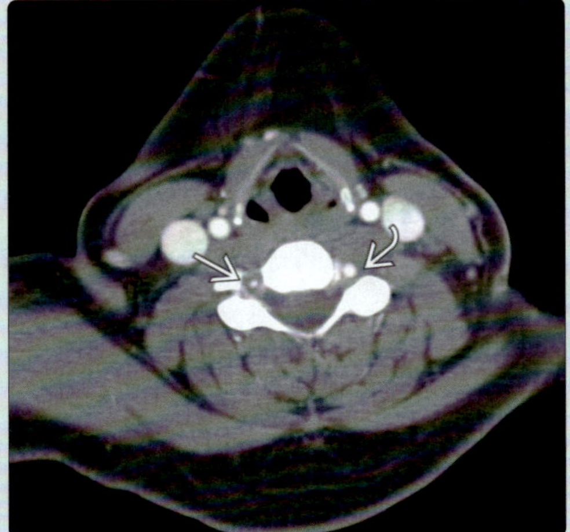

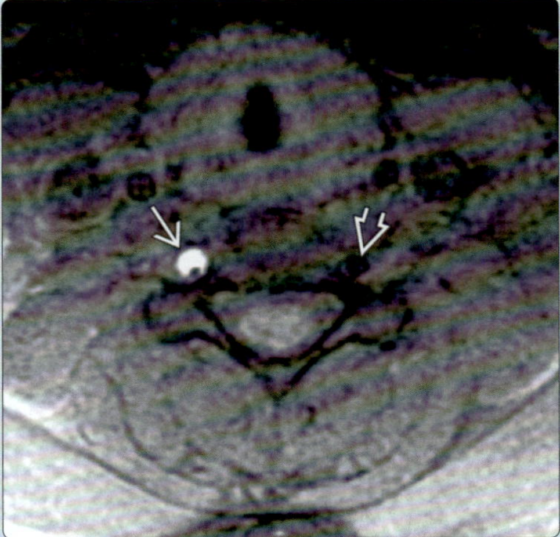

(Left) *Axial CTA shows the normal symmetric appearance of the common carotid arteries with adjacent jugular veins. The left vertebral artery (VA) is patent ➔ and normal in caliber. Right VA shows markedly diminished lumen caliber ➔ and wall thickening representing mural hematoma.* **(Right)** *Axial T1WI FS MR in a patient with vertebral dissection reveals a hyperintense crescent within the wall of the right VA ➔ significantly narrowing the VA lumen. This is typical of an intramural hematoma. Note normal left VA flow void ➔.*

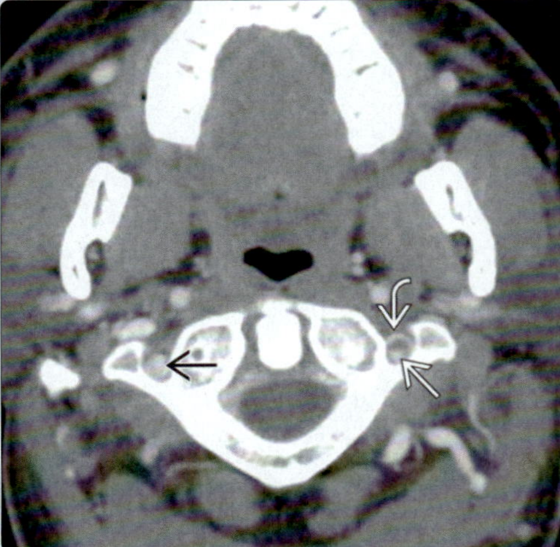

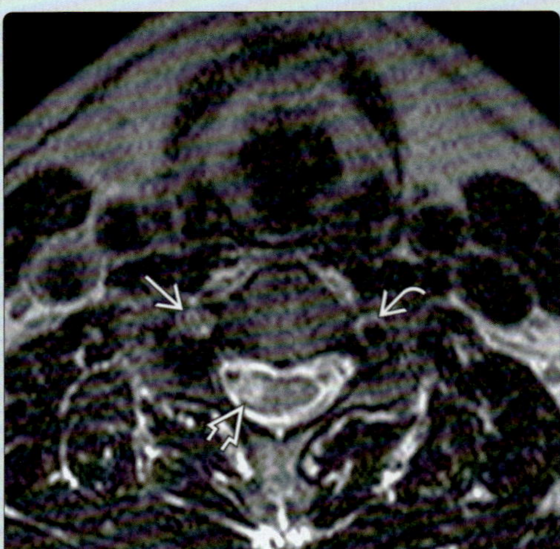

(Left) *Axial CTA shows rim enhancement of the left VA ➔ with a low-density mural hematoma and contrast filling the narrowed lumen ➔. Subtle linear lucency in the right VA proved not to be a dissection flap ➔.* **(Right)** *Axial T2 MR in a different patient with neck trauma and cervical fractures reveals traumatic VA dissection as loss of right vertebral flow void ➔ as compared to the normal left side ➔. Note right cervical hemicord hyperintensity from infarction ➔.*

KEY FACTS

TERMINOLOGY

- Brachial plexus schwannoma: Benign Schwann cell neoplasm that **arises from brachial plexus** (BP)

IMAGING

- General imaging features
  - Well-circumscribed, **fusiform mass** along course of BP
  - Occur along course of BP in any segment
    - Intradural → extradural → neural foramen → perivertebral space (PVS) → axillary apex
  - In PVS between anterior & middle scalene muscles
- CECT & enhanced MR findings
  - Larger schwannomas show **intramural cysts**
  - MR better for depicting nerve branch of origin
  - 3D STIR to produce MR neurography depicts BP normal anatomy and schwannomas

TOP DIFFERENTIAL DIAGNOSES

- Systemic nodal metastases
- Neurofibroma
- Lateral meningocele

PATHOLOGY

- 5% of benign soft tissue neoplasms
- Firm, encapsulated, fusiform mass
- Cystic degeneration & hemorrhage common
- Attaches to and displaces nerve
- Multiple schwannomas occur with multiple inherited schwannomas, meningiomas, ependymomas, & schwannomatosis

CLINICAL ISSUES

- Clinical presentation
  - Painless, slow-growing mass in lateral neck
  - ± radiculopathy
- Treatment options
  - Surgical resection curative
  - Observation or XRT other options

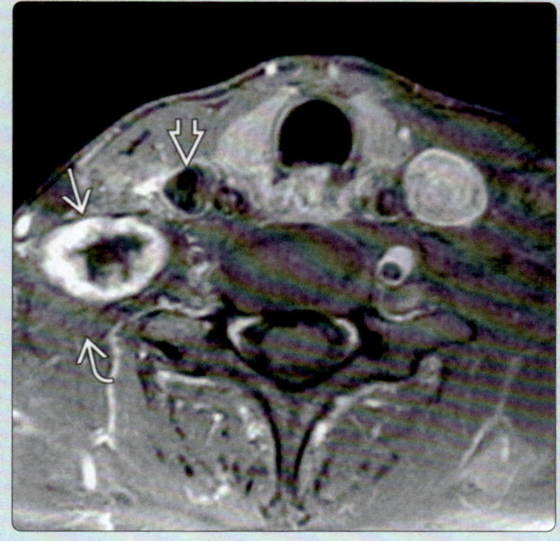

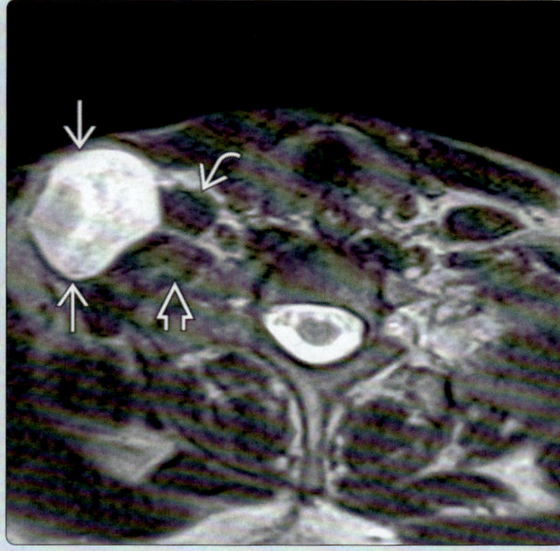

(Left) *Axial T1WI C+ FS MR demonstrates a large schwannoma ➡ in the lower right neck overlying the middle scalene muscle ➡ with intense, irregular peripheral enhancement. Central nonenhancement represents cystic degeneration. The lesion is more lateral in location than expected for lower cervical nodes, which typically abut the internal jugular vein ➡.* **(Right)** *Axial T2WI MR shows heterogeneously hyperintense schwannoma in lower neck ➡ splaying & deforming anterior ➡ & middle ➡ scalene muscles in perivertebral space.*

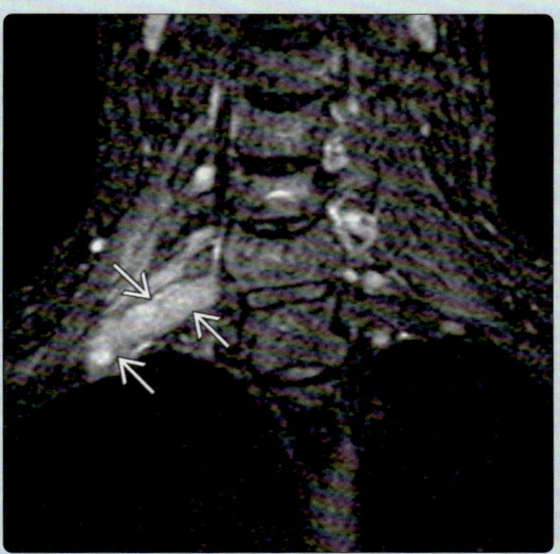

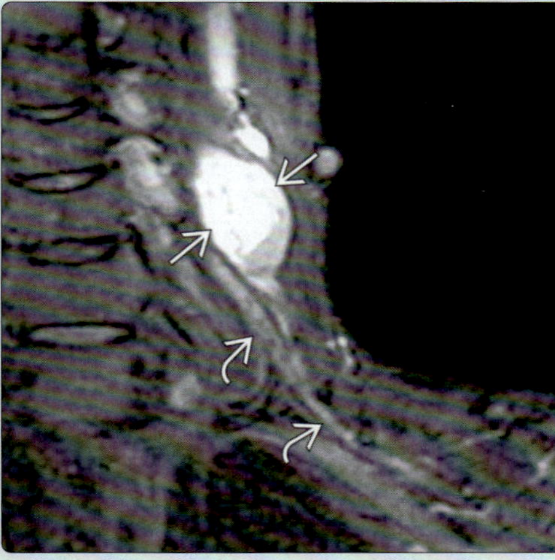

(Left) *Coronal STIR MR (MR neurography technique) demonstrates an asymmetrically enlarged right CNVIII nerve root ➡ extending from the CNVII-T1 neural foramen.* **(Right)** *Coronal STIR MR in a different patient shows a fusiform, heterogeneously hyperintense schwannoma ➡ of the lower neck. Note marked hyperintensity as compared to the adjacent brachial plexus elements ➡ that the lesion parallels. Needle biopsy caused arm twitching but did confirm diagnosis.*

Chordoma in Perivertebral Space

KEY FACTS

TERMINOLOGY

- Chordoma definition: Rare low-grade primary malignant tumor of notochord origin

IMAGING

- General imaging findings
  - Upper cervical spine C2-5 most often
  - Lytic vertebral body (VB) lesion without collapse
- CT findings
  - Lobulated low-density mass emanating from VB
  - Coarse, amorphous **calcifications** in **30%**
- MR findings
  - **Marked T2 hyperintensity**, similar to CSF
  - Typically heterogeneous enhancement
- FDG PET: Heterogeneous, increased uptake

TOP DIFFERENTIAL DIAGNOSES

- VB metastasis
- Prevertebral space infection
- Brachial plexus schwannoma
- Vertebral chondrosarcoma

PATHOLOGY

- Arises from embryonic notochord
  - Sacrococcygeal > clival > vertebral
- 5% all chordomas arise in cervical spine
- Lobulated, soft, grayish mass with pseudocapsule
- Characteristic **physaliphorous** and **epithelioid chief cells**

CLINICAL ISSUES

- Clinical presentation
  - 3rd-6th decade, peaks in 5th decade
  - Local pressure effects on cord or prevertebral structures
  - Nonspecific neck pain ± mass
    - Myelopathy ± radiculopathy
- Treatment issues
  - Surgery, then follow with radiotherapy
  - Late local recurrence common

(Left) *Sagittal T2 MR in a patient with neck swelling & a palpable mass demonstrates a large, multilevel, markedly hyperintense chordoma arising from the cervical vertebral body (VB) with a large soft tissue component extending into the perivertebral space (PVS)* ➡. **(Right)** *Axial T2* image demonstrates cervical chordoma that erodes the VB* ➡, *extending into the epidural space and spinal canal* ➡, *with bulky tumor in the PVS* ➡. *Tumor is contiguous with right vertebral artery* ➡. *Lobulated configuration is well shown.*

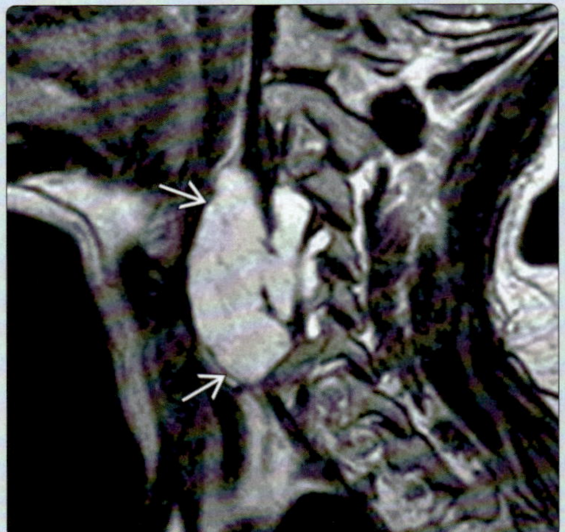

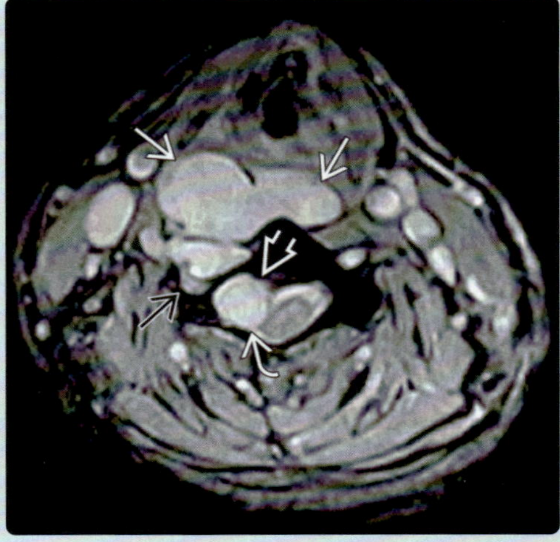

(Left) *Coronal CT reformat demonstrates cervical chordoma involving contiguous C2 and C3 levels. The mass has extensive bone destruction with relatively well-defined margins* ➡ *and with no discernible matrix. The lesion extends into and involves the neural foramen* ➡. **(Right)** *Axial T2WI MR of typical cervical chordoma with PVS extension* ➡ *without VB destruction is shown. The mass extends into the neural foramen with epidural extension* ➡ *and nearly encases the left vertebral artery* ➡.

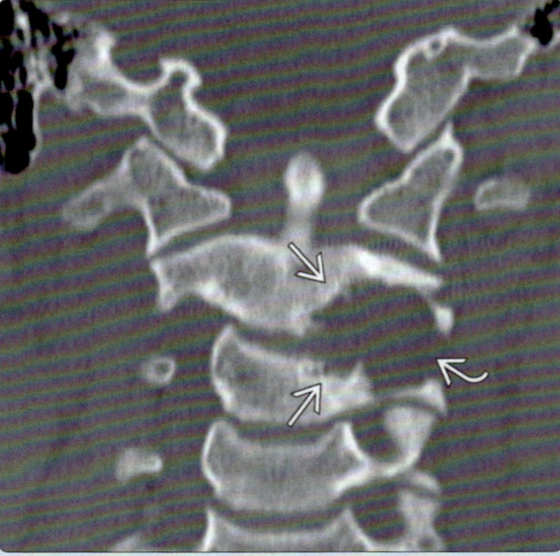

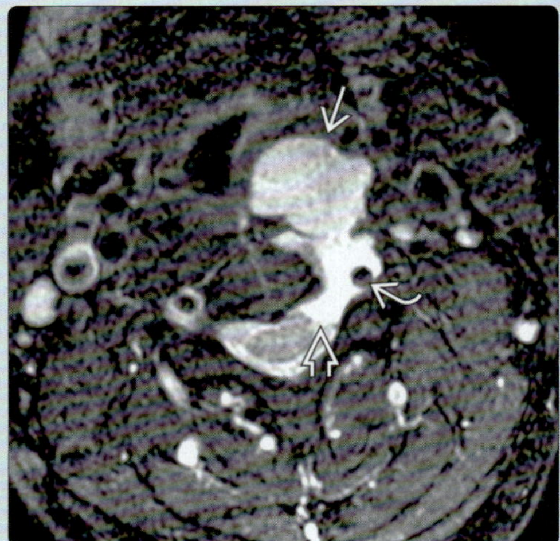

KEY FACTS

TERMINOLOGY

- Definition: Metastatic tumor to cervical vertebral body (VB) ± invasion of perivertebral space (PVS)

IMAGING

- CECT or enhanced MR
  - Destructive VB mass
  - Infiltrated or anteriorly displaced prevertebral muscles
  - > 50% have multiple level involvement

TOP DIFFERENTIAL DIAGNOSES

- PVS infection
- Longus colli tendinitis
- PVS chordoma

PATHOLOGY

- Vertebral metastases may be confined by **prevertebral fascia**, directing tumor to **epidural space**
  - Lumbar > thoracic > cervical spine
- Most VB metastases from hematogenous spread
  - Spinal metastases proportionate to red marrow
- VB metastasis is most common malignant spine lesion
  - Vertebra is most common site of bone metastasis
- In adults is most often lung, breast, prostate, kidney, GI
- In children is most often hematologic malignancies & neuroblastoma

CLINICAL ISSUES

- Clinical presentation
  - Adult with known primary tumor presenting with spine pain & neurological compromise
- Treatment depends on tumor type, symptomatology, and neurological complications
  - Radiation therapy ± stereotactic radiotherapy
  - Endovascular tumor embolization
  - Vertebroplasty
  - Surgical resection for cord decompression ± spine stabilization

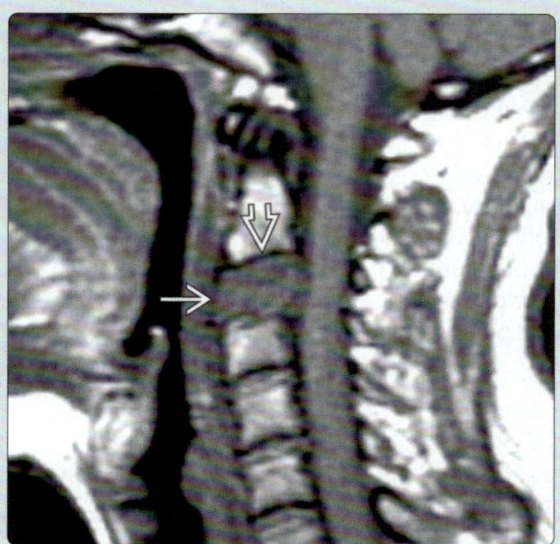

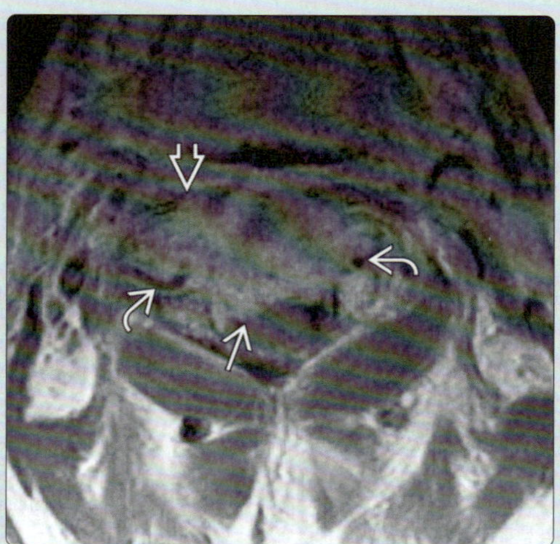

(Left) *Sagittal T1WI MR reveals a C3 vertebral body (VB) replaced by renal cell carcinoma metastasis. There is anterior extension into the perivertebral space (PVS) ➡. Note diffusely hypointense VB marrow with preservation of adjacent disc space ➡.* **(Right)** *Axial T1WI C+ MR in a patient with upper limb symptoms and a past history of breast cancer shows enhancing C2 vertebra with epidural ➡ and prevertebral ➡ extension. Note that the tumor abuts and partially surrounds the vertebral arteries ➡.*

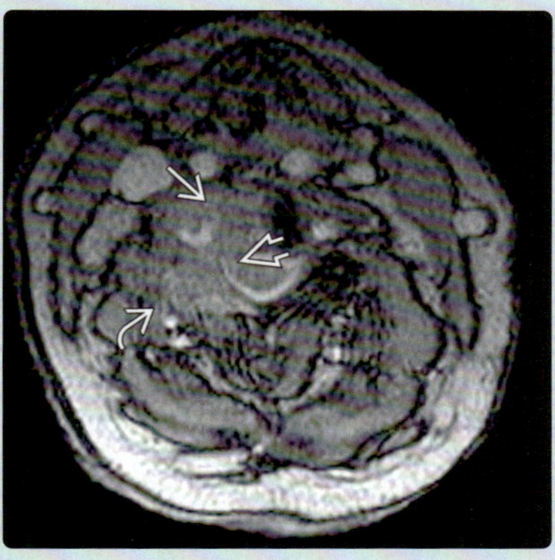

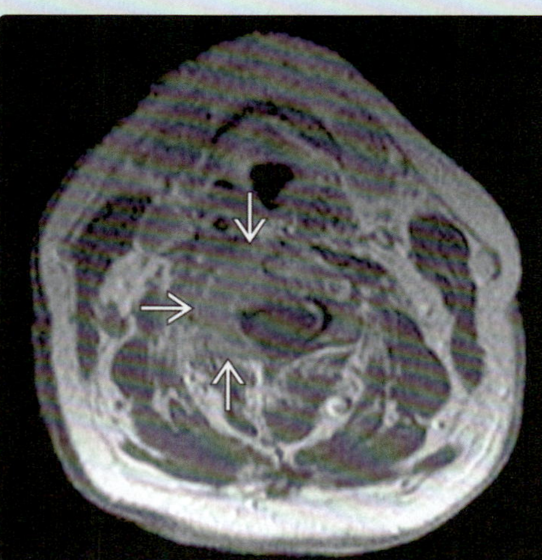

(Left) *Axial T2 GRE shows high signal intensity of osseous metastases involving the VB, posterior elements, and extending into the prevertebral ➡ and paraspinal ➡ portions of the PVS. Minimal epidural tumor ➡ is present.* **(Right)** *Postcontrast axial T1 MR shows diffuse enhancement throughout the C4 lesion ➡ with better depiction of the tumor interface with the muscle and subarachnoid space.*

Summary Thoughts: Posterior Cervical Space

The **posterior cervical space** (**PCS**) lies in the lateral neck deep to the sternocleidomastoid (SCM) and trapezius muscles and includes the triangle of fat between them. This triangle of fat is superficial to the paraspinal muscles and is known clinically as the **posterior triangle** of the neck. The PCS is small superiorly, encompassing just a region of tissue around the mastoid tip, but it expands inferiorly to encompass most of the lateral neck.

The most frequent pathology to affect the PCS is inflammatory or malignant **lymphadenopathy** in the spinal accessory chain. Identifying the likely source of the primary tumor is of great importance. Other pathology in the PCS is often related to CNXI, which runs obliquely across the PCS, or the brachial plexus, which traverses the lower PCS.

Imaging Approaches and Indications

Masses and inflammation of the PCS may be imaged either with CECT or MR of the neck, depending on regional preferences. Be sure to evaluate the entire PCS, from the mastoid tip to the clavicles.

Imaging Anatomy

Superficial PCS **anatomic boundaries** include the SCM and trapezius muscles and the superficial space (platysma and subcutaneous fat). Deep to the PCS lies the prevertebral (more anteriorly) and paraspinal (more posteriorly) portions of the perivertebral space (PVS). Anteromedial to the PCS, the carotid space (CS) is found.

The PCS has complex **fascial boundaries**. The deep margin of the PCS is separated from the PVS by the deep layer of the deep cervical fascia (DCF); the superficial margin of the PCS is separated from the SCM and trapezius, as well as from the superficial space, by the superficial (investing) layer of the DCF. The PCS is separated from the CS by all 3 layers of the DCF that make up the carotid sheath.

The main **PCS contents** are fat, lymph nodes, and the spinal accessory nerve (CNXI). The nerve lies along the floor of the space, running obliquely from anterosuperior to posteroinferior. The nodes included are predominantly from the **spinal accessory chain**, along with portions of the transverse cervical chain. This corresponds to **level V** if the nodes are strictly posterior to the posterior border of the SCM or **levels IIB, III, and IV** if the nodes are deep to the SCM.

Segments of the **brachial plexus** run through the PCS. After the trunks of the brachial plexus emerge from the scalene triangle between the anterior and middle scalene muscles, they ramify into divisions and then cords within the PCS before continuing into the axilla.

The dorsal scapular nerve and segmental cervical nerve roots also traverse the PCS, as does the 3rd portion of the subclavian artery, but the bulk of the PCS is filled with **fat**.

While radiologists divide the neck into fascial-lined spaces, clinicians divide the neck into muscular triangles. The triangle that corresponds to the PCS is the **posterior triangle** of the neck, between the SCM and trapezius muscles. The posterior triangle can be subdivided into the occipital and subclavian triangles using the inferior belly of the omohyoid muscle as the dividing line. The occipital triangle is superior to the omohyoid, whereas the subclavian triangle is inferior.

- Occipital triangle contains fat, CNXI, dorsal scapular nerve, and spinal accessory nodes
- Subclavian triangle contains 3rd portion of subclavian artery and brachial plexus

Approaches to Imaging Issues of Posterior Cervical Space

Multiple imaging findings help answer the question, "What defines a mass as being in the PCS?" First, the lesion should arise within the PCS fat. Larger PCS masses will displace the CS anteromedially, elevate the SCM (aggressive malignancies may invade into SCM, obliterating the intervening fat), and flatten the deeper prevertebral and paraspinal muscles.

The PCS contains nodes from both level V and levels II through IV. This situation yields the question, "How can these nodal stations be distinguished?" Draw an imaginary line from the posterior border of one SCM to the posterior border of the other SCM. If the center of the affected node is posterior to this line, the node is assigned to level V. If it is anterior to this line, it is a level II-IV internal jugular node. The level II-IV nodes are sorted by horizontal landmarks. If the node is above the hyoid bone, it belongs to level II. If it is below the cricoid cartilage, it belongs to level IV, while between these landmarks lies level III.

Clinical Implications

PCS masses can affect function of CNXI, but the most frequent source of CNXI dysfunction is prior surgery in the PCS. When CNXI is injured or resected, the SCM and trapezius muscles atrophy. Acutely, the muscles may enlarge and enhance, but, chronically, the muscles shrink and undergo fatty infiltration. In postsurgical patients, the SCM has often been resected, so atrophy of the trapezius muscle may be the only radiologic clue to prior CNXI injury.

When the trapezius muscle is dysfunctional, the **levator scapulae muscle** takes over its function in elevating the scapula. The levator scapulae muscle is one of the lateral paraspinal muscles. When it hypertrophies, it may be mistaken for a pathologic mass (such as recurrent tumor) both clinically and radiologically.

Differential Diagnosis

PCS Differential Diagnosis by Pathology Category

- Pseudolesion: Cervical rib, levator scapulae hypertrophy
- Congenital: Lymphatic malformation, 3rd branchial cleft cyst
- Inflammatory: Reactive or sarcoid adenopathy
- Infectious: TB adenitis, suppurative adenitis, abscess
- Benign tumor: Lipoma, CNXI or brachial plexus schwannoma or neurofibroma
- Malignant primary tumor: Sarcoma, primary non-Hodgkin lymphoma (NHL) of PCS nodes
- Metastatic nodes: H&N squamous cell carcinoma, NHL, differentiated thyroid cancer, melanoma

Selected References

1. Parker GD et al: Radiologic evaluation of the normal and diseased posterior cervical space. AJR Am J Roentgenol. 157(1):161-5, 1991

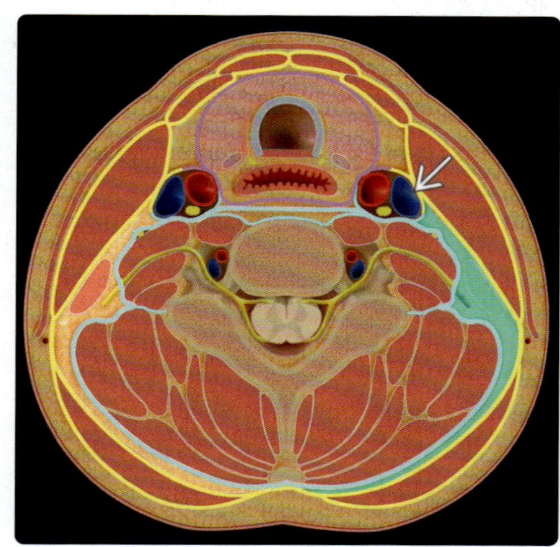

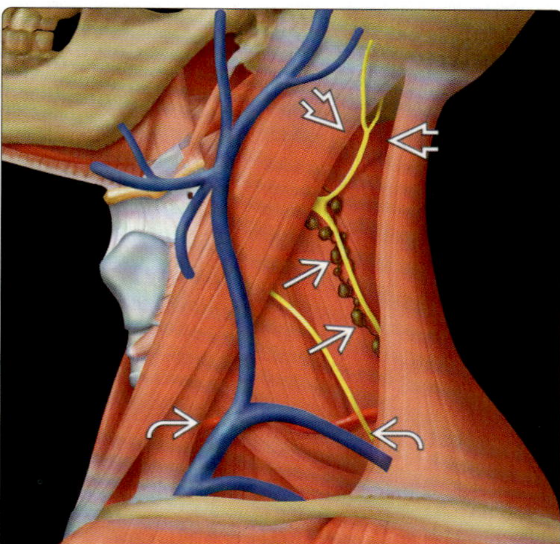

(Left) *Axial graphic depicts the normal posterior cervical space (PCS) (blue-green shading) below the level of the hyoid bone. Complex fascial margins include the superficial layer of the deep cervical fascia (DCF) (yellow line), the deep layer of the DCF (blue line), and the tricolored carotid sheath* ➡ *(containing all 3 layers of DCF).* **(Right)** *Lateral graphic shows that the spinal accessory nodal chain* ➡ *follows the general course of the spinal accessory nerve (CNXI). The PCS is smaller superiorly* ➡ *than inferiorly* ➡*.*

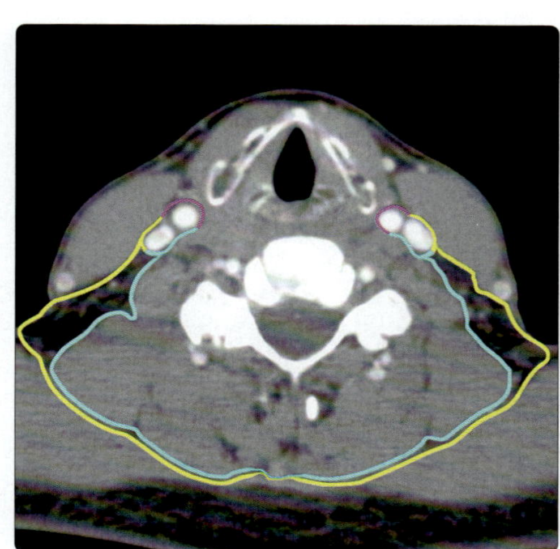

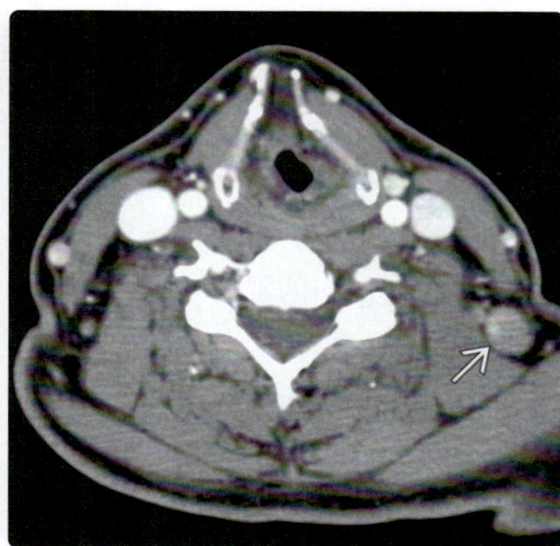

(Left) *Normal axial CECT has the PCS fascial boundaries drawn onto it. The portions of the superficial (yellow) and deep (light blue) layers of the DCF that surround the PCS are depicted.* **(Right)** *Axial CECT of the infrahyoid neck shows a typical PCS mass. This enlarged lymph node* ➡ *lies strictly posterior to the posterior margin of the sternocleidomastoid, so it is classified as level V. Clinically, this mass would be within the posterior triangle.*

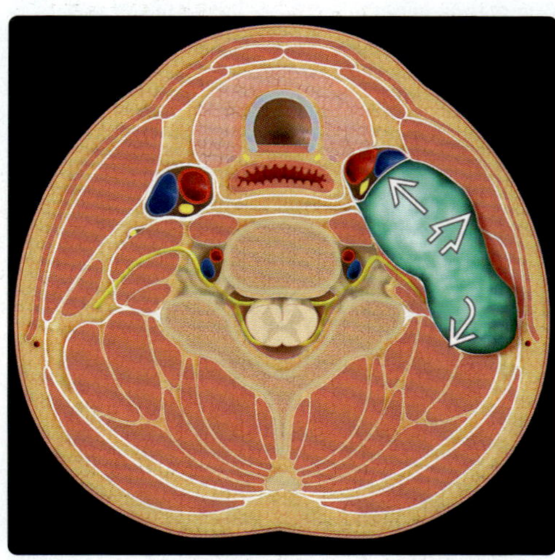

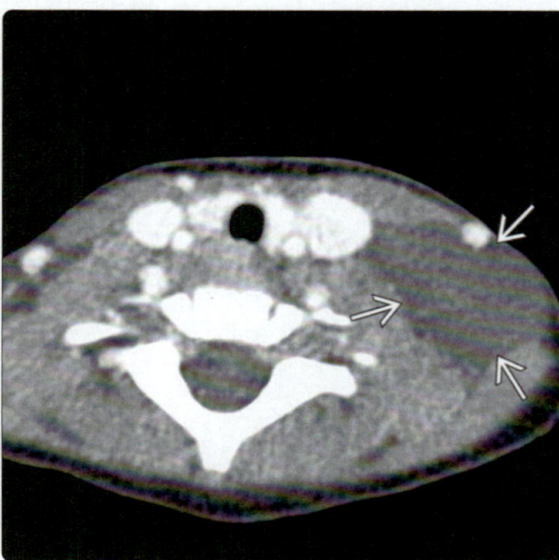

(Left) *Axial graphic of a generic PCS mass reveals compression of the deep paraspinal muscles* ➡*, elevation of the sternocleidomastoid muscle* ➡*, and anteromedial displacement of the carotid sheath* ➡*.* **(Right)** *Axial CECT demonstrates an ill-defined, low-density mass* ➡ *filling the infrahyoid PCS. The conformational configuration, uniform low density (fluid), and lack of enhancement are strongly suggestive of the diagnosis lymphatic malformation.*

Posterior Cervical Space Schwannoma

KEY FACTS

TERMINOLOGY

- Synonyms: Neuroma, neurinoma, neurilemmoma, nerve sheath tumor
- Schwannoma in PCS primarily from 3 sites
  - Distal brachial plexus root or trunk
  - Cervical sensory nerve
  - CNXI

IMAGING

- CT: Well-delineated, solitary, fusiform mass
  - Isodense to hypodense mass
- MR: Modality of choice for presurgical evaluation
  - Contrast-enhanced images critical
  - Large schwannomas often have **cystic** component
- US: Hypoechoic mass with posterior acoustic enhancement
  - Marked hypervascularity on color Doppler

TOP DIFFERENTIAL DIAGNOSES

- Spinal accessory reactive node
- Spinal accessory squamous cell carcinoma metastatic node
- Spinal accessory non-Hodgkin lymphoma node
- Lymphatic malformation

CLINICAL ISSUES

- Rapid enlargement suggests malignant degeneration
- Core biopsy needed for diagnosis
- Treatment options: Surgical resection most common
  - Excellent long-term results
  - Aim to preserve nerve function (frequently impossible)
  - Conservative imaging surveillance or XRT

DIAGNOSTIC CHECKLIST

- **Look for nerve or foramen of origin**
  - In upper neck from jugular foramen (CNXI), in lower neck from brachial plexus (C5-T1)
  - Mass pointing between anterior and middle scalene indicates brachial plexus origin
- Main differential is solitary PCS nodal mass

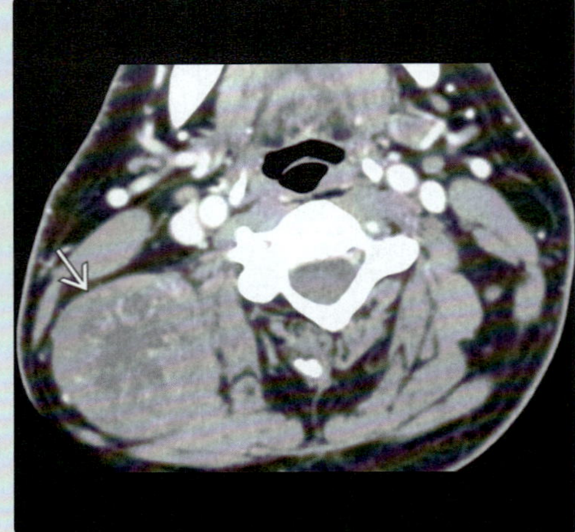

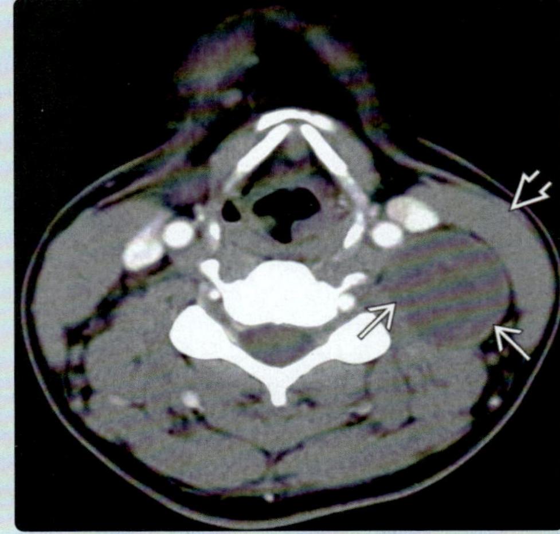

(Left) *Axial CECT demonstrates a large, well-defined mass ➡ in the posterior cervical space (PCS) with heterogeneous enhancement. This schwannoma arises from CNXI, which traverses the PCS.* **(Right)** *Axial CECT shows a round, well-defined, poorly enhancing mass ➡ in the PCS. Schwannomas in this location will sometimes be entirely cystic. Note lateral displacement of the overlying sternocleidomastoid muscle (SCM) ➡ but sparing of the surrounding fat planes.*

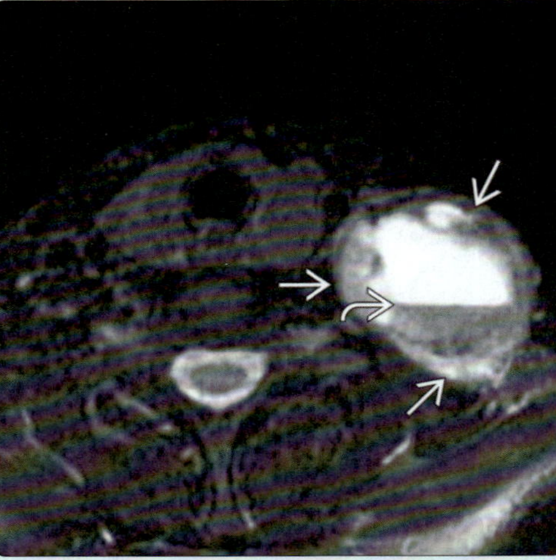

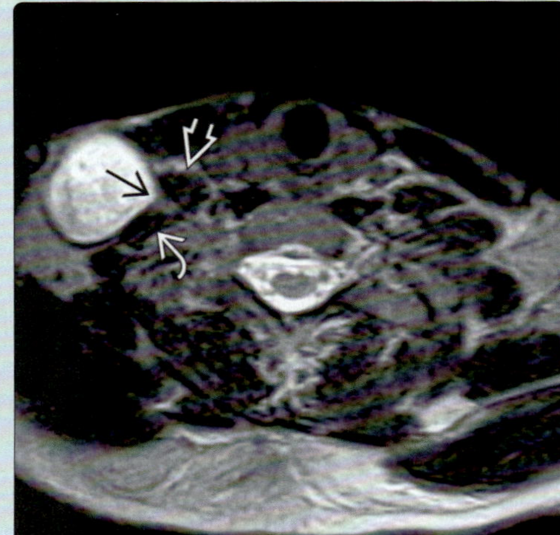

(Left) *Axial T2 FS MR shows a large mass ➡ in the PCS with well-defined margins. It is unusual for a schwannoma to have a fluid level ➡, but it does occur occasionally; this lesion shows internal hemorrhage.* **(Right)** *Axial T2 MR shows a uniformly hyperintense schwannoma in the low right neck with sternocleidomastoid muscle displaced anteromedially. The tumor projects ➡ between the anterior ➡ and middle ➡ scalene muscles, indicating it is from the brachial plexus.*

KEY FACTS

TERMINOLOGY

- Nodal chain accompanying spinal accessory nerve (CNXI)
- Spinal accessory chain divided into level IIB & level V nodes

IMAGING

- **Cervical nodes** concerning for **malignancy** if CECT shows
  - Central nodal **necrosis**
  - Ill-defined margins ± stranding of surrounding fat = **extracapsular spread** (most specific sign)
  - Shape: **Round** node more likely pathologic; uniform nodes likely benign
  - Number: Groups of **≥ 3** borderline enlarged nodes more likely pathologic
  - Size: > **1 cm** in diameter (least specific sign)
- Identification of 1° tumor is important when present
- US- or CT-guided biopsy for equivocal nodes
- CECT best 1st tool for indeterminate neck mass
- PET/CT most appropriate for unknown primary or for staging once SCCa diagnosis established

TOP DIFFERENTIAL DIAGNOSES

- Reactive adenopathy
- Suppurative adenopathy
- Non-Hodgkin lymphoma nodes
- Thyroid cancer node metastasis
- Skin cancer nodal metastasis from scalp/face

PATHOLOGY

- Often nasopharyngeal, oropharyngeal, & hypopharyngeal primaries; thyroid cancer
- Single nodal metastasis ↓ survival by 50%

CLINICAL ISSUES

- Clinical presentation
  - Posterior triangle mass in adult smoker
  - Check for mucosal SCCa primary; thyroid carcinoma
- Treatment options
  - Depends on primary site & nodal stage: Options include neck dissection, chemo, XRT

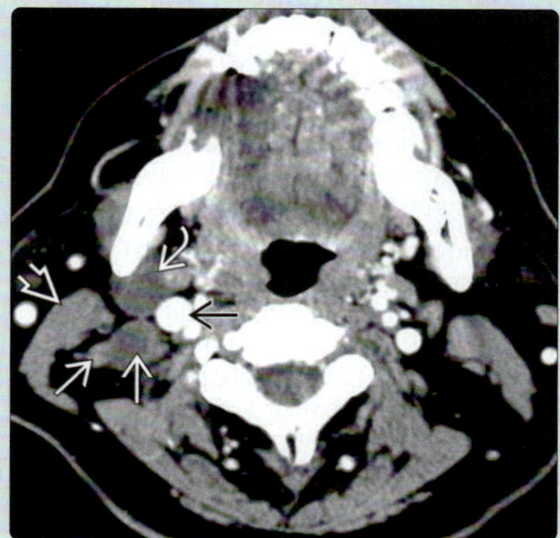

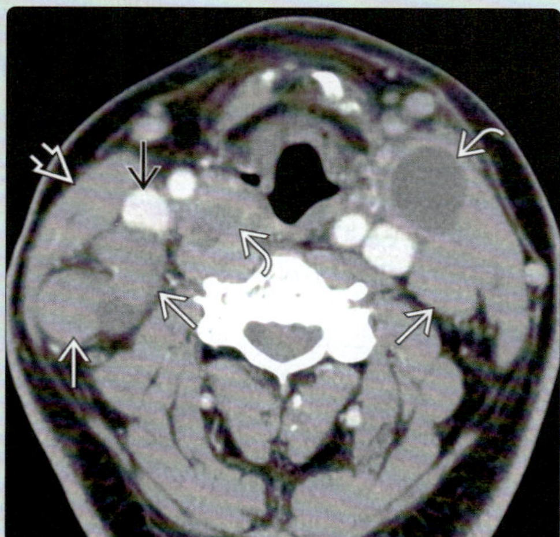

(Left) *Axial CECT shows spinal accessory metastases ➡ from SCCa in level IIB. Note that the nodes are deep to the sternocleidomastoid muscle (SCM) ➡ and posterior to the internal jugular vein (IJV) ➡. Level IIA nodes ➡ are also present, but they are not part of the spinal accessory chain. Central necrosis gives the nodes a cystic appearance.* **(Right)** *Axial CECT shows solidly enhancing nodes ➡ in the spinal accessory chain (level IIB, deep to the SCM ➡ and posterior to the IJV ➡). Other nodal stations are also represented ➡.*

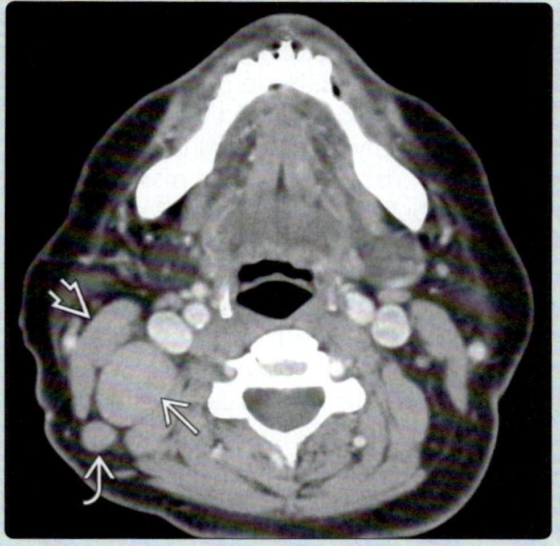

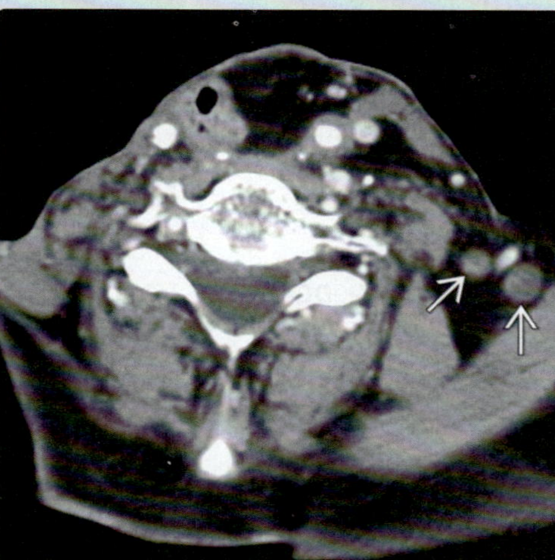

(Left) *Axial CECT shows SCCa in the spinal accessory chain, involving both level IIB ➡ and level V ➡. Note that the level V node lies strictly posterior to the SCM ➡, while the level IIB node is deep to the muscle.* **(Right)** *Axial CECT shows recurrent contralateral spinal accessory nodes ➡ after laryngectomy and right neck dissection. These nodes are low in the neck, such that the spinal accessory nerve is along the posterior aspect of the posterior cervical space.*

Summary Thoughts: Visceral Space

The visceral space (VS) is a tubular space that occupies the midline anterior aspect of the infrahyoid neck. Extending to the superior mediastinum, the VS lies between the laterally placed carotid spaces (CS) and is completely encircled by the **middle layer of deep cervical fascia** (ML-DCF), also known as the **visceral fascia**.

While the largest VS components are the hypopharynx-larynx, trachea, and esophagus, the **thyroid gland** most often necessitates imaging of this space. The other key anatomic elements of the VS are not normally identifiable on routine imaging; the **parathyroid glands** are only evident if hyperplastic or neoplastic, and the **recurrent laryngeal nerves** (RLN) cannot be seen, although their course through the VS must be carefully evaluated whenever vocal cord paralysis is present. The larynx and hypopharynx are covered elsewhere.

Imaging Techniques & Indications

Either CT or MR are excellent modalities for demonstrating the **thyroid** and its relationship to other VS and neck structures. As there is no inferior fascial limit to the VS, any cross-sectional imaging should continue into the superior mediastinum and preferably to the level of the aortopulmonic window. This will encompass the entire course of the left RLN and all of the superior mediastinal nodes. CT is preferred for evaluation of the left RLN as it allows better review of any pulmonary pathology.

If there is clinical suspicion of **thyroid neoplasia**, iodinated contrast should **not** be administered for CT. **Iodinated contrast** is taken up by differentiated thyroid carcinoma (DTCa) and **may delay therapeutic ^{131}I for up to 6 months**.

Ultrasound allows excellent high-resolution evaluation of the thyroid, its adjacent nodes, and, when enlarged, the parathyroid glands. **Color Doppler** should always be used when evaluating a thyroid nodule as increased vascularity is a frequent finding in malignant lesions. It is also important when searching for hypervascular parathyroid adenomas.

Tc-99m-sestamibi is the most sensitive and specific **nuclear medicine** technique for localizing **parathyroid adenomas** and is often supplemented with preoperative ultrasound. When these studies are equivocal or discordant, or in a postoperative patient with recurrent hyperparathyroidism, MR or multidetector CECT techniques may be useful to identify ectopic adenomas. Several different CECT protocols have been described, aiming to capitalize on the arterial phase enhancement of parathyroid adenomas. Some protocols advocate imaging from the skull base to the left pulmonary artery, although suprahyoid ectopic adenomas are rare.

Imaging Anatomy

The VS is the anterior tubular space in the midline of the infrahyoid neck. It is completely encircled by the **ML-DCF**. The VS shares a common fascial wall with the retropharyngeal space, which is immediately posterior and contains only fat in the infrahyoid neck (no nodes). The VS is surrounded anteriorly and anterolaterally by the strap muscles, sternocleidomastoid muscles, and the anterior cervical fat. Both muscle groups are enclosed by the superficial layer of the deep cervical fascia. The CSs are at the lateral margin of the VS, with all 3 layers of the deep cervical fascia contributing to the **carotid sheaths**.

The **larynx** and **hypopharynx** are infrahyoid continuations of the oropharynx, and these structures are contiguous with the **trachea** and **esophagus**, respectively, which then traverse the VS to the mediastinum.

The paired thyroid lobes are joined by a midline isthmus. The **thyroid** lobes "cup" the cricoid cartilage and 1st tracheal rings. It is this intimate relation that allows thyroid tumors to invade the trachea.

There are 2 pairs of **parathyroid glands**. The superior glands are consistently found at the posterosuperior aspect of the thyroid, in the lateral aspect of the tracheoesophageal groove (TEG). The inferior lobes are in a similar position near the inferior aspect of the thyroid; however, they are less reliably found in this location. They are often found lower in the neck or within the superior mediastinum.

Paratracheal nodes are found in the TEG and are commonly referred to as **level VI nodes**.

Also located in the TEG, the **RLNs** ascend in the neck to the level of the cricothyroid joint, where they enter the larynx to supply the vocal cords. The **right RLN** arises from the vagus nerve in the low neck then loops around the subclavian artery to enter the inferior VS. The **left RLN** arises more inferiorly, looping beneath the aortic arch before ascending to the VS.

Approaches to Imaging Issues of Visceral Space

Infrahyoid neck lesions differ from suprahyoid masses in that their **space of origin** is typically not an imaging dilemma. The VS has carotid sheaths on either side but is not otherwise surrounded by sources of pathological processes in the same way that the suprahyoid neck spaces are. The VS does, however, have several common diagnostic dilemmas.

The **"nonspecific" thyroid mass** incidentally found on CT or MR is the most common imaging dilemma in the VS. This type of lesion is a well-defined round or oval mass within the thyroid gland, with or without calcifications, cystic change, or hemorrhage, and is not associated with adenopathy. Sharply delineated contours are found with benign colloid cysts and thyroid adenomas; however, they may also be seen with DTCa (papillary and follicular) and with medullary thyroid carcinoma.

- **Calcifications** are not an uncommon feature in **adenomas**, whereas fine, speckled calcifications are a frequent finding in DTCa, particularly the papillary type. Coarse calcifications may be found in **medullary thyroid carcinoma**. **Hemorrhage** or **cystic degeneration** within a thyroid adenoma results in a very heterogeneous appearance of a mass, which mimics malignant necrotic change. Finally, the size of thyroid lesion does not indicate any particular pathology. Benign thyroid adenomas can grow to many centimeters in size, whereas malignant thyroid papillary carcinomas may only be several millimeters but already metastatic to nodes.
- Clearly there is a large overlap of benign and malignant features with **CT** and **MR**. The most concerning characteristics on these modalities are invasive features, such as extrathyroidal extension with infiltration of adjacent tissues or associated neck adenopathy. Such cases do not pose a significant imaging dilemma and should all be referred for fine-needle aspiration (FNA).
- **Ultrasound** is able to identify unique imaging features that are most concerning for malignancy and hence is often the 2nd-line study after a lesion is found on CT or MR. Thyroid ultrasound will frequently identify

Differential Diagnosis: Visceral Space

Pseudolesion	**Metabolic**
Thyroid pyramidal lobe	Multinodular goiter
Patulous cervical esophagus	**Benign tumor**
Inflammatory	Thyroid adenoma
Chronic lymphocytic thyroiditis (Hashimoto)	Parathyroid adenoma
Infectious	Recurrent laryngeal nerve schwannoma
Suppurative thyroiditis	**Malignant tumor**
Congenital	Differentiated thyroid carcinoma (DTCa)
Infrahyoid thyroglossal duct cyst (± 4th branchial cleft anomaly)	Paratracheal node from DTCa
Degenerative	Thyroid anaplastic carcinoma
Colloid cyst of thyroid	Thyroid non-Hodgkin lymphoma
Parathyroid cyst	Systemic metastasis to thyroid
Esophagopharyngeal diverticulum (Zenker)	Parathyroid carcinoma
Lateral cervical esophageal diverticulum	Tracheal adenoid cystic carcinoma
Tracheal diverticulum	Cervical esophageal carcinoma

characteristics of a **multinodular goiter (MNG)** when only 1 nodule was originally evident on clinical or CECT evaluation. Ultrasound also allows differentiation between a **cystic**, and therefore benign, thyroid lesion from a **solid lesion** and allows image-guided FNA of the latter.

- On **PET/CT** imaging, diffuse thyroid uptake is not an uncommon finding and may be due to **thyroiditis**. Thyroid function tests can determine whether the patient has subclinical hypothyroidism. **Focal** thyroid FDG **uptake** has ~ **20%** chance of **malignancy**. FNA should be obtained if this is incidentally found during PET imaging.

TEG lesions may also prove to be a VS diagnostic dilemma. TEG lesions reside in or efface the triangle of fat between the posterior wall of the trachea and the anterior margin of the esophagus. Well-defined nodules (< 1 cm and clearly distinct from the thyroid, trachea, and esophagus) may be **level VI lymph nodes**. These are a drainage site for thyroid malignancies but also squamous cell carcinoma of the larynx, hypopharynx, and esophagus and are often involved in non-Hodgkin lymphoma. Searching for other nodes and a primary source is helpful in making this diagnosis. **Parathyroid adenomas** may mimic nodes unless arterial-phase imaging is performed, in which most appear **hypervascular** with distinctive avid enhancement. **Schwannomas** here are rare and are difficult to diagnose prospectively. The differential for these well-defined lesions is an exophytic thyroid or esophageal mass, such as an adenoma or diverticulum, respectively. Multiplanar imaging may clarify these relationships.

- When soft tissue **infiltrates the TEG** and effaces its fat triangle, the differential favors a **malignant process**, such as thyroid, parathyroid, or esophageal carcinoma or thyroid lymphoma. These neoplastic processes more often present clinically with disruption of the RLN and **vocal cord paralysis**.

Clinical Implications

Patients may be referred for cross-sectional imaging with either a **midline neck mass** ± **lateral neck mass(es)** from **adenopathy**. When protocoling such a study, it is important to remember that, if DTCa is a possible cause, consideration should be given to ultrasound, MR, or even NECT rather than CECT. Iodinated contrast can delay therapeutic ^{131}I up to 6 months. Clinical indicators of possible thyroid cancer include young women with neck masses, particularly low neck masses &/or cystic lymph nodes, and masses associated with vocal cord paralysis.

There are 3 main considerations for a **rapidly growing VS mass**: (1) Hemorrhage or cystic degeneration of thyroid adenoma, (2) anaplastic thyroid carcinoma, and (3) thyroid lymphoma. The latter 2 lesions can appear quite similar on imaging, although lymphoma is more frequently a homogeneous lesion. Calcifications, cystic change, and hemorrhage are much less common in lymphoma than anaplastic carcinoma, which is typically heterogeneous and has a greater tendency to invade the trachea.

When imaging is required for preoperative evaluation of the complete extent of a **MNG**, 2 considerations must be kept in mind: (1) The scan is performed with the patient's arms by his or her side so as not to exaggerate the substernal extension that occurs with the patient's arms are positioned over their head, and (2) up to 5% of MNGs harbor a focus of DTCa. While most often these are small foci that have not metastasized, the neck should be carefully evaluated for adenopathy and any invasive features of the thyroid contours that might make surgery complex.

Selected References

1. Sofferman RA et al. Ultrasound of the thyroid and parathyroid glands. New York: Springer, 2012
2. Loevner LA et al: Cross-sectional imaging of the thyroid gland. Neuroimaging Clin N Am. 18(3):445-61, vii, 2008
3. Parker EE et al: MR imaging of the thoracic inlet. Magn Reson Imaging Clin N Am. 16(2):341-53, x, 2008
4. Babbel RW et al: The visceral space: the unique infrahyoid space. Semin Ultrasound CT MR. 12(3):204-23, 1991

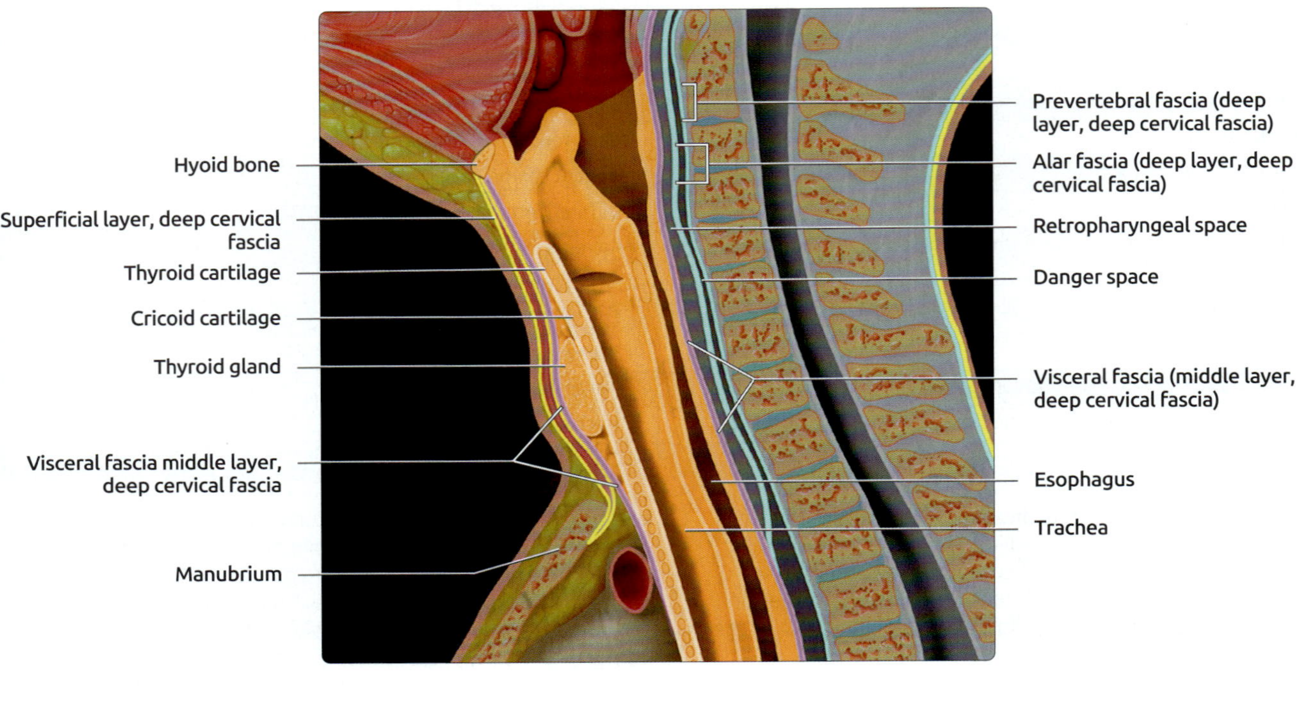

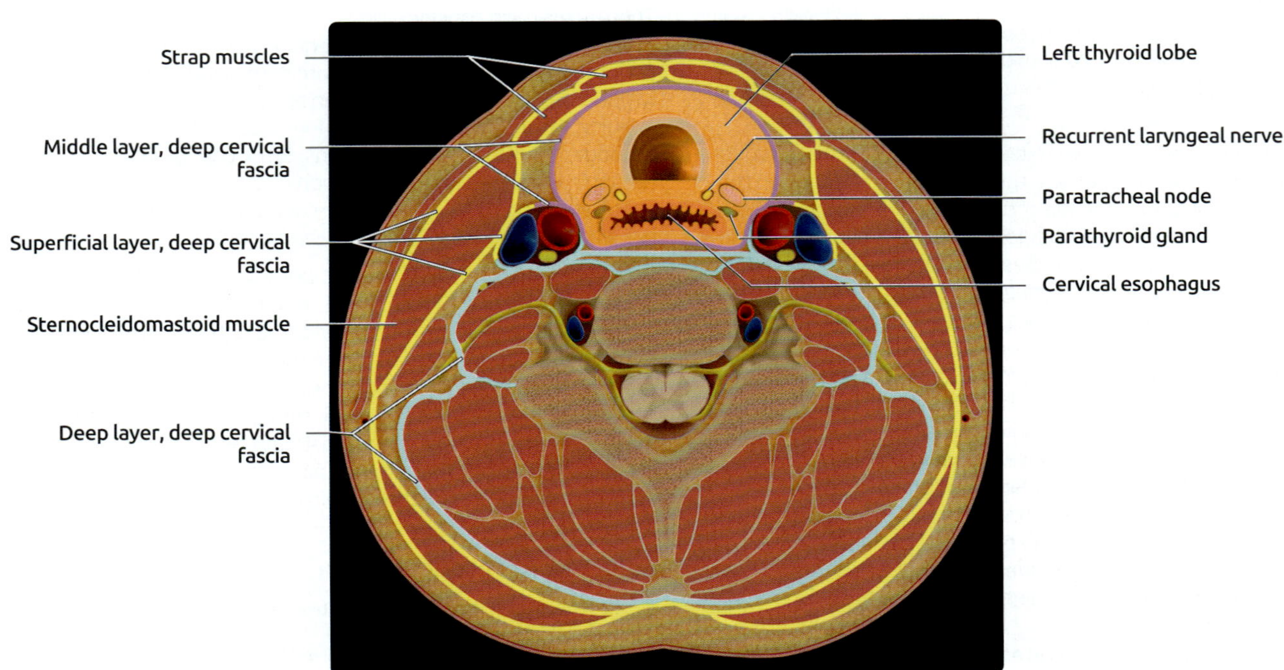

(Top) *Sagittal graphic illustrates the craniocaudal extent of the visceral space (VS) in the anterior aspect of the neck. At the hyoid bone, the superficial and middle layers of deep cervical fascia (DCF) insert. The superficial layer encloses the strap muscles of the anterior neck and sternocleidomastoid muscles of the lateral neck. These muscles surround but are separate from the VS. The middle layer of DCF surrounds the VS. The larynx and cervical trachea and the hypopharynx and cervical esophagus form longitudinal columns within this space from the hyoid to the mediastinum.* **(Bottom)** *Axial graphic depicts the anterior central location of the VS in the infrahyoid neck, between the carotid sheaths. Other important VS structures surround the larynx/trachea and the hypopharynx/esophagus, such as the thyroid gland, superior and inferior parathyroid glands, and level VI lymph nodes. The recurrent laryngeal nerves (RLNs) course superiorly to the larynx in the tracheoesophageal grooves.*

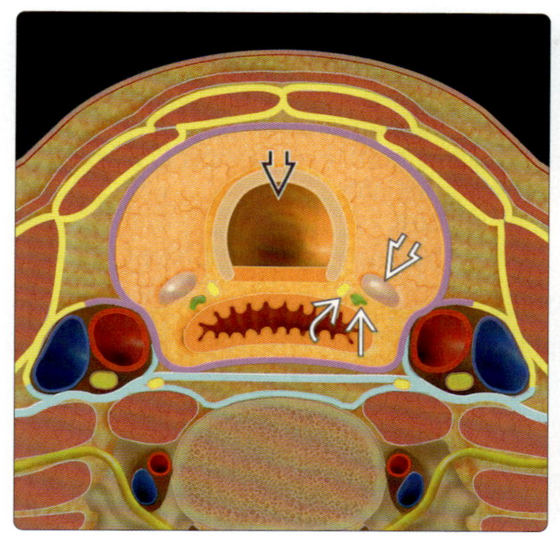

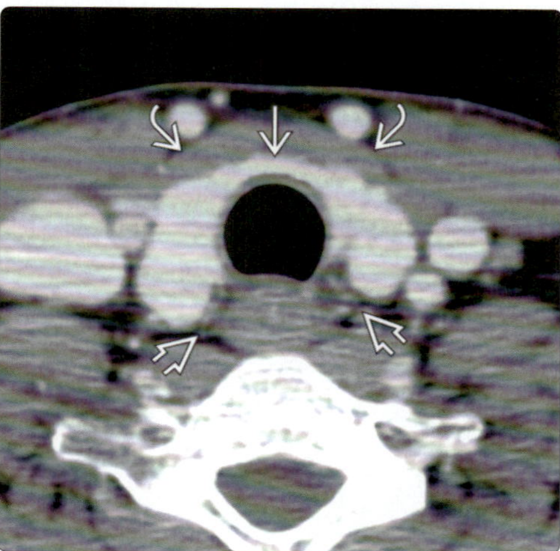

(Left) *Axial graphic depicts the thyroid gland in the anterior VS wrapping around the trachea ⇨. Graphic also illustrates 3 key structures found in the tracheoesophageal groove: the RLN ➡, paratracheal lymph nodes ➡, and parathyroid gland ➡.* **(Right)** *Axial CECT at the level of the thyroid gland isthmus ➡ (which crosses the anterior surface of trachea beneath the strap muscles ➡) shows normal fat, small vessels, and tiny lymph nodes in the tracheoesophageal groove ➡.*

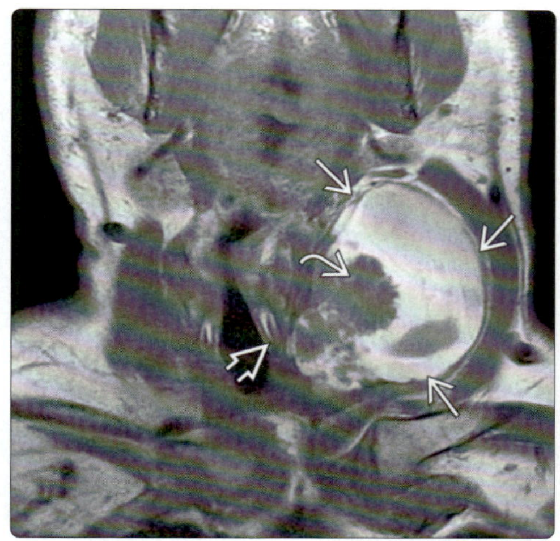

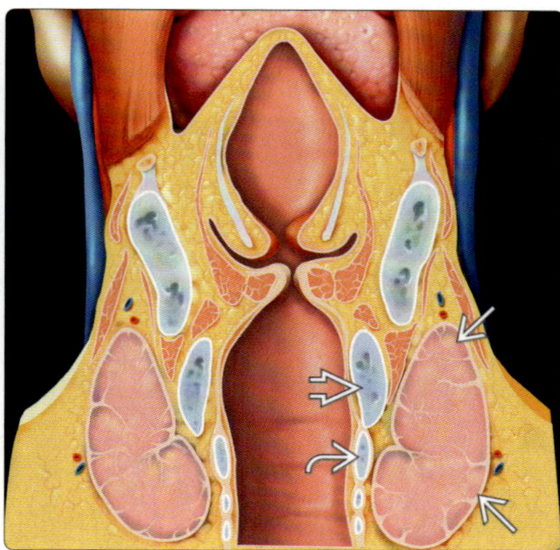

(Left) *Coronal T1 MR shows a heterogeneous solid ➡ and cystic ➡ infrahyoid neck mass arising from the left thyroid. Note the intrinsic hyperintensity within the cystic component from thyroglobulin. This was found to be papillary thyroid carcinoma, displacing the larynx without cricoid ➡ invasion.* **(Right)** *Coronal graphic shows the relationship of thyroid ➡ to cricoid cartilage ➡ & the 1st tracheal ring ➡. It is important to carefully examine cricoid and proximal trachea for invasion of malignant thyroid tumor.*

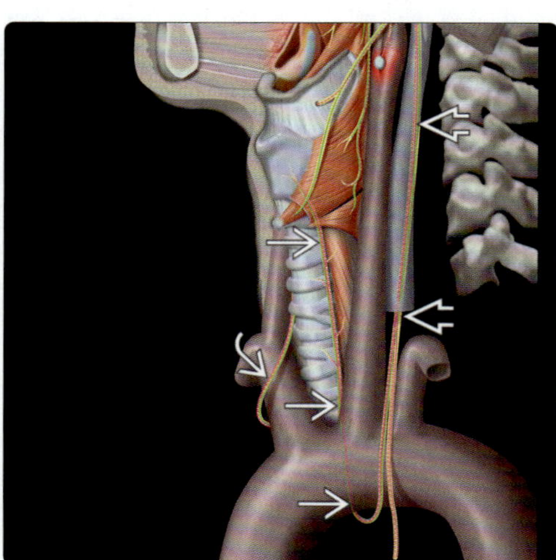

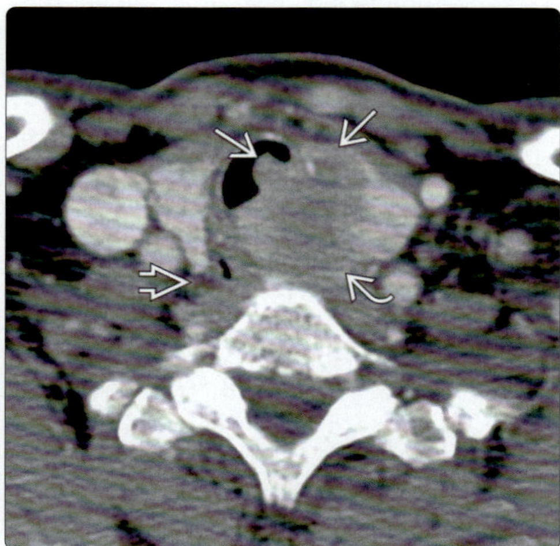

(Left) *Lateral graphic illustrates the ascending course of the RLNs in the tracheoesophageal groove of the VS. Left RLN ➡ arises from the left vagus ➡ in the superior mediastinum. Right RLN ➡ arises from the vagus at the level of the subclavian artery.* **(Right)** *Axial CECT in a patient with left RLN paralysis shows a heterogeneous mass within the left thyroid lobe ➡ that invades trachea & is inseparable from esophagus. Fat of left tracheoesophageal groove appears infiltrated ➡ compared with normal right side ➡.*

Chronic Lymphocytic Thyroiditis (Hashimoto)

KEY FACTS

TERMINOLOGY

- Hashimoto thyroiditis, chronic/sclerosing lymphocytic thyroiditis

IMAGING

- Best imaging modality is US for diagnosis & monitoring
  - US: Early stage shows enlarged lobulated thyroid, decreased echogenicity, & marked hypervascularity
  - US: Late stage shows small echogenic fibrosed gland with absent flow signals
- CECT: Diffuse moderately **enlarged**, **low-density thyroid** without calcifications, cysts, or necrosis

TOP DIFFERENTIAL DIAGNOSES

- Multinodular goiter
- Invasive fibrous (Riedel) thyroiditis
- Thyroid non-Hodgkin lymphoma (NHL)
- Thyroid anaplastic carcinoma

PATHOLOGY

- Some chronic lymphocytic thyroiditis (CLT) occurs in setting of isolated or systemic **Immunoglobulin G4 (IgG4)**-related disease
- Antithyroid autoantibodies in serum
- Micro: Atrophic follicles, Hürthle cell metaplasia, fibrosis, lymphocyte & plasma cell infiltration
- 60-80x risk of thyroid **NHL**
- > 90% of patients with primary thyroid NHL have CLT

CLINICAL ISSUES

- Clinical presentation
  - Most commonly in women 30-50 years old
  - Gradual painless enlargement of thyroid
  - Patients most often euthyroid
- Treatment options
  - Nonsurgical unless large gland compresses airway
  - Thyroid hormone replacement as necessary
  - Long-term follow-up watching for NHL

(Left) *Axial CECT in a patient with CLT shows an enlarged thyroid gland ➡ with inhomogeneous hypodense enhancement & lobulated texture. Heterogeneity & moderate enlargement mimic small multinodular goiter; however, there are no calcifications, hemorrhage, or cystic changes evident.* **(Right)** *CECT in 68-year-old woman with a rapidly enlarging left neck mass shows an ill-defined hypodense left thyroid mass ➡ that was a large B-cell lymphoma developing in background of preexisting CLT at histopathology.*

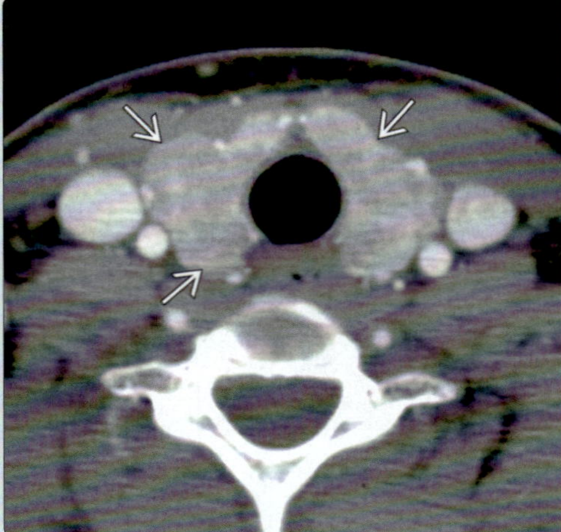

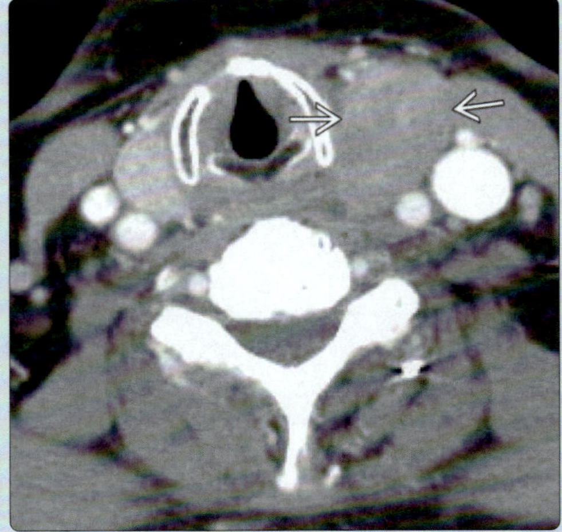

(Left) *Transverse color Doppler US in the early phase of CLT shows diffusely enlarged, hypoechoic left & right ➡ thyroid lobes & thyroid isthmus ➡. Moderate parenchymal hypervascularity is evident.* **(Right)** *Axial T1 C+ MR in a patient with a long history of hypothyroidism and biopsy-proven CLT reveals chronic phase changes with markedly atrophic thyroid so that only the right lobe is evident ➡. This has little appreciable contrast enhancement.*

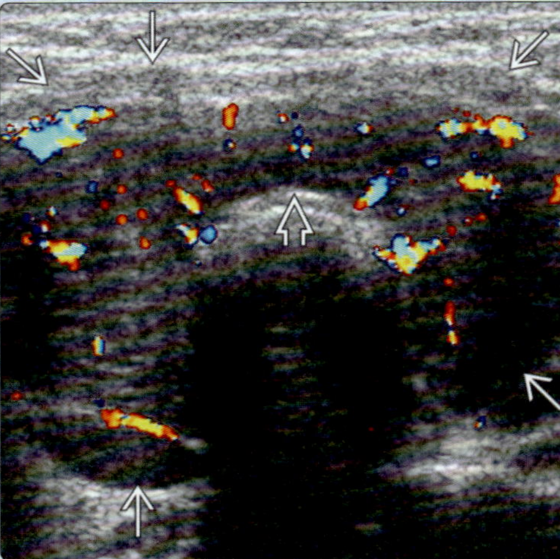

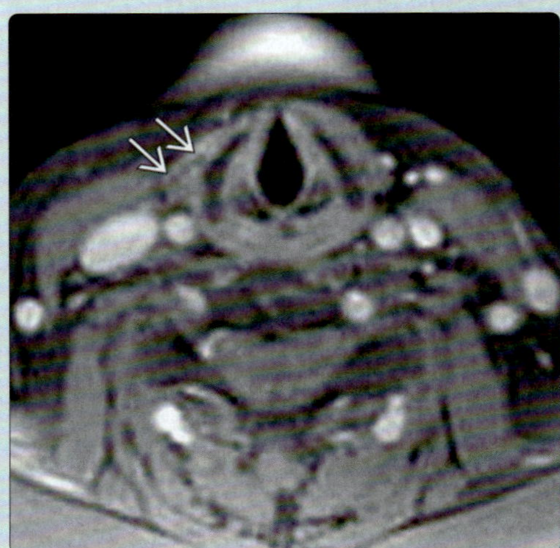

KEY FACTS

TERMINOLOGY

- Diffuse, multinodular thyroid enlargement in response to chronic thyroid stimulating hormone stimulation

IMAGING

- General: Diffuse enlargement of thyroid gland with heterogeneous, multinodular appearance
  - **40%** have **retrosternal extension**
  - Sharp thyroid edge despite bizarre imaging appearance
  - CECT with arms at side; scan to aortic arch
- CT findings: Calcifications, degenerative cysts, & hemorrhage; multinodular goiter (MNG) shows clear delineation from displaced structures
- MR: Heterogeneous signal and enhancement

TOP DIFFERENTIAL DIAGNOSES

- Thyroid colloid cyst or adenoma
- Thyroid differentiated carcinoma
- Thyroid anaplastic carcinoma

PATHOLOGY

- **Sporadic goiter**: Etiology unknown; rarely drug-induced (3-5% of population in developed countries)
- **Endemic goiter**: Associated with iodine deficiency (> 13% of world population affected)
- 5% have malignant focus at surgery
- **Anaplastic thyroid carcinoma** may arise from MNG

CLINICAL ISSUES

- Clinical presentation
  - Large, multinodular lower neck mass
  - Most patients euthyroid, rarely hypothyroid
  - Toxic goiter = MNG + hyperthyroidism; uncommon
  - Plummer disease = toxic adenoma within MNG
- Treatment options
  - Incidental imaging finding, no symptoms: Surveillance
  - Large, nontoxic, compressive MNG: Surgical removal
  - Sternotomy rarely required for retrosternal component but needs to be considered

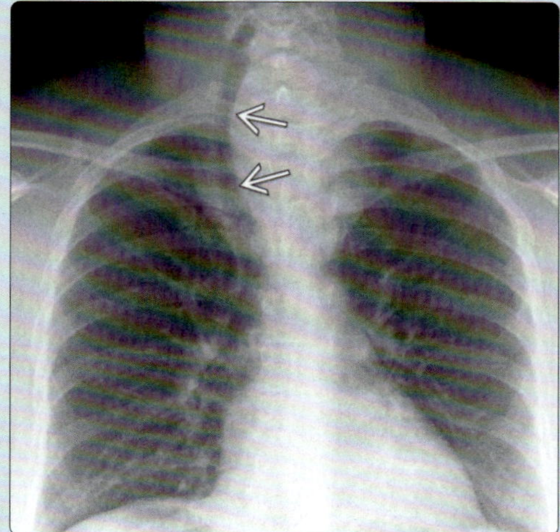

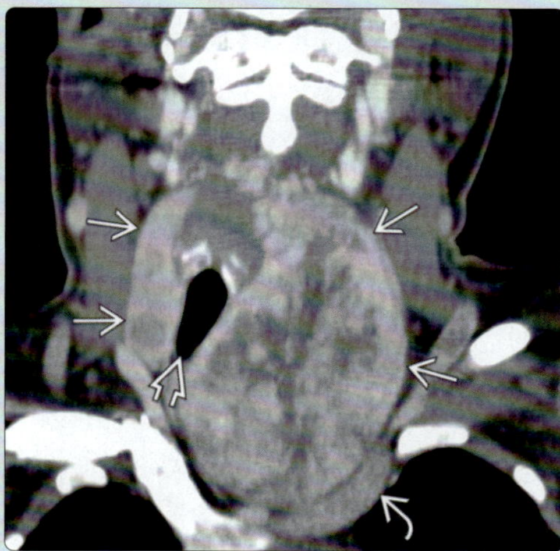

(Left) *PA chest radiograph demonstrates marked displacement of the cervical & thoracic trachea ➡ by a large, left-sided neck & superior mediastinum mass.* **(Right)** *Coronal reformatted CECT in the same patient illustrates craniocaudad extent of the multinodular goiter ➡ with heterogeneous thyroid tissue bilaterally but more markedly left lobe enlargement. Marked displacement of the subglottic larynx & trachea is evident ➡. The left brachiocephalic vein ➡ is displaced inferiorly but not compressed by the left lobe.*

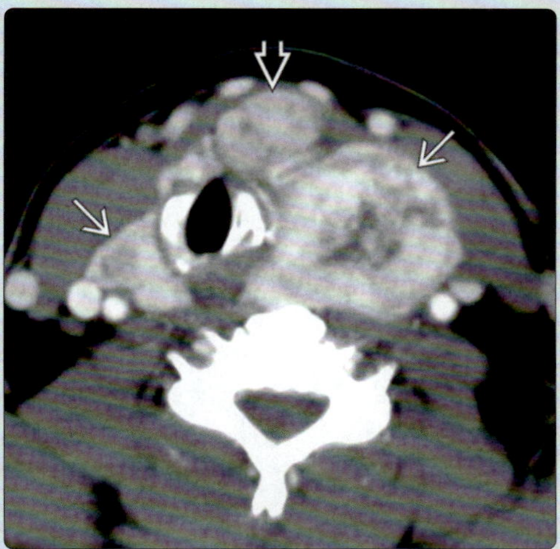

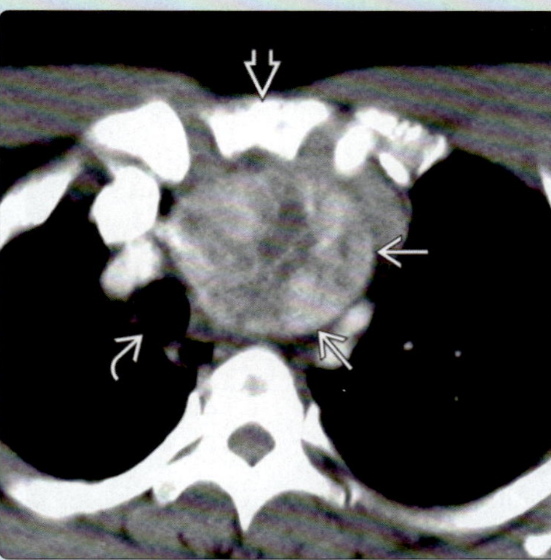

(Left) *Axial CECT at level of cricoid shows markedly heterogeneous, lobulated, & enlarged thyroid lobes ➡ as well as thyroid isthmus ➡. No calcifications or frank cysts are evident. Despite heterogeneity of the thyroid, gland margins are well defined & adjacent structures merely displaced.* **(Right)** *Axial CECT through the cervicothoracic junction in the same patient reveals inferior extension of the enlarged left lobe ➡ into the superior mediastinum, posterior to the manubrium ➡. The trachea is displaced to the right ➡.*

KEY FACTS

TERMINOLOGY

- 2 benign categories that present as thyroid nodule
  - **True adenoma** and **adenomatous nodule**

IMAGING

- General imaging findings
  - Thyroid adenoma
    - Well-defined nodule compresses adjacent gland
  - Adenomatous nodule
    - Less distinct lesion contours; ± multiple lesions
  - Calcifications or cystic change may be seen
  - No invasive features or neck adenopathy
- Enhanced CT or MR
  - Large adenomas often have heterogeneous enhancement with degeneration
- FDG/PET: Uptake may be seen in adenomas
- Nuclear scintigraphy (Tc-99m pertechnetate or iodine-123)
  - Hot nodules are usually benign adenomas (99%)
  - 20% cold nodules are malignant

TOP DIFFERENTIAL DIAGNOSES

- Thyroid colloid cyst
- Multinodular goiter
- Thyroid differentiated carcinoma

PATHOLOGY

- Adenomatous nodule > follicular adenoma
- Hürthle cell adenoma least common

CLINICAL ISSUES

- Clinical presentation
  - Most commonly incidental imaging finding
  - US used as 1st-line study; guides FNA
  - Do not evaluate suspected thyroid mass with CECT
    - Contrast can delay treatment with radioactive iodine
- Treatment options
  - Nodules with "malignant" US features need excised
  - While FNA can suggest adenoma, only resection can distinguish from carcinoma

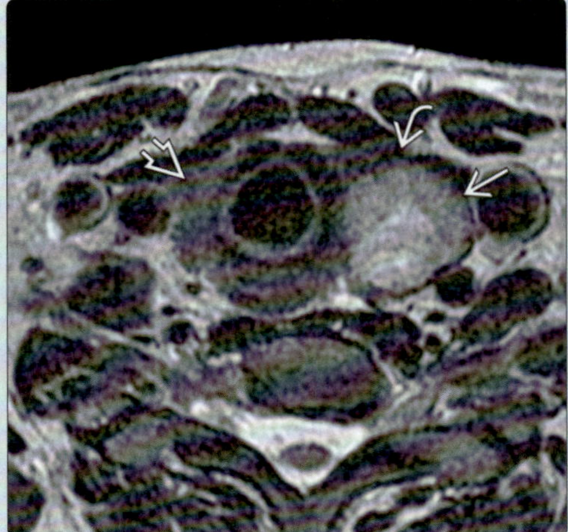

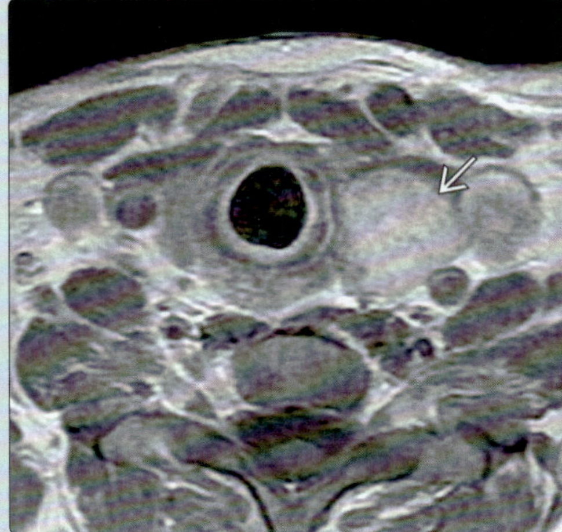

(Left) *Axial T2 MR reveals mildly hyperintense adenoma ➡ replacing much of the left thyroid lobe with only a thin rim of normal gland evident at the anterior margin ➡. The mass is well circumscribed and clearly delineated from strap muscles and the adjacent carotid artery and jugular vein. The right thyroid lobe appears small ➡.* **(Right)** *Axial T1 C+ MR in the same patient reveals diffusely homogeneous enhancement of the lesion ➡. There is no neck adenopathy. At resection, the lesion was determined to be follicular adenoma.*

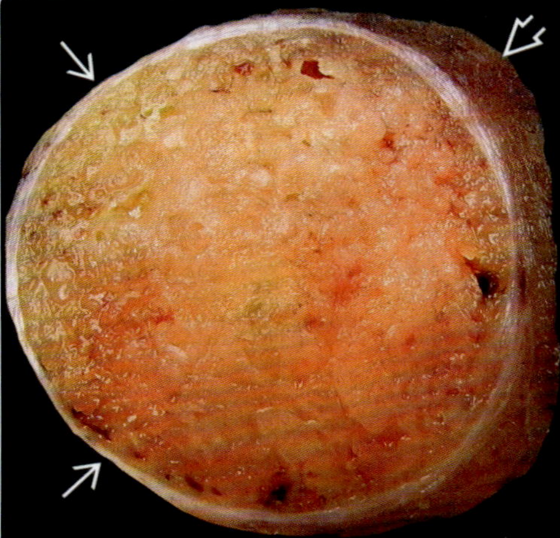

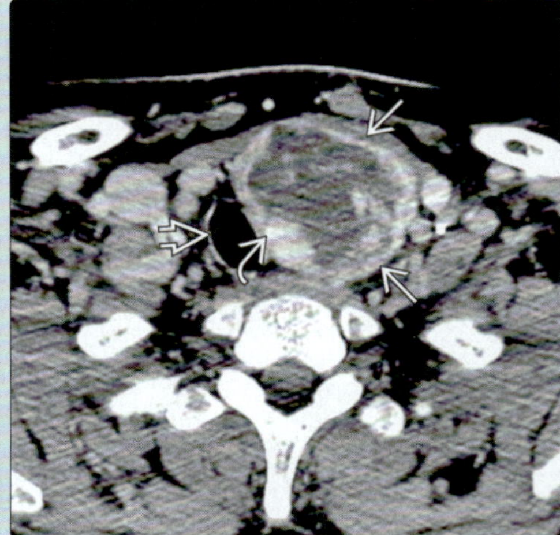

(Left) *Gross pathology shows follicular adenoma. There is a thick, well-formed fibrous connective tissue capsule ➡ separating the adenoma from the surrounding thyroid parenchyma. There is compression of the adjacent thyroid ➡, which is more beefy red.* **(Right)** *Axial CECT shows a large, heterogeneous adenoma ➡ with central low density arising within the left thyroid lobe. Focal calcification is evident ➡. The mass abuts the trachea ➡, but there is no evidence of invasion.*

KEY FACTS

TERMINOLOGY

- Benign neoplasm of parathyroid gland producing excess parathyroid hormone (PTH), resulting in hypercalcemia

IMAGING

- General imaging findings
  - Adenoma 10-30 mm; normal gland 5 x 3 x 1 mm
  - Round or oval, well-circumscribed solid mass
  - Hypervascular compared to nodes
- Imaging approach
  - 1st look: US neck only
  - No adenoma found, persistent symptoms
    - Sestamibi exam + CT localization
- US: Homogeneous, **hypoechoic, hypervascular**
- Nuclear scintigraphy: Usual 1st-line imaging study
  - **Tc-99m sestamibi** > 90% sensitive & > 90% specific
    - **Focal increased uptake** on early & **delayed** images
    - May perform as SPECT ± CT to localize
  - Nuclear subtraction scans helpful if thyroid mass
- CECT: **Arterial-phase** (30 sec) avid enhancement helps distinguish from lymph node
- MR: T2 iso- to hyperintense compared to thyroid

TOP DIFFERENTIAL DIAGNOSES

- Reactive lymph nodes (level VI)
- Thyroid adenoma
- Parathyroid cyst
- Parathyroid carcinoma

CLINICAL ISSUES

- Most patients have **asymptomatic hypercalcemia**
- Hypercalcemia symptoms: "Stones, bones, groans, & psychiatric overtones"
- Surgical treatment
  - Indications: < 50 y/o, Ca^{++} >1mg/dL above upper limit of normal, DEXA < 2.5 standard deviations (by T-score); ↓ Cr clearance, 24-hour urinary Ca^{++} is > 400mg/dL
  - Intraoperative PTH useful, > 50% decline from baseline

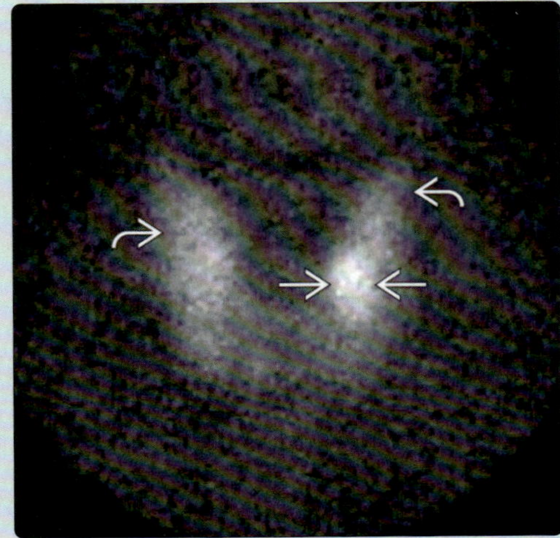

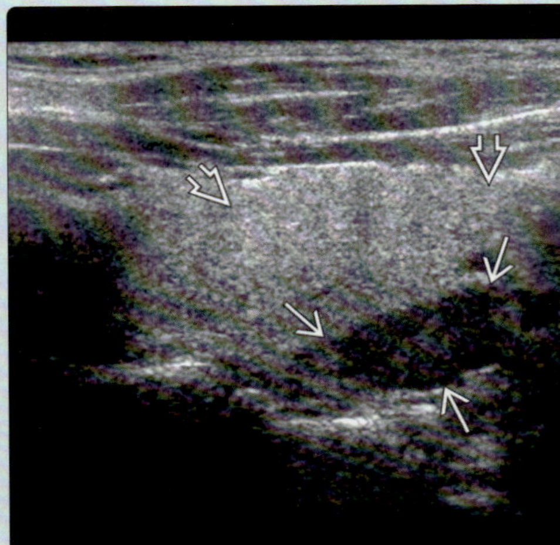

(Left) *AP delayed Tc-99m sestamibi scan demonstrates parathyroid adenoma with persistent focal uptake ➡ in the lower aspect of the left thyroid. Only faint residual tracer is evident in the thyroid ➡.* **(Right)** *Longitudinal US in the same patient reveals a hypoechoic, solid ovoid lesion ➡ that measures 15 x 9 x 7 mm posterior to the left thyroid lobe ➡. Color Doppler also showed the lesion to be hypervascular. Parathyroid adenoma was resected with normalization of parathyroid hormone levels and resolution of hypercalcemia.*

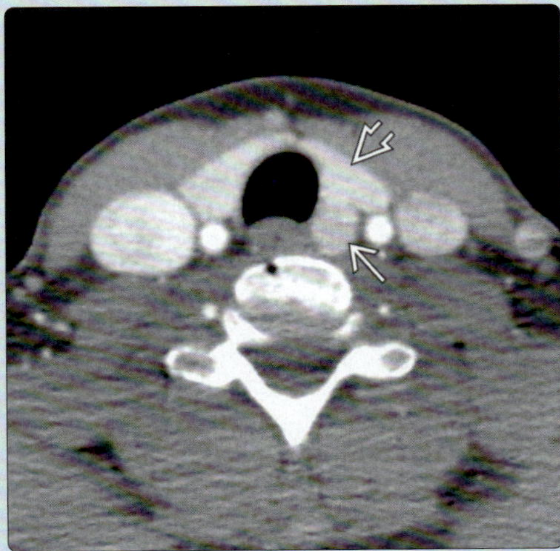

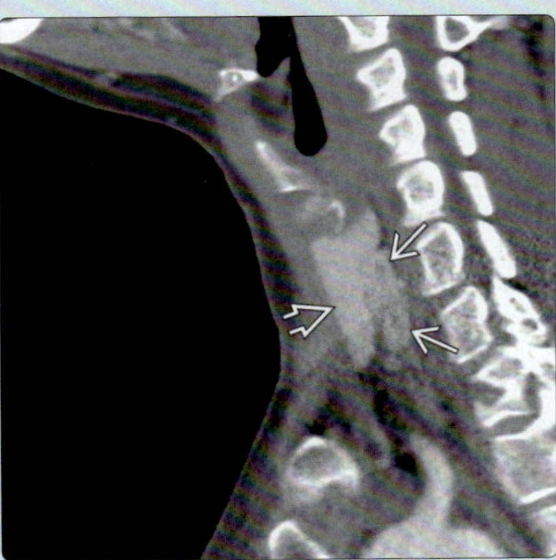

(Left) *Axial CECT in a patient with acute hoarseness shows a well-defined round lesion ➡ in the left tracheoesophageal groove. The mass is distinct from the posterior aspect of the left thyroid lobe ➡ and appears slightly less enhancing than the thyroid on this delayed scan.* **(Right)** *Sagittal CECT shows a heterogeneous oval mass ➡ immediately posterior to the left thyroid ➡. There is internal heterogeneity from degeneration that led to adenoma enlargement. Vocal cord paralysis resolved postoperatively.*

Differentiated Thyroid Carcinoma

KEY FACTS

IMAGING

- Thyroid mass ± extracapsular invasion ± metastatic nodes
  - Rarely in ectopic thyroid, thyroglossal duct cyst
- CT: Variable size, texture, Ca^{++}, invasive features
  - Nodal metastases **cystic** or solid, small or large, ± **Ca^{++}** (**psammoma bodies**)
  - **Do not give iodinated contrast if suspected differentiated thyroid carcinoma**
    - Delays I-131 therapy up to 6 months
- MR: Variable signal reflects intrinsic T1 signal of thyroglobulin &/or hemorrhage (methemoglobin)
- US: **Concerning features**: Hypoechoic, ill defined, microcalcification, taller than wide, hypervascular
- PET/CT: Use if tumor does not take up I-131

TOP DIFFERENTIAL DIAGNOSES

- Benign: Follicular adenoma, multinodular goiter
- Malignant: Medullary carcinoma, anaplastic carcinoma, non-Hodgkin lymphoma

PATHOLOGY

- **Papillary = 80%, follicular = 10%** of thyroid cancers;
- **Papillary** prefers **nodal** spread; **follicular** prefers **hematogenous** spread
- 5-year survival: Stages I & II > 90%, stage IV 40%; if < 45 y/o, cannot be greater than stage II, even with metastasis

CLINICAL ISSUES

- Painless, palpable, solitary thyroid nodule
- 3x more common in women; peaks in 2nd & 3rd decades
- **Rising serum thyroglobulin** is indicator of recurrence
- FNA results: Benign, malignant, nondiagnostic, suspicious
- Treatment options
  - Total thyroidectomy with level VI nodal dissection; ± I-131
  - Selective neck dissection for other nodal metastases
  - I-131 scintigraphy to diagnose & treat recurrent or metastatic disease

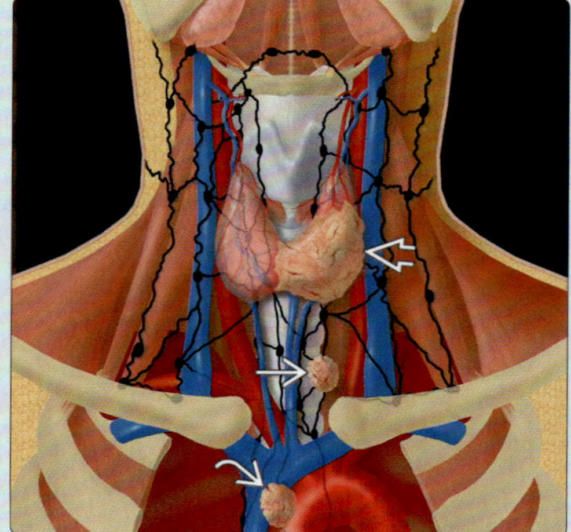

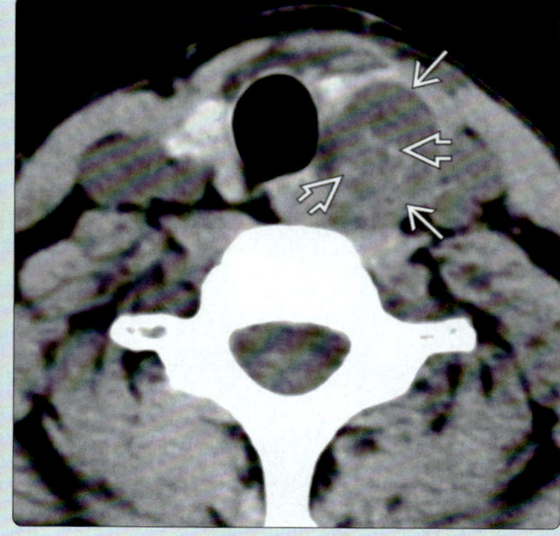

(Left) *Coronal graphic illustrates a left thyroid lobe differentiated thyroid carcinoma (DCTa) primary tumor ➲ with metastatic nodal disease in the left paratracheal chain ➲ and superior mediastinum ➲.* **(Right)** *Axial NECT shows a well-defined mass ➲ arising from the left thyroid lobe with fine, speckled microcalcifications ➲ centrally. Small calcifications such as these are a suspicious finding for DTCa and especially papillary carcinoma. Intrathyroid tumor is < 4 cm = T2.*

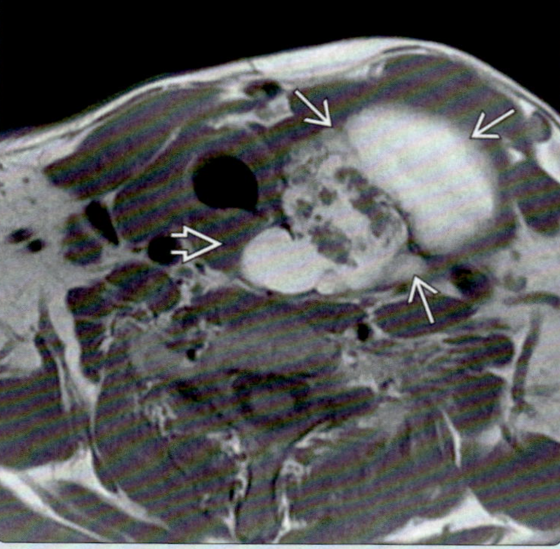

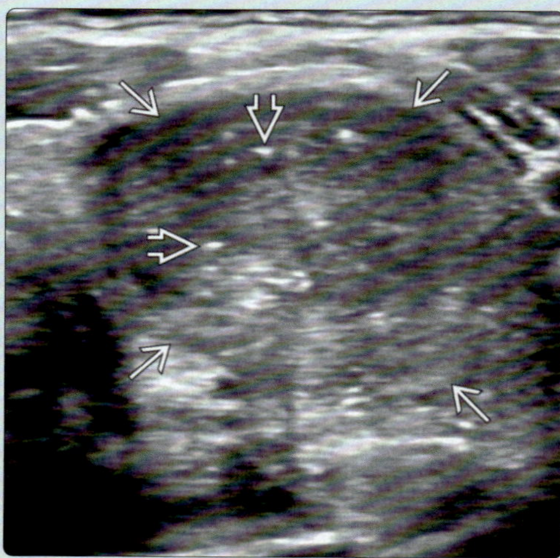

(Left) *Axial T1 MR in a 49-year-old man with an enlarging neck mass shows a heterogeneous solid and cystic mass arising in the left thyroid lobe ➲, displacing the esophagus ➲. Note the intrinsic hyperintensity from thyroglobulin. This feature is also present in multiple nodes; tumor was determined to be papillary thyroid carcinoma.* **(Right)** *Longitudinal thyroid ultrasound in a different patient reveals a well-defined mass ➲ with multiple tiny, hyperechoic microcalcifications ➲, found to be a papillary carcinoma.*

KEY FACTS

TERMINOLOGY

- Medullary thyroid carcinoma (MTCa)
- Rare neuroendocrine malignancy arising from thyroid **parafollicular C cells** that produce calcitonin

IMAGING

- CECT findings
  - Heterogeneous, well-circumscribed thyroid mass
    - Familial: Multifocal, invasive
  - Similar-appearing nodal metastases (50%)
  - ± calcifications in tumor &/or nodes
  - Intravenous iodine not contraindicated for MTCa
- Ultrasound findings
  - Hypoechoic, irregular mass
  - Color Doppler hypervascularity evident
- PET/CT not used (**not** reliably FDG avid)
- I-131 MIBG or octreotide scintigraphy for metastases

TOP DIFFERENTIAL DIAGNOSES

- Multinodular goiter
- Thyroid adenoma
- Thyroid differentiated carcinoma

PATHOLOGY

- *RET* protooncogene mutations involves 10q11.2
- MTCa = 3% of all thyroid carcinoma
- Most MTCa sporadic; 25% MTCa inherited
- Strong inherited association with MEN type 2A & 2B

CLINICAL ISSUES

- Clinical presentation: Thyroid mass; 50% nodal mass
  - Sporadic: Presents in 5th to 6th decades
  - Familial: Presents in 3rd decade; multifocal tumors
  - Serum calcitonin & CEA levels elevated
- Treatment options
  - Primarily surgical ± radiotherapy
  - Prophylactic thyroidectomy if *RET*(+) gene mutation

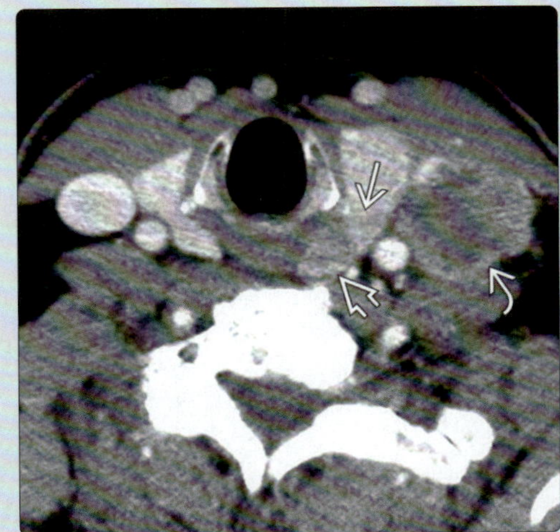

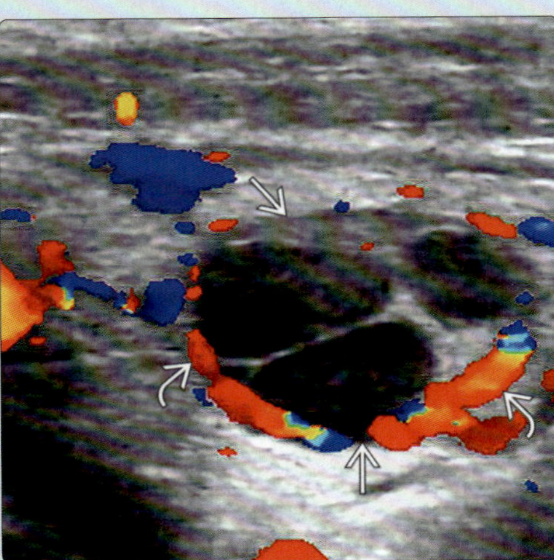

(Left) *Axial CECT shows a small left posterior thyroid mass ➡ with a malignant node in the tracheoesophageal groove ➡ & low internal jugular chain ➡. Although differentiated thyroid carcinoma was suggested, this thyroid cancer turned out to be the sporadic form of medullary carcinoma.* **(Right)** *Longitudinal color Doppler US through the thyroid shows a mixed cystic & solid mass ➡ with peripheral vascularity ➡. Ultrasound features of medullary carcinoma are variable, but increased vascularity is typical.*

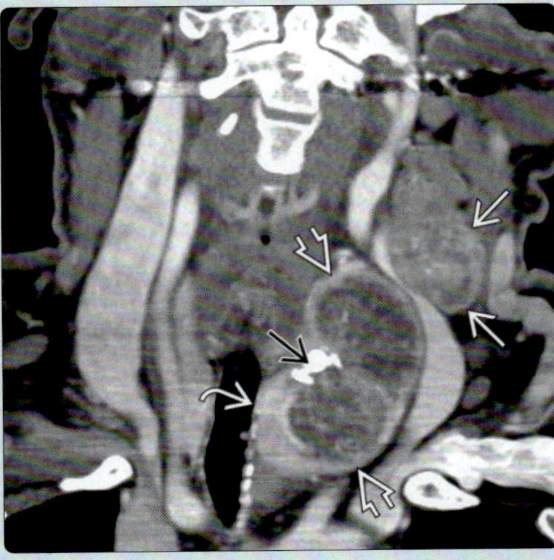

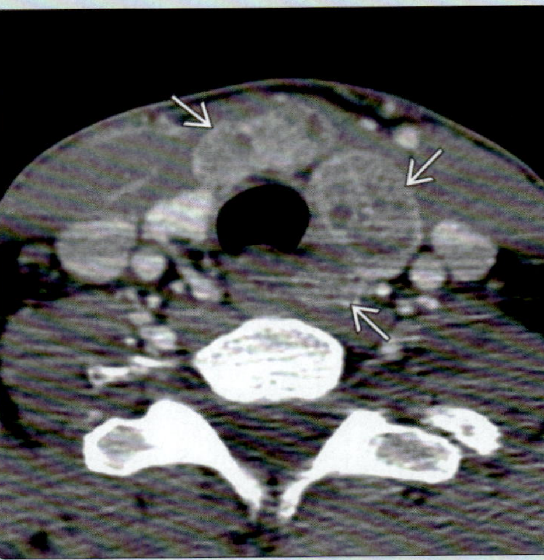

(Left) *Coronal CECT shows a heterogeneous but well-defined thyroid mass ➡ with coarse calcifications ➡ & ipsilateral similarly heterogeneous adenopathy ➡. At surgery, medullary carcinoma was found to have infiltrated the tracheal wall ➡.* **(Right)** *Axial CECT shows multiple left thyroid & isthmus lesions ➡ found to be multifocal medullary thyroid carcinoma (MTCa). Lesions are all similarly heterogeneous but well defined & not calcified. Familial MTCa often presents earlier with multifocal disease.*

KEY FACTS

TERMINOLOGY

- Synonym: Undifferentiated thyroid tumor
- May arise from **differentiated thyroid carcinoma** or **multinodular goiter** (MNG)

IMAGING

- General findings
  - Large, heterogeneous, infiltrating thyroid mass
  - Necrosis, hemorrhage, calcifications
  - Invades surrounding structures and spaces
  - Common to have nodal metastases at presentation
- CECT for suspected anaplastic thyroid carcinoma (ATCa)
  - Iodinated contrast not issue with ATCa
- US: Inadequate for staging purposes
- PET/CT: FDG avid; may help identify metastasis
- Bone scan: Bone metastases evaluation for staging
- I-123 and I-131 scintigraphy not useful due to lack of iodine concentration

TOP DIFFERENTIAL DIAGNOSES

- Thyroid non-Hodgkin lymphoma
- Thyroid differentiated carcinoma
- MNG

PATHOLOGY

- Undifferentiated cells with extrathyroidal extension, lymph-vascular invasion, significant necrosis, and hemorrhage
- **50% distant metastasis**: Lungs, bone, brain
- Automatically staged as T4, stage IV tumors
- 1-2% of thyroid malignancies 39% of thyroid deaths
- Lethal tumor; mean survival: 6 months

CLINICAL ISSUES

- Clinical presentation
  - Tumor of elderly; mean age: 71 years
  - Rapidly growing, large, painful neck mass
- Early presentation: Aggressive, multimodality treatment
- Late presentation: Typically palliative

(Left) *Axial CECT demonstrates a large, heterogeneous, predominantly right-sided thyroid mass ➡ with large pools of low-density necrosis ➡. Mass cannot be separated from strap muscles and infiltrates cricothyroid membrane to tracheal lumen ➡.* **(Right)** *Doppler US shows the right thyroid lobe appearing completely replaced by a large heterogeneous lobulated solid mass ➡ with irregular margins. No internal calcifications are evident; however, color Doppler shows prominent peripheral vascularity ➡.*

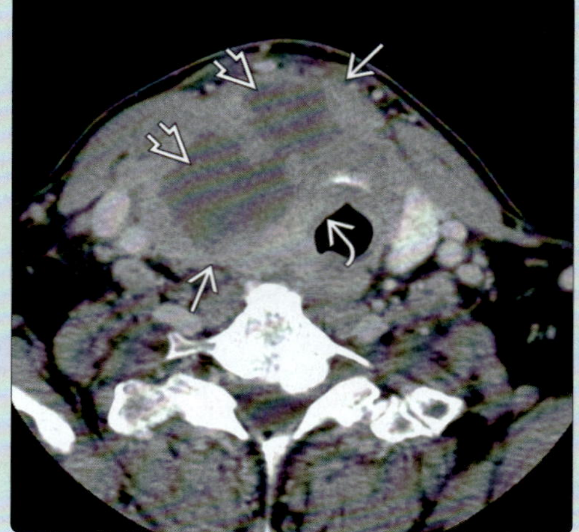

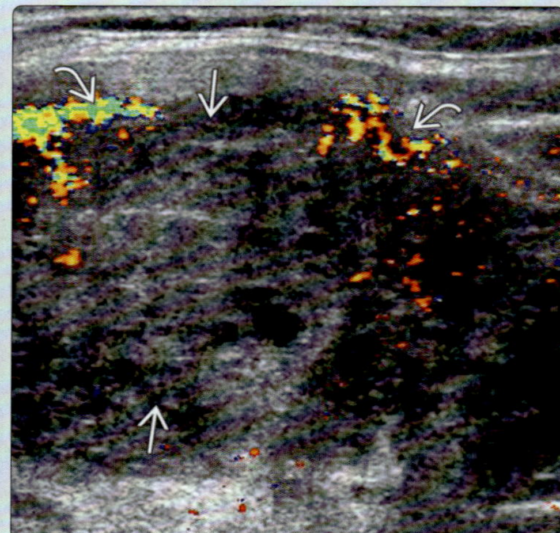

(Left) *Axial T2 MR in a patient with stridor imaged after tracheostomy shows extensive areas of marked signal loss ➡ suggesting either fibrosis, calcifications (that were not evident on CT), or hemosiderin deposition. T2 signal surrounding the tube represents both secretions and infiltrative tumor ➡.* **(Right)** *Axial T1 C+ MR in the same patient illustrates the infiltrative nature of this aggressive, heterogeneously enhancing neoplasm ➡, which involves strap muscles and other extrathyroidal tissues.*

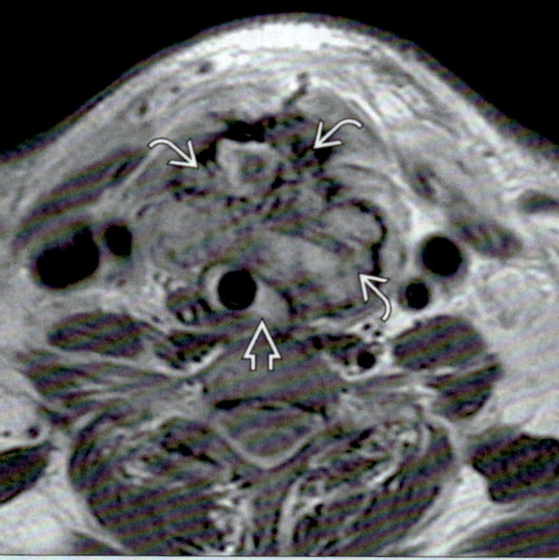

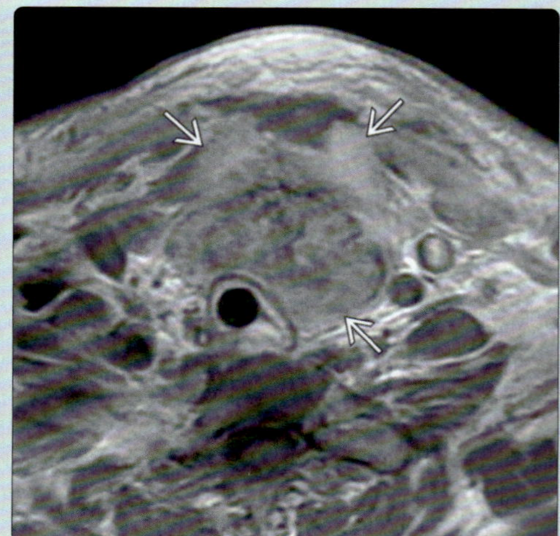

KEY FACTS

TERMINOLOGY

- Thyroid non-Hodgkin lymphoma (NHL)
  - Lymphoma arising in thyroid gland

IMAGING

- Rapidly enlarging, solid, noncalcified thyroid mass in elderly woman with history of chronic lymphocytic thyroiditis
- 80% solitary homogeneous thyroid mass
- 20% multiple masses or diffuse infiltration
- CECT: Necrosis and calcification uncommon
- US: Well-defined, homogeneous, hypoechoic
- PET/CT generally useful except if MALT lymphoma

TOP DIFFERENTIAL DIAGNOSES

- Anaplastic thyroid carcinoma
- Multinodular goiter
- Chronic lymphocytic (Hashimoto) thyroiditis
- Thyroid differentiated carcinoma

PATHOLOGY

- Most often diffuse large **B-cell lymphoma**
- 40-80% of cases occur in patients with **chronic lymphocytic (Hashimoto) thyroiditis**
  - Hashimoto has 70x increased risk of thyroid NHL

CLINICAL ISSUES

- Presents as rapidly enlarging neck mass
- 2-5% of all thyroid malignancies
- 5-yr survival: 75-95%
  - Extrathyroidal spread: ↓ 5-yr survival to 35%
- Nonsurgical disease, unless acute relief of airway obstruction is required

DIAGNOSTIC CHECKLIST

- Main differential is **anaplastic thyroid carcinoma**
- NHL more homogeneous; no necrosis, hemorrhage
- NHL less likely to invade tissues such as trachea

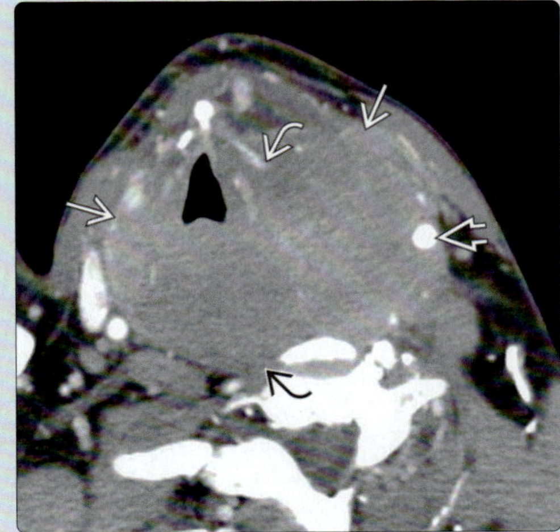

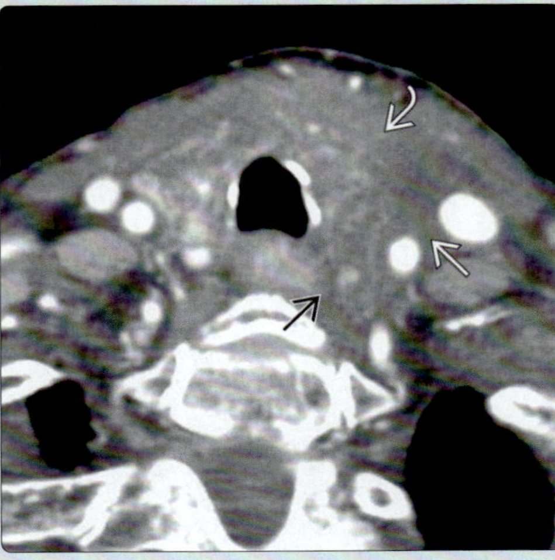

(Left) *Axial CECT shows a large, minimally enhancing mass ➡ centered in the thyroid gland. The mass invades laryngeal cartilages ➡ and prevertebral muscles ⇨ and surrounds the carotid artery ➡. The homogeneous density of the mass suggests lymphoma, but anaplastic thyroid cancer is the main differential.* **(Right)** *Axial CECT shows infiltrative non-Hodgkin lymphoma of the left thyroid with invasion of the carotid sheath ➡, esophagus ⇨, and overlying strap muscles ➡.*

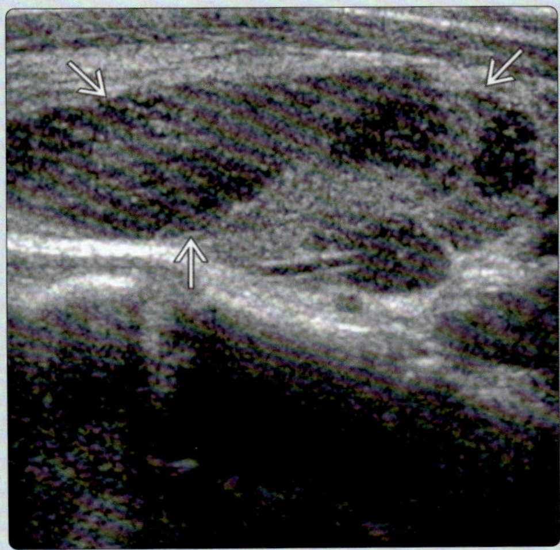

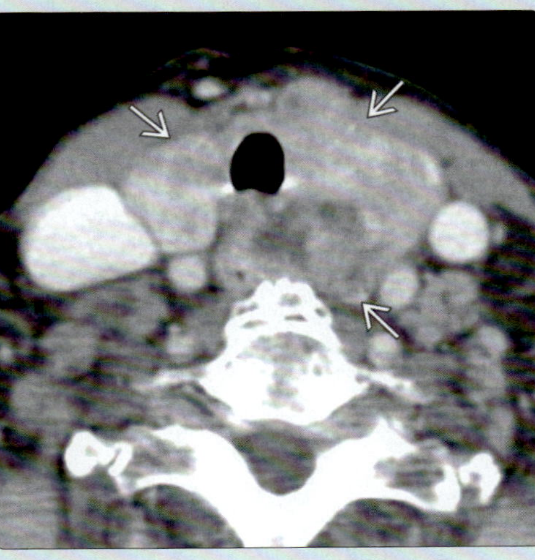

(Left) *Longitudinal ultrasound of the thyroid gland shows a low-echogenicity lobular mass ➡. The uniform nature of lymphoma can result in low echogenicity on ultrasound, which may be mistaken for a cyst.* **(Right)** *Axial CECT shows multifocal masses ➡ in the thyroid. Although this primary lymphoma might be mistaken for a multinodular goiter, focal loss of definition of the thyroid margins and absence of calcification suggest an alternate diagnosis. The loss of clarity of the borders is particularly suspicious for malignancy.*

Thyroglossal Duct Cyst Carcinoma

KEY FACTS

TERMINOLOGY

- Definition: Malignant tumor arising from remnants of embryologic thyroglossal duct (TGD)

IMAGING

- CECT or enhanced MR
  - **Solid component** ± **calcifications** within TGD cyst
  - May occur as tumor within solid ectopic thyroid tissue from tongue base to lower neck
  - CECT more likely to show calcifications
    - MR relatively blind to calcifications
  - Lymph node metastases rare
    - If present, confirms TGD cyst + carcinoma suspicion
- US: Look for solid components ± calcifications with TGD cyst
- PET/CT: Carcinoma may be FDG avid

TOP DIFFERENTIAL DIAGNOSES

- Thyroglossal duct cyst
- Lingual thyroid
- Thyroid remnants along TGD

PATHOLOGY

- **95%** TGD carcinoma are **papillary thyroid**
  - Papillary thyroid carcinoma often contains **psammoma** bodies, which can result in calcifications evident on CT
- < 5% are squamous carcinoma
  - Clinical behavior & CT appearance more aggressive
- < 2% of TGD cysts have carcinoma

CLINICAL ISSUES

- Enlarging midline neck mass
  - No symptoms to distinguish from benign TGD cyst
- Most commonly adults; mean = 40 years
- Treatment options
  - FNA prior to TGD resection
  - Complete resection of TGD (Sistrunk procedure)
  - Treatment often necessitates thyroidectomy, ± neck dissection

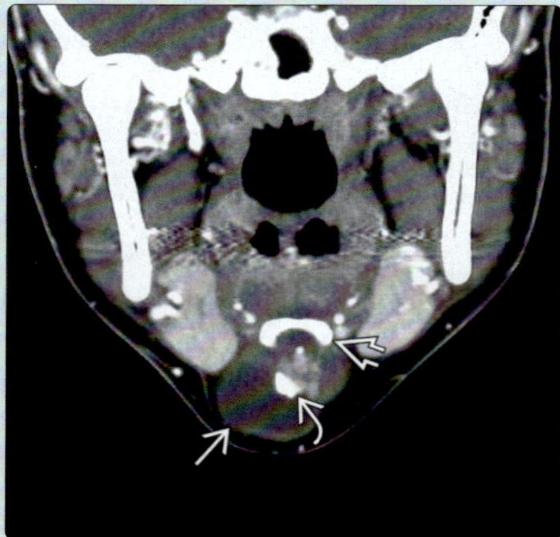

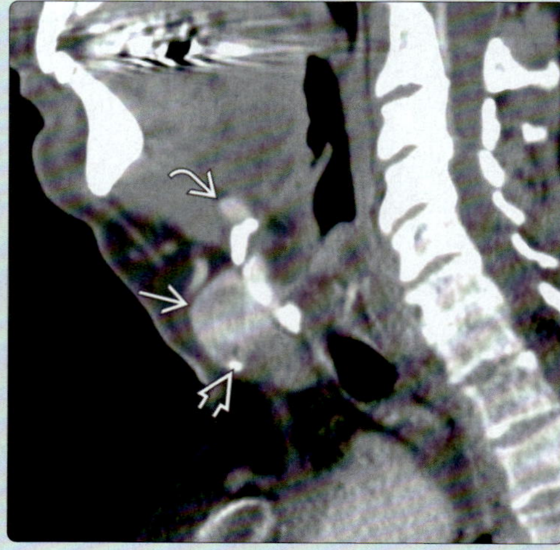

(Left) *Coronal CECT reveals a midline neck cystic mass ➡ that is intimately related to the hyoid bone ➡. At the superior aspect of the cyst, there is enhancing soft tissue and dense calcifications ➡ suggesting a thyroglossal duct (TGD) cyst with carcinoma present.* **(Right)** *Sagittal CECT of a TGD cyst carcinoma shows a solid heterogeneous mass ➡ just below hyoid bone & containing focal calcification ➡. An additional small solid rest of ectopic tissue is present above the hyoid ➡. There was no normal-appearing thyroid in lower neck.*

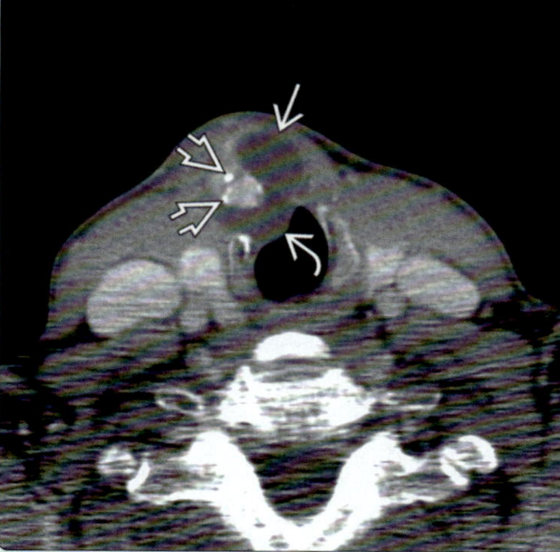

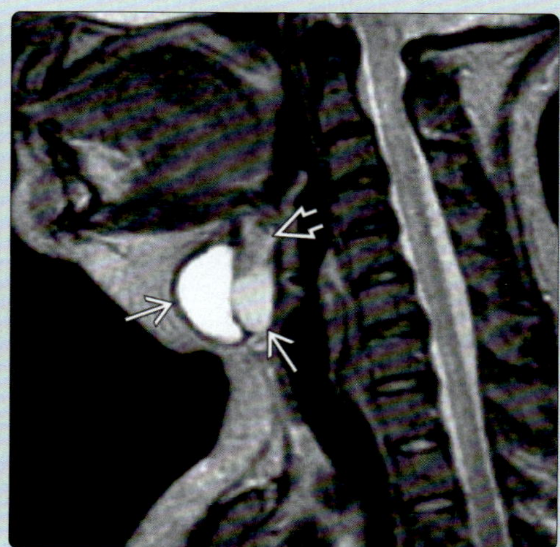

(Left) *Axial CECT shows a subglottic paramedian complex cystic TGD cyst with carcinoma ➡ within infrahyoid strap muscles. The cystic component of the mass is submucosal in the subglottic endolarynx ➡. Within the extralaryngeal cystic mass, an enhancing nodule with punctate calcifications is visible ➡.* **(Right)** *Sagittal T2 MR shows an infrahyoid, hyperintense, multilobulated TGD cyst with carcinoma ➡ with intermediate to low intensity of the superior solid nodule ➡.*

KEY FACTS

TERMINOLOGY

- Definition: Carcinoma affected cervical portion of esophagus
  - > 95% are squamous cell carcinoma (SCCa)

IMAGING

- Cervical esophagus = lower cricoid to thoracic inlet
- **Posterior midline** visceral space focal or invasive mass
- CECT/MR: Both adequate to evaluate invasive extent of tumor
  - Esophageal wall thickened + ill-defined margin
  - Frequent extension to hypopharynx, larynx, thyroid
  - Look for paratracheal (level VI) and mediastinal nodes
  - Cord paralysis from recurrent laryngeal nerve injury
- PET/CT best tool for staging, monitoring, and surveillance

TOP DIFFERENTIAL DIAGNOSES

- Hypopharyngeal SCCa
- Thyroid anaplastic carcinoma
- Thyroid non-Hodgkin lymphoma
- Thyroid differentiated carcinoma

PATHOLOGY

- Strong association with tobacco & alcohol abuse
- AJCC staging as for all esophagus
  - **T1-T3**: Depth of wall invasion
  - **T4**: Invasion of adjacent structures
- Nodal disease present in **70%** at diagnosis
- 5-year survival = 10% (late diagnosis)

CLINICAL ISSUES

- Clinical presentation
  - Late; presents with dysphagia, weight loss
  - Increased risk of 2nd primary malignancy
- Treatment options
  - Chemoradiotherapy when advanced presentation
  - Radical resection of esophagus & hypopharynx with jejunal interposition or gastric pull-up

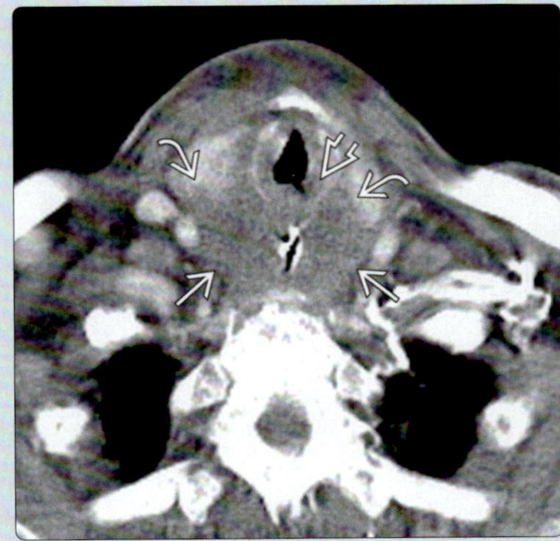

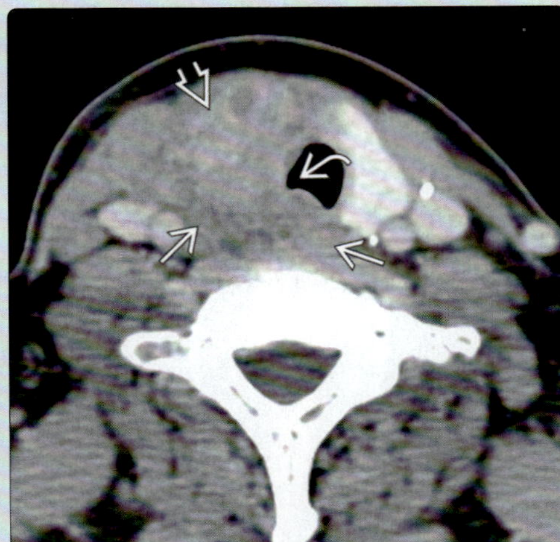

(Left) *CECT shows infiltrative, aggressive-appearing midline mass ➡ in the posterior visceral space invading the thyroid gland ➡ and cricoid cartilage ➡. A nasogastric tube is in the center of this posterior midline esophageal SCCa.* **(Right)** *Axial CECT shows a heterogeneous mass ➡ filling posterior & right side of visceral space. Right thyroid lobe is replaced ➡ & trachea ➡ is invaded. This esophageal SCCa mimics anaplastic thyroid carcinoma or thyroid lymphoma. This primary tumor is T4 due to invasion of adjacent structures.*

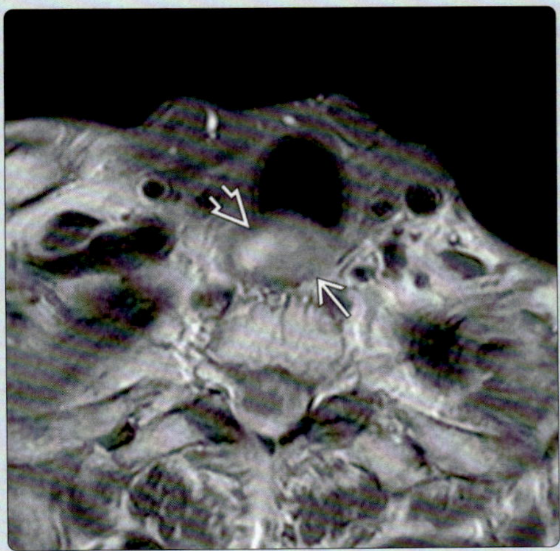

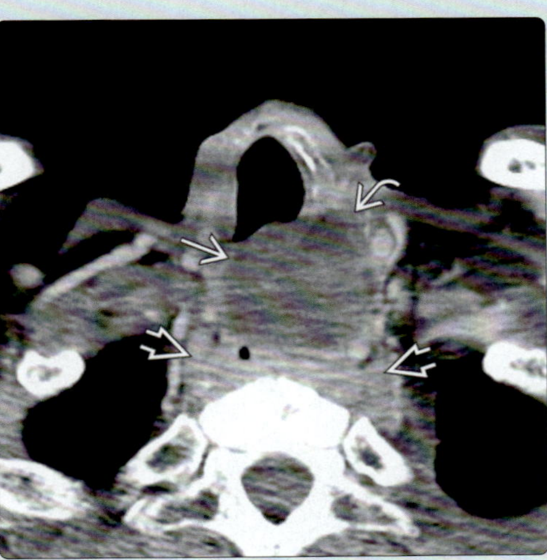

(Left) *Axial T2 MR in a 62-year-old man who had chemoradiation for tongue base SCCa 7 years prior shows eccentric thickening of the cervical esophageal wall ➡, outlined by hyperintense obstructed secretions ➡. This was proven to be a small esophageal SCCa.* **(Right)** *Axial CECT at the level of the cervical thoracic junction shows a large posterior midline esophageal SCCa ➡. Anterior invasion on the left ➡ is visible with retropharyngeal-danger space invasion seen posteriorly ➡.*

Esophagopharyngeal Diverticulum (Zenker)

KEY FACTS

TERMINOLOGY

- Mucosa-lined outpouching of posterior hypopharynx
- Posterior pulsion diverticulum **above** cricopharyngeus

IMAGING

- Sac arising from posterior pharynx at C5-6 level
- Extends posteroinferiorly and to **left** side
- **Barium esophagram** is best imaging tool
  - Confirms diagnosis and shows diverticular neck
  - Evaluates associated reflux and hiatal hernia
- CECT: Well-defined mass posterior and to left of esophagus
  - Nonenhancing mass with air, fluid, ± food debris
- MR: Sagittal plane best delineates sac
  - May have air-fluid level
  - Food debris results in heterogeneous signal
  - May see linear enhancement of mucosa

TOP DIFFERENTIAL DIAGNOSES

- Lateral cervical esophageal diverticulum
- Paratracheal air cyst
- Parathyroid cyst

PATHOLOGY

- Herniation occurs at Killian dehiscence
- Multiple causes proposed; likely multifactorial
- Almost all have hiatal hernia
- Many have reflux esophagitis

CLINICAL ISSUES

- Dysphagia as pouch compresses esophagus
- Regurgitation of contents ± aspiration
- Treatment options
  - Elderly patients with minimal symptoms are frequently treated by observation alone
  - Symptomatic diverticula can be treated by endoscopic or external surgical techniques
  - Endoscopy: Bivalved laryngoscope; common wall parted by electrocautery, laser, ultrasonic shears, or staples

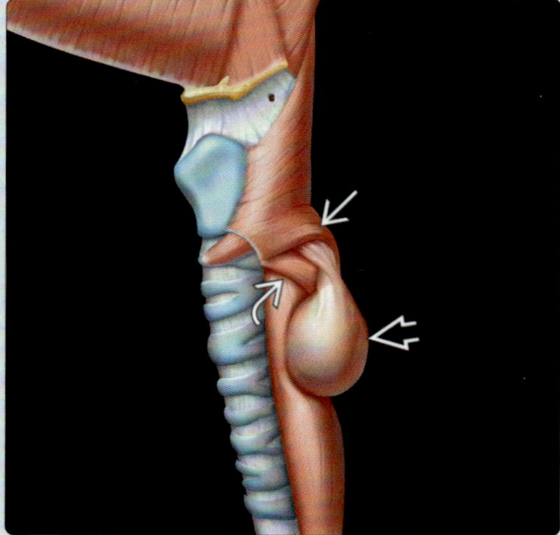

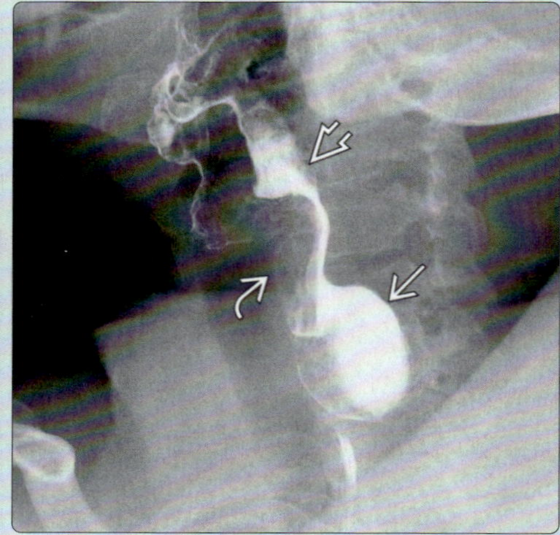

(Left) *Graphic depicts Zenker diverticulum ➡ with herniation at the Killian dehiscence between the thyropharyngeal ➡ and cricopharyngeal ➡ fibers of the inferior constrictor muscle.* **(Right)** *Barium esophagram demonstrates a large diverticulum with retained layering contrast ➡ from the posterior lateral junction of the hypopharynx ➡ and the cervical esophagus ➡. The posterior lateral projection confirms this lesion as an esophagopharyngeal (Zenker) diverticulum.*

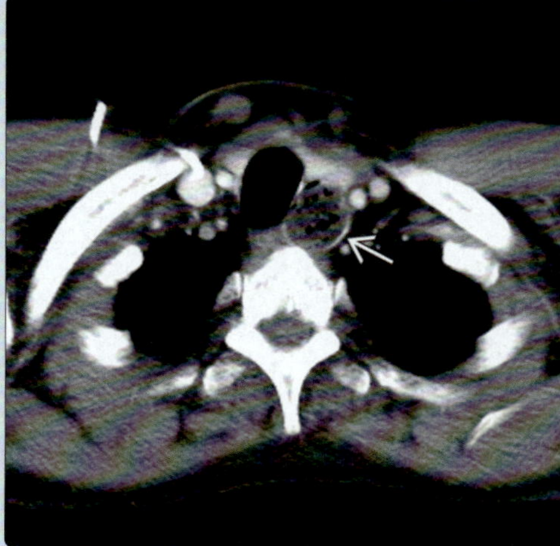

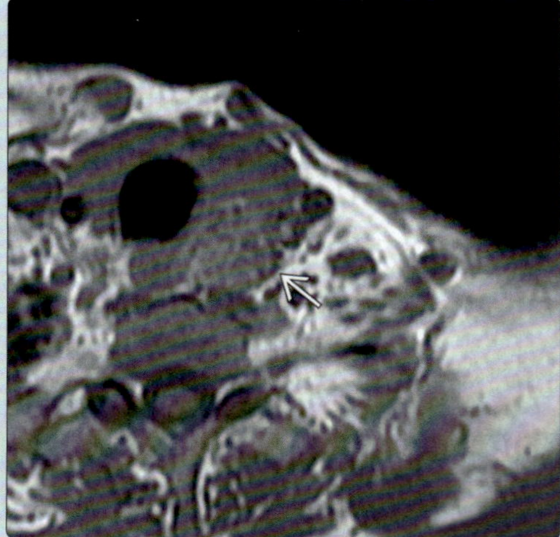

(Left) *Axial CECT shows gas and debris within the left paraesophageal ovoid lesion ➡. Differential considerations would include a esophagopharyngeal diverticulum and lateral esophageal diverticulum. Esophagram revealed it to be the more common esophagopharyngeal diverticulum.* **(Right)** *Axial T1 MR through the thyroid bed shows a left esophagopharyngeal diverticulum ➡.*

KEY FACTS

TERMINOLOGY

- Synonym: Colloid nodule
- Definition: Fluid lesion of thyroid containing stored form of thyroid hormone (colloid)

IMAGING

- Typically 1-4 cm; when large, usually hemorrhagic
- Sharply defined, fluid-filled lesion
- CECT: Low-density, round to oval lesion
  - Thyroid tissue "beaks" around cyst
- MR: T2 hyperintense, well-defined lesion
  - T1 frequently hyperintense, may be iso- or hypointense to thyroid
- Ultrasound is key modality for determining nature
  - Shows **thin wall with smooth margins**
  - Typically anechoic, ↑ through transmission
  - Colloid crystals may be suspended in fluid with **posterior comet tail artifact**

TOP DIFFERENTIAL DIAGNOSES

- Thyroid adenoma
- Simple thyroid cyst
- Thyroid differentiated carcinoma
- Thyroglossal duct cyst

CLINICAL ISSUES

- 15-25% thyroid nodules
- May rapidly enlarge from hemorrhage
- Often incidental imaging finding
  - Smaller cysts commonly seen during thyroid ultrasound
- Benign lesion without malignant potential
- Surgery, typically hemithyroid lobectomy, for cosmesis or compressive symptoms

DIAGNOSTIC CHECKLIST

- Important to carefully evaluate "cystic" lesion on ultrasound
- Complex thyroid "cyst" may be malignant degenerating lesion

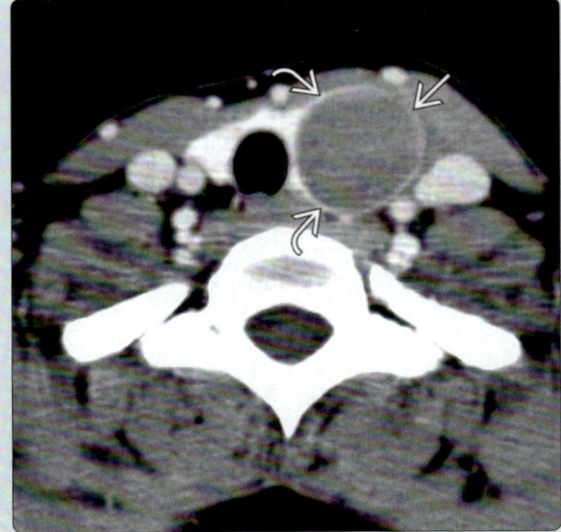

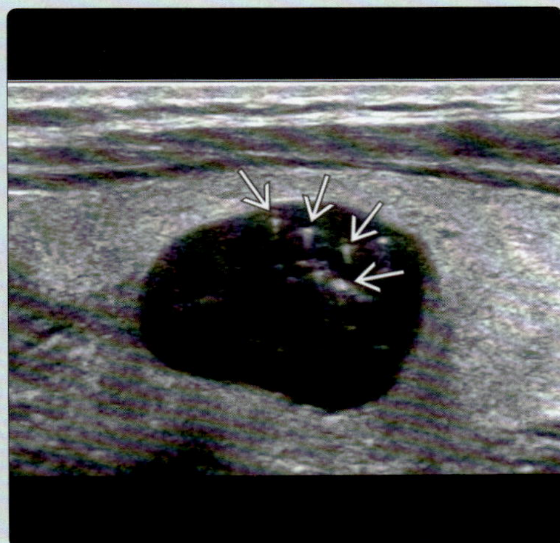

(Left) *Axial CECT demonstrates an ovoid, sharply defined, low-density mass ➡ in the left thyroid lobe with thyroid tissue "beaking" around anterior & posterior margins of the mass ⮕. Needle aspiration of lesion revealed a hemorrhagic colloid cyst.* **(Right)** *Longitudinal grayscale US demonstrates a typical colloid nodule with multiple characteristic echogenic foci & comet tail artifacts suspended in the cyst ➡. These represent colloid particles in the viscous fluid concentrated with thyroglobulin.*

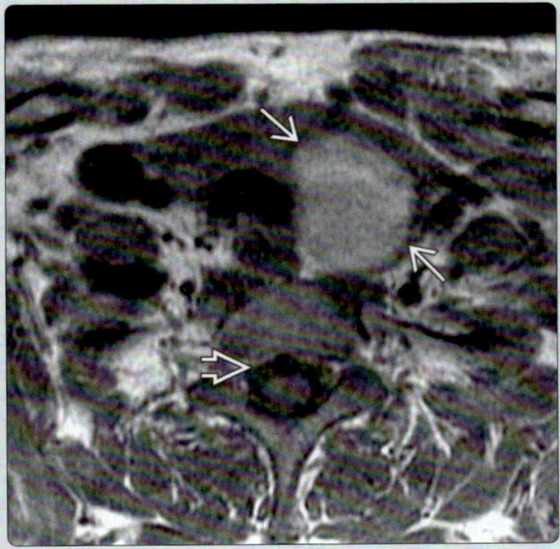

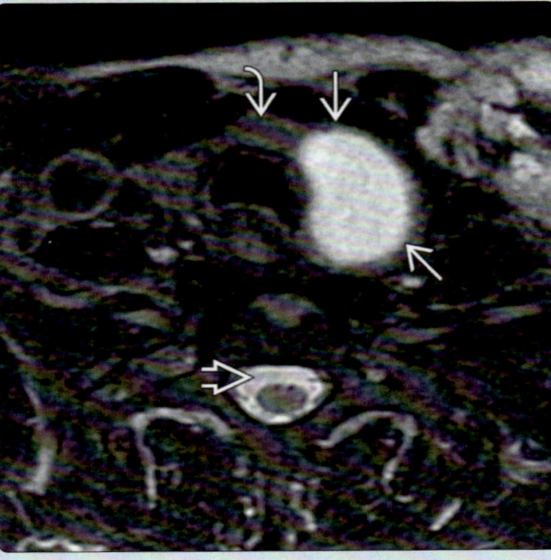

(Left) *Axial T1 MR demonstrates a large, well-defined mass ➡ within the left thyroid lobe that is hyperintense to CSF ⮕. Mass abuts & displaces the left strap muscles anteriorly, but there are no aggressive features to suggest an invasive mass.* **(Right)** *Axial T2 FS MR shows the mass ➡ to be uniformly & markedly hyperintense, similar to intensity of CSF ⮕. The lesion clearly resides within the left thyroid lobe & is sharply demarcated from the normal adjacent thyroid isthmus ⮕. No adenopathy is evident in the neck.*

Lateral Cervical Esophageal Diverticulum

KEY FACTS

TERMINOLOGY

- Synonym: Killian-Jamieson diverticulum
- **Lateral outpouching** from **proximal cervical esophagus below cricopharyngeus muscle**

IMAGING

- Small, smoothly marginated lateral sac
- **Usually unilateral**, **left sided**
- Bilateral in 25%; rarely unilateral, right sided
- Diameter: 0.2-5.0 cm; average: 1.4 cm
- Barium swallow (frontal & lateral) best imaging tool
  - Lateral sac; overlaps anterior esophageal wall
- Incidental finding on CECT/MR
  - Round or oval mass lateral to esophagus
  - Abuts and may displace left thyroid lobe &/or common carotid artery anteriorly
  - Contents may be air, fluid, food debris, or mixed

TOP DIFFERENTIAL DIAGNOSES

- Esophago-pharyngeal (Zenker) diverticulum
- Thyroid carcinoma nodal metastasis
- Parathyroid cyst

PATHOLOGY

- Protrusion through **Killian-Jamieson triangle** in **anterolateral wall** of cervical esophagus
  - Zenker at posterior midline Killian dehiscence

CLINICAL ISSUES

- Rare, usually asymptomatic, incidental imaging finding
- May have dysphagia from pharyngeal dysmotility
- Respiratory symptoms uncommon
  - Cricopharyngeus prevents reflux to hypopharynx
- Most not surgically treated due to asymptomatic nature
  - Diverticulectomy ± esophagomyotomy if symptomatic

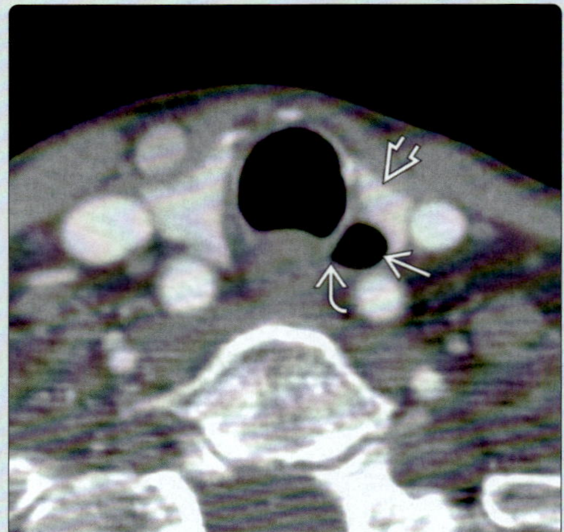

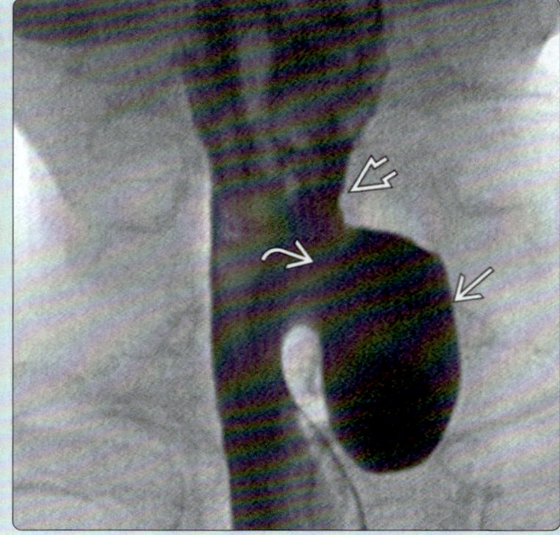

(Left) *Axial CECT shows an air-filled diverticulum ➡ interposed between the cervical esophagus, left thyroid lobe ➡, and common carotid. Note the air "points" ➡ toward esophagus, a clue to its origin.* **(Right)** *Frontal esophagram shows a prominent diverticular outpouching ➡ from the left lateral cervical esophageal wall ➡ compatible with a lateral cervical esophageal diverticulum (Killian-Jamieson). This lesion is below the level of the indentation from the cricopharyngeus muscle ➡.*

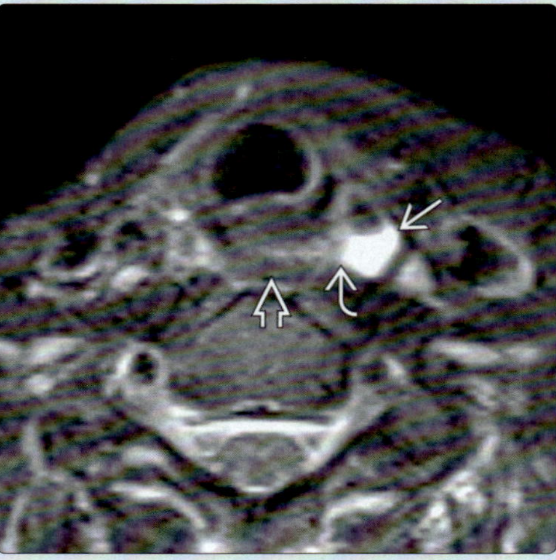

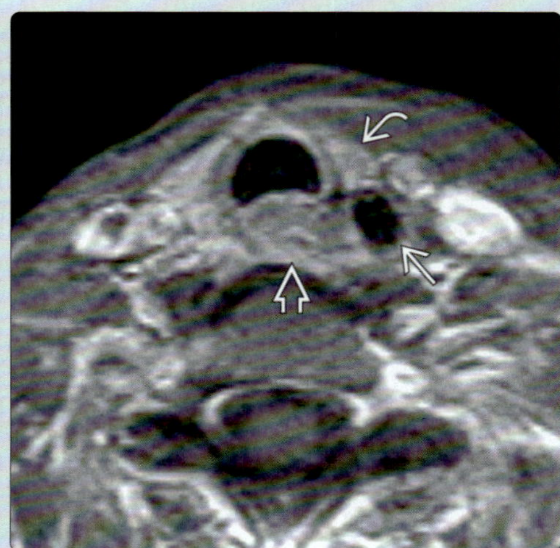

(Left) *Axial T2 FS MR shows an irregular mass ➡ lateral to the cervical esophagus ➡. The mass has an air-fluid level with hyperintense fluid layering posteriorly and subtly "points" toward the cervical esophagus ➡, suggesting its organ of origin.* **(Right)** *Axial T1 C+ FS MR reveals an esophageal diverticulum as an air-filled hypointense structure ➡ in the lower neck posterior to the left thyroid lobe ➡ and lateral to the cervical esophagus ➡. The left common carotid artery is also displaced anteriorly, lateral to the thyroid.*

TERMINOLOGY

Synonyms

- Killian-Jamieson diverticulum, proximal lateral cervical esophageal diverticulum
- Lateral pharyngoesophageal diverticulum

Definitions

- Lateral outpouching from proximal cervical esophagus

IMAGING

General Features

- Location
  - **Usually unilateral, left sided**
  - Bilateral up to 25%
  - Rarely unilateral, right sided
- Size
  - Average diameter: 1.4 cm
  - Range: 0.2-5.0 cm
- Morphology
  - Smoothly marginated round-oval sac

Imaging Recommendations

- Best imaging tool
  - Barium swallow best for confirming diagnosis
- Protocol advice
  - True lateral and frontal views should be obtained

Radiographic Findings

- Barium swallow findings
  - Frontal view: Small outpouching from proximal cervical esophagus
  - Lateral view: Arises below cricopharyngeus impression
    - Diverticulum overlaps anterior esophageal wall
- Aspiration rare as cricopharyngeus closes above diverticulum preventing reflux to larynx

CT Findings

- CECT
  - Well-defined round or oval mass lateral to proximal esophagus
  - May see air "pointing" toward esophagus
  - Abuts and may displace anteriorly, left thyroid lobe and common carotid artery
  - Density may be air, fluid, food debris, or mixed

MR Findings

- T2WI
  - Signal varies depending on luminal contents
  - Well-defined mass lateral to cervical esophagus
    - Abuts/displaces left thyroid and common carotid artery

DIFFERENTIAL DIAGNOSIS

Esophagopharyngeal (Zenker) Diverticulum

- Arises from **posterior midline above cricopharyngeus**

Thyroid Carcinoma Nodal Metastasis

- Level VI adenopathy from differentiated carcinoma
- Variable density (CT) or intensity (MR)
- Does not contain air

Parathyroid Cyst

- Degenerative or congenital along parathyroid tract
- Fluid density/intensity
- Does not contain air

PATHOLOGY

General Features

- Etiology
  - Protrusion through muscular gap (Killian-Jamieson triangle) in anterolateral wall of cervical esophagus
    - Inferior to cricopharyngeus and lateral to longitudinal muscle of esophagus just below insertion on posterior cricoid cartilage
    - Note Zenker diverticulum through Killian dehiscence in posterior portion of cricopharyngeus
  - Develops from refluxed pressure against competent cricopharyngeus
- Associated abnormalities
  - May see in association with esophageal-pharyngeal (Zenker) diverticulum

CLINICAL ISSUES

Presentation

- Most common signs/symptoms
  - Vast majority asymptomatic, incidental imaging finding
  - Dysphagia from pharyngeal dysmotility
- Other signs/symptoms
  - Respiratory symptoms uncommon as diverticulum below cricopharyngeus, preventing reflux to hypopharynx and larynx

Demographics

- Age
  - Usually > 60 years
- Epidemiology
  - Uncommon diverticulum
  - Less common than esophagopharyngeal (Zenker) diverticulum

Treatment

- Typically not treated if asymptomatic
- Diverticulectomy ± esophagomyotomy if symptomatic

DIAGNOSTIC CHECKLIST

Consider

- Arises from lateral cervical esophagus **below cricopharyngeus**
  - Zenker arises just above cricopharyngeus in midline

Image Interpretation Pearls

- Lateral barium swallow best for distinguishing from Zenker
  - On lateral swallow overlaps anterior esophageal wall

Reporting Tips

- Less common than Zenker and more likely to be asymptomatic

SELECTED REFERENCES

1. Bock JM et al: Clinical conundrum: Killian-Jamieson diverticulum with paraesophageal hernia. Dysphagia. 31(4):587-91, 2016

Summary Thoughts: Hypopharynx & Larynx

The hypopharynx and larynx both begin at the lower margin of the oropharynx and end at the lower margin of the cricoid cartilage. The **hypopharynx** is part of the digestive tract, carrying food and liquids to the esophagus. The **larynx** is part of the respiratory tract, connecting to the trachea, creating speech, and preventing aspiration.

Imaging of the **hypopharynx** and **larynx** is commonly performed for evaluation and staging of **squamous cell carcinoma (SCCa)**. Other common pathologies include laryngocele, thyroglossal duct cyst, and trauma. **Important tracheal lesions** include stenosis from intubation or tracheostomy, extrinsic compression or invasion by mass, and, less commonly, tracheal inflammatory diseases.

The **larynx** and **hypopharynx** are intimately related anatomically, sharing 2 common walls. This means that pathology in 1 location readily involves the other. One should be able to distinguish the 2 sites and define their anatomical subsites, particularly when **staging SCCa**.

Imaging Techniques & Indications

CECT with sagittal and coronal reformations is the study of choice for the hypopharynx, larynx, and trachea. A standard protocol covers from the alveolar mandible to the clavicles at 2.5- to 3.0-mm intervals during quiet respiration, 90 seconds after contrast bolus. For hypopharyngeal or laryngeal SCCa, a **2nd pass** may help assess vocal cord motion. This is performed from the hyoid to cricoid during a breath hold, which opens the pyriform sinuses while the cords adduct.

MR is less commonly used because of breathing artifacts, but it is a useful adjunctive modality for staging of SCCa because of better detection of laryngeal **cartilage invasion**.

FDG-PET/CT can help identify 2nd primary malignancies of the lung and upper aerodigestive tract in SCCa patients. It is useful for evaluation of recurrent or residual SCCa but is subject to false-positive results in the 2-3 months after radiation therapy. It increases nodal detection in advanced T tumors but does not consistently identify subcentimeter nodes due to camera resolution limitations.

Embryology

The **laryngeal ventricle** marks the division of 2 embryologically distinct laryngeal components. The **supraglottic larynx** forms from primitive buccopharyngeal anlage and the **glottic** and the **subglottic larynx** form from tracheobronchial buds. The buccopharyngeal anlage has a much richer lymphatic network compared with the tracheobronchial buds. As a result, **supraglottic SCCa** has a much higher incidence of **nodal metastases** at presentation compared with **glottic** and **subglottic SCCa**. Moreover, the lack of a midline fusion plane of the embryologic supraglottic larynx allows for the possibility of bilateral nodal metastasis.

Imaging Anatomy

The **hypopharynx** is part of the digestive tract, connecting the oropharynx to the esophagus. At its superior limit, the hyoid bone, the glossoepiglottic fold, and the pharyngoepiglottic fold demarcate the valleculae, which are part of the oropharynx. The cricopharyngeus muscle defines the inferior limit of the hypopharynx, just below the cricoid cartilage.

The **3 major hypopharyngeal subsites** are the pyriform sinus, posterior wall, and postcricoid region. The **pyriform sinuses** are symmetric pouches hanging behind the larynx. The anteromedial margins of the pyriform sinuses are the posterolateral walls of the supraglottic **aryepiglottic (AE) folds**. The pyriform sinus inferior tip, or pyriform apex, is at the level of the true vocal cords (TVC).

The **posterior hypopharyngeal wall** is the inferior continuation of the posterior oropharyngeal wall, extending from the hyoid to the inferior cricoid margin. Mucosa covering the posterior surface of the cricoid cartilage is the **postcricoid region**. This is 1 of the shared "walls" of the hypopharynx and larynx but is considered hypopharyngeal.

As part of the respiratory tract and the junction between the upper and lower airways, the **larynx** lies between the oropharynx and the trachea. The thyroid, cricoid, and arytenoid cartilages make up the framework over which the laryngeal soft tissues are draped.

As the largest of the laryngeal cartilages, the **thyroid cartilage** "shields" the larynx. Two laminae meet anteriorly at an acute angle in the midline to form an inverted V appearance on axial images. The posteriorly located **superior cornua** attach to the thyrohyoid membrane, and **inferior cornua** articulate medially with the cricoid cartilage sides, forming the cricothyroid joint. This is a useful imaging landmark for the entry of the recurrent laryngeal nerve to the larynx.

The **cricoid cartilage** provides structural integrity to the larynx as the only complete ring. It has a **signet ring** shape with a shorter anterior arch and the quadrate lamina forming the signet posteriorly. Paired pyramidal **arytenoid cartilages** perch atop the posterior lamina with true synovial cricoarytenoid articulations. The arytenoid **vocal processes** project anteriorly and are attachments for the posterior margins of the **TVC**. The inferior limit of the cricoid marks the junction between the larynx and the trachea.

There are **3 areas** of the **larynx** with components that become important when staging SCCa. These are the supraglottic, glottic, and subglottic larynx. The **supraglottic larynx** (supraglottis) extends from the tip of the epiglottis above to the laryngeal ventricles below. **Important components** include the vestibule (supraglottic airway), epiglottis, preepiglottic space, arytenoid cartilages, false vocal cords, and paraglottic (paralaryngeal) spaces.

- The **epiglottis** is a leaf-shaped cartilage that serves as a lid to the endolaryngeal "box," which closes to prevent aspiration during swallowing. It has a superior **free margin** that projects above the hyoid bone and inferiorly is fixed to the thyroid cartilage by the thyroepiglottic ligament, just below the midline notch. Anterior to the epiglottis and posterior and inferior to the hyoid bone lies the fat-filled, preepiglottic space, a clinical blind spot for submucosal tumor.
- The **false vocal cords** are the mucosal surfaces of the laryngeal vestibule. Deep to the false vocal cords are the paired **paraglottic spaces**. These fat-filled spaces merge superiorly into the preepiglottic space and extend inferiorly deep to the TVC in the glottis.
- The **AE folds** extend from the cephalad tips of the arytenoid cartilages to the inferolateral free margin of the epiglottis. The AE folds form the superolateral borders of the supraglottis and also form the anteromedial margin of the pyriform sinuses (part of the hypopharynx). They are the 2nd shared "wall." An AE fold SCCa is called a "marginal supraglottic laryngeal tumor."

Hypopharynx, Larynx, & Trachea Lesion Differential Diagnosis

Congenital	Trauma
Laryngomalacia	Arytenoid cartilage dislocation
Laryngeal web	Cricoid or thyroid cartilage fracture
Thyroglossal duct cyst	Hematoma
Degenerative/acquired	Laceration
Laryngocele (saccular cyst)	**Benign neoplasms**
Retention cyst	Hemangioma
Infectious/inflammatory	Chondroma
Laryngotracheobronchitis (croup)	Lipoma
Epiglottitis/supraglottitis	Squamous papilloma
Recurrent respiratory papillomatosis	**Malignant neoplasms**
Tuberculosis	Squamous cell carcinoma
Sarcoid	Sarcoma (chondrosarcoma)
Rheumatoid arthritis	Minor salivary gland tumor
Amyloid	Lymphoma
Wegener granulomatosis	Thyroid cancer invasion

The **glottic larynx** (glottis) consists of the TVCs and their mucosal covering. The **TVCs** are comprised of thyroarytenoid muscle, with medial fibers called the "vocalis muscle." Medially, there are thick elastic bands known as the vocal ligaments. TVCs meet in the midline anteriorly at the **anterior commissure**, which is only adequately imaged during quiet respiration. The **posterior commissure** is the mucosal surface between the arytenoid cartilages anterior to the cricoid. The mucosa over these areas normally is ≤ 1 mm in thickness.

The **subglottic larynx** (subglottis) includes the undersurface of the TVCs to the lower border of the cricoid cartilage. Its lateral walls are formed by the **conus elasticus**, a fibroelastic membrane extending from the vocal ligaments above to the cricoid below, which is not visible on imaging. Similar to the commissures of the glottis, the mucosa of the subglottis is normally < 1 mm in thickness.

The **trachea** connects the larynx to the lungs, beginning just below the cricoid and ending in the chest at the carina. Each "imperfect" cartilaginous ring surrounds the anterior 2/3 of the trachea, with a fibromuscular membrane covering the flat posterior portion. **Important anatomic relationships** include the thyroid lobes laterally, thyroid isthmus anteriorly from the 2nd-4th tracheal rings, and esophagus posteriorly. Posterolaterally, the tracheoesophageal grooves contain the recurrent laryngeal nerves, paratracheal nodes, and parathyroid glands.

Approaches to Imaging Issues of Hypopharynx, Larynx, & Trachea

It is important to be able to distinguish laryngeal and hypopharyngeal anatomical structures when evaluating pathology in this region, especially when **staging SCCa**. Two key shared "walls" are the **postcricoid region**, which is part of the hypopharynx, and the **AE folds**, which are considered supraglottic larynx.

There are **clinical blind spots** in the hypopharynx and larynx where imaging plays a critical role in tumor detection. In the hypopharynx, the **pyriform sinus apex** is a major site to search in patients presenting with "unknown primary" adenopathy.

In the larynx, the normally fat-filled preepiglottic and paraglottic spaces are clinical blind spots for submucosal spread of SCCa. As no fascia divides these spaces, SCCa can travel freely from one to the other.

Cartilage involvement with SCCa is an important clinical blind spot and an area of imaging complexity. Irregular cartilage ossification makes determination of cartilage involvement difficult. The diagnosis of invasion should not be made lightly, as it changes the tumor staging and is an indicator for total laryngectomy, as opposed to organ preservation surgery or chemoradiation. Cartilage invasion is determined when there is clear medullary invasion, cartilage destruction, or tumor mass on the outer extralaryngeal side of cartilage.

The endoscopic exam provides information that may be essential for imaging evaluation, particularly for early stage glottic tumors. Conversely, imaging is very important for staging SCCa and especially important for guiding surgeons to biopsy sites when a patient has an unknown primary tumor.

Clinical Implications

Hoarseness is a common presentation for tumors of the **larynx**. Glottic SCCa usually presents at an early stage with hoarseness because minor perturbations of the vocal mucosal wave create symptoms. Subglottic SCCa is often discovered at an advanced stage with extralaryngeal spread. Supraglottic SCCa is often diagnosed in an advanced stage because hoarseness does not develop until the tumor grows down to the vocal cords. Supraglottic and hypopharyngeal SCCa often present with or from nodal metastases. Other symptoms include sore throat, dysphagia, and referred otalgia.

Tracheal lesions present with **shortness of breath** and **stridor** and may carry the diagnosis of "asthma." Primary tracheal tumors are rare; one is more likely to see displacement, compression, or invasion of the trachea by an extrinsic mass.

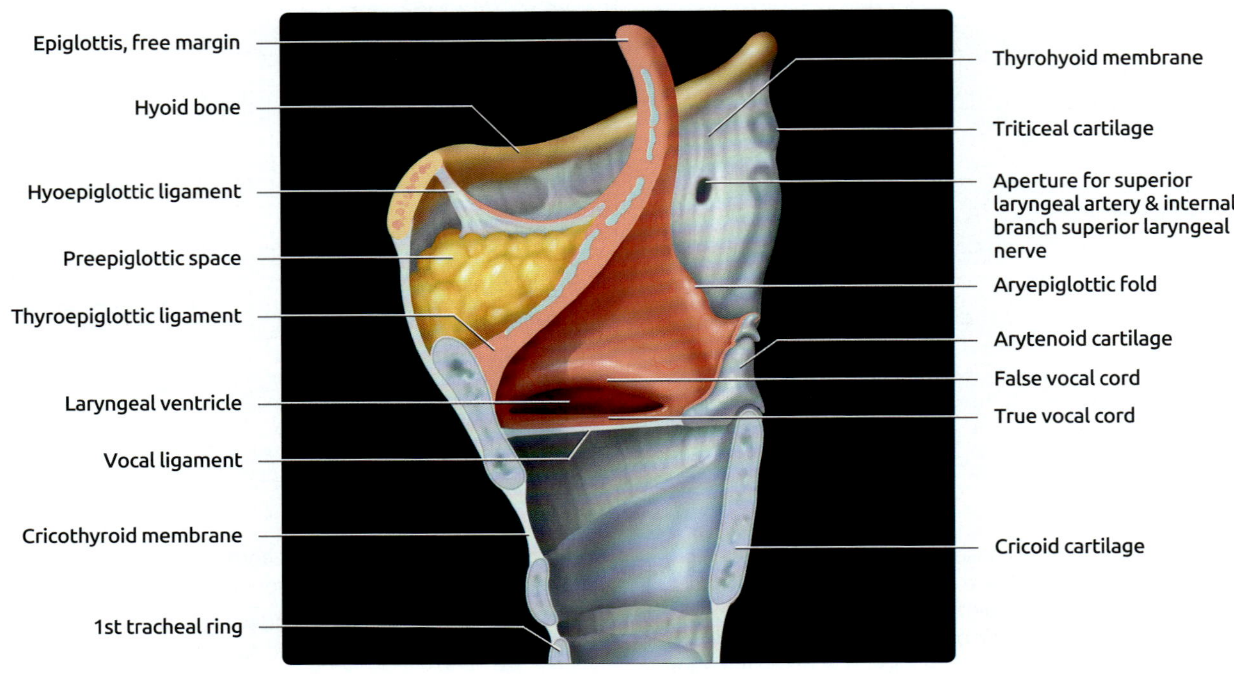

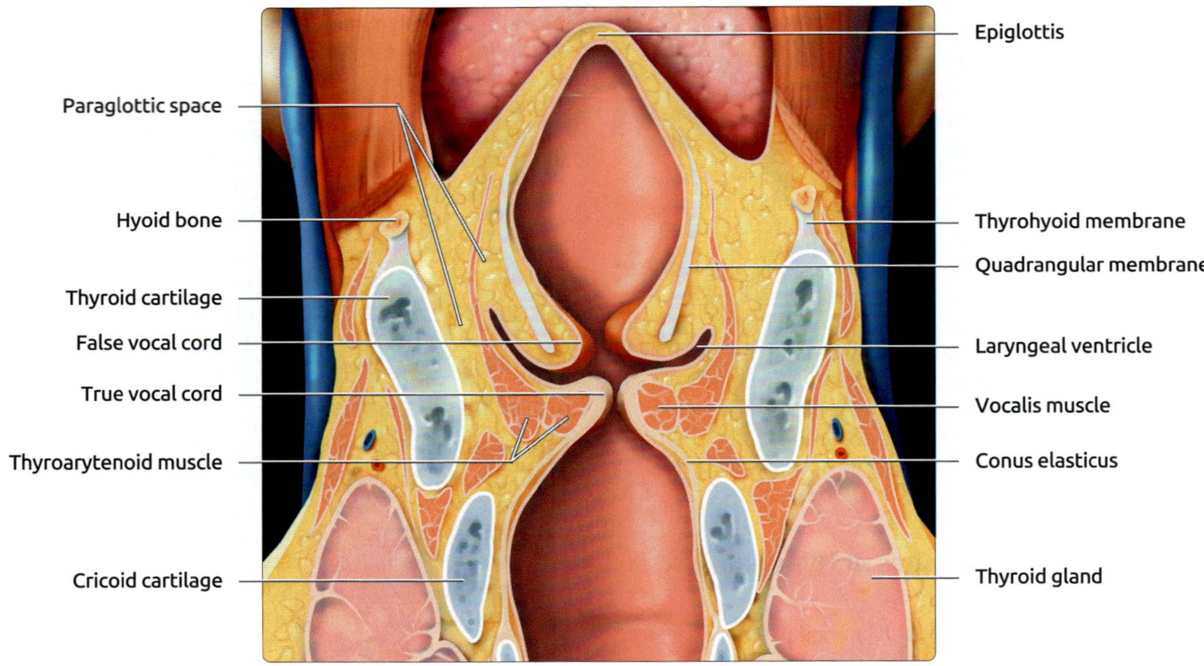

(Top) *Sagittal graphic of midline larynx shows laryngeal ventricle, the airspace that separates false vocal cords above and true vocal cords below. Aryepiglottic (AE) folds project from tip of arytenoid cartilage to inferolateral margin of epiglottis and represent a junction between the supraglottic larynx and hypopharynx. The epiglottis attaches to thyroid cartilage by thyroepiglottic ligament and to hyoid bone by hyoepiglottic ligament. Note the aperture in the thyrohyoid membrane for passage of superior laryngeal vessels and the internal branch of the superior laryngeal nerve.* **(Bottom)** *Coronal graphic posterior view of the larynx shows false and true vocal cords separated by laryngeal ventricle. Quadrangular membrane is a fibrous membrane that extends from upper arytenoid and corniculate cartilages to lateral epiglottis. Conus elasticus is a fibroelastic membrane that extends from vocal ligament of true vocal cord to cricoid. These membranes represent a relative barrier to tumor spread but are not seen on routine imaging.*

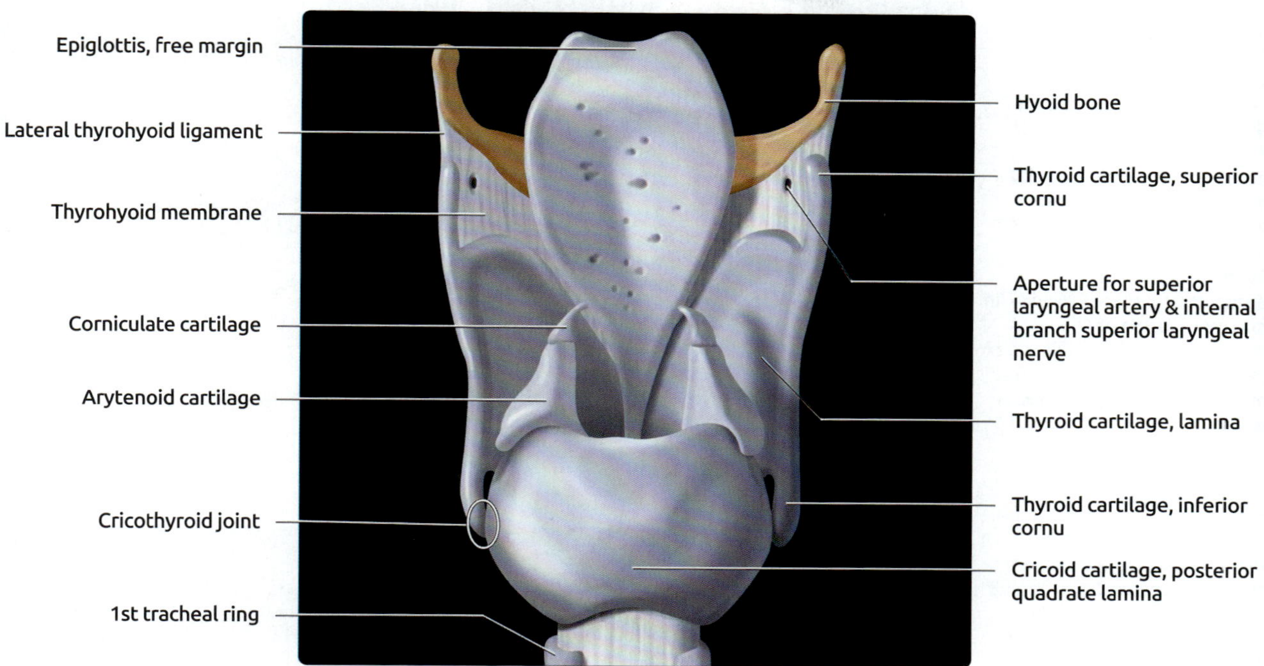

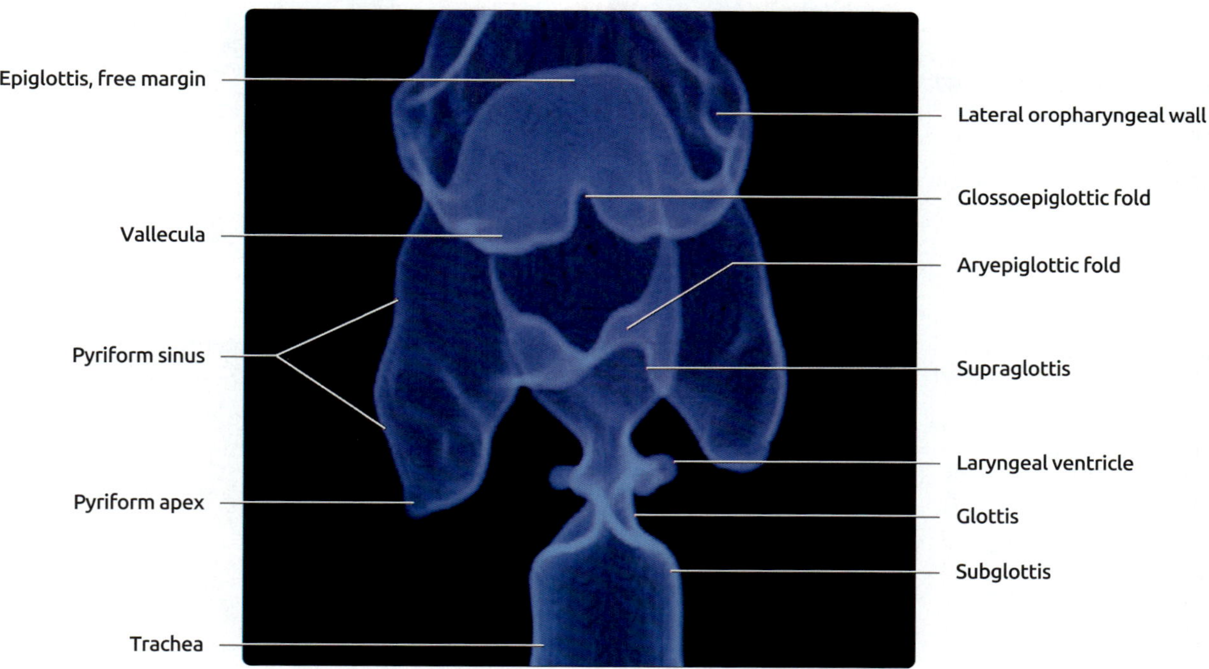

(Top) *Posterior view shows the epiglottis, a leaf-shaped cartilage containing fixed and free margins. The fixed portion has a narrow stem that attaches by thyroepiglottic ligament to internal aspect thyroid cartilage, just below the superior thyroid notch. Arytenoid cartilages perch on and articulate with the superior aspect of posterior cricoid cartilage. Inferior thyroid cornu articulates with cricoid in synovial-lined cricothyroid joint. Cricoid cartilage is the only complete ring in endolarynx and provides structural integrity. It is comprised of the anterior arch and taller posterior quadrate lamina. Lower border of cricoid represents junction between larynx and trachea. Thyroid, cricoid, and most of arytenoids are hyaline cartilage and ossify with age. Epiglottis, corniculate, and vocal process of arytenoid are yellow fibrocartilage and do not tend to ossify.* **(Bottom)** *Frontal view of 3D surface-rendered CT shows normal mucosal surfaces of oropharynx, hypopharynx, larynx, and trachea when distended during phonation.*

(Left) *Axial graphic at the level of the hyoid bone through the roof of the hypopharynx shows anterior preepiglottic space filled with fat ➾. Midline glossoepiglottic fold ➡, free margin of epiglottis ➡, and lateral pharyngoepiglottic folds ➡ delineate contours of the valleculae.* **(Right)** *Axial CECT at the same level reveals a hypodense fat-filled preepiglottic space ➾ and the anterior margin of the glossoepiglottic fold ➡, which separates valleculae. The free margin of the epiglottis ➡ is visible.*

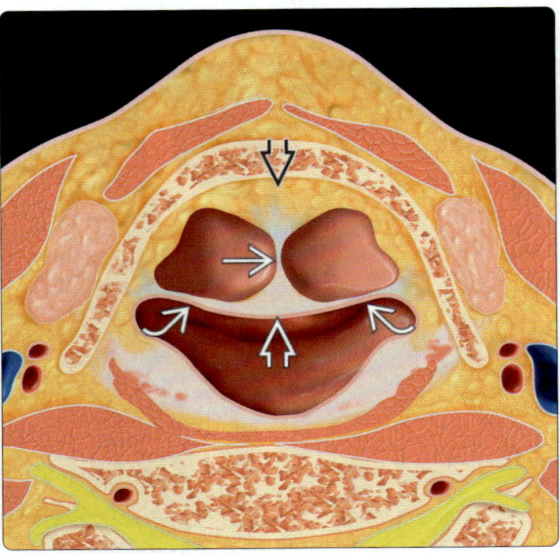

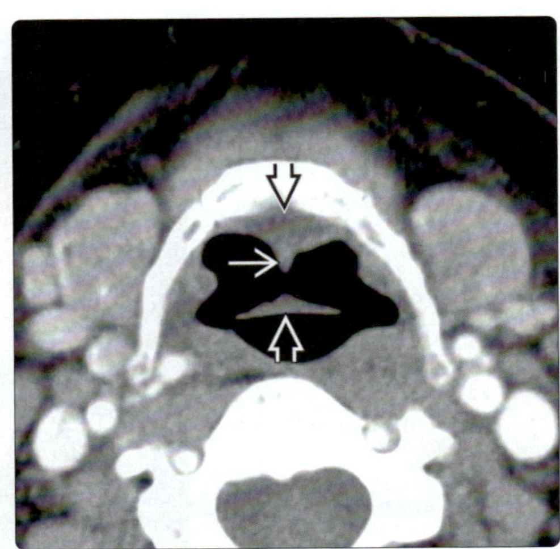

(Left) *Axial graphic at the midsupraglottic level shows the hyoepiglottic ligament ➾ to the fixed portion of the epiglottis ➾. AE folds ➡ are part of the supraglottic larynx but also form the anterior wall of the pyriform sinuses ➡ and therefore form a junction between larynx and hypopharynx.* **(Right)** *Axial CECT at the same level shows the hyoepiglottic ligament ➡ and the fixed portion of the epiglottis ➾ anteriorly. The posterior wall of the AE folds ➡ forms the anterior wall of the pyriform sinuses ➡.*

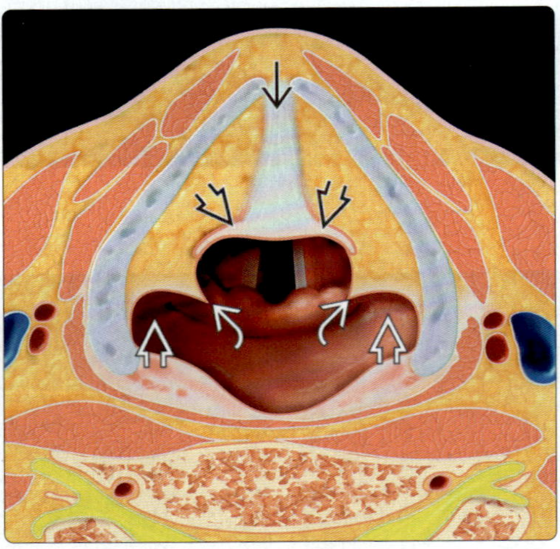

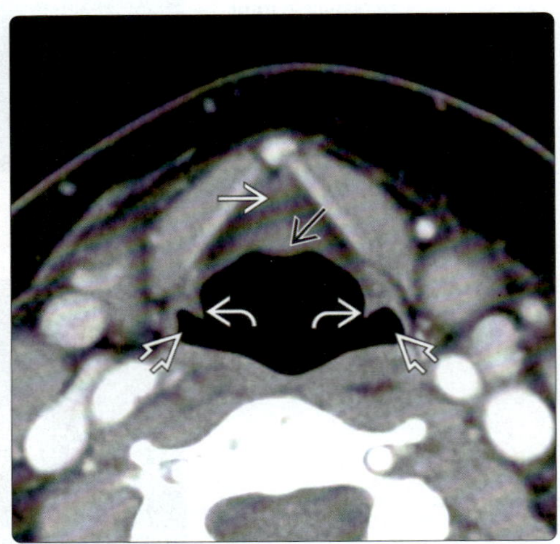

(Left) *Axial graphic depicts glottis or true vocal cord level where vocalis ➡ and thyroarytenoid ➾ muscles are evident deep to vocal ligaments ➡. Pyriform sinus apex ➾ reaches the level of true vocal cord and cricoarytenoid joints ➡.* **(Right)** *Axial CECT shows cricoarytenoid joints ➡, indicating that the scan is at the level of the glottis. The true vocal cords ➡ are abducted as the study was performed during quiet respiration. Note the thin normal anterior commissure ➡ during this phase.*

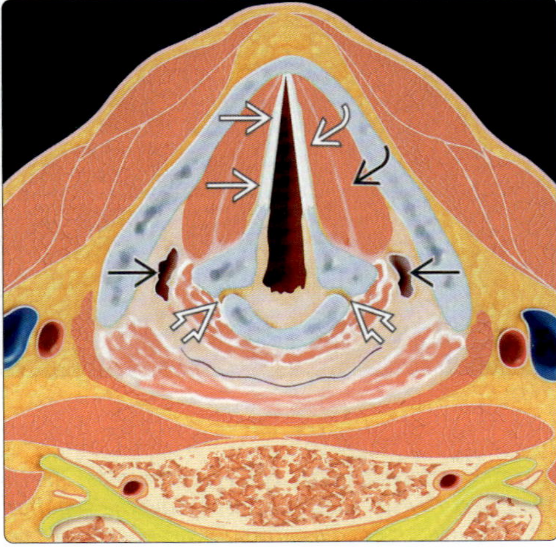

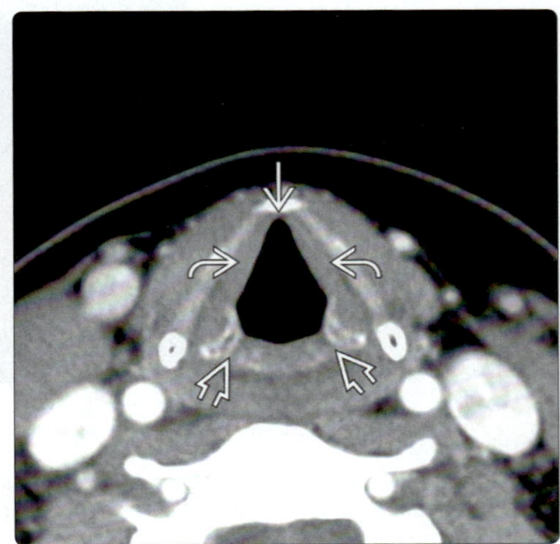

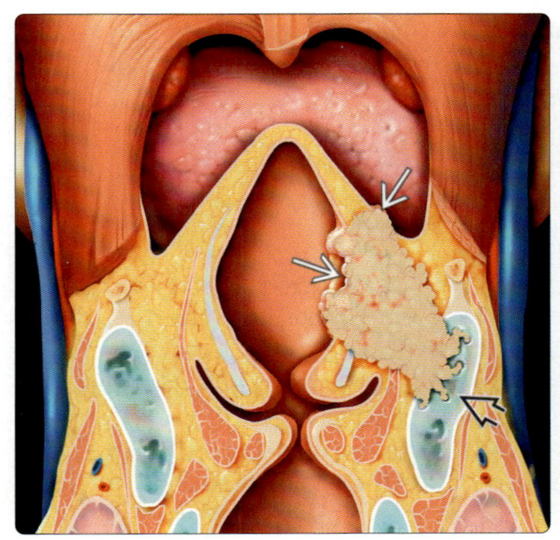

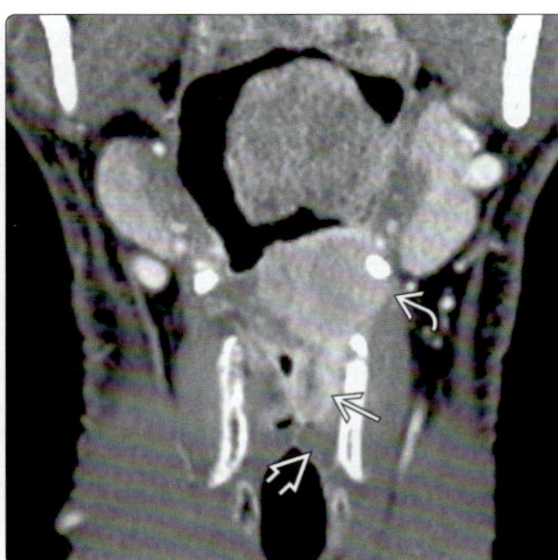

(Left) *Coronal graphic viewed from behind depicts supraglottic squamous cell carcinoma (SCCa) ➡ centered in the right AE fold & false cord, laterally invading thyroid cartilage ⇨.* **(Right)** *Coronal CECT reformatted image demonstrates a large enhancing mass arising in the left supraglottic larynx and extending inferiorly down paraglottic fat to false cord ➡. There is no evidence of extension to true cord ➡. Superiorly, the mass extends up to the valleculae, and laterally, it protrudes through the thyrohyoid membrane ➡.*

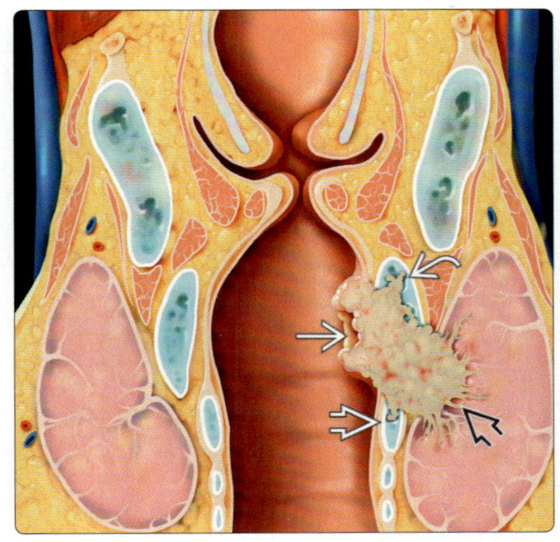

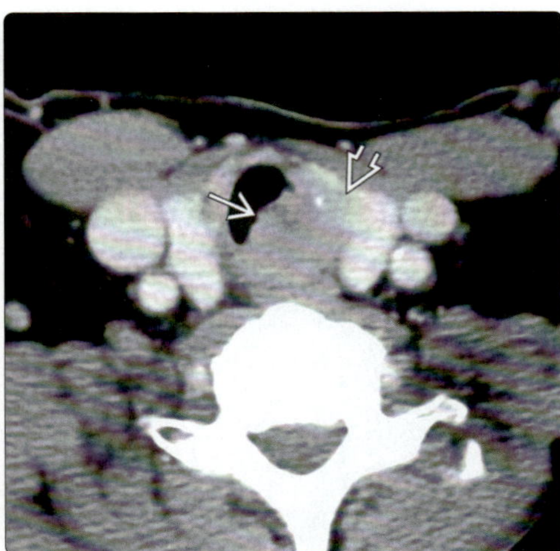

(Left) *Coronal graphic depicts subglottic SCCa ➡ invading laterally through cricoid cartilage ➡ into the thyroid gland ⇨. First tracheal ring cartilage is also involved ➡. Nodal drainage for subglottic tumors is to levels IV and VI nodes initially.* **(Right)** *Axial CECT through the lower neck reveals the inferior aspect of subglottic SCCa ➡ as it invades laterally into the left thyroid gland ➡. Approximately 50% of subglottic tumors present at this T4 stage.*

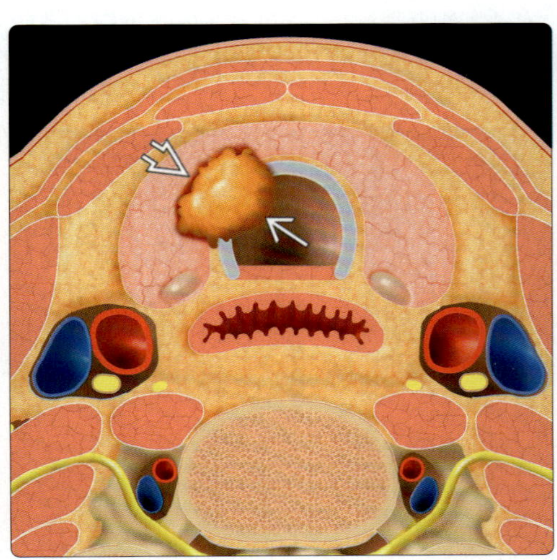

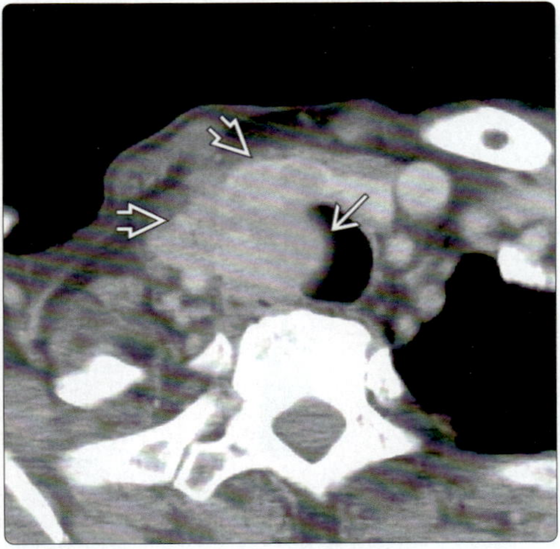

(Left) *Axial graphic through the thyroid bed illustrates a tracheal wall mass protruding into the tracheal lumen ➡ and laterally invading the thyroid gland ➡. Cervical tracheal wall lesions are rare, but diagnosis is often delayed due to nonlocalizing symptoms that may be misinterpreted as asthma.* **(Right)** *Axial CECT shows a tracheal wall carcinoma invading laterally and anteriorly into the thyroid gland ➡. Patient presented with stridor from tumor encroachment on tracheal lumen ➡.*

Croup

KEY FACTS

TERMINOLOGY

- Benign, self-limited viral inflammation of upper airway
- Symmetric subglottic edema results in stridor & characteristic "barky" cough

IMAGING

- Radiographs used to exclude more serious causes of stridor (rather than diagnosing croup)
- Frontal view: Often more revealing than lateral view
  - Gradual, symmetric tapering of subglottic trachea from inferior to superior
    - Steeple, pencil tip, or inverted V configuration
    - Loss of normal "shoulders" (focal lateral convexities) of subglottic trachea secondary to edema
- Lateral view: Best for excluding other diagnoses
  - Relatively mild narrowing of AP dimension
  - Haziness with loss of subglottic tracheal wall definition
  - ± hypopharyngeal overdistention

TOP DIFFERENTIAL DIAGNOSES

- Foreign body
- Epiglottitis
- Exudative tracheitis
- Angioedema
- Infantile hemangioma
- Iatrogenic subglottic stenosis

CLINICAL ISSUES

- Acute clinical syndrome characterized by "barky" or seal-like ("croupy") cough, inspiratory stridor, hoarseness
  - Age range: 6 months to 3 years; peak: 1 year
- ± prodrome of low-grade fever, mild cough, rhinorrhea
- Affected child usually well otherwise
- Most cases successfully treated with corticosteroids ± nebulized epinephrine with < 4-hour observation
- Recurrent episodes or atypical age suggest alternate diagnosis

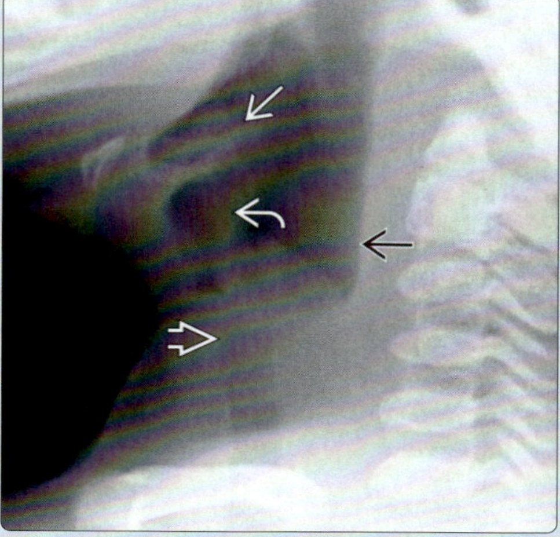

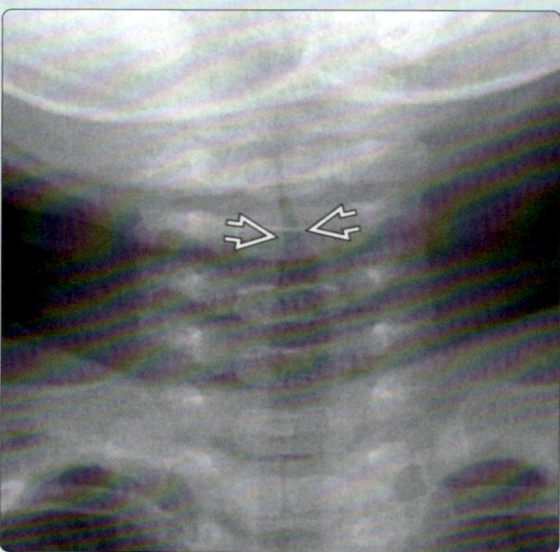

(Left) *Lateral radiograph in a 9 month old with stridor shows haziness of the subglottic airway ➡. Overdistention (ballooning) of the hypopharynx is noted ⇒. The epiglottis ➡ & aryepiglottic folds ➡ are normal.* **(Right)** *AP radiograph in the same patient shows symmetric narrowing of the subglottic trachea ➡, typical of croup. The loss of the normal abrupt subglottic/glottic shouldering with gradual tapering of the subglottic airway lumen from inferior to superior is referred to as the steeple sign.*

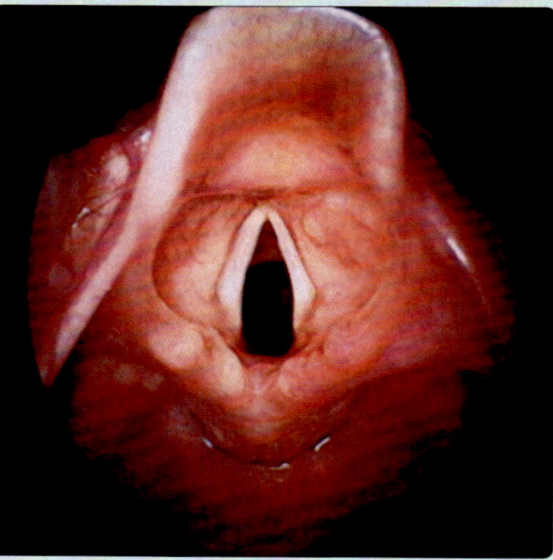

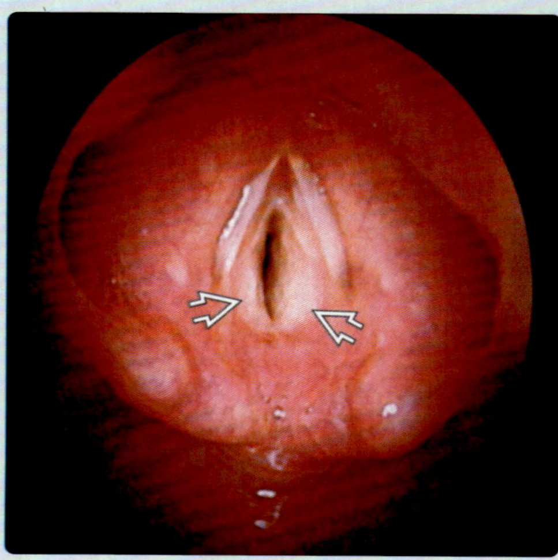

(Left) *Endoscopic photograph shows a normal appearance of the subglottic airway. The subglottis is widely patent such that the mucosa is actually hidden beneath the vocal cords.* **(Right)** *Endoscopic photograph in a child with viral croup shows edematous subglottic mucosa ➡, which is visualized through the vocal cords. There is marked narrowing of the subglottic airway lumen, predominantly in the transverse dimension.*

KEY FACTS

TERMINOLOGY

- Infectious inflammation of epiglottis and supraglottic larynx → airway obstruction

IMAGING

- Lateral radiograph
  - Enlarged epiglottis (**thumb sign**)
  - Aryepiglottic folds thick and convex superiorly
  - Ballooning of hypopharynx
- Frontal radiograph
  - May see symmetric subglottic narrowing
- CECT usually not required
  - Rarely see phlegmon or abscess

TOP DIFFERENTIAL DIAGNOSES

- Croup
- Exudative tracheitis
- Retropharyngeal abscess

PATHOLOGY

- Most often *Haemophilus influenzae* type b (Hib)
- Decreased incidence after Hib vaccination

CLINICAL ISSUES

- **Acute life-threatening disease**, often requires emergent intubation
- **Toxic child** with difficulty breathing and swallowing
- Mean age 14.6 years after Hib vaccine introduced
  - May also occur in adults
- Treatment options
  - Intubation; steroids + intravenous antibiotics

DIAGNOSTIC CHECKLIST

- Life-threatening emergency
  - May not be time to image
- For radiograph: Child should be upright, comfortable
  - Do not agitate or place in supine position
  - MD escort with equipment to secure airway if necessary

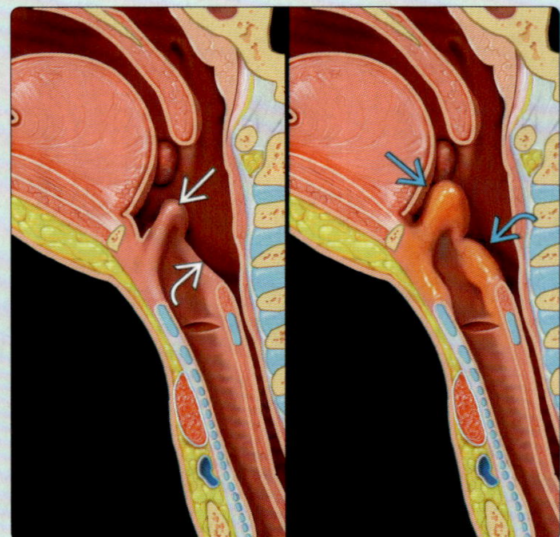

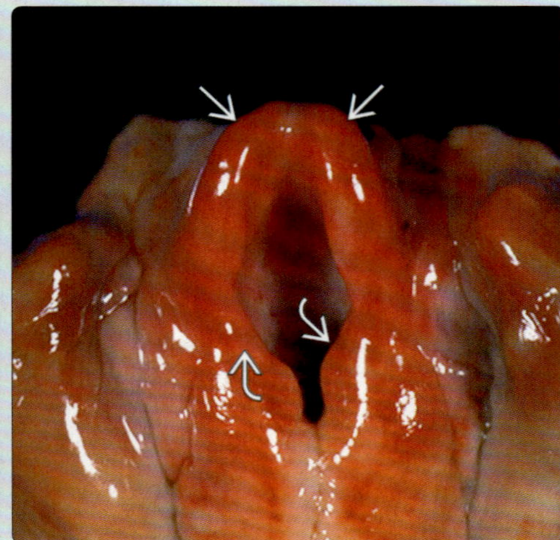

(Left) *Lateral graphic shows a normal supraglottic larynx on the left with a sharply defined epiglottis ➡ and straight or slightly concave aryepiglottic (AE) folds ⮫. Graphic on right shows epiglottitis with a thick, swollen epiglottis ➡ and convex, inflamed AE folds ⮫.* **(Right)** *Gross pathology specimen shows a markedly swollen, reddened epiglottis ➡ and similarly inflamed AE folds ⮫, narrowing the supraglottic lumen.*

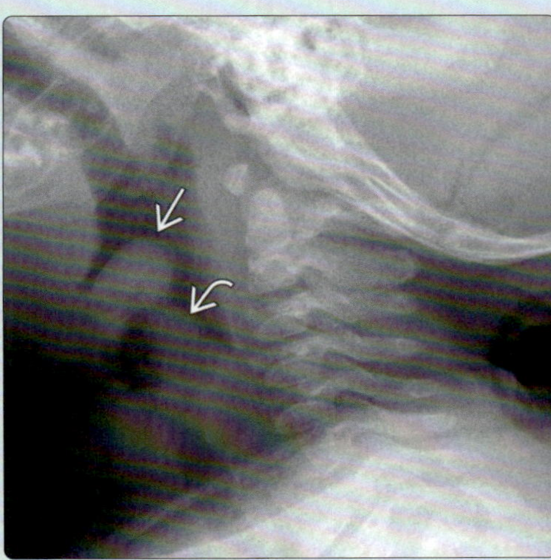

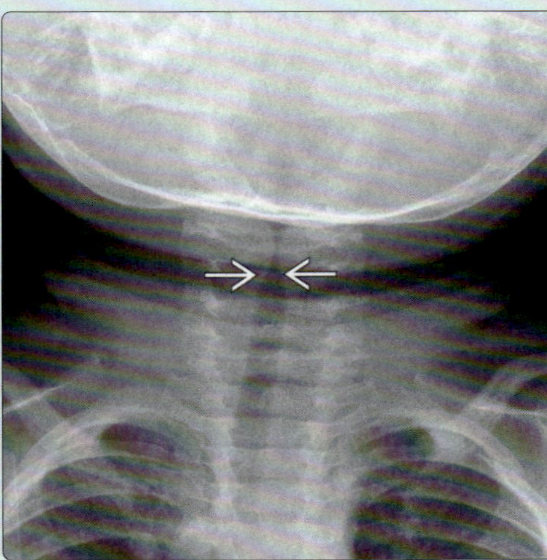

(Left) *Lateral radiograph in a 6-month-old infant with epiglottitis shows diffuse swelling of the epiglottis ➡, resulting in the thumb sign. AE folds ⮫ are thick with a convex contour indicating supraglottic inflammation.* **(Right)** *AP radiograph in a different child with epiglottitis demonstrates a mildly steepled appearance of the subglottic trachea ➡ that only on AP radiograph is indistinguishable from croup. With epiglottitis, this appearance is due to accompanying subglottic edema.*

KEY FACTS

TERMINOLOGY

- Definition: Relatively uncommon, potentially life-threatening infection/inflammation of supraglottic larynx in adult presenting with sore throat & dysphagia

IMAGING

- CECT: Thickened epiglottis, aryepiglottic folds, obliterated preepiglottic fat
  - Mucosal enhancement may be seen
  - Often involves tonsils and base of tongue
- CECT **not for diagnosis** but to evaluate complications or patients with difficult clinical exam
  - Contraindicated if airway compromise

TOP DIFFERENTIAL DIAGNOSES

- Supraglottic squamous cell carcinoma
- Radiated larynx
- Epiglottitis in child
- Caustic or thermal laryngeal injury

PATHOLOGY

- Adult epiglottitis now more common than pediatric
- Etiology: Usually *Streptococcus* or *Staphylococcus* species

CLINICAL ISSUES

- Clinical presentation
  - Sore throat, dysphagia; ↑ fever, ↑ WBC
- Most resolve with IV antibiotics ± steroids
- Airway management: Observation, intubation, or tracheostomy (15%); early intubation when clinically indicated may prevent emergent trach
  - Less likely to require airway intervention than children

DIAGNOSTIC CHECKLIST

- Inflammation affects entire supraglottic larynx ± posterior oropharynx & tongue base
  - **Not** just epiglottis
- Evaluate for abscess (ring-enhancing fluid collection) or emphysematous changes (multiple air dots)

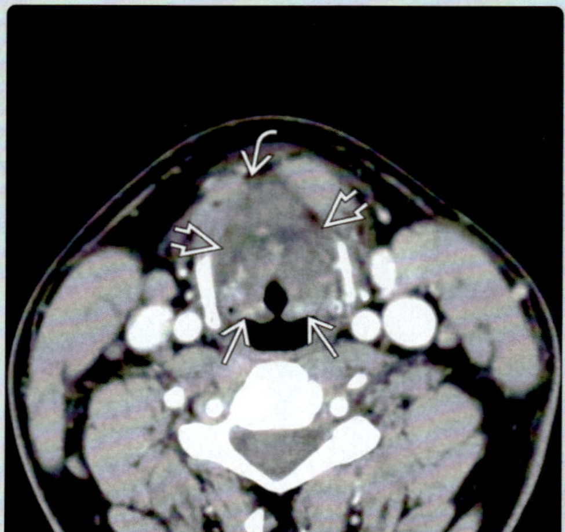

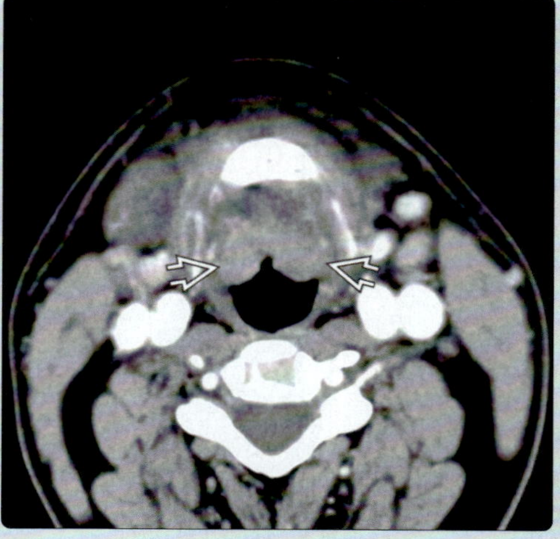

(Left) *Axial CECT in an adult patient with a sore throat and dysphagia reveals the typical findings of supraglottitis. There is thickening and enhancement of the epiglottis ➡ with soft tissue obliteration of the preepiglottic ➡ and superior paraglottic fat ➡.* **(Right)** *Axial CECT in the same patient shows enlargement and enhancement of the lingual tonsils ➡. Supraglottitis can also involve the soft palate, base of tongue, valleculae, uvula, and prevertebral soft tissues.*

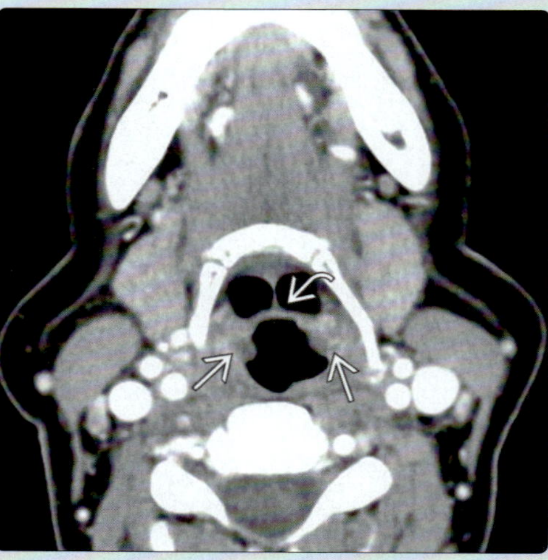

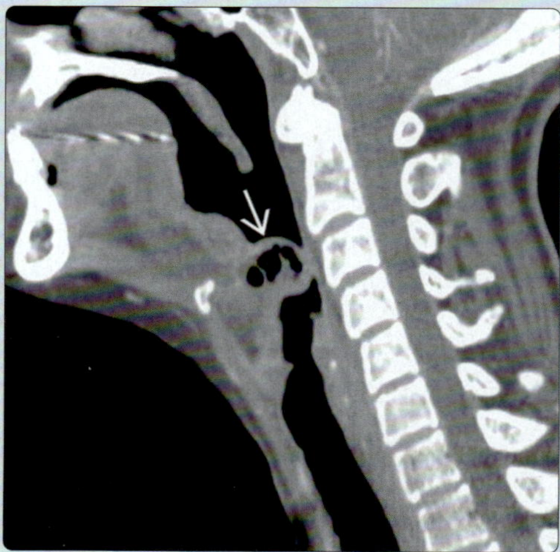

(Left) *Axial CECT shows a variant case of supraglottitis with thickening and enhancement of the aryepiglottic folds ➡ with relative sparing of the epiglottis ➡. Variable involvement of the epiglottis decreases the sensitivity of plain films in making the diagnosis.* **(Right)** *Sagittal CECT reformat demonstrates epiglottic enlargement with central air density ➡, characteristic of emphysematous supraglottitis. Emphysematous supraglottitis is more common in AIDS patients.*

Laryngeal Trauma

KEY FACTS

TERMINOLOGY

- Laryngeal trauma includes
  - Mucosal injury, fracture, or dislocation
  - External blunt trauma or penetrating injury
  - Internal iatrogenic injury scope or tube

IMAGING

- Nonenhanced CT best in suspected laryngeal trauma
  - Vascular injury considered, CTA
  - CT soft tissue windows best evaluate cartilage
    - Child's larynx not ossified; fractures may be missed
- CT findings to look for
  - Soft tissue air suggests mucosal laceration; site of aerodigestive track injury should be identified
  - Endolaryngeal hematoma
  - Thyroid cartilage fracture (vertical or horizontal)
  - Cricoid ring fracture (often 2 or more)
  - Arytenoid cartilage dislocation
    - May mimic paralyzed vocal cord
  - Cricothyroid joint dislocation (CNX injury)
  - Hyoid bone fracture
- May see 1 or multiple cartilage abnormalities
- Airway deformity from fracture or hematoma
- If larynx trauma seen, check for C-spine fracture

TOP DIFFERENTIAL DIAGNOSES

- Vocal cord paralysis

CLINICAL ISSUES

- Initial aim of therapy is to stabilize airway
- Endoscopy ± surgical exploration to evaluate
- Nonoperative management
  - Less severe mucosal tears, hyoid bone fractures, nondisplaced thyroid cartilage fractures
- Endoscopic reduction: Arytenoid cartilage dislocation
- Open reduction & fixation: Displaced, comminuted laryngeal fractures
- Airway stenting: Massive laryngeal injury and collapse

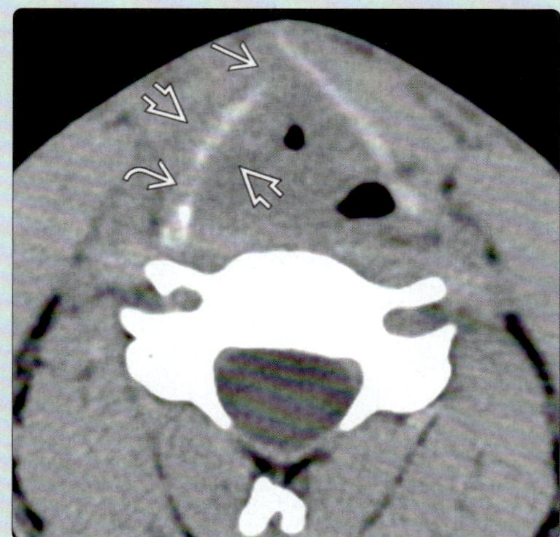

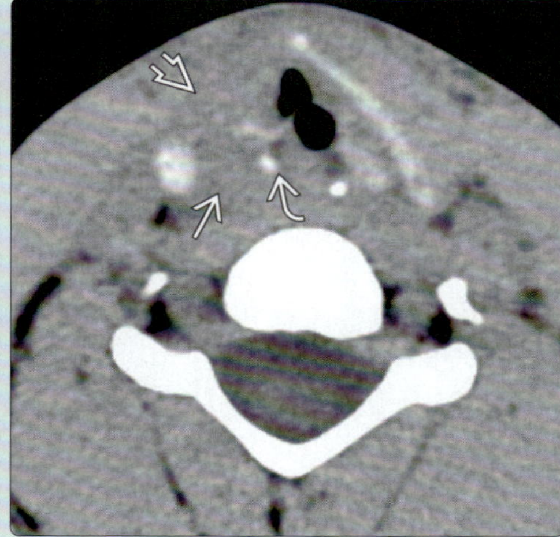

(Left) *Axial NECT through the supraglottic larynx shows step-off at the superior thyroid notch ➡. There is a subtle fracture of the right thyroid lamina with internal rotation ➡ of fractured cartilage and diffuse edema ➡ of the larynx and extralaryngeal tissues.* **(Right)** *Axial NECT more inferiorly in same patient, just above the cricoarytenoid joints, shows the anteromedial displacement of the right arytenoid cartilage ➡ and widening of right cricothyroid space ➡. Extensive laryngeal and paralaryngeal edema ➡ is evident.*

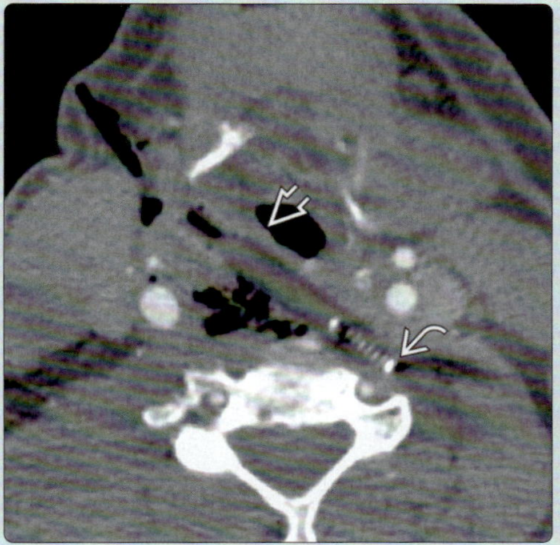

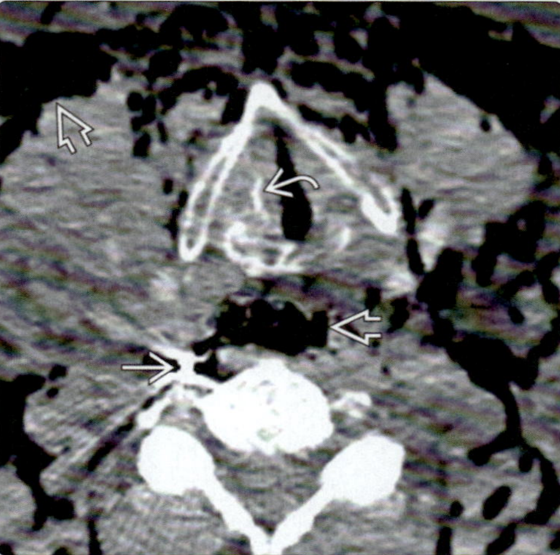

(Left) *Axial CTA performed for a pen stabbing through the supraglottic larynx shows a displaced edematous right aryepiglottic fold ➡. The pen tip ➡ terminates adjacent to the left vertebral artery, illustrating the importance of CTA in penetrating injuries.* **(Right)** *Axial CTA from gunshot victim shows diffuse soft tissue emphysema ➡ and shrapnel ➡ adjacent to the cervical vertebra. There are comminuted fractures of cricoid cartilage and the right arytenoid with displaced fragment into the right true vocal cord ➡.*

Upper Airway Infantile Hemangioma

KEY FACTS

TERMINOLOGY

- Definition: Hemangioma involving subglottic airway

IMAGING

- **Asymmetric** subglottic narrowing in young child
  - Classically subglottic, may be transglottic
- **Enhancing submucosal mass** on CT/MR
  - May be circumferential, bilateral, or unilateral
  - Usually asymmetric or affecting only 1 side, L > R

TOP DIFFERENTIAL DIAGNOSES

- Congenital subglottic-tracheal stenosis
  - **Symmetric** tracheal narrowing
- Iatrogenic subglottic-tracheal stenosis
  - Prior history of intubation or tracheostomy
- Croup
  - **Symmetric** subglottic tracheal narrowing
- Tracheomalacia
  - Abnormal **dynamic collapse** of intrathoracic trachea
- Exudative tracheitis
  - **Intraluminal filling defects**/inflammatory exudates

PATHOLOGY

- Benign **vascular neoplasm**
- **PHACES** syndrome
- 3 phases of growth and regression
  - Proliferative phase begins few weeks after birth
  - Involuting phase shows gradual regression
  - Involuted phase complete by late childhood
- **GLUT1(+)** in all phases

CLINICAL ISSUES

- **Inspiratory stridor** in infants < 6 months
- Usually symptomatic prior to 6 months of age
- Treatment
  - Conservative monitoring, propranolol, corticosteroids, laser therapy, surgical excision rarely required
  - Combination of therapies used in 75% of children

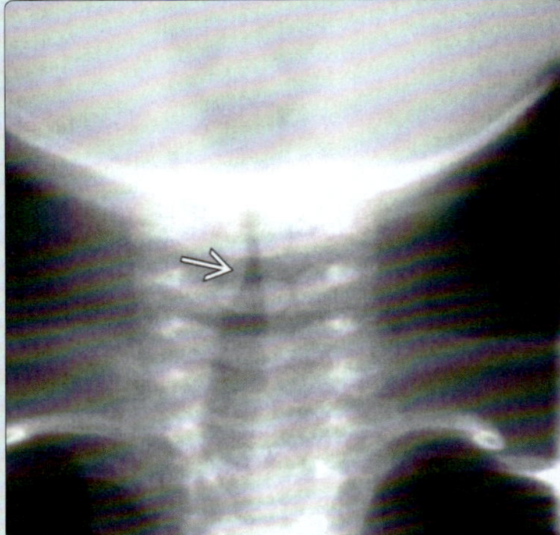
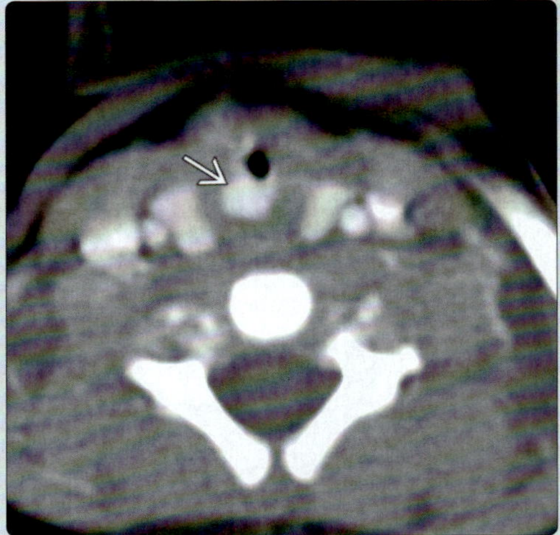

(Left) *AP radiograph shows asymmetric subglottic tracheal narrowing → in a 2-week-old infant presenting with stridor. Asymmetric narrowing is always concerning for hemangioma, as opposed to symmetric subglottic narrowing that is typical of croup.* **(Right)** *Axial CECT in the same patient shows a well-defined, enhancing hemangioma → along the dorsolateral aspect of the subglottic airway.*

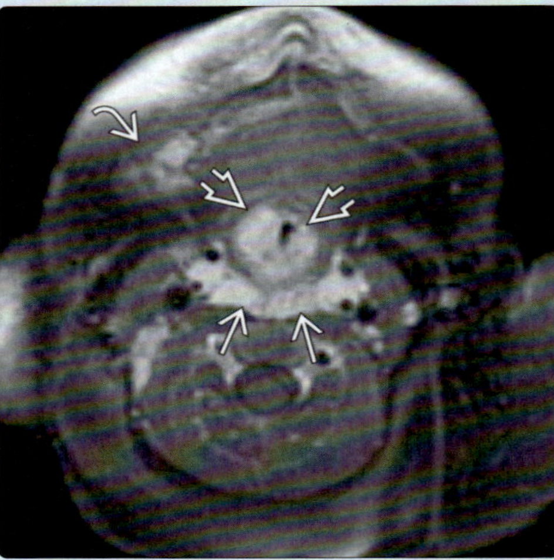
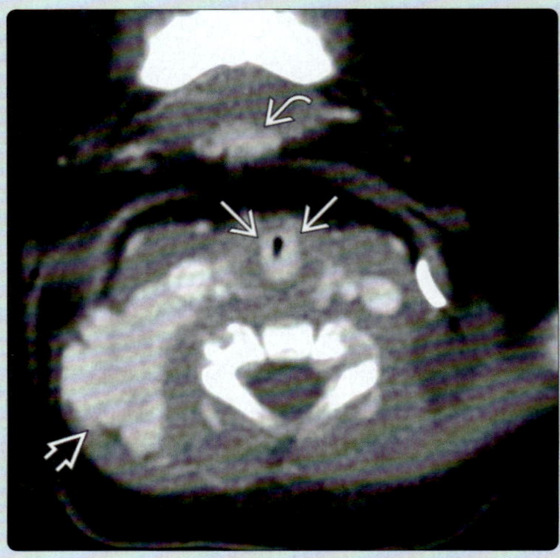

(Left) *Axial T1WI C+ FS MR in a child with PHACES syndrome demonstrates multiple enhancing hemangiomas in the retropharyngeal space → surrounding the subglottic trachea → and in the right submental space →.* **(Right)** *Axial CECT in an 11-week-old girl demonstrates a circumferential, well-defined subglottic hemangioma →. Notice also the posterior cervical space → and submental infantile hemangiomas → that should raise the question of PHACES syndrome.*

Laryngeal Chondrosarcoma

KEY FACTS

TERMINOLOGY

- Definition: Cartilage-producing chondrocytic neoplasm with cellular atypia, bone destruction, or local invasion

IMAGING

- **Expansile mass within laryngeal cartilage** with intact mucosal surfaces, chondroid matrix
- Cricoid >> thyroid cartilage origination
- CT: **Ring-like or "popcorn" calcifications** (chondroid matrix) in expansile intracartilage mass
  - Noncalcific component of mass hypodense to muscle
  - Cartilage/bone destruction or local invasion
- MR: **T2-hyperintense** mass, best seen with T2 FS, STIR
  - T1WI C+: Heterogeneous enhancement

TOP DIFFERENTIAL DIAGNOSES

- Chondroma
- Other sarcoma: Osteosarcoma bone forming
  - Synovial cell sarcoma, fibrosarcoma, malignant fibrous histiocytoma: No calcified matrix
- Metastasis to laryngeal cartilage

PATHOLOGY

- Arise from hyaline cartilage: Cricoid (85%), thyroid (15%), and, very rarely, arytenoid cartilage

CLINICAL ISSUES

- M:F = 4:1; mean age: 60 years
- Dysphagia or palpable neck mass (with exophytic growth pattern), dysphonia, stridor
- Symptoms often present for long duration, suggesting indolent process
- Submucosal mass on endoscopy
- Treatment options
  - Initial approach: Voice conservation surgery, when possible, with complete lesion removal
  - Salvage laryngectomy if recurs

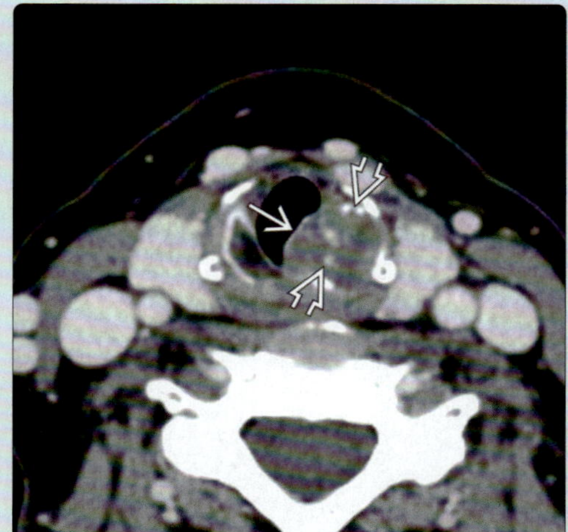

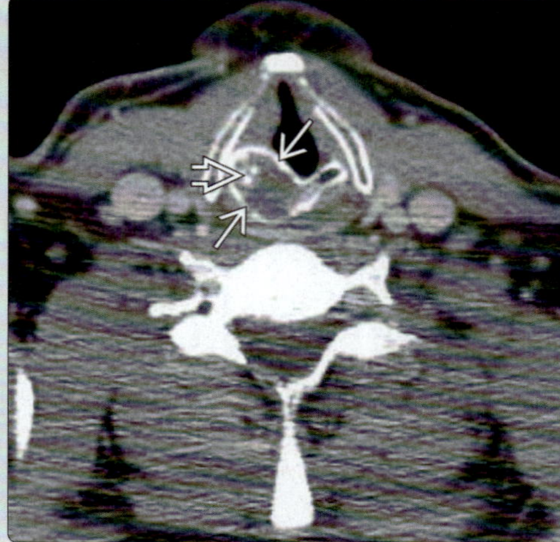

(Left) *Axial CECT in a 55-year-old woman with hoarseness shows a predominantly hypodense chondrosarcoma (CSa) ➡ arising from the left cricoid cartilage with internal calcifications ➡.* **(Right)** *Axial CECT shows a well-defined, expansile mass involving the right cricoid cartilage ➡. Small foci of internal calcified chondroid matrix are present ➡ in this grade I CSa.*

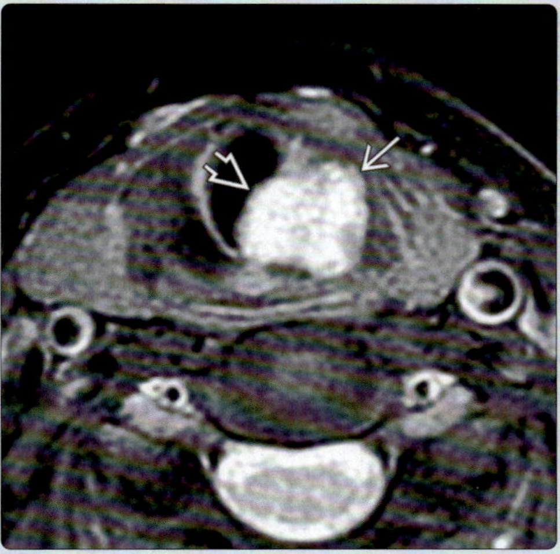

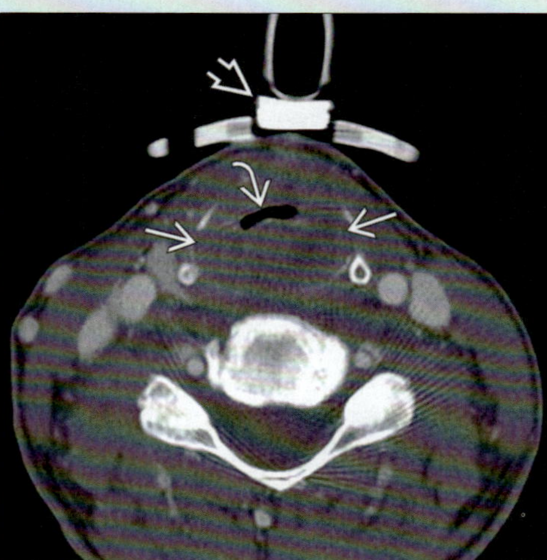

(Left) *Axial T2 FS MR shows this CSa as a homogeneously hyperintense mass ➡ impinging on the subglottic lumen ➡.* **(Right)** *Axial bone CT shows a noncalcified, low-grade CSa ➡. In such a case, imaging cannot differentiate CSa and benign chondroma. Note the tracheostomy apparatus ➡, necessitated by airway compromise ➡ and caused by the tumor.*

Postradiation Larynx

KEY FACTS

TERMINOLOGY

- Spectrum of soft tissue and cartilage changes following radiation therapy (XRT) for H&N tumors
- Changes may be XRT **effects** or **complications**
  - XRT effects seen in nearly all patients
  - Complications seen in minority

IMAGING

- Radiation effects: Expected findings
  - Acute-subacute: Submucosal edema, increased linear mucosal enhancement
  - Chronic: Fibrosis and atrophy
- Radiation complications
  - Persistent edema > 6 months
  - **Chondronecrosis**: Cartilage fragmentation/collapse, sclerosis, adjacent gas
- Treatment failure
  - Persistent mass, solid enhancement, deep ulcer

TOP DIFFERENTIAL DIAGNOSES

- Transglottic squamous cell carcinoma
- Supraglottitis
- Laryngeal trauma

CLINICAL ISSUES

- Clinical presentation
  - Hoarseness, mucosal dryness, dysphagia after XRT
  - Pain and dyspnea with more severe changes
- ↑ XRT dose ↑ severity of XRT effects and complications
- Baseline CT/MR should be done ~ 8 weeks post XRT
- Treatment options
  - Supportive therapy: Humidifier, voice rest, smoking cessation, reflux treatment
  - Severe dysphagia/odynophagia: Temporary gastrostomy
  - Radiation chondronecrosis: Hyperbaric oxygen therapy initially; laryngectomy or tracheostomy in nonresponsive cases or in chronic aspirators with pulmonary complications

(Left) *Axial CECT in a patient radiated after left modified neck dissection shows marked edema of both aryepiglottic (AE) folds ➡ with thin, linear enhancement of mucosa ➡. Note hazy edema of paraglottic ➡ and preepiglottic fat and subcutaneous soft tissues ➡ with platysma thickening ➡.* **(Right)** *Axial T2 FS MR 8 weeks following chemo/XRT for tonsillar SCCa reveals extensive symmetric edema of all soft tissues. Hyperintense, edematous, thick AE folds ➡ efface pyriform sinuses. Note hazy preepiglottic fat ➡.*

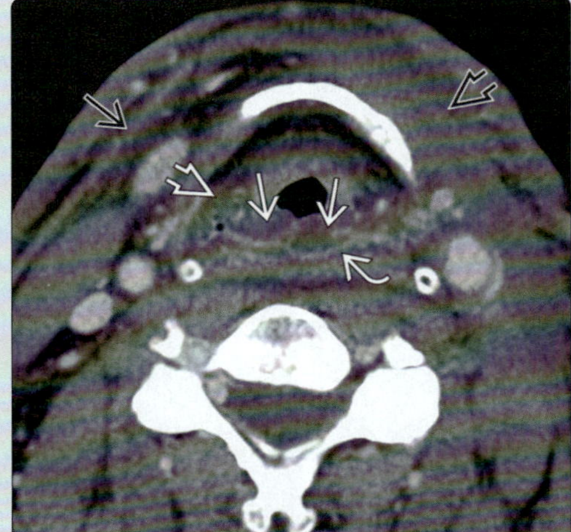

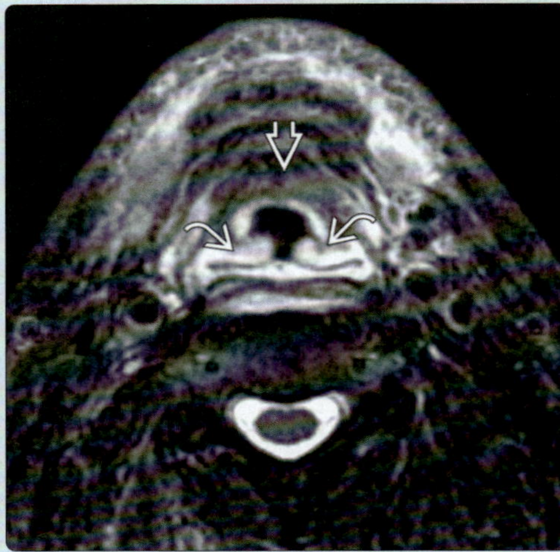

(Left) *Following XRT for laryngeal SCCa, there is particularly prominent mucositis manifested as thick but regular enhancement of the mucosal surfaces of the larynx ➡ and hypopharynx ➡. Absence of nodularity or discrete mass is reassuring.* **(Right)** *Gross pathology following laryngectomy with the larynx opened from a midline posterior incision demonstrates diffuse laryngeal swelling ➡ particularly affecting the AE folds ➡. Note focal hemorrhagic necrosis at the left cricothyroid joint ➡.*

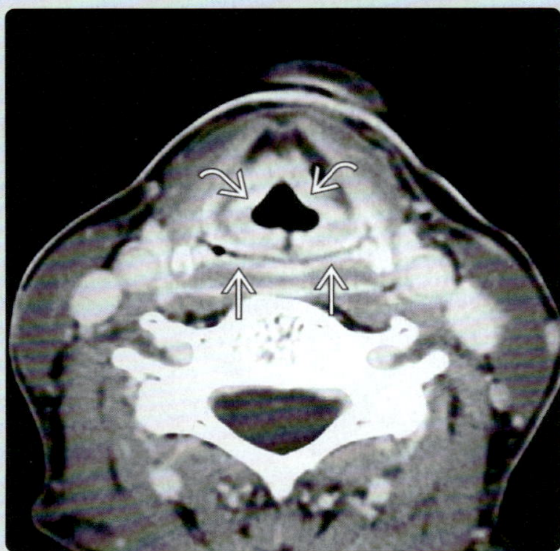

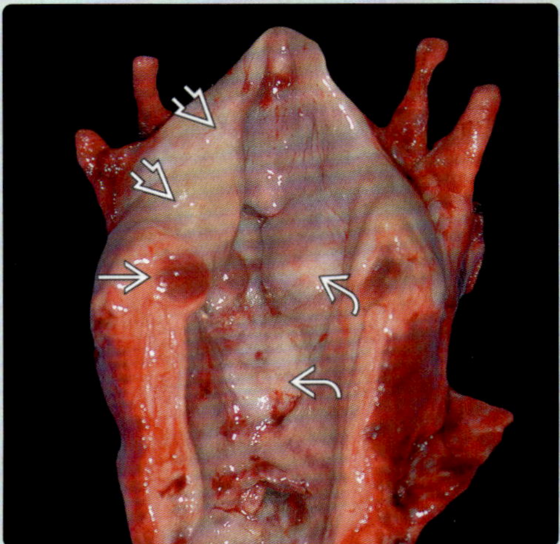

KEY FACTS

TERMINOLOGY

- Internal laryngocele: Dilated, air- or fluid-filled laryngeal saccule; located in paraglottic region of supraglottis
- Mixed laryngocele: Extends laterally through thyrohyoid membrane to low submandibular space
- Pyolaryngocele: Pus-containing superinfected laryngocele
- Secondary laryngocele: Glottic or inferior supraglottic lesion obstructs laryngeal ventricle (5% all laryngoceles)

IMAGING

- Best diagnostic clue with CECT
  - **Internal laryngocele**: Thin-walled, air- or fluid-filled cystic lesion communicating with laryngeal ventricle
  - **Mixed laryngocele**: Internal + extralaryngeal extension through thyrohyoid membrane
  - **Pyolaryngocele**: Pus-filled laryngocele with thick, enhancing walls
  - **Secondary laryngocele**: Glottic or inferior supraglottic lesion causal

TOP DIFFERENTIAL DIAGNOSES

- Thyroglossal duct cyst
- 2nd branchial cleft cyst
- Lateral hypopharyngeal pouch
- Supraglottitis with abscess
- Laryngeal saccule (normal ventricular appendix)

CLINICAL ISSUES

- Clinical presentation
  - Internal laryngocele: Voice change; hoarseness
  - Mixed laryngocele: Upper lateral neck mass
  - Caused by chronic increase in intraglottic pressure
    - Glass blowers, instrument players, chronic coughers
- Treatment options
  - Isolated internal laryngocele: Microlaryngoscopic CO_2 laser resection
  - Mixed laryngocele: External transthyrohyoid membrane surgical approach
  - Secondary laryngocele: Treat laryngeal SCCa

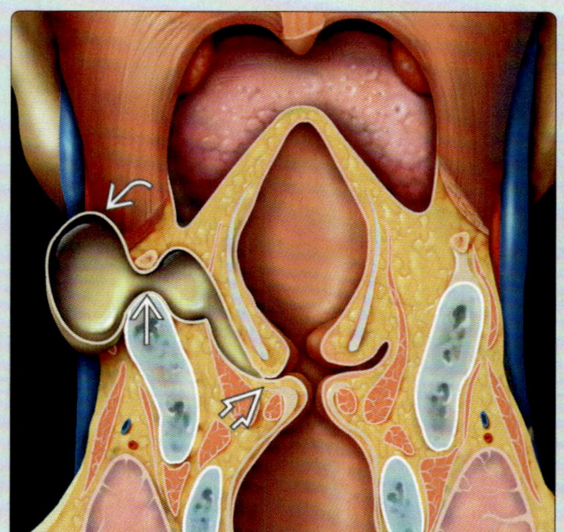

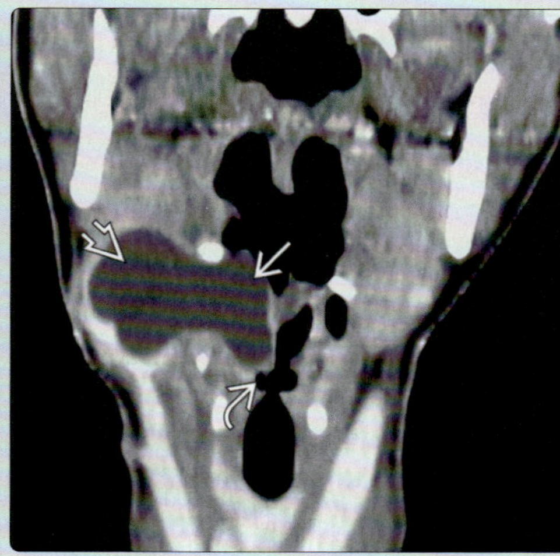

(Left) *Coronal graphic shows a laryngocele with extralaryngeal extension. There is an isthmus ➡ where the lesion squeezes through the thyrohyoid membrane to the low submandibular space ➡. Note stenosis at the laryngeal ventricle ➡.* **(Right)** *Coronal CECT reformat shows a similar lesion. This is also known as a "mixed" laryngocele because it contains internal ➡ (intralaryngeal) and external ➡ (extralaryngeal) portions. It can be followed to the laryngeal ventricle ➡.*

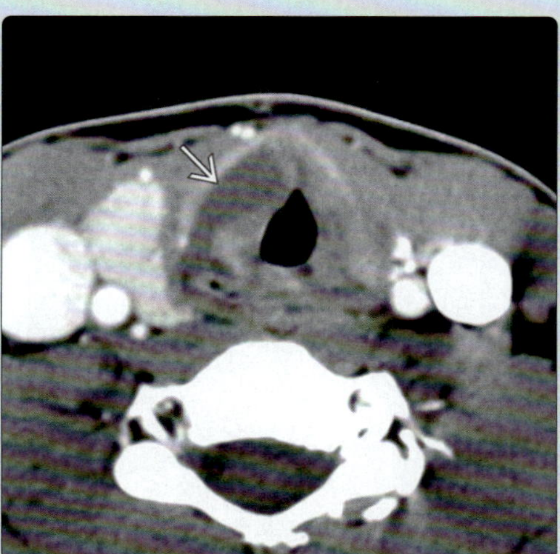

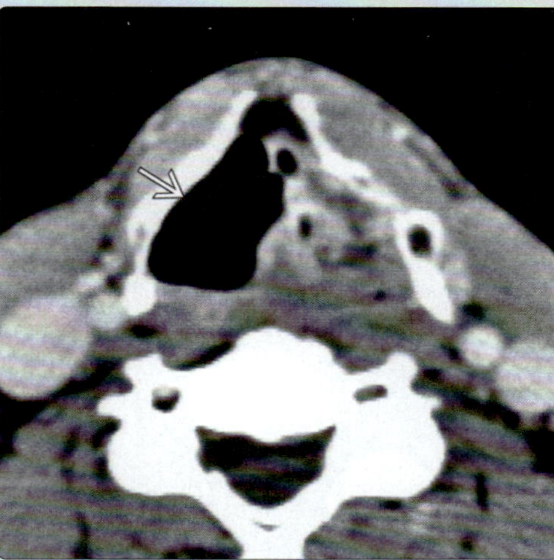

(Left) *Axial CECT demonstrates the typical findings of a fluid-filled, internal (simple) laryngocele. There is a nonenhancing, fluid density lesion ➡ confined to the right paraglottic region of the supraglottis, lateral to the false vocal cord.* **(Right)** *Axial CECT in a professional trumpet player shows an air-filled sac confined to the right paraglottic region ➡. Findings are typical of an air-filled, internal (simple) laryngocele.*

Vocal Cord Paralysis

KEY FACTS

TERMINOLOGY

- Definition: Immobilization of true vocal cord by ipsilateral vagus (CNX) or recurrent laryngeal nerve dysfunction

IMAGING

- Constellation of unilateral laryngeal CECT findings
  - Paramedian position of affected true vocal cord or
    - Ballooning of laryngeal ventricle = **sail sign**
  - Anteromedial rotation of arytenoid cartilage
  - Medially displaced, thickened aryepiglottic fold
  - Enlarged pyriform sinus
- Imaging **must cover entire course of CNX** and recurrent laryngeal nerve
  - This requires imaging from medullary nuclei to point of recurrent nerve branch
  - On **right** recurrent laryngeal nerve arises from CNX at **subclavian artery**
  - On **left** recurrent laryngeal nerve arises from CNX at **aortopulmonary window**
  - Specific areas along CNX need viewed for causal lesion
    - Jugular foramen, carotid space, mediastinum, & tracheoesophageal groove

TOP DIFFERENTIAL DIAGNOSES

- Neoplasm: Laryngeal SCCa; jugular foramen tumors
- Laryngeal trauma, including iatrogenic postsurgical (thyroid, patent ductus arteriosus ligation, etc.)
- Laryngocele

PATHOLOGY

- Most common etiologies: Neoplasm, trauma, congenital, iatrogenic, idiopathic & nonmalignant thoracic pathology

CLINICAL ISSUES

- Hoarseness, dysphonia, "breathy voice," dysphagia, aspiration, pneumonia
- Before ordering CECT from medulla to mediastinum
  - Clear larynx of tumor causing mechanical fixed cord
  - Obtain CXR to rule out thoracic cause

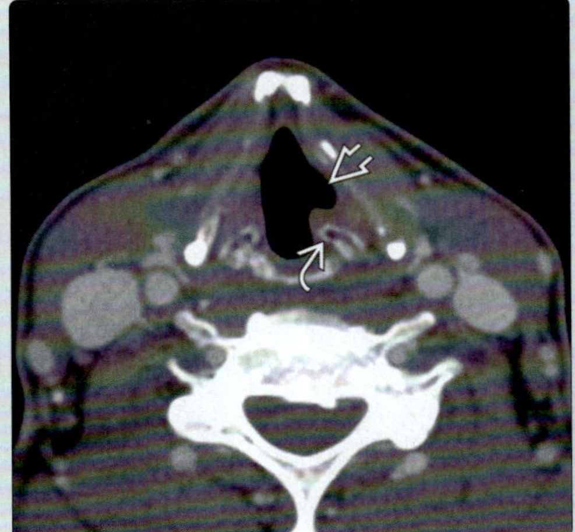

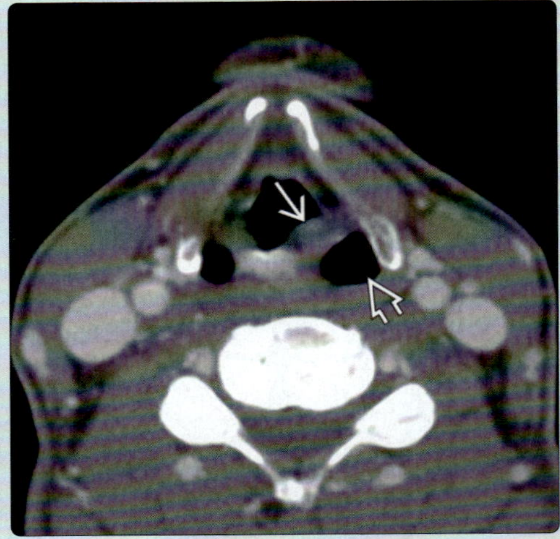

(Left) *CECT in a patient with new-onset hoarseness shows slightly medially rotated left arytenoid cartilage* ➡ *and a more prominent dilated left laryngeal ventricle* ➡*. This is sometimes referred to as the sail sign, as it mimics the spinnaker of a boat.* **(Right)** *Axial CECT in the same patient demonstrates asymmetrically enlarged left pyriform sinus* ➡ *& a medial position of the left aryepiglottic fold* ➡*, which also appears thickened. Imaging features are consistent with clinical finding of left vocal cord paralysis (VCP).*

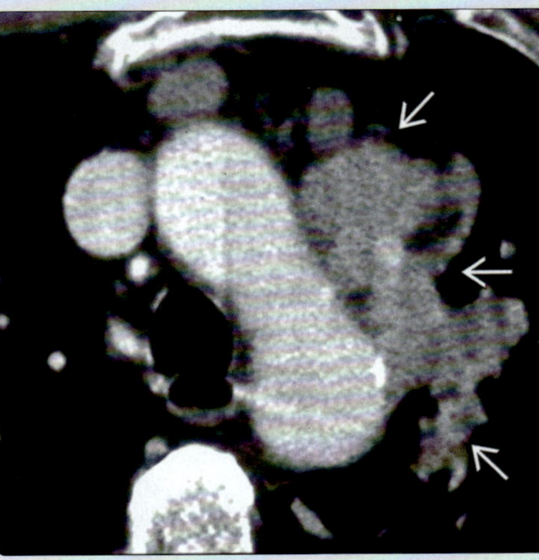

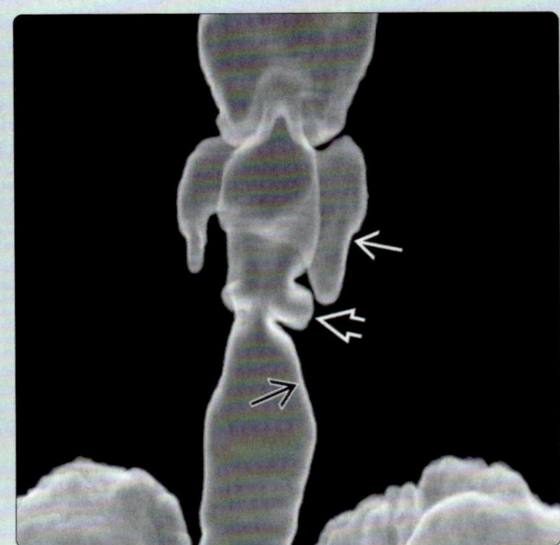

(Left) *Axial CECT in the same patient stresses the importance of scanning the aortopulmonary window for left VCP. A mediastinal mass (lung carcinoma)* ➡ *involves the left recurrent laryngeal nerve as it courses under the aortic arch.* **(Right)** *Anteroposterior 3D volume rendering of the airway in a patient with left VCP shows an enlarged ipsilateral laryngeal ventricle* ➡ *and pyriform sinus* ➡ *with flattening of the subglottic arch* ➡*.*

KEY FACTS

TERMINOLOGY

- Synonyms: Subglottic or laryngotracheal stenosis
- Definition: Nondevelopmental narrowing of cervical airway below vocal cords
  - Due to intrinsic pathology or extrinsic process compressing or invading airway

IMAGING

- **Intrinsic stenosis** usually iatrogenic from **intubation** or tracheostomy
  - Soft tissue narrows lumen
  - May see irregular, fragmented cartilage
- **Extrinsic stenosis** usually due to thyroid mass
  - Multinodular goiter: Enlarged heterogeneous lobes, ± calcifications, hemorrhage, cysts
  - Thyroid carcinoma or non-Hodgkin lymphoma: May compress or invade airway

TOP DIFFERENTIAL DIAGNOSES

- Subglottic infantile hemangioma
- Vascular rings and slings
- Congenital subglottic-tracheal stenosis

CLINICAL ISSUES

- Clinical presentation
  - Dyspnea, stridor: Biphasic (subglottic) or expiratory (tracheobronchial)
    - **50%** stenosis before dyspnea on exertion
    - **> 75%** airway narrowing before symptoms at rest
- Treatment options
  - Tracheal repair often needs redone
  - Endoscopy: Balloon dilatation; stenting; laser; posterior cricoid split
  - Surgical: Resection with reanastomosis; laryngotracheoplasty; slide tracheoplasty; cartilage grafts
    - Recurrent stenosis common

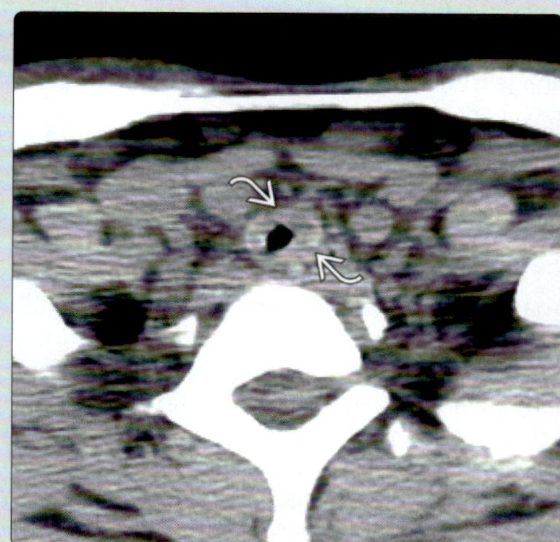

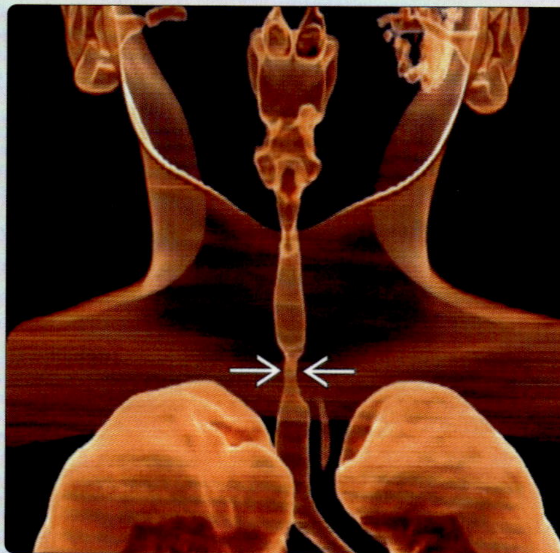

(Left) *Axial NECT at the thoracic inlet in a patient with a history of prolonged intubation shows smooth, noncalcified, circumferential thickening ➩ of the cervical tracheal wall with significant narrowing of the airway lumen.* **(Right)** *Volume-rendered 3D image from axial helical NECT demonstrates tracheal stenosis at the thoracic inlet related to a cuffed tube injury. Note the abrupt shelf of stenosis but with smooth edges ➡.*

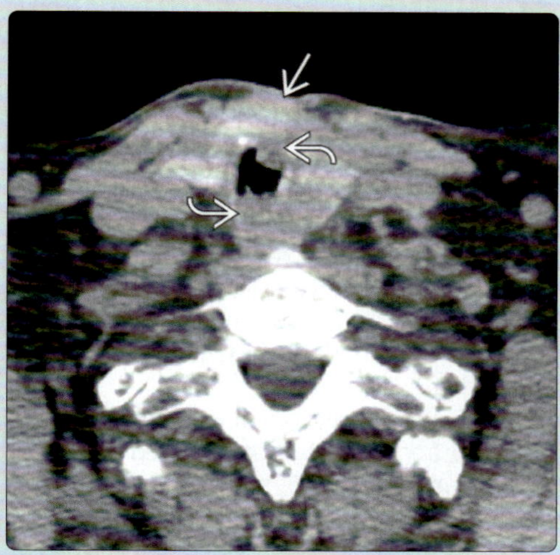

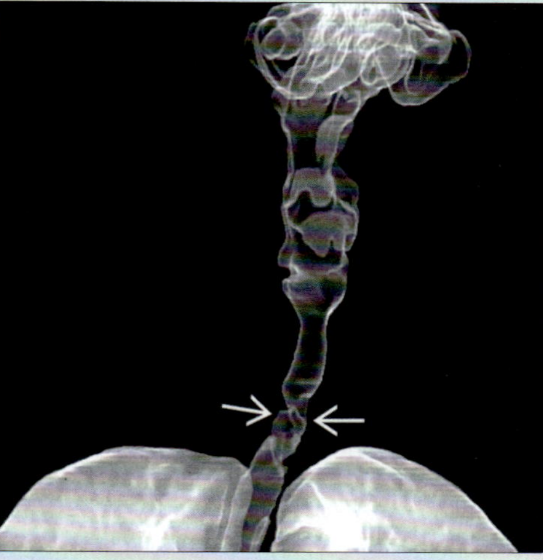

(Left) *Axial NECT in a patient with previous tracheostomy reveals subglottic-tracheal narrowing with marked luminal irregularity due to exuberant granulation tissue ➩. Note skin thickening with increased density of subcutaneous fat from scarring along the tracheostomy tract ➡.* **(Right)** *Volume-rendered 3D image from axial helical NECT demonstrates irregular subglottic tracheal stenosis over multiple centimeters due to granulation tissue at prior tracheostomy site ➡.*

Lymph Nodes Differential Diagnosis

Inflammatory	Infectious	Regional metastases
Reactive nodes	Viral upper respiratory infection	Squamous cell carcinoma
Castleman disease	Tuberculosis	NHL
Kimura disease	Atypical *Mycobacterium* species	Melanoma
Kikuchi disease	Cat-scratch disease	Salivary neoplasms
Rosai-Dorfman disease	HIV adenopathy	Thyroid carcinoma
Inflammatory pseudotumor	**Malignant primary tumor**	Lung cancer
	Hodgkin lymphoma	
	Non-Hodgkin lymphoma (NHL)	**Systemic metastases**

Summary Thoughts: Cervical Nodes

Cervical lymph nodes can be classified based on anatomic distribution or surgical levels used for neck dissection.

The key decision when assessing a lymph node is deciding whether it is **abnormal**. Traditionally, size criteria have been employed, but a multifactorial approach (size, homogeneity, morphology, enhancement, and borders) is more useful.

If a lymph node appears abnormal, one must decide whether it harbors inflammation (reactive), infection (suppurative), or tumor [usually squamous cell carcinoma (SCCa)]. This distinction is often quite difficult, especially with uncommon inflammatory diseases.

It is important for radiologists to understand the typical patterns of nodal spread of disease. Particular attention must be paid to subclinical lymph nodes (e.g., retropharyngeal).

Imaging Anatomy

Anatomically, the cervical lymph nodes are organized into groups (submental, submandibular, parotid, facial, occipital, and retropharyngeal) and chains (internal jugular, spinal accessory, transverse cervical, paratracheal, and external jugular).

- **Submental** group: Midline, between anterior bellies of digastric muscles
- **Submandibular** group: Anterior to posterior margin of submandibular gland, lateral to anterior belly of digastric muscles
- Parotid group: Within parotid gland itself
- Facial group: Scattered across face (includes mandibular, buccal, infraorbital, malar, and retrozygomatic)
- Occipital group: Posterior and inferior to calvarium
- Retropharyngeal group: In retropharyngeal space
- **Internal jugular** chain (IJC): Surrounding IJ vein from skull base to thoracic inlet
- **Spinal accessory** chain (SAC): Along course of CNXI across posterior cervical space of neck
- **Transverse cervical** chain (TCC): Along transverse cervical artery, in supraclavicular fossa; connects inferior aspects of IJC and SAC
- Paratracheal (juxtavisceral) chain: Anterior (midline, overlying strap muscles) and lateral to trachea (tracheoesophageal groove)
- External jugular chain: Superficial to sternocleidomastoid (SCM)
- Major chains (IJC, SAC, TCC) form triangle of nodes in lateral neck

Surgically, the cervical lymph nodes are organized into **6 levels** (or zones) based on surgical landmarks. Radiologic landmarks are used to approximate the surgical boundaries on imaging.

- Level I: Submental (level Ia) and submandibular (level Ib) clusters, located inferior to mandible; receives drainage from lips, floor of mouth, and oral tongue; drains into level II
- Level II: Upper portions of IJC (level IIa) and SAC (level IIb); anterior or deep to SCM, superior to **hyoid bone**; receives drainage from all nodal clusters and from pharynx; drains into level III
- Level III: Mid 1/3 of IJC; anterior or deep to SCM, inferior to hyoid but superior to bottom of **cricoid cartilage**; receives drainage from larynx and level II; drains into level IV
- Level IV: Bottom of IJC and medial 1/2 of TCC; anterior or deep to SCM, inferior to cricoid cartilage; receives drainage from level III and chest and abdomen
- Level V: Bottom of SAC (level Va) and posterior 1/2 of TCC (level Vb); lies in posterior cervical space, strictly posterior to back edge of SCM; receives drainage from occipital, retropharyngeal, periauricular, and parotid regions; drains into level IV and mediastinum
- Level VI: Paratracheal chain; superficial to strap muscles, between carotid arteries and lateral to trachea in tracheoesophageal groove; receives drainage from visceral space (especially thyroid gland), drains into level IV, mediastinum
- In radiation oncology, "supraclavicular nodes" are considered distinct entity, but, in radiology scheme, they are part of levels IV and V
- Numerous sonographic classification schemes are available, only some of which correspond to formal radiologic classification

Many nodes found in anatomic classification scheme are not included in the surgical scheme because they are not included in routine neck dissections. These may be overlooked clinically and merit particular attention from radiologists.

- **Retropharyngeal nodes**, in particular, cannot be palpated or clinically visualized, thus relying on radiologic identification of pathology; lesions of sinonasal tract and nasopharynx drain to these nodes, which may also harbor metastatic thyroid carcinoma
- **Parotid nodes** receive drainage from periauricular region and scalp; most common tumors involved here are skin SCCa or melanoma
- **Facial and occipital** metastases are less frequent but still important when they occur

A few cervical lymph nodes have been singled out and named because of clinical importance or radiologic appearances.

- **Signal (Virchow) node**: Lowest IJC node; if no neck primary tumor, consider chest or abdomen primary with metastasis carried via thoracic duct; left > right
- **Rouvière node**: Highest node in retropharyngeal group; lies within 2 cm of skull base; site of spread for nasopharyngeal carcinoma, esthesioneuroblastoma
- **Jugulodigastric (sentinel) node**: Lies within IJC just above hyoid bone; larger than surrounding nodes

Imaging Techniques and Indications

CECT is the 1st-line imaging modality to evaluate an adult patient with a neck mass of uncertain etiology. In children, US or MR should be considered 1st in order to minimize ionizing radiation. If the mass turns out to be metastatic, CECT usually can identify the primary site of origin. In the setting of a known malignancy, CECT or MR can be used to stage the nodes or to search for recurrence. However, whole-body FDG PET/CT is the preferred modality for oncologic imaging, particularly the assessment of regional and distant disease.

Advanced imaging techniques, such as quantitative diffusion imaging (DWI), dynamic contrast-enhanced (DCE) MR perfusion, and dual-energy CT, show promise for improving the sensitivity and specificity of detecting nodal metastatic disease. While advanced imaging of cervical nodes has increased, larger multicenter studies are needed to establish reproducible diagnostic thresholds and imaging protocols. In current practice, these techniques remain investigational and are not yet considered standard of care.

Approaches to Lymph Node Imaging Issues

Deciding whether a mass arises within a lymph node can be difficult in a few specific locations. In the submandibular space, nodal masses lie anterior to the facial vein, whereas glandular masses lie posterior to the vein. In the lower left neck, the signal node and the distal thoracic duct have a similar location. A dilated distal thoracic duct may mimic an enlarged node. The duct is purely cystic and can be followed proximally into the superior mediastinum. In level II, 2nd branchial cleft anomalies and lymph nodes have a similar location, and metastatic disease from the oral cavity is often purely cystic. In adults, metastatic SCCa should be considered the diagnosis until proven otherwise.

Deciding whether a lymph node harbors malignancy is one of the most difficult (and important) issues in head and neck imaging. Traditionally, size criteria have been employed, but, when used in isolation, size criteria have poor accuracy. Furthermore, there is limited agreement on which axis of the node to measure and appropriate size thresholds. Instead, a multifactorial approach, including other imaging findings, should be used in addition to size criteria to improve the accuracy of assessment. None of these findings on its own is a perfect distinguishing characteristic, and all should be taken into consideration.

- **Homogeneity**: Central necrosis in untreated lymph node is highly suspicious for cancer; caveat: Do not mistake normal fatty hilum for necrosis when seen with partial volume averaging artifact
- **Morphology**: Normal nodes are reniform (i.e., kidney-shaped) with central hilum containing fat and vessels; malignant nodes are ovoid, round, or show focal cortical expansion
- **Enhancement**: Node that enhances more than its counterparts is worrisome
- **Borders**: Irregular borders with infiltration of surrounding fat are indicative of cancer and suspicious for **extracapsular spread**

Understanding the usual **patterns of lymphatic spread** from various primary sites is critical for several reasons: (1) Particular attention can be given to areas of likely spread (e.g., retropharyngeal space nodes in nasopharyngeal carcinoma or lower cervical nodes in lung cancer), (2) equivocal lymph nodes that are outside the usual pattern are less suspicious, (3) likely locations of the primary tumor can be suspected in patients presenting with a nodal mass, and (4) nodal disease outside the usual pattern can prompt a search for a 2nd primary.

The enhancement pattern of a lymph node can help to predict the site of origin. **Necrotic nodes** with a thick enhancing wall are most likely secondary to tonsillar or tongue base SCCa. **Cystic nodes** with imperceptible walls are associated with papillary thyroid carcinoma. Large, uniformly enhancing nodes are suggestive of lymphoma. Additionally, nodal **microcalcifications** or intrinsic **bright T1 signal** are suspicious for differentiated thyroid carcinoma, often showing a similar appearance to the primary thyroid malignancy.

Clinical Implications

One of the most vexing clinical problems in H&N oncology is the **unknown primary tumor**. This occurs when a patient presents with a nodal mass that proves to be metastatic SCCa. Because SCCa does not arise within a lymph node, a mucosal primary must be sought. There are different definitions regarding how thorough the search must be before declaring the primary to be unknown; usually, the patient must undergo physical examination, panendoscopy, conventional imaging (CECT or MR), and blind biopsies of likely sites of origin.

Unknown primary tumors are important because patients must undergo irradiation to all mucosal surfaces to ensure that the unseen primary is included. This is extremely morbid because of xerostomia and dry mouth. However, patients with unknown primary tumors have a relatively good prognosis. **FDG PET/CT** identifies the primary tumor in ~ 25% of patients who fit the definition of an unknown primary tumor and should be considered as routine work-up in these patients.

Patients with enlarged upper neck nodes and enlargement of Waldeyer lymphatic ring usually have an upper respiratory infection. Unfortunately, lymphoma and HIV adenopathy can have an identical appearance, so clinical or radiologic follow-up is needed to exclude these more troubling diseases.

The **signal node**, located at the medial neck base, has particular clinical significance. Although it is sometimes affected by metastatic disease from the neck or upper mediastinum, it may also receive metastatic disease from abdominal primaries without intervening nodes in the chest (presumably via the thoracic duct). Thus, when patients present with nodal disease in the signal node, whole-body imaging is warranted to discover the primary tumor.

Selected References

1. Eisenmenger LB et al: Imaging of head and neck lymph nodes. Radiol Clin North Am. 53(1):115-32, 2015
2. Mack MG et al: Cervical lymph nodes. Eur J Radiol. 66(3):493-500, 2008
3. Nakamura T et al: Nodal imaging in the neck: recent advances in US, CT and MR imaging of metastatic nodes. Eur Radiol. 17(5):1235-41, 2007

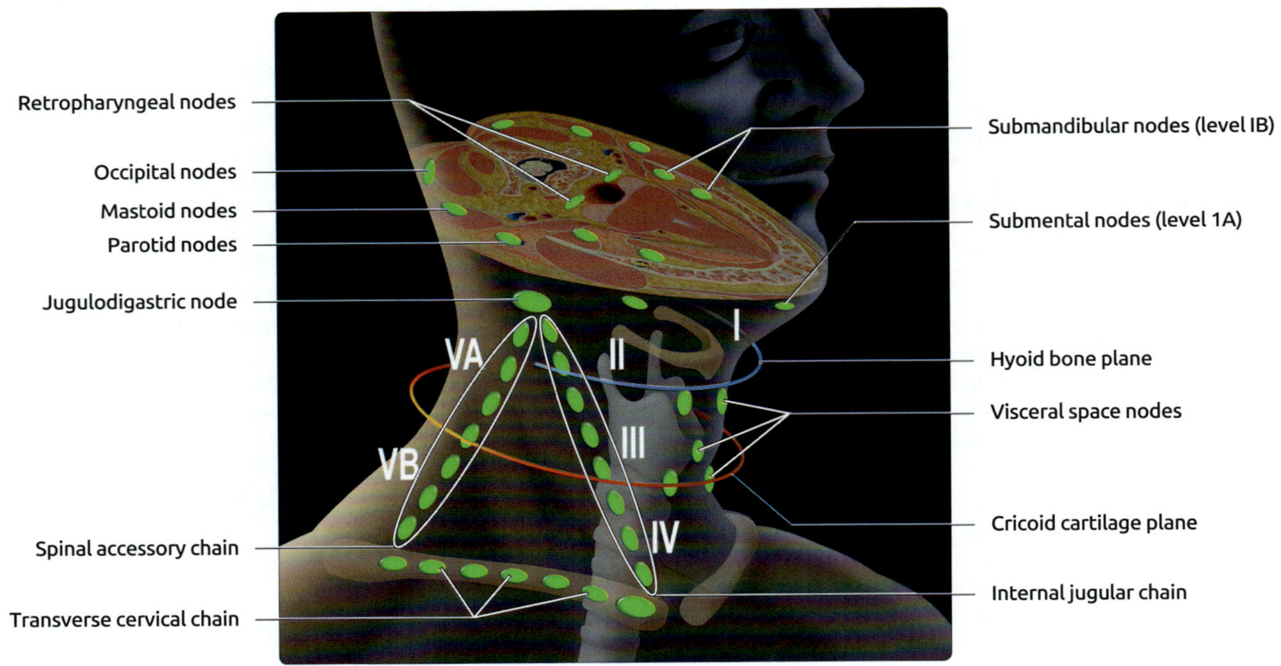

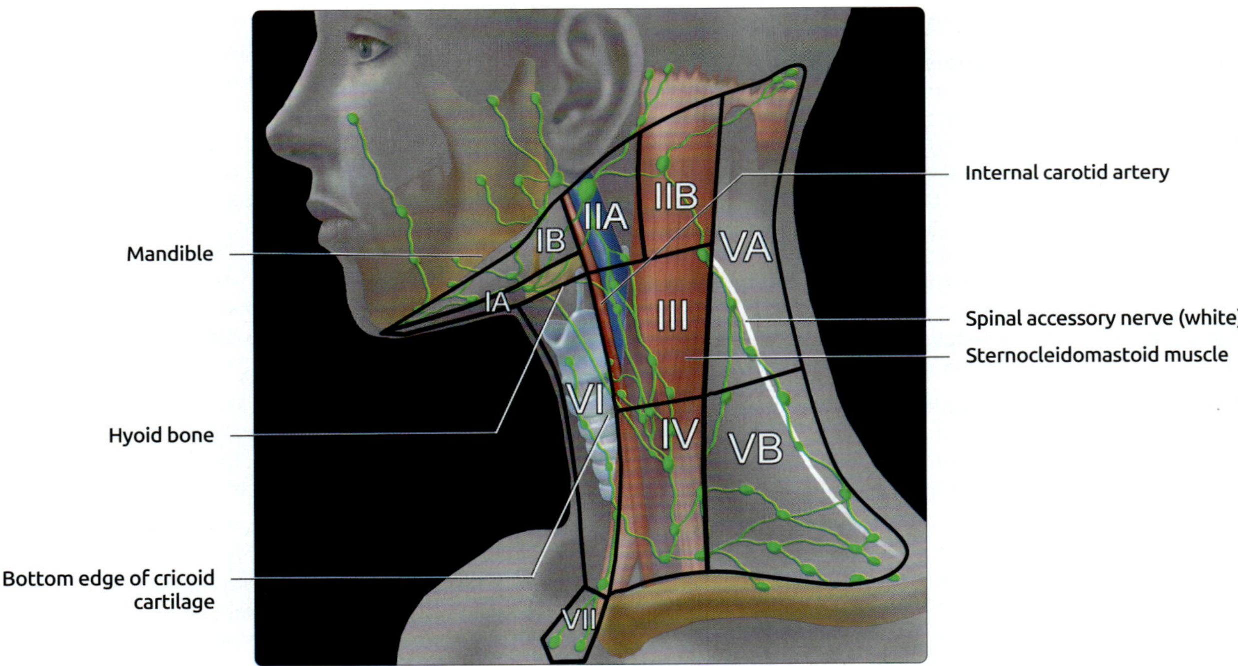

(Top) *Lateral oblique graphic of the cervical neck depicts an axial slice through the suprahyoid neck. Note that the major node chains [internal jugular chain (IJC), spinal accessory chain (SAC), transverse cervical chain] form a triangle in the lateral neck. The planes of the hyoid bone (blue arc) and cricoid cartilage (orange circle) divide the IJC and SAC into surgical levels.* **(Bottom)** *Lateral neck graphic shows the boundaries of the surgical levels. The chains and groups in this image are divided up not by their anatomic groups, as in the previous image, but by surgical landmarks. The hyoid bone separates level Ia from level VI and level II from level III. The inferior margin of the cricoid cartilage separates level III from level IV and level Va from level Vb. The posterior edge of the sternocleidomastoid muscle (SCM) separates levels II, III, and IV from level V. The carotid artery separates level VI from levels III and IV. The inferior margin of the mandible separates level Ib from the facial lymph nodes.*

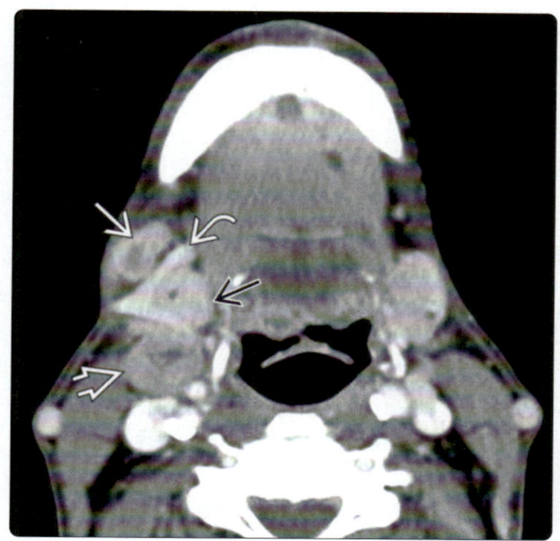

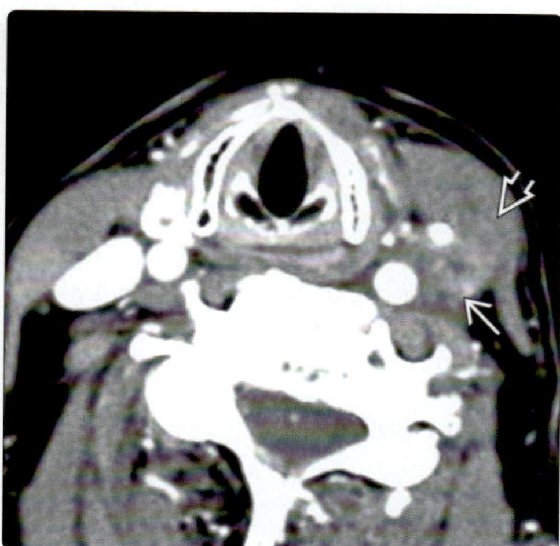

(Left) *Axial CECT shows an abnormal submandibular space mass ➡ anterior to the facial vein ➡, indicating it is a level Ib lymph node. The submandibular gland ➡ lies posterior to the vein. Nodes that lie posterior to the gland ➡ are in level II.* **(Right)** *Axial CECT shows a left lateral neck mass ➡ deep to the SCM muscle. Irregular margins and loss of the normal fat plane ➡ between the mass and the SCM indicate extracapsular spread, a definitive sign of malignancy.*

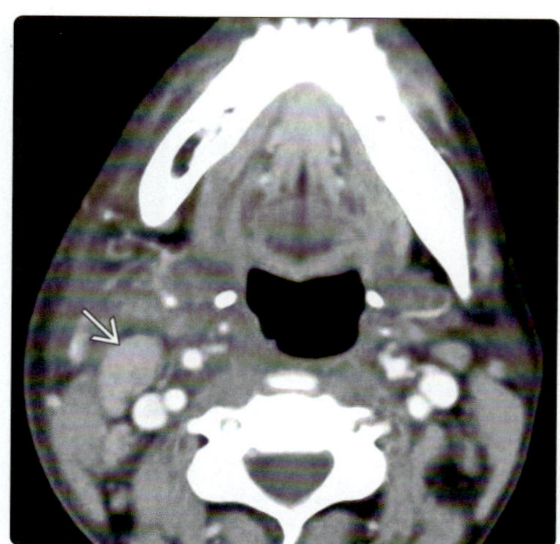

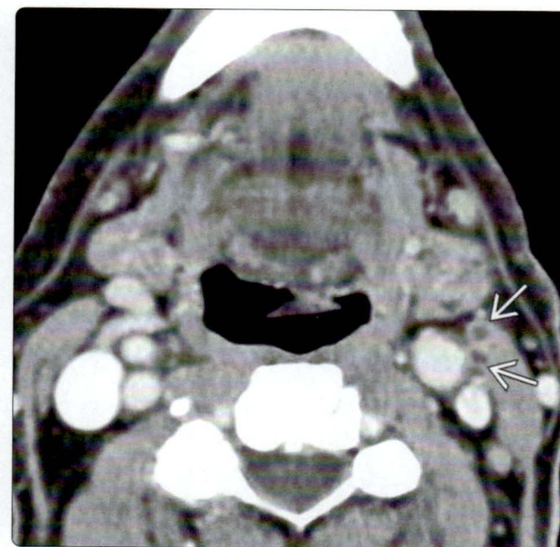

(Left) *Axial CECT shows a markedly enlarged level II lymph node ➡. By size criteria, this node would be considered malignant, but its kidney-shaped configuration is indicative of its benign nature (reactive node).* **(Right)** *Axial CECT shows multiple heterogeneously enhancing 2- to 4-mm level II lymph nodes ➡. By size criteria, this node would be normal. The presence of central necrosis, however, is a definitive sign of malignancy if seen prior to treatment.*

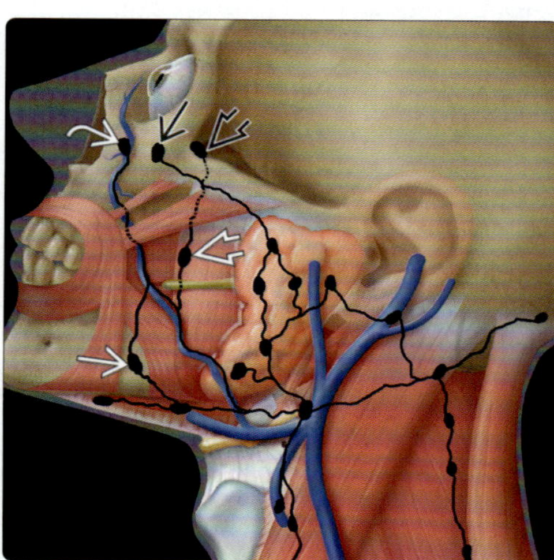

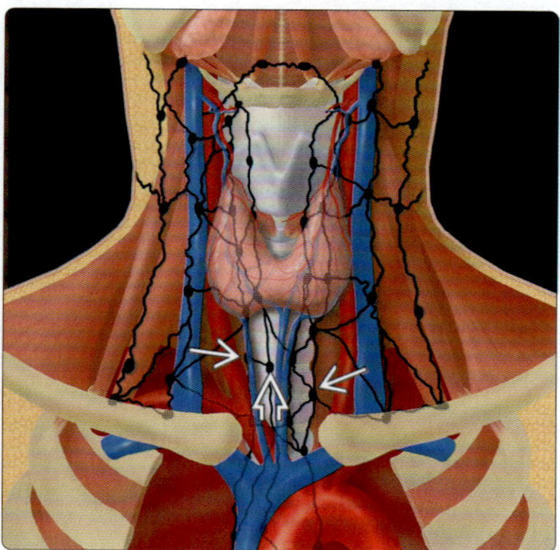

(Left) *Lateral graphic shows facial lymph nodes. Anteriorly, note the mandibular ➡ and infraorbital nodes ➡. The buccinator node ➡ is along the anterior margin of the buccinator muscle. The malar node ➡ and retrozygomatic node ➡ are superior.* **(Right)** *Frontal graphic reveals nodal drainage of the anterior neck. The thyroid gland drains into visceral space nodes (level VI), known as the pretracheal ➡ and paratracheal ➡ nodes.*

Reactive Lymph Nodes

KEY FACTS

TERMINOLOGY

- Definition: Benign, reversible enlargement of nodes in response to antigen stimulus

IMAGING

- Shape/number: Ovoid or reniform/multiple
- Size: Normal size or mildly enlarged
  - In children, reactive nodes may be ≥ 2 cm
- Ultrasound findings
  - Multiple solid, noncalcified, hypoechoic ovoid nodes with cortical hypertrophy and echogenic hilum
  - Power Doppler: Prominent, radiating hilar vascularity with no peripheral vascularity
  - Ultrasound elastography may differentiate benign, reactive nodes from malignancy
- CECT or enhanced MR
  - Enhancement minimal to mild, homogeneous
  - Linear enhancement within node is characteristic
  - If cystic, node is pathologic from infection or tumor

TOP DIFFERENTIAL DIAGNOSES

- Squamous cell carcinoma nodal metastases
- Systemic nodal metastases
- Non-Hodgkin lymphoma nodes
- Tuberculous adenitis

PATHOLOGY

- Node reaction seen as specific histologic patterns of hyperplasia: Follicular, sinus, diffuse, or mixed
- Lymph follicle hypertrophy common

CLINICAL ISSUES

- Children or young adults with multiple neck masses
- Upper respiratory tract infection may be present
- If in adult, consider malignancy or EBV or HIV infection
- Treatment options
  - Child: Manage clinically, most likely infectious; avoid CECT as possible; may take months to resolve
  - Adult: Ultrasound ± aspiration as needed

(Left) *Coronal CECT in a teenager with a palpable lump shows a solid, ovoid left IA lymph node ➡ subjacent to the skin marker. Note subtle intranodal linear enhancement ➡, an imaging feature commonly seen in reactive adenopathy. The enlarged node resolved with a short course of antibiotics.* **(Right)** *Sagittal CECT (same patient) shows benign, ovoid morphology of the reactive node ➡. Reactive nodes show homogeneous density without necrosis and can be followed clinically to resolution. Note bowed platysma muscle ➡.*

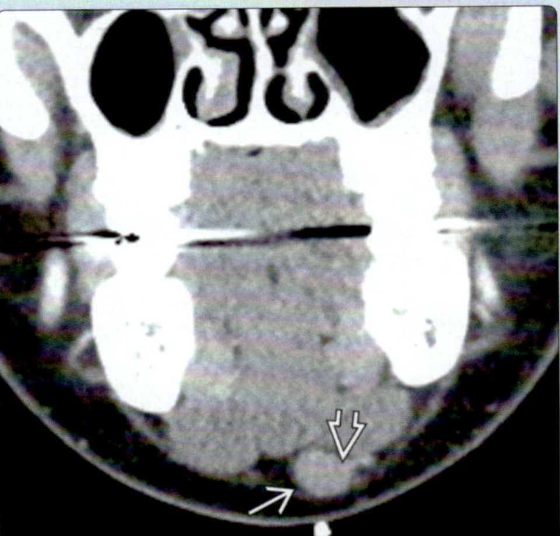

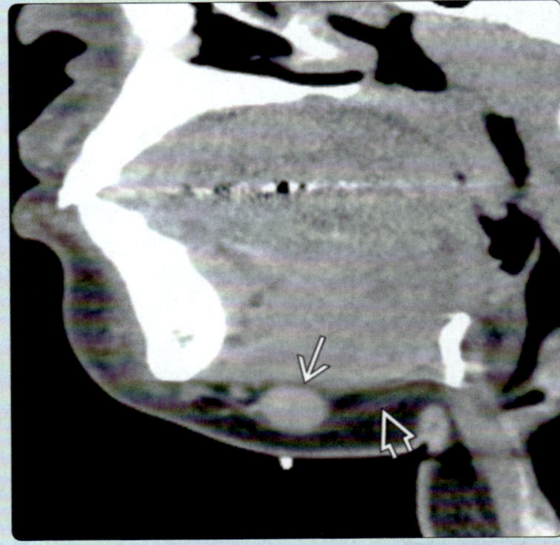

(Left) *Coronal T2 FS MR in a child with left otitis externa and media shows reactive adenopathy, including enlarged parotid ➡, retropharyngeal ➡, and high deep cervical ➡ nodes. Reactive nodes are solid, homogeneous, and reniform in shape.* **(Right)** *Axial CECT at the inferior aspect of enlarged palatine tonsils ➡ in a patient with clinical tonsillitis reveals bilateral reactive level IIA internal jugular nodes ➡. Note bilateral homogeneous mild enhancement of smaller level IIB reactive nodes in the neck ➡.*

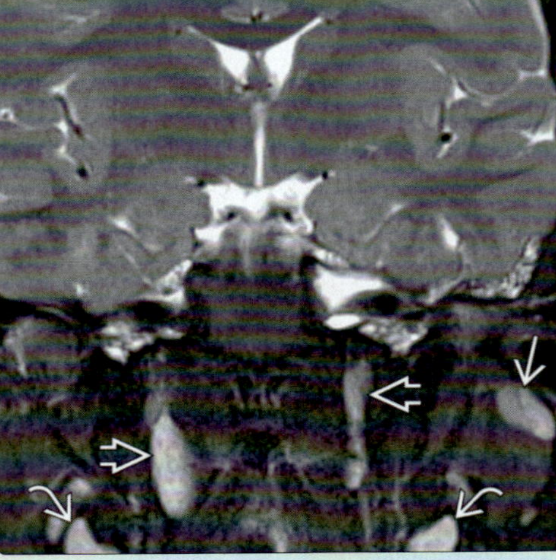

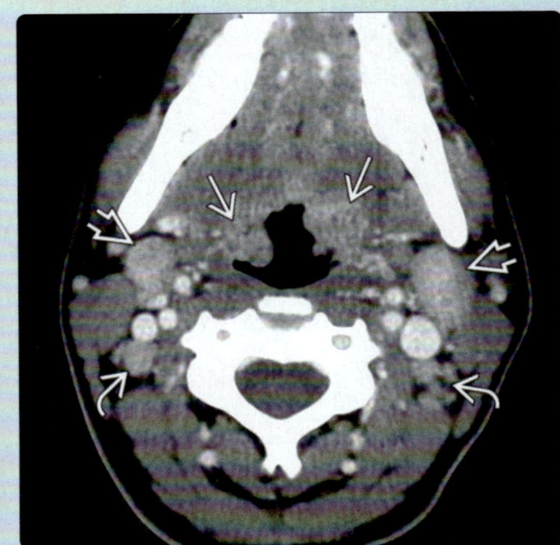

Suppurative Lymph Nodes

KEY FACTS

TERMINOLOGY

- Adenitis, acute lymphadenitis, intranodal abscess
- Pus formation within nodes from bacterial infection

IMAGING

- CECT findings
  - Enlarged node(s) with intranodal fluid and surrounding inflammation (cellulitis)
  - Most often jugulodigastric, submandibular, retropharyngeal nodes
- Contrast should be administered to best appreciate extent of suppurative changes
- Consider CT or US-guided aspiration for diagnosis and minimally invasive therapy

TOP DIFFERENTIAL DIAGNOSES

- Metastatic nodes
- 2nd branchial cleft anomaly
- Nontuberculosis *Mycobacterium* nodes
- Tuberculosis nodes

PATHOLOGY

- *Staphylococcus* and *Streptococcus* most frequent causative organisms
- Pediatric infections show clustering of organisms by age
- Dental infections are typically polymicrobial and predominantly anaerobic

DIAGNOSTIC CHECKLIST

- If no significant cellulitic changes around node
  - In children, consider nontuberculosis mycobacteria
  - In adults, consider squamous cell carcinoma or thyroid carcinoma nodal metastases
- Look for primary infectious source on images
  - Pharyngitis, dental infection, salivary gland calculi
- With any neck infection, must evaluate for airway compromise, thrombophlebitis, and pseudoaneurysm
- Treatment: Typically I&D followed by antibiotics

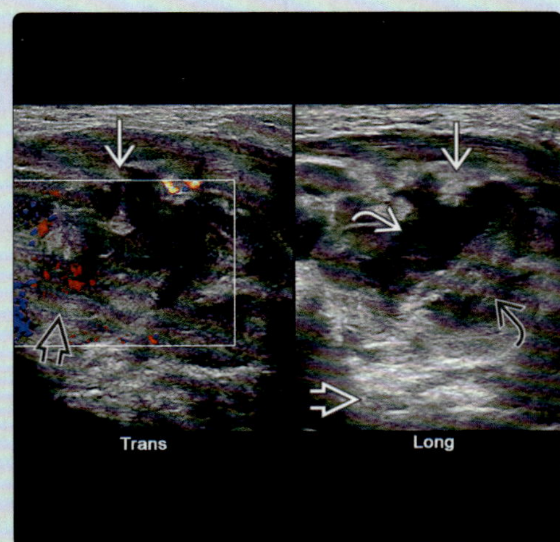

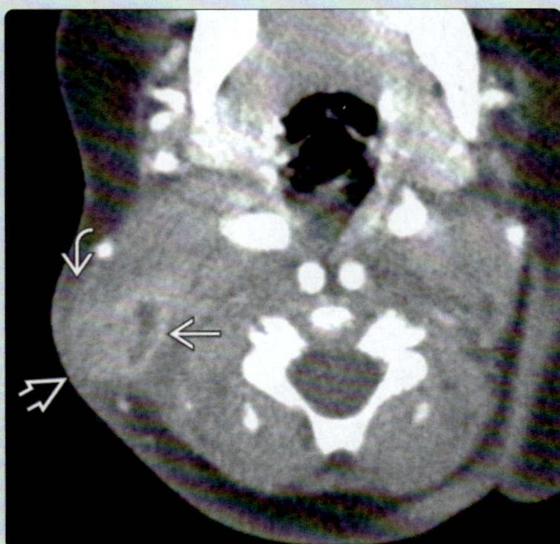

(Left) *Transverse (left) and longitudinal (right) color Doppler and grayscale US of an infant with suppurative adenopathy show an enlarged, heterogeneous echogenicity level II node with complex, cystic contents, internal debris, posterior acoustic enhancement, and peripheral hyperemia.* **(Right)** *Axial CECT in the same patient shows a rim-enhancing, centrally cystic/necrotic right level II suppurative lymph node. Note overlying cellulitis with skin thickening and edema.*

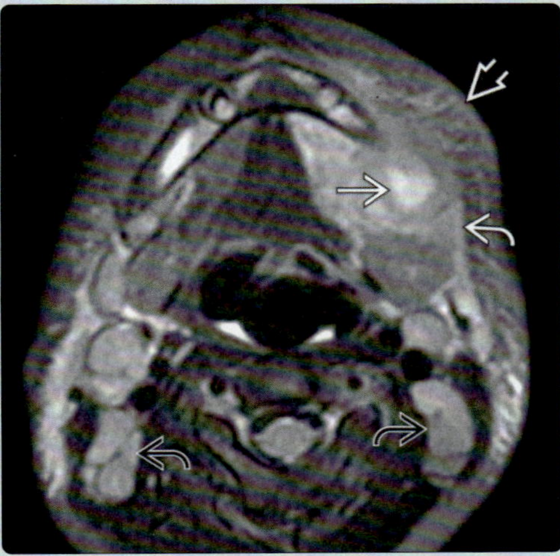

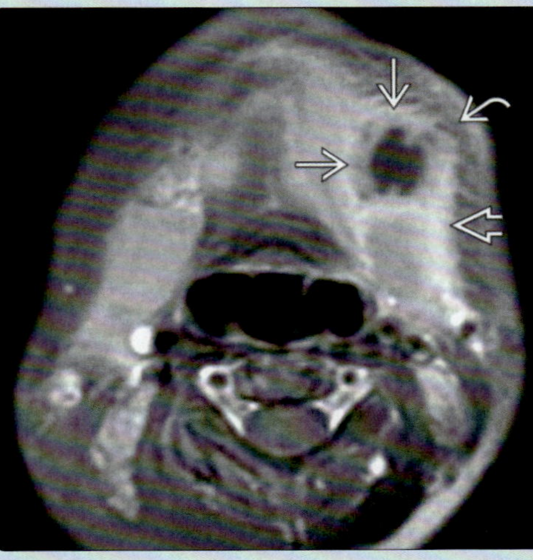

(Left) *Axial T2 FS MR shows an enlarged cystic/necrotic submandibular lymph node with central bright T2 signal. Note additional features of infection/inflammation, including edema in the left submandibular space and overlying cellulitis. Multiple solid reactive nodes are present.* **(Right)** *Axial T1 C+ FS MR in the same patient shows thick peripheral enhancement of the suppurative node. Note adjacent inflammatory changes with stranding of subcutaneous fat and thickened platysma.*

Tuberculous Lymph Nodes

KEY FACTS

TERMINOLOGY

- Synonym: Cervical TB adenitis
- Definition: *Mycobacterium tuberculosis* nodal infection

IMAGING

- CECT findings
  - Conglomerate nodal mass with **thick** enhancing rim and central necrosis
  - Inflammatory changes adjacent soft tissues
- Obtain CXR if TB suspected (other nonimaging diagnostic tests listed below)

TOP DIFFERENTIAL DIAGNOSES

- Suppurative nodes
- Non-TB *Mycobacterium* nodes
- Cat-scratch disease

PATHOLOGY

- **Caseating granulomas**; smear for acid-fast bacilli
- Excisional biopsy more sensitive than FNA
- Cervical nodes #1 site of extrapulmonary TB adenopathy

CLINICAL ISSUES

- Systemically unwell patients with pulmonary disease
  - Often immunosuppressed patient group
- Increasing incidence in USA
  - Increasing prevalence of AIDS, immunosuppressive drugs, immigrants from endemic countries
- 80-100% strongly **reactive skin test (PPD)**, interferon-γ release assay (blood) more sensitive
  - PPD may be negative with immunodeficiency
- Treat with 4-drug regimen: Rifampicin, isoniazid, pyrazinamide, ethambutol/streptomycin
- Surgery for medically unresponsive disease or large abscess

DIAGNOSTIC CHECKLIST

- Consider TB when inflammatory changes associated with necrotic nodal masses

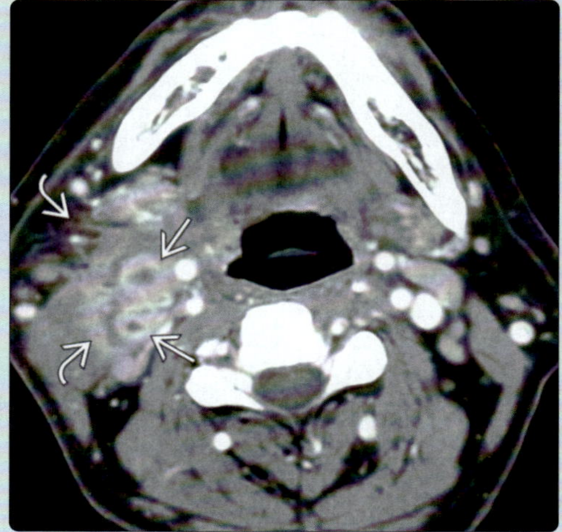
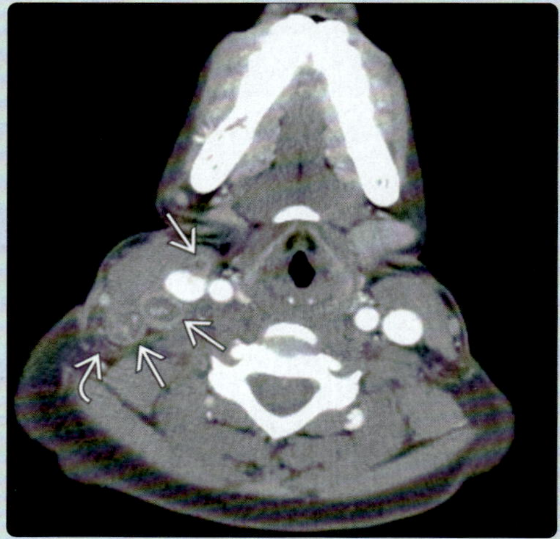

(Left) *Axial CECT shows multiple necrotic cervical nodes ➡ with thick rim enhancement, typical of TB. Marked extranodal inflammatory changes are also evident ➡.* **(Right)** *Axial CECT in a Sudanese woman with tuberculous lymphadenitis unresponsive to medical therapy demonstrates multiple necrotic cervical lymph nodes ➡. Note adjacent stranding/edema in the posterior cervical space ➡ related to active inflammation.*

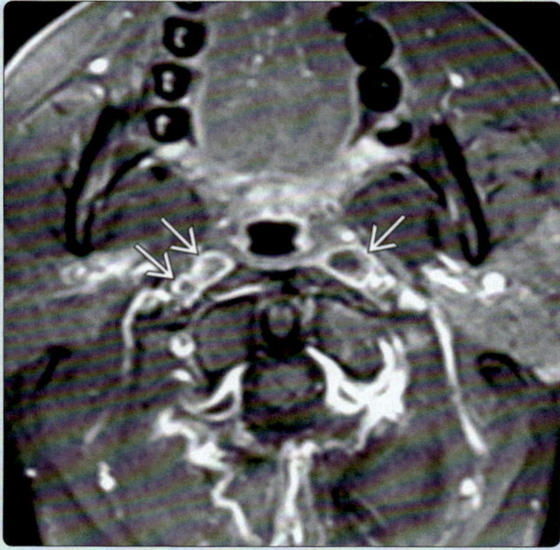
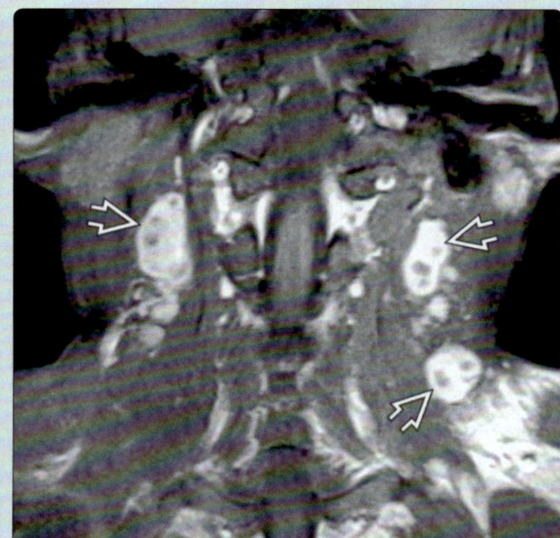

(Left) *Axial T1 C+ FS demonstrates bilateral intensely enhancing, but centrally necrotic, retropharyngeal nodes ➡.* **(Right)** *Coronal T1 C+ FS MR in the same patient shows markedly enhancing nodes ➡ in posterior cervical chains bilaterally but without significant surrounding inflammatory changes. Large nodes have focal areas of low signal intensity representing caseation necrosis. This patient was otherwise asymptomatic, but biopsy revealed granulomas and M. tuberculosis infection.*

KEY FACTS

TERMINOLOGY

- Non-TB *Mycobacterium* (NTM) nodes: Chronic neck infection with NTM
- Most often *Mycobacterium avium* **complex**

IMAGING

- Unilateral submandibular or preauricular painless mass in afebrile young child
- CXR: No pulmonary disease
- Ultrasound for neck mass evaluation and FNA
- CECT: Rim-enhancing, cystic-appearing node(s)
  - Minimal surrounding inflammatory changes

TOP DIFFERENTIAL DIAGNOSES

- Suppurative lymph nodes
- Tuberculosis lymph nodes
- Cat-scratch disease
- 2nd branchial cleft anomaly

PATHOLOGY

- Necrotizing granulomatous inflammation with acid-fast bacilli (Z-N stain)
- NTM creates fistula to skin surface if untreated

CLINICAL ISSUES

- Increasing incidence in immunosuppressed patients
- PPD test may be weakly reactive; **interferon γ release assay** usually negative (may effectively rule out TB)
- Antimycobacterial agents as adjuvant therapy
- Complete excision has > 90% success rate; I&D alone has 16-27% recurrence rate; risk of chronic draining fistula

DIAGNOSTIC CHECKLIST

- Always consider when cervical nodal mass not responding to standard treatment
- Consider if necrotic node with minimal surrounding inflammation
- Especially afebrile child < 5 years with painless mass

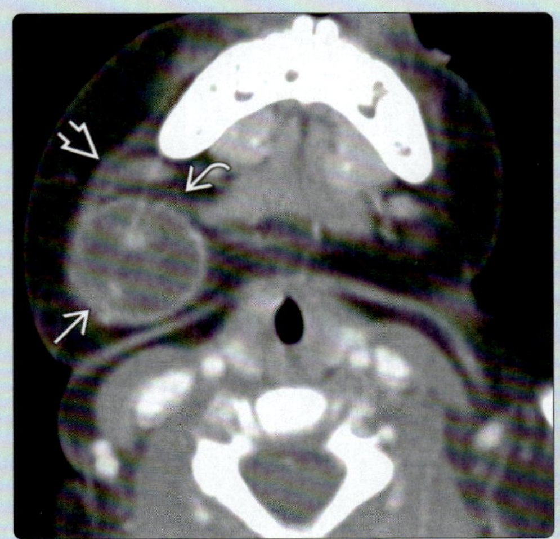

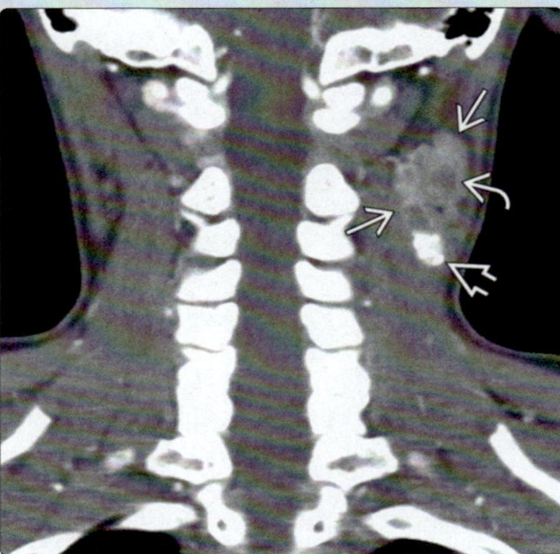

(Left) *Axial CECT of a child with non-TB Mycobacterium (NTM) adenitis shows a large, necrotic, submandibular nodal mass ➡. Stranding of adjacent fat ➡ and thickening of the platysma ➡ is minimal. When history is of short duration, fat stranding may be more conspicuous. Nodal calcification is not evident.* **(Right)** *Coronal CECT in a different child with chronic NTM adenitis shows a conglomerate nodal mass ➡ with internal cystic/necrotic regions ➡ and coarse calcification ➡.*

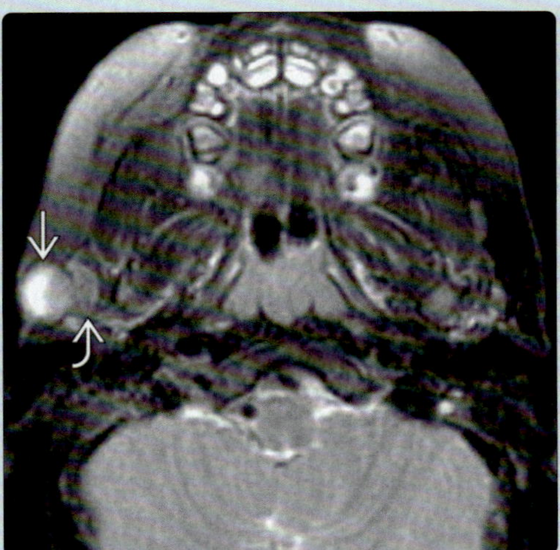

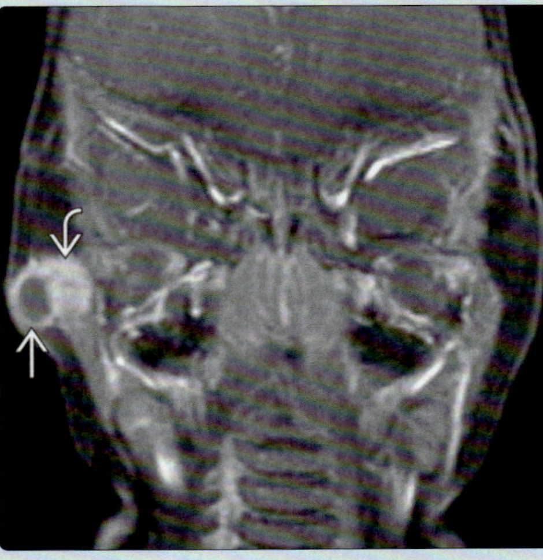

(Left) *Axial T2 FS MR in an 11 month old with a right preauricular mass demonstrates a well-defined, predominantly hyperintense lesion ➡ in the subcutaneous tissues of the right cheek, abutting superficial lobe of right parotid gland ➡. There is no evidence of infiltration of surrounding subcutaneous fat.* **(Right)** *Coronal T1 C+ FS MR in the same child reveals lesion ➡ to be cystic with peripheral enhancement and shows inflammation of adjacent superficial parotid lobe ➡. FNA revealed Mycobacterium avium complex.*

KEY FACTS

TERMINOLOGY

- Sarcoidosis definition: **Noncaseating granulomatous** inflammatory disease of unknown or autoimmune etiology

IMAGING

- CT, MR, ultrasound findings
  - Homogeneous, smoothly enlarged lymph nodes
  - Nodal calcification may be present on CT or ultrasound
  - Mild nodal enhancement with CECT or C+ MR
  - Nodes often in low neck and mediastinum
- PET/CT may be useful for assessing extent of systemic disease or determining site for biopsy
  - SUV frequently > 3.0; up to 15
- DWI may be of some value in differentiating FDG-avid sarcoidosis nodes from malignancy
  - Typically higher ADC value than malignant nodes
- CXR can show hilar lymphadenopathy, pulmonary infiltrate

TOP DIFFERENTIAL DIAGNOSES

- Reactive lymph nodes
- Non-Hodgkin lymphoma nodes

PATHOLOGY

- Unknown cause; may result from immune response to environmental triggers
- Histopathology: Multiple well-formed, **noncaseating granulomas**
  - Nodules of epithelioid histiocytes surrounded by mixed inflammatory infiltrate
  - **Langhans-type giant cells** with intracytoplasmic, star-shaped inclusions (asteroid bodies)

CLINICAL ISSUES

- Usually develops < 50 years, peak at 20-39 years; F > M
- > 90% of patients have thoracic nodes, pulmonary, skin, ± ocular sarcoid
- Fatigue, night sweats, and weight loss are common

(Left) *Axial CECT shows nonspecific enlargement of left supraclavicular lymph node ➡ without necrosis. Other enlarged cervical and mediastinal nodes (not shown) raise concern for lymphoma versus sarcoidosis.* **(Right)** *Fused axial FDG-PET/CT in the same patient shows increased FDG uptake in left supraclavicular node ➡ as well as other mildly FDG-avid nodes ➡. Biopsy revealed noncaseating granulomas, confirming sarcoidosis. Diffuse thyroid FDG uptake ➡ reflects thyroiditis, not uncommon in sarcoidosis.*

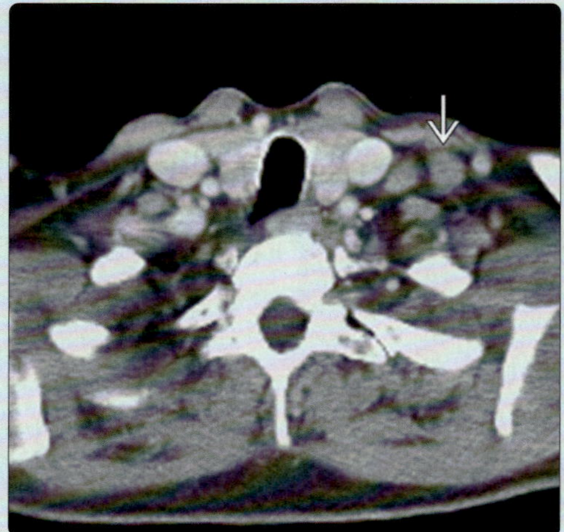

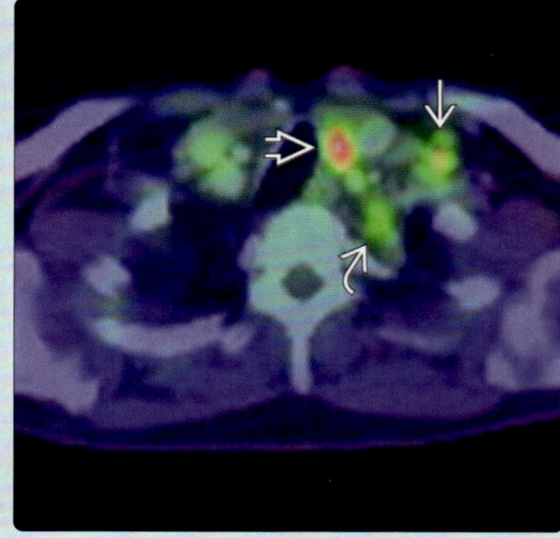

(Left) *Axial T1 MR reveals diffuse smoothly enlarged cervical sarcoidosis lymph nodes ➡ without evidence of necrosis. A left suboccipital node is evident ➡. Imaging differential of this appearance is non-Hodgkin lymphoma, reactive adenopathy, and, less commonly, sarcoidosis.* **(Right)** *Axial T1 C+ FS MR reveals bilateral enlarged, ovoid submandibular ➡ and upper jugular nodes ➡ in a patient with sarcoidosis. Central linear intranodal enhancement ➡, typically found in reactive nodes, is evident in multiple lymph nodes.*

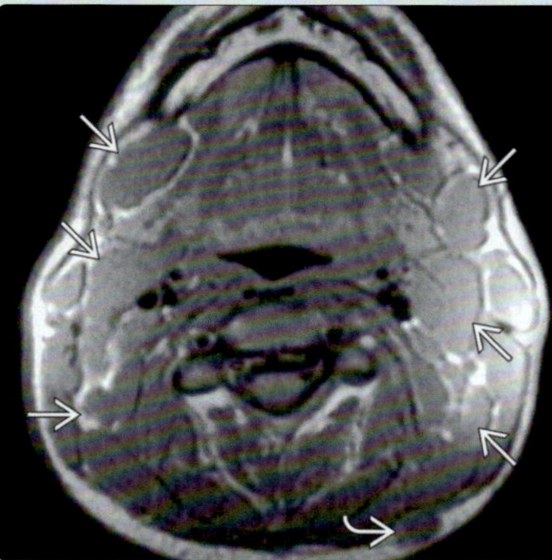

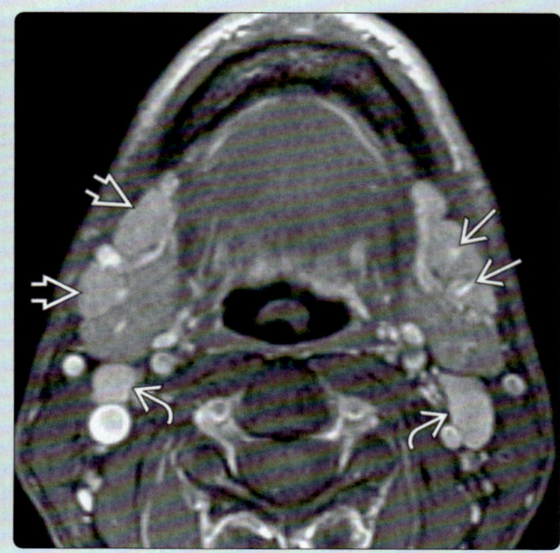

KEY FACTS

TERMINOLOGY

- Castleman disease (CD)
- Uncommon benign idiopathic hypervascular polyclonal lymphoid hyperplasia
- Histologic subtypes
  - Hyaline vascular (90%)
  - Plasma cell (10%)
    - Human herpesvirus 8 (HHV-8) related

IMAGING

- Most often mediastinum (70%), then H&N (15%)
- > 90% of H&N lesions are unifocal nodal disease
- CECT or enhanced MR findings
  - Moderate to markedly enhancing nodal mass
  - Central **nonenhancing scar**; uncommon (CECT)
  - Hypointense **striations** described; uncommon (T2 MR)
- Ultrasound: Hypoechoic single nodal mass
  - Intense hilar and peripheral vascularity (power Doppler)

TOP DIFFERENTIAL DIAGNOSES

- Non-Hodgkin lymphoma lymph nodes
- Reactive lymph nodes
- Differentiated thyroid carcinoma nodes

PATHOLOGY

- Unclear etiology, likely related to interleukin-6
- Most often unifocal, **hyaline vascular type** (90%)
- Multifocal form rare, **plasma cell type** (10%)
- Diagnosis requires core biopsy or node excision

CLINICAL ISSUES

- Clinical subtypes: **Unifocal** (90%) and **multicentric** (10%)
- Unifocal CD: Asymptomatic neck mass
  - Surgical removal curative
- Multicentric CD
  - B symptoms (fever, night sweats) occur in 95% patients
  - Hepatosplenomegaly, body cavity effusions, skin rash
  - Treatment: Surgery + chemotherapy and steroids

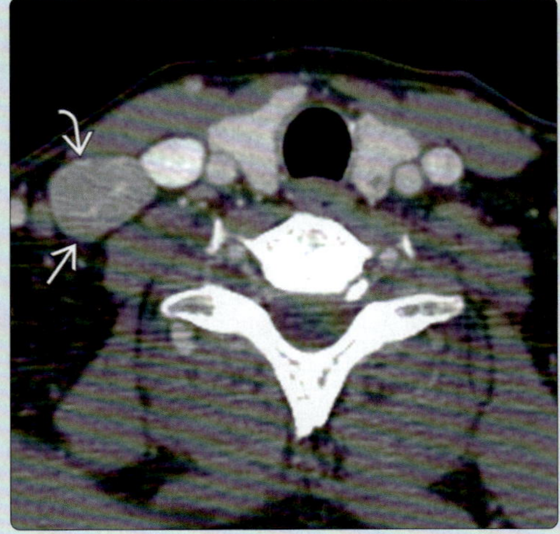

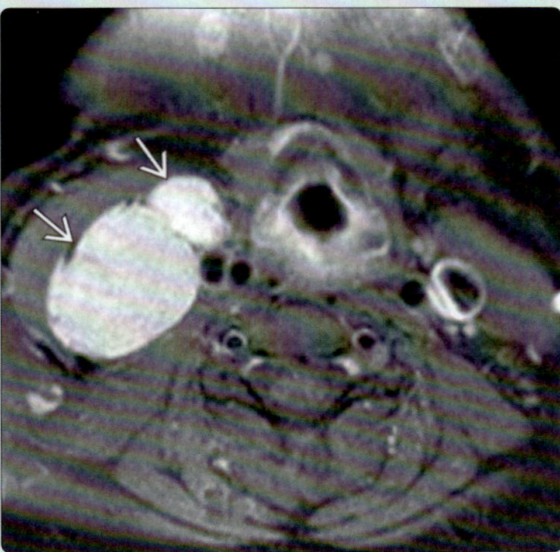

(Left) *Axial CECT for palpable neck mass shows a solitary, mildly enlarged lymph node ➡. There is homogeneous enhancement with associated prominent vessels ➡. This was unifocal hyaline vascular variant of Castleman disease (CD) cured with surgical resection.* **(Right)** *Axial T1 C+ FS MR in a different adult with hyaline vascular type of CD reveals right internal jugular chain nodes ➡ with uniform enhancement. The more posterior node is markedly enlarged. This is not evidence of extracapsular spread or inflammation.*

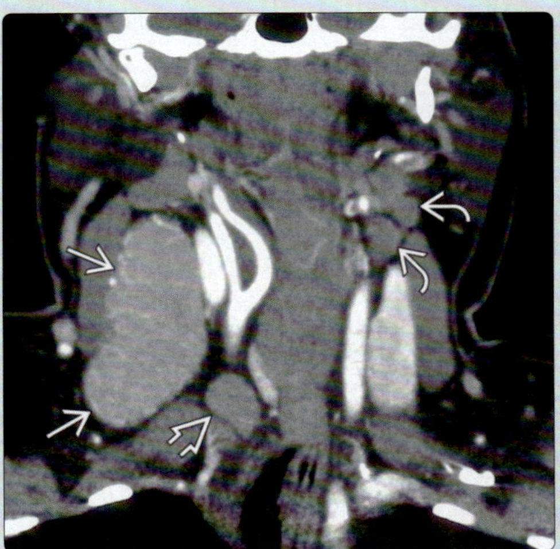

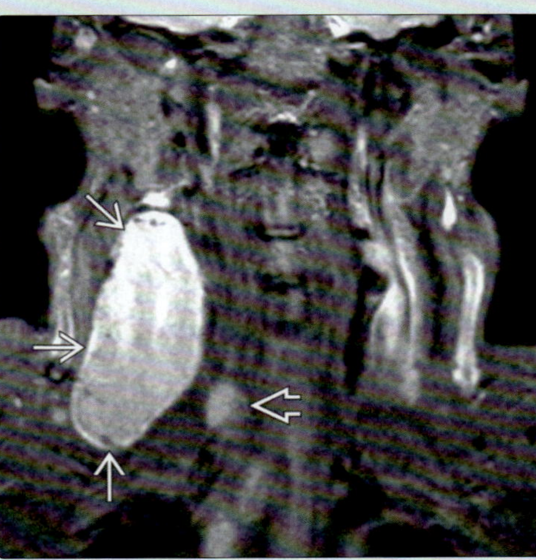

(Left) *Coronally reformatted CECT shows a large, homogeneous, moderately enhancing node ➡ along the right internal jugular chain. Also seen are additional smaller, less enhancing nodes in low-level VI ➡ and along contralateral jugular chain ➡.* **(Right)** *Coronal T2 FS MR in the same patient shows a large node ➡ to be markedly homogeneously hyperintense with no intranodal necrosis or inflammatory changes surrounding node. A smaller, moderately hyperintense node ➡ is also evident.*

Histiocytic Necrotizing Lymphadenitis (Kikuchi-Fujimoto)

KEY FACTS

TERMINOLOGY

- Definition: Benign idiopathic necrotizing cervical adenitis of **young Asian adults**
- Synonym: Kikuchi-Fujimoto disease

IMAGING

- CECT or enhanced MR findings
  - **Unilateral**, homogeneous, mildly enlarged nodes
    - With **inflammatory stranding** along margins
  - Posterior cervical and jugular chain nodes
  - Nodes appear solid or rim enhancing
- Ultrasound: Hypoechoic (100%) with hilar vascularity (90%)
  - Unsharp border (65%) due to inflammatory periadenitis

TOP DIFFERENTIAL DIAGNOSES

- Non-Hodgkin lymphoma lymph nodes
- Systemic nodal metastases
- Cat-scratch disease
- Reactive adenopathy
- Tuberculosis lymph nodes

PATHOLOGY

- Cortical and paracortical coagulative necrosis
- Cellular infiltrate of histiocytes and immunoblasts
- Possibly exuberant T-cell-mediated immune response to variety of nonspecific stimuli
- Associated with increased incidence of systemic lupus erythematosus
- Higher **Japanese** and other **Asian** incidence may be due to HLA genes

CLINICAL ISSUES

- Most commonly in Asian women in 3rd decade
- Tender unilateral neck nodes and high fever
- 30-50% have other systemic symptoms
- Usually resolves **without treatment** in 1-4 months
- Diagnosis requires excisional biopsy

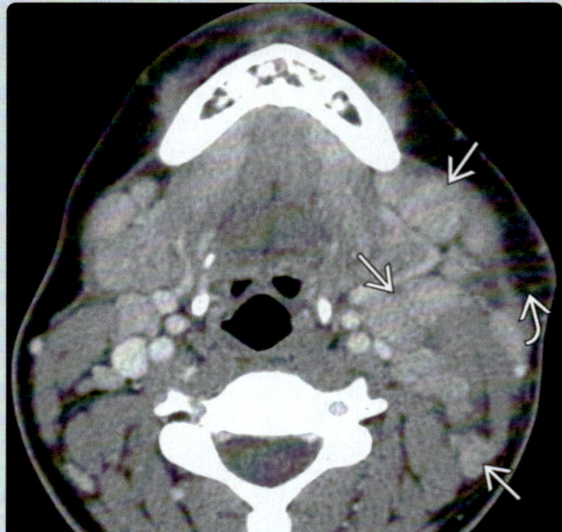

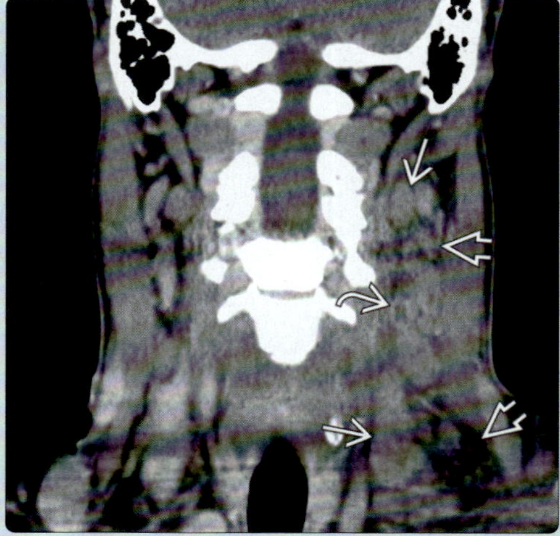

(Left) *Axial CECT shows predominantly left-sided, well-defined, noncalcifying nodes ➡. The nodes have homogeneous moderate enhancement, appear somewhat matted, and there is adjacent stranding of subcutaneous fat ➡.* **(Right)** *Coronal CECT depicts numerous enlarged left jugular chain lymph nodes ➡. Some demonstrate rim enhancement ➡. Inflammatory fat stranding is present adjacent to the nodes ➡.*

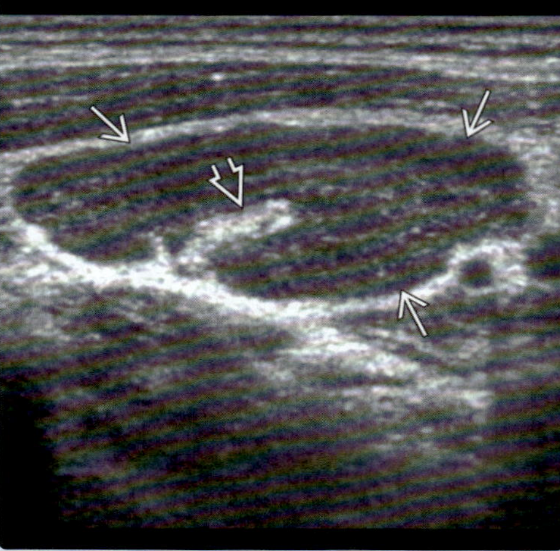

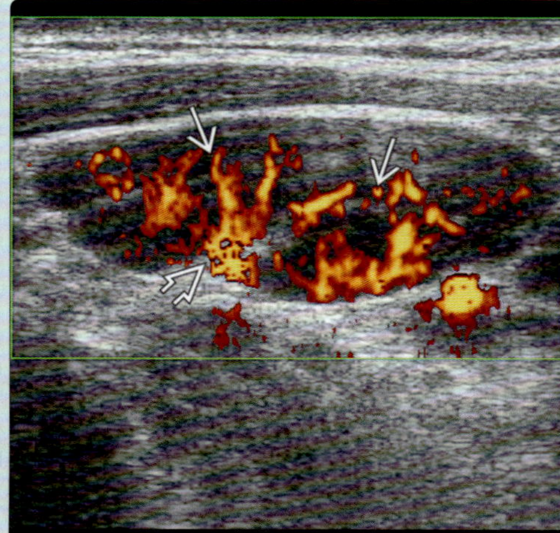

(Left) *Longitudinal US obtained in the posterior neck shows a hypoechoic enlarged node ➡ with a hypertrophied cortex but normal hilar architecture ➡ in a patient with histiocytic necrotizing lymphadenitis (Kikuchi-Fujimoto disease). Note the absence of associated soft tissue edema, intranodal necrosis, or matting of nodes.* **(Right)** *Power Doppler US in the same patient reveals prominent vascularity of the perihilar cortex ➡ and hilum ➡. This is a classic appearance of histiocytic necrotizing lymphadenitis.*

KEY FACTS

TERMINOLOGY

- Kimura disease (KD): Angiolymphoid proliferation with **serum eosinophilia** and **elevated IgE**
  - Inflammatory disorder with multiple H&N masses

IMAGING

- Classic triad
  - Subcutaneous and deep tissue H&N masses
  - Salivary gland masses: Parotid > submandibular
  - Solid cervical lymphadenopathy
- CT or MR findings
  - Variable enhancement (CT) and signal (MR)
  - Due to varying vascularity and fibrosis

TOP DIFFERENTIAL DIAGNOSES

- Nodal non-Hodgkin lymphoma
- Parotid carcinoma
- Nodal sarcoidosis
- Parotid metastatic nodal disease

PATHOLOGY

- Unknown etiology; allergic and autoimmune likely
- ~ 50% have renal dysfunction

CLINICAL ISSUES

- Most common in **young Asian male patients**
- Chronic, **slowly progressive** course over years
- Benign, can be self-limiting
- Diagnostic triad
  - Painless subcutaneous H&N masses + regional adenopathy
  - Blood and tissue **eosinophilia**
  - Markedly **elevated serum IgE**
- Treatment options
  - Observation alone if not symptomatic or disfiguring
  - Resection of mass lesion(s), morbidity is site specific; 25% recur
  - Cyclosporine A reported to induce remission
  - Consider radiotherapy for persistent/problematic lesions

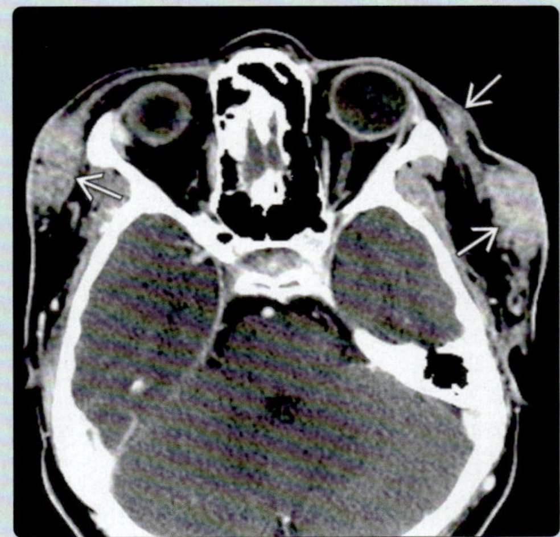

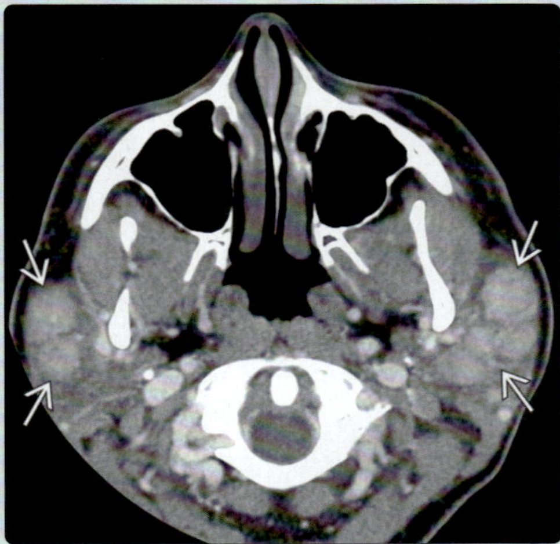

(Left) *Axial CECT in a young Asian female patient with a 9-year history of slowly enlarging forehead nodules reveals multiple bilateral subcutaneous plaque-like lesions ➡ with significant deformity of the scalp and facial contours.* **(Right)** *Axial neck CECT in the same patient shows multiple bilateral enhancing intraparotid nodules ➡. Numerous enlarged cervical nodes were also present bilaterally (not shown). Biopsy of forehead lesion revealed this to be Kimura disease (KD).*

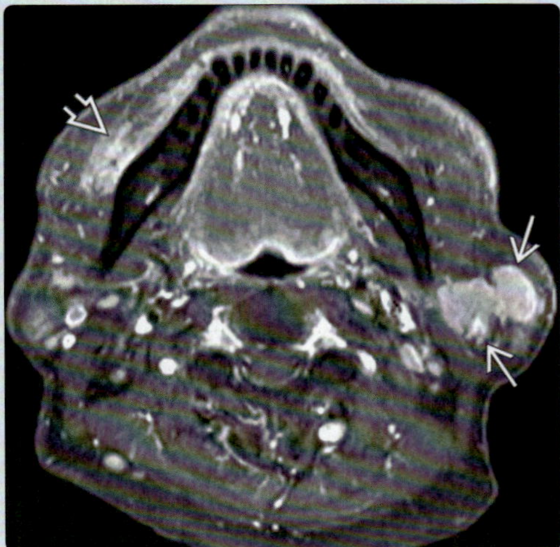

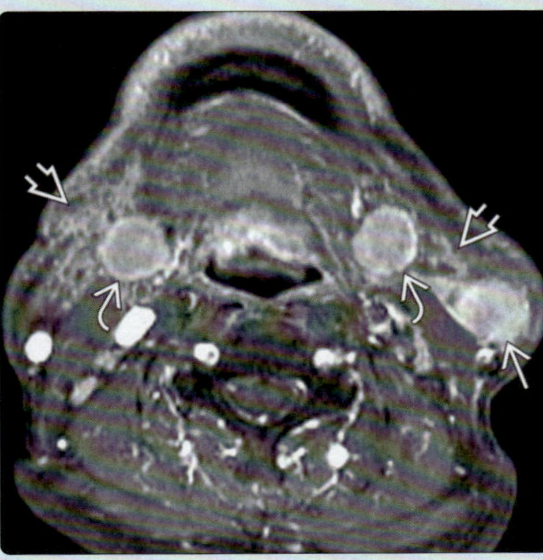

(Left) *Axial T1WI C+ FS MR in a patient with KD demonstrates intensely enhancing left intraparotid masses ➡ within the left parotid gland. Ill-defined, enhancing infiltration of right cheek deep soft tissues ➡ is evident on the contralateral side as well.* **(Right)** *More inferior axial T1WI C+ FS MR in the same patient shows bilateral enhancing submandibular lesions ➡ in addition to hazy, infiltrated appearance of deep and subcutaneous fat ➡ around them. The tail of the parotid enhancing node is evident on the left ➡.*

Nodal Hodgkin Lymphoma in Neck

KEY FACTS

TERMINOLOGY

- Abbreviation: Hodgkin lymphoma (HL)
- Definition: Lymphoma with **Reed-Sternberg cells**

IMAGING

- General findings
  - Enlarged **neck nodes**
  - Single nodal group or contiguous groups
  - Mediastinal nodes frequently also present
  - H&N HL is rarely extranodal
- CECT: Homogeneous solid nodal masses
  - Necrosis or calcification uncommon
  - CECT and FDG PET are basic staging modalities
- FDG PET shows **marked metabolic activity**
  - Persistently positive PET during treatment has high sensitivity for prediction of relapse
  - FDG PET differentiates posttreatment inactive scar from residual tumor

TOP DIFFERENTIAL DIAGNOSES

- Reactive lymph nodes
- Nodal non-Hodgkin lymphoma
- Nodal squamous cell carcinoma
- Nodal differentiated thyroid carcinoma

PATHOLOGY

- Neoplastic cells are **Reed-Sternberg cells**
- Most of tumor bulk is reactive inflammatory cells, not neoplastic cells
- 95% **classic HL**; more aggressive type
- 5% **nodular** lymphocyte-predominant HL

CLINICAL ISSUES

- 20- to-40 year old adult with enlarging, painless neck mass
- 40% have **B symptoms**: Fever, sweats, weight loss
- HL is potentially curable with chemoradiation
- 5-year survival: Stages I-III (≥ 85%), stage IV (80%)

(Left) *Axial CECT in a teen girl with palpable neck masses demonstrates bilateral adenopathy ➡, larger on the left. The modes are homogeneous and isodense to muscle without necrosis or calcifications.* **(Right)** *Coronal projection from FDG PET study in the same patient demonstrates marked nodal uptake in the lower neck bilaterally ➡ and the superior mediastinum ➡. PET study showed no evidence of infradiaphragmatic disease, although focal nodular lung disease was demonstrated (extranodal disease).*

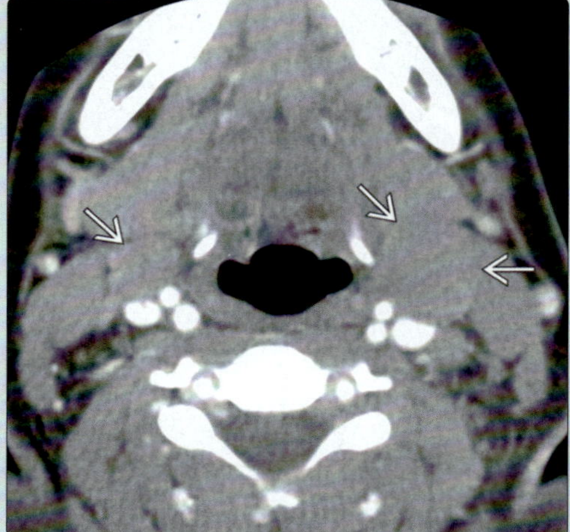

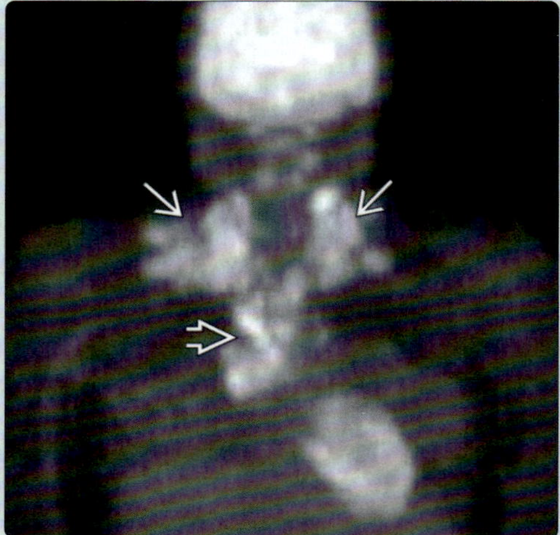

(Left) *Axial CECT more inferiorly demonstrates multiple solid large nodal masses isodense to muscle. On both sides, nodes splay the common carotid ➡ & internal jugular vein (IJV). The right IJV ➡ is flattened.* **(Right)** *Axial CECT at the cervicothoracic junction shows additional bilateral nodal masses ➡ abutting carotid sheaths with supraclavicular nodes ➡ also evident. This was nodular sclerosing Hodgkin lymphoma, determined to be stage IV. It was successfully treated with chemoradiation, without relapse at 4 years.*

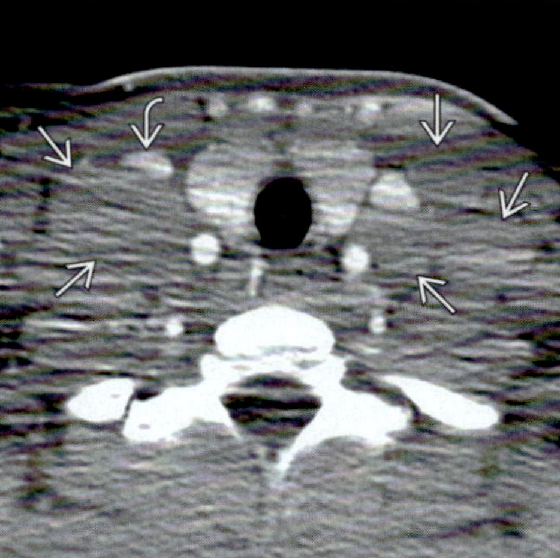

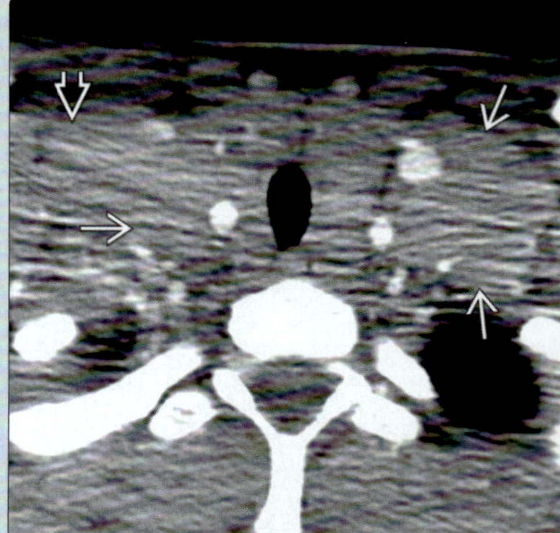

KEY FACTS

TERMINOLOGY

- Non-Hodgkin lymphoma (NHL) is lymphoreticular system malignancy
- Multiple different NHL subtypes
- Multiple manifestations of NHL in H&N
  - Nodal, nonnodal lymphatic (Waldeyer lymphatic ring), nonnodal extralymphatic NHL

IMAGING

- CT, MR, ultrasound findings
  - Multiple bilateral, enlarged nodes involving multiple nodal chains
  - Typically **large, solid**, round, or oval nodes
  - Enhancement may be variable, even in same patient
- May see different patterns of nodes
  - Multiple mildly enlarged, 1- to 3-cm nodes
  - Dominant, markedly enlarged nodes
- **Necrosis/extranodal spread** suggests **aggressive NHL**
- FDG PET shows variable avidity
  - High in aggressive NHL, lower in more indolent NHL

TOP DIFFERENTIAL DIAGNOSES

- Reactive adenopathy
- Sarcoidosis lymph nodes
- Hodgkin lymphoma nodes
- Nodal metastases from systemic primary

PATHOLOGY

- 80-85% B-cell tumors
  - Most common diffuse large B-cell lymphoma
- May be associated with AIDS

CLINICAL ISSUES

- Adult with painless neck masses
- May be indolent and progressive but not curable or aggressive but often curable
- Treat with XRT, chemotherapy, or both
- 5-year survival: Stages I-II (85%), stages III-IV (50%)
- FNA for flow cytometry; may require excisional biopsy

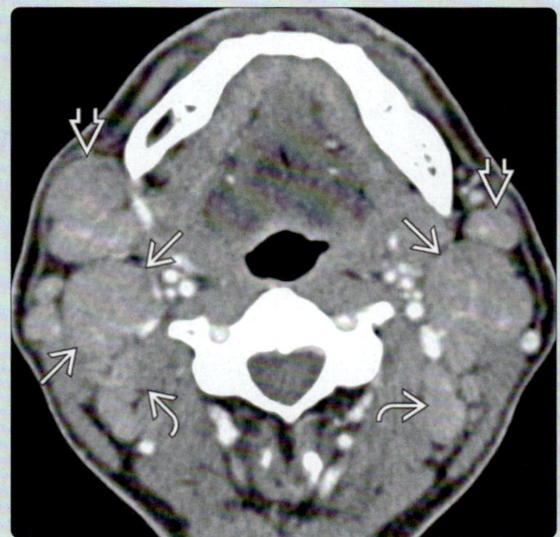

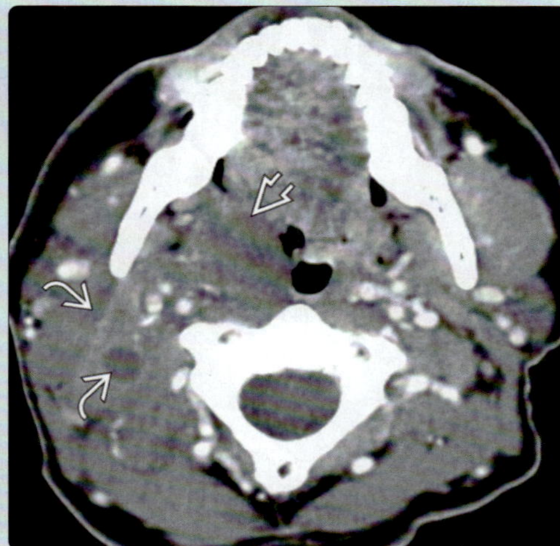

(Left) *Axial CECT shows multiple large, round, solid lymph nodes in every chain of the suprahyoid neck. Bilateral nodes are evident in levels IIA ➡, IIB ➡, and IB ➡. Absence of necrosis with such large nodes suggests that these are not metastases from H&N squamous cell carcinoma.* **(Right)** *Axial CECT shows nodal and tonsillar lymphoma. This level II nodal mass is partially necrotic ➡ with extranodal infiltration of fat and paraspinal muscles. The right tonsil is homogeneously enlarged ➡.*

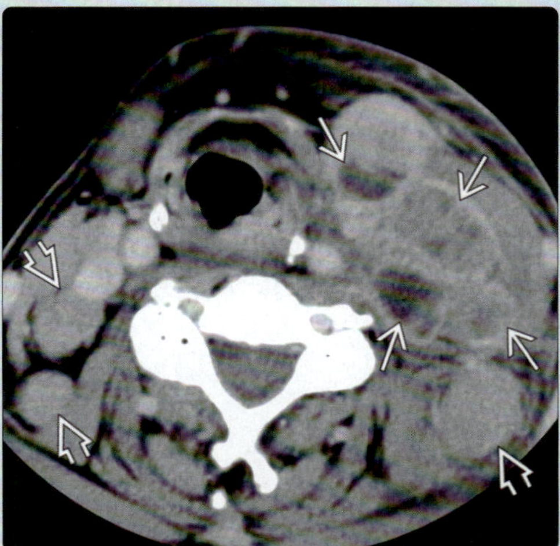

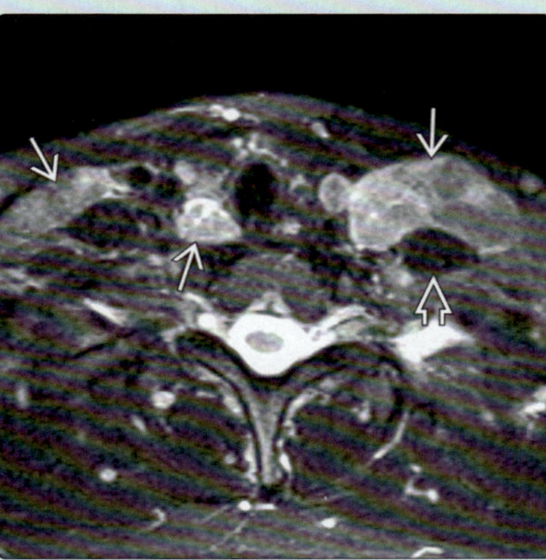

(Left) *Axial CECT demonstrates a massive left nodal conglomerate, some with necrosis ➡. Surrounding induration and stranding of fat in the left neck suggests inflammatory response. Other large nonnecrotic nodes ➡ are seen bilaterally.* **(Right)** *Axial T2 FS MR reveals multiple heterogeneous and predominantly hyperintense nodal masses ➡. Despite the large size, nodes insinuate around structures with little mass effect and no arterial compression. The largest node wraps around the anterior scalene muscle ➡.*

KEY FACTS

TERMINOLOGY

- Abbreviation: Differentiated thyroid carcinoma (DTCa)
- Definition: Metastatic node(s) from papillary or follicular thyroid carcinoma

IMAGING

- Ultrasound: Look for cystic change, hyperechoic calcifications, loss of hilar architecture
  - Peripheral vascularization on power Doppler
- CECT may be done but delays ^{131}I-radioablation
  - Nodes heterogeneous: Solid, cystic, calcified
- MR: Nodes heterogeneous in size and signal
- FDG PET: Not useful for DTCa
  - Best for **recurrence** when ↑ **thyroglobulin** with negative iodide scan
- I-123 and I-131 scans show low sensitivity, high specificity

TOP DIFFERENTIAL DIAGNOSES

- Nodal squamous cell carcinoma
- Nodal non-Hodgkin lymphoma
- Nodal tuberculosis
- Systemic nodal metastases

PATHOLOGY

- Extranodal extension may be poor prognostic characteristic

CLINICAL ISSUES

- Nodal metastases common; however, prognostically significant only if > 45 years of age
- Tumor may present as slow-growing nodal mass does
- Treatment: Thyroidectomy, neck dissection, adjuvant RAI

DIAGNOSTIC CHECKLIST

- If patient presents with nodal mass, some features highly suggestive of DTCa
  - Heterogeneous nodes
  - **Calcifications** on CT or ultrasound
  - Variable T1 intensity on MR
- Primary thyroid tumor may not be evident on CT/MR

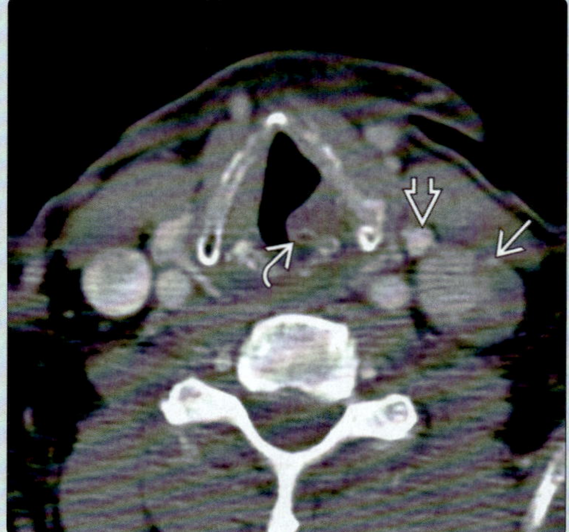

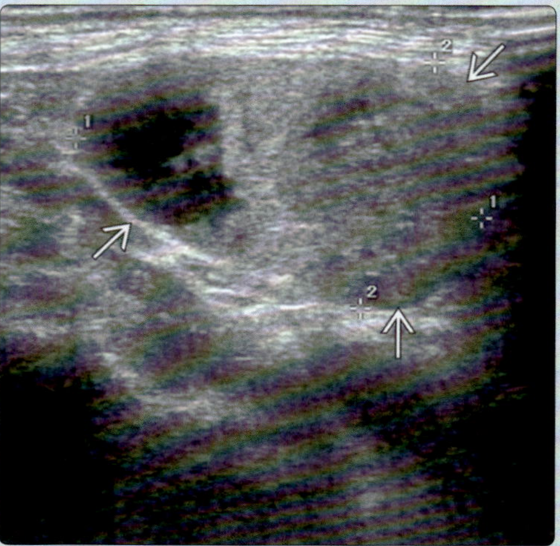

(Left) *Axial CECT shows a large, heterogeneous, left level III node ➡ displacing the jugular vein ➡ anteriorly. Nodal calcifications were present more inferiorly. Note medially rotated left arytenoid cartilage ➡, indicating left vocal cord paralysis, which was secondary to invasive left differentiated thyroid carcinoma.* **(Right)** *Longitudinal ultrasound in the same patient shows marked internal heterogeneity of an enlarged level III node ➡, which on FNA aspiration revealed papillary thyroid carcinoma.*

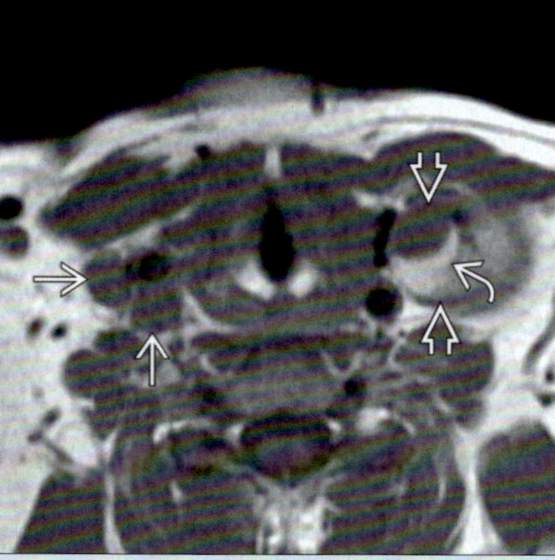

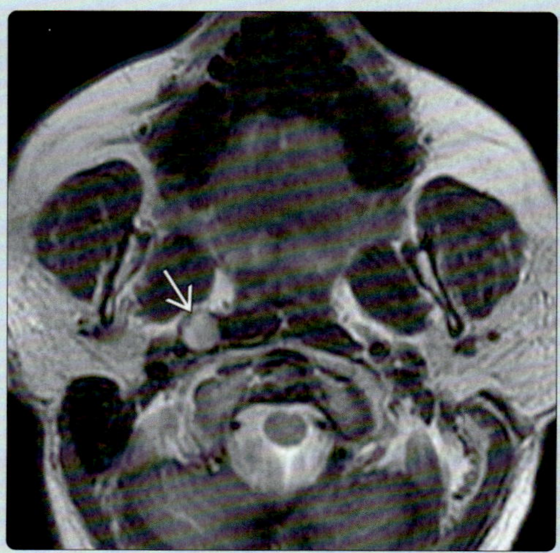

(Left) *Axial T1WI MR through the lower neck shows a cluster of round, minimally enlarged homogeneous nodes on the right at level III ➡ and a more complex cystic and solid mass in the lower left neck ➡. T1 hyperintensity within posterior cystic component ➡ makes papillary thyroid carcinoma the most likely primary diagnosis.* **(Right)** *Axial T2WI MR more superiorly (same patient) shows an enlarged, round, right retropharyngeal node ➡. Thyroidectomy revealed thyroid papillary carcinoma in nonenlarged heterogeneous gland.*

KEY FACTS

TERMINOLOGY

- Definition: Cervical metastatic adenopathy from infraclavicular primary tumor
- Virchow nodal metastasis: Left supraclavicular nodal lesion

IMAGING

- CT/MR findings of systemic nodal metastases in neck
  - Nodes generally in lower neck, especially on **left**
  - Variable size nodes, often > 1.5 cm
  - May be cluster of small nodes
  - May form conglomerate mass > 5-6 cm
  - If calcification present, consider primary tumor may be systemic adenocarcinoma or thyroid carcinoma

TOP DIFFERENTIAL DIAGNOSES

- Reactive lymph nodes
- Sarcoidosis nodes
- Squamous cell carcinoma metastatic nodes
- Non-Hodgkin lymphoma nodes

PATHOLOGY

- Common primary tumors: Esophageal, breast, and lung
- May be unknown primary tumor
- Focal nodal parenchyma nonenhancement on CT/MR corresponds to nest of tumor cells or necrosis

CLINICAL ISSUES

- Adult with new left supraclavicular mass FNA positive for cancer
  - FNA can direct sites for further imaging
  - Known chest, abdomen, or pelvis cancer usually
  - If no known tumor, imaging may begin with neck CECT
  - If neck CECT shows no other upper neck nodes, primary tumor is in chest, abdomen, or pelvis
- If no known primary tumor, scan request may be to look for pharyngeal primary tumor
  - If nodes only in left supraclavicular neck, primary is not in pharynx or larynx
  - Recommend CT chest, abdomen, and pelvis or PET/CT

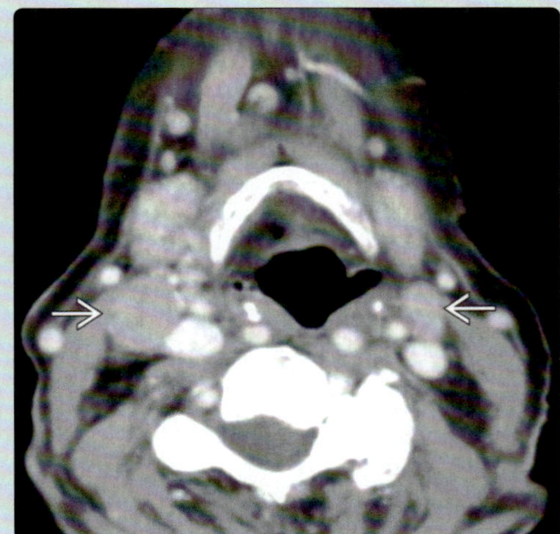

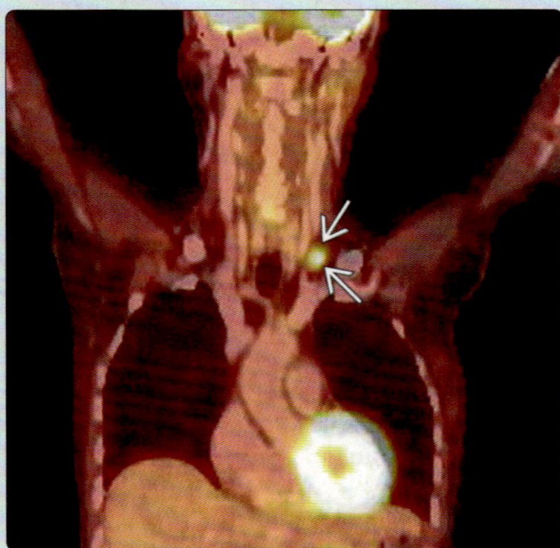

(Left) *Axial CECT shows enlarged, noncalcified, solidly enhancing bilateral level IIA neck nodes ➡. No primary source was present in the head and neck, but the patient was found to have primary lung carcinoma.* **(Right)** *Coronal PET/CT in a patient with ovarian carcinoma reveals a single enlarged left supraclavicular node ➡ with FDG avidity. This patient had been previously treated for abdominal metastases and had known pulmonary metastases at the time of study.*

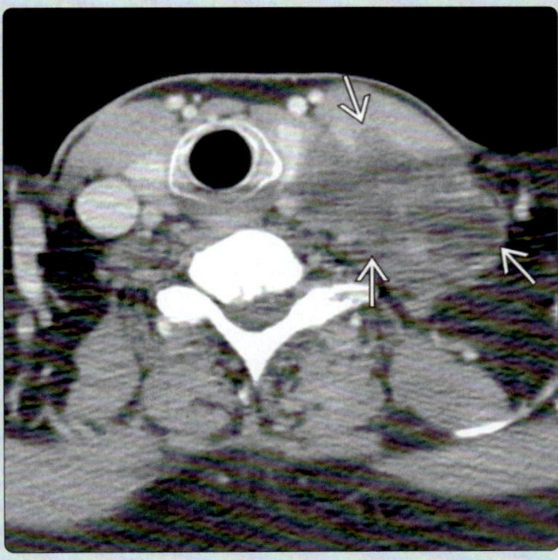

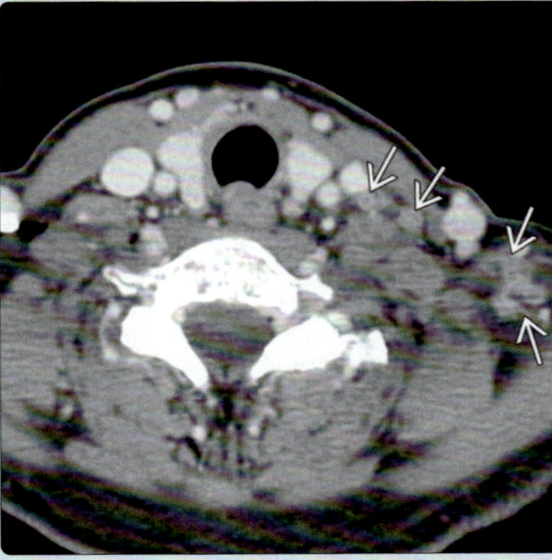

(Left) *Axial CECT shows a large complex conglomerate left supraclavicular nodal mass ➡ with extensive necrosis and infiltration of the scalene and sternocleidomastoid muscles. This patient had neural deficits from invasion of brachial plexus. FNA revealed metastatic colonic adenocarcinoma.* **(Right)** *Axial CECT reveals multiple small nodes ➡ in the lower left neck in a patient with known metastatic breast carcinoma. The nodes are heterogeneous; many have focal eccentric low density, indicating necrosis.*

Summary Thoughts: Trans- and Multispatial Lesions

Transspatial and multispatial terms are used to describe specific subsets of lesions found in the head and neck. The **transspatial** descriptor is used to describe a lesion that involves multiple **contiguous** spaces or areas of the extracranial head and neck. **Multispatial** is applied to a lesion that is found in multiple **noncontiguous** spaces or areas.

Approaches to Imaging Issues in Trans- and Multispatial Lesions

Transspatial Lesions

Transspatial lesions are defined as involving multiple contiguous spaces or areas in the neck. In the soft tissues of the suprahyoid neck, infrahyoid neck, and oral cavity, where the anatomy can be defined by fascia-circumscribed spaces, this term is directly applicable. In the skull base, sinuses, nose, and orbit where the anatomic areas are distinct but not fascia defined, the term can still be used to describe lesions that involve multiple contiguous areas.

Transspatial lesions generally fall into 4 major pathologic categories: Congenital, inflammatory-infectious, benign tumor, and malignant tumor.

- **Congenital lesions** form at the same time or prior to fascia in extracranial head and neck. As a result, they do not always stay within spatial boundaries and are often transspatial. Congenital lesions, such as venous and lymphatic malformation, commonly appear transspatial when first imaged.
- **Inflammatory-infectious lesions** fall within the transspatial group when cellulitis, phlegmon, or abscess involves multiple contiguous spaces. In the case of abscess, defining each space involved for the surgeon ensures that each space is entered with either a probe or a drain.
- **Benign tumors**, such as infantile hemangioma and schwannoma, often involve multiple contiguous spaces. In the case of schwannoma, this is because the nerves that they form from normally run through multiple spaces as they course through head and neck.
- **Malignant tumors** invade contiguous spaces as they enlarge; in fact, squamous cell carcinoma (SCCa) of pharynx and oral cavity initially arises from mucosal space/surface and immediately invades deeply into surrounding soft tissue spaces. Larger SCCa primary tumors are almost always transspatial at presentation. Along with perineural tumor, the exact spaces invaded by primary SCCa determine tumor resectability and radiation ports.

Multispatial Lesions

The term **multispatial** is helpful in describing lesions of the head and neck that occupy multiple noncontiguous spaces or areas. These lesions generally are identified as 1 of 3 pathologic categories: Congenital, inflammatory-infectious, and malignant neoplasms.

- **Congenital lesions** that may be multispatial include neurofibromatosis types 1 and 2, PHACES syndrome, and other syndromes that have multiple noncontiguous manifestations.
- **Inflammatory-infectious nodal lesions** are commonly multispatial at presentation; reactive nodes may progress to suppurative nodes (intranodal abscesses); tuberculous adenopathy may also be multispatial; any of the many rarer nodal diseases of head and neck may also present as multispatial.
- **Malignant tumors** of head and neck are often transspatial in their primary site and multispatial in their nodal spread; oral cavity and pharyngeal SCCas and non-Hodgkin lymphoma (NHL) (of Waldeyer lymphatic ring) are both prone to this behavior; Hodgkin lymphoma neck nodes and systemic nodal metastases may also be multispatial in head and neck.

Transspatial Diseases of H&N

Congenital Lesions
- Venous malformation
- Lymphatic malformation
- Branchial cleft cysts
- Thyroglossal duct cyst
- Thymic cyst
- Neurofibromatosis type 1 (plexiform neurofibroma)

Inflammatory and Infectious Lesions
- Cellulitis
- Phlegmon
- Abscess
- Invasive fungal sinusitis
- Sinonasal Wegener granulomatosis
- Fibromatosis

Benign Tumors
- Schwannoma
- Neurofibroma
- Infantile hemangioma
- Hemangiopericytoma

Malignant Tumors
- Pharyngeal & laryngeal SCCa
- Extranodal NHL
- Rhabdomyosarcoma
- Anaplastic carcinoma of thyroid
- Sinonasal SCCa
- Sinonasal undifferentiated carcinoma
- Esthesioneuroblastoma of nose
- Chondrosarcoma of skull base
- Chordoma of skull base

Multispatial Diseases of H&N

Congenital Lesions
- Neurofibromatosis type 1
- Neurofibromatosis type 2
- PHACES association

Inflammatory and Infectious Lesions
- Reactive adenopathy
- Suppurative adenopathy
- Tuberculous adenopathy

Malignant Tumors
- Pharyngeal SCCa + malignant nodes
- NHL extranodal + nodal
- Systemic metastases
- Metastatic neuroblastoma

Selected References

1. Aiken AH et al: Imaging Hodgkin and non-Hodgkin lymphoma in the head and neck. Radiol Clin North Am. 46(2):363-78, ix-x, 2008
2. Vogelzang P et al: Multispatial and transpatial diseases of the extracranial head and neck. Semin Ultrasound CT MR. 12(3):274-87, 1991

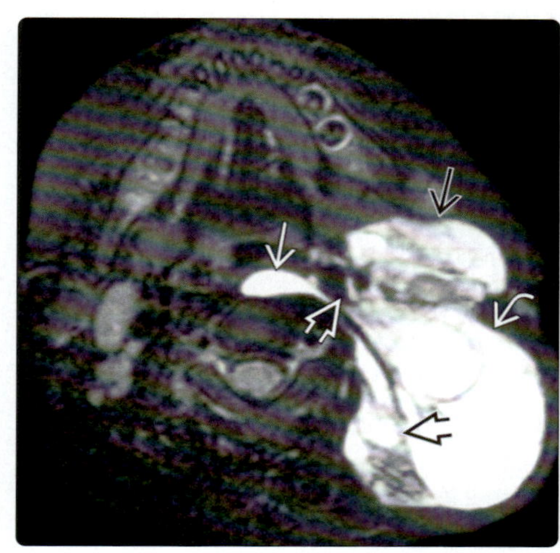

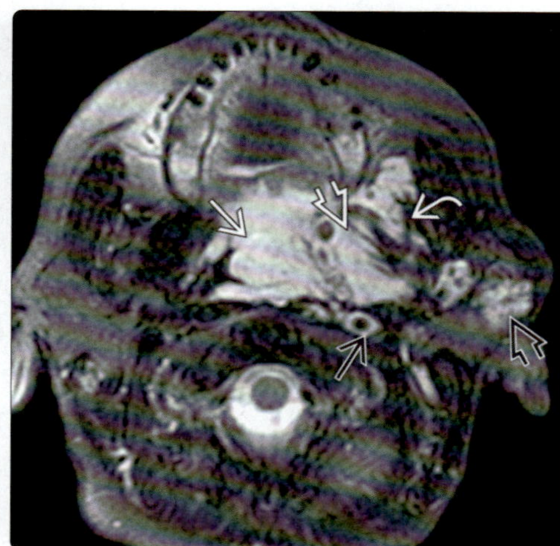

(Left) *Axial T2 FS MR demonstrates a large, hyperintense lymphatic malformation of the neck, which is multilocular and transspatial. Multiple contiguous space involvement includes the retropharyngeal, carotid, posterior cervical, submandibular, and perivertebral spaces.* **(Right)** *Axial T2 FS MR in a patient with a large venous malformation shows transspatial involvement of the pharyngeal mucosal, parapharyngeal, masticator, carotid, and parotid spaces.*

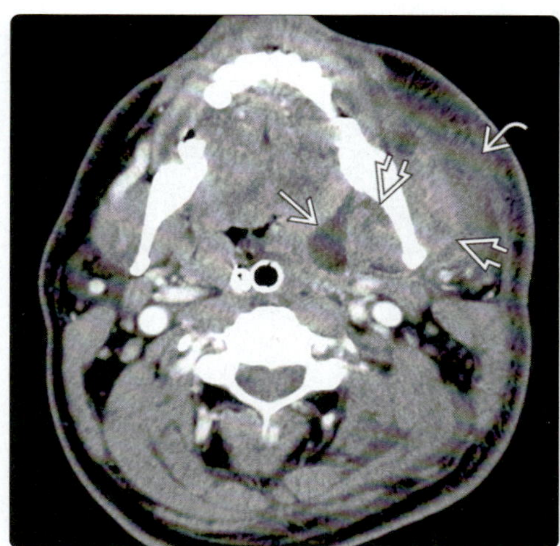

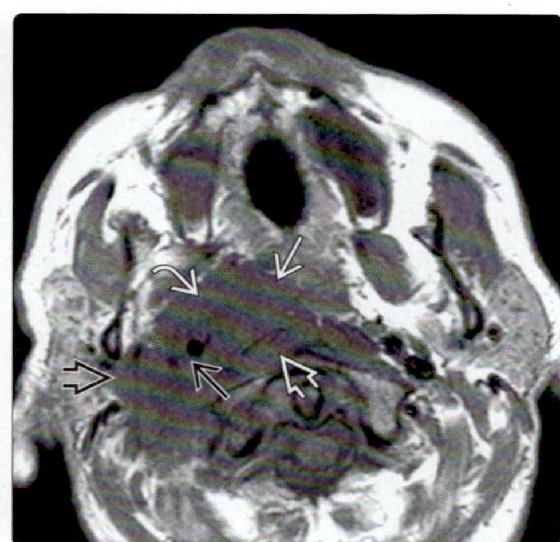

(Left) *Axial CECT in a septic patient with trismus reveals a transspatial infection in the deep face. Abscess in the parapharyngeal and masticator spaces is accompanied by contiguous, superficial space cellulitis.* **(Right)** *Axial T1 MR demonstrates an invasive, transspatial nasopharyngeal carcinoma. This nasopharyngeal mucosal space carcinoma has directly invaded the parapharyngeal, perivertebral, carotid, and parotid spaces.*

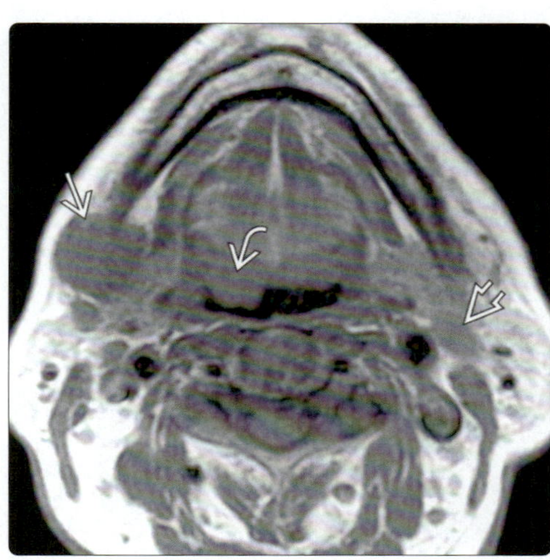

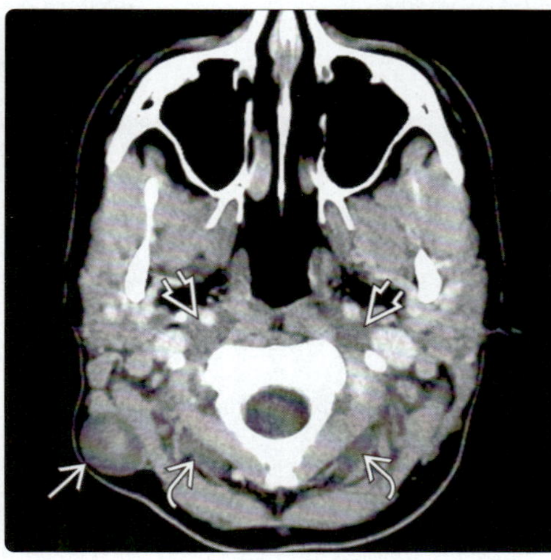

(Left) *Axial T1 MR in a patient with multiple H&N lesions shows abnormal lymph node in submandibular & parotid spaces accompanied by a focal mass in the pharyngeal mucosal space (lingual tonsil). This example of multispatial disease is caused by non-Hodgkin lymphoma.* **(Right)** *Axial CECT in a 31-year-old woman with neurofibromatosis type 1 reveals multispatial low-density neurofibromas. In this image, the neurofibromas can be identified in the superficial, carotid, and perivertebral spaces.*

Prominent Thoracic Duct in Neck

KEY FACTS

TERMINOLOGY

- Synonym: Prominent, normal left lymphatic duct
- Definition: Normal anatomical structure draining lymph and chyle from abdomen and left chest

IMAGING

- General findings
  - Courses cranially in **left** lower neck posterior to common carotid artery
  - Drains into junction of internal jugular & subclavian veins
- CECT & MR findings
  - Tubular structure with same density/intensity as CSF
  - Average diameter: 4-5 mm
  - May be prominent, bulbous in lower neck

TOP DIFFERENTIAL DIAGNOSES

- Differentiated thyroid carcinoma node
- Nodal metastasis from systemic disease
- Squamous cell carcinoma node
- Lymphocele

PATHOLOGY

- Drains lymph and chyle from abdomen and left chest to venous circulation
- Right-sided thoracic duct uncommonly also found
  - Ends in right subclavian vein
- Obstruction results in pleural effusion
- Source of metastasis to left supraclavicular node
  - Virchow node

CLINICAL ISSUES

- Incidental normal finding on CT or MR

DIAGNOSTIC CHECKLIST

- Key imaging features
  - Tubular structure in left neck
  - Isointense/isodense to CSF
- May be mistaken for cystic level IV or VI node

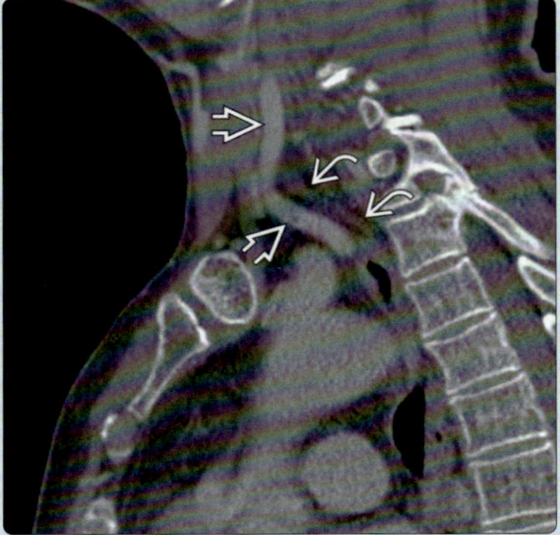

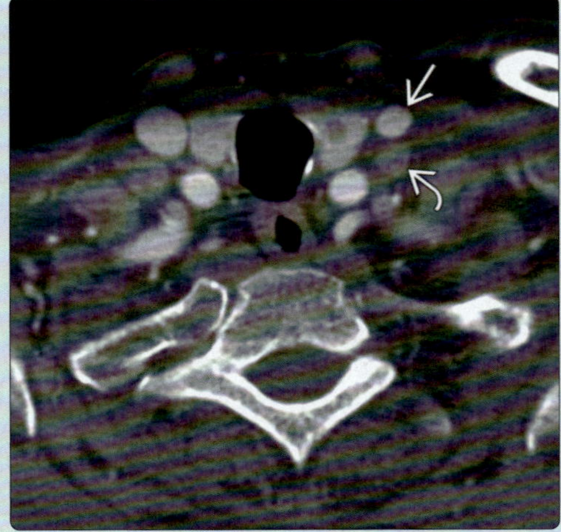

(Left) *Sagittal reformat CECT demonstrates a tubular, low-density thoracic duct ➡ ascending from the chest posterior to the left carotid artery ➡, which may be mistaken for a thrombosed vessel in the sagittal plane.* **(Right)** *Axial CECT shows a more lateral location of the thoracic duct ➡ as it courses toward the terminus at the junction of the internal jugular vein (IJV) ➡ and subclavian vein. The thoracic duct mimics a cystic node in its axial cross section contour.*

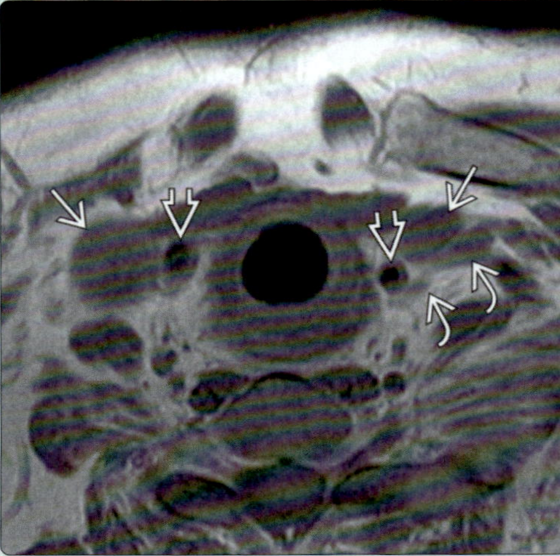

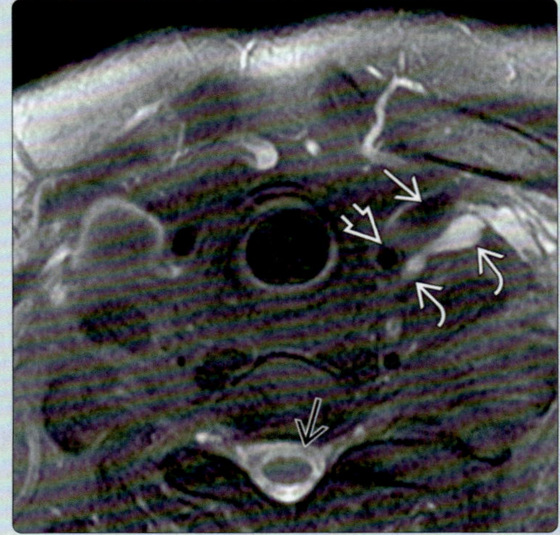

(Left) *Axial T1 MR shows normal carotid arterial flow voids ➡ and mixed signal in the IJVs ➡, as is frequently seen on MR. The right jugular vein is dominant in this patient. The thoracic duct is evident at the subtle tubular structure posterior to the left jugular vein ➡.* **(Right)** *Axial T2 fat-saturated MR shows the thoracic duct ➡ as a markedly intense varicose structure posterior to the left carotid artery ➡ and IJV ➡. The thoracic duct appears isointense to CSF ➡ on all sequences.*

KEY FACTS

TERMINOLOGY

- Benign neoplasm composed of mature fat

IMAGING

- 15% of lipomas occur in H&N
- 5% are multiple, more often in female patients
- May occur in any H&N space & may be transspatial
- Well-circumscribed, homogeneous mass composed of fat and displacing normal structures
- Homogeneous fat with minimal internal stranding
  - 8% have small nonfatty soft tissue component
- CT: Homogeneous, well-defined, low-density mass
- MR: Homogeneous signal of subcutaneous fat
- CT or MR: Any enhancement or soft tissue raises concern for liposarcoma
- FDG PET: No uptake in bland benign lipoma
  - Uptake suggests sarcoma or lipoma variant

TOP DIFFERENTIAL DIAGNOSES

- Dermoid
- Teratoma
- Lymphatic malformation
- Liposarcoma

CLINICAL ISSUES

- Asymptomatic lump in neck, more often in male patients
- Clinical differential is lymphatic malformation
- Most often found in 5th-6th decade
- Often does not require treatment; may treat surgically if symptomatic

DIAGNOSTIC CHECKLIST

- CT: Measure density to determine fat content
- MR: Use chemical-selective fat saturation techniques, not STIR, to prove fat content
- If lipoma has soft tissue or enhancement, cannot distinguish from well-differentiated liposarcoma

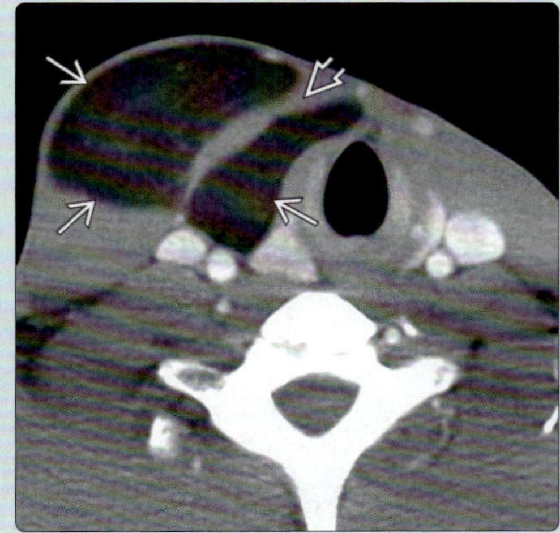

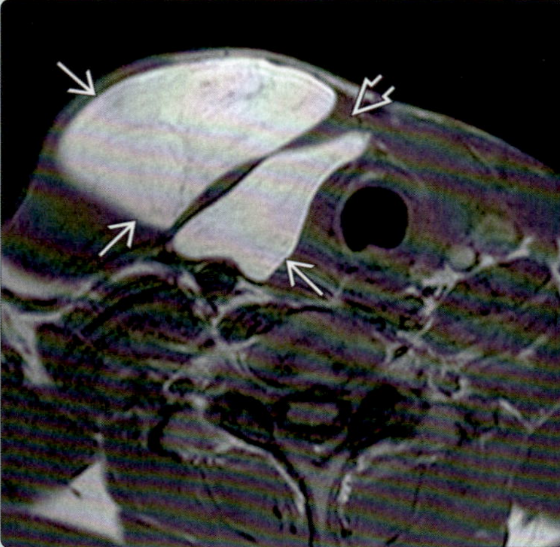

(Left) *Axial CECT through the lower neck of a young adult with a prominent neck mass demonstrates a well-defined, low-density right neck mass ➡. A mass herniates around the anterior portion of the omohyoid muscle ➡, displacing tissues with no evidence of infiltration.* **(Right)** *Axial T1 MR 6 weeks later shows an intrinsically hyperintense mass ➡ enveloping the omohyoid ➡ without invasion of adjacent tissues. The mass was thought to have enlarged clinically.*

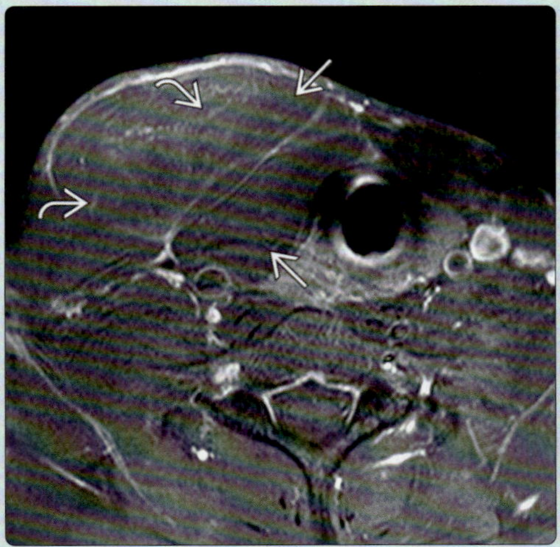

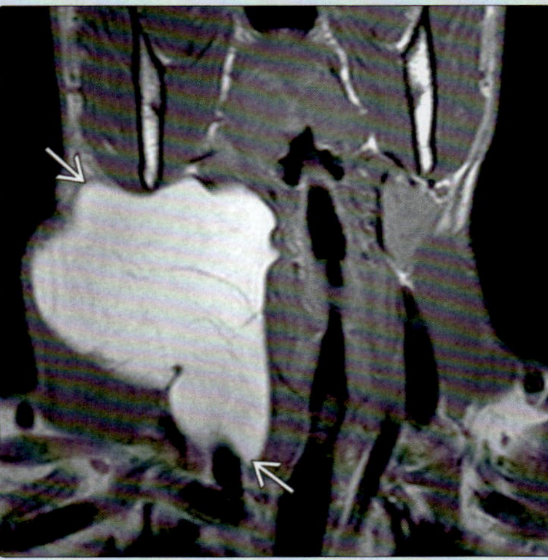

(Left) *Axial T1 C+ FS MR reveals suppression of the high-intensity fat within the mass ➡ while also showing mildly complicated fibrous internal architecture ➡.* **(Right)** *Coronal T1 MR illustrates the craniocaudad extent of the mass ➡. The scan also shows mass effect on the larynx, which was deviated to a greater extent across midline than on prior CT, raising concern for liposarcoma rather than lipoma. Resection of the mass showed mature adipose tissue of benign lipoma.*

KEY FACTS

TERMINOLOGY

- Plexiform neurofibroma: Architecturally complex neurofibroma involving multiple nerve fascicles
  - **Pathognomonic** for **neurofibromatosis type 1 (NF1)**

IMAGING

- **Lobular, serpiginous infiltrative transspatial mass**
- CECT has nonspecific infiltrative appearance
  - Mild contrast enhancement
- MR best characterizes and delineates complete extent
  - Lobulated T2 hyperintensity
  - Central T2 hypointense foci: **Target sign**

TOP DIFFERENTIAL DIAGNOSES

- Vascular (venous or lymphatic) malformation
- Sarcoma

PATHOLOGY

- Deletion in *NF1* gene on long arm of **chromosome 17**
- Autosomal dominant inheritance
- Decreased production of neurofibromin (tumor suppressor) protein

CLINICAL ISSUES

- Present at birth or develops with age
- "Bag of worms" on clinical exam
- PNFs in **~ 30% of NF1** patients
- 5-10% risk of malignant transformation
- Gross total resection often not possible, may incur significant morbidity
  - Debulking may be necessary when symptomatic, depending on location

DIAGNOSTIC CHECKLIST

- On CECT appears as infiltrative solid mass
- On MR may mimic venous malformation; distinguish with target sign
- Look for other manifestations of NF1

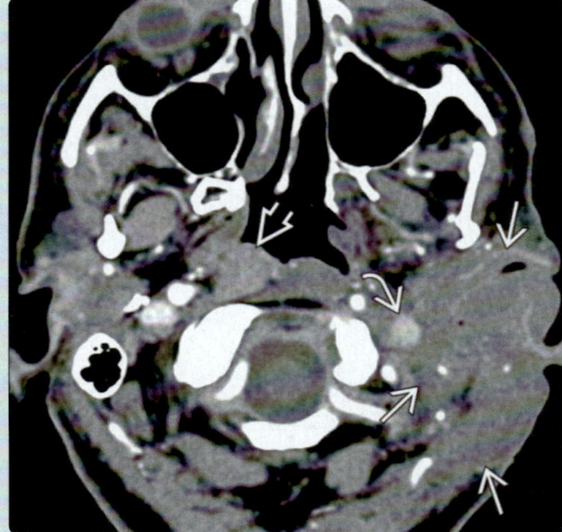

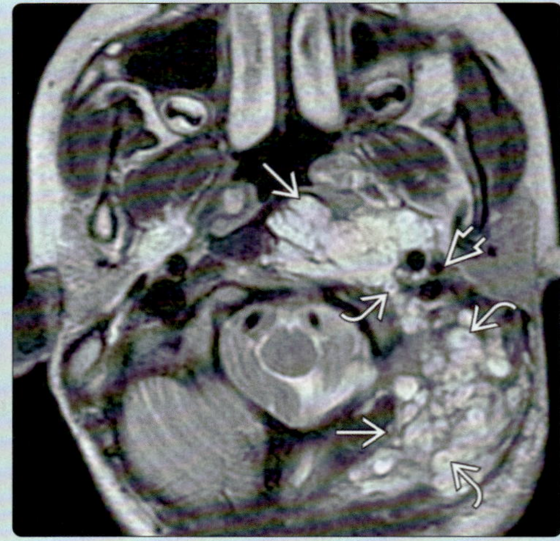

(Left) *Axial CECT demonstrates a minimally enhancing infiltrative soft tissue mass ➡ involving subcutaneous and deep tissues. The mass abuts and surrounds the left internal jugular vein ➡. Notice the mildly enhancing lesion of the right prevertebral muscle ➡.* **(Right)** *Axial T2 MR reveals characteristic MR findings of plexiform neurofibroma ➡ in prevertebral and paraspinous tissues and around the carotid sheath ➡. The multilobulated mass is hyperintense except for the central areas of low T2 signal ➡.*

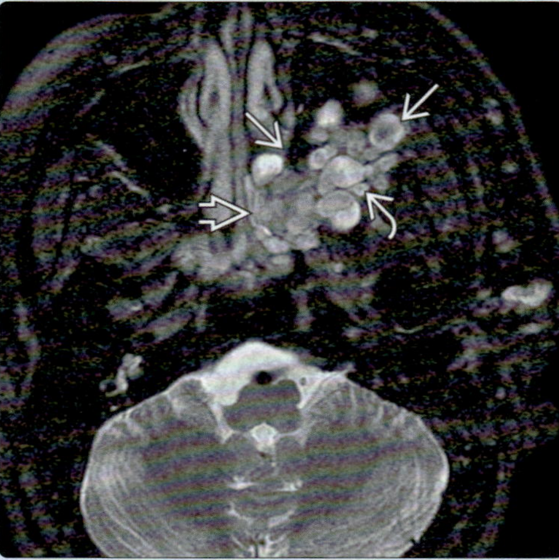

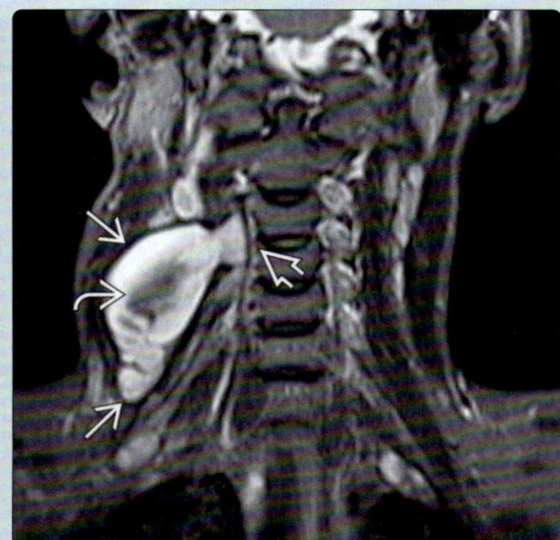

(Left) *Axial T2 FS MR in a patient with neurofibromatosis type 1 shows a multilobulated mass ➡ distending the left pterygopalatine fossa & extending into the posterior nasal cavity ➡ through the sphenopalatine foramen. The target sign of focal low signal ➡ suggests plexiform neurofibroma.* **(Right)** *Coronal STIR MR shows a large right neck plexiform neurofibroma ➡ from the right C3-C4 neuroforamen ➡. This multilobulated mass shows the classic target sign of central T2 hypointensity ➡.*

KEY FACTS

TERMINOLOGY

- Posttransplantation lymphoproliferative disorder (PTLD)
- Uncontrolled lymphoid growth in transplant recipient on immunosuppressive therapy
- Disease spectrum ranges from hyperplasia to malignancy
  - Reactive hyperplasia → polymorphic PTLD → monomorphic PTLD → Hodgkin disease & non-Hodgkin lymphoma-like PTLD

IMAGING

- Mimics H&N lymphoma seen in nontransplant patients
- May also mimic pharyngeal infection and abscesses
- Consider when history of transplant plus any nodal or extranodal enlargement, or H&N mass
  - Adenotonsillar &/or nodal enlargement
  - Sinonasal masses or infiltrating tissue to skull base
  - Orbital or oral cavity mass
- Increased FDG uptake on PET/CT

TOP DIFFERENTIAL DIAGNOSES

- Tonsillar inflammation
- Tonsillar/peritonsillar abscess
- Reactive lymph nodes
- Invasive fungal sinusitis

PATHOLOGY

- Therapeutic T-cell suppression allows proliferation of B cells infected with Epstein-Barr virus

CLINICAL ISSUES

- Solid organ transplant > > bone marrow transplant
- More common in pediatric transplant patients
- Up to 80% 1st year posttransplant

DIAGNOSTIC CHECKLIST

- Consider PTLD with every transplant patient when imaging suggests infection or lymphoma-like lesions

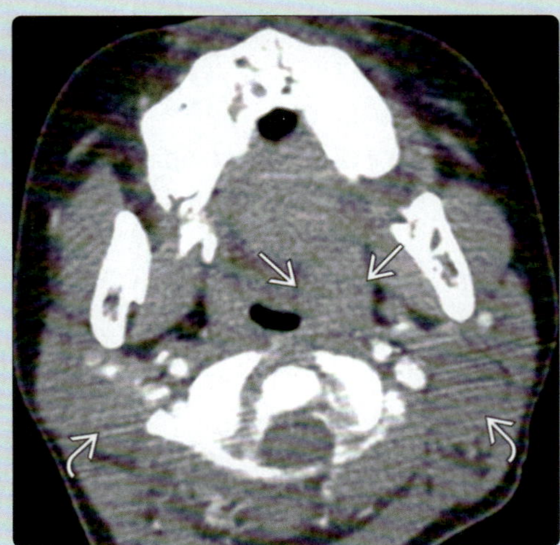

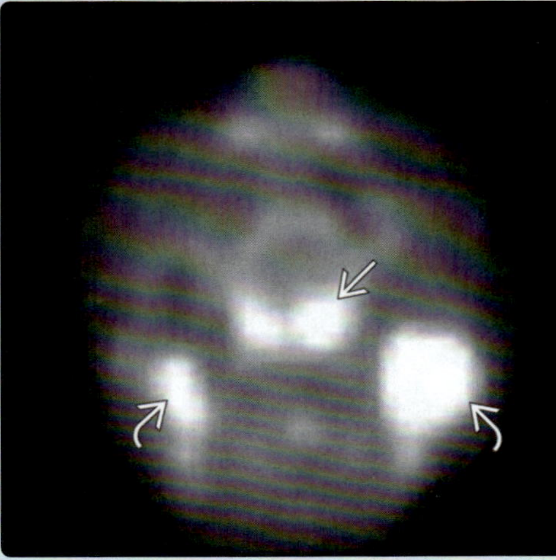

(Left) *Axial CECT shows an asymmetrically enlarged left palatine tonsil ➡ but no abnormal enhancement or peritonsillar collection. Multiple enlarged, homogeneous neck nodes are apparent ➡ in high jugular chains.* **(Right)** *Axial PET in the same patient reveals marked FDG avidity in bilateral neck nodes ➡ with asymmetric FDG uptake in the left palatine tonsil ➡. PTLD can mimic tonsillitis with reactive adenopathy, but transplant history is key. Biopsy distinguishes these processes.*

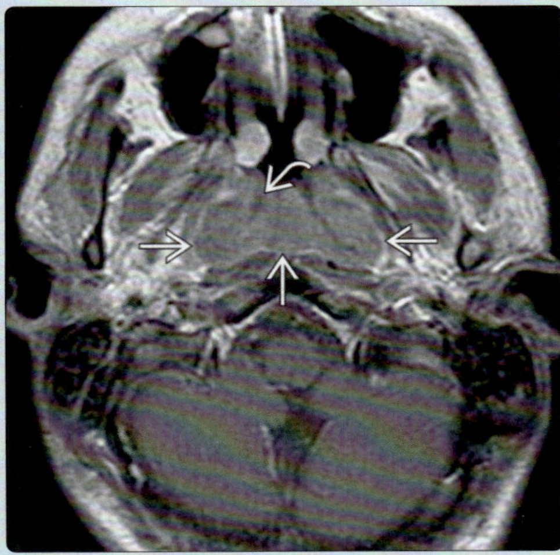

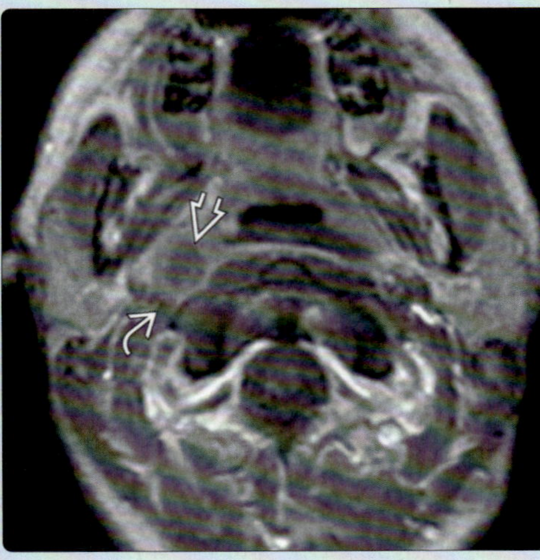

(Left) *Axial T1 C+ MR shows enlarged enhancing nasopharyngeal adenoidal tissue ➡. The tonsil has endophytic growth and an irregular mucosal margin ➡.* **(Right)** *Inferiorly, note the enlarged right retropharyngeal node ➡ anteromedial to the right internal carotid artery ➡. The retropharyngeal node is centrally necrotic with peripheral enhancement. No retropharyngeal edema is seen, as might be expected with suppurative node and tonsillitis.*

KEY FACTS

TERMINOLOGY

- **N**on-**H**odgkin **L**ymphoma (NHL)
- Heterogeneous lymphoreticular system malignancy
- H&N NHL has multiple forms
  - Nodal, nonnodal lymphatic (Waldeyer lymphatic ring), extralymphatic (e.g., skull base, thyroid, sinuses)

IMAGING

- **Nodal NHL**
  - Multiple 1- to 3-cm solid nodes
  - Dominant large node up to 5 cm
  - Aggressive NHL may have necrosis
- **Nonnodal lymphatic NHL (palatine, lingual, & adenoidal tonsils)**
  - Enlarged, homogeneously enhancing tonsils ± adenoids ± enlarged ipsilateral nodes
  - May be heterogeneous & infiltrative
- **Extralymphatic NHL**
  - Focal or infiltrative mass in any tissue in neck

TOP DIFFERENTIAL DIAGNOSES

- Wide differential diagnosis depending on form of NHL: Nodal, nonnodal lymphatic, extralymphatic
- Lymphoma is one of great mimickers

PATHOLOGY

- WHO is favored classification (2016)
- Modified Ann Arbor staging system is for clinical staging, treatment, and prognosis
- Lugano classification also used to assess interim and treatment response

CLINICAL ISSUES

- Treatment depends on cell type, stage, patient age
- Chemotherapy, radiation therapy, or combined modality therapy
- May be indolent, progressive but not curable, or aggressive but often curable
- 5-year survival: Stage I/II 85%, III/IV 50%

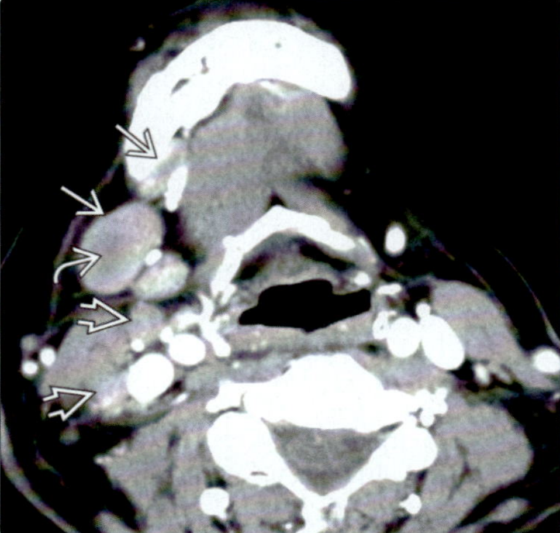
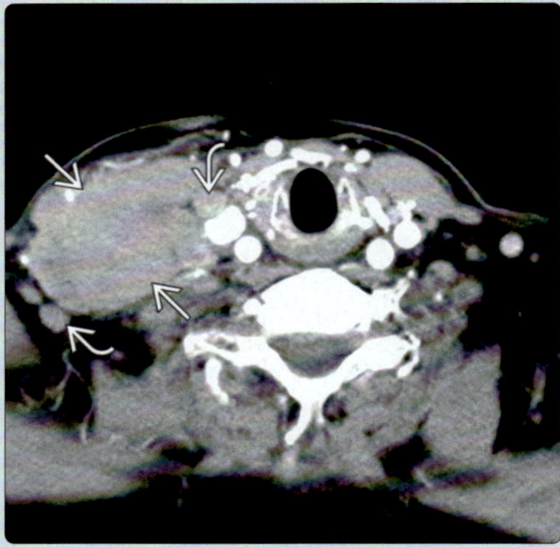

(Left) *Axial CECT in 66-year-old patient shows multiple nodal masses in right levels IB ➡ and IIA ➡ nodal locations. Submandibular nodes are heterogeneous with eccentric low density ➡, suggesting necrosis, and the posterior IIA node is irregular and poorly defined.* **(Right)** *Axial CECT in the infrahyoid neck demonstrates a homogeneous mass ➡ inseparable from the right sternocleidomastoid muscle with multiple smaller abnormal nodes ➡. Biopsy showed diffuse large B-cell lymphoma.*

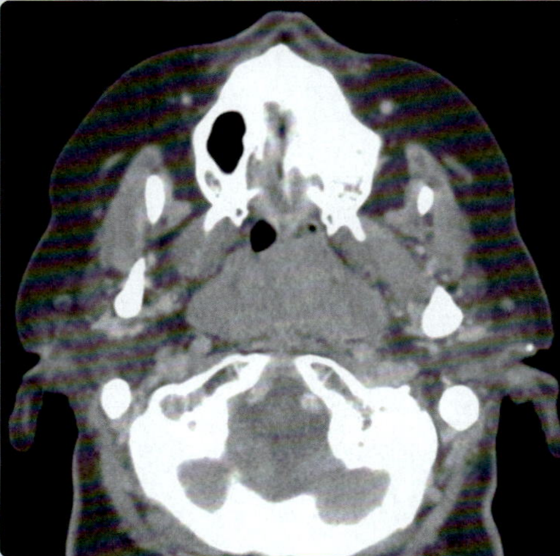
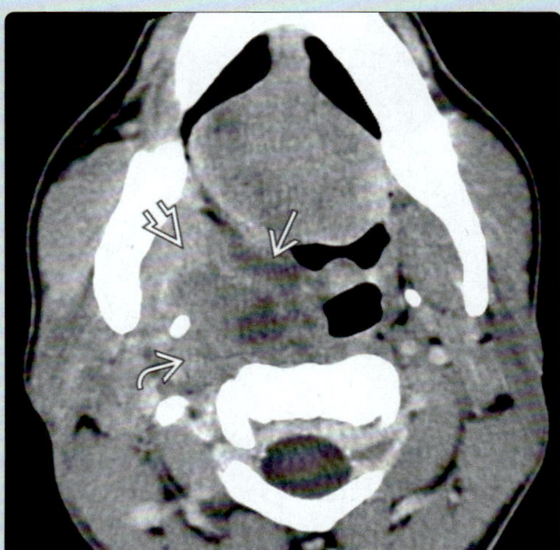

(Left) *Axial CECT in an adult reveals a nasopharyngeal mucosal space mass filling the airway but not invading the adjacent deep tissue spaces. Biopsy revealed non-Hodgkin lymphoma (NHL). This is an example of nonnodal, lymphatic NHL.* **(Right)** *Axial CECT in HIV(+) patient with facial pain shows a large necrotic right tonsillar mass ➡ infiltrating the masticator ➡, parapharyngeal, retropharyngeal, and carotid spaces ➡. Biopsy showed atypical Burkitt lymphoma. This is an example of extralymphatic NHL.*

Lymphocele of Neck

KEY FACTS

TERMINOLOGY

- Benign lymph-filled cyst due to leaking lymphatic channels
- Synonyms: Lymphatic cyst, lymphocyst, chylocele, chyloma, chylous cyst, (distal) thoracic duct cyst

IMAGING

- Best imaging tools are CECT and ultrasound
- Characteristic location is low posterior cervical space in **supraclavicular fossa**
  - Between scalene and sternocleidomastoid muscles
  - Cyst often "points" toward confluence of internal jugular and subclavian veins
- Unilocular, well-circumscribed cyst with **no visible cyst wall**, enhancement, or septa
  - Cyst wall thickened ± enhancing if complicated by infection/treatment
  - Fluid density (CT HU usually 0-20) or signal (MR)
- Ultrasound: Used to guide FNA to confirm diagnosis

TOP DIFFERENTIAL DIAGNOSES

- Congenital neck cysts
  - Lymphatic malformation
  - Branchial cleft
  - Thymic cyst
- Postoperative seroma, hematoma, or pseudomeningocele
- Suppurative lymph nodes
- Systemic nodal metastases

PATHOLOGY

- Endothelial-lined cyst with acellular fluid and **fat droplets**

CLINICAL ISSUES

- Growing painless neck mass without signs of infection
  - Patient may be **postoperative** with history of lower neck surgery
- Treatment options
  - Complete surgical removal is curative
  - Percutaneous sclerotherapy if surgery not possible

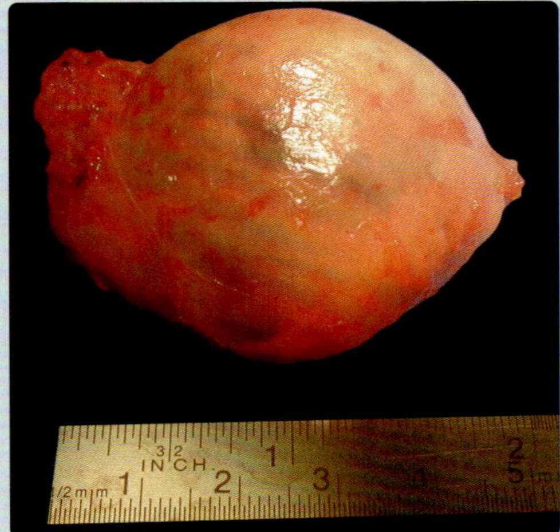

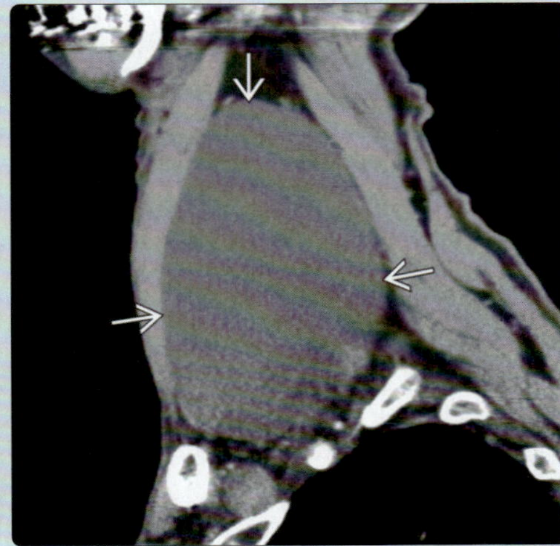

(Left) *Gross specimen of a lymphocele shows its typical encapsulated appearance. These masses are usually easy to remove surgically, with subsequent cure.* **(Right)** *Sagittal CECT multiplanar reconstruction demonstrates the typical CT characteristics of a lymphocele: A unilocular nonseptated round or ovoid water density cyst in the posterior cervical space-supraclavicular fossa with no perceptible cyst wall ➔ or enhancement.*

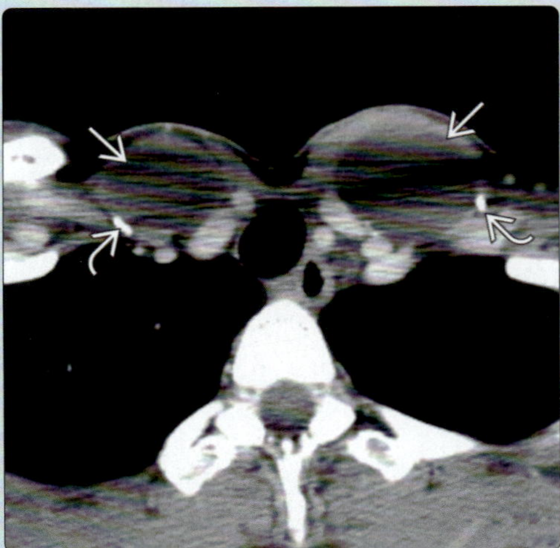

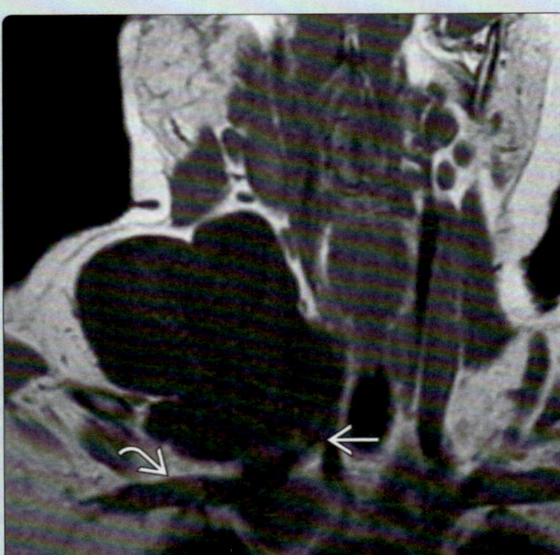

(Left) *Axial CECT shows bilateral lymphoceles ➔ in a patient post thyroid resection for cancer. Clips from prior node dissection ➥ are a clue to postsurgical origin from lymphatic duct iatrogenic injury.* **(Right)** *Coronal T1 MR shows a spontaneously occurring, lobulated, unilocular, fluid signal intensity lymphocele in the right supraclavicular fossa just above the subclavian ➥ and internal jugular ➔ venous confluence.*

Sinus Histiocytosis (Rosai-Dorfman) of Head and Neck

KEY FACTS

TERMINOLOGY

- Sinus histiocytosis: Benign pseudolymphomatous clinicopathologic entity of unknown etiology

IMAGING

- **Massive, bilateral cervical lymphadenopathy**
- H&N extranodal sites ~ **50%**
  - Skin, sinonasal area, orbit, eyelids, bone, salivary glands, & dura
- Rare other extranodal sites
  - Oral cavity, pharynx, trachea, bronchi, & mediastinal lymph nodes
- CT or MR findings
  - Homogeneously enhancing large lymph nodes
  - Enhancing extranodal infiltrates
  - **T2 low signal** of nodal or extranodal lesions common

TOP DIFFERENTIAL DIAGNOSES

- Non-Hodgkin lymphoma
- Reactive lymph nodes
- Skull base meningioma
- Langerhans cell histiocytosis

PATHOLOGY

- Unknown pathophysiology

CLINICAL ISSUES

- Clinical presentation
  - Painless neck masses
- Age at presentation
  - < 20 years old (80%)
- Natural history
  - Long history of benign disease involvement common
  - ↑ morbidity when immunologic dysfunction present (arthritis, circulating autoantibodies)
- Treatment
  - Clinical observation preferred
  - Surgical debulking if vital structure compression

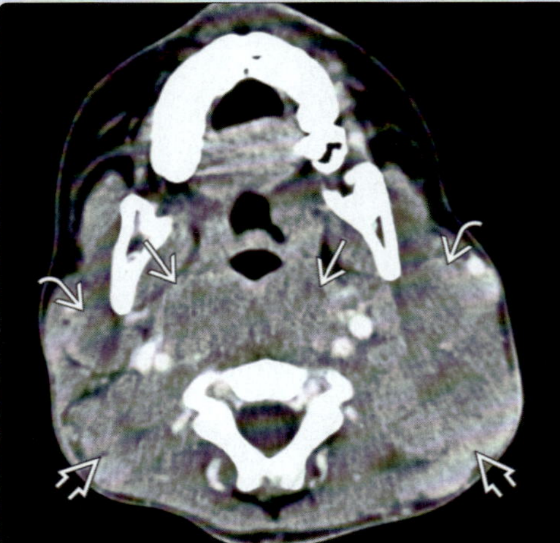

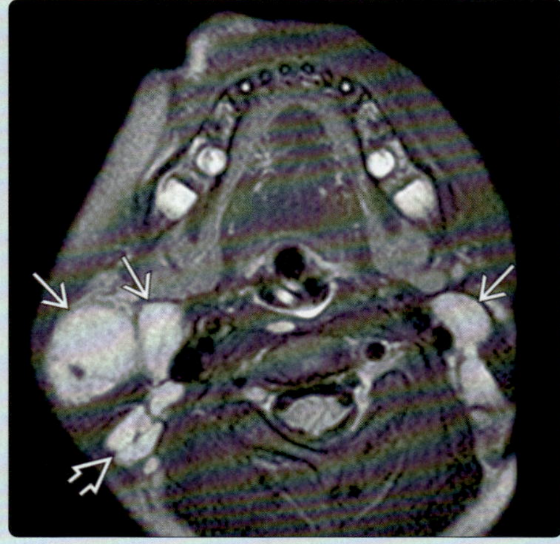

(Left) *Axial CECT shows very large bilateral retropharyngeal nodes ➡ in association with massive adenopathy in the internal jugular vein ➡ and spinal accessory nodal chains ➡. Non-Hodgkin lymphoma nodes were suspected before biopsy revealed sinus histiocytosis.* **(Right)** *Axial STIR MR in a child reveals large jugulodigastric ➡ and spinal accessory ➡ lymph nodes. Notice the right parotid tail large nodal focus as well. Nodal biopsy showed sinus histiocytosis.*

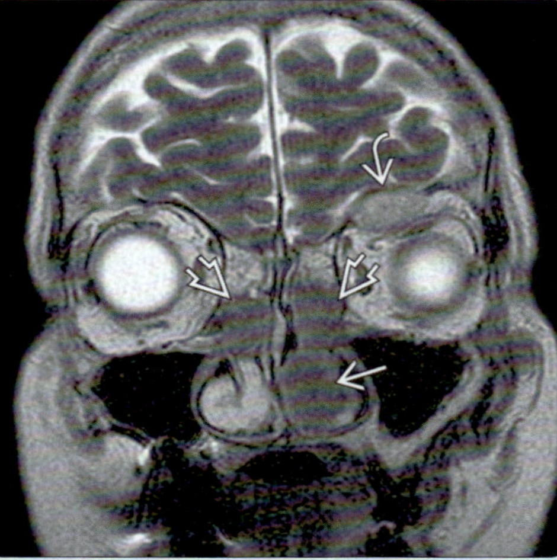

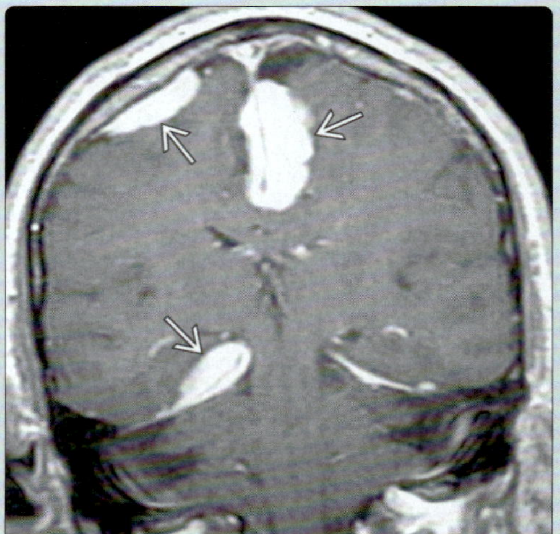

(Left) *Coronal T2 MR shows multifocal low-signal nasal ➡ and ethmoid sinus ➡ masses. Note also the slightly higher signal left extraconal orbital ➡ sinus histiocytosis lesion.* **(Right)** *Coronal T1 C+ MR demonstrates multiple dural-based, strongly enhancing masses ➡ originally thought to be multiple meningiomatosis. Surgical pathology revealed sinus histiocytosis.*

KEY FACTS

TERMINOLOGY

- Synonyms: Aggressive fibromatosis, extraabdominal desmoid, desmoid fibromatosis, infantile fibromatosis
- Definition: Rare infiltrative mass of benign monoclonal fibroblast proliferation that never metastasizes

IMAGING

- Ill-defined, nonnecrotic transspatial (spreads into multiple contiguous spaces) enhancing mass in any H&N space(s)
- Variable appearance: May be both **sharply circumscribed and infiltrative**
- CT: No tumor matrix calcification or ossification
- MR: T1 iso- to hypointense compared to muscle
  - T2 hyperintense ± hypointense bands
  - Generally avid enhancement on MR
  - Contrast-enhanced MR is study of choice, as it best shows relationship to critical structures
- If image-guided biopsy performed, always get **core sample** for histology and stains

TOP DIFFERENTIAL DIAGNOSES

- Non-Hodgkin lymphoma
- Rhabdomyosarcoma
- Soft tissue fibrosarcoma
- Soft tissue metastases

PATHOLOGY

- Infiltrative unencapsulated growth with sweeping **uniform spindle cell** fascicles and **collagenous stroma**
- In adults, more likely to be associated with **Gardner syndrome** (familial adenomatous polyposis)
- Infantile fibromatosis differs in demographics, genetics, behavior, and treatment
- No metastatic potential but high local recurrence rate

CLINICAL ISSUES

- 15- to 40-year-old adults; firm, fixed mass
- **Complete resection** is treatment of choice
- Radiation ± chemotherapy as adjuvant treatment

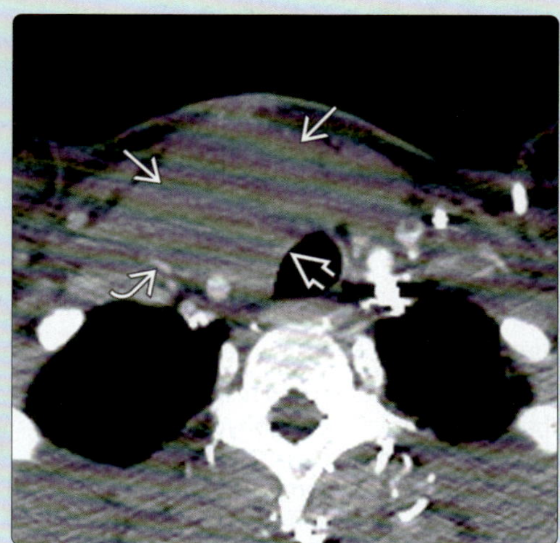

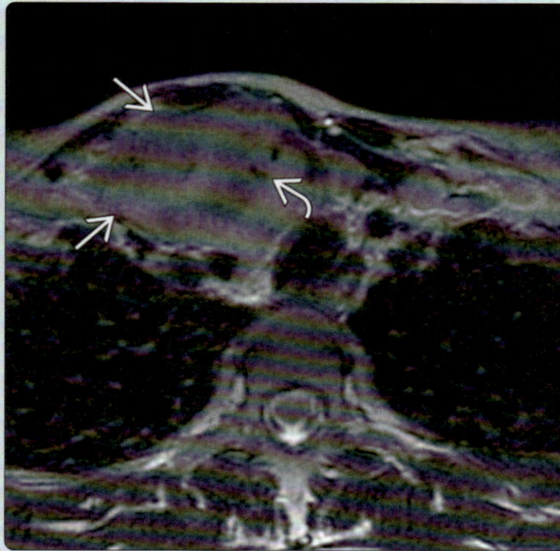

(Left) *Axial CECT through the low neck in a young adult shows a homogeneous, nonenhancing mass ➡ isodense to and indistinguishable from neck muscles. The mass abuts and displaces the trachea ➡ and displaces and compresses the right jugular vein ➡.* **(Right)** *Axial T2 MR in the same patient better delineates the hyperintense mass ➡ from the adjacent strap and sternocleidomastoid muscles and shows focal and linear areas of low signal ➡. The mass is clearly separate from the trachea and vessels.*

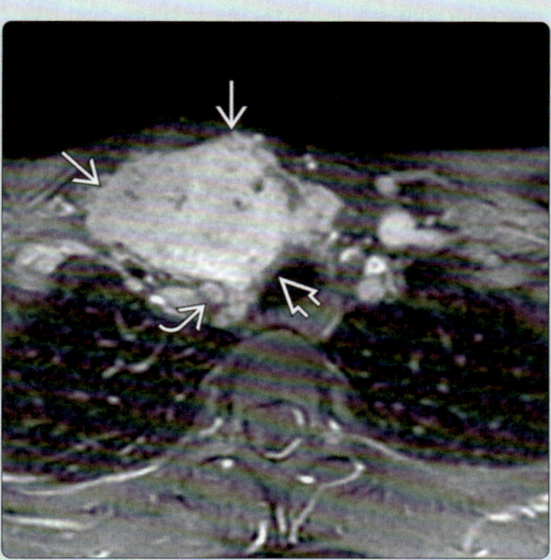

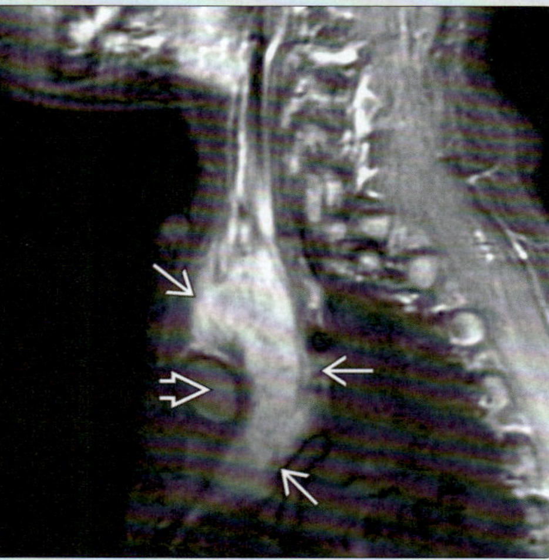

(Left) *Axial T1 C+ FS MR shows diffuse marked enhancement of the mass ➡. Fibromatosis abuts the trachea ➡ in the superior mediastinum but does not infiltrate the tracheal wall. Note the clear plane between the mass and right common carotid artery ➡.* **(Right)** *Sagittal T2 FS MR illustrates craniocaudal extent of the mass ➡, from the infrahyoid neck, posterior to the clavicle ➡, into superior mediastinum. At resection, it was distinct from the thymus & thyroid but encased the right recurrent laryngeal nerve, which was transected.*

Summary Thoughts: Oral Cavity

The oral cavity (OC) is the area of the suprahyoid neck anterior to the oropharynx and inferior to the sinonasal region. Imaging indications for the OC are usually highly refined because the referring physician can see all mucosal surfaces and palpate most lesions found here. The role of imaging for the clinician is to assess the deep tissue extent of OC tumors and space-based differential diagnoses when a deep tissue lesion is discovered. Three indications drive the vast majority of CT and MR exams of the OC: (1) Staging OC squamous cell carcinoma (SCCa), (2) evaluating for abscess and its etiology, and (3) differentiating submandibular nodal and gland mass.

Imaging Techniques & Indications

Tumor Assessment

Both CECT and enhanced MR are used to stage SCCa. Primary tumor and nodal metastases are assessed simultaneously in either case. CT is often compromised by dental amalgam artifact. MR is less affected by dental amalgam and better delineates soft tissue extent of tumor and perineural spread. As a result, enhanced fat-saturated MR is considered a superior tool for staging OC SCCa.

Infection Assessment

In the clinical setting of suspected OC infection, CECT with mandible and maxilla with bone windows is the preferred imaging exam. Abscess of any OC space is easily assessed with CECT. Infectious causes, like **mandibular teeth decay** with associated apical cyst or mandibular osteomyelitis and submandibular duct **stone**, are more easily seen on bone CT images.

Imaging Anatomy

The OC is the area above the hyoid bone, anterior to the oropharynx, and inferior to the sinuses and nose. Its borders are defined superiorly as the hard palate and maxillary alveolar ridge, laterally by the cheek, posteriorly by the oropharyngeal lingual tonsil and soft palate, and inferiorly by the platysma. The OC contains the oral tongue, mandible body and teeth, maxillary ridge and teeth, and the hard palate. The mandible and maxilla and their associated teeth will be covered in the mandible and maxilla overview module.

The OC can be subdivided into 4 distinct imaging areas: (1) **Oral mucosal space/surface** (OMS), (2) **sublingual space** (SLS), (3) **submandibular space** (SMS), and (4) **root of tongue** (ROT). Each area contains unique structures and provides its own space-specific differential diagnosis.

The **OMS** is covered by a continuous mucosal sheet of nonkeratinized stratified squamous epithelium. Since primary SCCa tumors arise within the OMS, the mucosal components are defined according to **SCCa subsites**. These include the mucosa overlying the oral tongue, floor of mouth (FOM), alveolar ridge, retromolar trigone (RMT), buccal (cheek), and hard palate. Subepithelial collections of **minor salivary glands** are most commonly located in the inner surface of the lip, buccal mucosa, and palate.

The **SLS** is an area within the deep oral tongue superomedial to mylohyoid muscles and lateral to the genioglossus muscle that is **not** encapsulated by fascia. Anteriorly, the SLS runs into the mandible. The SLS is horseshoe-shaped with the 2 sides communicating anteriorly under the frenulum of the tongue. Posteriorly, the SLS empties into the superior SMS and the inferior parapharyngeal space (PPS). No fascia separates the posterior SLS from the SMS and inferior PPS. All 3 spaces communicate at the posterior edge of the mylohyoid muscle.

The SLS contains multiple oral tongue structures. SLS nerves include the **lingual nerve** (sensory branch of CNV3 + chorda tympani branch of CNVI with taste fibers from anterior 2/3 of tongue) and distal **CNIX** and **CNXII**. The tongue's vascular pedicle (lingual artery and vein) passes through the SLS. The sublingual glands and ducts as well as the deep portion of the submandibular gland and submandibular gland duct are all found in the SLS. Finally, the anterior margin of the hyoglossus muscle projects into the posterior SLS from below.

The **SMS** (surgical synonym is submaxillary space) is located inferolateral to the mylohyoid muscle, superior to the hyoid bone, and deep to the platysma muscle. It is the only fascia-lined OC space. The superficial layer of deep cervical fascia lines its deep and superficial surfaces. The deep slip of fascia is found along the external surface of the mylohyoid muscle, and the superficial slip of fascia lines the deep margin of the platysma muscle. Posteriorly, no fascia separates the SMS from the inferior PPS or posterior SLS spaces.

The SMS can be conceptualized as a horseshoe-shaped space between the mylohyoid above and the hyoid bone below. There is no fascia blocking the spread of disease from side to side in the SMS.

The SMS contains the **submandibular gland** and submental (level IA) and submandibular (level IB) **nodes**. These 2 structures are responsible for most SMS masses. Other critical structures within the SMS include the facial vein and artery, the caudal loop of CNXII, the anterior belly of the digastric muscle, and fat.

The **ROT** is a term used by surgeons to describe the deep midline oral tongue above the mylohyoid sling and below the extrinsic tongue muscles. The ROT ends anteriorly at the mandibular symphysis. It is made up of the **genioglossus muscle** and the fibrofatty **lingual septum**.

There are 4 additional structures that require specific mention when reviewing the OC anatomy: The **mylohyoid** and **geniohyoid muscles**, the **oral tongue**, and the **RMT**. The **mylohyoid** and **geniohyoid** muscles form the **FOM**. The mylohyoid muscle arises from the mylohyoid line of the medial mandibular body. Anterior and middle fibers insert into median fibrous raphe extending from the symphysis menti to the hyoid bone to its posterior margin. Posterior mylohyoid fibers pass inferomedially to insert into the hyoid bone body. The mylohyoid muscle has been described as the **muscular "sling"** separating the SLS or SMS.

The OC component of the tongue is referred to as the **oral tongue** and represents the anterior 2/3 of the entire tongue. The posterior 1/3 is called the **base of tongue (lingual tonsil)** and is part of the oropharynx. The **extrinsic tongue muscles** of the oral tongue include the genioglossus, hyoglossus, styloglossus, and palatoglossus. The **genioglossus** is the large, fan-shaped muscle arising anteriorly from the superior mental spine on the inner surface of the symphysis menti of the mandible. It inserts along the entire length of the undersurface of the intrinsic tongue muscles. The **hyoglossus** is a thin, quadrilateral-shaped muscle arising from the body and cornu of the hyoid bone, from there passing vertically upward to insert into the side of the tongue. The **styloglossus** arises from the styloid process and stylomandibular ligament and passes anteroinferiorly between the external and internal

Differential Diagnosis: Oral Cavity

Pseudolesion	Congenital	Inflammatory-Infectious	Benign Tumor	Malignant Tumor
CNXII atrophy (SLS, ROT)	Lymphatic malformation (SLS, SMS, ROT)	Phlegmon or abscess (SLS, SMS, ROT)	BMT, sublingual gland (SLS)	SCCa (OMS)
CNV3 atrophy (SMS)	Venous malformation (SLS, SMS, ROT)	Dilated submandibular duct + stone (SLS)	BMT, submandibular gland (SMS)	Oral tongue SCCa
Accessory salivary gland (SMS)	Dermoid/epidermoid (SLS, SMS, ROT)	Submandibular gland sialadenitis (SMS)	BMT, hard palate (OMS)	Floor of mouth SCCa
	Lingual thyroid (ROT, SMS, PMS-BOT)	Sublingual gland sialadenitis (SLS)	Lipoma (SMS)	Retromolar trigone SCCa
	Thyroglossal duct cyst (ROT, SMS, PMS-BOT)	Submandibular gland mucocele (SMS)		Alveolar ridge SCCa
	Cellulitis (SLS, SMS, ROT)	Chronic sclerosis sialadenitis (SMS)		Hard palate SCCa
	2nd branchial cleft cyst (SMS)	Simple (SLS) or diving (SLS-SMS) ranula		Buccal mucosa SCCa
		Sialocele (SLS)		Submandibular gland (SMS) or sublingual gland (SLS) carcinoma
		Reactive or suppurative nodes (SMS)		Nodal SCCa or NHL nodes (SMS, level IA or IB)

OMS = oral mucosal space; PMS = pharyngeal mucosal space; SLS = sublingual space; SMS = submandibular space; ROT = root of tongue; BOT = base of tongue (lingual tonsil); BMT = benign mixed tumor; SCCa = squamous cell carcinoma; NHL = non-Hodgkin lymphoma.

carotid arteries to insert into the side of the tongue. Finally, the **palatoglossus** is a thin muscle arising from the anterior surface of the soft palate. From there, it passes anteroinferiorly in front of the palatine tonsil to insert into the side of the tongue. The palatoglossus underlies the anterior tonsillar pillar, which serves as the dividing line between the OC and the oropharynx.

The **RMT** is a small, triangular-shaped region of OC mucosa behind the last mandibular molar. SCCa of the RMT can spread early into critical proximal locations, such as the masticator space and PPS. Since the **pterygomandibular raphe** (fibrous band at the intersection of the buccinator muscle and the superior constrictor muscle) extends from the hamulus of the medial pterygoid plate above to the medial aspect of the RMT below, RMT SCCa can spread readily in a superior direction along this perifascial route.

Approaches to Imaging Issues in Oral Cavity

There are 3 main OC imaging indications: (1) Staging of primary SCCa and nodes, (2) searching for abscess and its cause, and (3) evaluating an SMS mass to determine if the mass is nodal or glandular. Knowing the clinical context can affect the type of exam (CECT vs. MR) and facilitate the creation of a highly relevant radiology report. Without clinical history, assigning a lesion to a space of origin (OMS, SLS, ROT, SMS) and comparing its radiologic features to those of the **space-specific differential diagnoses** is an alternative approach to analyzing OC images.

OMS SCCa is known at the time of imaging. The mucosal extent of the SCCa is best determined by the clinician. Imaging is critical to evaluate deep soft tissue extent, bone involvement, perineural tumor, and nodal spread. Small tumors may be extremely subtle or even occult to imaging, and for this reason it is very helpful to know the primary subsite when reading OMS SCCa scans. This allows careful evaluation for features that are key to surgical management, such as cortical bone erosion. Each OC primary SCCa subsite has its own set of imaging questions that should be considered at the time of primary tumor staging. Refer to the module on each of these primary sites in the SCCa content area to review these imaging questions.

SMS masses usually arise from either the submandibular gland or the submandibular nodal chain (levels IA and IB). Making this distinction allows the imager to develop a differential diagnosis based on glandular disease or nodal disease. Note that a smaller submandibular gland tumor may be difficult to see on CECT. US or MR may be used in the cases where the clinician is certain a lesion is present and CECT is equivocal.

ROT lesions are rare. The differential diagnosis of ROT lesions is short, as can be seen by the global differential diagnosis table. If a lesion appears to bow the genioglossus muscles laterally away from each other, then it should be considered primary to the ROT.

Differential Diagnosis

When a lesion is found within the OC, assigning it a space of origin and reviewing that space-specific differential diagnosis can be a very useful strategy for evaluating the imaging exam findings. Review of the global differential diagnosis table provided here shows the space or spaces where the OC lesions are found. This global differential diagnosis can be subdivided into 4 distinct differential diagnoses lists based on the 4 major OC anatomic areas (OMS, SLS, SMS, and ROT).

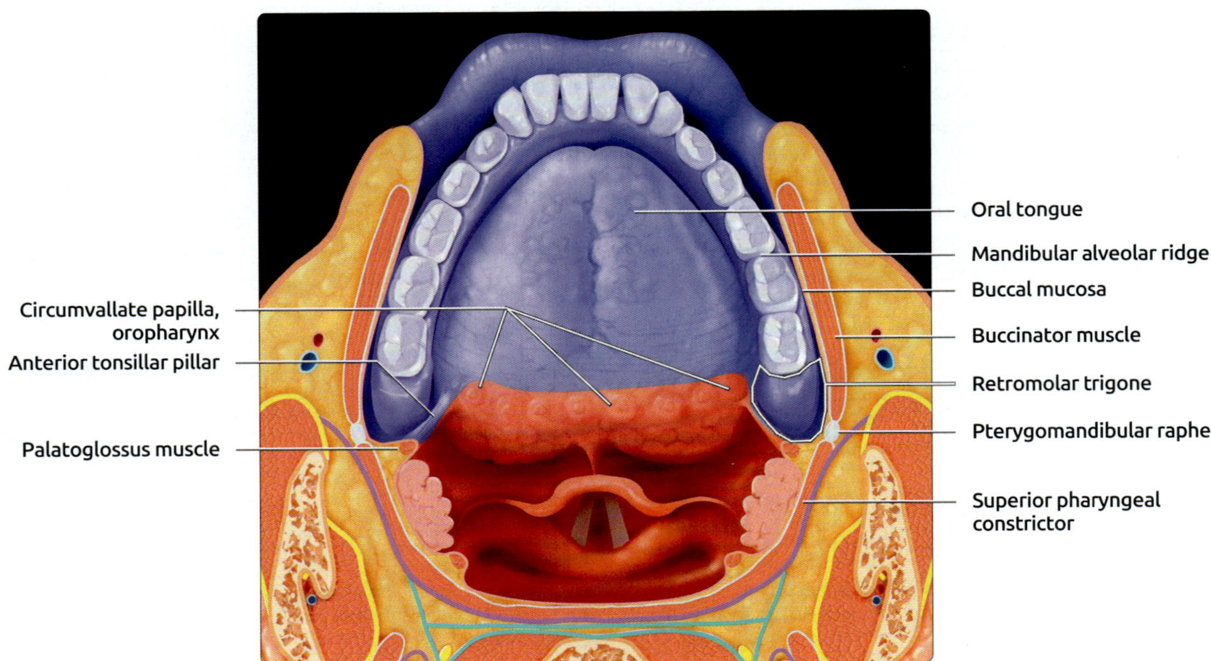

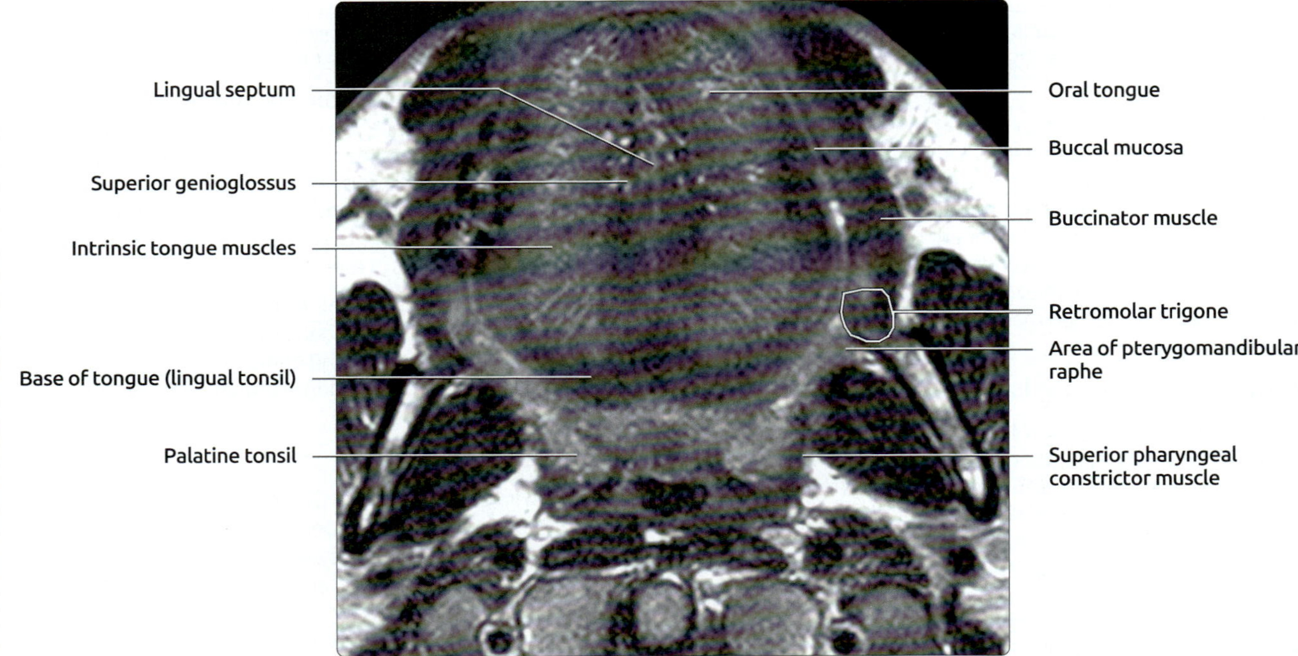

(Top) *Axial graphic shows oral mucosal space &/or surface (OMS) shaded in blue. Notice that the circumvallate papilla, a superficial line of taste buds, divides anterior oral cavity (OC) from posterior oropharynx. The lingual tonsil is part of oropharynx, not the OC. Four of the 6 squamous cell carcinoma (SCCa) subsites are labeled on the right, including the oral tongue, alveolar ridge, buccal mucosa, and retromolar trigone (RMT). The floor of mouth (FOM) and hard palate subsites are not shown. Note that the pterygomandibular raphe (PMR) connects the posterior margin of buccinator muscle to anterior margin of the superior pharyngeal constrictor muscle. The RMT represents a key route of perifascial spread of SCCa of the RMT.* **(Bottom)** *Axial T2 MR through the superior tongue shows the mucosal subsites on the right along with the buccinator, PMR, and superior constrictor adjacent to the RMT. Note the oropharyngeal palatine and lingual tonsils labeled on the left.*

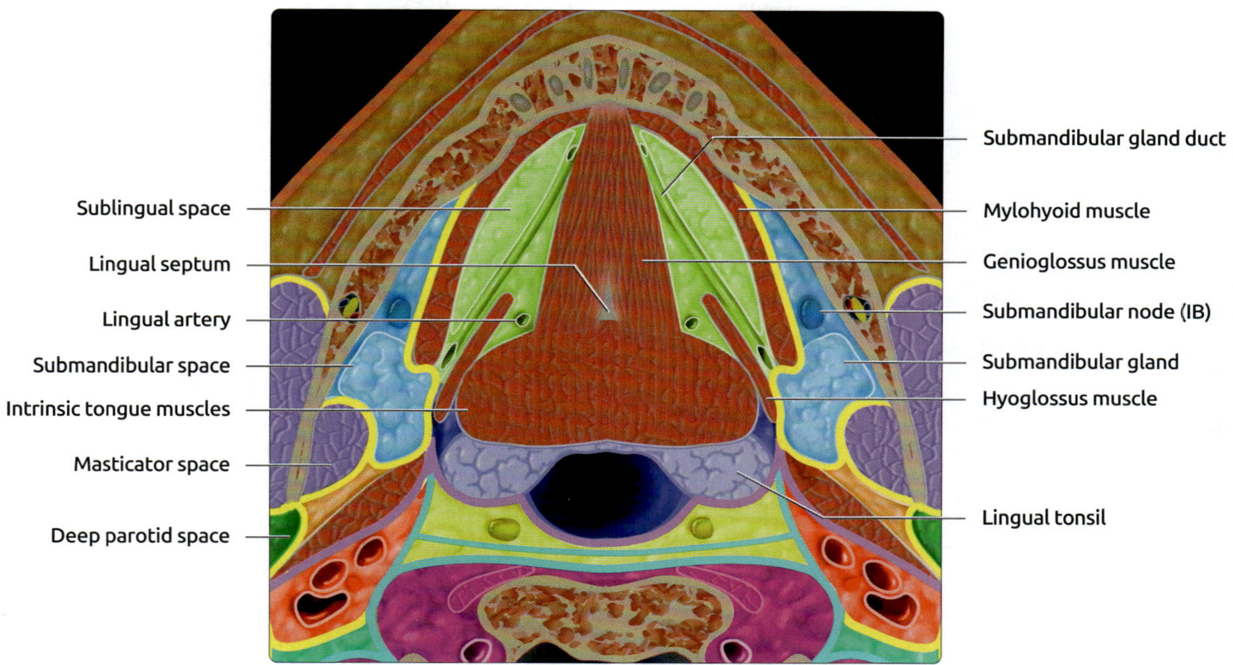

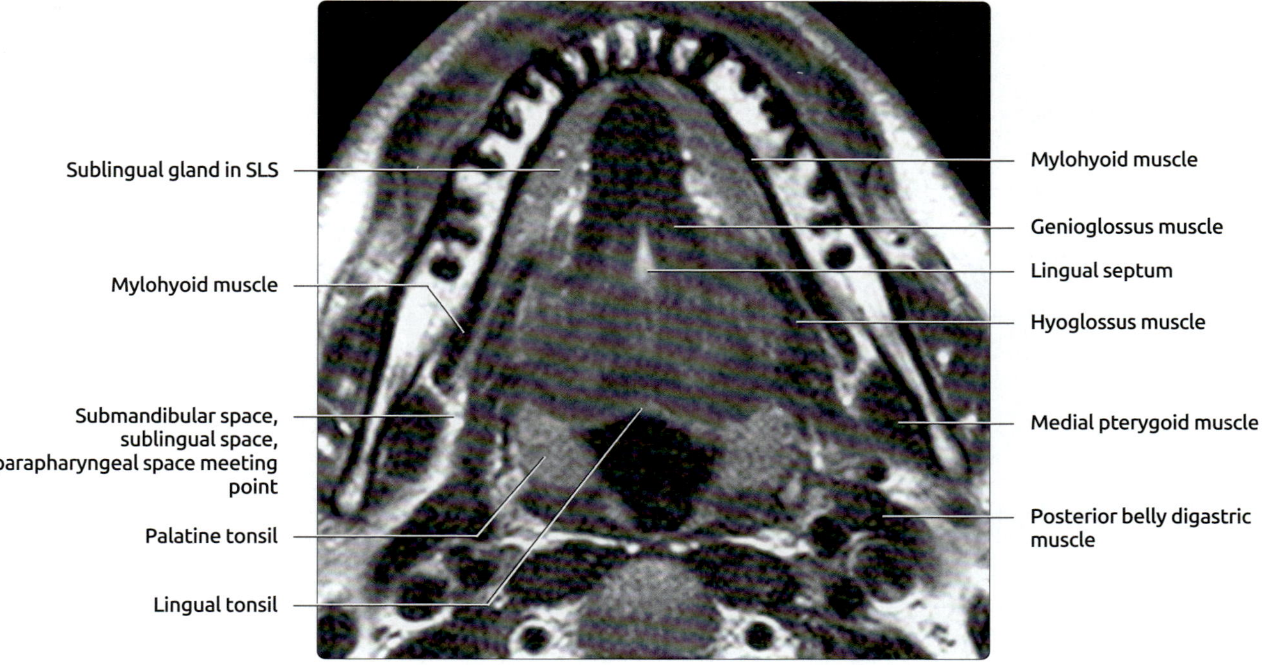

(Top) *Axial graphic through mid-OC shows superficial layer of deep cervical fascia (yellow line) circumscribing the masticator and parotid spaces posteriorly and defining deep margin of submandibular space (SMS) (colored in blue). Notice the principal occupants of SMS are submandibular gland and level I nodes. The green sublingual space (SLS) has many structures within it, including the sublingual gland, submandibular duct, lingual artery, and the anterior margin of hyoglossus muscle.* **(Bottom)** *Axial T2 MR shows the structures of the FOM and root of tongue (ROT). Notice the symmetric paired genioglossus muscles separated by a fatty lingual septum. The hyoglossus muscles insert into the lateral aspect of the tongue and delineate the location of the submandibular duct, which courses between hyoglossus and mylohyoid and terminates in the anterior aspect of the FOM. The sublingual glands are also nestled anteriorly in the FOM.*

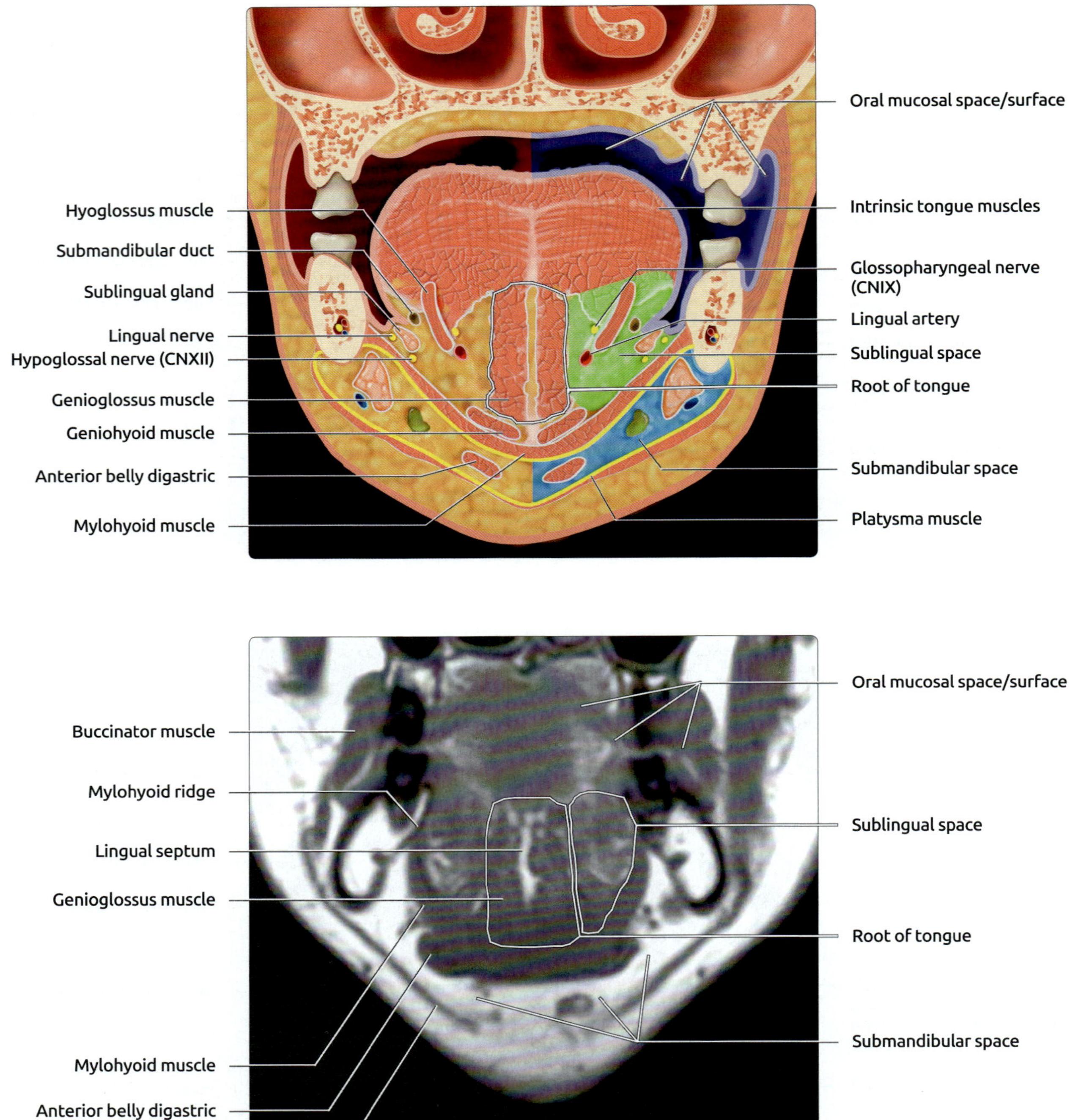

(Top) *Coronal graphic through OC shows the mylohyoid muscle inserting on each side of the OC along the mylohyoid ridges of the medial mandible. This muscle separates the superomedial SLS (green) from inferolateral SMS (blue). The SLS contains the lingual nerve and artery, submandibular duct, CNIX, CNXII, and sublingual gland. The SMS contains the submandibular gland, facial vein and artery, level I nodes, and anterior belly of the digastric muscle. Genioglossus and the lingual septum form the ROT. The OMS lines the surface of the OC (purple).* **(Bottom)** *Coronal T1 MR depicts the mylohyoid muscular sling (FOM) "strung" between the mylohyoid ridges of the mandible. The OMS is difficult to identify on a closed-mouth image, while the SLS, SMS, and ROT are all well delineated. Notice that the neurovascular contents of the SLS and SMS cannot be identified.*

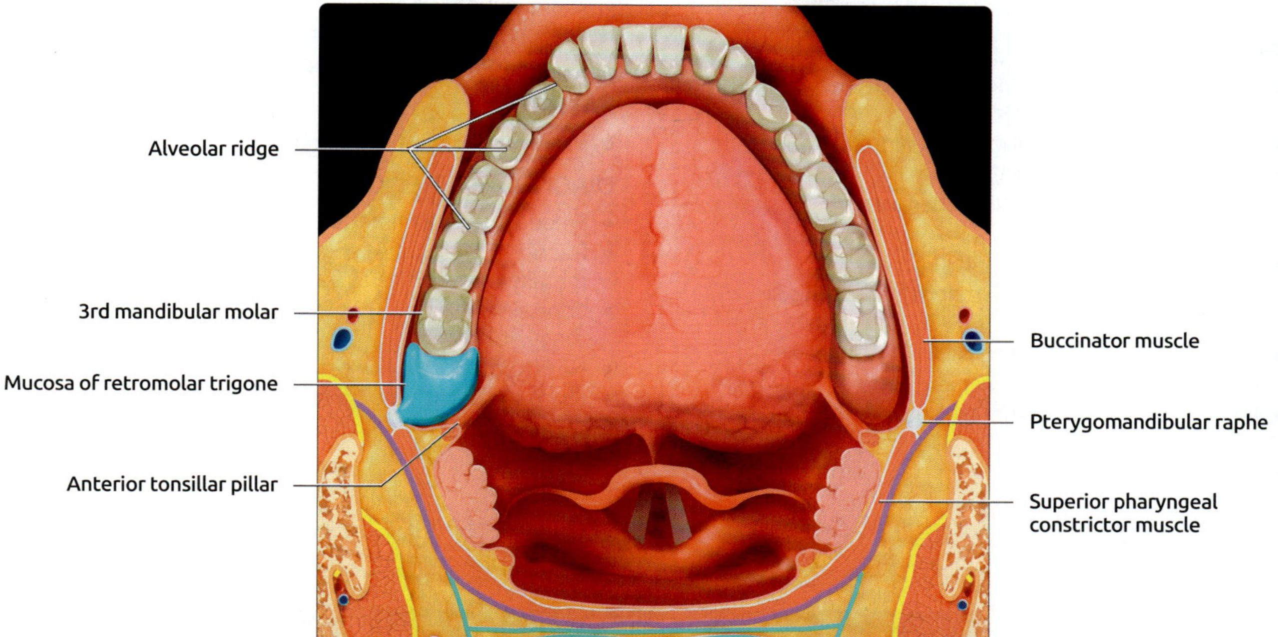

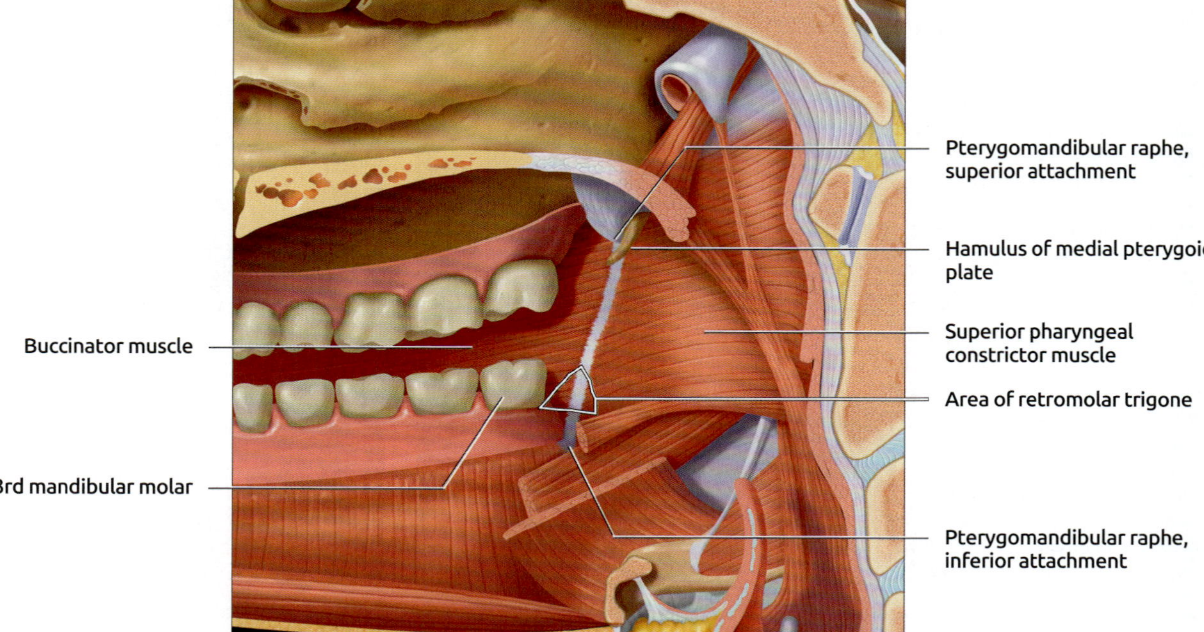

(Top) *Axial graphic highlights the RMT (shaded in light blue on the left) and the PMR. Notice that the mucosal surface of the RMT is found directly behind the mandibular 3rd molar. The RMT is designated as its own OC subsite for SCCa, but it is really just the most posterior portion of the alveolar ridge. The proximity to the PMR (fascial band connecting buccinator and superior constrictor muscles) is important when SCCa occurs in the RMT because it gives the tumor access to the pterygoid plate above via this perifascial spread route.* **(Bottom)** *Sagittal graphic viewed from inside the mouth delineates the full extent of the PMR. Note the cephalad PMR attachment to the hamulus of the medial pterygoid plate and its inferior attachment to the posterior aspect of the mylohyoid ridge on the inner mandibular cortex. The PMR "connects" the buccinator muscle to the superior pharyngeal constrictor muscle.*

Hypoglossal Nerve Motor Denervation

KEY FACTS

TERMINOLOGY

- Hypoglossal nerve (CNXII)
- Loss of nerve supply to muscles of 1/2 tongue

IMAGING

- Asymmetry of tongue appearance with linear demarcation of abnormality; varies over time
- CT density and MR signal intensity vary over time
- Acute (typically < 1 month)
  - 1/2 tongue initially swollen, then atrophies
  - Enhancement variable
- Subacute (typically 1-20 months)
  - Loss of volume and fatty change of 1/2 tongue
  - Decreasing enhancement
- Chronic (typically > 20 months)
  - Fatty atrophy, no enhancement
- Image course of CNXII from skull base to hyoid

TOP DIFFERENTIAL DIAGNOSES

- Lingual tonsil squamous cell carcinoma (SCCa)
- Oral tongue SCCa
- Oral cavity lymphatic malformation
- Oral cavity venous malformation

PATHOLOGY

- Many causes; may be isolated or with CNIX-XI

DIAGNOSTIC CHECKLIST

- Frequent source of mistaken identity
- Flaccid 1/2 of tongue hangs posteriorly into oropharynx, mistaken for (ipsilateral) tongue base tumor
- Contralateral larger 1/2 of tongue may be mistaken for tongue tumor
- No FDG uptake may be called contralateral tumor
- Sharp line delineating unilateral changes is key

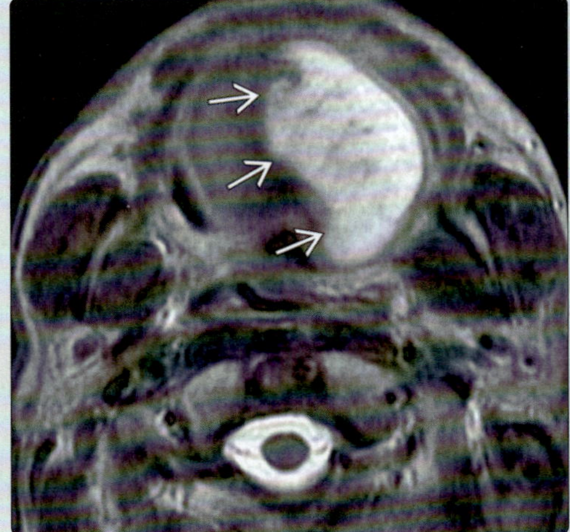

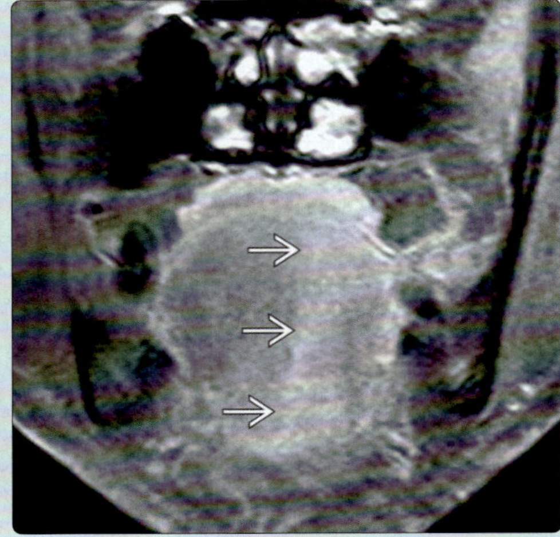

(Left) *Axial T2 MR shows the acute stage of tongue denervation with swollen left hemitongue and markedly increased T2 signal from edema* ➡. *Note sharp delineation of the abnormality. Denervation was due to perineural tumor spread along CNXII.* **(Right)** *Coronal T1 C+ FS MR shows subacute denervation changes with heterogeneous enhancement of unilateral left tongue musculature* ➡. *Note sharp demarcation of changes; finding was secondary to skull base metastatic focus involving hypoglossal canal.*

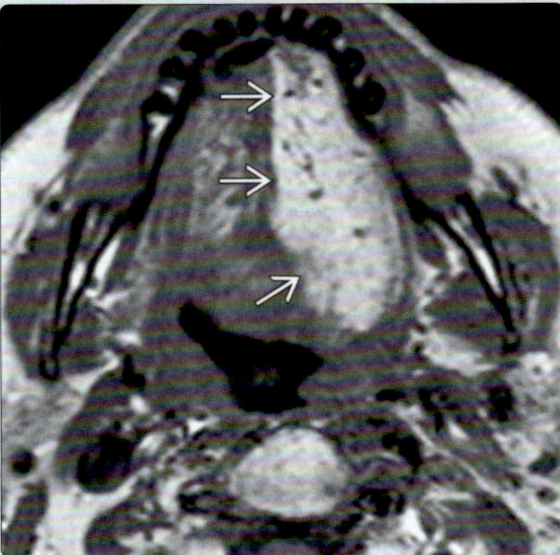

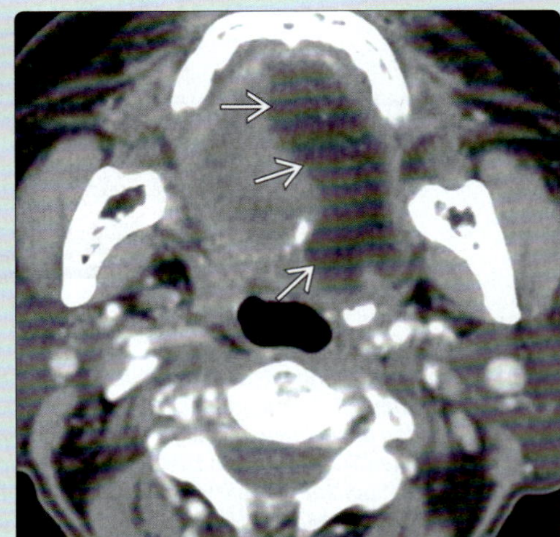

(Left) *Axial T1 MR shows chronic changes of tongue denervation with markedly increased signal* ➡ *in the left hemitongue, consistent with fatty replacement. Hypoglossal denervation was due to jugular foramen paraganglioma (not shown).* **(Right)** *Axial CECT shows fatty atrophy from chronic left hypoglossal nerve denervation* ➡. *The right 1/2 of the tongue appears larger than the left and can be mistaken for a tongue tumor. Denervation was found to be secondary to destructive bone lesion at hypoglossal canal.*

KEY FACTS

TERMINOLOGY

- Accessory salivary tissue in **mylohyoid boutonnière**
- Definition: Normal salivary tissue in variant position within submandibular space (SMS)

IMAGING

- CECT or enhanced MR
  - Benign-appearing SMS mass, with density/intensity following normal salivary glands
  - SMS; inferior to mylohyoid, most commonly anterior to submandibular gland

TOP DIFFERENTIAL DIAGNOSES

- SMS reactive nodal disease
- SMS lymphatic malformation
- SMS abscess
- Diving ranula
- Submandibular gland mucocele

PATHOLOGY

- Ectopic sublingual or submandibular gland tissue in SMS

CLINICAL ISSUES

- Most commonly **incidental** & discovered on imaging for unrelated indications
- May occasionally present as SMS mass
- Subject to same spectrum of disease as other salivary tissue, including sialadenitis and sialolithiasis, though these occur only rarely

DIAGNOSTIC CHECKLIST

- Include diagnosis of accessory salivary tissue when evaluating submandibular masses
- Accessory SMS salivary tissue focus, when discovered, is **"leave alone" lesion**
- Look for density/intensity that follows normal submandibular gland parenchyma

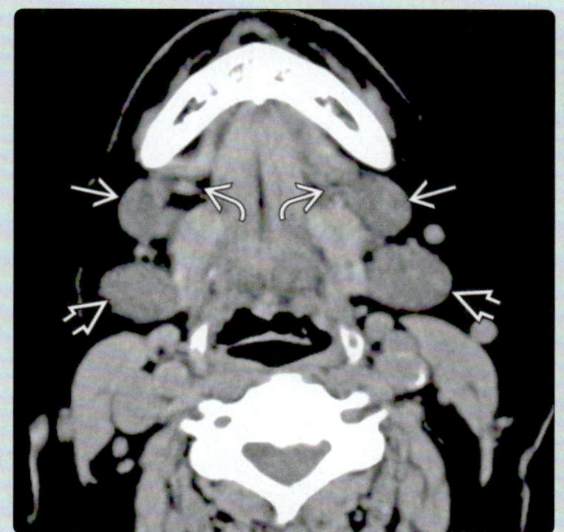

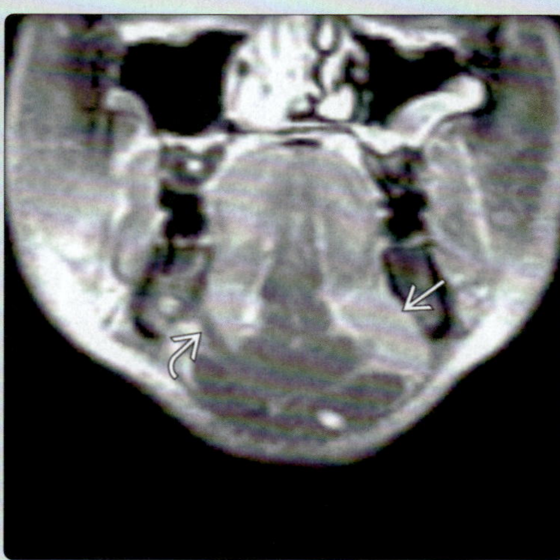

(Left) *Axial NECT demonstrates bilateral accessory salivary tissue in the submandibular space ➡. Bilateral mylohyoid dehiscence is evident ➡. Note the density of the accessory salivary tissue is identical to that of the native submandibular glands ➡.* **(Right)** *Coronal T1 postcontrast MR reveals the left sublingual gland ➡ extending into the submandibular space through a defect in the left mylohyoid. The right mylohyoid is intact ➡.*

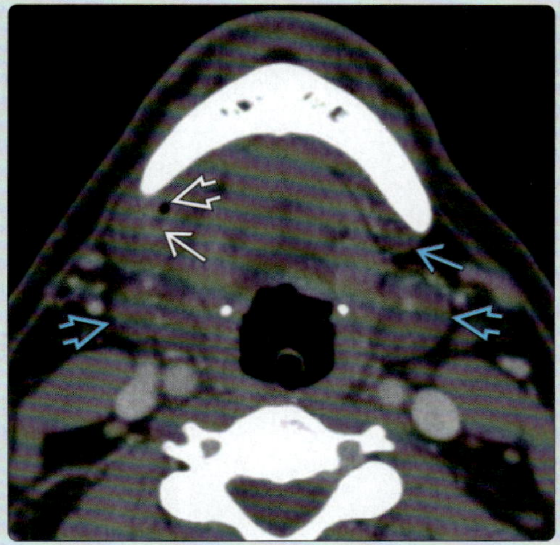

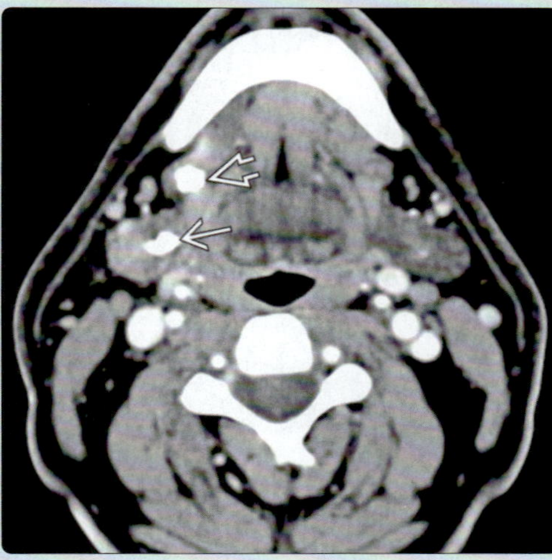

(Left) *Axial CECT shows relative enhancement of the inflamed right accessory salivary tissue, particularly of its duct ➡, which contains gas ➡. Compare to normal density of the left accessory tissue ➡. Note the normal submandibular glands ➡.* **(Right)** *Axial CECT shows a calcified mass in hyperdense right submandibular gland ➡. Accessory salivary tissue is present anteriorly & medially with an additional stone ➡. This appearance is consistent with sialolithiasis within both native & accessory salivary tissue.*

Oral Cavity Dermoid and Epidermoid

KEY FACTS

TERMINOLOGY

- Cystic oral cavity (OC) lesion resulting from congenital epithelial inclusion or rest
- Dermoid: Epithelial elements plus dermal adnexa
- Epidermoid: Epithelial elements only

IMAGING

- General imaging findings
  - Dermoid and epidermoid appear as well-demarcated cysts in OC
  - Dermoid more often midline
  - Dermoid: Complex cystic mass, often with fat ± calcification
  - Epidermoid: Fluid contents only
  - Sublingual and submandibular spaces most affected
- MR imaging findings
  - Best reveals foci of fat with chemical shift artifact
  - Fat also bright on T1WI and low signal with fat saturation
  - Both may have restricted diffusion on DWI

TOP DIFFERENTIAL DIAGNOSES

- Lymphatic malformation
- Thyroglossal duct cyst
- Ranula
- Submandibular cystic squamous cell carcinoma node

CLINICAL ISSUES

- Clinical presentation
  - Average age at presentation: 30 years
  - Painless subcutaneous or submucosal mass (85-90%)
  - Dermoid grows rapidly during puberty when sebaceous glands activated
- Treatment options: Surgical resection curative; care to not injure lingual nerve, sublingual duct

DIAGNOSTIC CHECKLIST

- Sublingual space epidermoid, ranula, and lymphatic malformation may appear indistinguishable

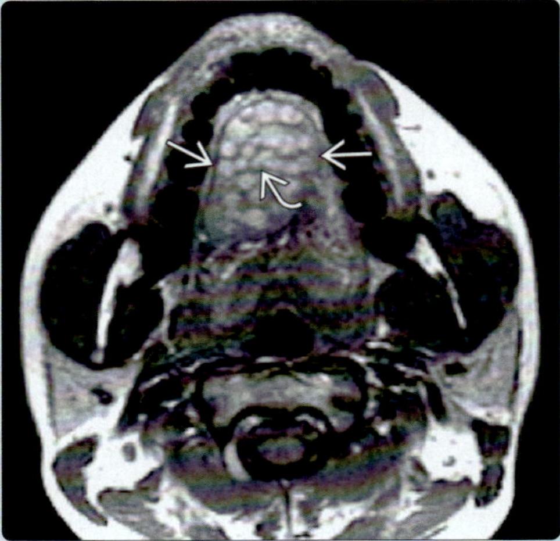

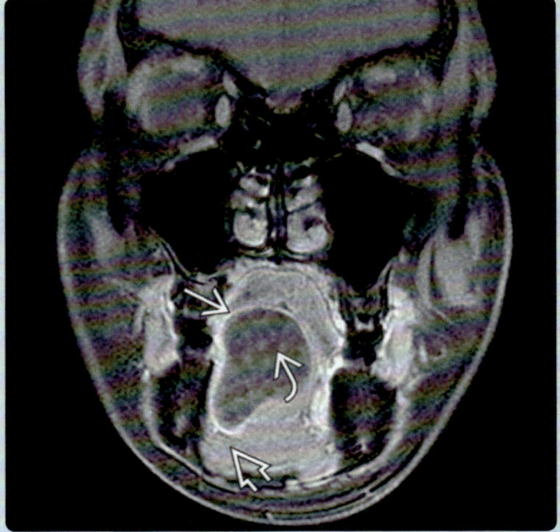

(Left) *Axial T1WI MR through the floor of mouth shows an ovoid, well-circumscribed mass ➡. There are internal hyperintense globules with chemical shift artifact ➡ that indicate fatty content, consistent with dermoid cyst.* **(Right)** *Coronal T1WI C+ FS MR shows a well-circumscribed mass with thin rim enhancement ➡ superior to the mylohyoid muscle ➡, consistent with sublingual location. Internal fat globules ➡ are markedly hypointense with fat-saturation technique and confirm dermoid cyst.*

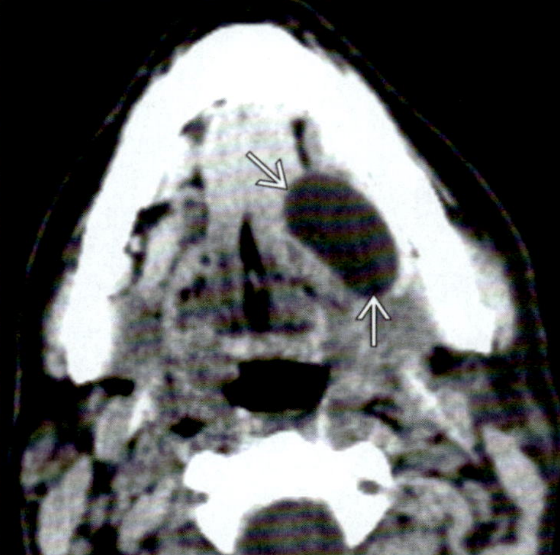

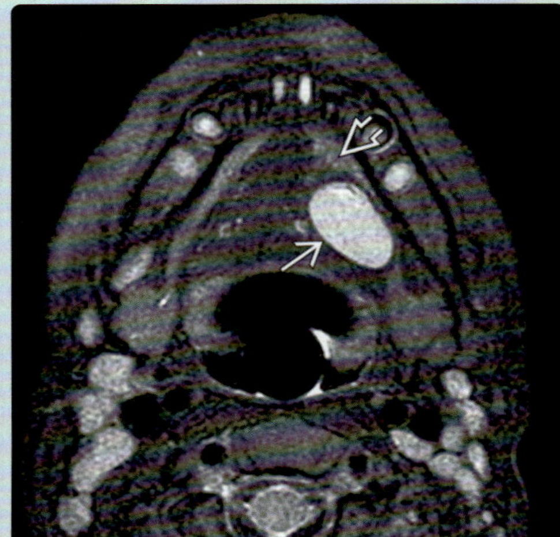

(Left) *Axial NECT shows a well-circumscribed cystic mass in the left sublingual space ➡, pathologically proven to be a dermoid. A sublingual space dermoid, without visible complex elements, mimics an epidermoid, simple ranula, and lymphatic malformation.* **(Right)** *Axial STIR MR in a different patient reveals a well-circumscribed, hyperintense epidermoid in the left sublingual space ➡, posterior to the sublingual gland ➡. With simple fluid content, an epidermoid is indistinguishable from ranula or lymphatic malformation.*

KEY FACTS

TERMINOLOGY

- Synonyms: Lymphangioma, cystic hygroma
- Lymphatic malformation (LM): Congenital slow-flow lymph vessel tissue rest

IMAGING

- General findings
  - Macrocystic (**uni- or multilocular**) or microcystic
    - Microcystic LM more often transspatial
  - Submandibular & posterior cervical spaces common
- CT, MR or US findings
  - Cystic, uni- or multilocular
  - Relative paucity of mass effect given size
  - Fluid-fluid levels indicate prior hemorrhage
    - Wall thin without significant enhancement
- Contrast-enhanced MR best for characterization
- Cysts + solid enhancement or phleboliths suggest venous or mixed venolymphatic malformation

TOP DIFFERENTIAL DIAGNOSES

- Venous vascular malformation
- Ranula

PATHOLOGY

- 1 type of **slow-flow vascular malformation**
- Classified into macrocystic & microcystic forms

CLINICAL ISSUES

- Diffuse microcystic malformations often have significant functional/cosmetic impairment
  - Potential for airway obstruction
- Dramatic enlargement if hemorrhages
- Enlargement may occur with upper respiratory infection
- Treatment options
  - Percutaneous sclerosing agents of macrocystic LM include OK-432, alcohol, & doxycycline
  - Surgical resection if lesion is isolated, unilocular, & not associated with major vessels or nerves

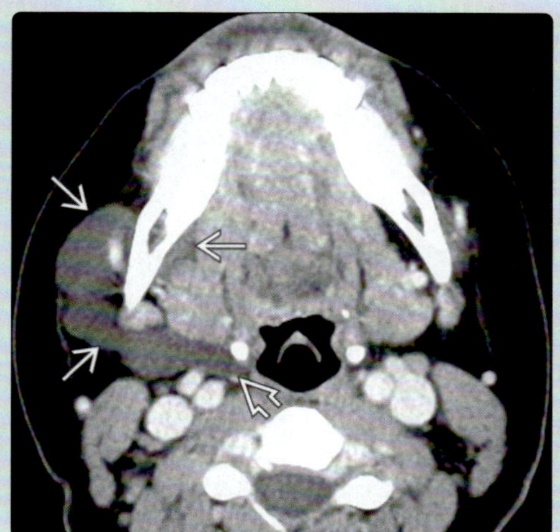

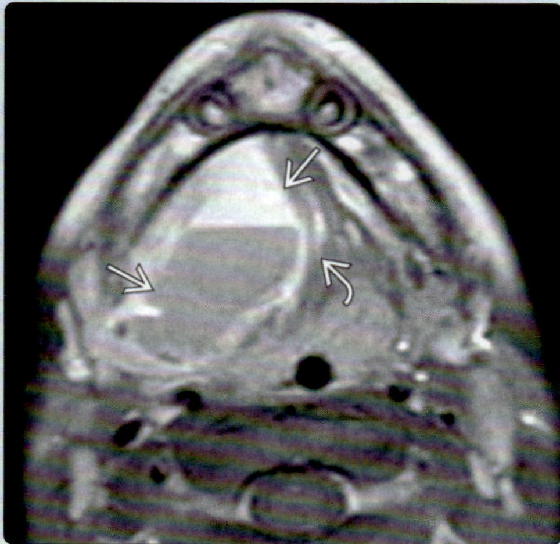

(Left) *Axial CECT reveals a multilobulated cystic mass ➡ predominantly in the right submandibular space but insinuating around posterior margin of submandibular gland & into parapharyngeal space ➡. Note no perceptible soft tissue, wall, or evidence of contrast enhancement.* **(Right)** *T1WI C+ FS MR in a different patient depicts well-demarcated, path-proven lymphatic malformation (LM) ➡ in the right sublingual space displacing genioglossus muscles medially ➡. Complex signal with fluid-fluid level indicates prior hemorrhage.*

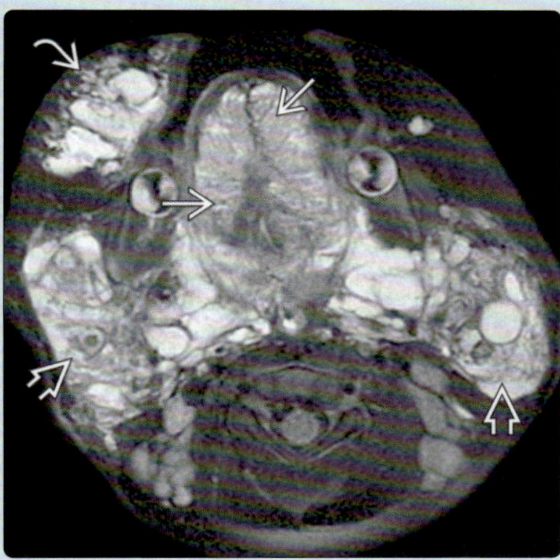

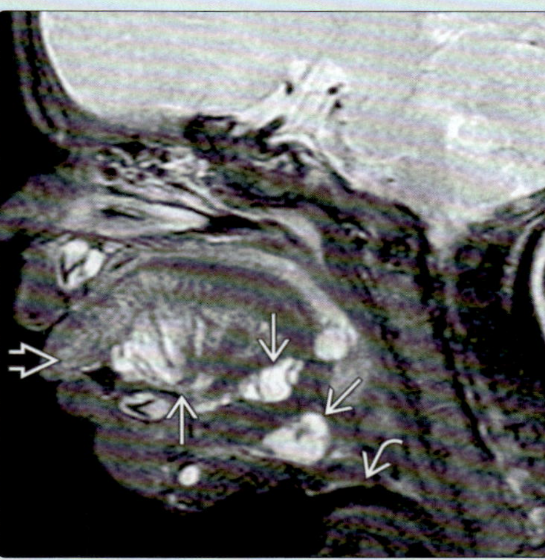

(Left) *Axial T2WI FS MR illustrates extensive diffuse microcystic & macrocystic LM involving many spaces of neck & oral cavity. Hyperintense components are evident in tongue ➡, parapharyngeal, carotid, retropharyngeal, parotid ➡, & buccal ➡ spaces.* **(Right)** *Sagittal STIR MR delineates LM infiltration ➡ of the root & base of tongue through to the submandibular space. Sagittal MR assesses degree of tongue protrusion ➡, which is useful for assessing therapy response. Note tracheotomy ➡ for airway management.*

Lingual Thyroid

KEY FACTS

TERMINOLOGY

- Lingual thyroid definition: Thyroid tissue in abnormal location in base of tongue or floor of mouth
- Synonym: Ectopic thyroid tissue

IMAGING

- Nonenhanced CT findings
  - Intrinsic high density on NECT characteristic
    - Due to native iodine content
  - Imaging features similar to normal thyroid tissue
- Enhanced CT findings
  - Well-circumscribed ovoid midline base of tongue mass
    - Usually at site of **foramen cecum**
    - Less commonly in sublingual space or tongue root
  - Usually avid homogeneous enhancement
- Tc-99m pertechnetate or radioiodine scan
  - Confirms diagnosis + determines other sites of thyroid

TOP DIFFERENTIAL DIAGNOSES

- Venous malformation
- Upper airway hemangioma
- Prominent lingual tonsillar tissue

PATHOLOGY

- Arrest of thyroid precursor descent along thyroglossal duct in 1st trimester
- In **75%** of patients lingual thyroid is **only** functioning tissue
- Lingual location most common (90%)

CLINICAL ISSUES

- More common in female patients (4x male patients)
- Thyroid hormone production may be insufficient, resulting in ectopic thyroid gland enlargement
  - Goiter in ectopic gland causes obstructive symptoms
- Treatment options
  - 1st shrink lesion with thyroid hormone replacement
  - Surgical resection if obstructive symptoms

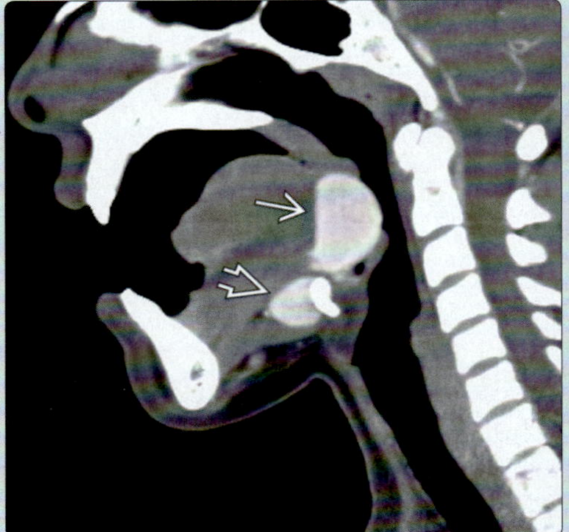

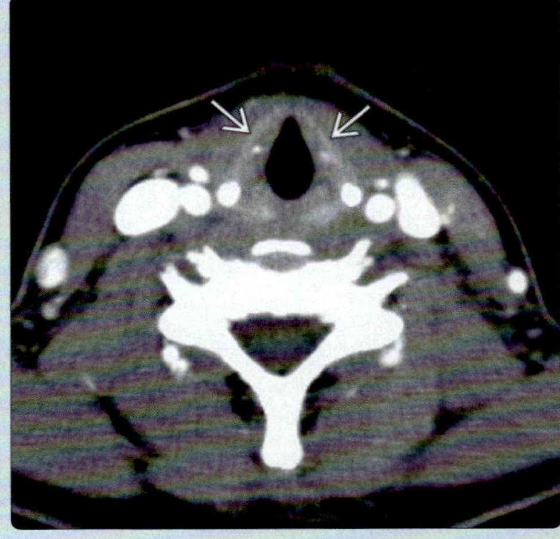

(Left) *Sagittal CECT shows a young woman with a tongue base mass. This multifocal midline hyperdense mass is consistent with lingual thyroid ➡. An additional component of the ectopic thyroid anterior to the hyoid body ➡ is shown. Thyroid ectopic tissue may occur anywhere along the thyroglossal duct tract.* **(Right)** *Axial CECT of a patient with lingual thyroid, at the level of thyroid cartilage ➡, shows no visible thyroid tissue on either side. This is the case in 75% of patients with lingual thyroid.*

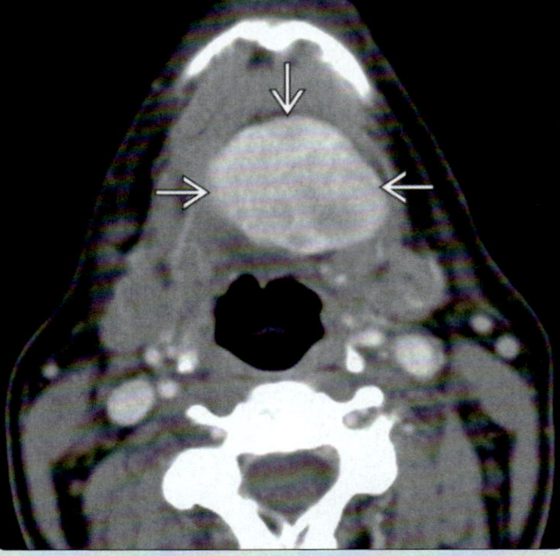

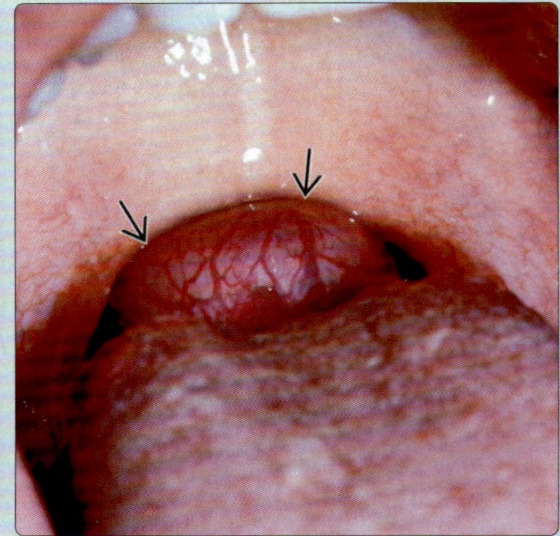

(Left) *Axial CECT demonstrates a sharply defined submucosal mass ➡ in the midline floor of the mouth. Heterogeneous density suggests development of a goiter. As 60% of patients presenting with lingual thyroid are hypothyroid, goitrous enlargement of this lesion is common.* **(Right)** *Clinical photograph shows a lingual thyroid ➡ that presents as a smooth, sessile, hyperemic mass on the dorsal tongue just posterior to the circumvallate papillae.*

Ranula

KEY FACTS

TERMINOLOGY

- Definitions: Simple ranula (SR), diving ranula (DR)
  - SR: Sublingual gland (SLG) retention cyst in sublingual space (SLS)
    - Initially true cyst; may become small pseudocyst
  - DR: SR ruptured to form pseudocyst that spreads into submandibular space (SMS)

IMAGING

- CECT findings
  - Unilocular water density cyst, thin wall enhancement
  - **SR**: Unilocular SLS cyst
    - Unilateral oval or bilateral horseshoe shape
  - **DR**: Comet-shaped unilocular cyst
    - "Body" in SMS and "tail" in SLS
    - **Tail sign** = collapsed SLS portion
    - DR may "dive" through mylohyoid muscle boutonniere or around posterior margin
      - Through boutonniere, tail tracks anteriorly
      - Posterior to margin, tail tracks posterolaterally
- MR findings: Signal intensity follows water/CSF
- US findings: Hypoechoic cysts of SLS ± SMS
  - SLG herniation through mylohyoid defect in DR common

TOP DIFFERENTIAL DIAGNOSES

- Oral cavity lymphatic malformation; oral cavity dermoid & epidermoid

PATHOLOGY

- Etiology: Retention cyst resulting from trauma or inflammation of SLG or SLS minor salivary gland
- Histologic findings
  - SR before rupture: Retention cyst with epithelial wall
  - Pseudocyst: Mucin spillage with granulation tissue wall

CLINICAL ISSUES

- Bluish cyst under tongue (SR) ± SMS swelling (DR)
- Treatment: Transoral excision of SLG & cyst evacuation
  - Transcervical excision less common

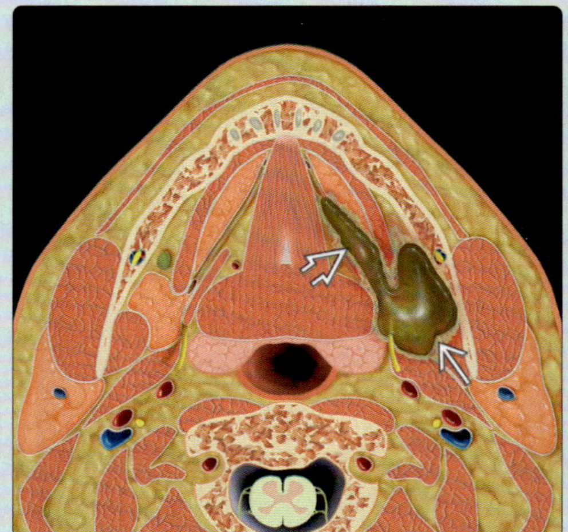

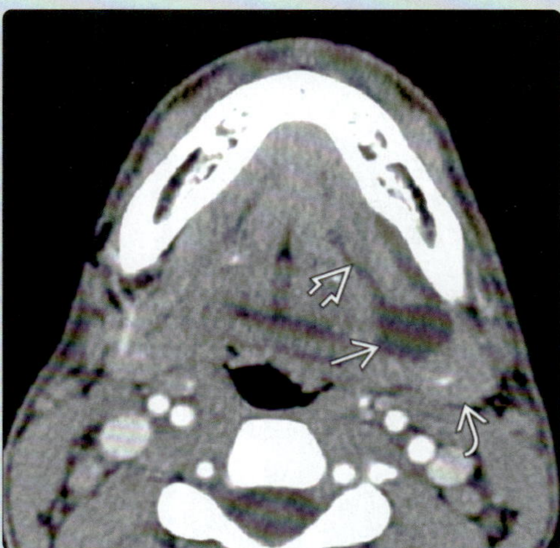

(Left) *Axial graphic depicts a diving ranula herniating posteriorly from the sublingual space into the submandibular space ➡. The tail sign ➡ is the collapsed portion of the cyst in the sublingual space.* **(Right)** *Axial CECT demonstrates a rounded cystic mass ➡ in the submandibular space abutting the posterior margin of the mylohyoid muscle and displacing the submandibular gland ➡ posterolaterally. A linear, low-density tail ➡ of the collapsed ranula extends anteriorly within the left sublingual space (tail sign).*

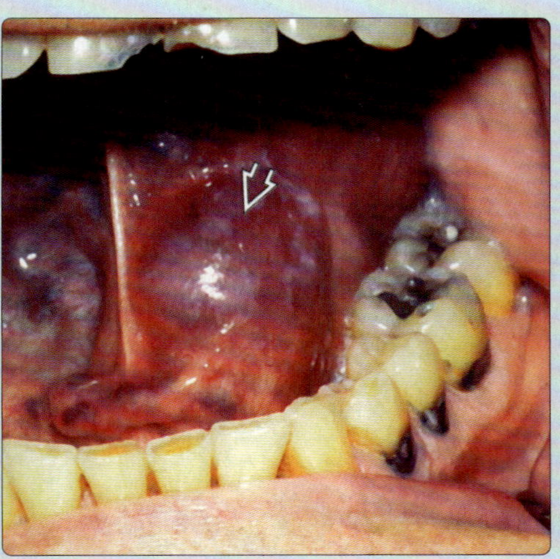

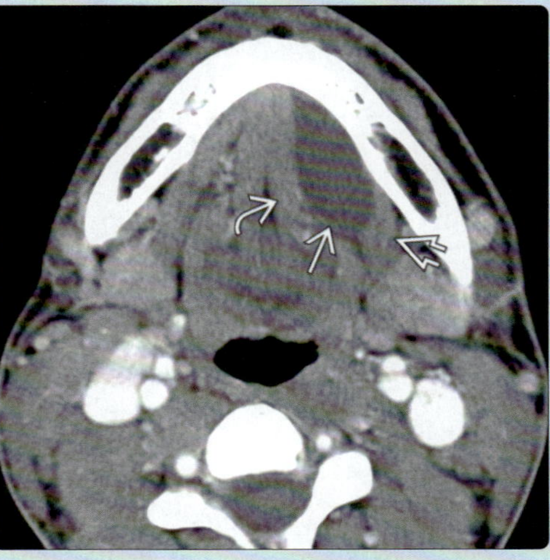

(Left) *A blue, dome-shaped lesion in the floor of the mouth is the typical presentation of a ranula ➡. The spilled mucin is usually of sublingual gland origin but can arise from minor salivary glands in the area.* **(Right)** *Axial CECT shows a simple unilateral ranula as an ovoid, low-density lesion in the left anterior sublingual space ➡. There is no perceptible thickening or enhancement of the wall. The mylohyoid is displaced posterolaterally ➡ and the genioglossus ➡ bowed medially.*

KEY FACTS

TERMINOLOGY

- Definition: Ruptured submandibular duct (SMD) extravasates saliva into sublingual space (SLS)

IMAGING

- CECT findings
  - SLS fluid density lesion ± enhancing adjacent inflammatory soft tissues
    - Rarely extends into posterior submandibular space
  - If associated with SMD **calculus**, SMD enlargement with enhancing, enlarged submandibular gland
  - Fluid collection is distinct from SMD
- When cystic SLS lesion is identified, always look closely for possible obstructing calculi
- CECT best delineates sialocele & calculus if present

TOP DIFFERENTIAL DIAGNOSES

- Ranula
- Abscess in SLS
- Lymphatic malformation in SLS

PATHOLOGY

- Etiology: **SMD injury** with leakage of saliva into SLS
  - Submandibular duct calculus with rupture > > rupture from trauma or surgery
- Pocket of saliva with fibrous pseudocapsule

CLINICAL ISSUES

- Clinical presentation
  - Fluctuant, soft, painless sublingual mass
  - Patient with SMD stone, recent oral cavity surgery, or trauma presents with new SLS mass
- Treatment options
  - Surgical excision with associated gland; sialendoscopy
  - Local injection of botulinum toxin type A (30-50 U)
  - Multiple aspirations, antisialagogic agents
  - Propantheline bromide: Interrupts parasympathetic control of salivary secretion

(Left) *Axial CECT shows calculus obstructing the submandibular duct ➲ at terminal papilla, causing the submandibular duct to dilate ➲. Duct rupture has occurred with sialocele ➲ visible in the medial sublingual space.* **(Right)** *Axial CECT reveals an ovoid cystic lesion in the right sublingual space ➲. Dependent calculus is seen posteriorly ➲. This patient most likely began with a stone obstructing the submandibular duct. When the duct ruptured, the stone fell into the sialocele.*

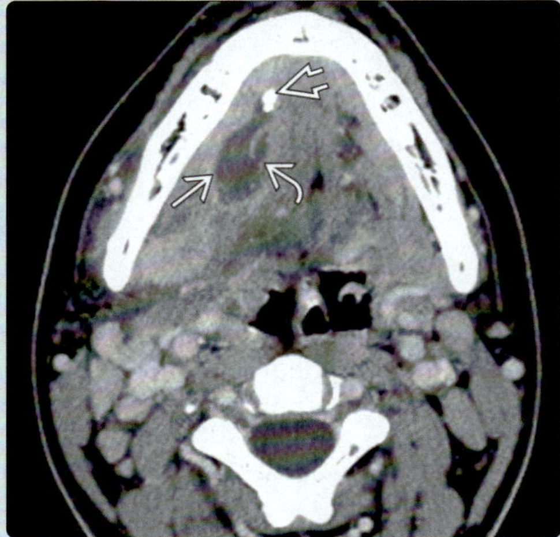

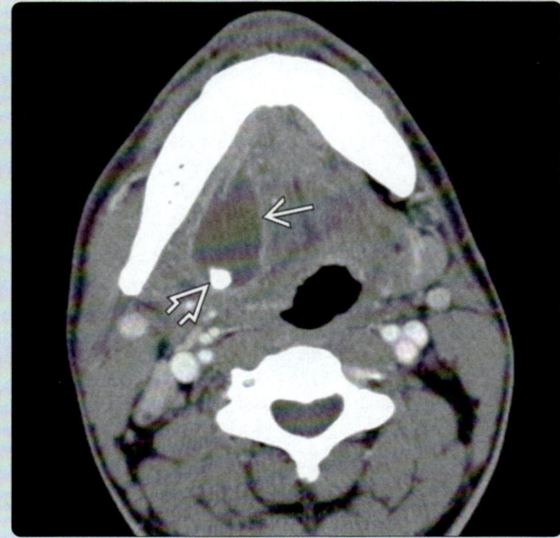

(Left) *Axial CECT demonstrates a small cystic mass in the posterior sublingual space ➲. Ranula, sialocele, and epidermoid were all considered. At surgery, a small pocket of saliva with a fibrous pseudocapsule was found.* **(Right)** *Axial CECT in a patient with history of facial trauma and floor of mouth swelling shows a cystic lesion in the left sublingual space ➲. Both ranula and sialocele were considered; sialocele was found at surgery. History of facial trauma supported sialocele diagnosis.*

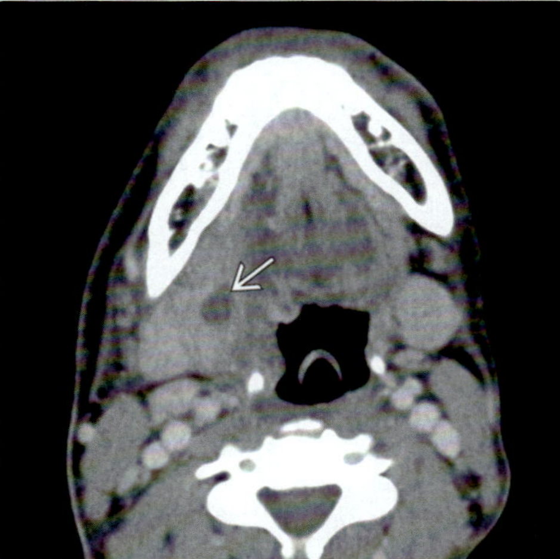

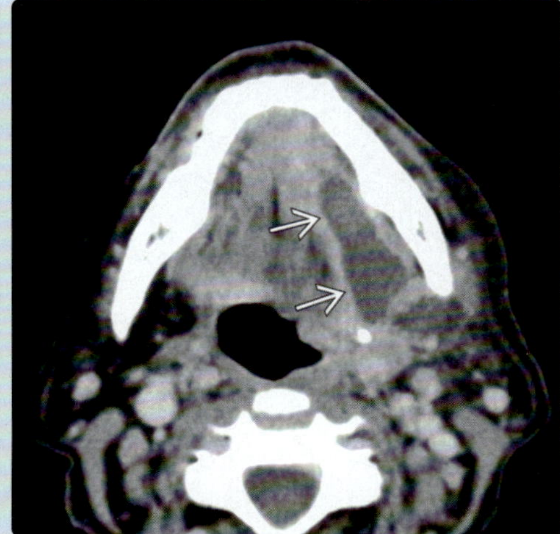

KEY FACTS

TERMINOLOGY

- Inflammation of submandibular gland (SMG)

IMAGING

- Most often **acute inflammation** + obstructed duct
  - **Duct calculus** or stenosis, floor-of-mouth tumor
  - 90% calculi opaque on occlusal view x-ray
  - Submandibular sialography rarely used
- **CECT** recommended to evaluate gland ± calculus
  - Ductal dilatation ± **calculus**, **stenosis**, or tumor
    - SMG calculi more often within duct than gland
    - Caveat: Calculi may be obscured by dental amalgam
  - Ipsilateral enlarged SMG + cellulitis
- NECT unnecessary; calculus & vessel densities differ
- **Chronic recurrent sialadenitis** less common
  - Ipsilateral atrophic SMG, ± fatty change
- Autoimmune disease (Sjögren) uncommon in SMG
- Fibroinflammatory disease (Küttner tumor) rare
- MR more sensitive for gland parenchymal changes

TOP DIFFERENTIAL DIAGNOSES

- Dental infection
- SMG carcinoma
- SMG benign mixed tumor
- Suppurative submandibular adenopathy

CLINICAL ISSUES

- Presentation: Tender floor of mouth swelling
  - Fever, ↑ WBC, purulence from duct
- Treatment options
  - If calculus in anterior duct, may remove by sialendoscopy or intraoral approach without SMG resection
    - If in SMG hilum, sialendoscopy vs. gland resection
  - If intrinsic to gland, no calculus, stenosis, or tumor
    - Antibiotics, sialogogues, hydration, warm compress
    - Treat cause of primary gland inflammatory disease (Sjögren syndrome, sialadenosis, Küttner tumor)

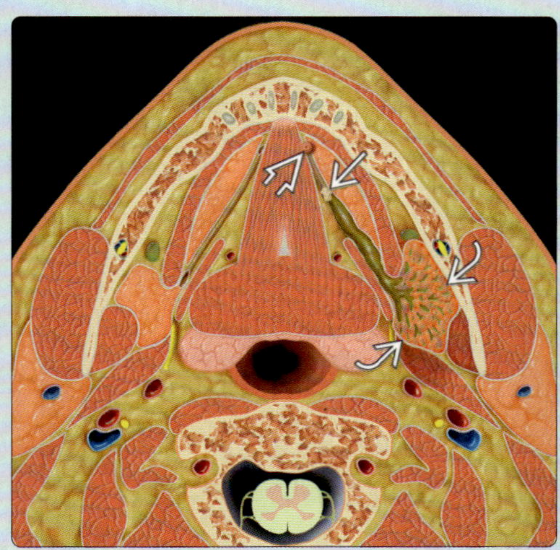

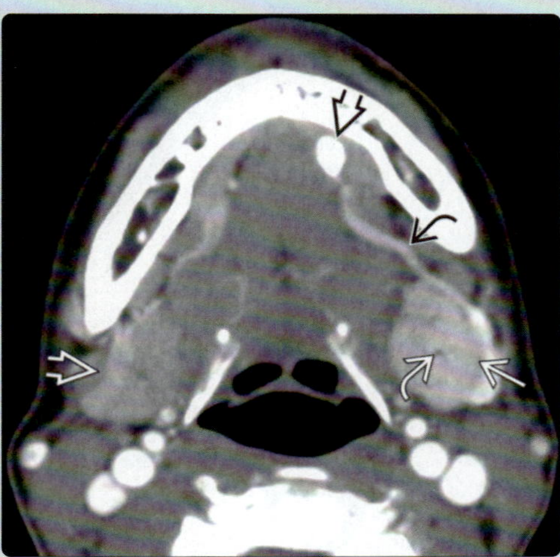

(Left) *Axial graphic depicts a calculus ➡ near the papilla of Wharton duct ➡. Proximal duct and intraductal radicles are enlarged. The submandibular gland (SMG) is inflamed and enlarged ➡.* **(Right)** *Axial CECT demonstrates an asymmetrically enhancing, enlarged left SMG ➡ compared to the right ➡. Calculus is evident in the distal submandibular duct at the level of the ductal papilla ➡. Only mild prominence of the duct at hilum is evident ➡. A prominent vessel in floor of mouth is also noted ➡.*

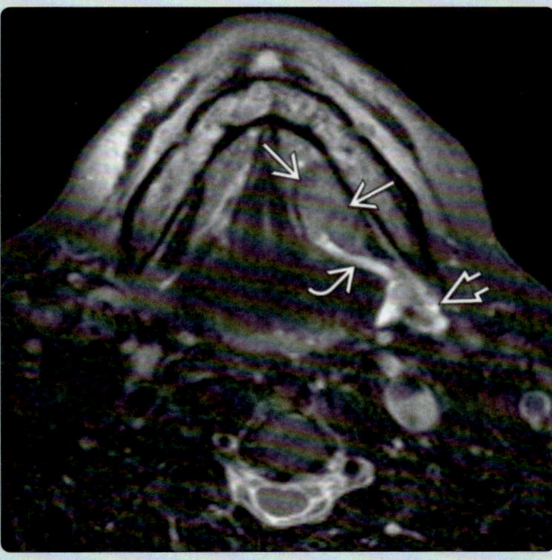

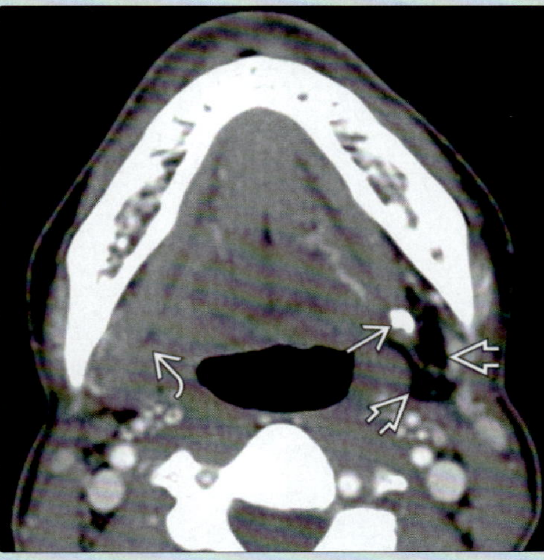

(Left) *Axial T2 FS MR demonstrates a well-circumscribed mass in the left floor of mouth ➡ in a patient with mucosal squamous cell carcinoma. Mass is obstructing the left submandibular duct ➡, & there is secondary inflammation of the left SMG ➡, which is hyperintense.* **(Right)** *Axial CECT through the floor of mouth in a patient with a right submandibular "mass" shows dense calculus ➡ in a proximal duct at the SMG hilus. Note marked fatty atrophy with left chronic sialadenitis ➡. The right "mass" was a normal SMG ➡.*

Oral Cavity Abscess

KEY FACTS

TERMINOLOGY

- Synonyms: Sublingual space (SLS), submandibular space (SMS), root of tongue (ROT), or oral cavity (OC) transspatial abscess
- OC abscess: Focal collection of pus within OC space(s)
- May be in 1 space or multiple contiguous spaces (transspatial)

IMAGING

- CECT findings
  - Abscess: Rim-enhancing, fluid collection in OC space(s)
  - Found within anatomic spaces (SMS, SLS, &/or ROT)
  - Phlegmon: Enhancing inflammatory tissue without focal fluid/pus
  - Cellulitis: Adjacent soft tissue stranding ± dermal thickening
  - Reactive or suppurative nodes
- CECT = best exam for OC abscess examination

TOP DIFFERENTIAL DIAGNOSES

- OC squamous cell carcinoma
- Simple or diving ranula
- OC dermoid/epidermoid
- Sialocele of submandibular duct

CLINICAL ISSUES

- Clinical presentation
  - Sublingual or submandibular swelling
  - Painful tongue with dysphagia, dysphonia
- Treatment: Surgical drainage + antibiotics; airway management as needed

DIAGNOSTIC CHECKLIST

- Consider abscess mimics (see differential above)
- Define space(s) with abscess: SLS, SMS, ROT
- Find underlying cause: Tooth abscess ± mandibular osteomyelitis, submandibular duct calculus, pharyngitis + suppurative node

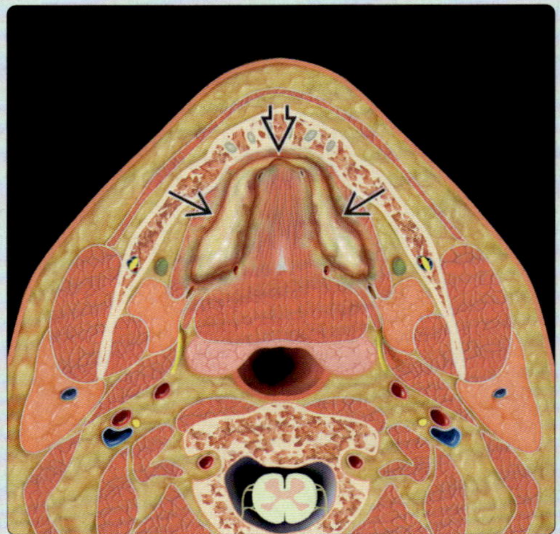

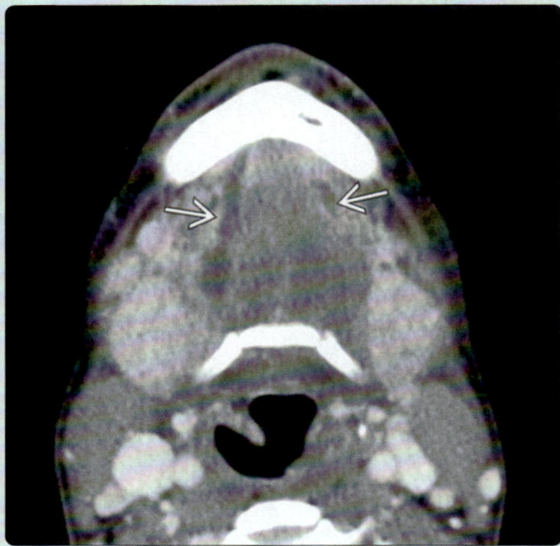

(Left) *Axial graphic depicts a bilateral sublingual space abscess ➾. The walled-off infected fluid collection is seen superomedially to the mylohyoid muscles and has a characteristic midline isthmus ➾ anteriorly at the midline.* **(Right)** *Axial CECT demonstrates an axial plane horseshoe-shaped sublingual space abscess with a fluid collection with surrounding enhancement within both ➔ sublingual spaces. The sublingual spaces connect anteriorly under the frenulum of the tongue (not seen).*

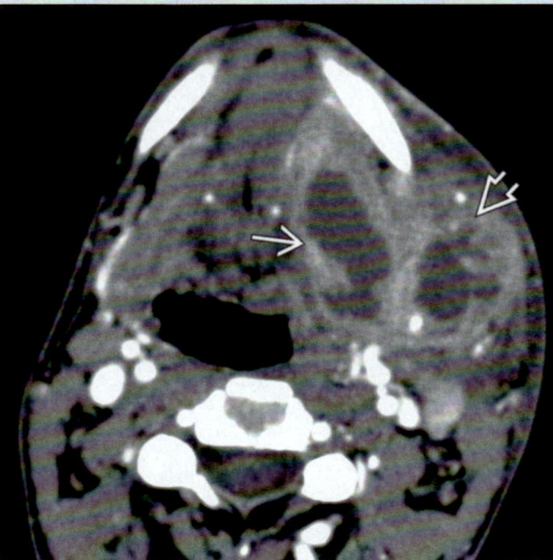

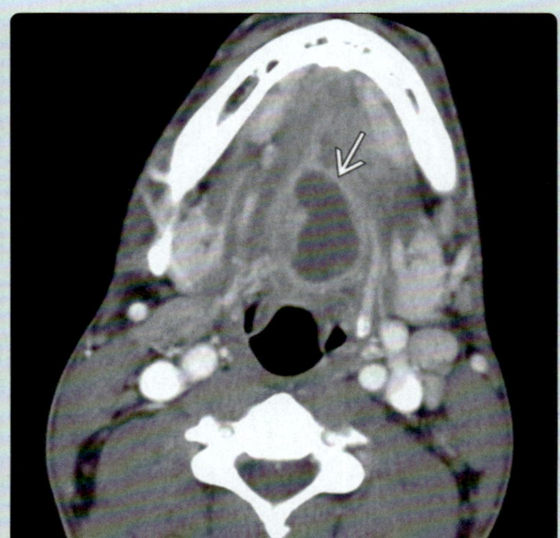

(Left) *Axial CECT shows mandibular infection spread inferomedially into the sublingual space ➔ and inferolaterally into the submandibular space ➔.* **(Right)** *Axial CECT in a patient with painful tongue swelling and fever shows a root of tongue midline rim-enhancing abscess pocket ➔. Such abscesses begin in the midline lingual septum area between the genioglossus muscles.*

KEY FACTS

TERMINOLOGY

- Synonym: Pleomorphic adenoma

IMAGING

- CECT
  - Enlarged submandibular gland (SMG) with focal or diffuse heterogeneous mass ± calcification
  - Isodense lesions may be "invisible"
  - Dual-phase CECT improves conspicuity
- MR
  - Small lesion: Low T1, high T2 intensity, homogeneous enhancement
  - Large lesion: More heterogeneous, ± focal areas of very high T2 signal, signal loss with calcification
  - Variable low T2 intensity "capsule"
- US
  - Well-defined, solid, intraglandular lesion
  - Large lesion may show focal cysts, calcification
- Best imaging tool: **MR > CECT** (some poorly seen on CECT)
  - **US affords excellent SMG evaluation**

TOP DIFFERENTIAL DIAGNOSES

- SMG sialadenitis
- SMG mucocele
- SMG carcinoma
- Submandibular space lymphadenopathy
- Chronic sclerosing sialadenitis (Kuttner tumor)

PATHOLOGY

- Epithelial, myoepithelial, and stromal components

CLINICAL ISSUES

- Most common neoplasm of SMG
- Treatment: Surgical excision with care not to spill tumor

DIAGNOSTIC CHECKLIST

- If patient presents with palpable submandibular mass
  - Determine if mass is in SMG or extrinsic (node)
  - If no mass found on CECT, recommend US or MR

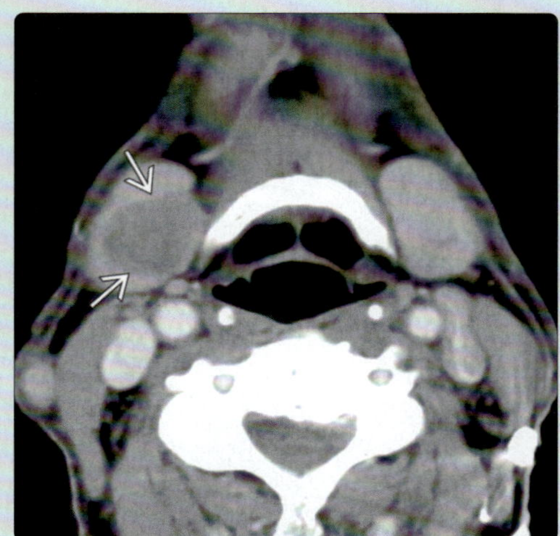

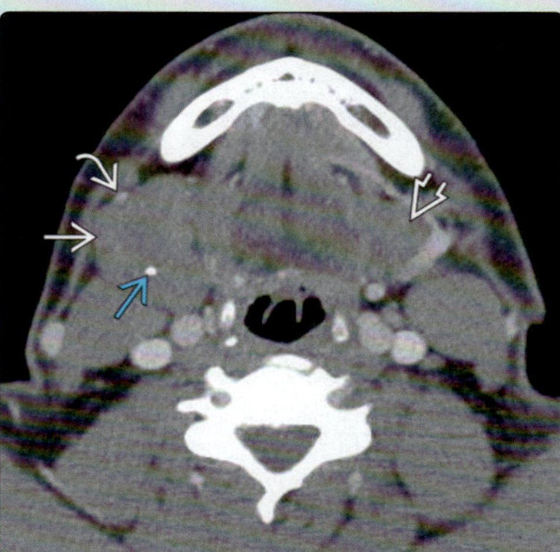

(Left) *Axial CECT shows a hypodense focal mass ➡ enlarging the right submandibular gland (SMG). This lesion is well defined, favoring a benign nature, but requires pathology confirmation.* **(Right)** *Axial CECT shows an enlarged right SMG ➡ compared to the left gland ➡. The displaced anterior facial vein ➡ confirms an intraglandular mass origin. This benign mixed tumor was nearly "invisible" due to isodensity, except for mass-related gland asymmetry and a focal calcification ➡.*

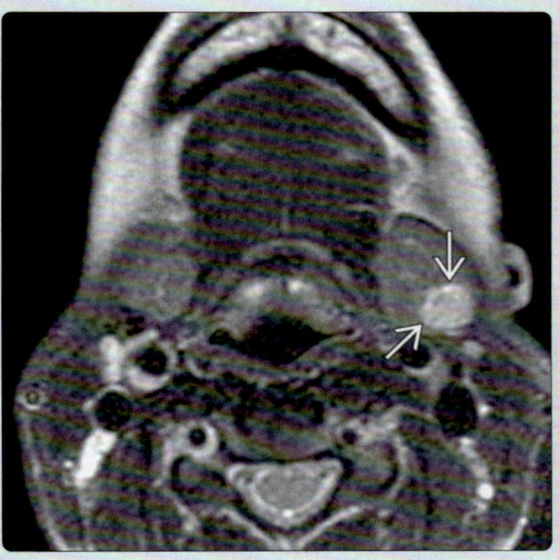

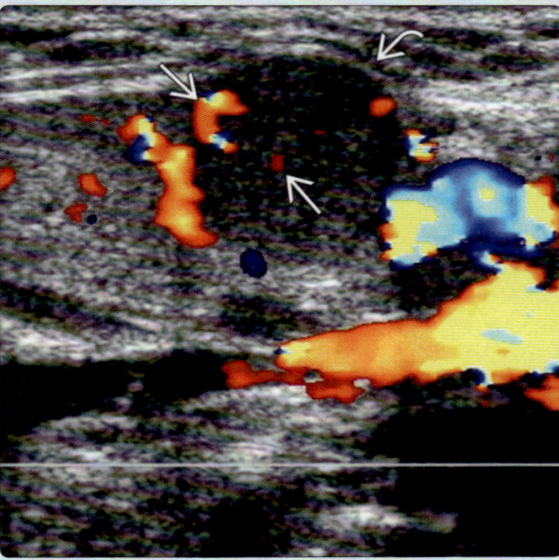

(Left) *Axial T2 MR in a young woman with a palpable submandibular mass shows a well-circumscribed and hyperintense oval lesion within the left SMG ➡ with no evidence of extension outside of the gland.* **(Right)** *Longitudinal oblique color Doppler ultrasound in the same patient shows a well-defined solid structure within the left SMG, distorting its external contour ➡. No internal calcifications or cystic change are evident. Vascular flow is evident at the periphery and internal aspect of this solid lesion ➡.*

KEY FACTS

TERMINOLOGY

- Definition: Benign minor salivary gland tumor of palate
- Abbreviation: Benign mixed tumor (BMT)
- Synonym: Palate pleomorphic adenoma

IMAGING

- General imaging findings
  - Most commonly found at soft-hard palate juncture
  - Small BMT: Well-defined palatal mass with homogeneous avid enhancement
  - Large BMT: Lobulated, heterogeneous C+
- Bone CT: Larger BMT remodels bony hard palate
- MR findings
  - Intermediate-high T2 signal ovoid palatal mass
  - Very high T2 signal suggests BMT
  - Larger BMT often with inhomogeneous signal (necrosis, blood products, calcification)
- Sagittal and coronal plane T2 and T1 C+ FS MR sequences best (orthogonal to palate)

TOP DIFFERENTIAL DIAGNOSES

- Palatal minor salivary gland neoplasms
- Palatal squamous cell carcinoma

PATHOLOGY

- Arise in minor salivary glands of palate
  - Hard-soft palate junction = most common site glands
- Interspersed epithelial, myoepithelial, and stromal cellular components must be identified to diagnose BMT

CLINICAL ISSUES

- Typical presentation is painless palatal mass
- BMT is 40% of all tumors of palate
- Most common site, minor salivary gland BMT (~ 10%)
- Risk factors for malignant transformation (carcinoma ex pleomorphic adenoma) are longevity and recurrence (3%)
- Treatment: Complete resection of encapsulated mass
  - Adequate soft tissue margins critical to avoid cellular "spillage" and future seeding of surgical bed

(Left) *Clinical photo of a patient with a submucosal mass ⇨ at the junction of the hard-soft palate. The tumor was resected and found to be a minor salivary gland benign mixed tumor (From DP: Head & Neck).* **(Right)** *Midline sagittal T1 MR shows a large ovoid mass at the junction of the soft and hard palate ➡ causing mild remodeling of the osseous hard palate ➡, with preserved normal T1 hyperintensity (indicating no invasion). This is the most common location for oral cavity benign mixed tumor (BMT).*

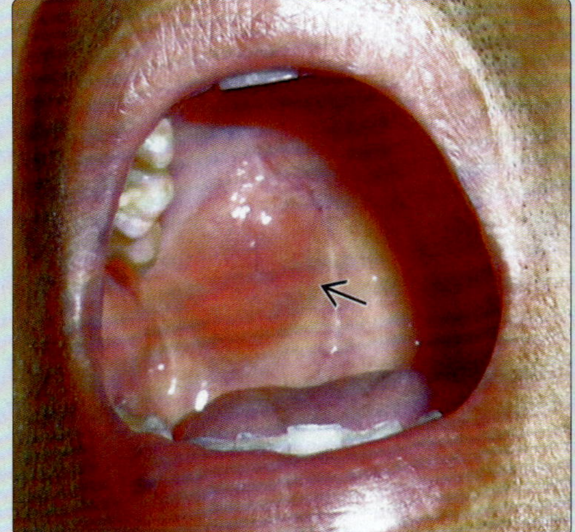

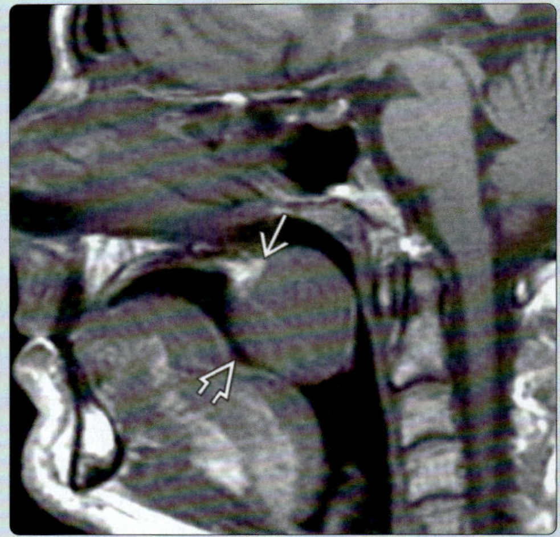

(Left) *Axial CECT demonstrates a well-circumscribed, somewhat heterogeneous, mildly enhancing soft tissue mass ➡ in the soft palate. Surgical removal revealed this to be a BMT.* **(Right)** *Sagittal CECT near the midline reveals a well-circumscribed, mildly enhancing heterogeneous mass ➡ in the soft palate. BMT and dermoid were both initially considered in the imaging differential diagnosis.*

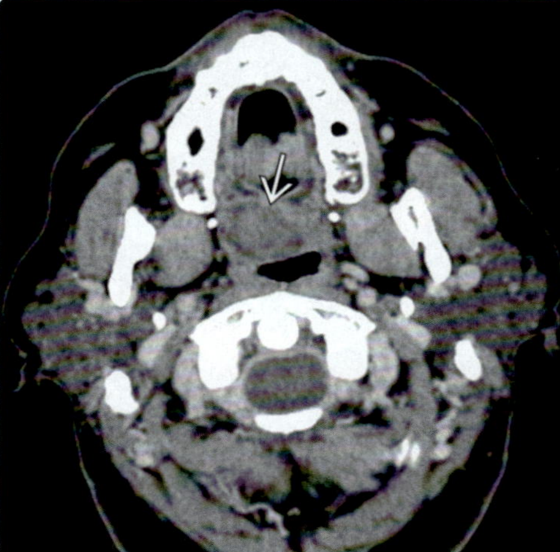

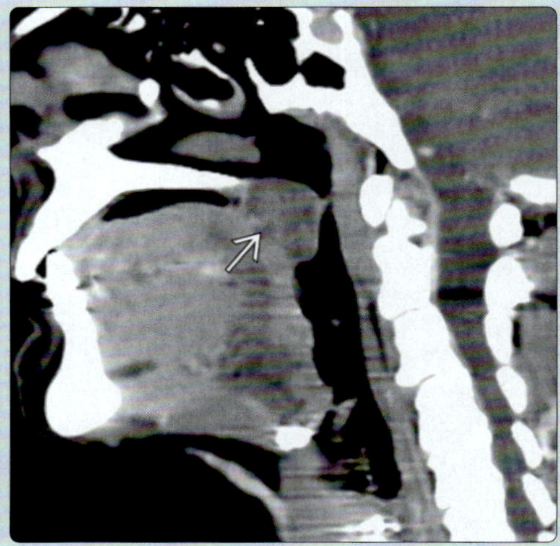

KEY FACTS

TERMINOLOGY

- Primary salivary malignancy of sublingual gland (SLG)

IMAGING

- CECT: Well-defined or invasive sublingual space (SLS) mass
  - Mild to moderately enhancing; may be subtle
  - Look for evidence of mandible erosion
    - Invasive margins signal malignancy
- MR: Variable signal and contrast enhancement
  - Well-differentiated tumors may have ↑ ↑ T2 signal
  - FS & STIR improve conspicuity
  - Evaluate for perineural invasion
- Look for invasion of extrinsic tongue muscles
- PET: Generally low FDG avidity unless high grade

TOP DIFFERENTIAL DIAGNOSES

- Floor of mouth squamous cell carcinoma
- Ranula
- Oral cavity abscess

PATHOLOGY

- **Adenoid cystic carcinoma**
  - Strong propensity for perineural spread
  - Tends to hematogenously spread to lungs
  - Slow-growing; may metastasize many years later
- **Mucoepidermoid carcinoma**
  - Tends to spread to lymph nodes
- Malignant degeneration of benign mixed tumor

CLINICAL ISSUES

- Painless, hard anterior floor of mouth mass on palpation
- 30-60 years of age
- **80%** of SLG masses are **malignant**
- Prognosis depends on stage > histologic grade
- Treatment primarily surgical ± XRT

DIAGNOSTIC CHECKLIST

- Aggressive-appearing lesions within SLS should be considered malignant until proven otherwise

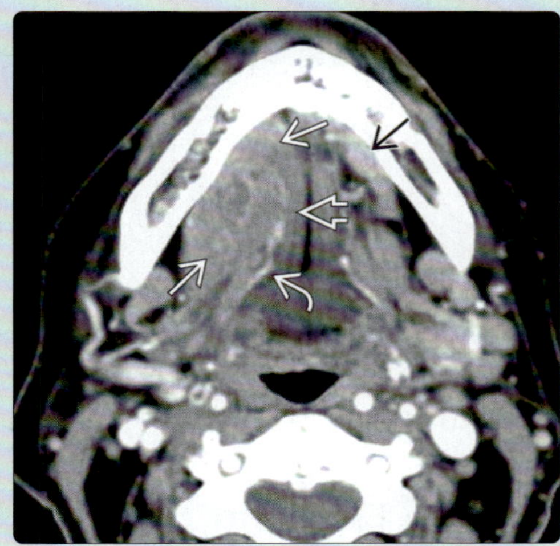

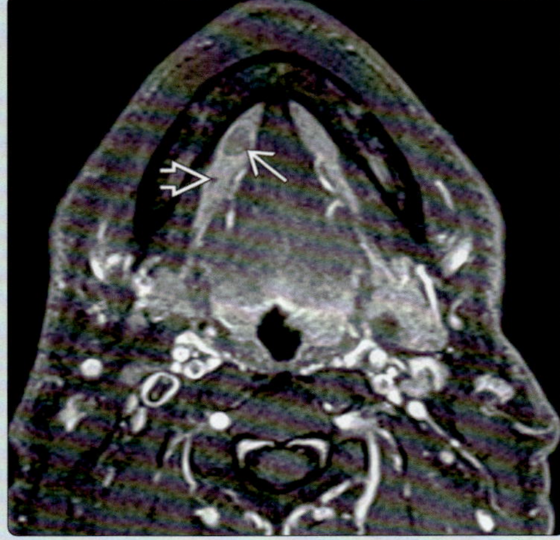

(Left) *CECT shows asymmetric floor of mouth from a large infiltrative adenoid cystic carcinoma ➡ in the right sublingual gland (SLG). Tumor extends into the genioglossus muscle ➡ & neurovascular bundle ➡, allowing ready access to CNV3 & CNXII. Note normal left SLG ➡.* **(Right)** *Axial T1 C+ FS MR shows a well-defined small mass ➡ in right SLG representing early mucoepidermoid carcinoma (MECa). Tumor is hypointense to normal SLG ➡ but can have variable enhancing characteristics. There is no evidence of mandible invasion.*

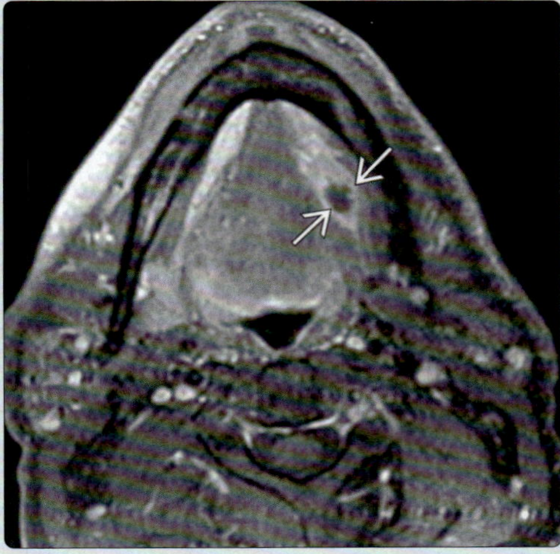

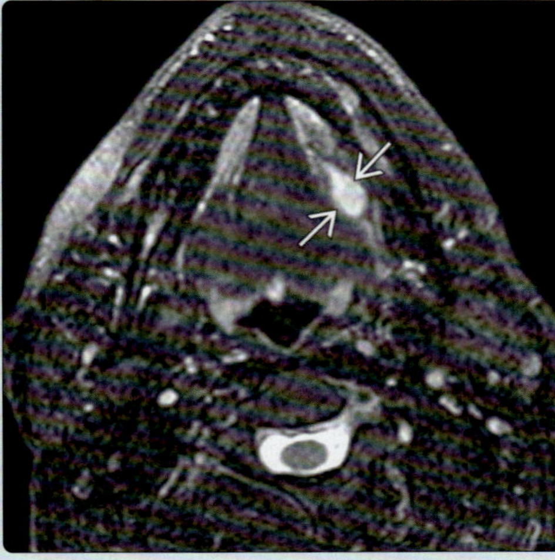

(Left) *Axial T1 C+ FS MR demonstrates a small heterogeneous left SLG mass ➡ with ill-defined borders. The irregular contours suggest this mass may be malignant; however, even well-defined lesions are statistically more likely to be malignant in SLG.* **(Right)** *Axial T2 FS MR in the same patient shows the mass ➡ to be markedly hyperintense. More differentiated salivary malignancies produce fluid/mucin and have high signal. This was found to be MECa.*

Submandibular Gland Carcinoma

KEY FACTS

TERMINOLOGY

- Primary malignancy arising in submandibular gland (SMG)
- Most commonly adenoid cystic (ACCa), mucoepidermoid (MECa), adenocarcinoma (AdCa)

IMAGING

- Focal or irregular SMG mass ± adjacent soft tissue invasion
- CECT: Asymmetric &/or heterogeneous SMG
  - Well-defined or ill-defined mass
  - Gland may be focally or diffusely hypodense
  - Mild to moderate contrast enhancement
- MR: Intermediate to high mixed T2 signal
  - Heterogeneous gadolinium enhancement
  - MR: Use fat saturation (FS) on T2 & T1 C+
- PET/CT: Low FDG avidity, unless high grade
- US: Ill-defined, spiculated, hypoechoic lesion

TOP DIFFERENTIAL DIAGNOSES

- SMG sialadenitis
- SMG benign mixed tumor
- Reactive lymph nodes
- Nodal squamous cell carcinoma in submandibular space

PATHOLOGY

- Beware FNA sampling & interpretive errors

CLINICAL ISSUES

- Painless submandibular swelling or focal mass
- **45%** SMG neoplasms are **malignant**
- ACCa: Early perineural spreads, also to lungs
- MECa & AdCa: Nodal & hematogenous spread
- Treatment: En bloc complete resection of tumor
  - Postoperative XRT for high stage, high grade

DIAGNOSTIC CHECKLIST

- 1st determine whether mass is **within SMG or extrinsic**, such as node
- **Beware subtle or occult SMG mass** on CECT
  - If none found on CECT, recommend US or MR

(Left) *Axial CECT shows asymmetric enlargement of the right submandibular gland (SMG) compared to the left ➡ with a hypodense ill-defined mass ➡ in posterior aspect. On resection, the mass was found to be adenocarcinoma confined to SMG.* **(Right)** *Axial CECT in adult with fluctuating neck fullness shows asymmetric fullness & poorly marginated enhancement in the lateral right SMG ➡. The image was interpreted as vascular malformation but patient age & MR did not support this. Fine-needle aspiration revealed ACCa.*

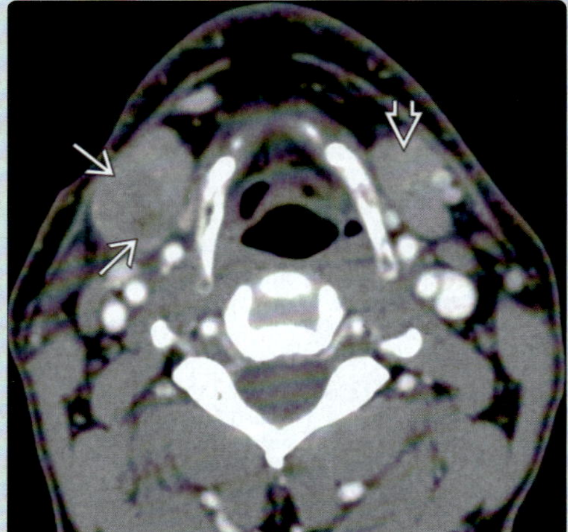

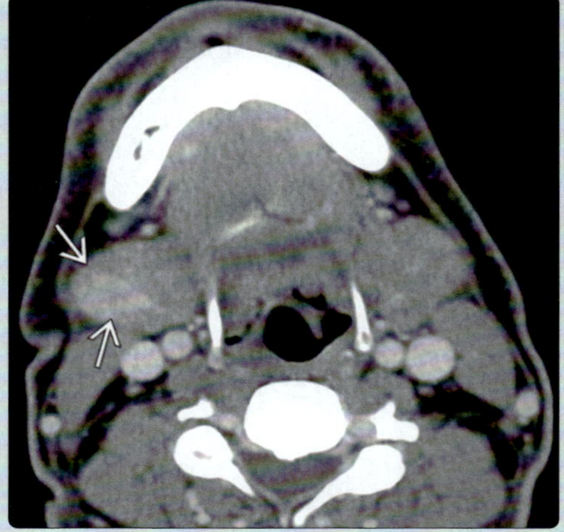

(Left) *Axial T1 MR demonstrates a fuller and more hypointense right SMG ➡ compared to the left ➡ in a patient with a palpable abnormality; this was misinterpreted as gland asymmetry. No adenopathy is present.* **(Right)** *Coronal T1 C+ FS MR in the same patient 2 years later reveals ill-defined, heterogeneous right SMG ➡ with infiltration of the tumor medially through mylohyoid muscle ➡. Note involvement of the mandible and inferior alveolar nerve ➡. Tumor was found to be adenocarcinoma with metastatic nodes.*

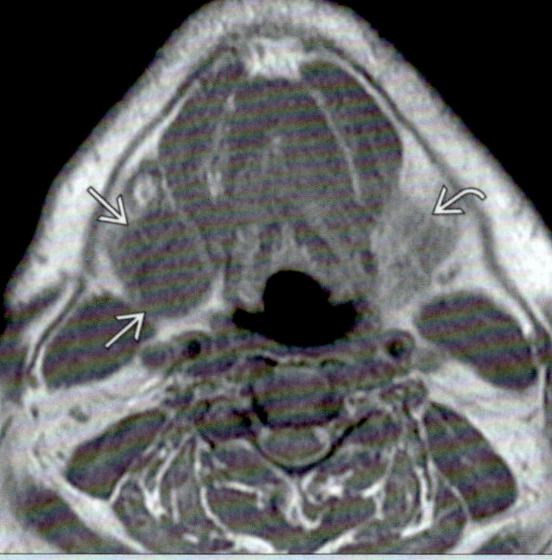

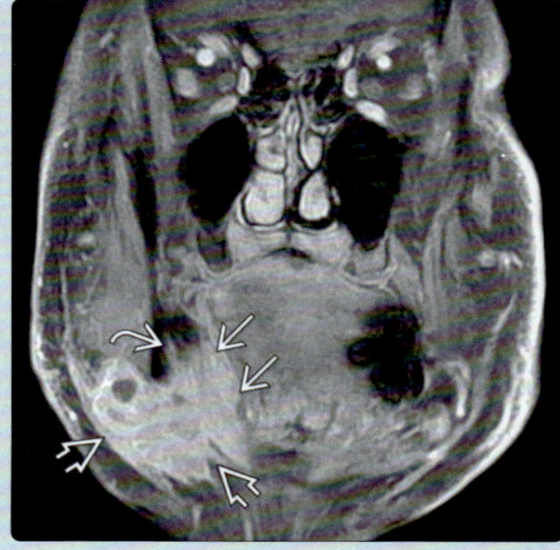

Oral Cavity Minor Salivary Gland Malignancy

KEY FACTS

TERMINOLOGY

- Abbreviation: Minor salivary gland malignancy (MSGM)
- Most common MSGM: Adenoid cystic carcinoma (ACCa) & mucoepidermoid carcinoma (MECa)

IMAGING

- General imaging findings
  - MSGM location: Submucosa of upper aerodigestive tract
    - Hard-soft palate junction > > buccal mucosa
  - Oral cavity well defined, smooth submucosal mass
- Bone CT findings
  - Bone erosion: Palate, mandible
  - Greater and lesser palatine foramen enlargement
- MR findings
  - T1: Low signal tumor replaces hard palate marrow fat
  - T1 C+ fat-saturated to **look for perineural tumor spread**
- PET imaging best for staging/restaging

TOP DIFFERENTIAL DIAGNOSES

- Squamous cell carcinoma
- Benign mixed tumor of palate
- Dentigerous cyst

PATHOLOGY

- Prognosis depends on **stage > histologic grade**

CLINICAL ISSUES

- **ACCa**: Tendency for **perineural tumor**, lung metastases
- **MECa**: Tendency for regional **nodal** metastasis
- Treatment: Surgical resection ± postoperative radiation

DIAGNOSTIC CHECKLIST

- Long-term (> 10 year) imaging follow-up recommended for ACCa given **tendency to recur late**
- Check for perineural tumor in MSGM
  - CNV2 & CNV3 biggest culprits
- Noncontrast T1 MR may offer best inherent contrast

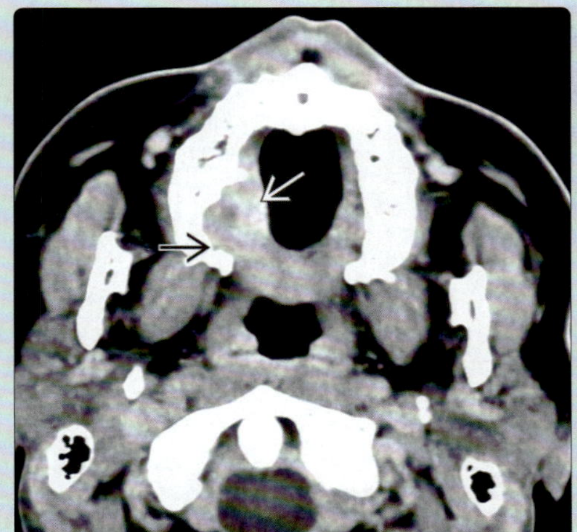

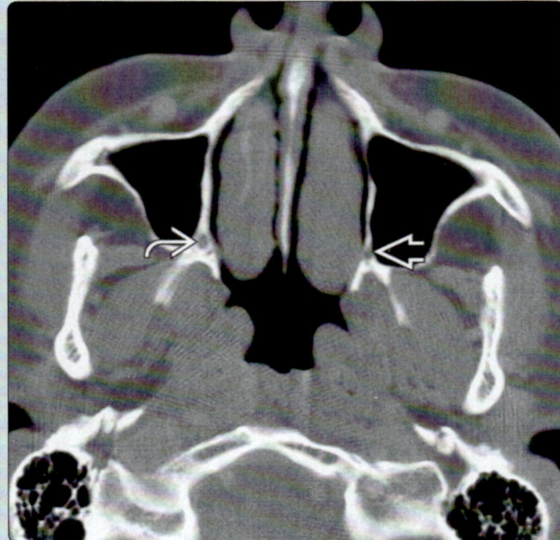

(Left) *Axial CECT shows a classic example of an adenoid cystic carcinoma (ACCa) in the right hard palate ➡ invading adjacent bone & thus gaining access to the greater palatine nerve in the greater palatine canal ➡.* **(Right)** *Axial bone CT shows widening of the right greater palatine canal ➡, indicating perineural tumor spread along the greater palatine nerve. Note the normal left canal ➡. Tumor can now spread to the pterygopalatine fossa giving access to V2, vidian nerve, orbit, nasal cavity, & infratemporal fossa.*

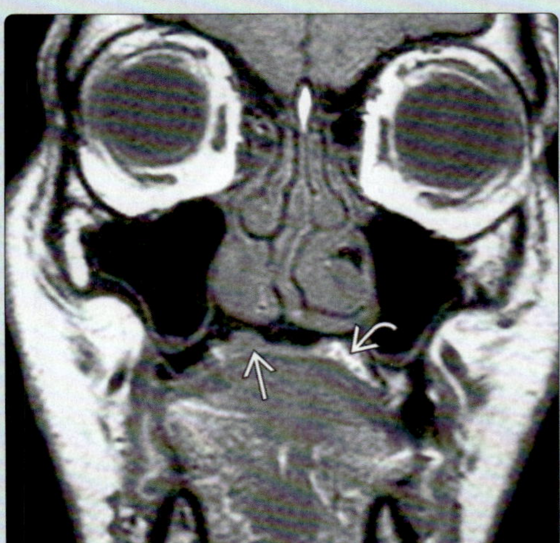

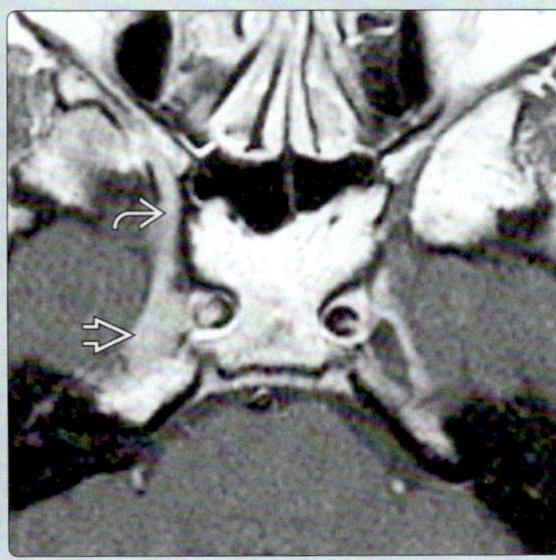

(Left) *Coronal T1 MR shows dark tumor ➡ infiltration of the right hard palate marrow in this patient with ACCa. Note normal fat signal ➡ in the contralateral hard palate. Noncontrast T1 MR may offer better inherent tumor contrast in areas with fat.* **(Right)** *Axial T1 C+ MR in a different patient with hard palate ACCa shows perineural tumor along the right maxillary division of the trigeminal nerve (V2) in the foramen rotundum ➡ & cavernous sinus ➡, from the contiguous greater palatine nerve & pterygopalatine fossa involvement (not shown).*

Submandibular Space Nodal Non-Hodgkin Lymphoma

KEY FACTS

TERMINOLOGY

- Submandibular space (SMS) nodal non-Hodgkin lymphoma (NHL)
- NHL develops in lymphoreticular system

IMAGING

- CECT findings
  - Multiple, bilateral, nonnecrotic enlarged level I SMS nodes
  - May see only dominant, single large node
  - Usually large, solid, round nodes
  - Necrosis/extranodal spread indicate aggressive NHL
- PET/CT increasingly used to determine disease extent

TOP DIFFERENTIAL DIAGNOSES

- Reactive lymph nodes
- Nodal squamous cell carcinoma of SMS
- Nodal metastases from systemic primary
- Sarcoidosis lymph nodes
- Tuberculosis lymph nodes

PATHOLOGY

- Unregulated malignant monoclonal lymphocytes in lymphoreticular system
- Multiple different NHL subtypes
  - Most common (> 30%) diffuse large B-cell lymphoma
  - Multiple other subtypes

CLINICAL ISSUES

- Presentation: Painless multiple SMS masses
- Treatment: Radiotherapy, chemotherapy, or both
- 5% all H&N cancers
- Prognosis
  - 5-year survival: Stage I-II (85%), stage III-IV (50%)

DIAGNOSTIC CHECKLIST

- Consider NHL if imaging reveals multiple 1- to 3-cm cervical nodes in multiple nodal chains, especially if nonnecrotic

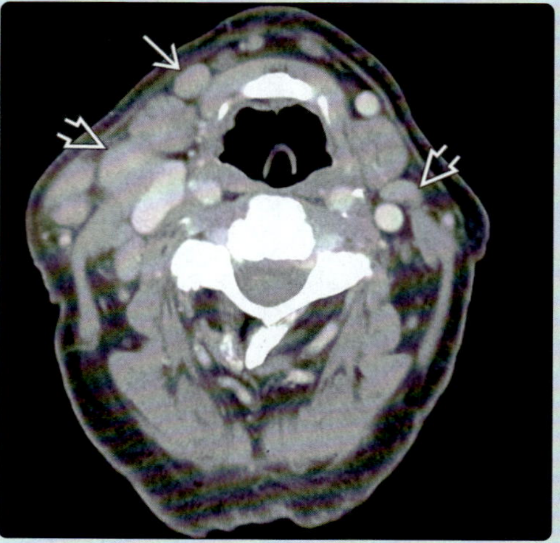

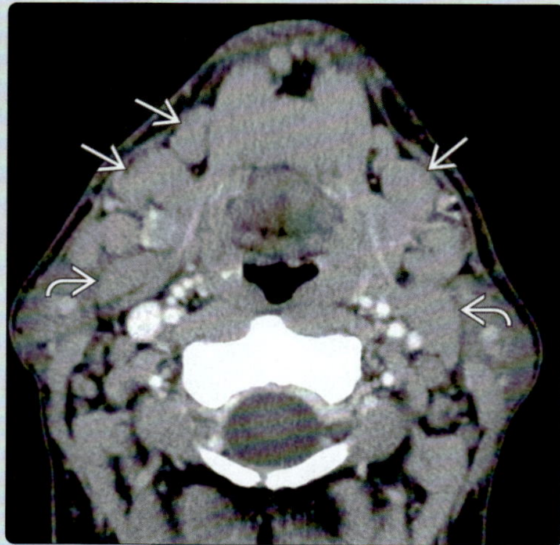

(Left) *Axial CECT at the level of the hyoid bone in a patient with non-Hodgkin lymphoma (NHL) demonstrates diffuse adenopathy in the upper neck, with a prominent right submandibular IB node and bilateral level II nodes.* **(Right)** *Axial CECT reveals multiple smoothly marginated, enlarged level IB nodes in the submandibular space bilaterally along with large, solid level II nodes in a patient with NHL.*

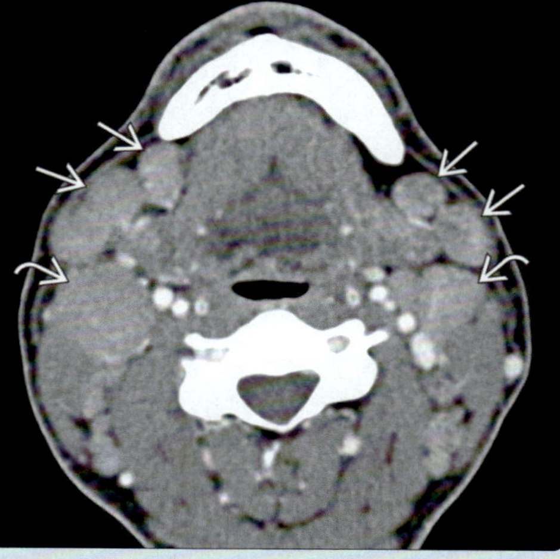

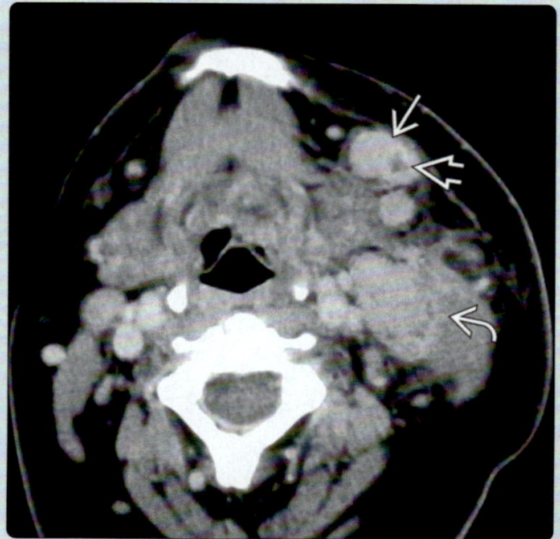

(Left) *Axial CECT at the level of the inferior mandible shows large nonnecrotic NHL nodes in the level IB submandibular chain and bilateral level II jugulodigastric group.* **(Right)** *Axial CECT in this HIV(+) patient with NHL shows a prominent left level IB submandibular space node with a small focus of cystic change. A larger level II jugulodigastric node appears to invade the adjacent sternocleidomastoid muscle. Nodal necrosis and extranodal NHL spread usually indicate a high-grade NHL is present.*

KEY FACTS

TERMINOLOGY

- Submandibular space (SMS), nodal squamous cell carcinoma (SCCa)

IMAGING

- SMS level IA & IB nodes
  - Level IA: Suprahyoid node(s) between anterior belly of digastric muscles
  - Level IB: Suprahyoid node(s) located lateral' & immediately anterior to a line tangent to posterior border of submandibular glands
- CECT or MR findings
  - CECT generally preferred over MR for nodal staging
  - CECT improves N staging accuracy over clinical staging
  - SMS nodes **> 1.5 cm** considered malignant in context of H&N SCCa
  - **Central nodal necrosis** considered sign of malignant involvement in any size node
  - Irregular enhancing margin invades adjacent soft tissues implies **extracapsular spread**
- PET/CT
  - Superior to CT/MR in clinical N0 neck
- Ultrasonographic findings
  - Round node with loss of hilar echogenicity
  - Main limitation is some nodes are inaccessible

TOP DIFFERENTIAL DIAGNOSES

- Suppurative lymph nodes
- Nodal non-Hodgkin lymphoma

CLINICAL ISSUES

- Treatment: Primary tumor resection vs. chemoradiotherapy ± nodal dissection
- Prognostic implication of malignant adenopathy
  - Single unilateral node ↓ prognosis by 50%
  - Bilateral nodes ↓ prognosis by 75%
  - Extracapsular spread ↓ prognosis by further 50%

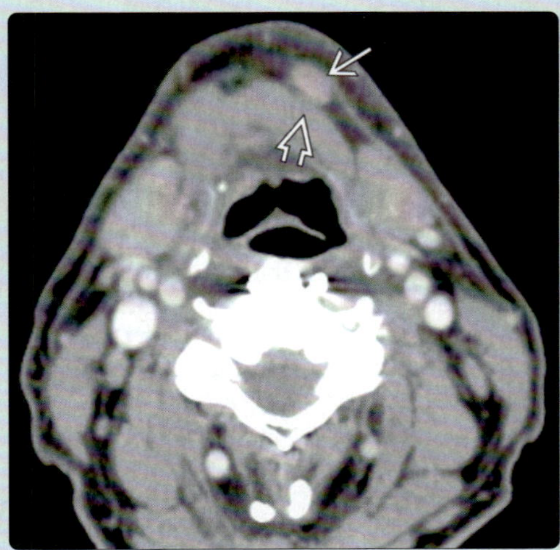

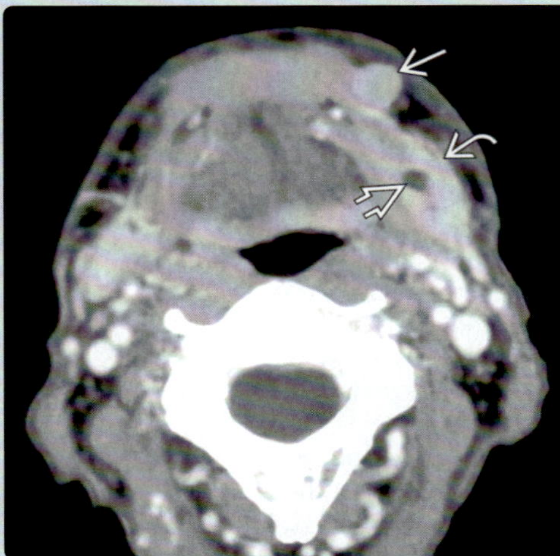

(Left) *Axial CECT in a patient with a lower lip squamous cell carcinoma (SCCa) shows a single pathologic (subtle low-density center) submandibular space (SMS) node ➡ lateral to the anterior belly of the digastric muscle ➡, making it a level IB node.* **(Right)** *Axial CECT through the suprahyoid neck reveals an enlarged, round, enhancing metastatic level IB SCCa node ➡. The left submandibular gland (SMG) ➡ is enlarged and enhancing with a dilated hilar duct ➡. Anterior floor of mouth SCCa (not shown) has obstructed the submandibular duct.*

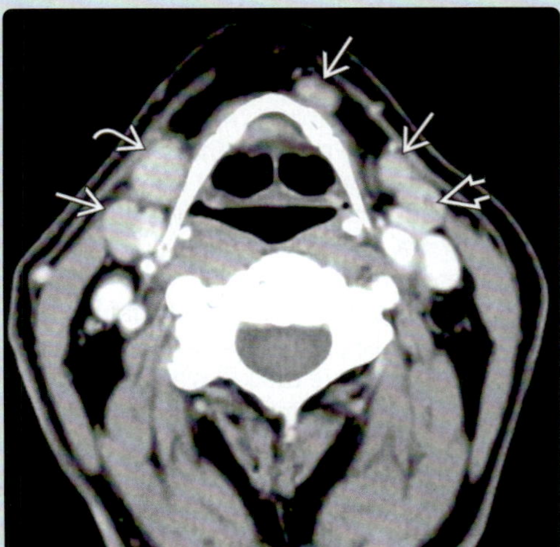

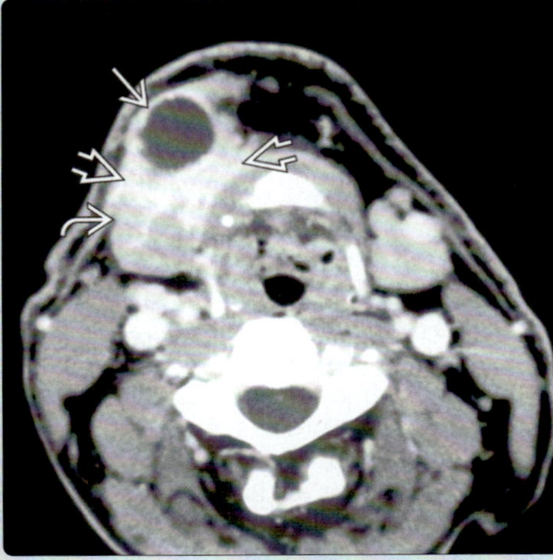

(Left) *Axial CECT in a patient with anterior floor of mouth primary SCCa shows multiple level IB nodes. A few enhance ➡, but not all are malignant by CT criteria. Two nodes meet criteria for malignancy: One on right based on size > 1.5 cm ➡, and one on left due to central low density ➡.* **(Right)** *Axial CECT reveals a large cystic level IB SMS nodal mass ➡ in a patient with lateral tongue SCCa. Enhancing spreading nodal margins ➡ inseparable from surrounding tissues suggest extracapsular extension. The SMG ➡ is engulfed by spreading tumor.*

Imaging Techniques and Indications

Mandible and Maxilla

The study of choice for evaluating the mandible and maxilla is **thin-section bone algorithm CT** and **CECT**. A standard protocol consists of coverage from the orbits to the hyoid at ≤ 1-mm intervals following contrast administration and postprocessing with both bone and soft tissue algorithm. Axial images should be acquired parallel to the inferior border of the mandible. Acquiring the maxilla and mandible angled separately so as to avoid artifact from dental restorations assists in evaluation of the alveolar ridge and adjacent structures. Multiplanar reformats should be performed in the coronal and sagittal planes. In addition, it is frequently helpful to the referring clinician to reformat in a panoramic view.

MR of the maxillofacial complex is used to assess marrow changes, involvement of the inferior alveolar nerve, and soft tissue involvement of adjacent structures. T1-/T2-weighted and contrast-enhanced images should be acquired from the orbits to the hyoid at 3 mm and ideally should be acquired with high-resolution/small-FOV techniques. As with CT, axial images should be acquired parallel to the inferior border of the mandible. STIR or T2 fat-saturation sequences along with contrast enhancement are sensitive for marrow/nerve changes associated with inflammation or neoplastic involvement.

TMJ

MR is the tool of choice for evaluating the TMJ. Small surface, circular (3-inch), or TMJ coils are ideally used, although multichannel coils (12 channels or greater) provide adequate signal. Sagittal images are acquired perpendicular to the long axis of the condyle ("corrected sagittal oblique") at 3-mm intervals. T1-weighted or proton density sagittal images are acquired in the closed- and open-mouth positions. Cine images provide the most accurate assessment of condylar rotation and translation and the associated disc function. Sagittal T2-weighted images are acquired to assess for joint effusion. Coronal T1-weighted images in the closed-mouth position are used to assess medial or lateral disc displacements as well as multiplanar views of the condyle. Contrast-enhanced images are generally reserved for the evaluation of synovitis or tumors.

CT imaging of the TMJ is generally reserved for the evaluation of **trauma**, assessment of bony abnormalities or **calcified masses**, or **joint reconstruction** with metallic prosthesis. Thin-section bone algorithm images are acquired at 1-mm intervals from the sella to the hyoid and reformatted in the coronal and sagittal planes.

Imaging Anatomy

Mandible and Maxilla

The **maxilla** consists of a **body** containing the maxillary sinus and 4 processes: **Zygomatic**, **frontal**, **alveolar**, and **palatine**. The maxilla forms the boundaries of 3 cavities: The roof of the oral cavity, the floor and lateral wall of the nasal cavity, and the floor of the orbit. In addition, the maxilla forms the anterior boundary of the infratemporal and pterygopalatine fossae and contributes to the formation of the infraorbital and pterygomaxillary fissures. The zygomatic (**malar**) process contributes to the inferior pillar of the zygomatic buttress. The frontal (nasal) process articulates with the nasal bones on the lateral surface with the medial surface forming the lateral wall of the nasal cavity and articulating with the ethmoid bone to enclose the agger nasi cells and anterior ethmoidal cells. The posterior border of the frontal process forms the lacrimal fossa and the anterior lacrimal crest. The **alveolar process** is the thickest and most spongy part of the maxilla and forms the alveolar arches containing the dentition and their supporting periodontal structures. The 3D U-shaped configuration of the maxillary alveolus is such that benign expansile inflammatory or neoplastic processes will typically expand it concentrically. Innervation of the teeth and gingiva is via the anterior and posterior superior alveolar nerves.

The **maxillary tuberosity** is the rounded most posterior eminence of the alveolar arch, which articulates with the pyramidal process of the palatine bone. The palatine process is a relatively thick horizontal bone that forms the roof of the mouth and the floor of the nasal cavity. The incisive foramen lies in the anterior midline of the premaxilla and transmits the nasopalatine nerves and descending palatine artery. The premaxillary suture, posterior to the incisive foramen, separates the anterior premaxilla from the more posterior palatine process, which forms the anterior 75% of the hard palate. The remainder of the hard palate is formed by the horizontal plate of the palatine bone and contains foramina for the **greater and lesser palatine nerves**. The blood supply to the palate is formed from the descending palatine artery emerging through the greater palatine foramen and running in a shallow groove along the lateral aspect of the palate to the incisive foramen. The blood supply to the maxillary alveolus is via the posterior superior alveolar artery, which supplies the gingiva, premolar, and molar teeth. The incisors and canines are supplied by the anterior &/or middle superior alveolar arteries, which are branches of the infraorbital artery.

The **mandible** consists of a horseshoe-shaped body and vertical rami joining in the anterior midline symphysis. On the external surface of the mandible, at roughly the level of the 1st premolar, is the mental foramen for the mental nerve and vessels. Emerging anterosuperiorly from the ramus is the triangular eminence of the coronoid process to which the temporalis and masseter muscles attach. At the posterior-superior termination of the ramus is the condyloid process consisting of the condyle supported by the more constricted neck. On the medial (lingual) surface of the ramus is the **mandibular foramen** for intraosseous passage of the neurovascular supply, namely the inferior alveolar nerve and artery. The mandibular foramen is bounded by a small bony spine, the lingula. The coronoid process and condyle are separated by a depression, the mandibular (coronoid) notch, through which the masseteric vessels and nerves pass.

Permanent dentition consists of 32 teeth: 2 central incisors, 2 lateral incisors, 2 canines, 4 premolars, and 6 molars in each jaw. These are numbered 1-16 in the maxilla right to left and 17-32 in the mandible left to right. **Primary dentition** consists of 20 teeth: 2 central incisors, 2 lateral incisors, 2 canines, and 4 molars in each jaw. These are numbered A-J in the maxilla and K-T in the mandible. Dental infection in the form of dental caries or periodontal disease spreads into the alveolus through the root apex or through the **periodontal ligament** (PDL) space. The PDL is a potential conduit for development of infection following alveolar fracture as well as direct intraosseous extension of gingival squamous cell carcinoma.

TMJ

The **TMJ complex** consists of the diarthrodial osseous articulation between the mandibular condyle and the glenoid fossa and articular eminence of the temporal bone. The TMJ is the only joint in which articulating surfaces are covered by

Mandible-Maxilla Differential Diagnosis

Inflammatory/infectious	Cysts	Malignant neoplasms
Apical rarefying osteitis	**Odontogenic**	**Nonodontogenic**
Radicular cyst	Dentigerous cyst	Gingival squamous cell carcinoma
Osteomyelitis	Glandular odontogenic cyst	Osteosarcoma/chondrosarcoma
Osteonecrosis	Calcifying epithelial odontogenic cyst	Multiple myeloma or metastasis
Osteoradionecrosis	**Benign neoplasms**	**Odontogenic**
Congenital/developmental	**Nonodontogenic**	Odontogenic carcinoma
Solitary median maxillary central incisor	Osteoma	Odontogenic sarcoma
Acquired	Ossifying fibroma	**Fibroosseous lesions**
Stafne bone cavity	**Odontogenic**	Periapical osseous dysplasia
Simple bone cyst	Odontoma	Florid osseous dysplasia
Central giant cell granuloma	Keratocystic odontogenic tumor	Fibrous dysplasia
Cysts	Ameloblastoma	Cherubism
Nonodontogenic	Odontogenic myxoma	**Other**
Nasopalatine duct cyst	Adenomatoid odontogenic tumor	Neurofibroma, schwannoma
Nasolabial cyst	Calcifying epithelial odontogenic tumor	Eosinophilic granuloma

TMJ Differential Diagnosis

Meniscal dislocation	Anterior, medial, lateral, or (rarely) posterior displacement of articular disc
Juvenile idiopathic arthritis	Bilateral flattened, deformed mandibular condyles, joint effusion, synovial enhancement
Synovial chondromatosis	Multiple calcified small nodules in superior joint space
Pigmented villonodular synovitis	Locally destructive mass with peripheral hypointense rim on MR
Calcium pyrophosphate dihydrate deposition disease	Chunky, diffuse, calcified mass

fibrocartilage. The articular disc is a biconcave, dense, avascular fibrous connective tissue with 3 segments: The anterior band, which is attached to the capsule and fibers of the superior belly of the lateral pterygoid muscle, the thin intermediate zone, and the posterior band. The bilaminar zone or retrodiscal tissues attach to the posterior band and provide neurovascular innervation.

Approaches to Imaging Issues of Mandible and Maxilla

As lesions of the mandible and maxilla may arise from a myriad of odontogenic and nonodontogenic tissues, it is best to use a systematic approach to evaluate lesions of the jaw. The 1st step is to try to determine whether the lesion is odontogenic or nonodontogenic in origin. Infectious and inflammatory lesions usually have a dental origin, even if remote. **Odontogenic** cysts and benign and malignant neoplasms usually arise from, or are centered within, tooth-bearing areas of the alveolus. The major exception to this is gingival squamous cell carcinoma extending through the gingiva or PDL space. **Nonodontogenic lesions** often arise at the tooth root apices or superior (maxilla) or inferior (mandible) to them.

Once an assessment of odontogenic vs. nonodontogenic is achieved, an evaluation of lesion features, such as location, cystic vs. solid, presence of internal calcification, loculation, bony expansion or erosion, and enhancement, will narrow the differential. Most odontogenic lesions are cystic, cystic-appearing, or relatively hypodense on CT. They are distinguished by their location, loculation, presence of internal calcification, and expansion/erosion of bone. Most dentigerous cysts and keratocystic odontogenic tumors do not become loculated until large; most ameloblastomas demonstrate multiple loculations. The only odontogenic lesions with internal calcification are the odontoma, calcifying epithelial cyst/tumor, and adenomatoid odontogenic tumor. Malignant neoplasms generally demonstrate more enhancement than benign lesions.

There are **3 key pieces of information** the referring clinician needs to know.

- Does lesion or fracture involve lamina dura and PDL space or tooth roots.
- Does lesion or fracture in mandible involve inferior alveolar canal.
- Does lesion extend to adjacent structures or spaces, including maxillary sinus, orbit, pterygopalatine fossa, buccal vestibule and space, masticator space, or sublingual or submandibular space.

Selected References

1. Mosier KM: Lesions of the jaw. Semin Ultrasound CT MR. 36(5):444-50, 2015
2. Mosier KM: Magnetic resonance imaging of the maxilla and mandible: signal characteristics and features in the differential diagnosis of common lesions. Top Magn Reson Imaging. 24(1):23-37, 2015
3. Aiken A et al: MR imaging of the temporomandibular joint. Magn Reson Imaging Clin N Am. 20(3):397-412, 2012
4. Curé JK et al: Radiopaque jaw lesions: an approach to the differential diagnosis. Radiographics. 32(7):1909-25, 2012

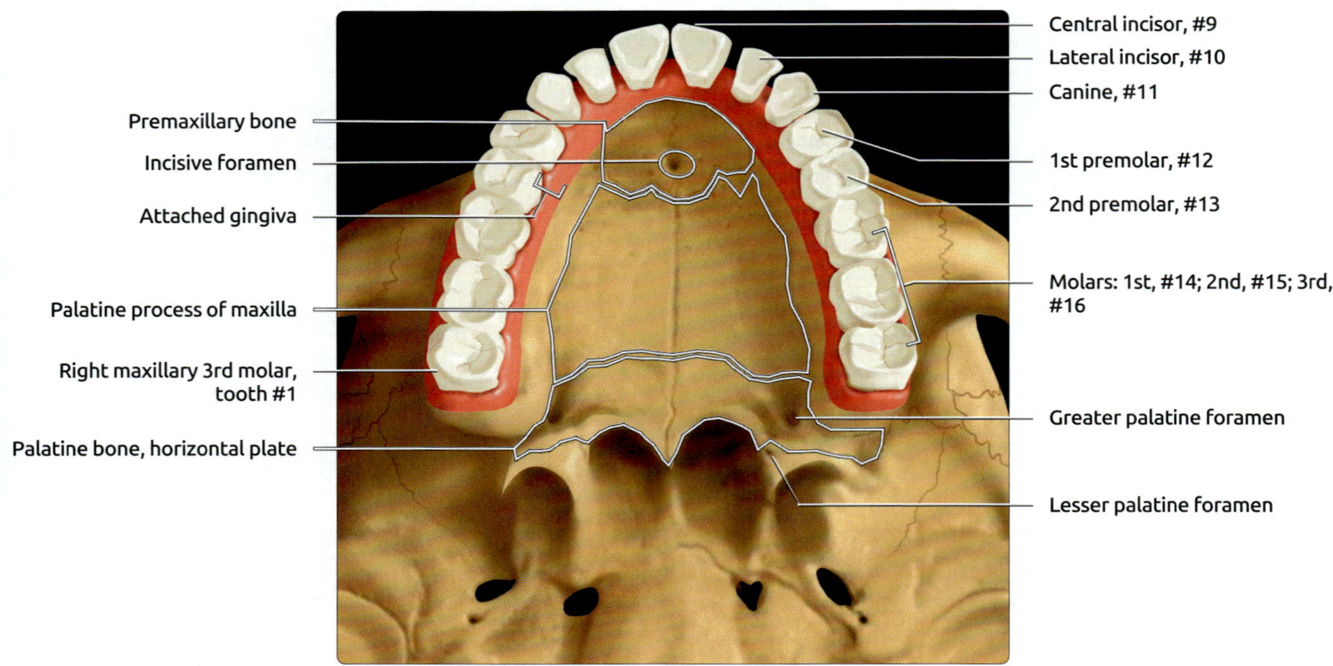

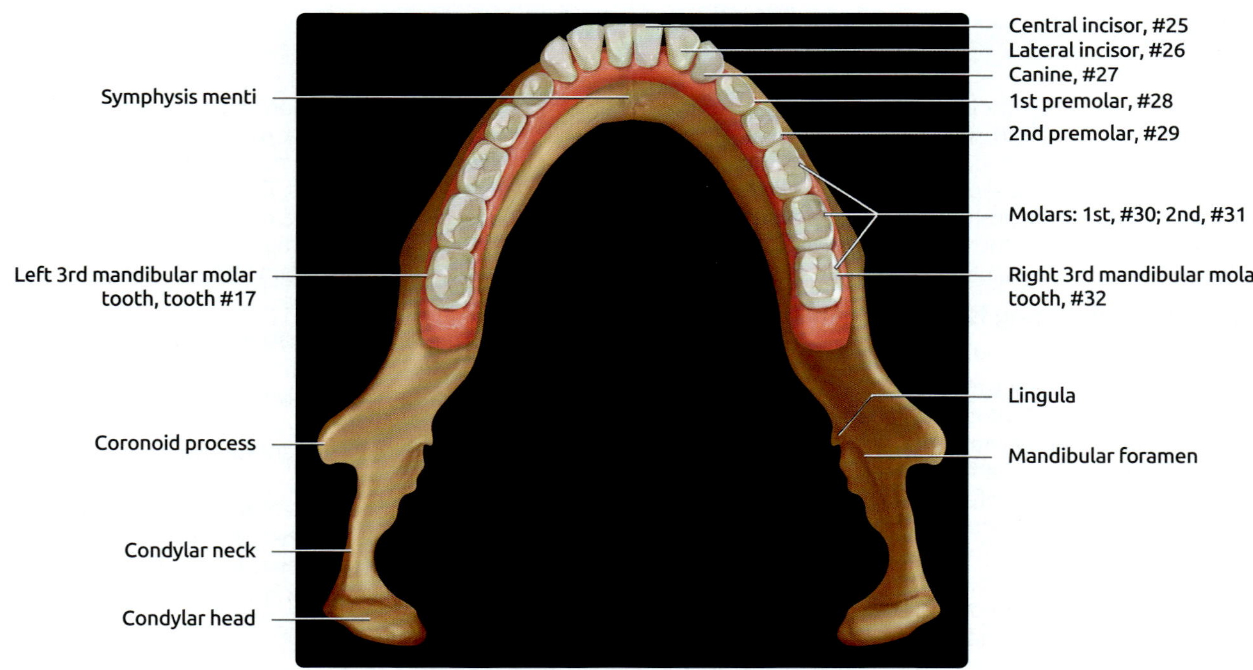

(Top) *Axial graphic of hard palate and maxillary alveolar ridge viewed from below shows the anterior premaxillary bone and the larger palatine process of the maxillary bone. Posteriorly is the horizontal plate of the palatine bone. Note the anterior midline incisive canal and the posterolateral greater and lesser palatine foramina. The alveolus is covered by attached gingiva, which is the oral mucous membrane bound to the tooth and the alveolus. The maxilla has 16 permanent teeth; numbering begins with the right 3rd molar.* **(Bottom)** *Axial graphic of mandible seen from above demonstrates the cephalad condylar head and neck leading to the more inferior ramus. The mandibular foramen is seen on the inner surface of the mandibular ramus. The cephalad projecting coronoid processes attach to the temporalis muscle tendons. The U-shaped mandibular bodies fuse in the midline at the symphysis menti. There are 16 permanent teeth, numbered beginning at the left 3rd molar from 17-32 (right 3rd molar tooth).*

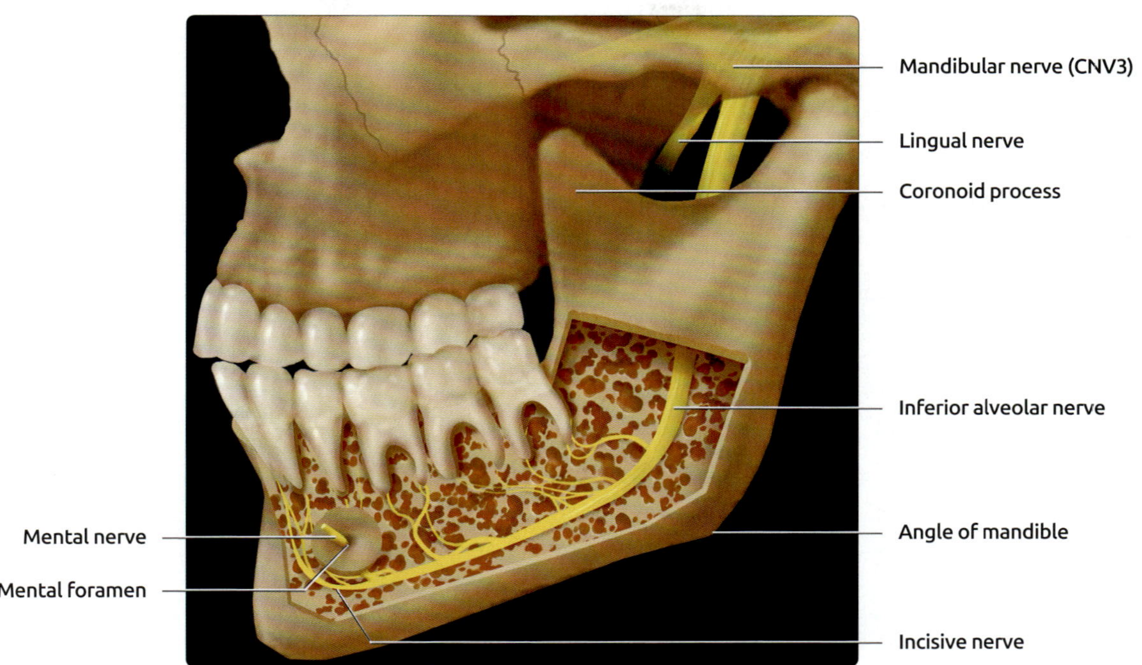

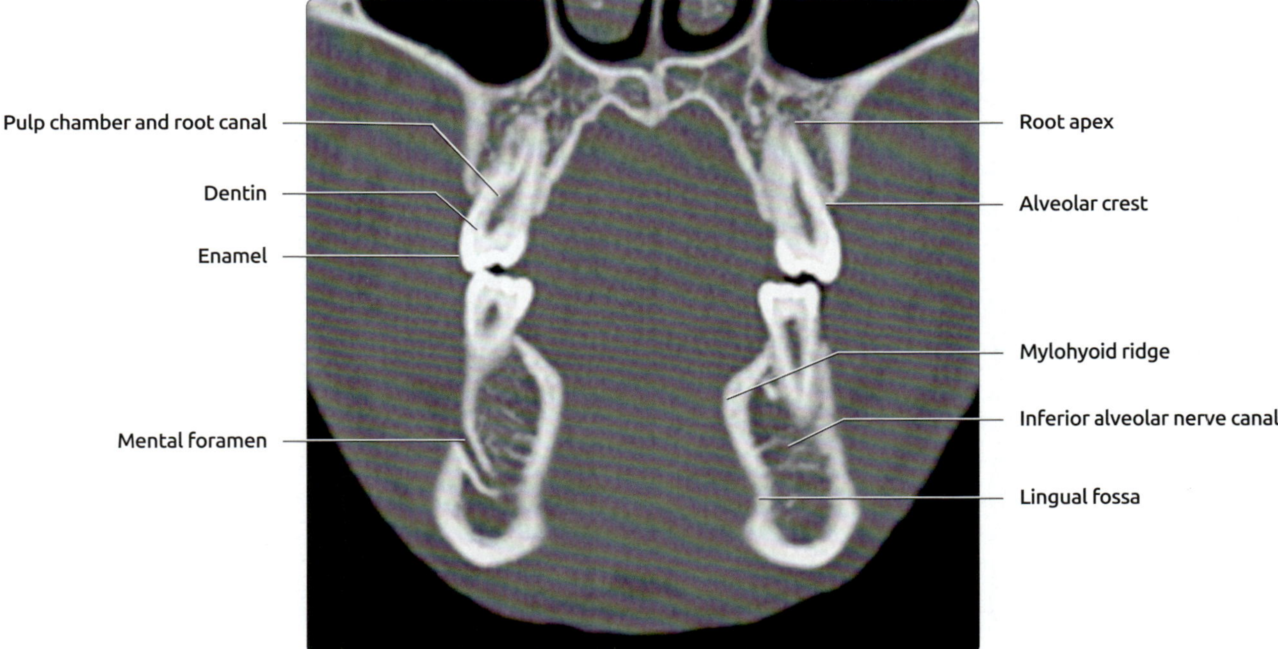

(Top) *Lateral drawing of mandible with its lateral cortex removed reveals that the mandibular nerve divides into lingual and inferior alveolar nerves. The inferior alveolar nerve divides distally into mental and incisive branches. The mental nerve branch reaches the superficial chin through the mental foramen.* **(Bottom)** *Coronal bone CT through the anterior mandible is shown. The most common lesion of the maxilla and mandible is dental infection, primarily through carious lesions involving the enamel and dentin with or without extension to the pulp. Lesions at the root apex typically result from infection transgressing the pulp. Apical lesions may also arise from infection of the periodontium with loss of bone at the alveolar crest. The jaws are the only bones with direct exposure to the external environment via the teeth. Infection from teeth may extend through the buccal or lingual cortex to adjacent spaces. The proximity of the lingual fossa to premolar or molar roots predisposes to involvement of the sublingual and submandibular space.*

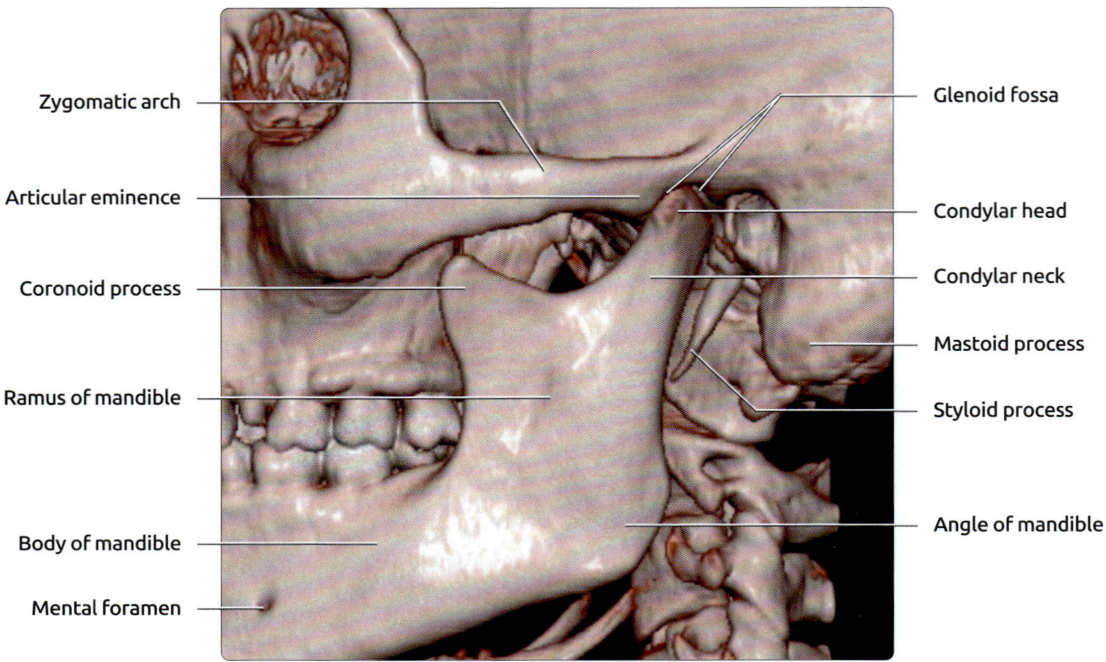

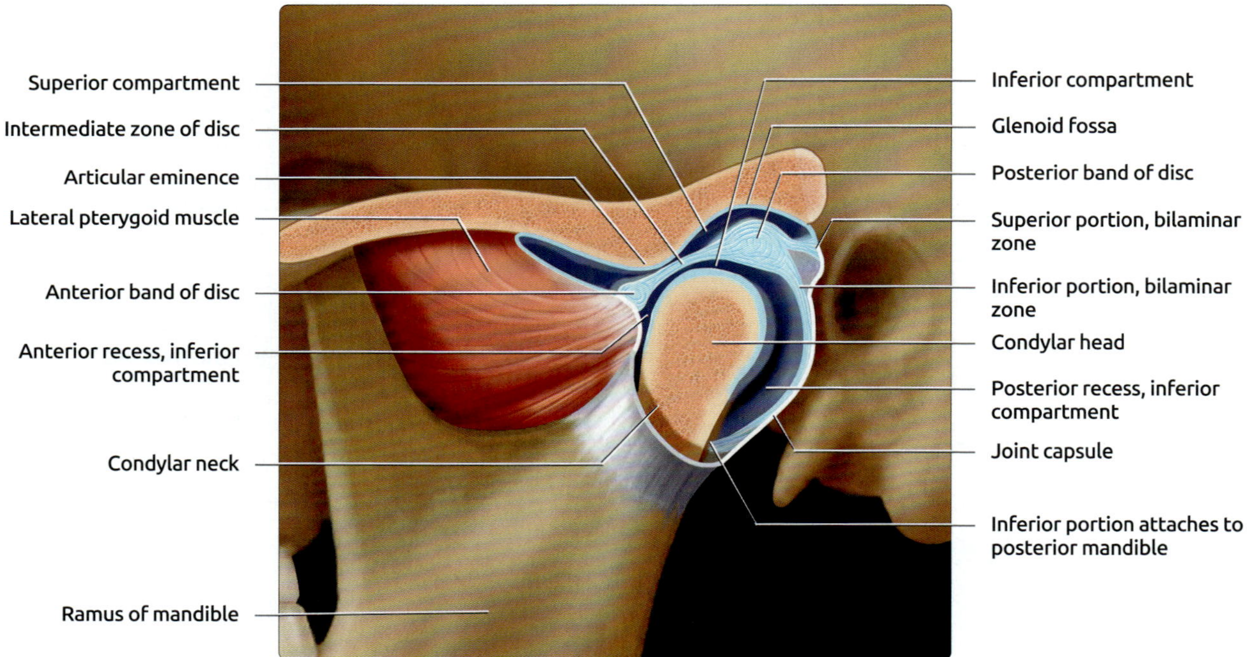

(Top) *Sagittal 3D VRT image shows the osseous anatomy of TMJ. The condylar head is situated in the glenoid fossa deep to the posterior zygomatic arch. The zygomatic arch provides some protection laterally for the TMJ in the setting of trauma. The TMJ must be fully evaluated on all mandibular trauma cases to ensure that no dislocation of the mandibular condyle has occurred.* **(Bottom)** *Magnified lateral graphic of the TMJ shows the articular disc with its anterior and posterior bands. The thinner part of the disc connecting these bands is called the intermediate zone. The disc separates the joint into a superior and an inferior compartment. Note the lateral pterygoid muscle inserting anteriorly on the joint capsule and anterior band. The posterior margin of the posterior band is referred to as the bilaminar zone, with the superior strut attaching to the posterior mandibular fossa, while the inferior strut attaches to the posterior margin of the mandibular condyle.*

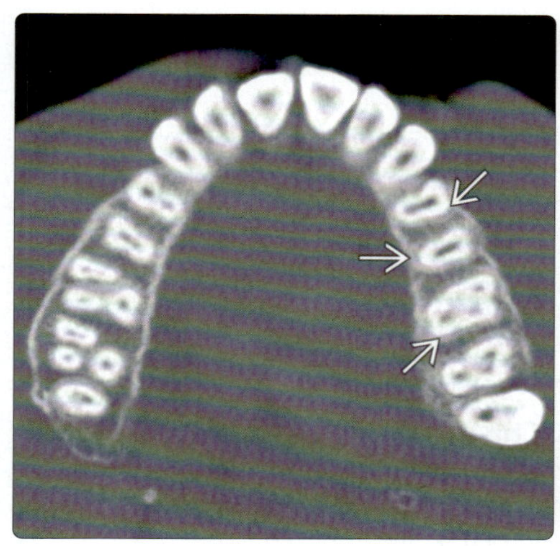

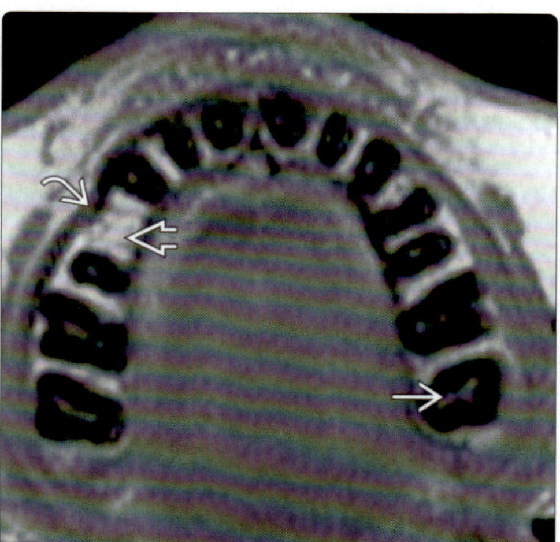

(Left) *Axial bone CT shows normal adult maxilla. Each tooth is surrounded by the periodontal ligament space containing fibers of the periodontal ligament and the lamina dura (cortical bone forming the tooth socket)* ➡. **(Right)** *Axial T1 MR shows the normal adult maxilla. Note the slightly hyperintense vascular tissue of the pulp chamber* ➡, *the normal yellow marrow* ➡, *and the attached gingiva* ➡.

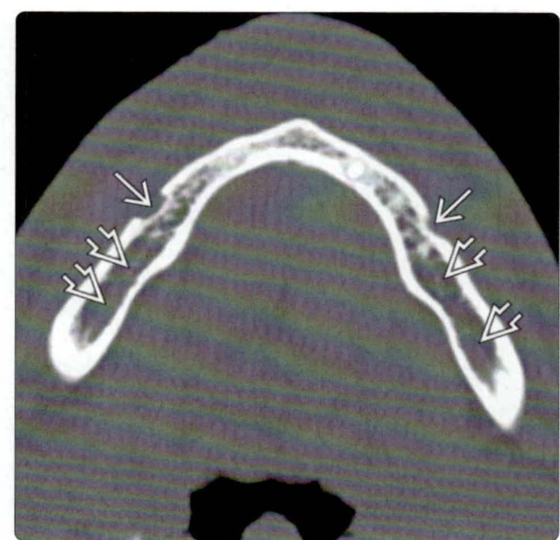

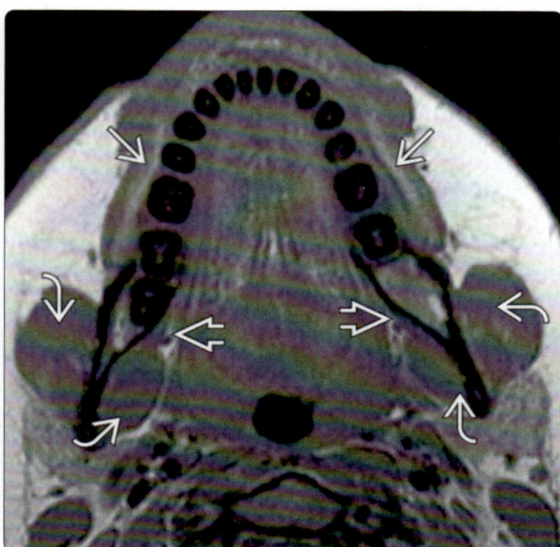

(Left) *Axial bone CT of the mandible shows bilateral mental foramen* ➡ *with inferior alveolar canals* ➡ *containing inferior alveolar nerves and arteries. The mandible is an end-artery system with ↑ risk relative to the maxilla for development of osteomyelitis, osteonecrosis, or osteoradionecrosis.* **(Right)** *Axial T1 MR shows the relationship of the mandible to the buccal vestibule/space* ➡, *masticator space* ➡, *and submandibular space* ➡, *all routes for spread of infection or tumor.*

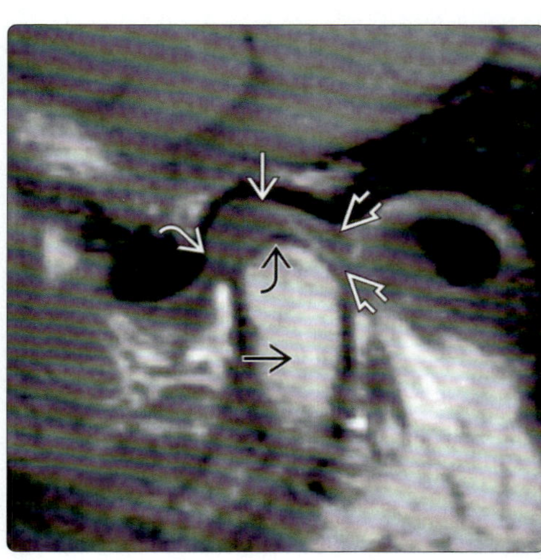

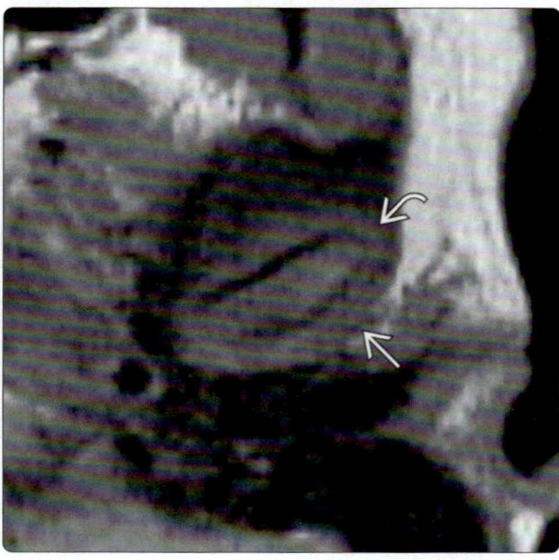

(Left) *Sagittal T1 MR shows the posterior band in normal position at about the 11 to 12 o'clock position relative to the condyle* ➡, *the intermediate zone* ➡, *and the superior and inferior struts of the bilaminar zone (retrodiscal tissue)* ➡. *Note the normal marrow signal* ➡ *and intact cortex* ➡. **(Right)** *Axial T1 MR through the left TMJ demonstrates the joint capsule surrounding the joint* ➡. *Note the auriculotemporal nerve exiting the joint space posterolaterally* ➡.

Solitary Median Maxillary Central Incisor

KEY FACTS

TERMINOLOGY

- Solitary median maxillary central incisor (SMMCI) syndrome

IMAGING

- Small, **triangle-shaped hard palate**
- **Single maxillary central incisor** in midline
- Congenital nasal pyriform aperture stenosis (CNPAS), midnasal stenosis, or choanal atresia in 90%
- ± **holoprosencephaly (HPE)**

TOP DIFFERENTIAL DIAGNOSES

- Congenital nasal pyriform aperture stenosis
  - Solitary central maxillary incisor in 60%
- Choanal atresia
  - Rarely with solitary central maxillary incisor
- Mesiodens
  - Supernumerary midline tooth develops between 2 maxillary central incisors

PATHOLOGY

- Associated with mutations in human sonic hedgehog (*SHH*) gene & deletions on chromosomes 7 & 18
- *SHH* mutations are most frequent etiology of HPE
  - SMMCI can be considered predictor or risk factor for HPE or gene carrier status

CLINICAL ISSUES

- Respiratory distress during feeding
- Hypotelorism, microcephaly, short stature, hypopituitarism
- Treatment directed toward relief of associated nasal stenosis
  - Surgical enlargement and stenting

DIAGNOSTIC CHECKLIST

- Look for SMMCI, CNPAS, or choanal atresia when imaging neonates with feeding/breathing difficulties
- If SMMCI diagnosed, be sure to check for findings of HPE

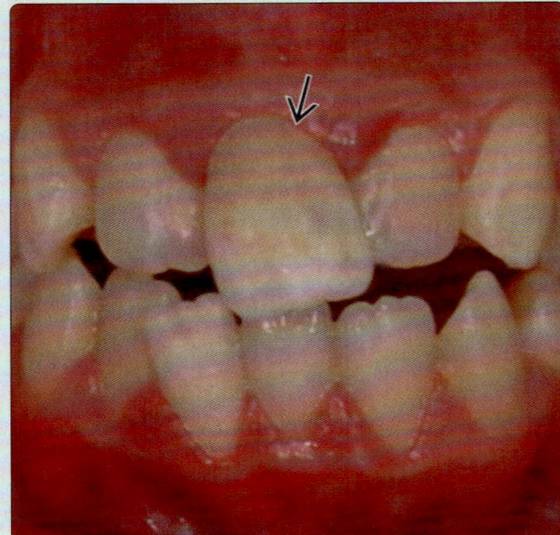

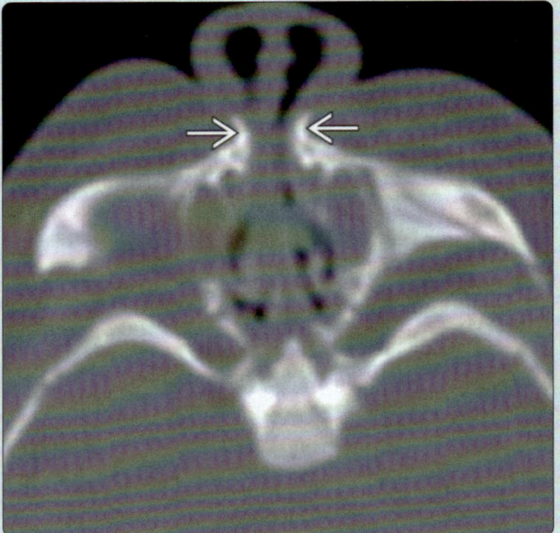

(Left) *Clinical photo is shown in a patient with a solitary median maxillary central incisor ⇨. These patients also have a small triangular hard palate (not seen) and a propensity for associated holoprosencephaly.* **(Right)** *Axial bone CT at the level of the anterior nasal inlet demonstrates pyriform aperture stenosis ➡.*

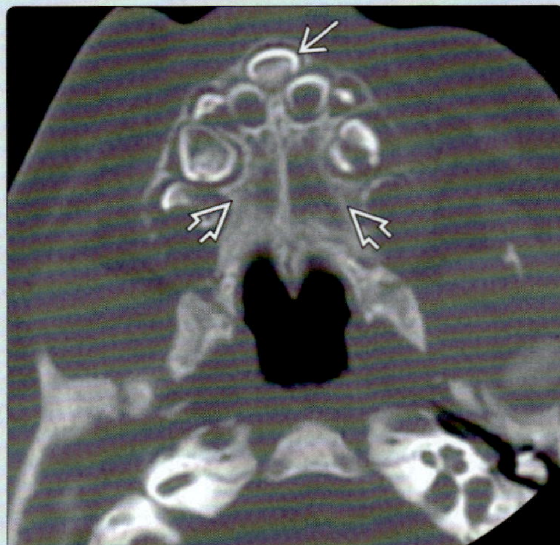

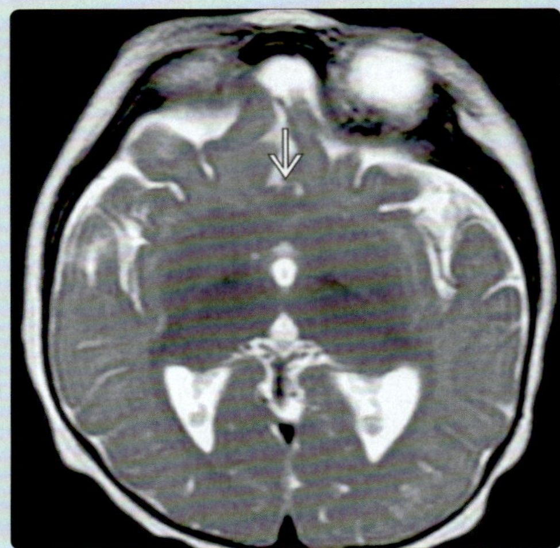

(Left) *Axial bone CT in the same patient at the level of the hard palate shows a solitary median maxillary central incisor ➡ and a small, triangle-shaped hard palate ➡.* **(Right)** *Axial T2 brain MR in the same infant shows very mild lobar holoprosencephaly with incomplete separation of hemispheres ➡.*

KEY FACTS

TERMINOLOGY

- Rare, benign, developmental cyst in nasal ala
- Synonyms: Nasoalveolar cyst, Klestadt cyst

IMAGING

- Typically < 2 cm; ≤ 10% bilateral
- Pyriform rim, between upper lip & nasal vestibule
- CT: Nonenhancing hyperdense ± dense fluid levels
  - May cause bone remodeling of maxilla as enlarges
- MR: T2 hyperintense cyst with variable T1 intensity
  - No contrast enhancement of lesion

TOP DIFFERENTIAL DIAGNOSES

- Nasopalatine duct cyst
- Nasolacrimal duct mucocele
- Periapical (radicular) cyst
- Dermoid and epidermoid of oral cavity

PATHOLOGY

- Developmental; 2 theories of pathogenesis
  - Persistence of anlage of nasolacrimal duct or inclusion cyst from formation of facial skeleton
  - Former is favored theory

CLINICAL ISSUES

- Mean age: 40 years; M:F = 1:3
- Presents as facial swelling ± nasal obstruction
- Smooth fluctuant mass, loss of nasolabial fold
- 30% present with infection: Swelling, pain, erythema
- Surgical excision is definitive treatment

DIAGNOSTIC CHECKLIST

- Extraosseous origin distinguishes from odontogenic lesions
- Look for bone erosion, extension to turbinate, or nasolacrimal duct obstruction

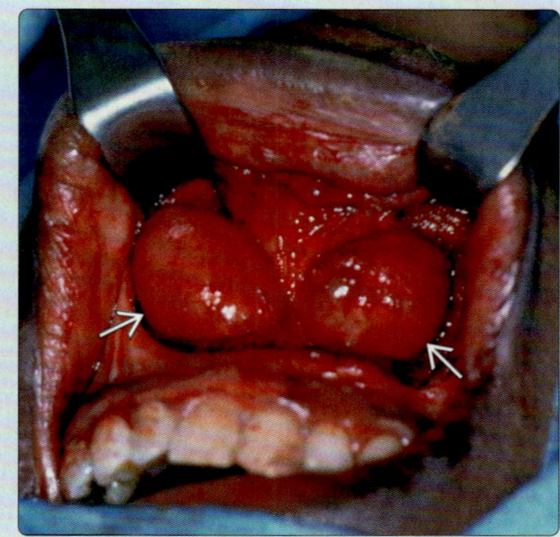

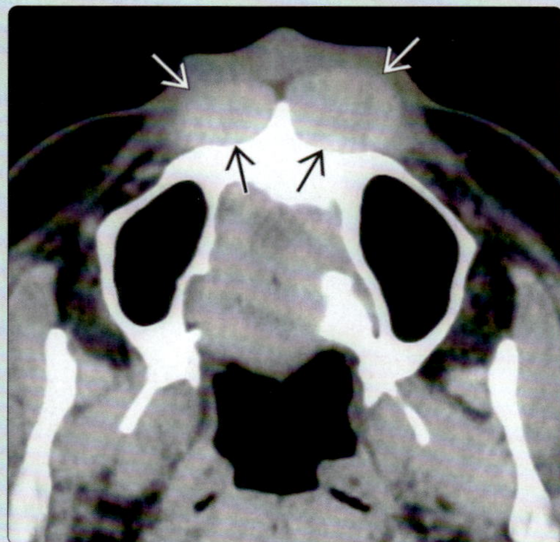

(Left) *Intraoperative photograph reveals surgically exposed bilateral nasolabial cysts ➡.* **(Right)** *Axial NECT demonstrates bilateral, well-demarcated, hyperdense rounded lesions ➡ anterior to the premaxilla. Lesions result in subtle, left greater than right, remodeling of the maxilla ⇨. Fewer than 10% of nasolabial cyst cases are bilateral.*

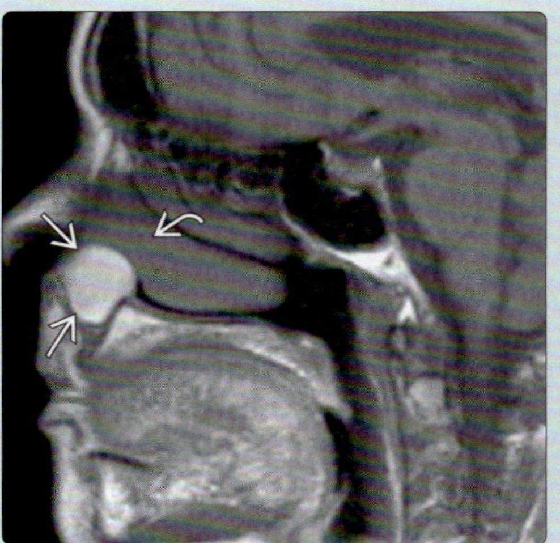

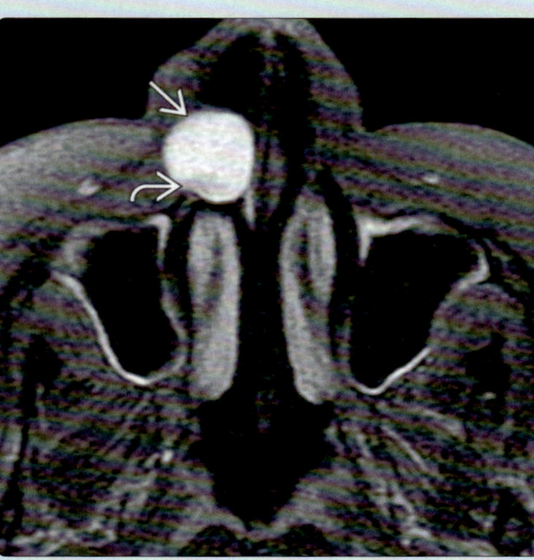

(Left) *Sagittal T1 MR shows a sharply marginated, diffusely hyperintense nasolabial cyst ➡. Note the proximity of the superior aspect of the lesion to the inferior turbinate ➡ and floor of the nasal vestibule. On exam, these were submucosal masses.* **(Right)** *Axial T2 FS MR reveals typical homogeneous round T2 hyperintensity of the nasolabial cyst ➡ with subtly hypointense proteinaceous debris ➡.*

Periapical Cyst (Radicular)

KEY FACTS

TERMINOLOGY

- Synonym = radicular cyst
- **Most common odontogenic cyst**
- Periapical rarefying osteitis = newer term to include periapical cyst, periapical granuloma, and periapical abscess

IMAGING

- Bone CT findings
  - **Ovoid cyst at apex of nonvital tooth**
  - Millimeters to ≤ 1 cm usually
  - Ovoid to round corticated lucency associated with tooth apex
  - May see dental caries: Enamel ± crown erosion
  - If infected in maxillary tooth, may see odontogenic sinusitis

TOP DIFFERENTIAL DIAGNOSES

- Lateral periodontal cyst
- Keratocystic odontogenic tumor
- Dentigerous (follicular) cyst

PATHOLOGY

- Develops after inflammation and necrosis of pulp ("nonvital" tooth)
  - Most often from dental caries, periodontal disease
  - Less often posttraumatic
- Pulp necrosis → growth of epithelial rests of Malassez in periodontal ligament

CLINICAL ISSUES

- Most commonly found on dental radiographs
- Usually asymptomatic unless secondary infection
- Infection → intermittent intense jaw pain
- May progress to periapical abscess ± cellulitis

DIAGNOSTIC CHECKLIST

- Report relationship of lesion to important structures
  - Maxillary teeth: Maxillary sinus
  - Mandible: Inferior alveolar nerve canal

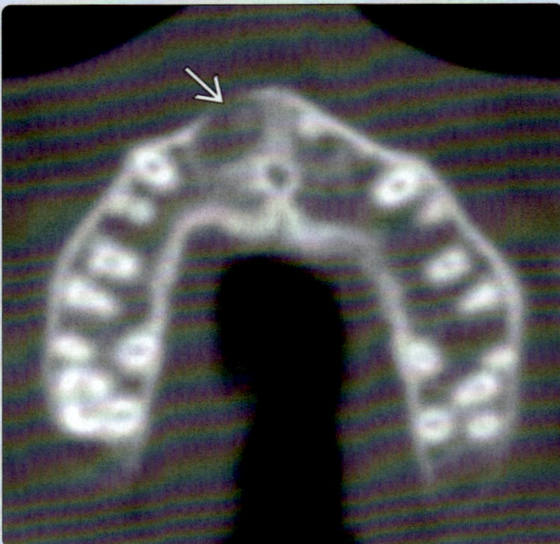
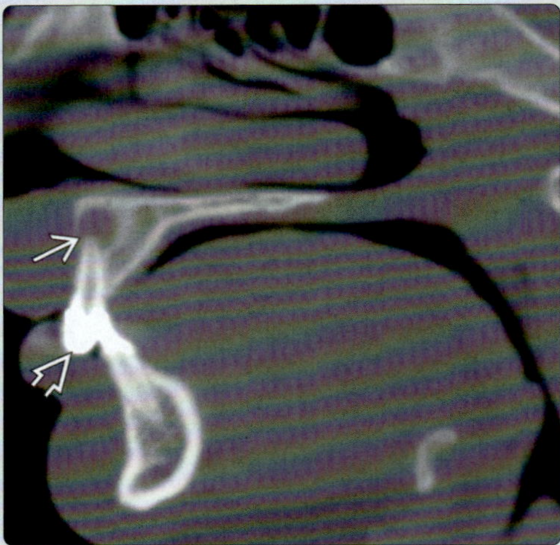

(Left) *Axial bone CT demonstrates a small periapical radicular cyst ➡ associated with the right maxillary central incisor, without periosteal reaction or extraosseous soft tissue mass.* **(Right)** *Sagittal reformatted bone CT in the same patient shows the periapical cyst ➡ and dental amalgam ➡ in the same tooth.*

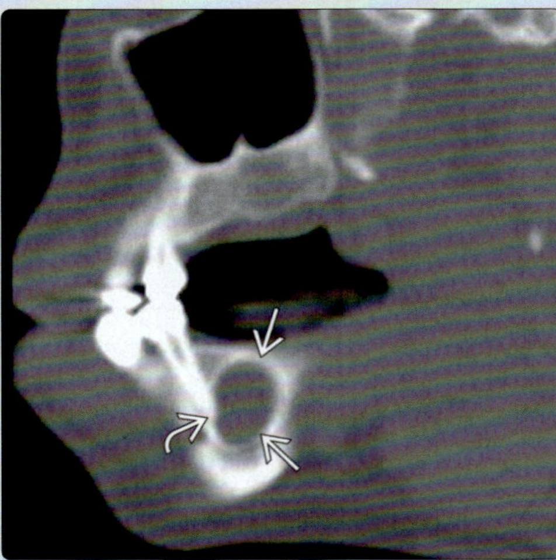
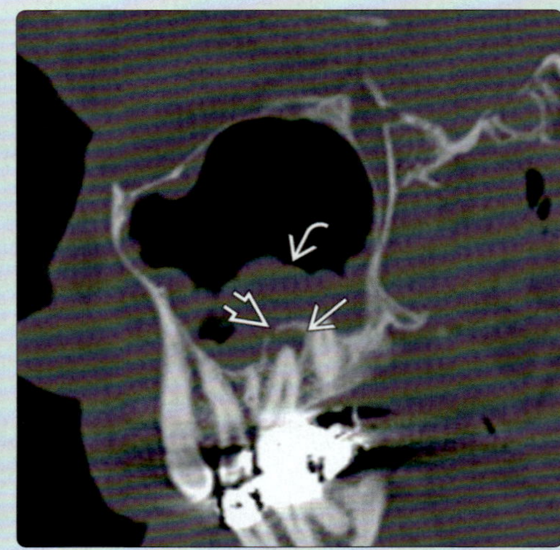

(Left) *Sagittal reformatted bone CT shows a well-corticated unilocular cyst ➡ at the root apex of the right mandibular 1st premolar tooth. The cyst is contiguous with lamina dura and periodontal ligament space ➡, indicating it is likely of inflammatory origin.* **(Right)** *Sagittal reformatted bone CT shows a moderate-sized maxillary periapical cyst ➡ with a focal dehiscence ➡ in the cyst roof and associated inferior maxillary sinus odontogenic sinusitis ➡.*

Dentigerous Cyst

KEY FACTS

TERMINOLOGY

- Definition: Benign developmental jaw cyst associated with crown of unerupted tooth
- Synonym: Follicular cyst

IMAGING

- Well-circumscribed, expansile cyst **surrounding crown of unerupted or impacted tooth**
- **Unilocular** cyst even when large
- Sclerotic border spares osseous cortex
- Typically displaces teeth, rarely resorbs
- 75% found in mandible
  - Mandibular 3rd molars > maxillary 3rd molars > maxillary canines

TOP DIFFERENTIAL DIAGNOSES

- Keratocystic odontogenic tumor
- Ameloblastoma
- Periapical (radicular) cyst

PATHOLOGY

- Arises after developmental anomaly during formation of enamel (amelogenesis)
- Cyst wall attached to tooth at cementoenamel junction and forms collar
- Slow-growing benign cyst
- 20% of all odontogenic cysts

CLINICAL ISSUES

- Clinical presentation
  - Most patients asymptomatic
  - Symptomatic if cyst infection or fracture
  - Ameloblastomas may develop in cyst wall
- Treatment options
  - Enucleation of cyst & extraction of unerupted tooth
  - Recurrence rare following complete resection
  - Marsupialization or fenestration of cyst may preserve permanent tooth in children

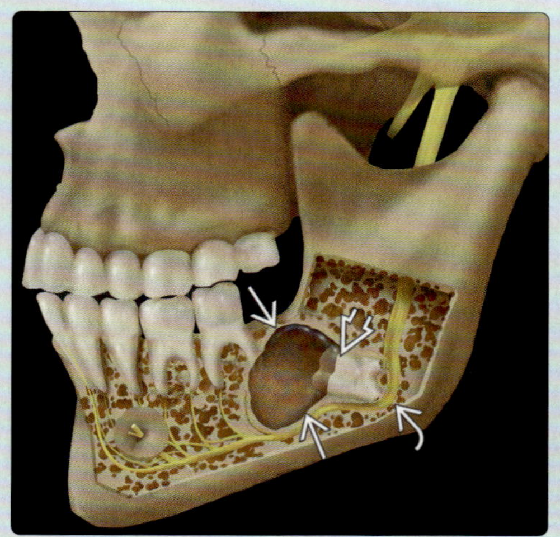

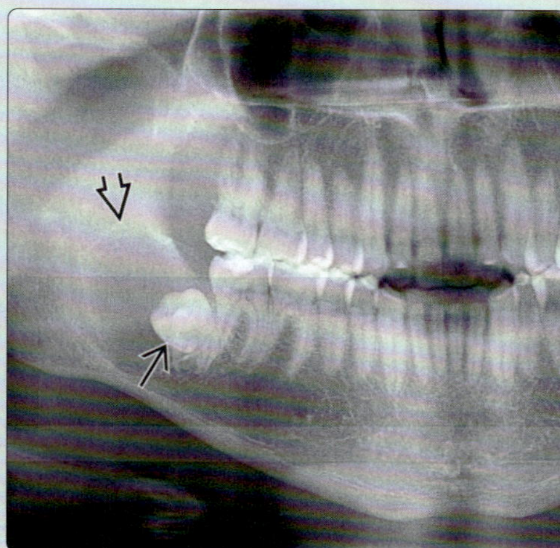

(Left) *Lateral graphic of the mandible with the lateral cortical surface removed depicts a classic unilocular dentigerous cyst ➡ intimately related to the crown ➡ of the unerupted 3rd mandibular molar tooth. The inferior alveolar nerve ➡ is displaced by the molar.* **(Right)** *This orthopantomograph shows a misplaced mandibular 3rd molar (#32) ➡ with a radiolucent unilocular cyst ➡ originating near the crown-root junction and surrounding the tooth crown. This is the typical appearance of a dentigerous cyst.*

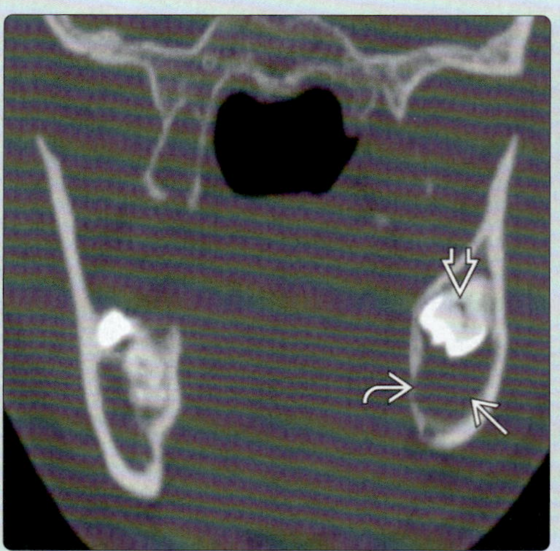

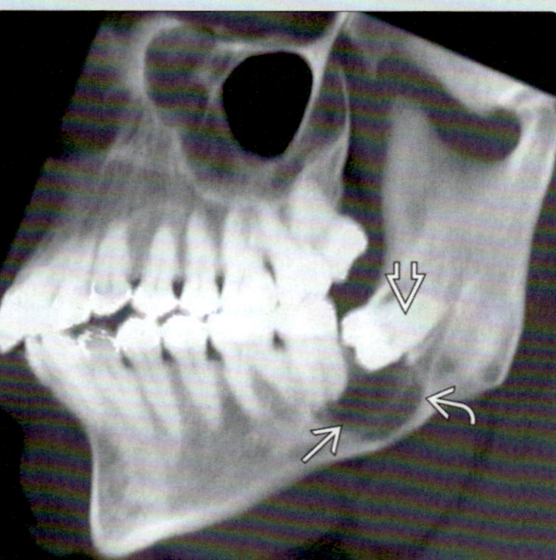

(Left) *Coronal bone CT demonstrates an impacted left 3rd mandibular molar ➡ associated with the smooth-walled cyst ➡ that expands the mandible and thins the lingual cortex ➡. The cyst abuts the crown and has no calcifications or periosteal reaction.* **(Right)** *Ray-sum CT rendering depicts the appearance of a classic dentigerous cyst. The impacted mandibular molar ➡ has a well-defined unilocular cyst ➡ adjacent to the crown. The cyst and molar displace the inferior alveolar canal ➡ inferiorly.*

Simple Bone Cyst (Traumatic)

KEY FACTS

TERMINOLOGY

- Solitary bony cavity; "cyst" designation is misnomer

IMAGING

- CT: Solitary well-corticated, lucent area in body, ramus, or condyle of mandible
  - Homogeneously iso- to hypodense with no internal calcification or matrix
- T2 MR: Hyperintense; no fluid-fluid levels
- T1 C+ MR: Delayed enhancement key

TOP DIFFERENTIAL DIAGNOSES

- Aneurysmal bone cyst
- Periapical (radicular) cyst
- Giant cell granuloma of mandible-maxilla
- Keratocystic odontogenic tumor
- Unicystic ameloblastoma

PATHOLOGY

- Cystic cavity with connective tissue membrane; no epithelial lining
- "Traumatic" designation misnomer; < 1/2 associated with prior trauma
- May be found adjacent to osteomas, fibroosseous lesions, hypercementosis

CLINICAL ISSUES

- Incidental finding on imaging
- 10-30 years
- Variable but low recurrence rate reported
- Treatment: Surgical exploration to exclude other odontogenic lesions

DIAGNOSTIC CHECKLIST

- Look for association with teeth, cortical thinning and erosion, enhancement pattern to exclude other odontogenic lesions

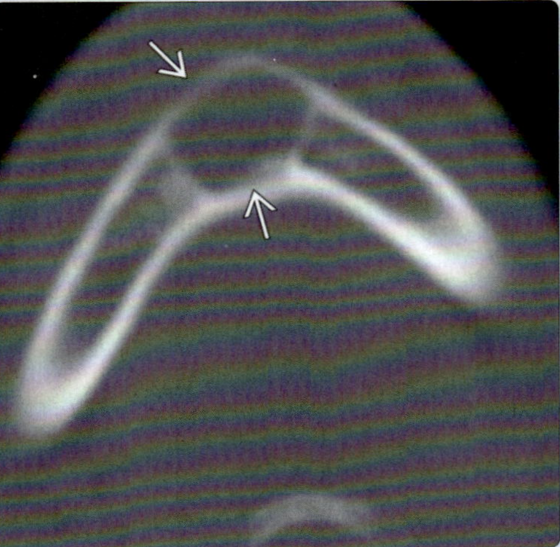

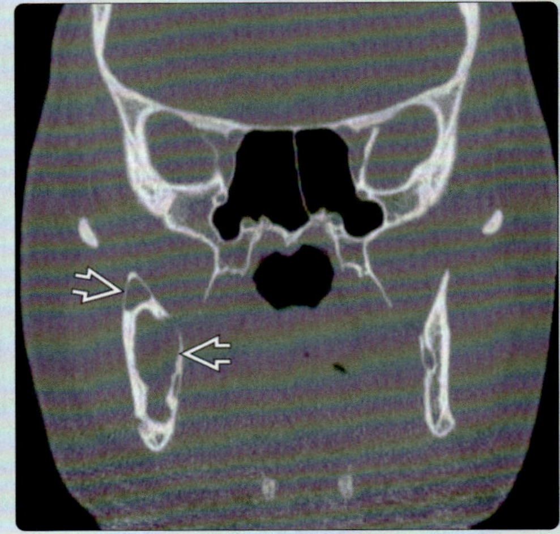

(Left) *Axial bone CT shows a unilocular simple bone cyst in the symphyseal mandible with a well-defined, corticated cortex ➡. Despite the size, there is no significant bony expansion.* **(Right)** *Coronal bone CT demonstrates a lucent ➡ right mandibular lesion involving/expanding the posterior mandibular body, angle, and ramus. The cortex is thinned over the lucent component but intact over the sclerotic component. There is a thin lucent zone surrounding the sclerotic component.*

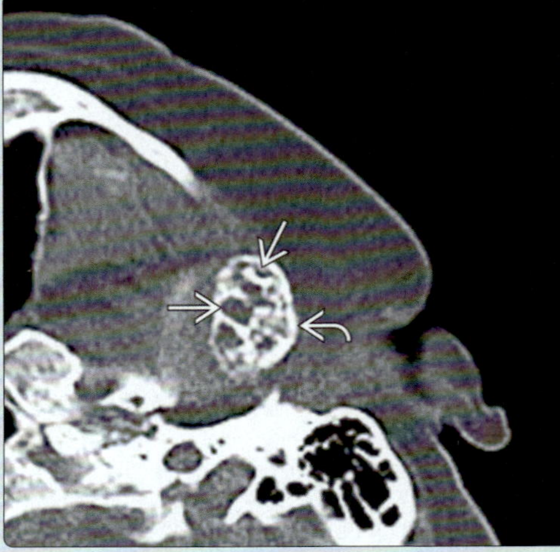

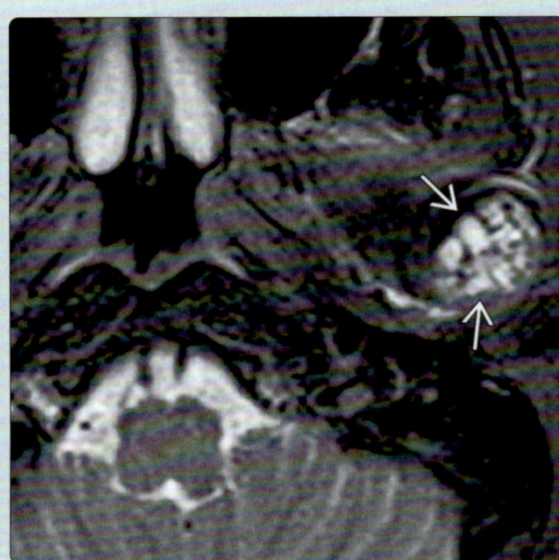

(Left) *Axial bone CT shows multiple cystic foci in the mandibular condyle ➡ with thickened and intact septations. Note the cortex is also intact ➡. The differential for this appearance necessarily includes aneurysmal bone cyst and central giant cell granuloma.* **(Right)** *Axial T2 FS MR in the same patient shows the typical hyperintensity of the cystic cavities ➡ without fluid-fluid levels. At surgical exploration, the diagnosis of simple bone cyst was made.*

KEY FACTS

TERMINOLOGY

- Definition: Developmental cyst arising from nasopalatine duct

IMAGING

- Bone CT findings
  - Well-circumscribed, rounded enlargement of maxillary incisive canal
  - Incisive canal with diameter **> 1 cm** is presumed nasopalatine duct cyst
  - Lamina dura and periodontal ligament space of adjacent teeth intact
- MR findings
  - Homogeneously iso- to hyperintense T1, hyperintense T2 signal
  - Typically nonenhancing

TOP DIFFERENTIAL DIAGNOSES

- Periapical (radicular) cyst
- Residual cyst
- Apical periodontitis
- Median palatal cyst
- Keratocystic odontogenic tumor
- Dentigerous (follicular) cyst

CLINICAL ISSUES

- Most common nonodontogenic fissural cyst
- Clinical presentation
  - Incidental finding on CT or MR
  - Less commonly pain, swelling of anterior maxilla
- Treatment: Enucleation via palatine or buccal approach
  - Recurrence rate very low

DIAGNOSTIC CHECKLIST

- Single rounded corticated lucent cyst in midline maxilla
- Look for widening along paired nasopalatine ducts
- Report extension to nasal cavity or displacement of teeth by larger lesions

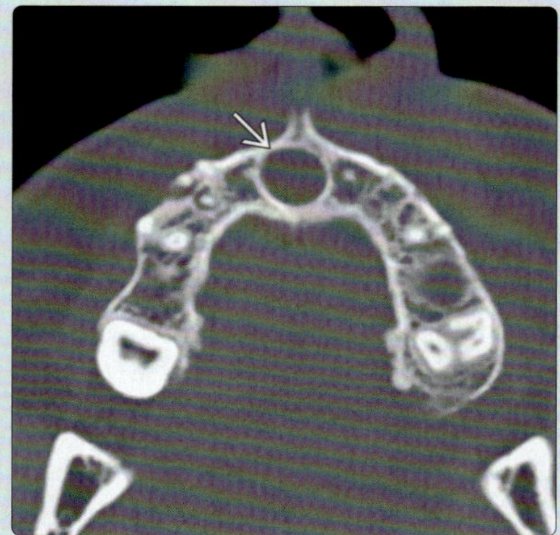

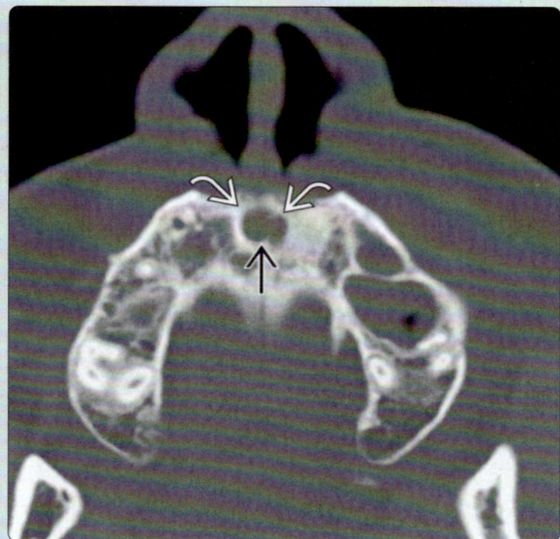

(Left) *Axial bone CT shows a corticated uniform and concentric expansion of the incisive canal in the midline maxillary alveolus ➡, typical of nasopalatine duct cyst.* **(Right)** *Axial bone CT shows an expansile nasopalatine duct cyst extending superiorly along the paired nasopalatine ducts ➡, which are seen separated here by a very thin bony septation ➡.*

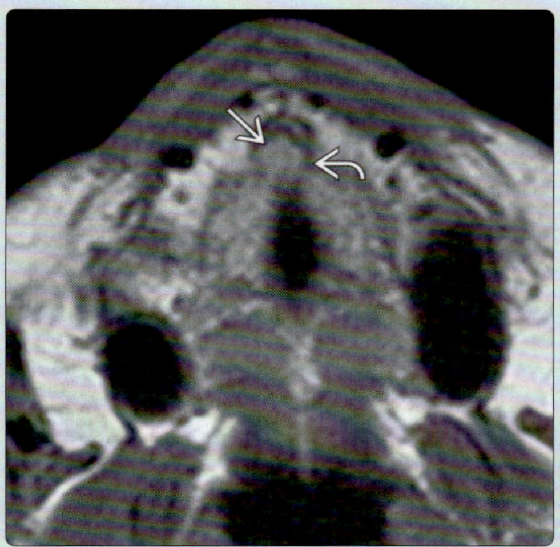

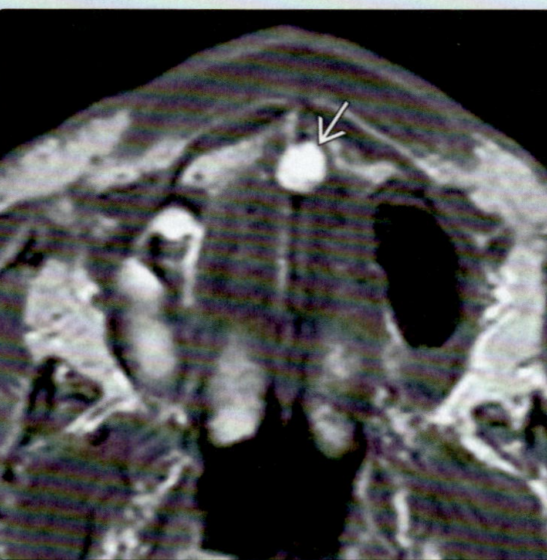

(Left) *Axial T1 MR shows an intermediate to slightly T1-hyperintense expansion of the incisive canal ➡ by a nasopalatine duct cyst. Note the thin but preserved cortex ➡.* **(Right)** *Axial T2 MR shows the classic MR appearance of a nasopalatine duct cyst. Note the uniformly round, homogeneously T2 hyperintense area in the midline maxilla ➡.*

TMJ Juvenile Idiopathic Arthritis

KEY FACTS

TERMINOLOGY

- Juvenile idiopathic arthritis (JIA)
- **Autoimmune** musculoskeletal synovial inflammatory disease of childhood

IMAGING

- Bone CT best demonstrates contours of TMJ
  - Flat, deformed mandibular condyles and wide, flat condylar fossae
  - Condyle concavity or bifid
  - Bilateral disease more common than unilateral
  - May have secondary osteoarthritis with osteophytes
- MR may show joint space enhancement and early inflammation before joint destruction
  - TMJ discs thin, perforated, or absent
- In cervical spine, may see atlantoaxial subluxation, vertebral fusion, and ↓ AP vertebral body dimension

TOP DIFFERENTIAL DIAGNOSES

- TMJ condylar hypoplasia
- TMJ degenerative disease
- TMJ synovitis/capsulitis

CLINICAL ISSUES

- JIA affects 1-22 per 1,000 children worldwide
- TMJ involved in 20-90% of children with JIA
  - More likely if systemic disease, young age at diagnosis, and long duration of activity
- TMJ and masticator muscle pain, decreased range of jaw motion, retrognathia, micrognathia
- **70% asymptomatic** when MR shows acute arthritis
- Treat with either or both local &/or systemic therapy
  - Local: Occlusal devices, arthrocentesis, intraarticular injections
  - Systemic: NSAIDs, methotrexate, sulfasalazine

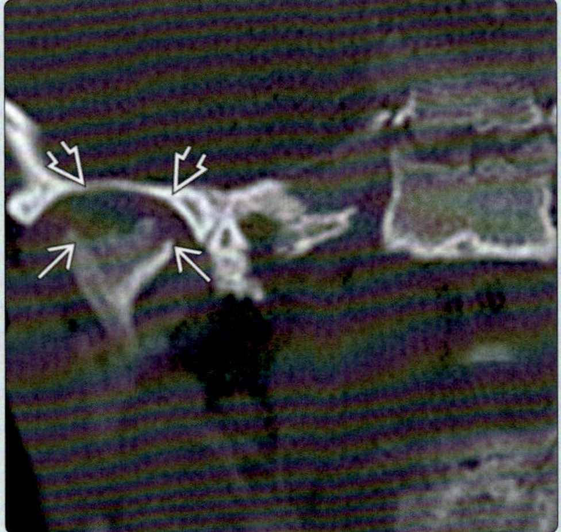

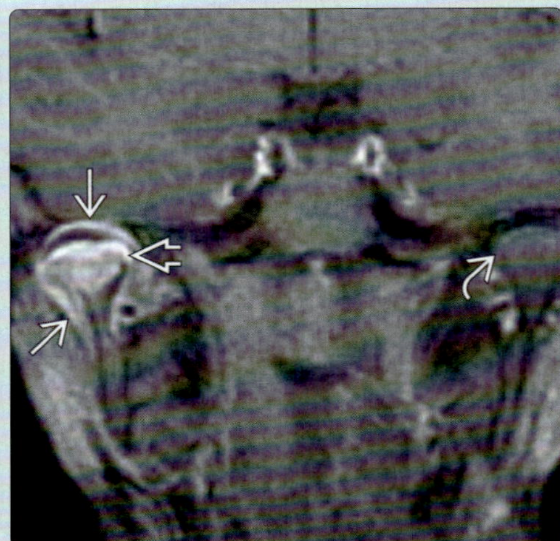

(Left) *Coronal bone CT in a 4-year-old girl with juvenile idiopathic arthritis (JIA) demonstrates irregular chronic erosion of the right mandibular condyle ➡. Note also the wide, flattened condylar fossa ➡.* **(Right)** *Coronal T1 C+ FS MR in the same child with JIA reveals marked inflammatory enhancement involving the joint ➡ and marrow space of the right mandibular condyle ➡. The left TMJ ➡ shows no inflammatory change, normal condyle, and normal condylar fossa.*

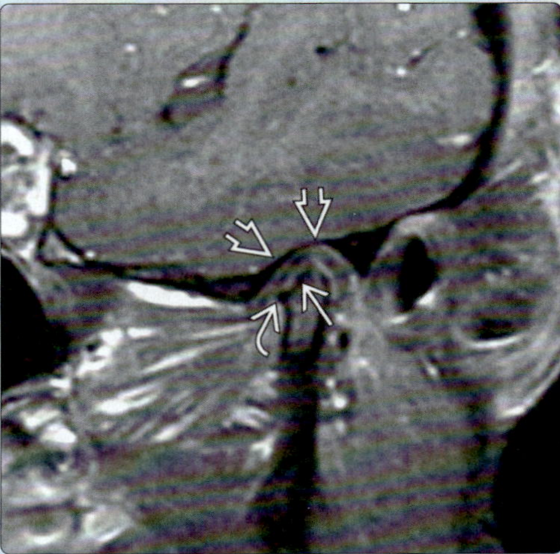

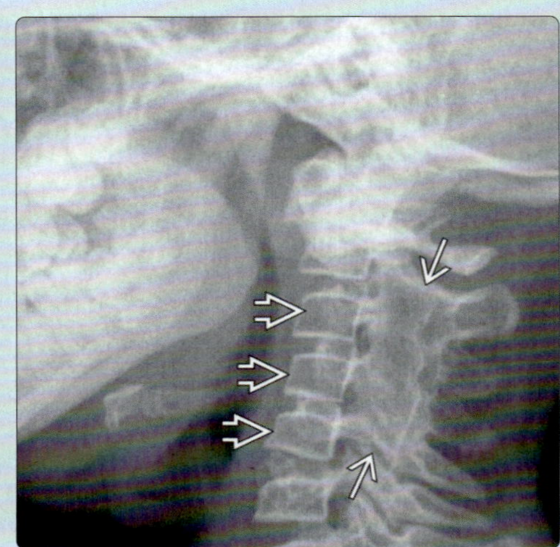

(Left) *Sagittal oblique T1 C+ FS MR in a 21-year-old woman with longstanding JIA reveals a small mandibular condyle with irregular, low-intensity sclerotic margins ➡ and a widened, flat condylar fossa ➡. There is no inflammatory enhancement but note the small anterior osteophyte ➡ from secondary osteoarthritis.* **(Right)** *Lateral radiograph in a 13-year-old girl with JIA demonstrates classic fusion of posterior elements of C2-C5 ➡ and decreased AP dimension of corresponding vertebral bodies ➡.*

KEY FACTS

TERMINOLOGY

- Definition: Polymicrobial bacterial infection, usually odontogenic, of mandible > maxilla

IMAGING

- CECT/bone CT findings
  - **Acute osteomyelitis**
    - Bone destruction, tooth/socket abnormality ± associated soft tissue abscess
      - Mandibular molar osteomyelitis → masticator space abscess
      - Body of mandible osteomyelitis → submandibular or sublingual space abscess
  - **Chronic osteomyelitis**
    - Bone sclerosis with periosteal reaction ± sequestrum
- Contrast-enhanced MR findings
  - MR sensitive for acute and chronic osteomyelitis
  - Shows full extent of mandible marrow involvement
  - If dental amalgam obscures CT, MR may show subtle abscess formation not seen by CT
- Serial exams may be necessary to confirm osteomyelitis and document positive clinical response

TOP DIFFERENTIAL DIAGNOSES

- Mandible-maxilla osteoradionecrosis
- Mandible-maxilla bisphosphonate osteochemonecrosis
- Infiltrative neoplasm invading mandible
- Primary chronic osteomyelitis
- Langerhans histiocytosis, mandible-maxilla

CLINICAL ISSUES

- Clinical presentation
  - Pain, swelling, and tenderness of jaw
- Treatment options
  - Acute: Oral ± IV antibiotics; abscess drainage
  - Chronic: Surgical debridement, may need free tissue transfer bony reconstruction, hyperbaric oxygen

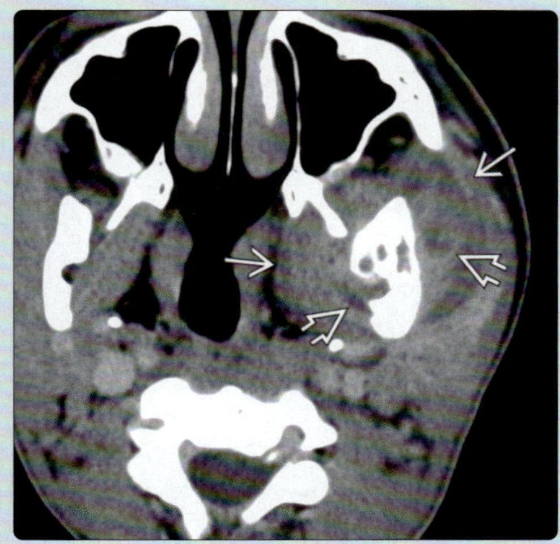

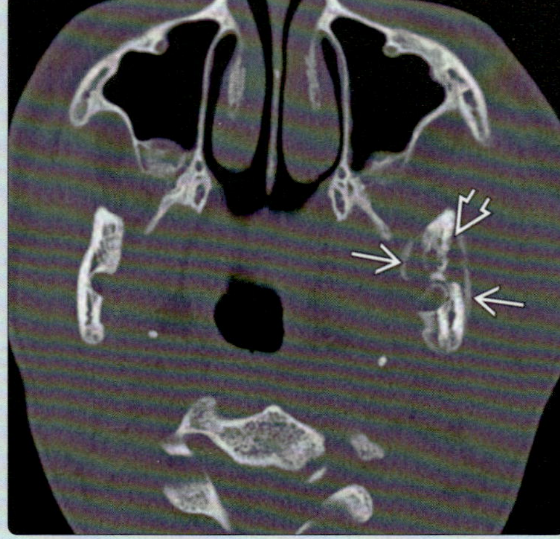

(Left) *Axial CECT in a 15 year old with previous surgical repair of a mandibular fracture, now with swelling and pain in the left cheek reveals marked inflammation of left masticator space ➡. The foci of low density represent early transformation of phlegmon to abscess ➡.* **(Right)** *Axial bone CT in the same patient shows periosteal reaction along the cortex of the mandibular ramus ➡ and both permeative and sclerotic bone changes centrally ➡. These findings suggest osteomyelitis.*

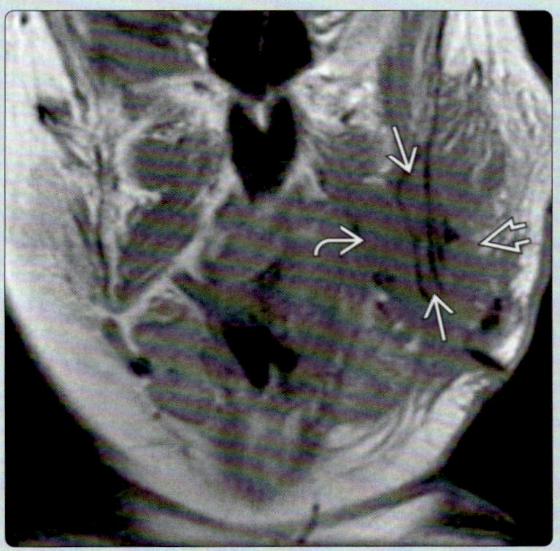

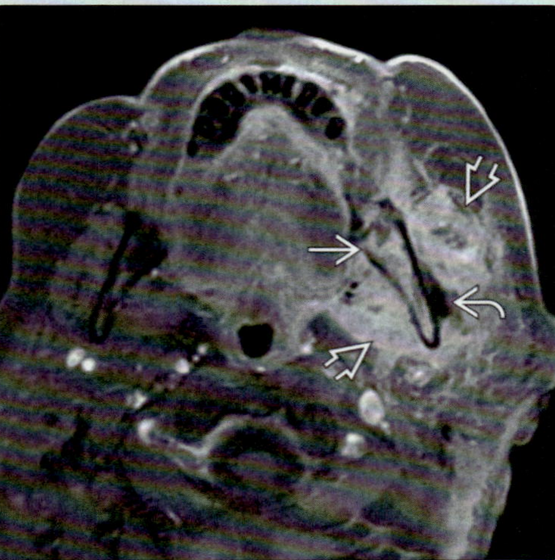

(Left) *Coronal T1WI MR shows a 79 year old with recurrent masticator space abscess 12 weeks after initial diagnosis and drainage. Normal high-signal marrow fat has been replaced ➡ in the left hemimandible, consistent with osteomyelitis. Note edema in the medial pterygoid ➡ and masseter ➡ muscles.* **(Right)** *Axial T1WI C+ FS MR in the same patient reveals diffuse enhancement of the left marrow space ➡ with masticator space enhancement (phlegmon) ➡ and small lateral compartment abscess ➡.*

KEY FACTS

TERMINOLOGY

- Calcium pyrophosphate deposition disease (**CPPD**)
- **Metabolic disease** resulting in peri- or intraarticular **chondrocalcinosis**
  - **Tophaceous (tumoral)** TMJ form most prevalent
- Synonym: Pseudogout

IMAGING

- Calcified TMJ lesion
  - May involve **masticator** or parotid space or adjacent skull base
- Bone CT
  - Mild/early CPPD: Subtle calcifications in TMJ
  - Late/severe CPPD →
    - Chunky **diffusely calcified** mass
    - Calcified mass may have **ground-glass** appearance
    - Associated remodeling, erosion, or mass effect on condyle
  - **50%** have involvement of **multiple joints**
- MR
  - T1: **Low-** to intermediate-signal lesion; capsule & joint space expansion
  - T2: **Hypointense**, somewhat heterogeneous mass
  - T1 C+: Heterogeneously enhancing TMJ lesion

TOP DIFFERENTIAL DIAGNOSES

- Synovial chondromatosis
- Pigmented villonodular synovitis
- Chondroblastoma
- Chondrosarcoma

PATHOLOGY

- **Calcium pyrophosphate crystals** in synovial fluid are **diagnostic**
  - In polarized light, crystals are **birefringent**

CLINICAL ISSUES

- Presenting symptoms: Preauricular pain & swelling
- Treatment: Surgical excision + arthrocentesis

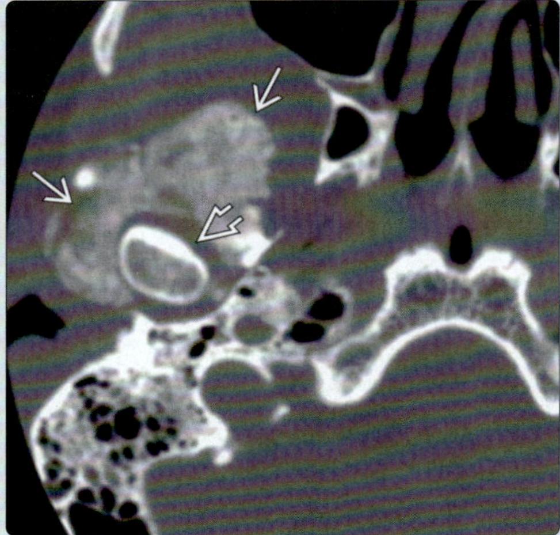

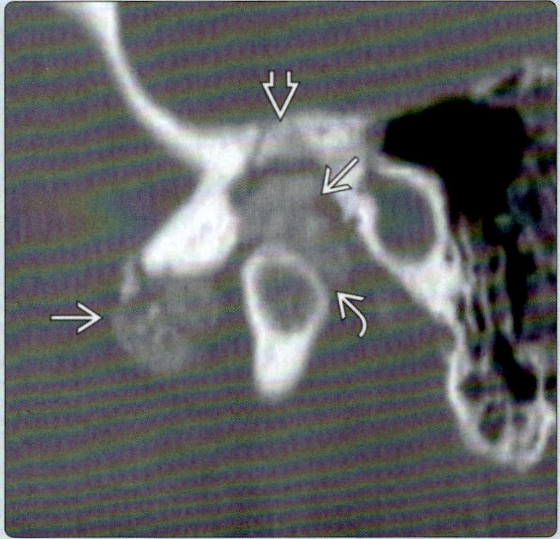

(Left) *Axial bone CT through the skull base reveals extensive calcific density surrounding the condyle and neck of the right mandible* ➡. *Note sparing of the joint space around the condyle* ➡. **(Right)** *Sagittal bone CT reformation in the same patient better delineates the calcifications* ➡ *in relation to the TMJ. Note condylar fossa demineralization and erosion* ➡, *resulting in a defect of the middle cranial fossa. The inferior joint space is compressed but spared* ➡.

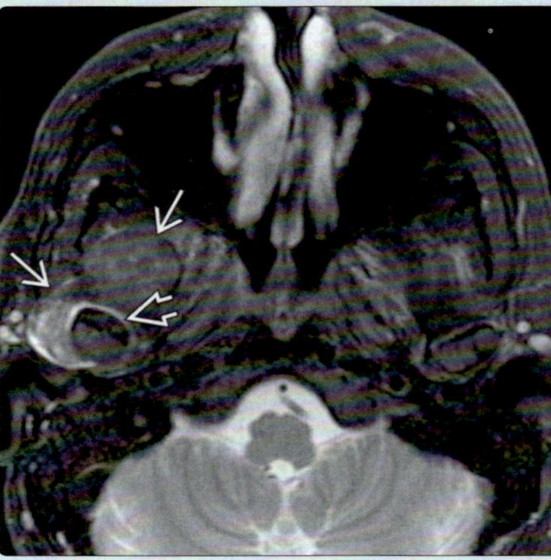

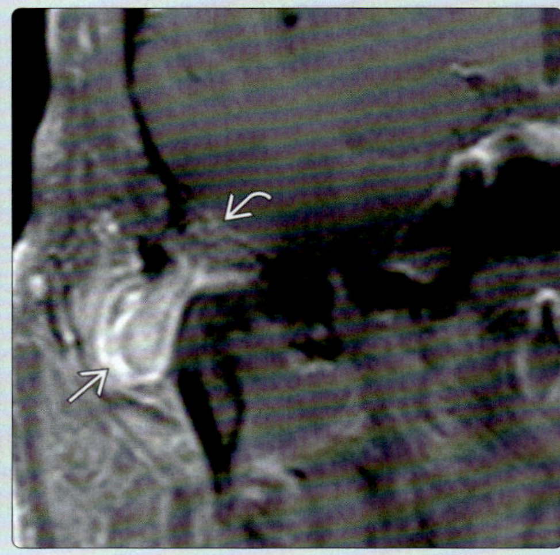

(Left) *Axial T2 FS MR in a patient with calcium pyrophosphate deposition disease in the right TMJ shows heterogeneous but predominantly low-signal intensity lesion* ➡ *along the margins of the TMJ. Note joint space fluid around the head of the mandibular condyle* ➡. **(Right)** *Coronal T1 C+ FS MR shows enhancement of the inferolateral mass* ➡. *Note the glenoid fossa defect and mild dural enhancement* ➡ *without overt intracranial extension.*

TMJ Pigmented Villonodular Synovitis

KEY FACTS

TERMINOLOGY

- Definition: Benign, locally aggressive, tumefactive disease of synovium

IMAGING

- CT: **Erosion** of mandibular **condyle** ± glenoid fossa
  - Lobulated, rounded lytic lesions
  - May extend to greater wing of sphenoid, temporal bone, intracranially
- T1 MR: **Hypointense** to isointense nodules with peripheral rim of low signal
- T2 MR: **Hypointense** lobulated nodules ± cystic areas of hyperintensity &/or joint effusion
  - Hypointensity due to **hemosiderin** deposition
    - Associated blooming artifact characteristic
- T1 C+ MR: Portions of mass may show mild enhancement
- Best imaging tool: Dedicated C+ MR & thin bone CT
- Interpretation pearl: T1/T2-hypointense joint nodules within TMJ are **noncalcified** on NECT

TOP DIFFERENTIAL DIAGNOSES

- Synovial chondromatosis
  - **Calcified nodules** in TMJ
- Calcium pyrophosphate dihydrate deposition disease
- Giant cell tumor
- Chondrosarcoma

PATHOLOGY

- Etiology: Unknown
  - Monarticular hyperplastic TMJ inflammation
- Plump histiocytes with **giant cells** + **hemosiderin**
- **Radiologic-pathologic correlation** important since histology may mimic sarcoma

CLINICAL ISSUES

- Presenting symptoms: Preauricular pain, swelling, trismus
- Age: 2nd-4th decades
- Gender: F:M = 3:1; recent data suggests F ~ M
- Treatment: Complete surgical resection

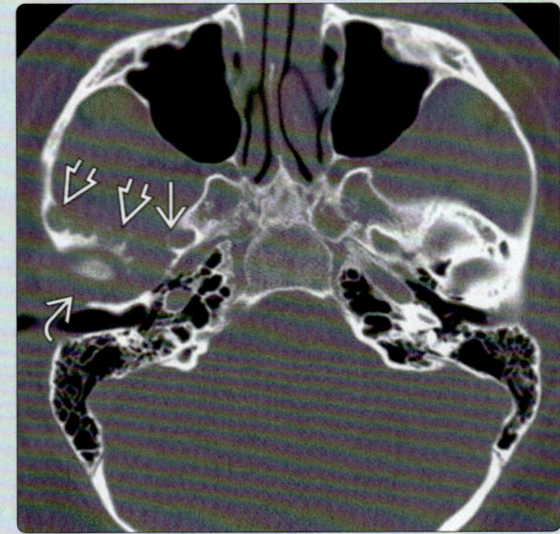

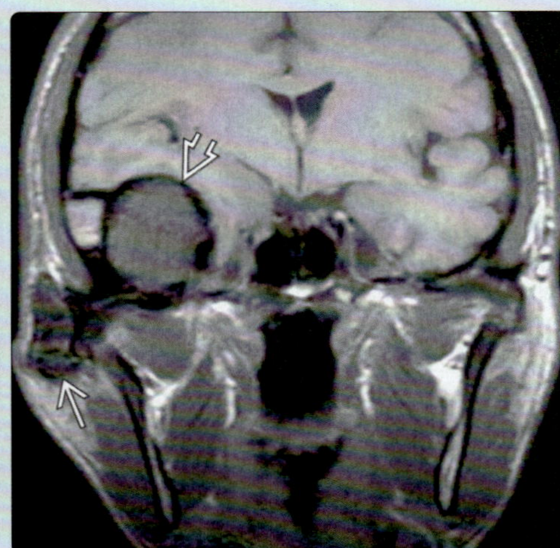

(Left) *Axial bone CT demonstrates widening of the right TMJ space ➡ and multiple rounded erosions of the adjacent skull base involving the internal aspect of the zygomatic arch ➡ and greater wing of the sphenoid up to the lateral margin of foramen ovale ➡.* **(Right)** *Coronal T1 MR shows a hypointense right TMJ mass ➡ with a periphery of lower signal intensity. A hypointense contiguous middle cranial fossa extraaxial mass ➡ is evident with similar markedly low-signal peripheral rim.*

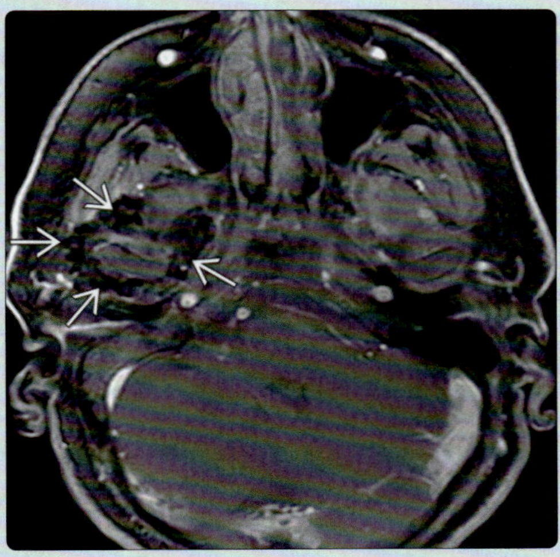

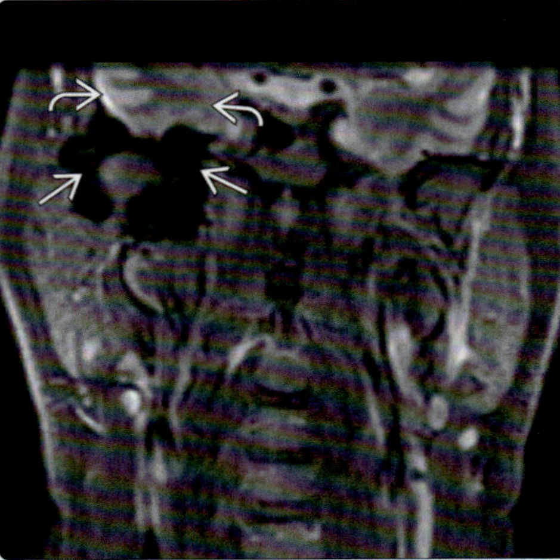

(Left) *Axial T1 C+ FS MR shows multiple nodular foci of hypointense signal ➡ in and surrounding the widened right TMJ space in this case of pigmented villonodular synovitis (PVNS). Note the minimal associated enhancement.* **(Right)** *Coronal STIR MR demonstrates nodular foci of markedly hypointense signal ➡ surrounding the right mandible condylar head in this case of PVNS. Note the blooming of the adjacent skull base from hemosiderin in these nodules ➡, a nearly pathognomonic finding.*

TMJ Synovial Chondromatosis

KEY FACTS

TERMINOLOGY

- **Synovial metaplasia** with foci of **hyaline cartilage**

IMAGING

- **Calcified nodules** in superior joint space (SJS)
- Location: Most commonly found in SJS of TMJ
  - Rarely may have extracapsular extension
  - Locations: Masticator space, parotid space, intracranial
- Protocol: Thin-section multiplanar bone CT + MR TMJ
- Bone CT findings
  - **Calcified nodules** surround **mandibular condyle**
  - Degenerative changes involving condyle common
- T1/proton density MR findings
  - Multiple **hypo-** to **isointense nodules** in SJS
  - Separate from articular disc
- T2 MR: Superior joint space **effusion** ± expansion; fluid surrounds collection of hypointense nodules
- T1 C+ MR: Enhancing synovium

TOP DIFFERENTIAL DIAGNOSES

- Osteochondritis dissecans
- Calcium pyrophosphate dihydrate deposition disease
- Pigmented villonodular synovitis
- Osteochondroma
- Chondrosarcoma

PATHOLOGY

- **Synovial inflammation** with lymphocytes, macrophages, giant cells
- Milgram staging
  - Phase 1: Synovial metaplasia with no chondroid nodules
  - Phase 2: Active synovial metaplasia & chondroid nodules
  - Phase 3: Chondroid nodules with no active synovial disease

CLINICAL ISSUES

- Presenting symptoms: Preauricular pain, swelling
- Treatment: Arthroscopy, synovectomy, condylectomy

(Left) *Axial bone CT demonstrates multiple small, calcified nodules ➡ within the right temporomandibular joint (TMJ). The condyle is sclerotic and slightly irregular ⇨ with anterior narrowing of the joint space due to degenerative change.* **(Right)** *Gross pathology specimen taken from TMJ affected by synovial chondromatosis shows calcified bodies exposed on a surgical towel. Notice the variable size of these nodules, from 2-10 millimeters.*

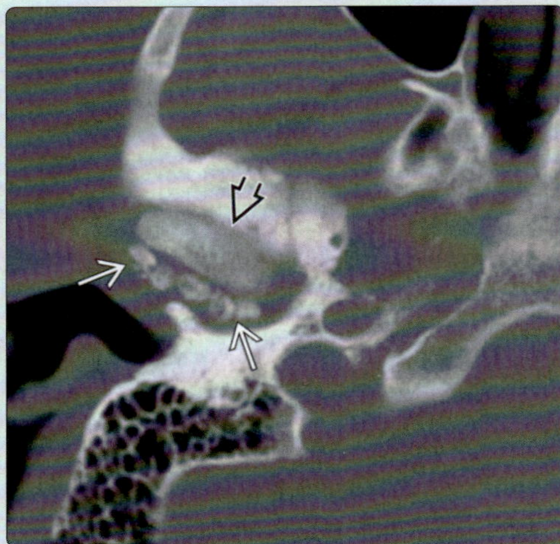

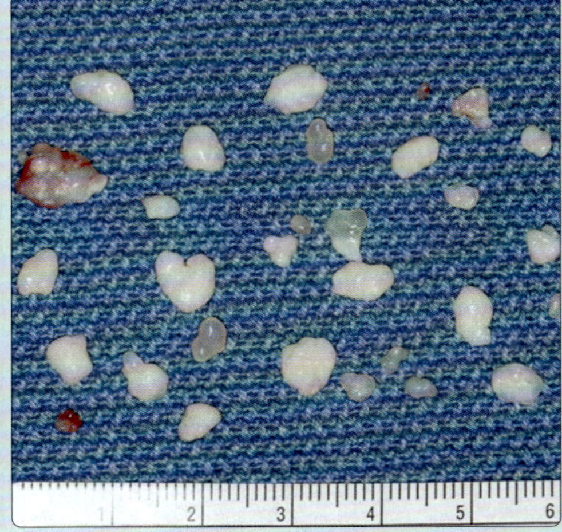

(Left) *Sagittal oblique T2 FS MR shows distension of the right TMJ capsule with hyperintense fluid ➡ surrounding the low-signal calcified loose bodies ➡.* **(Right)** *Sagittal T1 C+ FS MR reveals a rim-enhancing ➡ cystic lesion within the anterior aspect of the TMJ. The superior joint space is distended. The peripheral enhancement reflects enhancing synovium.*

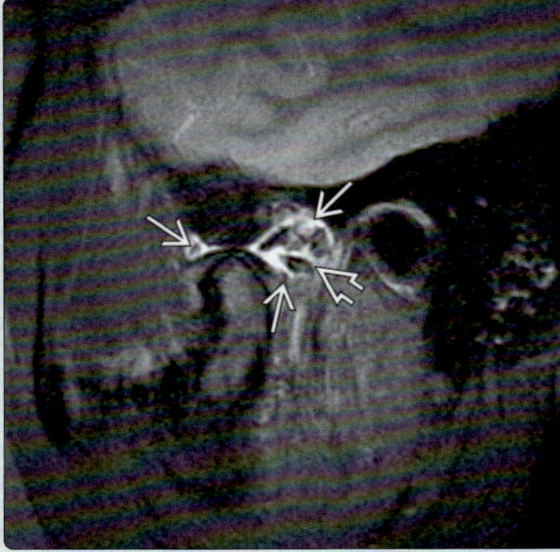

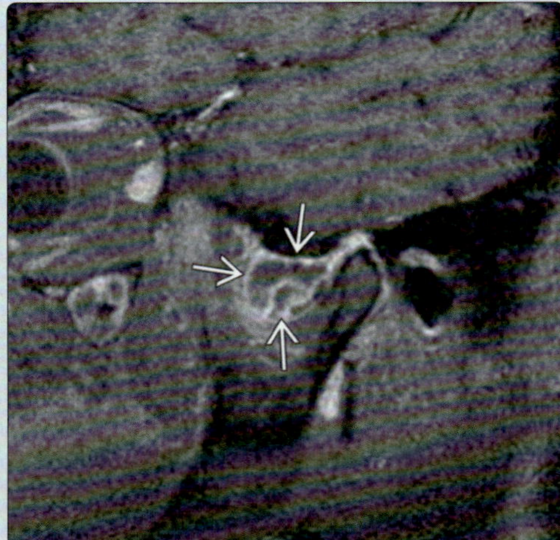

KEY FACTS

TERMINOLOGY

- Definition: Benign but locally aggressive neoplasm originating from odontogenic epithelium
  - Arises in tooth-bearing areas of mandibular or maxillary alveolus

IMAGING

- CT findings
  - **Expansile multiloculated** or multilobulated mixed cystic & solid posterior mandible mass, usually near 3rd molar
  - Lesions in maxilla usually arise near premolar-1st molar
  - Typically associated with **unerupted tooth**
- MR findings
  - T2: ↑ **signal intensity** of cystic areas
  - Smaller tumors: **Enhancing mural nodule**

TOP DIFFERENTIAL DIAGNOSES

- Periapical (radicular) cyst
- Dentigerous cyst
- Keratocystic odontogenic tumor
- Odontogenic myxoma
- Ossifying fibroma
- Aneurysmal bone cyst

CLINICAL ISSUES

- 3rd-5th decades; expansile, painless mass
- Progressive loosening of teeth; nonhealing "tooth abscess"
- Treatment: Complete surgical excision when small
  - En bloc removal for larger lesions, may require reconstructive or prosthetic options

DIAGNOSTIC CHECKLIST

- Larger dentigerous cyst (DC) & keratocystic odontogenic tumor (KOT) may mimic ameloblastoma
  - Ameloblastomas expand mandible more concentrically than DC or KOT
- High T2 signal intensity suggests ameloblastoma, rather than more aggressive neoplasm

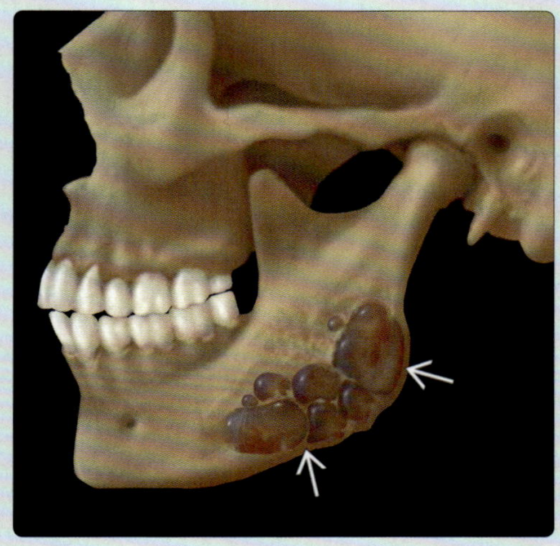

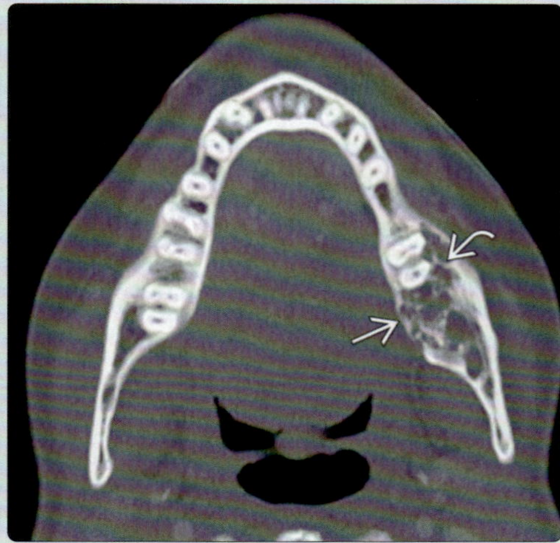

(Left) *Lateral graphic shows mandibular ameloblastoma ➡ as a bubbly, multilocular, expansile lesion. The location proximal to the 3rd molar is typical.* **(Right)** *Axial bone CT shows the classic appearance of solid/multicystic ameloblastoma as a multiloculated expansile mass in the 2nd-3rd molar region of the mandible ➡. Note the thinned overlying cortex and the characteristic multiple coarse septations ➡.*

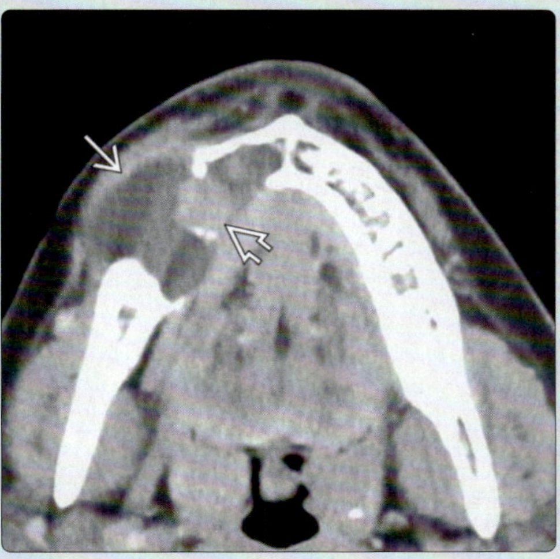

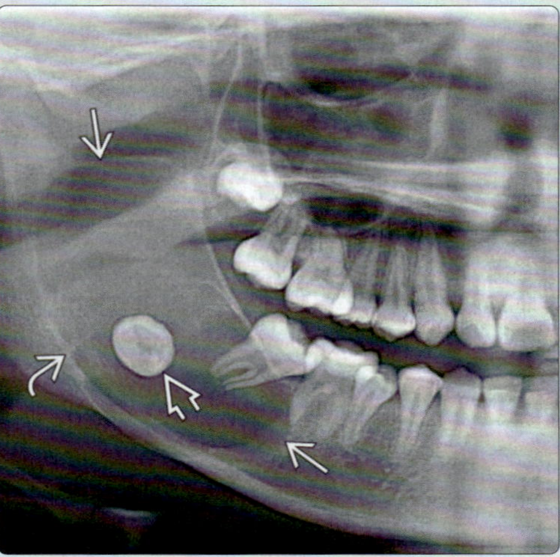

(Left) *Axial CECT of a unicystic ameloblastoma with a mural nodule shows the hypodense mass is nonenhancing and expansile ➡ with a central hyperdense and mildly enhancing nodule ➡. Note that the nodule lies adjacent to the eroded lingual cortex with potential for involvement of the sublingual space.* **(Right)** *AP radiograph of the jaw in a 12-year-old girl demonstrates an expansile cystic right mandible lesion ➡ associated with an unerupted right 3rd molar ➡, found to be ameloblastoma. A small septation is suggested ➡.*

Keratocystic Odontogenic Tumor (Odontogenic Keratocyst)

KEY FACTS

TERMINOLOGY

- Keratocystic odontogenic tumor (KOT)
  - Previously known as odontogenic keratocyst (OKC)
- Benign cystic neoplasm of jaw with aggressive behavior and high recurrence rate

IMAGING

- May displace developing teeth or resorb roots of erupted teeth
  - **Not** related to unerupted crown
- Bone CT: Unilocular cystic mass with sclerotic rim
  - Expansile solitary unilocular jaw lesion
    - Multilocular jaw cyst ↑ risk (12x) of KOT
  - 75% posterior mandible, often near 3rd molar
  - Extends longitudinally in mandible
- CECT: No solid enhancement
- C+ MR: Cystic with thin, enhancing rim
  - Greater enhancement with recurrent KOT

TOP DIFFERENTIAL DIAGNOSES

- Periapical (radicular) cyst
- Dentigerous (follicular) cyst
- Ameloblastoma

PATHOLOGY

- Thin-walled, friable cyst containing fluid and debris
- Viscosity of contents depends on keratinaceous debris
  - Straw-colored fluid → pus-like → "cheesy" mass

CLINICAL ISSUES

- 50% present with jaw swelling
  - Rapid growth and high recurrence rate
- Treatment: Enucleation with aggressive curettage

DIAGNOSTIC CHECKLIST

- If multiple KOTs (7% are multiple) ± basal cell carcinoma, consider **basal cell nevus (Gorlin) syndrome**
- Look for dural calcifications on same CT scan

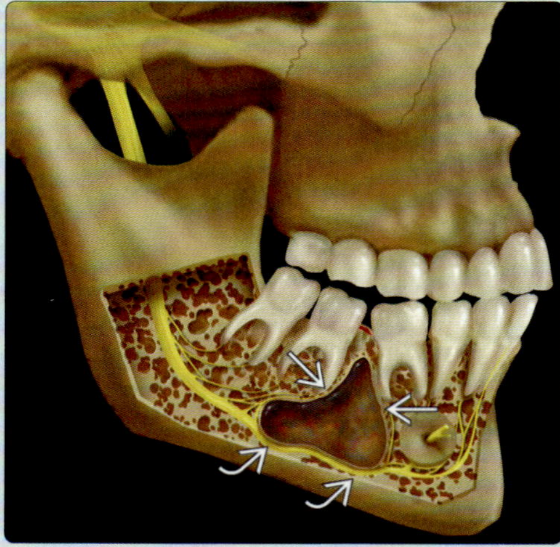

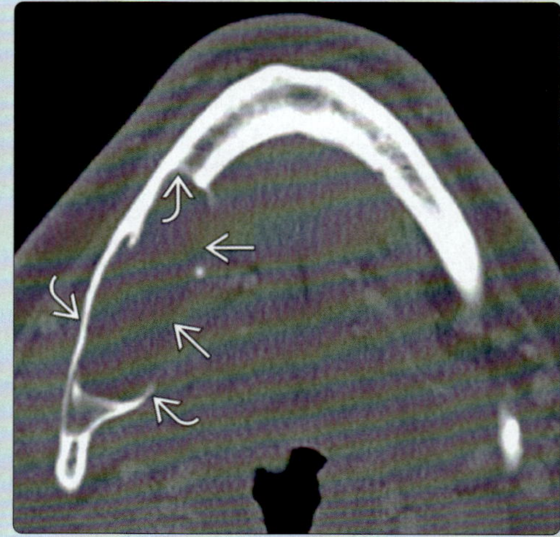

(Left) *Lateral graphic of the mandible with the buccal cortex removed illustrates features of classic keratocytic odontogenic tumor (KOT). A cystic lesion splays the roots of the 1st and 2nd molar teeth, enlarging the marrow space and displacing the inferior alveolar nerve.* **(Right)** *Axial bone CT in a patient with confirmed KOT demonstrates an expansile, unilocular cystic mass extending along long axis of mandible. Cortex is smoothly scalloped along most margins but is imperceptible at the lingual aspect.*

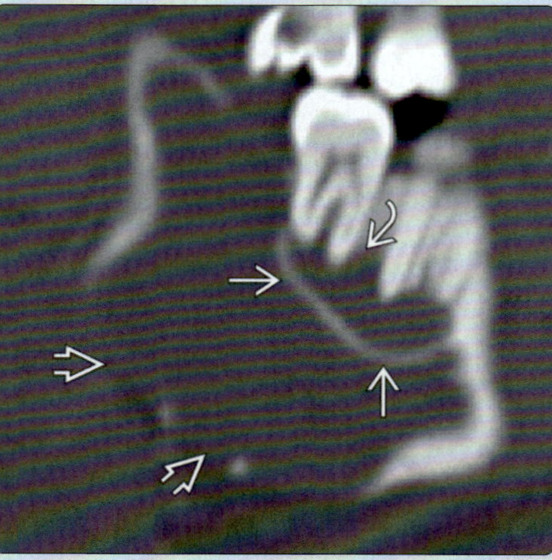

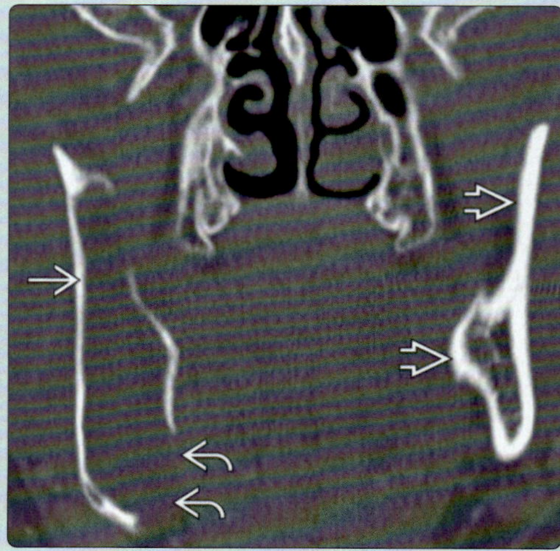

(Left) *Sagittal reconstruction of a mandible bone CT demonstrates an expansile mass with characteristic scalloping between roots of teeth. Note that the mylohyoid line of mandible is preserved despite marked thinning of the inferior mandibular cortex.* **(Right)** *Coronal reconstruction of a bone CT shows that KOT tends to expand through the ramus. The cortex is diffusely thinned, but the lingual cortex is imperceptible. The degree of bony expansion is evident in comparison to the normal left side.*

KEY FACTS

TERMINOLOGY

- Primary intramedullary high-grade malignant tumor of mesenchymal origin in which neoplastic cells produce osteoid, even if only in small amounts

IMAGING

- Bone CT findings
  - Bone destruction with **aggressive periosteal reaction** and **osteoid formation**
    - If not present, consider infection or metastasis
- MR findings
  - MR best evaluates soft tissue component of tumor
  - Intramedullary and extraosseous soft tissues
- Bone scan or PET/CT: Increased tracer uptake

TOP DIFFERENTIAL DIAGNOSES

- Mandible-maxilla osteomyelitis
- Mandible-maxilla osteoradionecrosis
- Mandible-maxilla metastasis
- Ewing sarcoma
- Langerhans cell histiocytosis

PATHOLOGY

- Heterogeneous mass with ossified and nonossified components
- Chondroblastic > osteoblastic > fibroblastic
- 5-year survival: **55%**
- If patient had remote radiation, XRT-induced osteosarcoma

CLINICAL ISSUES

- Clinical presentation
  - Mean age: 35 years; M:F = 1.5:1:0
  - Enlarging soft tissue mass over mandible with ↑ **pain**
  - Prognosis depends on pathologic type, size, location, and presence of metastases
- Treatment options
  - Complete resection affords best chance of survival
  - ± adjuvant chemotherapy, radiation

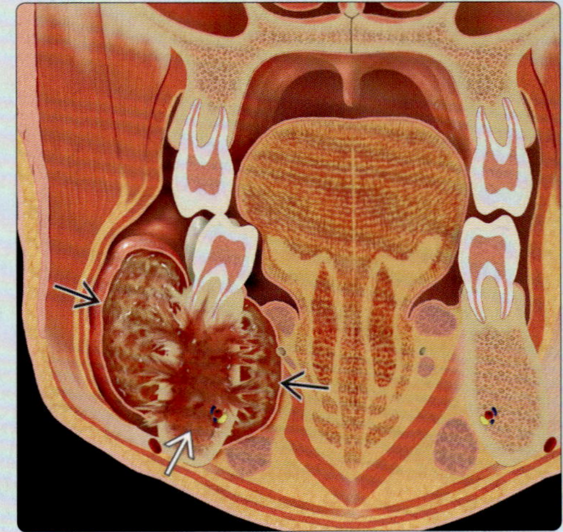

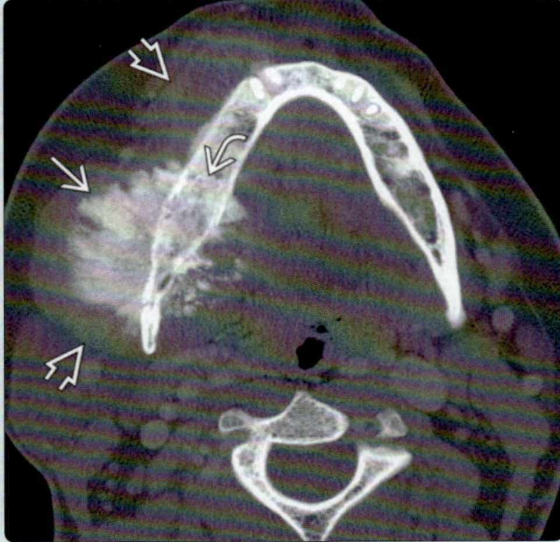

(Left) *Coronal graphic shows right mandible osteosarcoma. Note a soft tissue mass perforating through the cortex ⇨ & an intramedullary tumor ➡. **(Right)** Axial bone CT demonstrates a large, dense mass arising from the right mandible ➡ that has both osteoid matrix & periosteal reaction. This is classic periosteal reaction associated with osteosarcomas where periosteum is lifted off perpendicular to bone. Marrow within the involved portion of the mandible is sclerotic ➡. Note associated soft tissue mass ➡.*

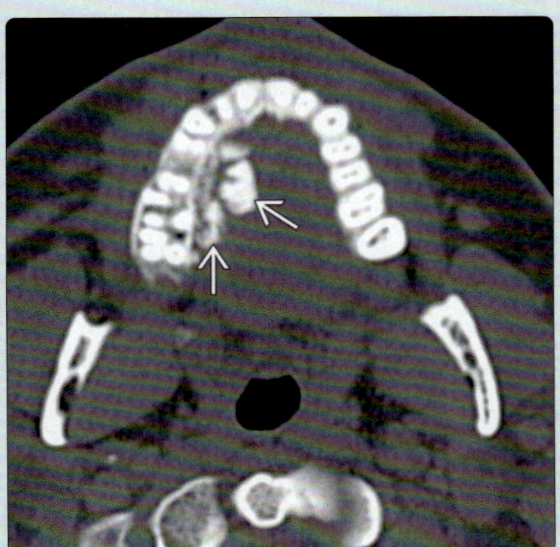

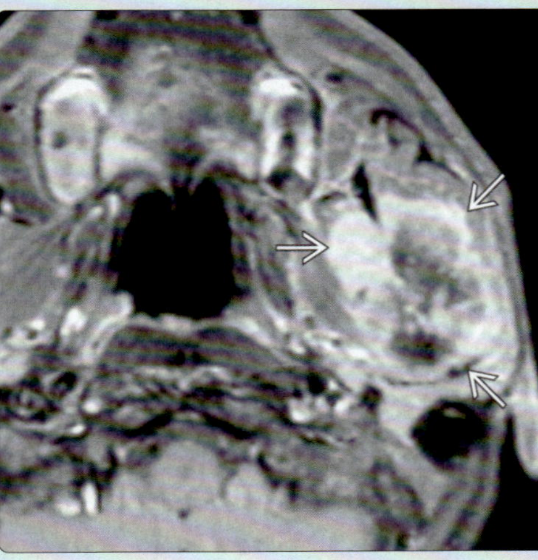

(Left) *Axial bone CT through the maxilla shows an exophytic mass with amorphous immature new bone ➡ & cortical breakthrough. This is the parosteal form of osteosarcoma. Note absence of a significant associated nonossified soft tissue mass.* **(Right)** *Axial T1 C+ FS MR shows heterogeneous enhancement of a soft tissue component of osteosarcoma arising in the mandible. Note that the tumor has infiltrated the parotid gland, masseter, & pterygoid muscles ➡.*

KEY FACTS

TERMINOLOGY

- Abbreviation: Osteoradionecrosis (ORN)
- Definition: Complication of radiation therapy (XRT) with necrosis of bone and failure to heal

IMAGING

- General imaging findings
  - Mandible > > maxilla or skull base
  - Soft tissue edema and induration common
  - Superinfection complication common
- CT: Mixed **lytic/sclerotic bone** with sequestra
  - Watch for **pathologic fracture** development
- MR: Diffuse low T1, high T2 signal from edema
- CECT/T1 C+ MR: Diffuse enhancement common

TOP DIFFERENTIAL DIAGNOSES

- Osteomyelitis
- Bisphosphonate osteonecrosis
- Alveolar ridge squamous cell carcinoma (SCCa)

PATHOLOGY

- Radiation results in damage to small blood vessels
  - **Hypovascular marrow** results
  - Impairs bone ability to resist infection or trauma
- May be precipitated by biopsy or tooth extraction
- **Pathologic fracture** through bone common

CLINICAL ISSUES

- Clinical presentation: Jaw pain, nonhealing ulcers
  - Most often follows XRT for oral cavity SCCa
    - Incidence peaks 6-12 months post XRT
  - Exposed bone from ulcerated mucosa
  - Must exclude recurrent SCCa as source of radiographic changes or persistent clinical symptoms
- Treatment options
  - Conservative treatment: Antibiotics and local irrigation
  - Hyperbaric oxygen therapy promotes angiogenesis
  - Sequestrectomy + primary wound closure if early
  - Bone resection + reconstruction if late in process

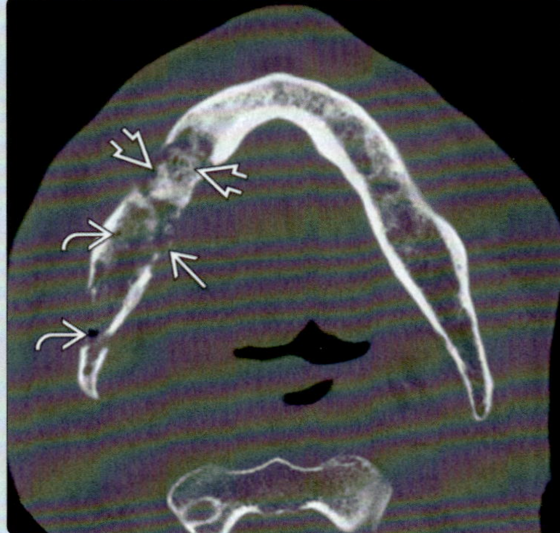

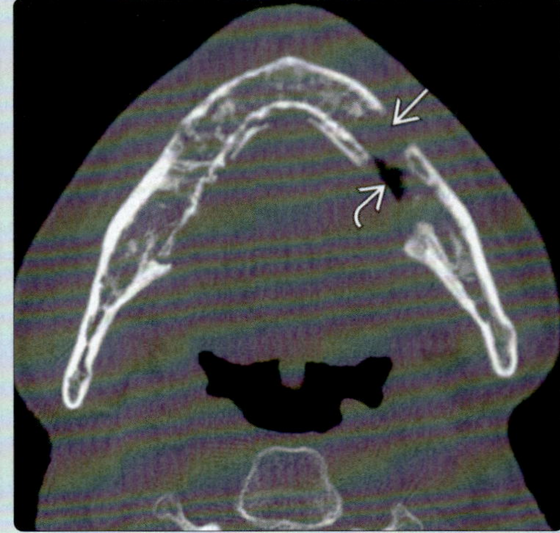

(Left) *Axial bone CT demonstrates typical mixed lytic/sclerotic changes and cortical bone interruption ➡ in the right hemimandible following XRT. Note the intraosseous gas bubbles ➡ and evolving bone-within-bone appearance ➡ due to intraosseous bone sequestra.* **(Right)** *Axial bone CT shows a primarily lytic pattern of osteoradionecrosis (ORN) with interrupted cortex ➡ and intraosseous gas ➡. There is also a pathologic fracture of the left mandibular body with off-setting of bone.*

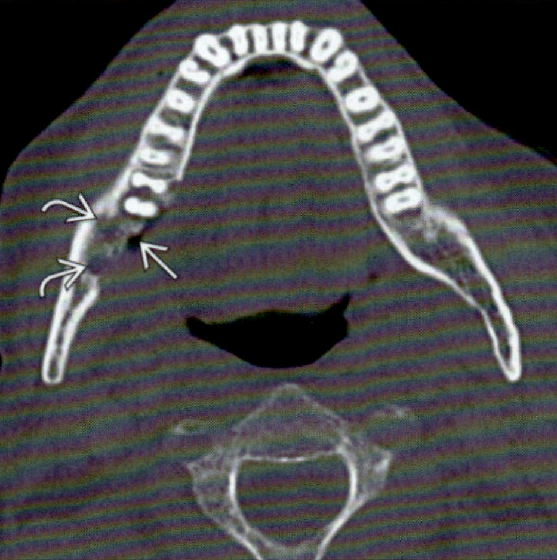

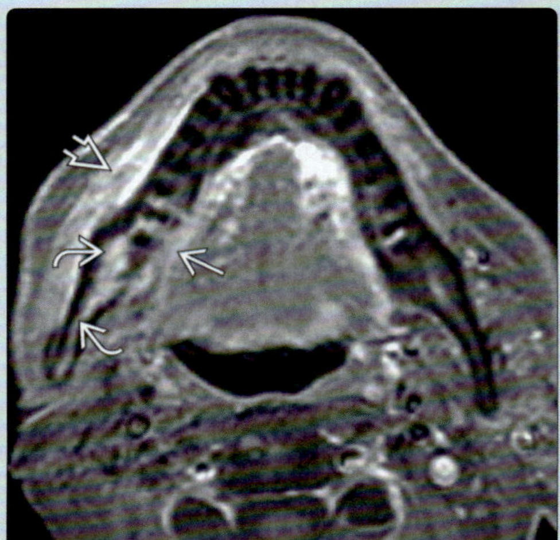

(Left) *Axial bone CT shows a mandibular extraction socket with a small bubble of gas ➡ indicating mucosal erosion with hazy lucency of the adjacent bone ➡. This patient had exposed bone on the physical exam.* **(Right)** *Axial T1 MR in the same patient shows enhancement in the mandible ➡ and diffusely in lingual ➡ and buccal ➡ soft tissues around the mandible. With a history of prior radiation therapy and now a swollen right face with exposed bone around the socket, imaging is most consistent with early ORN.*

Mandible-Maxilla Osteonecrosis

KEY FACTS

TERMINOLOGY

- Necrosis of mandible or maxilla associated with medications, often **bisphosphonates**

IMAGING

- General imaging issues
  - **Mandible much more common** than maxilla
  - Typically mixed lytic-sclerotic mandible-maxilla
    - ± edema in surrounding tissues
    - ± reactive adenopathy
  - Look out for pathologic fracture
    - ± extension of lytic process to inferior alveolar canal
    - ± abscess from secondary infection
- CT findings
  - Early: Nonhealing extraction socket
  - Late: Diffuse destructive changes in alveolar ridge
    - Widened periodontal ligament spaces
    - May be associated with pathologic fracture
  - Tissue swelling if severe, infected, pathologic fracture
- MR: Variable signal from edema & bone changes
  - Enhancement common & does not imply infection
- PET/CT: Typically FDG avid

TOP DIFFERENTIAL DIAGNOSES

- Mandible-maxilla osteomyelitis
- Mandible-maxilla osteoradionecrosis
- Mandible-maxilla metastasis

CLINICAL ISSUES

- Clinical presentation
  - Jaw pain ± localized swelling
  - Nonhealing exposed bone, after 8 weeks, in patient with no prior craniofacial radiation
  - Mimics dental infection & follows tooth extraction
  - Medication history (bisphosphonates) may be unknown
- Treatment options
  - Cease drug therapy & antibiotics if also infected
  - Surgical debridement of necrotic bony sequestra

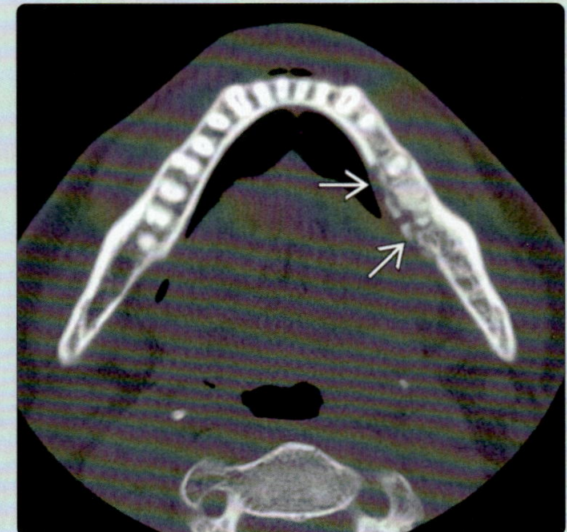

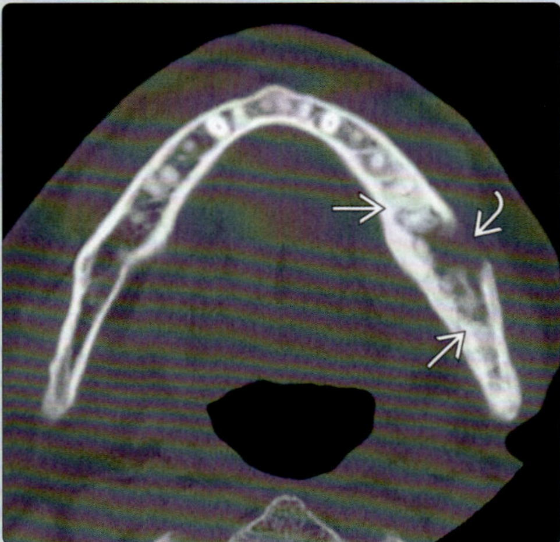

(Left) *Axial bone CT demonstrates a lytic cortical lesion → of the left mandible with periapical lucency of the left mandibular molars. Findings are diagnostic of osteonecrosis in a patient with a nonhealing ulcer, exposed bone, and bisphosphonate exposure.* **(Right)** *Axial bone CT shows a typical case of mandibular osteonecrosis related to intravenous bisphosphonates. Note the mixed sclerotic → and lytic → lesion in the left mandible body at the site of a recent tooth extraction.*

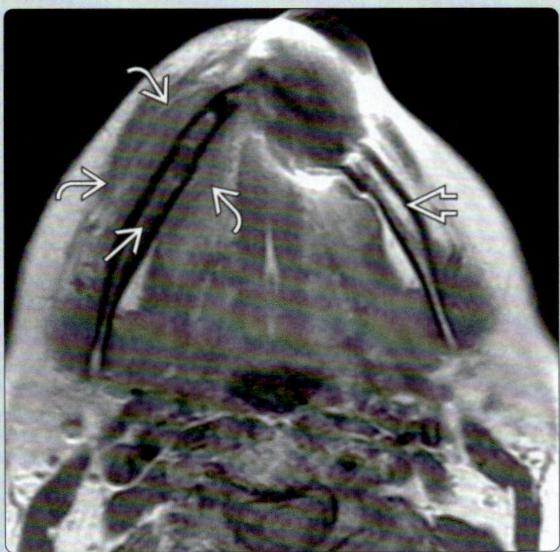

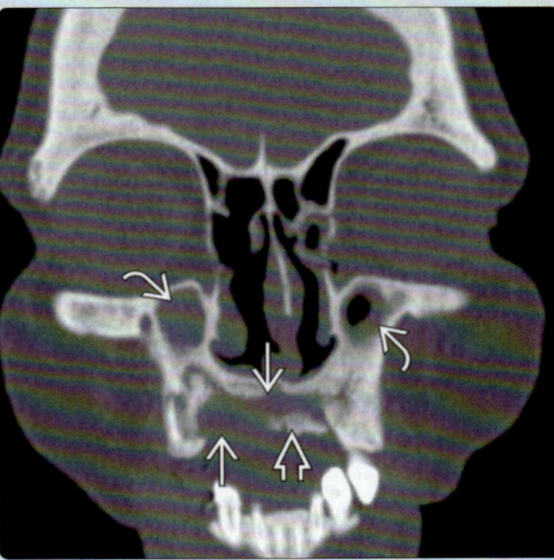

(Left) *Axial T1WI MR in a patient on bisphosphonates for metastatic breast cancer and new jaw pain shows normal marrow on the left → but low-signal edema in the right mandible →. Adjacent soft tissue inflammation → is noted. Distinguishing metastasis from osteonecrosis can be very difficult.* **(Right)** *Coronal bone CT shows severe maxillary osteonecrosis with destruction → in a patient with multiple myeloma and IV bisphosphonates. Note bone sequestrum →. Bilateral maxillary sinus opacification → is probably not associated.*

SECTION 2

Squamous Cell Carcinoma

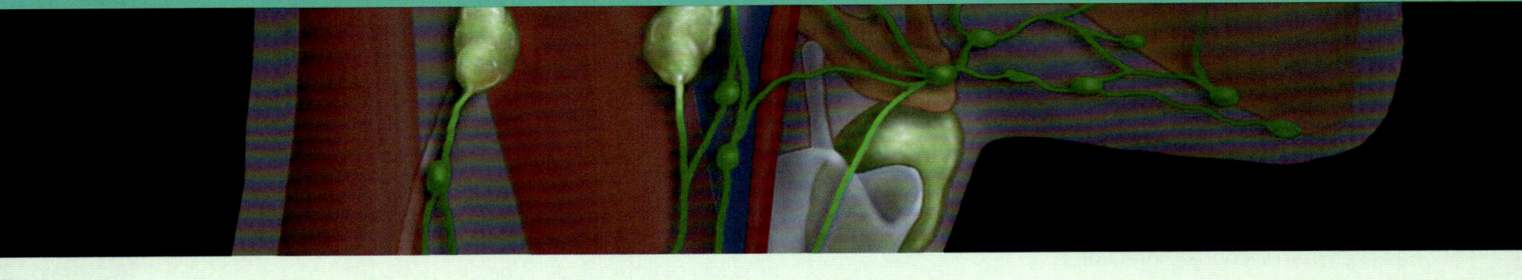

Primary Sites, Perineural Tumor, and Nodes

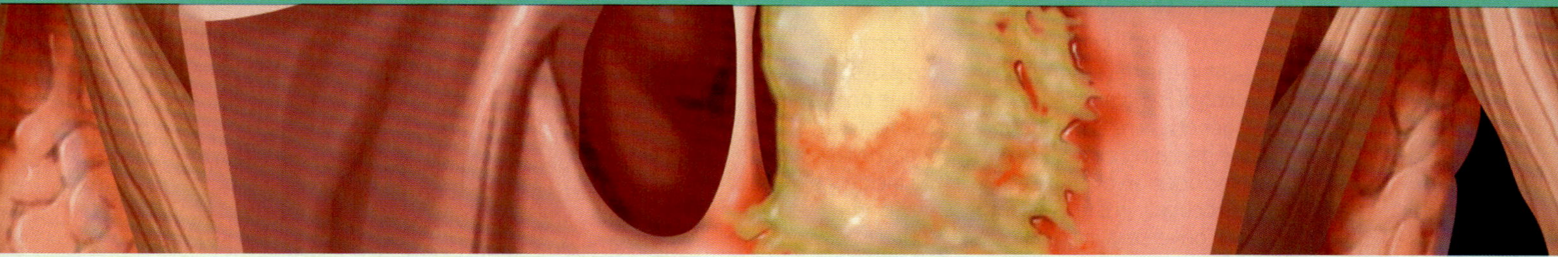

Posttreatment Neck

Summary Thoughts: Squamous Cell Carcinoma

Squamous cell carcinoma (SCCa) is, without question, the most common malignancy in the H&N. Recent developments in the understanding of the molecular nature and causes of SCCa now reveal it to be a heterogeneous malignancy.

In most sites of the H&N, **tobacco** is the most common causative agent in the development of mucosal dysplasia and neoplasia. **Alcohol** is a synergistic cofactor, while poor oral hygiene and genetics are also contributing risk factors. Paralleling the declining trend of smoking over the last 30 years, there has been an overall decline in the incidence of H&N SCCa, particularly in the oral cavity, larynx, and hypopharynx. Conversely, in the oropharynx there has been a rise in **base of tongue (BOT)** or **lingual** and **palatine tonsillar SCCa**, particularly in patients under 60 years, who may have a limited or no history of tobacco and alcohol use. This increasingly common group of SCCa tumors is positive for human papillomavirus (HPV), most commonly the HPV-16 subtype, which is also responsible for cervical and anogenital neoplasms. Currently in the United States, ~ **60%** of oropharyngeal SCCa (especially tonsil and BOT) are due to **HPV**. HPV(+) SCCa appears to be more responsive to chemoradiation than HPV(-) SCCa, and patients have an overall better survival. Patients with HPV(+) tumors who are also smokers carry an intermediate prognosis.

Nasopharyngeal carcinoma (NPCa) is a distinctly different neoplasm with the most common histopathologic subtypes associated with **Epstein-Barr virus** infection. The least common and most aggressive form (keratinizing NPCa) is related to tobacco and alcohol abuse, although some pathology literature has also suggested an association with HPV infection.

While the current understanding of SCCa is evolving through greater molecular interrogation of these tumors, the clinicians' roles remain largely unchanged. At the time of diagnosis, the clinician must determine details about the primary tumor to assign a **tumor stage**, including the **size** and **local extent** of the primary, detecting **perineural tumor** (PNT), and assessing regional **nodes** and **distant** spread of disease. Following treatment, both **baseline** and **surveillance** imaging require careful evaluation to detect **residual** or **recurrent SCCa, treatment complications**, and **2nd primary neoplasms**.

Imaging Approaches and Indications

There is no definitive best imaging modality for all H&N sites when staging SCCa. Some specific tumor sites are better served by either **CECT or MR or PET/CECT**. A patient with copious secretions or pain may not tolerate long MR sequences, and, in that instance, CECT or PET combined with CECT is preferred. Excellent quality neck imaging is more readily reproducible from patient to patient using CT than MR. Also, a large field of view, nonoptimized MR sequences, and lack of familiarity with basic neck anatomy make detection of key findings difficult. A poorly performed and inaccurately interpreted neck MR scan is an expensive, unsatisfactory alternative to CT imaging.

MR does offer specific utility in certain areas. For example, it is the preferred staging tool for NPCa because detection of skull base infiltration (T3) or intracranial disease (T4) is extremely important for staging and treatment planning. MR offers better soft tissue contrast for detecting small primary tonsillar tumors and evaluating the deep extent of a lesion when planning surgical resection or **intensity-modulated radiation therapy (IMRT)**. For this reason, MR may be used in the oral cavity and oropharynx. In the larynx, MR is so affected by motion artifact that it is largely reserved for determination of cartilage penetration (T4a) when CECT is equivocal. Finally, nodal disease at any site is almost equally well evaluated with either CECT or MR, but PET is superior to both anatomic studies.

Given the complexity of neck anatomy, **FDG PET** in the H&N is best performed as a combined PET/CECT examination. There are variable degrees of normal FDG uptake in muscles, brown fat, salivary and lymphoid tissue, and recent biopsy sites. These all are potential false-positive pitfalls in PET imaging, but routine measurement and reporting of standardized uptake values can obviate the pitfalls. A potential false-negative finding is absence of uptake in a cystic/necrotic node, but correlation with neck CECT imaging will allow correct identification of cystic/necrotic nodal metastases.

Ultrasound (US) has a limited role in H&N SCCa. Skilled ultrasonographers claim US is highly accurate for determining extracapsular spread of a nodal metastasis. US can also serve as imaging guidance for fine-needle aspiration.

Imaging Anatomy

SCCa arises from the mucosal surface of the upper airway and digestive tract, the pharynx and larynx. The pharynx is really a muscular tube encased by the middle layer of deep cervical fascia (ML-DCF) and attached to the skull base by the pharyngobasilar fascia. The **pharyngeal mucosal space** is a continuous sheet of tissue on the airway side of the ML-DCF. It is divided into separate sites anatomically. Staging of mucosal SCCa is individualized to each site or subsite.

The **nasopharynx**, posterior to the nasal cavity, extends from the most cranial pharynx at the skull base to the soft palate. Inferiorly, it is contiguous with the **oropharynx**, which extends caudally to the hyoid bone. The anterior tonsillar pillars and the circumvallate papillae of the tongue define the anterior limit of the oropharynx. The anterior 2/3 of the tongue lies in the oral cavity and is known as the oral tongue. The posterior 1/3 is called the tongue base and is part of the oropharynx.

Below the hyoid bone, the pharynx divides to form the **larynx**, which is continuous with the trachea, and the hypopharynx, which joins the cervical esophagus. The posterior wall of the hypopharynx is a continuation of the posterior wall of the oropharynx. Lateral "pockets" of the hypopharynx form the pyriform sinuses and are separated from the larynx by the aryepiglottic (AE) folds. Nearly 2/3 of hypopharyngeal SCCa arise in the pyriform sinuses. The larynx is anterior in the neck and has 3 subsites: The **supraglottic larynx**, which includes the epiglottis, AE folds, and false cords; the **glottis**, or true vocal cords; and the **subglottis**, which is contiguous with the cervical trachea. More than 1/2 of all laryngeal SCCa are glottic in origin.

Approaches to Imaging Issues in H&N SCCa

Staging SCCa is performed using the American Joint Committee on Cancer classification system, currently in its 8th edition (2017). Referral to the site-specific tumor (T) and nodal (N) features at the time of film review greatly enhances an imaging report. When the size of a T or N is important for tumor or nodal stage, respectively, the longest diameter is measured. Some superficial oral cavity tumors are best measured on clinical examination. The key role of cross-sectional imaging is to evaluate features that are not evident on exam, such as deep extent or bone infiltration, which may upstage a tumor or alter treatment options.

The detection of a PNT may significantly alter the surgical resection ± the radiation treatment field ± adjuvant chemotherapy. Both mucosal and skin SCCa exhibit neurotropism, as do some salivary gland tumors and lymphomas. PNT is usually more evident on MR but may be detected on CT with careful evaluation of skull base foramina and known routes of spread.

Metastatic **nodal disease** is the most important prognostic factor in H&N SCCa. For all sites but the nasopharynx, a single node < 3 cm in diameter is staged as N1, which automatically elevates staging to at least stage III disease. A larger node or multiple or bilateral nodes define N2 and stage IV disease. NPCa commonly has extensive, large nodal metastases; therefore, this tumor has separate, distinct nodal staging criteria. With any H&N SCCa, the neck should be evaluated for enlarged, heterogeneous, or frankly necrotic nodes. Extranodal spread is now to be recorded as part of formal nodal SCCa staging, and may change the treatment approach, as it is usually associated with a poorer prognosis and higher rate of tumor recurrence.

At the time of a staging neck CECT scan, the lung apices and the bones should also be evaluated for **metastases**. Finally, many SCCa H&N cancer patients have increased risk of a **2nd primary neoplasm**. Second primary tumors are most frequently found with hypopharyngeal SCCa, and 1/3 are synchronous with the initial SCCa.

Following surgery, radiation, ± chemotherapy, a **posttreatment baseline** imaging study should be obtained to confirm absence of **residual disease**. This also serves as a roadmap of an anatomically changed neck to aid in detection of **recurrent disease**. Often, the initial posttreatment study for SCCa is PET/CECT. PET/CECT should be delayed around 10-12 weeks to minimize false-positive FDG uptake from posttreatment inflammatory changes. A baseline CECT study may be obtained at 8-10 weeks following chemoradiation, while postsurgical studies are often obtained at 10-12 weeks.

The **posttreatment baseline** scan following radiation ± chemotherapy should show no evidence of residual disease. The presence of enlarged nodes or residual primary mass following treatment is of concern and is typically surgically resected. Posttreatment neck dissections are ideally performed before 10 weeks to minimize the complexity of surgery that results with neck fibrosis. So-called borderline soft tissue at baseline CT/MR may be carefully watched, may undergo US-guided aspiration, or may be resected.

Radiation therapy has changed enormously over the last 2 decades with increasing use of **IMRT** for H&N cancers. IMRT maximizes dose to the tumor, minimizes radiation to normal surrounding tissues, and requires accurate delineation of tumor margins. Greater input from radiologists and clinicians to ensure accurate treatment volumes may be needed, with MR, PET/CECT, or CECT alone. Radiation ± **chemotherapy** results in significant changes in the appearance of neck soft tissues. Radiation results in acute inflammation and edema of all tissues in the radiation field. Over time, this changes to fibrosis, atrophy, and altered appearances on CECT and MR. Both acute and chronic expected radiation changes can be confusing on CECT or MR.

Surgical resection of a primary tumor ± cervical neck nodes also results in changes to normal neck contours. Familiarity with the types of nodal **neck dissections** and common **flap reconstructions** helps to radiographically evaluate both complications and recurrence. Knowledge of what surgical procedure was performed prior to evaluating posttreatment imaging is critical. Some resections, such as selective neck dissections, can be subtle on imaging, while large resections with flap reconstructions can be quite complex. MR is less affected by hardware artifact and more sensitive for recurrent tumors; however, the muscular component of a flap reconstruction undergoes denervation changes resulting in variable MR signal intensity and enhancement. On the baseline scan following neck reconstruction, residual or progressive tumors should be described.

Recurrent SCCa most often occurs during the first 2 years following initial treatment. The frequency of **surveillance imaging** during this time is variable and may be performed in 3- to 6-month intervals, depending on the initial tumor stage, prognostic features, and the clinical course, including physical findings. At the follow-up imaging examination, the possibility of a **2nd primary tumor** must be considered. Remember to look for **residual, recurrent, and new** tumors on every follow-up study.

How to Stage New Tumor With CT or MR

- Determine site of primary; refer to TNM staging table for specific primary site
- Evaluate size and local extent of tumor; ask: What is deep extent? Is there bone marrow infiltration? Is there PNT? How far does it go in each direction?
- Evaluate regional drainage nodes and contralateral node(s); are there retropharyngeal nodes?
- Evaluate included lungs and bones for metastases
- PET or PET/CECT can greatly increase staging accuracy

Clinical Implications

When a patient presents with a new neck mass that is nodal SCCa, an initial clinical examination is performed either in a clinic or in the operating room with panendoscopy with biopsies. If a primary site is not evident, it is considered to be an **unknown primary tumor**, and imaging has an important role in finding the primary so that biopsy can be directed. There are 4 key sites to consider 1st when evaluating a neck CECT or MR in search of an unknown primary tumor: (1) Nasopharynx: **Fossa of Rosenmüller** (lateral pharyngeal recess), (2) oropharynx: **Palatine tonsil**, (3) oropharynx: **BOT or lingual tonsil**, and (4) hypopharynx: **Apex of pyriform sinus**. The fossa of Rosenmüller and pyriform sinus apex may be clinical "blind spots," either at the in-office examination or, if very small, even at the direct endoscopy. The palatine and lingual tonsils may harbor a tumor in the depths of crypts, so the mucosal tumor may not be evident visually or on palpation. In all 4 locations, asymmetric soft tissue on cross-sectional imaging is key.

The changing demographics of tonsillar and BOT lingual SCCa, due to the rising incidence of HPV(+) oropharyngeal SCCa, make it imperative that the clinician is vigilant when evaluating a younger, nonsmoking subset of patients presenting with a new neck mass, which may be a cystic/necrotic or solid metastatic node. **A new neck mass in an adult, unless obviously a thyroid goiter, should be assumed to be neoplastic until proven otherwise.**

Sites and Subsites of Head and Neck Squamous Cell Carcinoma

Nasopharynx	Oral Cavity	Hypopharynx
Fossa of Rosenmüller (lateral pharyngeal recess)	Oral tongue	Pyriform sinus
	Floor of mouth	Postcricoid region
Oropharynx	Alveolar ridge: Maxilla	Posterior hypopharyngeal wall
Palatine tonsil	Buccal mucosa	**Larynx**
Posterior oropharyngeal wall	Hard palate	Supraglottis
Soft palate	Lip	Glottis
Lingual tonsil/base of tongue	Retromolar trigone	Subglottis
	Alveolar ridge: Mandible	

Nasopharynx (AJCC 2017)

Anatomic Stage/Prognostic Groups	T Category	N Category	M Category
Stage 0	Tis (in situ)	N0	M0
Stage I	T1	N0	M0
Stage II	T2	N0	M0
	T1-T2	**N1**	M0
Stage III	**T3**	N0-N2	M0
	T1-T3	**N2**	M0
Stage IVA	**T4**	N0-N2	M0
Stage IVB	Any T	**N3**	M0
Stage IVC	Any T	Any N	**M1**

Adapted from 8th edition AJCC Staging Forms.

All Other Head and Neck Sites (AJCC 2017)

Anatomic Stage/Prognostic Groups	T Category	N Category	M Category
Stage 0	Tis (in situ)	N0	M0
Stage I	T1	N0	M0
Stage II	T2	N0	M0
Stage III	T3	N0	M0
	T1-T3	**N1**	M0
Stage IVA	T4a	N0-N1	M0
	T1-T4a	**N2**	M0
Stage IVB	**T4b**	Any N	M0
	Any T	**N3**	M0
Stage IVC	Any T	Any N	**M1**

Adapted from 8th edition AJCC Staging Forms.

Selected References

1. AJCC Cancer Staging Manual. Springer International Publishing, 2017
2. Landry D et al: Squamous cell carcinoma of the upper aerodigestive tract: a review. Radiol Clin North Am. 53(1):81-97, 2015
3. Hudgins PA et al: Introduction to the imaging and staging of cancer. Neuroimaging Clin N Am. 23(1):1-7, 2013
4. Genden EM et al: Human papillomavirus and oropharyngeal squamous cell carcinoma: what the clinician should know. Eur Arch Otorhinolaryngol. 270(2):405-16, 2012
5. Srinivasan A et al: Biologic imaging of head and neck cancer: the present and the future. AJNR Am J Neuroradiol. 33(4):586-94, 2012
6. Yoshizaki T et al: Current understanding and management of nasopharyngeal carcinoma. Auris Nasus Larynx. 39(2):137-44, 2012
7. Trotta BM et al: Oral cavity and oropharyngeal squamous cell cancer: key imaging findings for staging and treatment planning. Radiographics. 31(2):339-54, 2011
8. Ang KK et al: Human papillomavirus and survival of patients with oropharyngeal cancer. N Engl J Med. 363(1):24-35, 2010

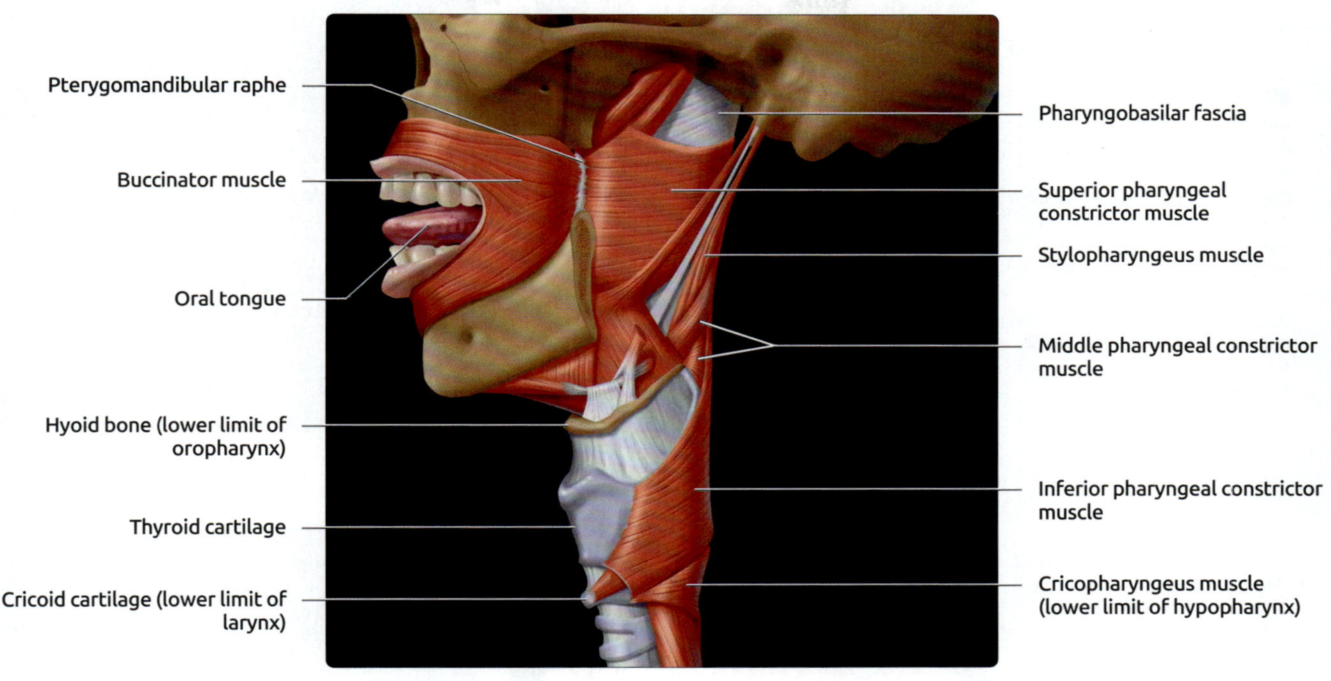

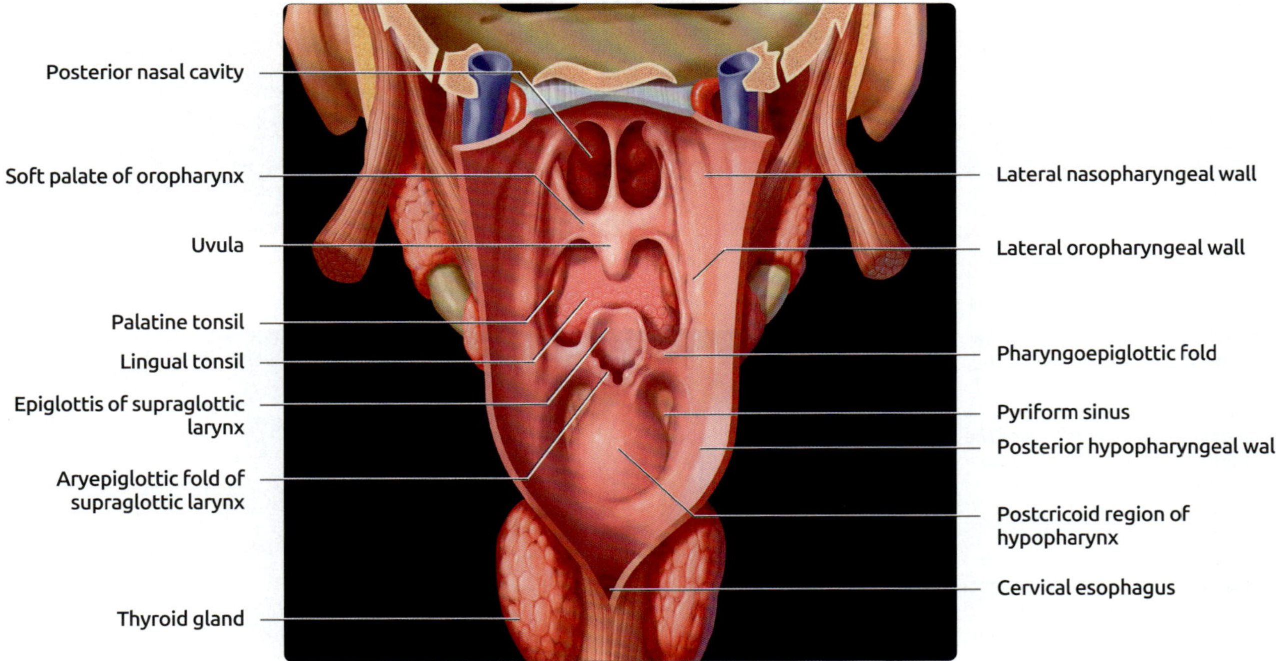

(Top) *Lateral graphic shows the major muscles of the pharyngeal mucosal space. Notice that the pharynx is essentially a tube attached superiorly to the skull base and formed from the superior, middle, and inferior pharyngeal constrictor muscles. The nasopharynx, oropharynx, and hypopharynx are contiguous segments of this tube with the oral cavity contiguous anteriorly with the oropharynx. The larynx is intimately related to the hypopharynx and originates at the lower aspect of the oropharynx.* **(Bottom)** *Graphic of the pharyngeal mucosal space/surface as if opened from behind shows that this space can be divided into nasopharyngeal, oropharyngeal, and hypopharyngeal areas. The lymphatic ring of the pharyngeal mucosal space (Waldeyer) contains the nasopharyngeal adenoids, the oropharyngeal palatine, and lingual tonsils or base of tongue.*

(Left) *Axial graphic of the nasopharyngeal mucosal space (blue) shows superior pharyngeal constrictor ➡ and levator veli palatini muscles ➡ within the space. The middle layer of deep cervical fascia (pink line) provides a deep margin to the space.* **(Right)** *Axial T1WI C+ FS MR in a 32-year-old Asian woman with trismus shows a large, mildly enhancing mass ➡ arising in the right nasopharynx & infiltrating the masticator space & clivus ➡. Involvement of cranial nerves found T4N2, stage IV NPCa. Note the levator veli ➡.*

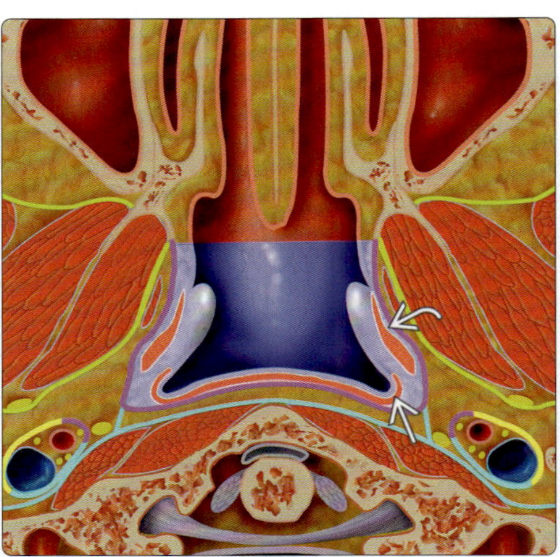

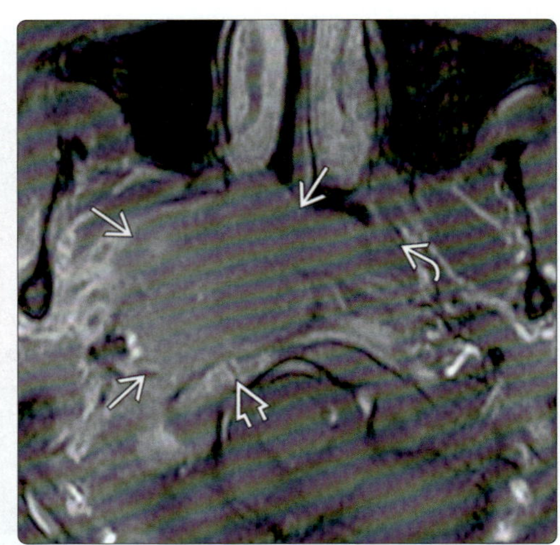

(Left) *Axial graphic of the oropharyngeal mucosal space (blue) viewed from above reveals distinction from a more anterior oral cavity. Anterior ➡ and posterior tonsillar pillars, palatine tonsils ➡, and lingual tonsil ➡, a.k.a. base of tongue, are the most common primary SCCa sites.* **(Right)** *Axial T1WI C+ FS MR in a 66 year old with asymmetry noted by dentist on examination shows a moderately enhancing mass ➡ in the tonsillar fossa. This case is unusual for the absence of adenopathy and is T1N0, stage I SCCa.*

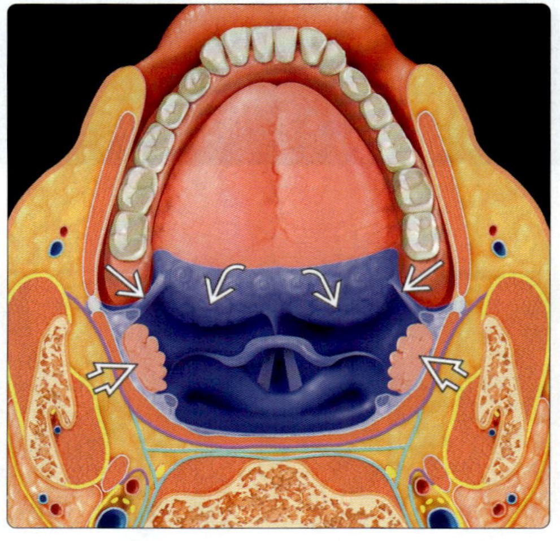

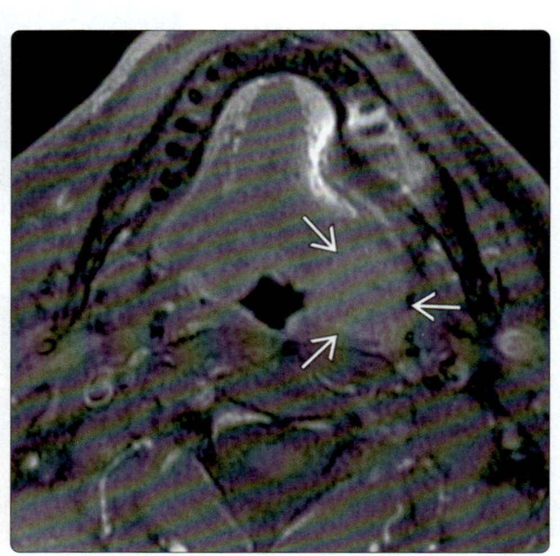

(Left) *Axial graphic shows the hypopharyngeal aspect of the pharyngeal mucosal space. At the supraglottis level, the hypopharynx is made up of the pyriform sinus ➡ & posterior wall ➡. Aryepiglottic (AE) folds ➡ are part of the supraglottis & separate the larynx from the hypopharynx.* **(Right)** *Axial CECT in a patient presenting with extensive matted bilateral adenopathy ➡ demonstrates an irregular, superficially spreading mass arising from the posterior hypopharyngeal wall ➡. This is T3N2c, stage IVA SCCa. Note the AE fold ➡.*

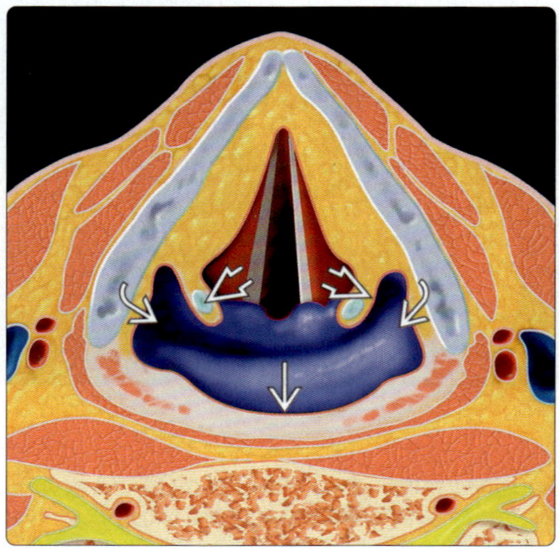

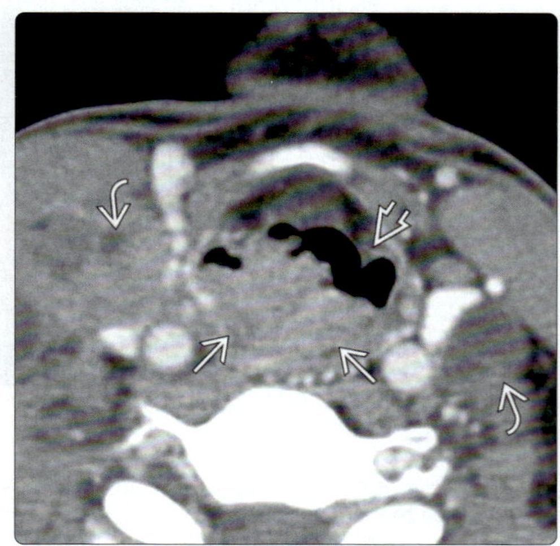

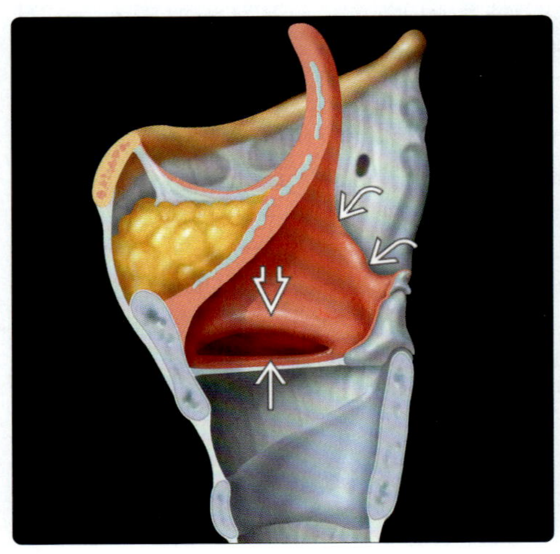

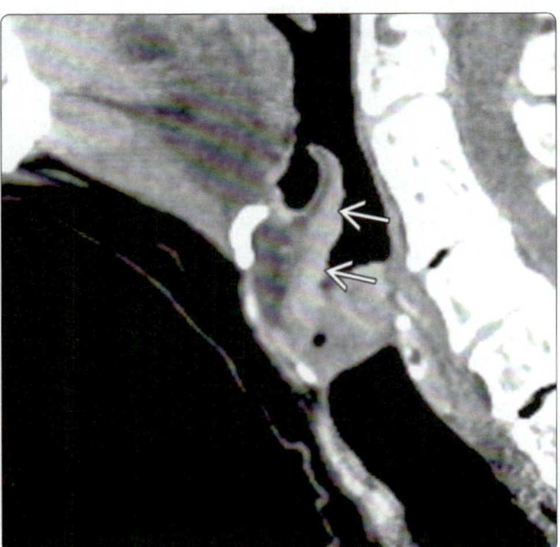

(Left) *Sagittal graphic of the larynx shows the true vocal cord ➡ of the glottic larynx. The false cord ➡ lies above and parallels this, while the AE fold ➡ projects from the tip of arytenoid cartilage to the inferolateral margin of the epiglottis. The subglottis extends from below the true cords to the inferior cricoid margin.* **(Right)** *Sagittal CECT reconstructed image in a 73-year-old woman demonstrates abnormal thickening of the laryngeal surface of the epiglottis ➡. This is T2N2c, stage IVA SCCa.*

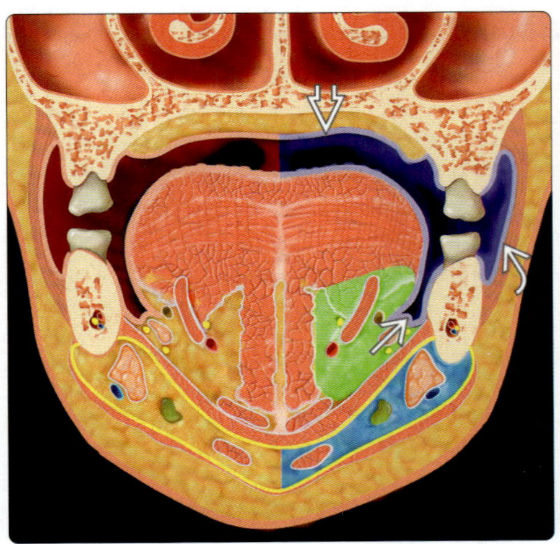

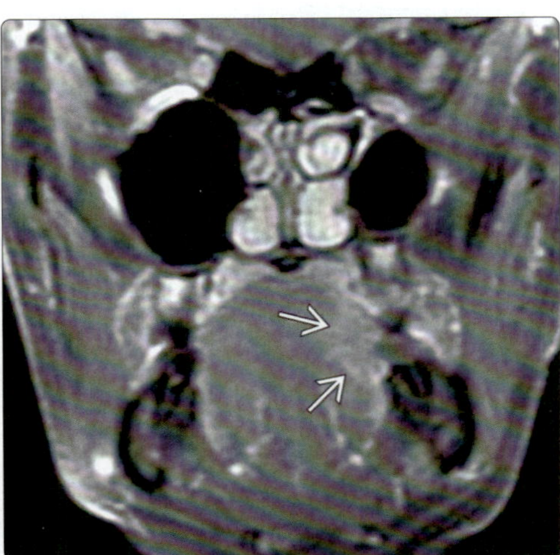

(Left) *Coronal graphic shows oral mucosal space/surface (blue) on the left. Hard palate ➡, oral tongue, upper & lower alveolar ridge, buccal ➡, & floor of mouth ➡ mucosal surfaces are seen. The coronal plane is helpful for deep involvement of the base of tongue, floor of mouth, & mandible.* **(Right)** *Coronal T1WI C+ FS MR in a 32-year-old woman with a remote history of cigarette and marijuana use shows a heterogeneous, mildly enhancing lesion of lateral tongue ➡. This is T2N2b, stage IVA SCCa.*

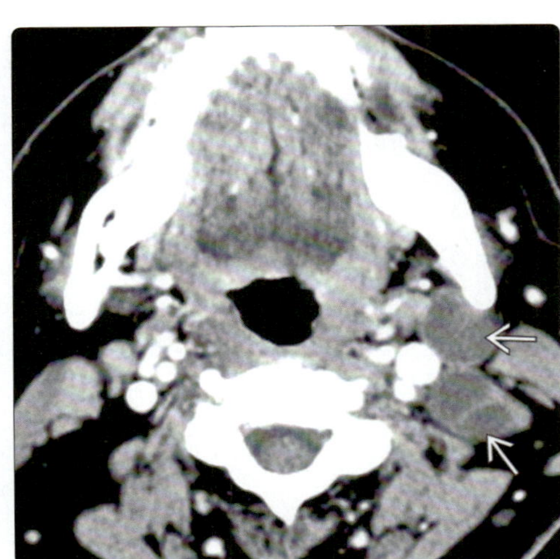

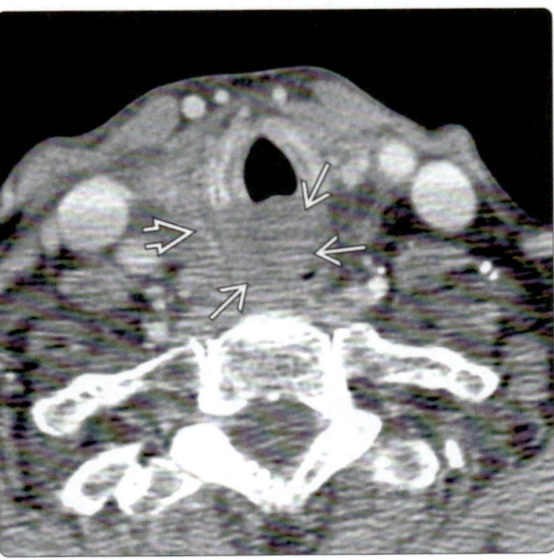

(Left) *Axial CECT in a 46-year-old woman with neck masses shows multiple necrotic/cystic nodes ➡. There was no primary on clinical exam or imaging, although tonsillectomy revealed a small primary tumor. This is T1N2b, stage IVA SCCa.* **(Right)** *Axial CECT in a 78-year-old man with new hoarseness 7 months following completion of radiation for T1 glottic SCCa shows ill-defined esophageal mass ➡ infiltrating the right tracheoesophageal groove ➡. The lesion was found to be a 2nd primary tumor (esophageal SCCa).*

T | Definition of Primary Tumor (T)

T Category	T Criteria
TX	Primary tumor cannot be assessed
Tis	Carcinoma in situ
T0	No tumor identified, but EBV-positive cervical node(s) involvement
T1	Tumor confined to nasopharynx or extension to oropharynx &/or nasal cavity without parapharyngeal extension[1]
T2	Tumor with parapharyngeal extension[1] &/or adjacent soft tissue involvement (medial pterygoid, lateral pterygoid, prevertebral muscles)
T3	Tumor with infiltration of bony structures at skull base, cervical vertebra, pterygoid structures, &/or paranasal sinuses
T4	Tumor with intracranial extension, involvement of cranial nerves, hypopharynx, orbit, parotid gland &/or extensive soft tissue infiltration beyond lateral surface of lateral pterygoid muscle (parotid; masseter &/or temporalis muscle)

[1]Parapharyngeal extension denotes posterolateral infiltration of tumor.

All tables adapted with permission from AJCC Cancer Staging Manual 8th ed., 2017.

N | Definition of Regional Lymph Node (N)

N Category	N Criteria
NX	Regional lymph nodes cannot be assessed
N0	No regional lymph node metastasis
N1	Unilateral metastasis in cervical lymph node(s) &/or unilateral or bilateral metastasis in retropharyngeal lymph node(s)[1], ≤ 6 cm in greatest dimension, above caudal border of cricoid cartilage (level II, III, or VA)
N2	Bilateral metastasis in cervical lymph node(s), ≤ 6 cm in greatest dimension, above caudal border of cricoid cartilage (level II, III, or VA)
N3	Unilateral or bilateral metastasis in cervical lymph node(s) > 6 cm &/or extension below caudal border of cricoid cartilage[2] (level IV &/or VB)

[1]Midline nodes are considered ipsilateral nodes; [2]nodal size > 6 cm &/or extension below caudal border of cricoid cartilage are associated with worst prognosis.

M | Definition of Distant Metastasis (M)

M Category	M Criteria
M0	No distant metastasis
M1	Distant metastasis

AJCC | Prognostic Stage Groups

When T is...	And N is...	And M is...	Then the stage group is...
Tis	N0	M0	Stage 0
T1	N0	M0	Stage I
T1, T0	N1	M0	Stage II
T2	N0	M0	Stage II
T2	N1	M0	Stage II
T1, T0	N2	M0	Stage III
T2	N2	M0	Stage III
T3	N0	M0	Stage III
T3	N1	M0	Stage III
T3	N2	M0	Stage III
T4	N0	M0	Stage IVA
T4	N1	M0	Stage IVA
T4	N2	M0	Stage IVA
Any T	N3	M0	Stage IVA
Any T	Any T	M1	Stage IVB

20-30% of patients will develop distant metastases typically within 2 years of diagnosis and treatment.

T1

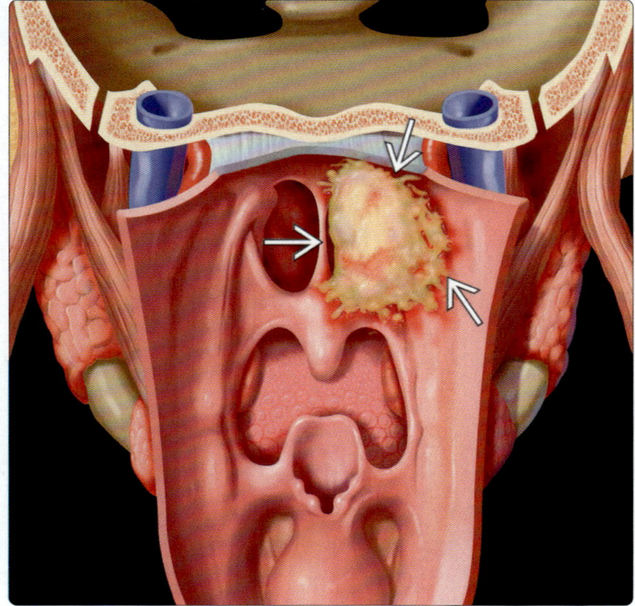

Graphic illustrates T1 nasopharyngeal carcinoma (NPC) that appears confined to the nasopharynx. A nasopharyngeal tumor may extend anteriorly to the nasal cavity or inferiorly to the oropharynx and still be T1 as long as there is no deep lateral infiltration to the parapharyngeal fat.

T2

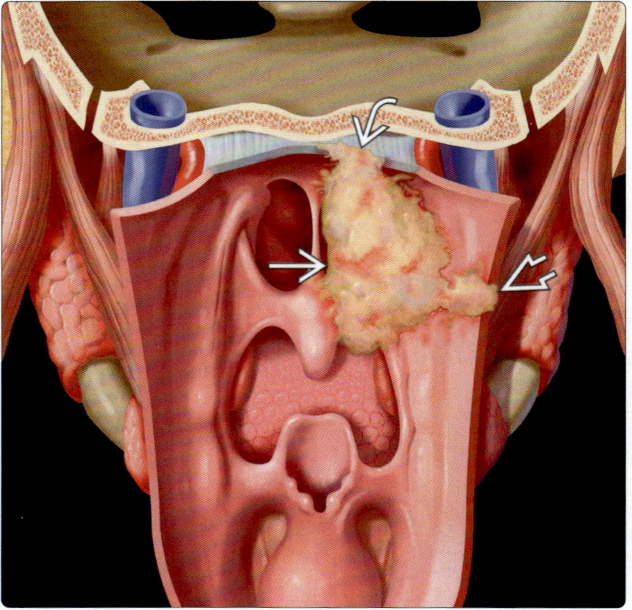

Graphic shows somewhat larger NPC that does not involve skull base. T2 designation is determined not by tumor size but by deep lateral infiltration to parapharyngeal fat infiltration &/or adjacent soft tissues (medial pterygoid, lateral pterygoid, prevertebral muscles).

T3

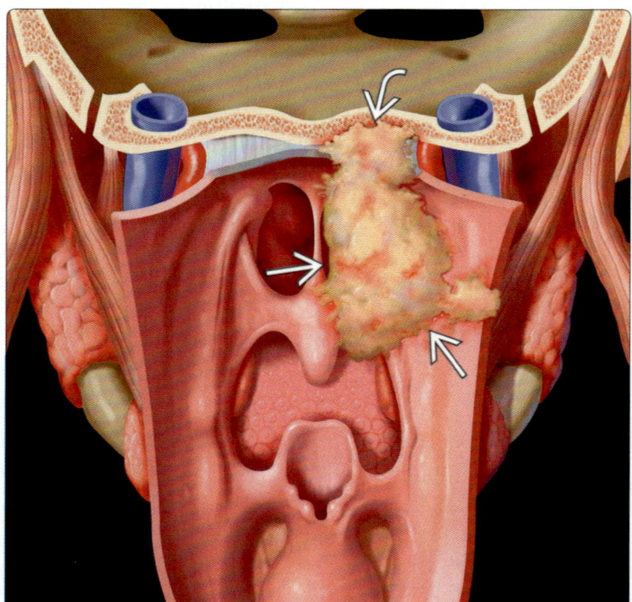

Graphic illustrates a larger T3 NPC extending superiorly to involve the bones of the skull base . Involvement of the cervical vertebra, pterygoid plates, &/or paranasal sinuses also denotes T3 tumor with NPC. T3 tumor is always at least stage III NPC.

T4

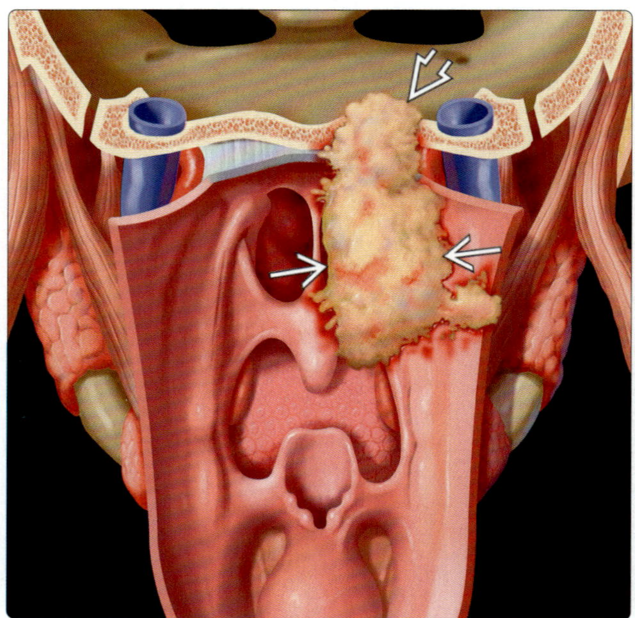

Graphic shows a more extensive T4 NPC that erodes through the skull base to the intracranial cavity . Involvement of the cranial nerves, hypopharynx, orbit, &/or extensive soft tissue infiltration beyond the lateral surface of the lateral pterygoid muscle (parotid, masseter, &/or temporalis muscles) are also T4.

N3

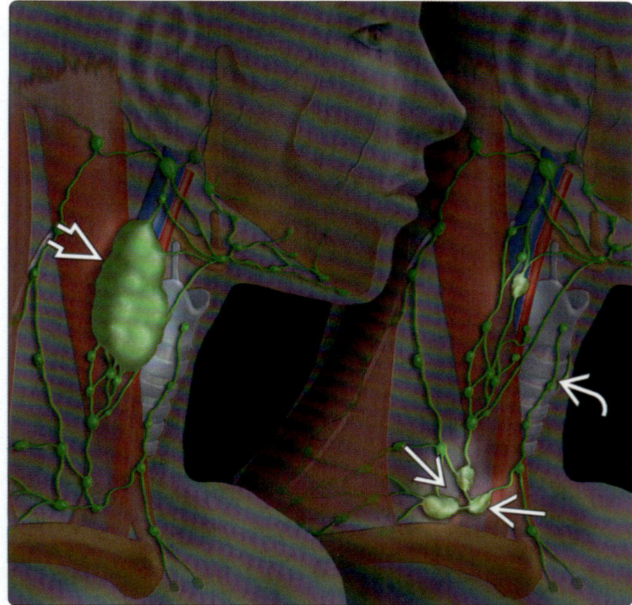

Graphic shows NPC N3 nodal staging illustrations. The patient on the left has N3 disease with a large nodal metastasis > 6 cm. The right drawing shows nodal disease below the caudal border of the cricoid cartilage in level IV nodes, which is denoted as N3 disease. N3 disease denotes at least stage IVA NPC.

N2

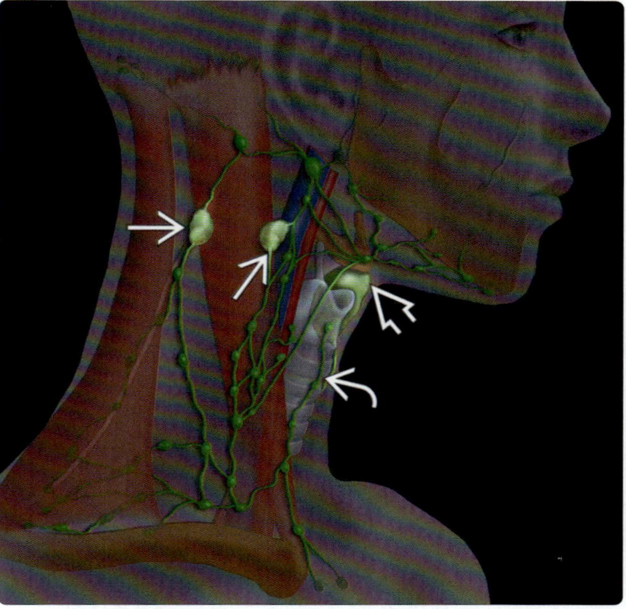

Graphic shows N2 nodal disease with both left and right neck nodes that are ≤ 6 cm in size. The TNM nodal staging for NPC is simplified relative to nodal staging for SCCa of the rest of the pharynx and larynx. N2 is not broken into substages as with SCCa elsewhere. Note the caudal border of cricoid cartilage.

Distant Metastases Sites

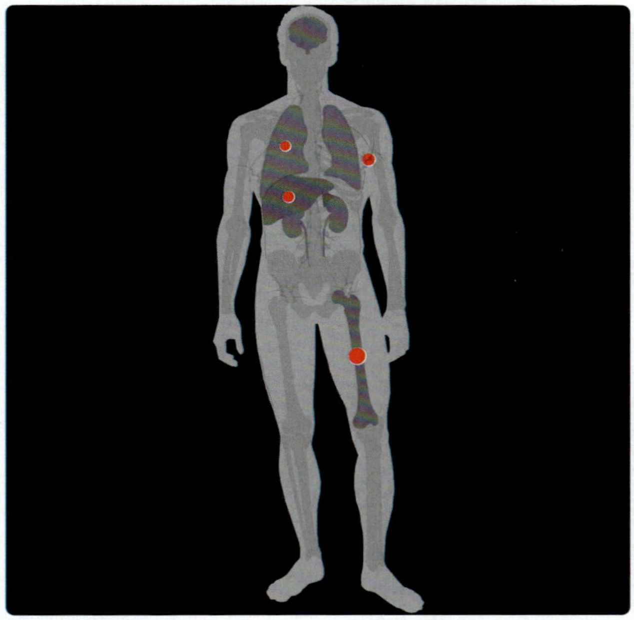

20-30% of patients will develop distant metastases within 2 years of diagnoses and treatment. The most common site of metastatic spread is to the bones followed by distant nodes, liver, and lung locations.

7th vs. 8th AJCC T2 and T4

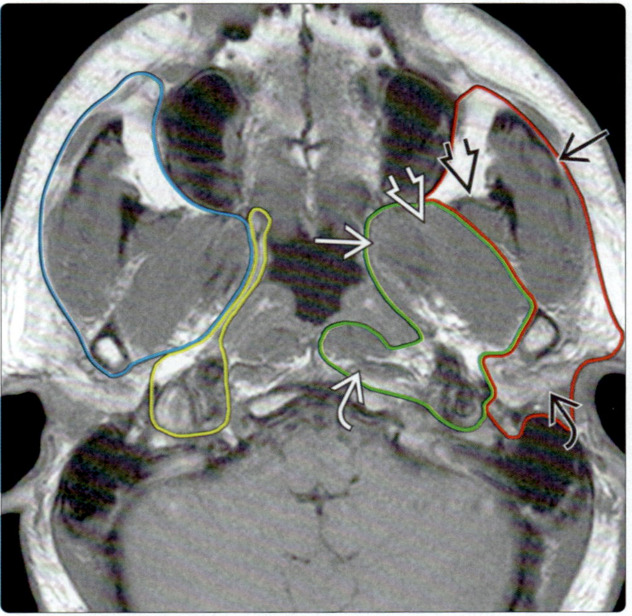

Comparison of T-stage criteria between 7th & 8th AJCC editions: 7th ed: T2 (yellow) & T4 (blue) vs. 8th ed: T2 (green) & T4 (red). T2 new (green) includes medial & lateral pterygoid & prevertebral muscles. T4 new (red) includes lateral to lateral pterygoid (parotid, masseter, ± temporalis).

KEY FACTS

TERMINOLOGY

- Nasopharyngeal carcinoma (NPCa)
- Mucosal tumor most commonly found in lateral pharyngeal recess (fossa of Rosenmüller), strongly associated with **EBV infection**

IMAGING

- MR best demonstrates parapharyngeal fat, skull base infiltration, and intracranial tumor
- Nodal disease in 90% at presentation: Retropharyngeal, levels II and V most common
- Metastatic nodes often large ± necrosis
  - Nodal staging NPCa unlike rest of pharyngeal SCCa
- NPCa is markedly FDG avid

TOP DIFFERENTIAL DIAGNOSES

- Adenoidal benign lymphoid hyperplasia
- Nasopharyngeal non-Hodgkin lymphoma
- Nasopharyngeal minor salivary gland malignancy

PATHOLOGY

- **25%: Keratinizing NPCa** (previously type I)
- **75%: Nonkeratinizing NPCa** (NK NPCa)
  - Strongly associated with **EBV infection**
  - **15% differentiated** (previously type II)
  - **60% undifferentiated** (previously type III)
- Rare: Basaloid squamous cell carcinoma

CLINICAL ISSUES

- Clinical presentations: 40-60 years; Asians
  - Bloody nasal discharge or epistaxis
  - Metastatic nodes: 50-70% at present
  - Serous otitis from eustachian tube obstruction
- NK NPCa has 5-year survival of **75%**
- Keratinizing NPCa has 5-year survival of **20-40%**
- Treatment options
  - Stage I (XRT alone); stage II-IV: Chemoradiation
  - M1 (Stage IVB): Chemotherapy; radiotherapy only if good response

(Left) *Coronal NECT of the paranasal sinuses performed in a 62-year-old Asian man for evaluation of nasal congestion and epistaxis demonstrates an asymmetric bulky mass of the nasopharynx ➡ with heterogeneous, mottled texture of the clivus ➡.* **(Right)** *Sagittal T1WI MR in same patient shows a large soft tissue mass in nasopharynx ➡ extending superiorly to the sphenoid & sella ➡ (T4, intracranial extension). Note replacement of normally hyperintense fatty marrow of the clivus ➡ without clival expansion.*

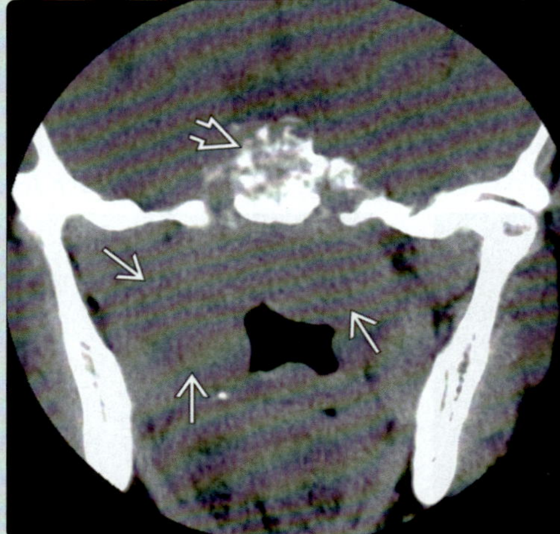

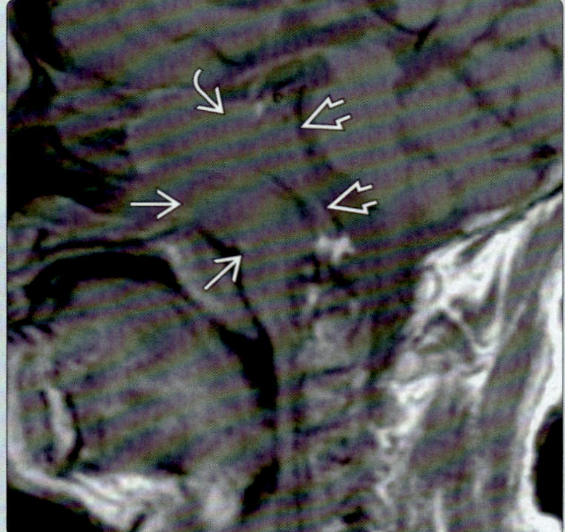

(Left) *Coronal T1WI C+ FS MR reveals moderate enhancement of a bulky mass ➡ filling the nasopharynx with an indistinct right lateral margin. Enhancing tumor extends cranially to infiltrate the sphenoid bone ➡. There is no abnormality of cavernous sinuses ➡.* **(Right)** *Axial T1WI C+ FS MR shows NPCa infiltration of parapharyngeal fat ➡. There is abnormal enhancement of basisphenoid ➡ consistent with marrow infiltration. There is abnormal right hypoglossal nerve enhancement ➡ (T4, cranial nerve involvement).*

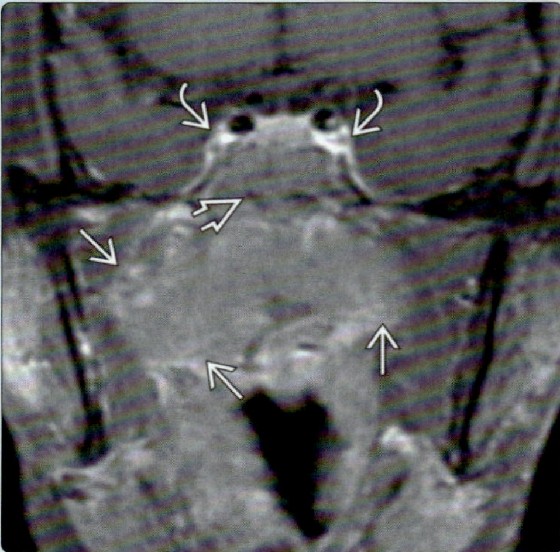

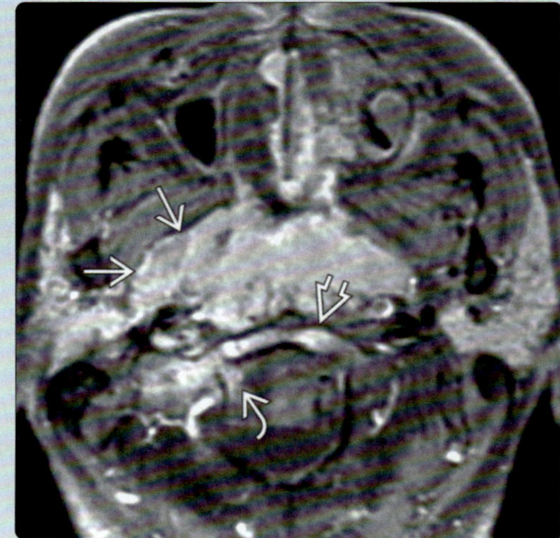

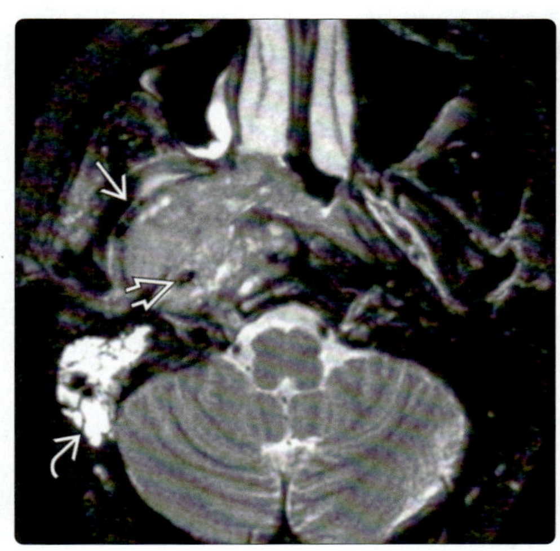

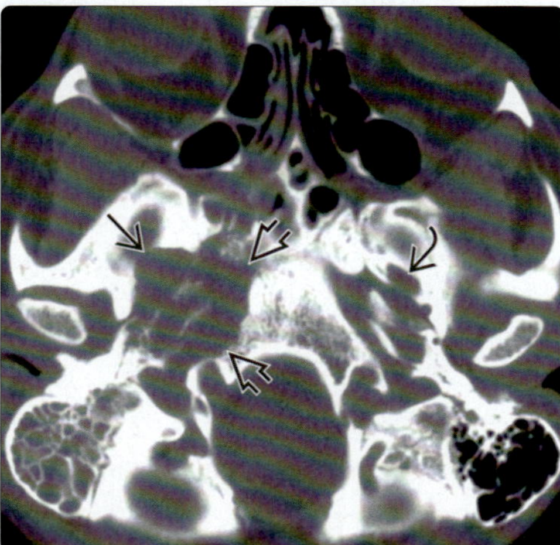

(Left) *Axial T2WI MR in a patient with a large NPCa shows a large right nasopharyngeal mass extending into the lateral pterygoid muscle & posteriorly to surround internal carotid artery. Note unilateral right mastoid fluid due to eustachian tube dysfunction.* **(Right)** *Axial bone CT in the same patient shows an enlarged right foramen ovale from perineural CNV3 spread with adjacent skull base destruction. Note the normal contralateral foramen ovale.*

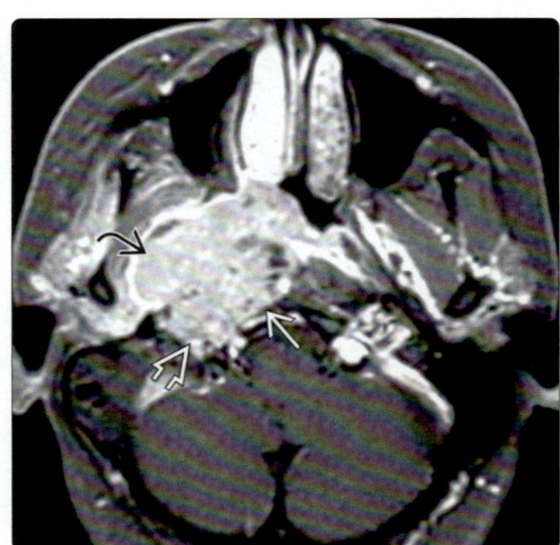

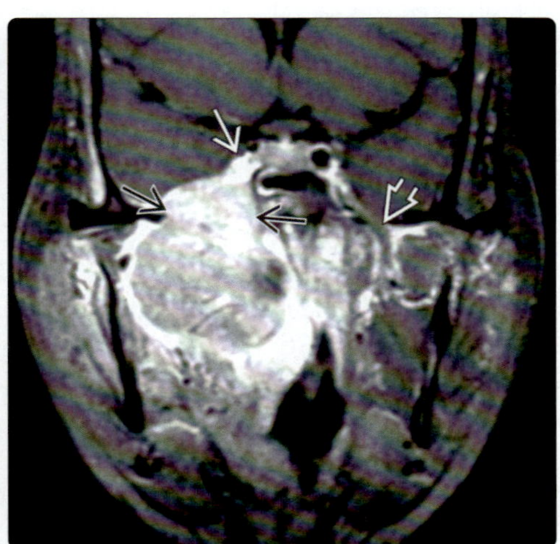

(Left) *Axial T1WI C+ MR in a patient with a large NPCa shows an enhancing, invasive right-sided nasopharyngeal mass. The tumor invades the prevertebral muscles, nasopharyngeal carotid space, and parapharyngeal space.* **(Right)** *Coronal T1WI C+ MR in a patient with a large nasopharyngeal carcinoma shows tumor destroying a large area of the skull base bone surrounding the foramen ovale. The tumor invades the right cavernous sinus. Notice the opposite normal foramen ovale with the CNV3 traversing it.*

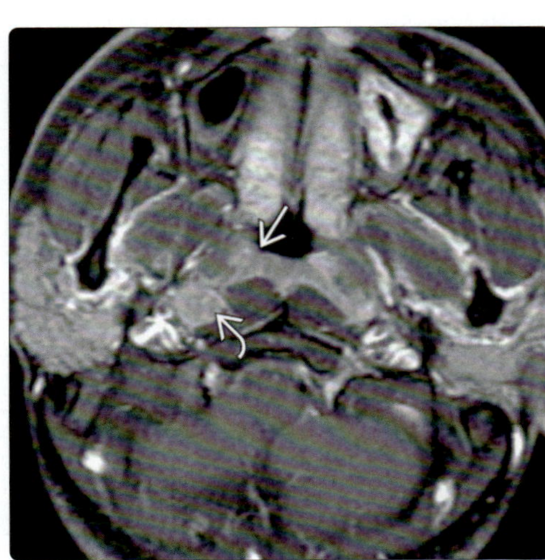

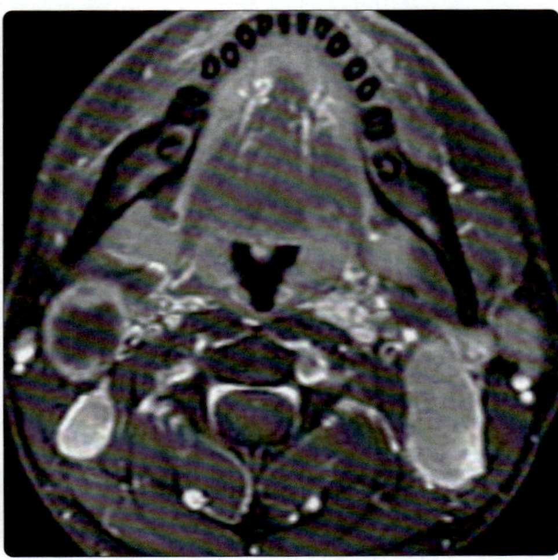

(Left) *Axial T1WI C+ FS MR in a 26-year-old Asian man presenting with neck masses demonstrates subtly asymmetric soft tissue fullness of nasopharynx mucosa found to be NPCa. No infiltration of the prevertebral muscles is seen. Malignant right retropharyngeal node is evident.* **(Right)** *Axial T1WI C+ fat-saturated MR in same patient shows bulky bilateral malignant lymph nodes typical of nasopharyngeal carcinoma.*

T | Definition of Primary Tumor (T)

T Category	T Criteria
TX	Primary tumor cannot be assessed
Tis	Carcinoma in situ
T1	Tumor ≤ 2 cm in greatest dimension
T2	Tumor > 2 cm but ≤ 4 cm in greatest dimension
T3	Tumor > 4 cm in greatest dimension or extension to lingual surface of epiglottis
T4a	Moderately advanced local disease: Tumor invades larynx, extrinsic muscle of tongue, medial pterygoid, hard palate, or mandible[1]
T4b	Very advanced local disease: Tumor invades lateral pterygoid muscle, pterygoid plates, lateral nasopharynx, or skull base or encases carotid artery

[1]Mucosal extension to lingual surface of epiglottis from primary tumors of base of tongue and vallecula does not constitute invasion of larynx.

All tables adapted with permission from AJCC Cancer Staging Manual 8th ed., 2017.

N | Definition of Regional Lymph Node (N[1]): Clinical N (cN)

N Category	N Criteria
NX	Regional lymph nodes cannot be assessed
N0	No regional lymph node metastasis
N1	Extranodal extension (ENE)(-)[2] metastasis in single ipsilateral lymph node, ≤ 3 cm
N2a N2b N2c	ENE(-) metastasis, single ipsilateral node > 3 cm but ≤ 6 cm ENE(-) metastasis in multiple ipsilateral lymph nodes, none > 6 cm ENE(-) metastasis in bilateral or contralateral lymph nodes, none 6 cm
N3a N3b	ENE(-) metastasis in lymph node > 6 cm Clinically overt ENE(+)[3] in any metastatic nodes

[1]Designation of "U" or "L" may be used for any N category to indicate metastasis above (U) or below (L) lower border of cricoid cartilage.
[2]ENE should be recorded as ENE(-) or ENE(+); however, clinically overt ENE (+) corresponds solely with cN3b.
[3]Clinically overt ENE(+) can be diagnosed by presence of "matted" nodal mass, overlying skin or adjacent soft tissue involvement, or clinical signs of cranial nerve, brachial plexus, sympathetic chain, or phrenic nerve invasion. CT/MR imaging signs of ENE are adjacent fat/muscle infiltration, indistinct nodal margin, or irregular nodal capsular enhancement. US, less accurate than CT/MR, suggests ENE by interrupted or undefined nodal contours.

N | Definition of Regional Lymph Node (N[1]): Pathological N (pN)

N Category	N Criteria
NX	Regional lymph nodes cannot be assessed
N0	No regional lymph node metastasis
N1	Extranodal extension(ENE)(-)[2] metastasis in single ipsilateral lymph node, ≤ 3 cm
N2a N2b N2c	ENE(+)[2] metastasis in single ipsilateral lymph node, ≤ 3 cm or ENE (-) metastasis in single ipsilateral lymph node, > 3 cm but ≤ 6 cm ENE(-) metastasis in multiple ipsilateral lymph nodes, none > 6 cm ENE(-) metastasis in bilateral or contralateral lymph nodes, none > 6 cm
N3a N3b	ENE(-) metastasis in lymph node > 6 cm ENE(+) metastasis in single ipsilateral lymph node, > 3 cm in greatest dimension; **or** multiple ipsilateral, single or multiple contralateral, or bilateral nodes with any ENE(+) nodes

[1]Designation of "U" or "L" may be used for any N category to indicate metastasis above (U) or below (L) lower border of cricoid cartilage.
[2]ENE should be recorded as ENE(-) or ENE(+). As above, pathological ENE(+) increases pN category by 1.

M | Definition of Distant Metastasis[1]

M Category	M Criteria
M0	No distant metastasis
M1	Distant metastasis

[1]Mediastinal lymph nodes are considered distant metastasis, except level VII nodes (anterior superior mediastinal nodes above inominate/brachiocephalic artery).

AJCC | Prognostic Stage Groups

When T is...	When N is...	And M is...	Then the stage group is...
Tis	N0	M0	0
T1	N0	M0	I
T2	N0	M0	II
T3	N0	M0	III
T1, T2, T3	N1	M0	III
T4a	N0, N1	M0	IVA
T1, T2,T3,T4a	N2	M0	IVA
Any T	N3	M0	IVB
T4b	Any N	M0	IVB
Any T	Any N	M1	IVC

G | Histologic Grade (G)

G	G Definition
GX	Grade cannot be assessed
G1	Well differentiated
G2	Moderately differentiated
G3	Poorly differentiated
G4	Undifferentiated

T1

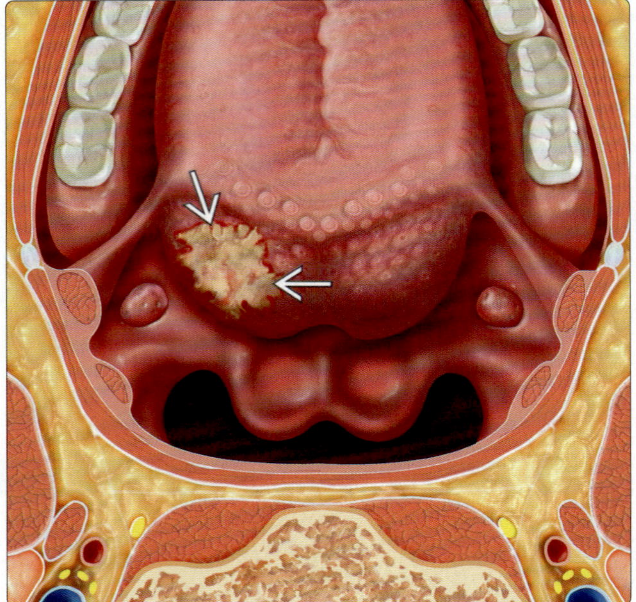

Graphic depicts a small, < 2-cm tumor confined to the right lingual tonsil ➡, which is considered T1. Oropharyngeal tumor subsites are specified as palatine/ lingual tonsil, tonsillar pillar, posterior oropharyngeal wall, and soft palate (AJCC 8th ed).

T2

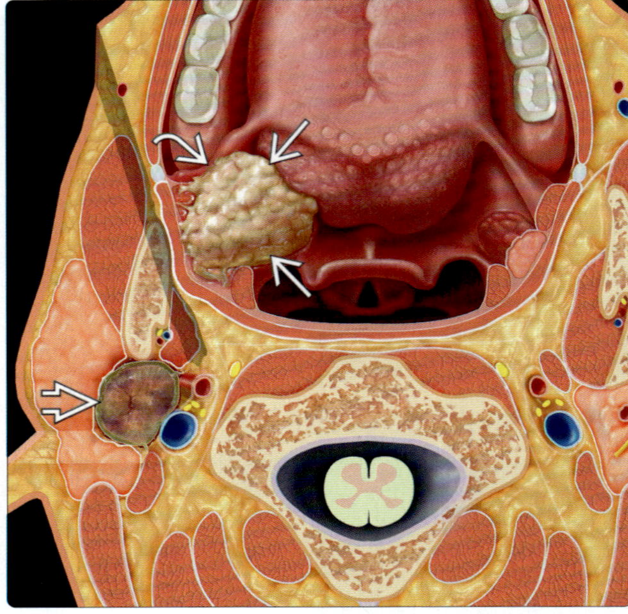

Graphic illustrates a larger tumor ➡, this time arising from the right palatine tonsil and involving the anterior tonsillar pillar ➡. The tumor is < 4 cm in greatest dimension and therefore staged as T2. Note ipsilateral level IIA node ➡, a frequent finding with oropharyngeal squamous cell carcinoma (SCCa).

T3

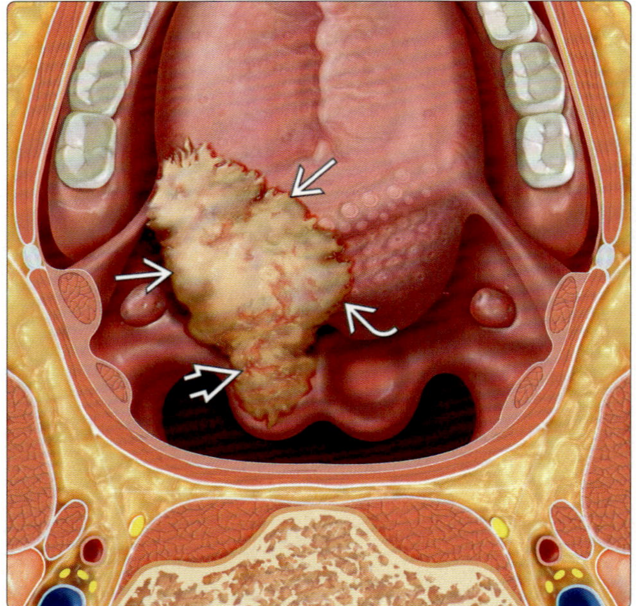

Graphic illustrates an even larger, > 4-cm, T3 lingual tonsil SCCa ➡, which extends inferiorly to the right vallecula ➡. Extension to the lingual surface of the epiglottis is still considered T3 disease. The tumor extends across the midline toward the left tongue base ➡, although that does not affect T staging.

T4a

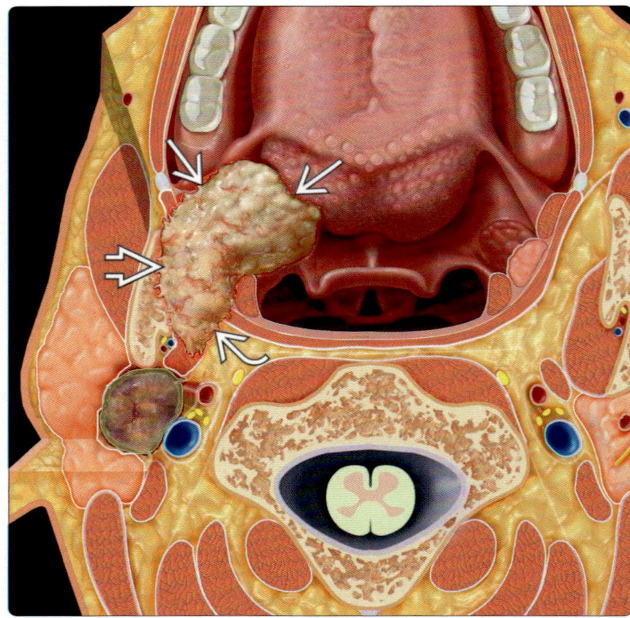

Graphic illustrates more extensive palatine tonsillar SCCa ➡, which infiltrates through the lateral oropharyngeal wall to invade both the medial pterygoid muscle ➡ and mandible ➡. Either area of invasion stages this tumor as T4a or moderately advanced local disease.

T4b

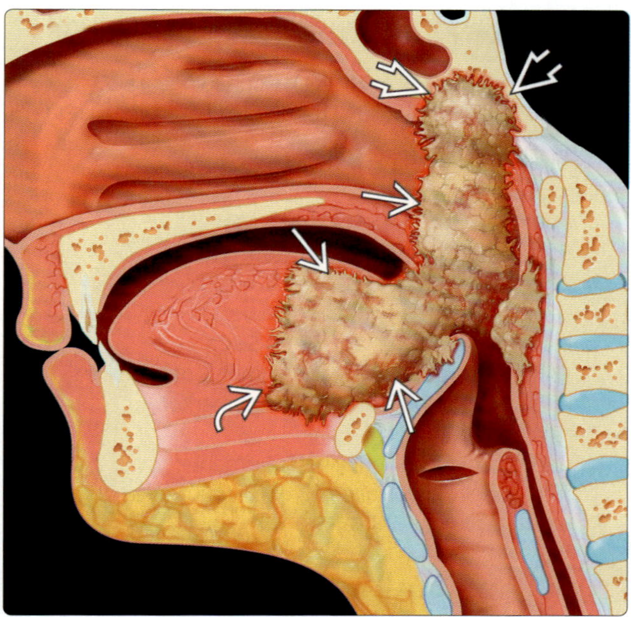

Graphic shows very advanced local disease with SCCa ➡ involving the tongue base and lateral pharyngeal wall extending anteriorly to the oral tongue and genioglossus muscle ➡ and superiorly to skull base ➡. Extrinsic tongue muscle involvement denotes T4a disease, but skull base invasion upstages this to T4b.

T4b

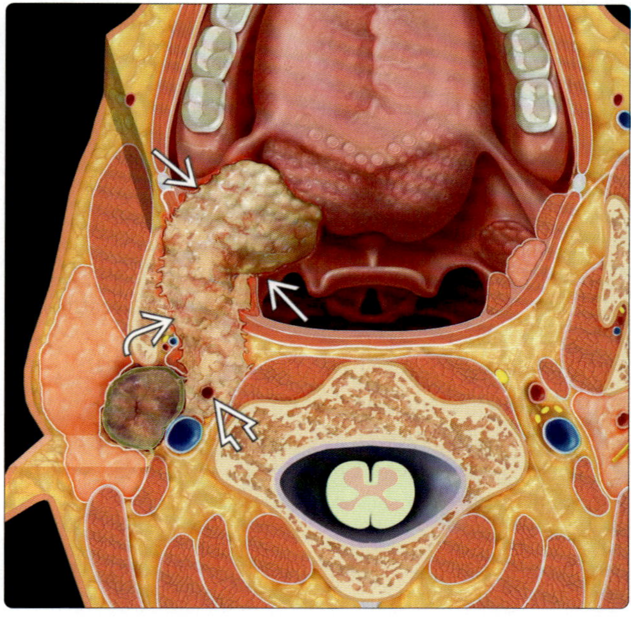

Graphic illustrates very advanced tumor ➡ arising from the right palatine tonsil, invading posteriorly through medial pterygoid muscle ➡ and mandible to encase the ICA ➡. T4b is determined by invasion of lateral pterygoid muscle, pterygoid plate, lateral nasopharynx, or skull base, or by encasement of carotid artery.

Metastases, Organ Frequency

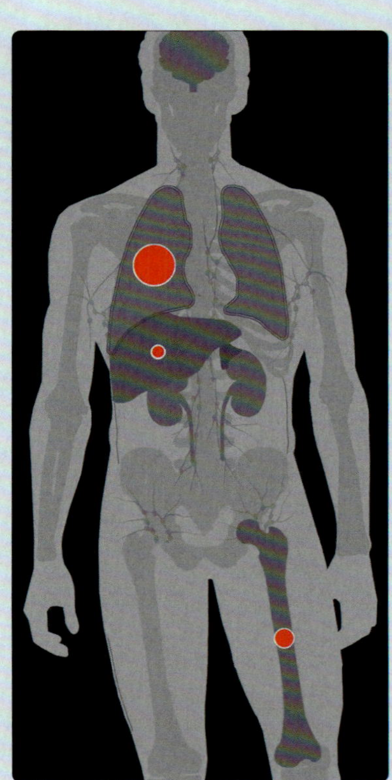

Lung	***83%***
Bone	***31%***
Liver	***6%***

Overall 12% of patients with oropharyngeal carcinoma develop distant metastases. Distant metastases are less common with HPV-related squamous cell carcinoma. The likelihood of distant metastasis is significantly reduced if local control is achieved in the neck.

Base of Tongue Squamous Cell Carcinoma

KEY FACTS

TERMINOLOGY

- Base of tongue (BOT) squamous cell carcinoma (SCCa)
- BOT: Tonsillar tissue at posterior 1/3 of tongue

IMAGING

- Primary tumor may be ulceroinfiltrative lesion or exophytic
- Nodal disease common even with small or subtle primary
- CECT most often used; MR more accurate for tumor extent
  - CECT protocol: Scan ≥ 90 seconds after IV contrast to maximize tumor and mucosal enhancement
  - MR: Fat-sat enhances soft tissue contrast: T2 and T1 C+
- PET/CT: Staging, unknown primary search, posttreatment baseline scan
  - Beware of FDG-negative cystic nodal metastasis

TOP DIFFERENTIAL DIAGNOSES

- Lingual tonsil lymphoid hyperplasia
- Lingual tonsil non-Hodgkin lymphoma
- Lingual tonsil minor salivary gland malignancy

PATHOLOGY

- Oropharyngeal SCCa classically associated with tobacco + alcohol abuse
- Increasing incidence of **HPV(+)** oropharyngeal SCCa
- Overall 5-yr survival = 50%, prognosis better when HPV(+)

CLINICAL ISSUES

- Clinical presentation
  - Adults; typically > 45 years; M > > F
  - Sore throat tongue mass sensation
  - Palpable level II node(s): ~ 50%, often cystic
    - 30% bilateral nodes at presentation
  - Increasing incidence of **HPV(+) SCCa**
    - Patients younger, more commonly nonsmokers
    - HPV is favorable prognostic biomarker
- Treatment options
  - Chemoradiation is principal treatment
  - Increasing role of transoral robotic surgery as primary modality, ± adjuvant treatment

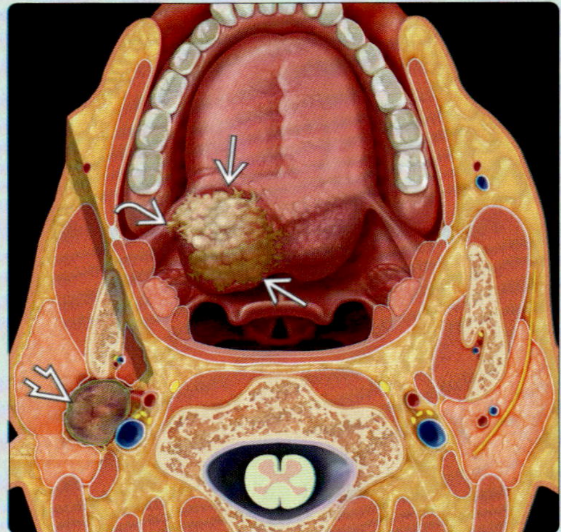

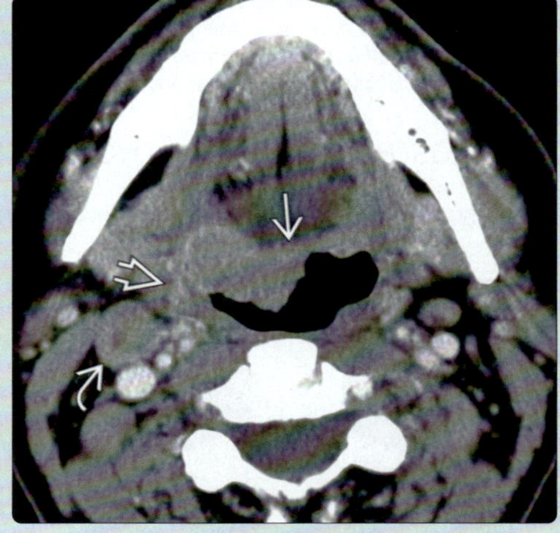

(Left) *Axial graphic depicts lingual tonsil squamous cell carcinoma (SCCa) ➡ with ipsilateral level IIA adenopathy ➡. The tongue base tumor has predominantly exophytic growth but infiltrates the inferior aspect of the anterior tonsillar pillar ➡.* **(Right)** *Axial CECT in a patient with a tongue base mass reveals exophytic lingual tonsil SCCa extending to the tongue base midline ➡ and lateral pharyngeal wall ➡. There is a metastatic IIA node ➡ with central necrosis.*

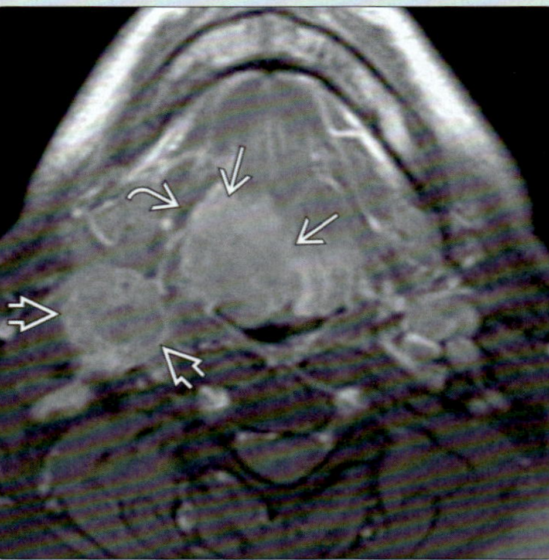

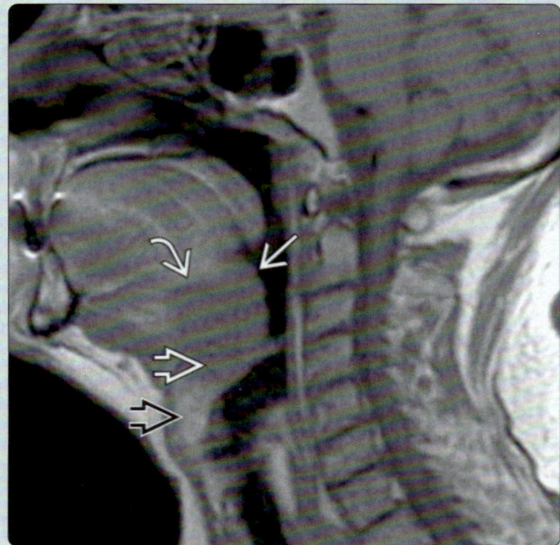

(Left) *Axial T1WI C+ FS MR in a 58-year-old alcoholic presenting with a right neck mass after a dental procedure demonstrates an enlarged, heterogeneous, right level IIA node ➡. The primary tumor is in the ipsilateral lingual tonsil ➡ and infiltrates the floor of mouth, medial to hyoglossus muscle ➡.* **(Right)** *Sagittal T1WI MR in the same patient shows the mass in the base of the tongue ➡. Infiltration of the subjacent floor of mouth ➡ is present. Tumor extends inferiorly to the valleculae ➡ but does not extend inferiorly into preepiglottic fat ➡.*

KEY FACTS

TERMINOLOGY

- Palatine tonsil squamous cell carcinoma (SCCa)
  - Most common oropharyngeal SCCa subsite

IMAGING

- Variable appearance and presentation of primary tumor
  - Small lesion may be occult on clinical ± imaging
  - Larger lesions often exophytic or deeply invasive
- Adenopathy common, most often ipsilateral level II
  - Nodes solid, cystic, or mixed
- PET/CECT, CECT alone, or MR used to stage primary and nodal extent
- PET/CECT: Confirms primary, detects smaller metastatic nodes, distant mets
- MR: Improves detection of small primary and delineation of tumor extent

TOP DIFFERENTIAL DIAGNOSES

- Tonsillar lymphoid hyperplasia
- Palatine tonsil non-Hodgkin lymphoma
- Palatine tonsil minor salivary gland carcinoma

PATHOLOGY

- **HPV** associated with tonsil SCCa, especially **HPV-16**
- Tobacco + alcohol abuse also associated with tonsil SCCa

CLINICAL ISSUES

- Presentation: Ipsilateral ear pain, dysphagia, neck node
  - If HPV(+), typically younger patient, smaller primary
  - If HPV(+), overall better treatment response and survival
  - **75%** have **adenopathy** at presentation
  - Small primary tumor may be clinically and imaging occult
- Most patients > 45 years; ↑ incidence in < 45 years [HPV(+)]
- Treatment options: Evolving with recognition that HPV(+) tumors have better prognosis
  - HPV(+) tumors: Resect primary via radical tonsillectomy & neck dissection with adjuvant radiation vs. chemoXRT
  - HPV(-) tumors: Chemoradiation

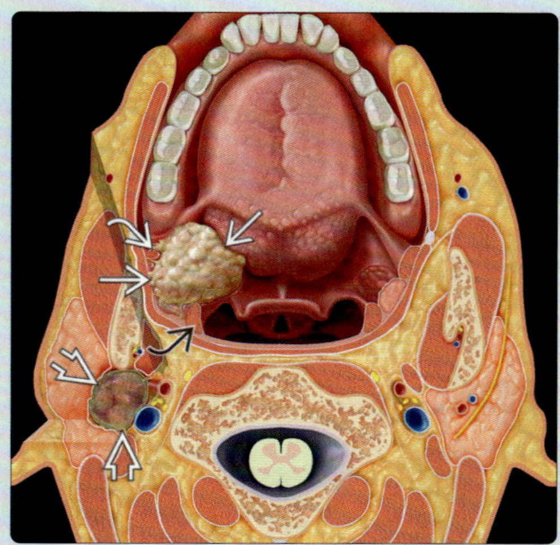

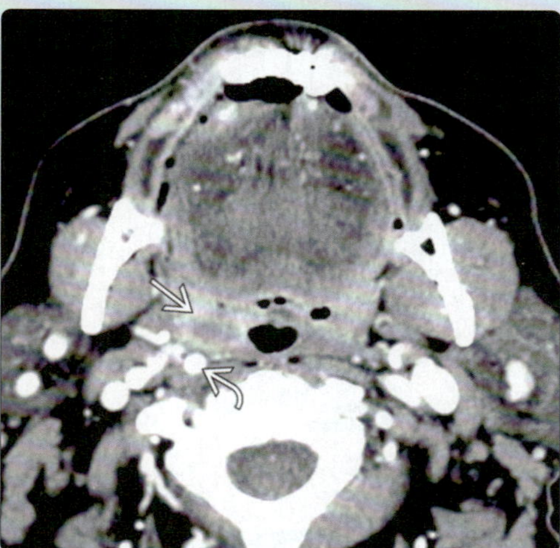

(Left) *Axial graphic shows palatine tonsillar primary squamous cell carcinoma (SCCa) ➡ in the lateral wall of the oropharynx with involvement of the anterior tonsillar pillar ➡. The posterior tonsillar pillar is not infiltrated ➡. Note ipsilateral level II adenopathy ➡.* **(Right)** *Axial CECT reveals an 1.8 x 1.0 cm centrally hypodense tonsil mass ➡, found to be well-differentiated SCCa. The primary tumor was staged as a T1. Patient received chemoradiation. A medialized right ICA ➡ precludes TORS.*

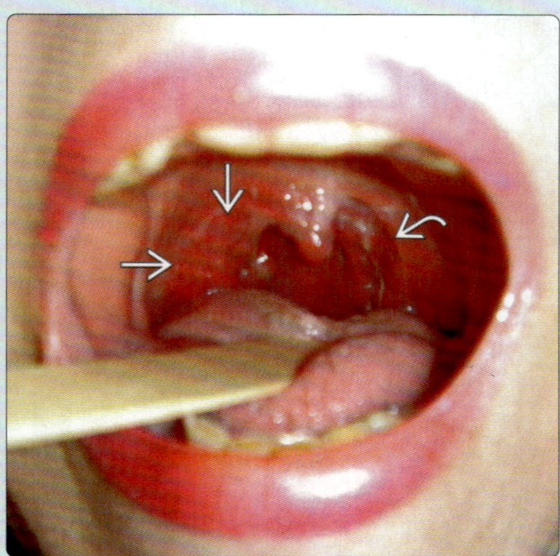

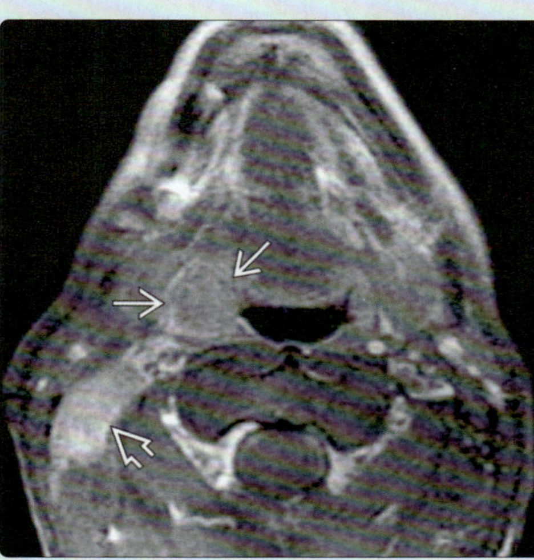

(Left) *Clinical photograph in a woman with dysphagia and right throat and ear pain demonstrates indurated ulcerated right palatine tonsil ➡. Note effacement of the anterior tonsillar pillar with normal comparison on the left ➡.* **(Right)** *Axial T1WI C+ FS MR in a patient presenting with a right neck mass demonstrates the superior aspect of a nodal conglomerate ➡; fine-need aspiration revealed SCCa. A well-defined primary palatine tonsillar tumor is evident ➡, measuring 2.2 x 1.8 cm. The primary tumor is staged as T2.*

Posterior Oropharyngeal Wall Squamous Cell Carcinoma

KEY FACTS

TERMINOLOGY

- Definition: Squamous cell carcinoma (SCCa) arising from posterior oropharyngeal wall
  - **Soft palate** is superior limit; **hyoid** is inferior limit

IMAGING

- Lobulated posterior oropharyngeal wall mass
  - Retropharyngeal nodal metastases common
    - Especially with prevertebral invasion
- CECT: Mild to moderately enhancing soft tissue
  - **Early invasion** of retropharyngeal/prevertebral spaces
- MR: Isointense to muscle on T1, moderate T2 signal
  - Moderate contrast enhancement
  - Intact retropharyngeal fat plane on MR has high negative predictive value for tumor invasion
- PET/CT: SCCa reliably FDG avid

TOP DIFFERENTIAL DIAGNOSES

- Nasopharyngeal carcinoma
- Posterior hypopharyngeal wall SCCa

PATHOLOGY

- **> 90%** of oropharyngeal cancers are **SCCa**
- Most posterior oropharyngeal SCCa are well differentiated

CLINICAL ISSUES

- Clinical presentation
  - Relatively rare compared to lingual-palatine tonsil SCCa
  - Strong association with tobacco and alcohol use
  - Typically relatively asymptomatic until late stage
  - Mucosal lesion seen on direct inspection
- Treatment options
  - Early deep invasion makes surgery difficult
    - Prevertebral invasion indicates unresectable tumor
    - If primary surgery considered, suggest MR to determine if prevertebral invasion
  - If small primary tumor, N0: Radiation alone
  - Larger tumors, ≥ N1: Chemoradiation ± neck dissection

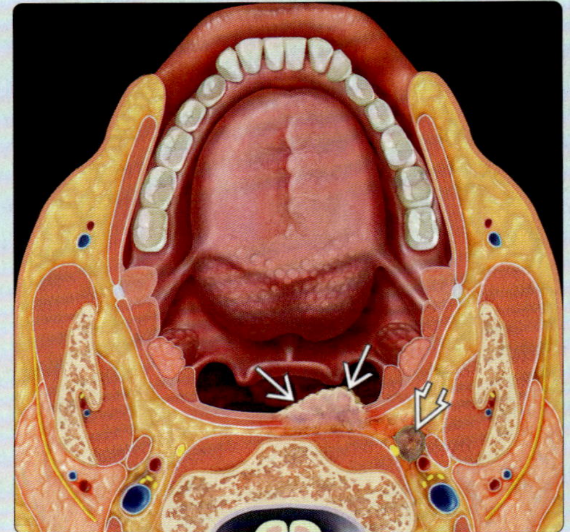

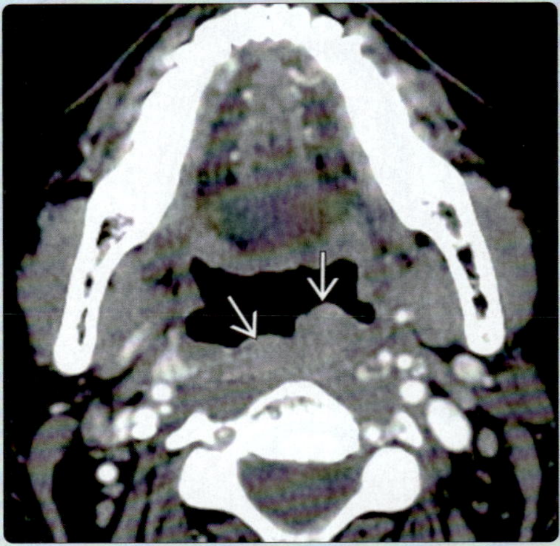

(Left) *Transverse graphic depicts irregular SCCa arising from the posterior oropharyngeal wall ➡ and invading retropharyngeal fat. Invasion of the prevertebral muscle indicates a T4b tumor. Note the ipsilateral necrotic metastatic retropharyngeal node ➡ medial to the carotid artery.* **(Right)** *Axial CECT demonstrates a mildly enhancing soft tissue mass in the left paramedian posterior oropharyngeal wall ➡. Prevertebral muscle invasion and adenopathy are not evident. Patient had extensive tobacco & alcohol use history.*

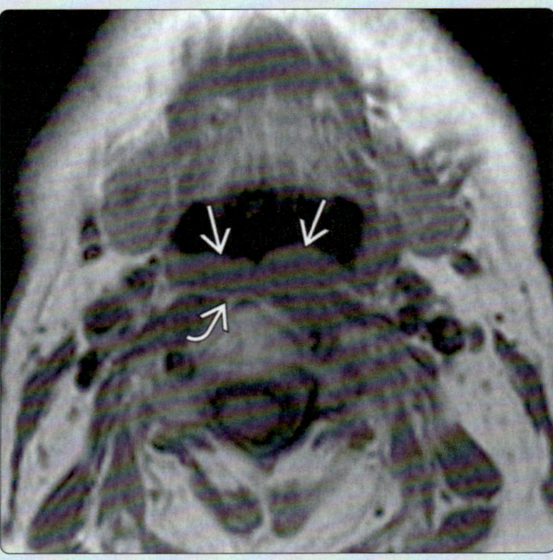

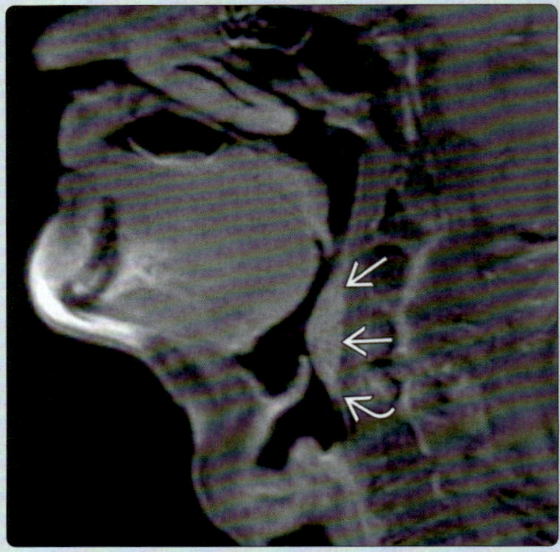

(Left) *Axial T1 MR in a patient with dysphagia shows irregular bilobed thickening of the posterior oropharyngeal wall ➡. Hyperintense retropharyngeal fat is seen on the right side ➡ but is indistinct on the left side. However, there is no evidence of prevertebral muscle invasion.* **(Right)** *Sagittal T1 C+ FS MR shows the left-sided component of a pharyngeal wall tumor bulging into the posterior oropharynx ➡. Inferiorly, it reaches superior aspect of the hypopharynx ➡ but does not extend superiorly to the nasopharynx.*

KEY FACTS

TERMINOLOGY

- Human papillomavirus-related [HPV(+)] oropharyngeal squamous cell carcinoma (SCCa)
  - Most often **HPV type 16**

IMAGING

- CECT or enhanced T1 MR imaging findings
  - C+ primary tumor site: Palatine or lingual tonsil
    - Identical to SCCa from tobacco and alcohol
  - Level II ± III adenopathy
    - Single or multiple, solid or necrotic/cystic nodes
    - Do not mistake cystic node for 2nd branchial cleft cyst
- PET/CECT may be helpful to determine unknown primary site, as often small; also useful for cancer surveillance

TOP DIFFERENTIAL DIAGNOSES

- 2nd branchial cleft cyst
- Non-Hodgkin lymphoma nodes
- Non-Hodgkin lymphoma lingual or palatine tonsil

PATHOLOGY

- No specific histologic characteristics distinguish HPV(+) SCCa from HPV(-) SCCa
- HPV causation determined by staining for HPV DNA or p16 kinase inhibitor
- Much better prognosis than oropharyngeal HPV(-) SCCa seen typically with tobacco and alcohol abuse
- Intermediate prognosis if smoker with HPV(+) SCCa

CLINICAL ISSUES

- Clinical presentation
  - Unilateral neck mass, level IIA nodes
  - Younger, mostly male, often nonsmokers
- Treatment options
  - Concurrent chemoradiation therapy
  - Transoral robotic surgery or transoral laser microsurgery ± XRT/chemoXRT
  - Prevention with HPV vaccines is likely effective if given before exposure

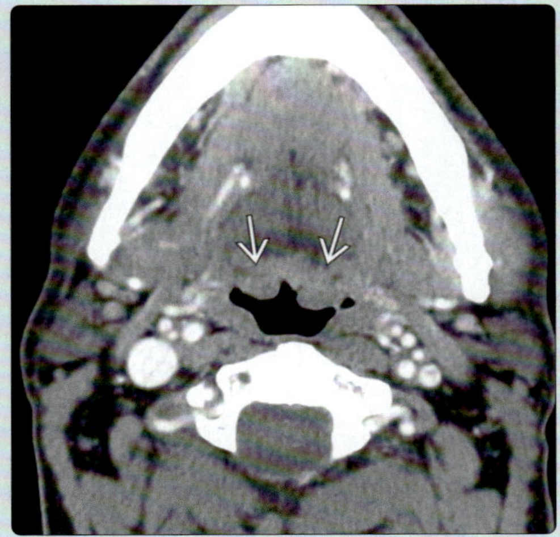

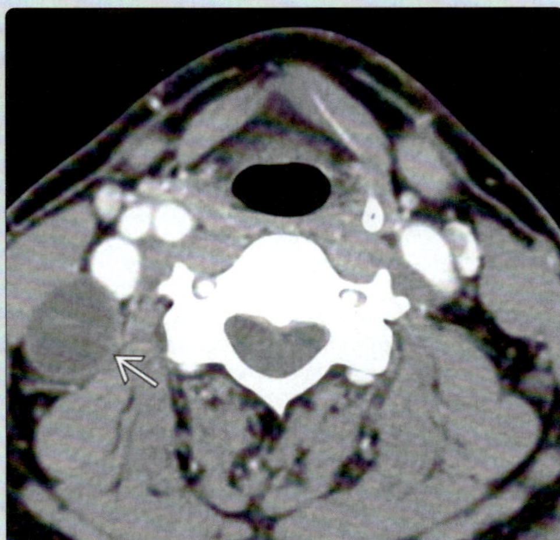

(Left) *Axial CECT shows a normal base of tongue bilaterally ➡ and no high IIA adenopathy.* **(Right)** *Axial CECT in the same patient shows a cystic septated mass in the right neck ➡. FNA of the node revealed squamous cell carcinoma (SCCa), and biopsy of the right base of tongue showed HPV(+) SCCa. Small tongue base primary neoplasms may be occult on cross-sectional imaging. HPV(+) oropharyngeal SCCas are notorious for small primary tumors but large and often cystic-appearing nodal metastases.*

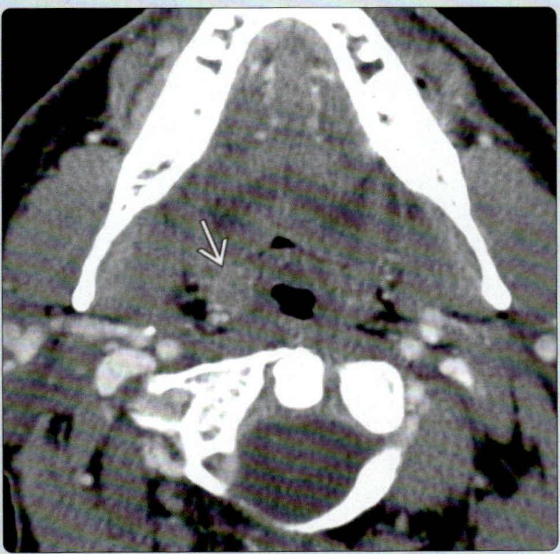

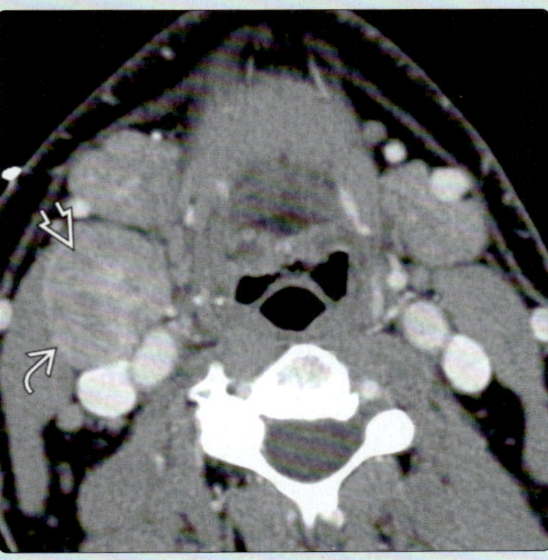

(Left) *Axial CECT in a patient with right ear pain and bulky cervical adenopathy shows a small, enhancing mass in the right palatine tonsil ➡. This CECT could be interpreted as normal if there was no adenopathy.* **(Right)** *Axial CECT in the same patient shows a large anterior right level IIA node ➡. Nodal necrosis is apparent as regions of low density ➡. In situ hybridization was positive for HPV-16 infection. With metastatic level IIA nodes, primary tumor is usually in the ipsilateral oropharynx, either the palatine or lingual tonsil.*

T | Definition of Primary Tumor (T)

T Category	T Criteria
TX	Primary tumor cannot be assessed
Tis	Carcinoma in situ
T1	Tumor ≤ 2 cm, ≤ 5-mm depth of invasion (DOI); DOI is not same as tumor thickness[1]
T2	Tumor ≤ 2 cm, DOI > 5 mm and ≤ 10 mm; or tumor > 2 cm but ≤ 4 cm and ≤ 10 mm DOI
T3	Tumor > 4 cm; or any tumor > 10 mm DOI
T4a	Moderately advanced local disease[2] Lip: Tumor invades through cortical bone, inferior alveolar nerve, floor of mouth, or skin of face (chin or nose) Oral cavity: Tumor invades adjacent structures only (e.g., mandible or maxilla cortical bone, or maxillary sinus or skin of face
T4b	Very advanced local disease: Tumor invades masticator space, pterygoid plates, or skull base &/or encases internal carotid artery

[1]DOI can be estimated clinically and is measured pathologically by dropping plumb line from level of closest intact squamous mucosal basement membrane (horizon) to deepest extent of tumor.
[2]Superficial erosion alone of bone/tooth socket by gingival primary is not sufficient to classify a tumor as T4.

All tables adapted with permission from AJCC Cancer Staging Manual 8th ed., 2017.

N | Definition of Regional Lymph Node (N[1]): Clinical N (cN)

N Category	N Criteria
NX	Regional lymph nodes cannot be assessed
N0	No regional lymph node metastasis
N1	Extranodal extension (ENE)(-)[2] metastasis in single ipsilateral lymph node, ≤ 3 cm
N2a N2b N2c	ENE(-) metastasis, single ipsilateral node > 3 cm but ≤ 6 cm ENE(-) metastasis in multiple ipsilateral lymph nodes, none > 6 cm ENE(-) metastasis in bilateral or contralateral lymph nodes, none > 6 cm
N3b	ENE(-) metastasis in lymph node > 6 cm Clinically overt ENE(+)[3] in any metastatic nodes

[1]Designation of "U" or "L" may be used for any N category to indicate metastasis above (U) or below (L) lower border of cricoid cartilage.
[2]ENE should be recorded as ENE(-) or ENE(+); however, clinically overt ENE(+) corresponds solely with cN3b.
[3]Clinically overt ENE(+) can be diagnosed by presence of "matted" nodal mass, overlying skin or adjacent soft tissue involvement, or clinical signs of cranial nerve, brachial plexus, sympathetic chain or phrenic nerve invasion. CT/MR imaging signs of ENE are adjacent fat/muscle infiltration, indistinct nodal margin, or irregular nodal capsular enhancement. US, less accurate than CT/MR, suggests ENE by interrupted or undefined nodal contours.

N | Definition of Regional Lymph Node (N[1]): Pathological N (pN)

N Category	N Criteria
NX	Regional lymph nodes cannot be assessed
N0	No regional lymph node metastasis
N1	Extranodal extension (ENE)(-)[2] metastasis in single ipsilateral lymph node, ≤ 3 cm
N2a N2b N2c	ENE(+)[2] metastasis in single ipsilateral lymph node, ≤ 3 cm or ENE(-) metastasis in single ipsilateral lymph node, > 3 cm but ≤ 6 cm ENE(-) metastasis in multiple ipsilateral lymph nodes, none > 6 cm ENE(-) metastasis in bilateral or contralateral lymph nodes, none > 6 cm
N3a N3b	ENER(-) metastasis in lymph node > 6 cm ENE(+) metastasis in single ipsilateral lymph node, > 3 cm in greatest dimension; or multiple ipsilateral, contralateral or bilateral nodes with any ENE(+) nodes

[1]Designation of "U" or "L" may be used for any N category to indicate metastasis above (U) or below (L) lower border of cricoid cartilage.
[2]ENE should be recorded as ENE(-) or ENE(+). As above, pathological ENE(+) increases pN category by 1.

M | M Stage

M Category	M Criteria
M0	No distant metastasis
M1	Distant metastasis[1]

[1]Mediastinal lymph nodes are considered distant metastasis, except level VII nodes (anterosuperior mediastinal nodes above innominate/brachiocephalic artery).

G | G Stage

G	G Definition
GX	Cannot be assessed
G1	Well differentiated
G2	Moderately differentiated
G3	Poorly differentiated

AJCC | Prognostic Stage Groups

When T is...	And N is...	And M is...	Then the stage group is...
T1	N0	M0	I
T2	N0	M0	II
T3	N0	M0	III
T1, 2, 3	N1	M0	III
T4a	N0, 1	M0	IVA
T1, 2, 3, 4a	N2	M0	IVA
Any T	N3	M0	IVB
T4b	Any N	M0	IVB
Any T	Any N	M1	IVC

T1 Oral Tongue

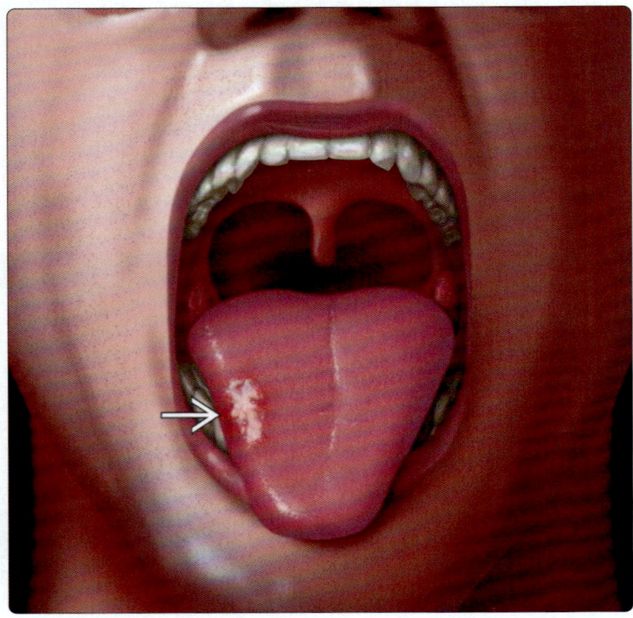

Graphic illustrates a small dorsolateral oral tongue SCCa ➡, which is ≤ 2 cm. Given the depth of invasion (DOI) is < 5 mm, this is a T1 oral cavity tumor. The oral tongue is described as having the tip, lateral, dorsal, and undersurface. The undersurface is often called the ventral surface.

T2 Oral Tongue

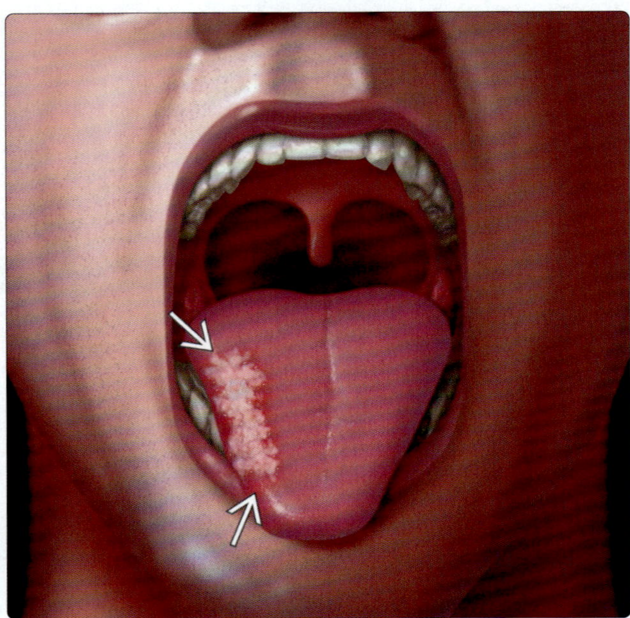

Graphic illustrates a larger primary SCCa of the oral tongue ➡. T2 primary tumor stage designation is applied if the lesion is > 2 cm but ≤ 4 cm and depth of invasion is ≤ 10 mm.

T3 Oral Tongue

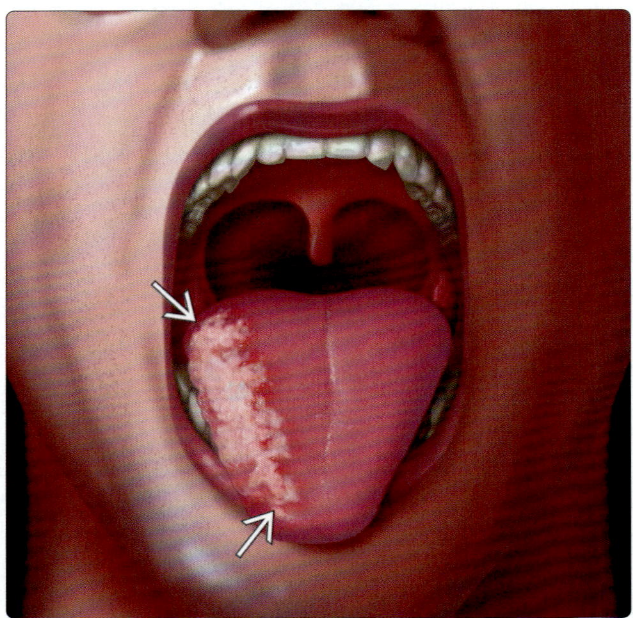

Graphic shows a larger tumor ➡ that is now > 4 cm and staged as T3 primary tumor stage SCCa. Without moderately advanced local disease spread, DOI of > 10 mm does not increase the T staging above T3.

T4a Oral Tongue

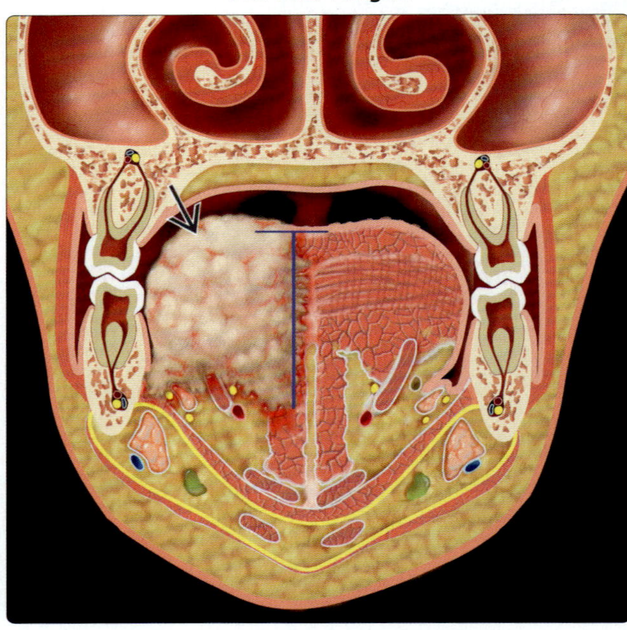

Coronal graphic shows DOI for oral tongue SCCa ➡. DOI can be estimated clinically, by imaging, &/or pathologically by dropping a plumb line (blue line) from nearest intact mucosal basement membrane to the deepest tumor margin. DOI > 5 mm & ≤ 10 mm, T2 stage rendered. DOI > 10 mm, T3 stage is assigned.

T4a Lower Alveolar Ridge

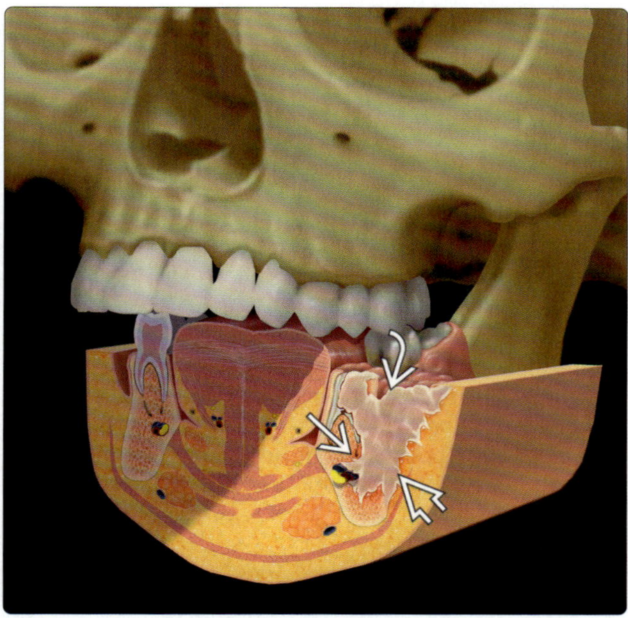

Graphic demonstrates an SCCa arising from the mucosa overlying the alveolar ridge ➬ and extending to the lower gingivobuccal sulcus ➡ and onto the buccal mucosa. There is invasion into the mandibular marrow ➡, which designates this as T4a oral cavity tumor.

T4b Retromolar Trigone

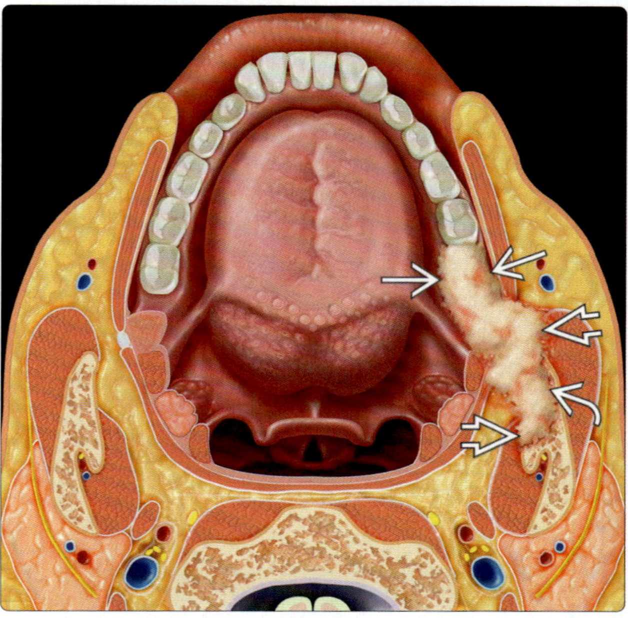

Graphic illustrates SCCa arising from the retromolar gingiva ➡ and extending posterolaterally to the mandible ➬ and masticator space ➡. The masticator space, pterygoid plate, skull base, &/or carotid artery encasement determine T4b staging.

Metastases, Organ Frequency

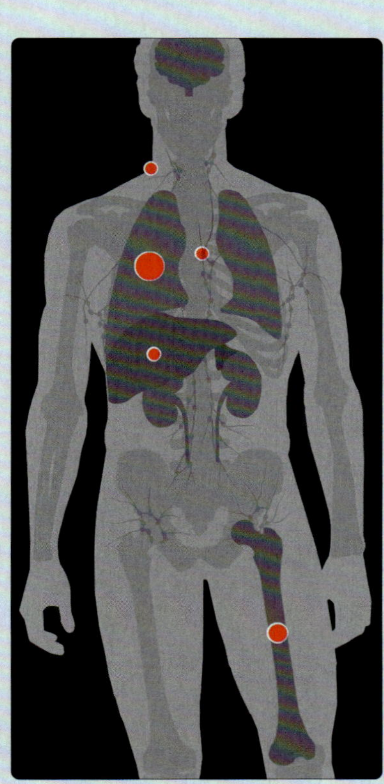

Lung/pleura	*47%*
Bone	*28%*
Skin	*10%*
Liver	*6%*
Distant nodes	*5%*

40% of patients with metastases have > 1 site of involvement. Overall incidence of distant metastases is ~ 10% and more likely if failure of local control of disease.

KEY FACTS

TERMINOLOGY

- Definition: Oral cavity mucosal malignancy arising from anterior 2/3 of tongue

IMAGING

- Imaging used to define deep extent and nodal status
- CECT: Variably enhancing invasive lesion
- MR less affected by dental amalgam artifact
  - T1WI C+: Variable enhancement, mild to moderate
- Imaging important for deep extent (T4a, T4b) and nodes
  - **T4a**: Still resectable local spread
  - **T4b**: Regional spread; unresectable
- 1st-order nodal drainage: Submandibular (IB), then jugulodigastric group (IIA)
- 35% have ≥ N1 disease at diagnosis
- 30% "N0" necks have microscopic nodal metastases

TOP DIFFERENTIAL DIAGNOSES

- Lingual tonsil squamous cell carcinoma
- Venous malformation of tongue

PATHOLOGY

- Strong association with tobacco and alcohol use
- Clinical assessment more accurate than imaging for mucosal size (T1-T3)
  - **T1**: 0-2 cm; **T2**: 2-4 cm; **T3**: > 4 cm

CLINICAL ISSUES

- Painful nonhealing ulcer of oral tongue
- Median age: 61 years; M:F = 4:1
- Overall 5-year survival: 60%
- Midline lesions have high likelihood for bilateral metastasis
- Treatment options: Surgery vs. chemoradiation
- Surgery includes wide local excision, partial or total glossectomy ± neck dissection
- Reconstructive options include healing by secondary intention, primary closure, skin graft, local-regional flap vs. free tissue transfer

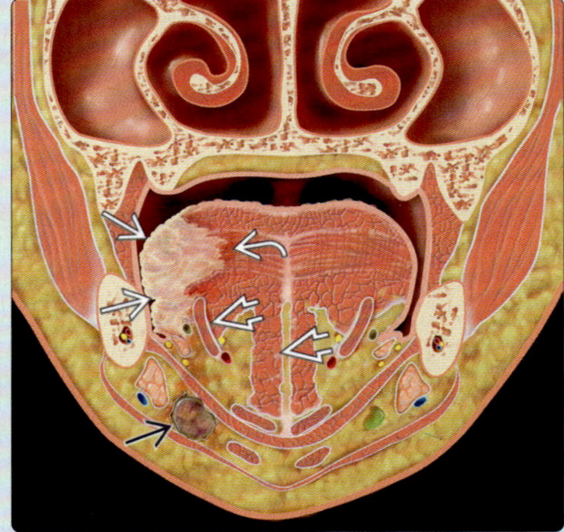

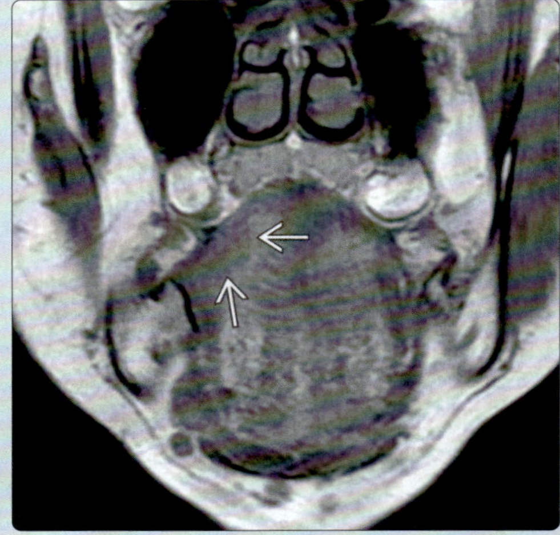

(Left) *Coronal graphic illustrates lateral oral tongue squamous cell carcinoma ➡ infiltrating intrinsic tongue muscles ➡. Coronal plane allows scrutiny of extrinsic tongue muscles ➡, which are not infiltrated by this tumor. T2 primary tumor stage is assigned (2-4 cm in size) nodal stage N1 (ipsilateral IB node ➡).* **(Right)** *Coronal T1WI MR in patient with a painful right tongue ulcer shows subtle low signal intensity at lateral tongue margin ➡. There is no evidence of involvement of extrinsic muscles or contralateral tumor spread.*

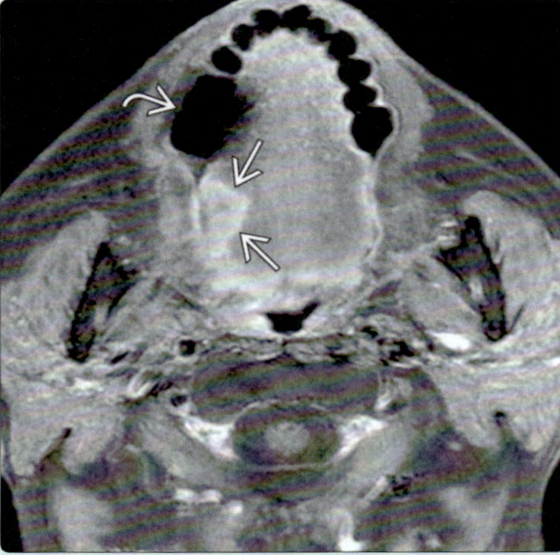

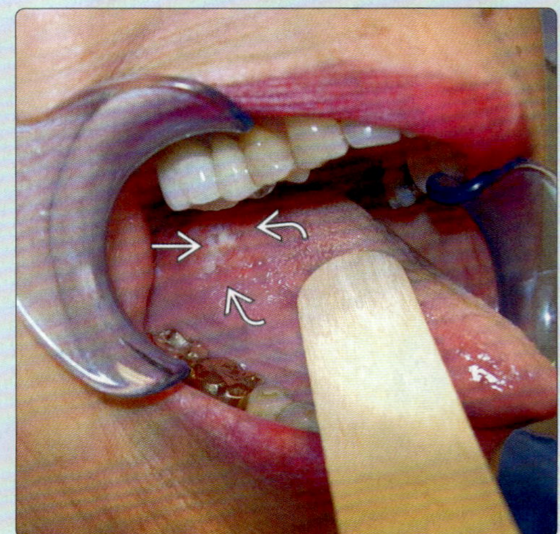

(Left) *Axial T1WI C+ FS MR (same patient) shows marked enhancement of a wedge-shaped ulcer at posterolateral tongue surface ➡. No neck nodes are present. Note that despite amalgam ➡, the tumor is still well seen.* **(Right)** *Clinical photograph shows a lateral tongue ulcer ➡ with indurated adjacent tissue ➡. Tumor was staged as T2 N0 by clinical exam and imaging and treated by hemiglossectomy with ipsilateral selective neck dissection (I-III). Final pathology concurred: pT2 N0 squamous cell carcinoma, stage II.*

KEY FACTS

TERMINOLOGY

- Floor of mouth (FOM) squamous cell carcinoma (SCCa)
  - Anatomic definition: FOM mucosa overlies mylohyoid and hyoglossus muscles, and body of tongue rests on it

IMAGING

- CECT: Irregular mild to moderately enhancing mass
- MR: Loss of normal FOM anatomical planes on T1
  - Increased T2 signal intensity and enhancement
- SCCa reliably FDG avid; increasing role in current practice
- May exactly mimic sublingual gland carcinoma
- Imaging important for deep extent and nodes: Question genioglossus, mylohyoid, base of tongue invasion; cortical bone erosion, marrow infiltration
- Clinical mucosal size more accurate than imaging

TOP DIFFERENTIAL DIAGNOSES

- Oral tongue SCCa
- Mandibular alveolar ridge SCCa
- Sublingual gland carcinoma
- Venolymphatic malformation

PATHOLOGY

- Strongly associated with tobacco (smoking and chewing) and alcohol use
- ≤ 35% have nodes at presentation: Levels I, II
- High incidence of occult nodal metastases; elective (staging) neck dissection may be indicated
- Overall 5-year survival = 60%

CLINICAL ISSUES

- Clinical presentation
  - Most commonly 50-70 years; M:F = 2:1
  - Painful hard ulcer/lesion, ± loose teeth
- Treatment options
  - Primary resection and reconstruction, ± neck dissection
  - Adjuvant postsurgical radiation ± chemotherapy (for high-risk histologic features, + surgical margins)

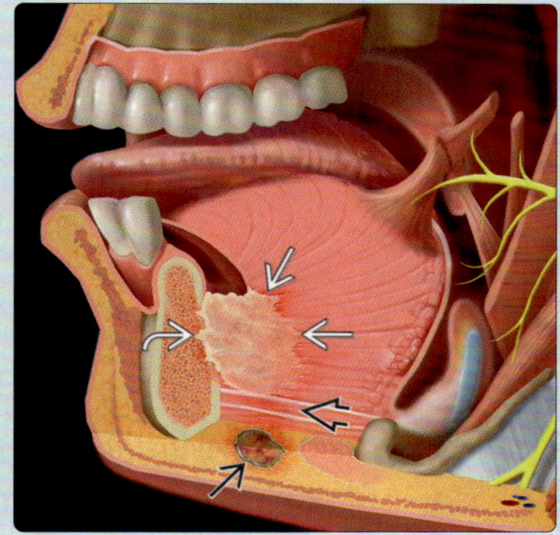

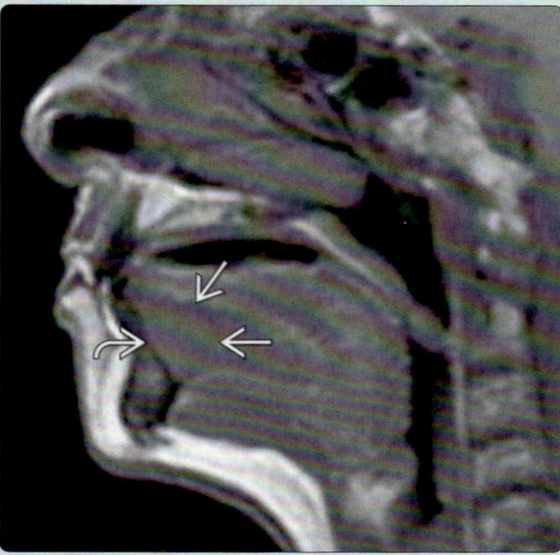

(Left) *Graphic illustrates the most common location of floor of mouth (FOM) squamous cell carcinoma ➡ within 2 cm of the midline anterior FOM. It is important to evaluate on imaging for invasion inferiorly to genioglossus & mylohyoid ➡ muscles, posteriorly to tongue base, & mandibular involvement anteriorly ➡ or laterally. This may require both MR & CT. The 2nd aim of imaging is evaluation of nodal disease ➡.* **(Right)** *Sagittal T1WI MR demonstrates a mass ➡ of low intensity compared to tongue muscles, abutting the midline mandible ➡.*

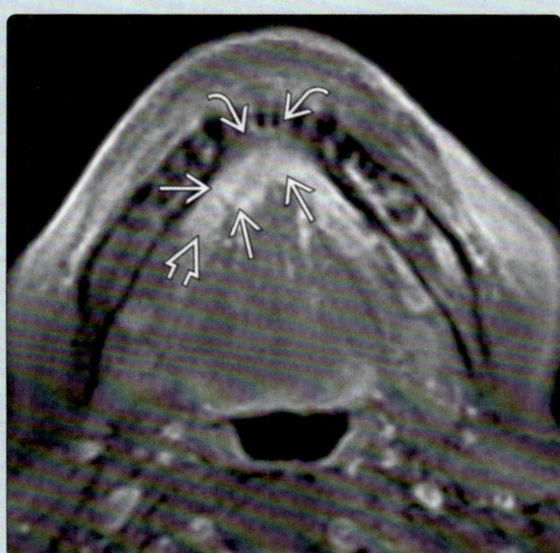

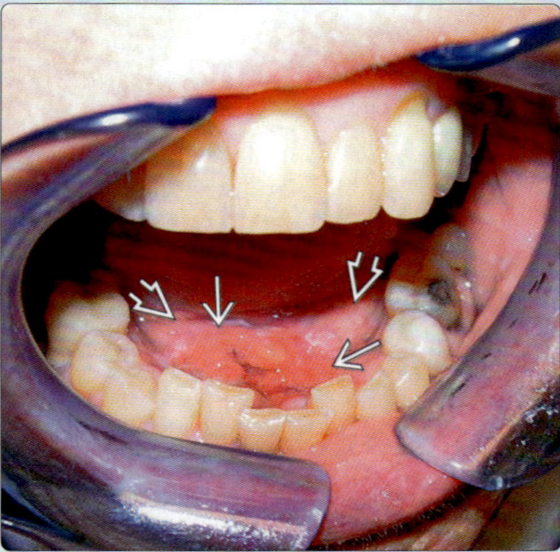

(Left) *Axial T1WI C+ FS MR in the same patient shows a subtle anterior midline FOM lesion ➡ that involves the anterior aspect of the right sublingual gland ➡. Note the loss of low-intensity cortex of the adjacent mandible ➡. This was confirmed on bone CT. No abnormal nodes were found.* **(Right)** *Clinical photograph in same patient reveals a tumor ➡ in anterior FOM & shows relation to the sublingual glands ➡. Composite resection & bilateral selective neck dissection (I-III) confirmed T4a N0 disease (mandible involvement).*

Alveolar Ridge Squamous Cell Carcinoma

KEY FACTS

TERMINOLOGY

- Squamous cell carcinoma (SCCa) arising from mucosa adjacent to teeth-bearing bone

IMAGING

- General imaging issues
  - Small, superficial lesions may be unseen by imaging
  - Larger lesions: **Enhancing, infiltrating mass** ± underlying **bone destruction**
  - Evaluate local spread, bone infiltration, nodes
    - Metastatic spread favors facial, levels I and II nodes
  - Mandible SCCa: Check buccal-masticator spaces
  - Maxillary SCCa: Check nasal cavity, maxillary sinus, palate
  - If in bone, evaluate for perineural tumor spread
    - **Inferior alveolar nerve** (mandible)
    - **Palatine nerves** (maxilla)
- CECT or enhanced MR imaging findings
  - Bone CT: Cortical destruction ± enlarged nerve canal
  - MR: Marrow signal and enhancement similar to tumor
- PET/CT: Increasing role in clinical practice
  - Detection of nodal and distant metastases
  - Complimentary to MR for detecting marrow invasion

TOP DIFFERENTIAL DIAGNOSES

- Osteoradionecrosis
- Osteonecrosis
- Osteosarcoma

PATHOLOGY

- **10%** oral cavity SCCa are from alveolar ridge
- Overall 5-year survival: ~ 60%

CLINICAL ISSUES

- Clinical presentation
  - Nonhealing ulcer of jaw
  - Pain, swelling, bleeding, ill-fitting dentures
  - Early bone marrow infiltration: **T4a**
- Treatment options: Surgical resection ± reconstruction; adjuvant radiation ± chemotherapy

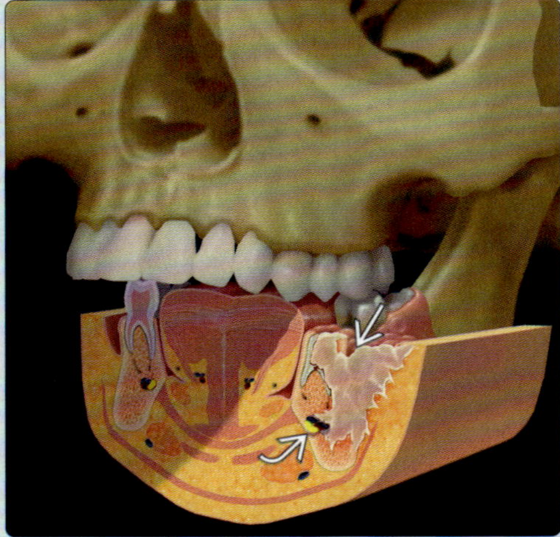

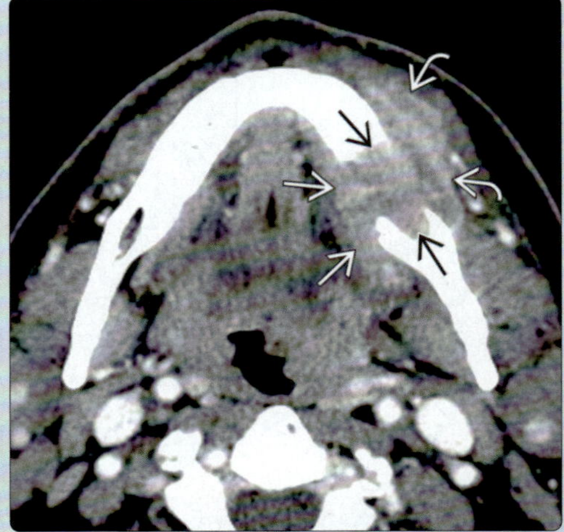

(Left) *Graphic illustrates SCCa ➡ arising from the mandibular alveolar ridge & invading mandible body, making it T4a. Note involvement of the inferior alveolar nerve ➡, which is important for complete resection.* **(Right)** *Axial CECT demonstrates heterogeneous mass with destruction of the left mandibular body ⇨. Mass extends laterally to involve the gingivobuccal sulcus & cheek ➡ & medially to involve the floor of mouth ➡. Lesion was T4AN1 & completely excised with reconstruction by composite flap.*

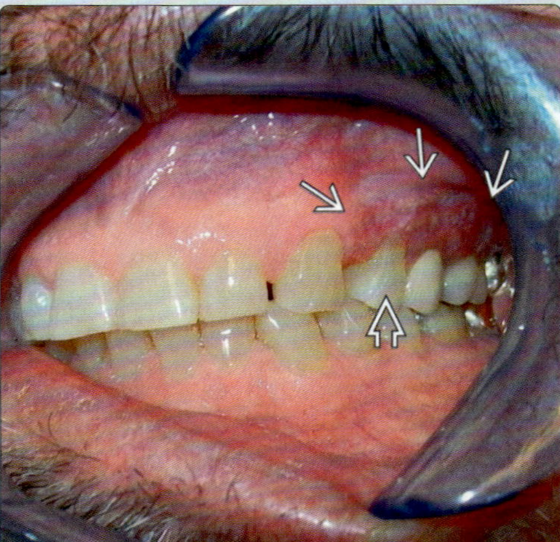

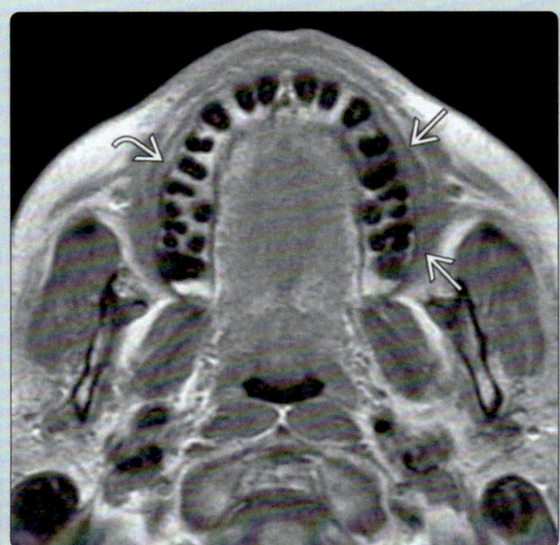

(Left) *Clinical photograph of a 66-year-old man depicts an irregular red, indurated, ulcerated lesion ➡ of the left maxillary alveolar ridge, from the 1st premolar ➡. Biopsy revealed invasive SCCa, & the clinical examination suspected it to be T2N0.* **(Right)** *Axial T1 MR in the same patient shows markedly subtle soft tissue fullness ➡ lateral to the maxillary alveolus with a loss of normal fat planes compared to contralateral side ➡. No convincing marrow infiltration was apparent by imaging, & partial maxillectomy concurred.*

KEY FACTS

TERMINOLOGY

- Oral cavity subsite
- Complex shape: Mucosa over mandibular body and ramus posterior to molars, ascending to maxillary tuberosity

IMAGING

- Retromolar trigone (RMT) contiguous with anterior tonsillar pillar, buccal mucosa, and alveolar ridge mucosa
  - Squamous cell carcinoma (SCCa) primary site may be difficult to determine
- RMT site results in complex tumor spread patterns
  - Via **pterygomandibular raphe** to pterygoid plate
  - Mandible, maxilla, inferior alveolar nerve
  - Buccal and masticator spaces, oral cavity, and oropharynx
- CECT: Mildly enhancing mass, may be occult if small
  - Look for asymmetry of fat planes
  - Puffed-cheek technique may improve visualization of mucosal space tumor in RMT
  - Dental amalgam artifact may obscure primary tumor or tumor spreading via pterygomandibular raphe
- MR: Allows most accurate delineation of primary tumor, marrow infiltration, perineural and perifascial tumor
  - Less affected by dental amalgam artifact
- SCCa reliably FDG avid in PET/CT

TOP DIFFERENTIAL DIAGNOSES

- Buccal mucosa SCCa
- Oral minor salivary gland malignancy

CLINICAL ISSUES

- Tumor often indolent with late presentation
- Bone/masticator muscle involvement → pain, trismus
  - Both indicate T4 disease; poorest prognosis
- Treatment options
  - Surgical resection ± adjuvant XRT for advance stage; single modality may be appropriate in early stage tumors
  - Surgery + radiation = best 5-year survival

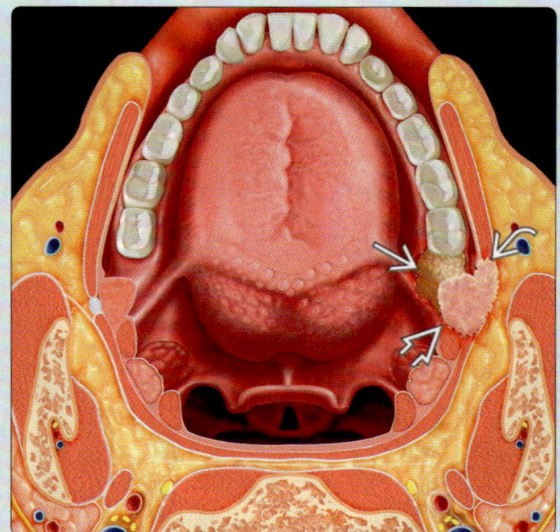

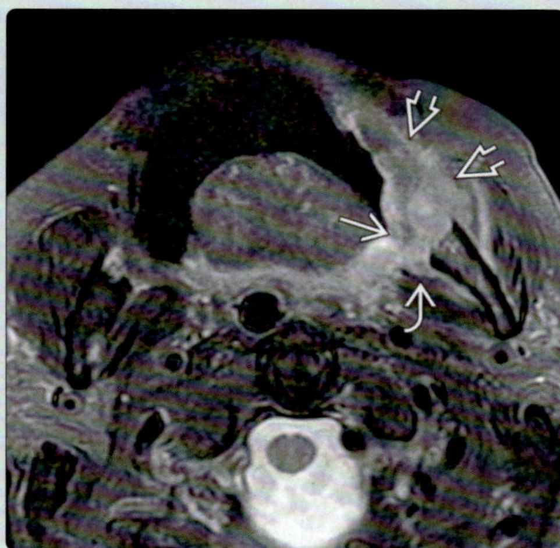

(Left) *Graphic illustrates SCCa ➡ arising posterior to the 3rd molar & extending superiorly along the pterygomandibular raphe & laterally onto the buccinator ➡. Tumor encroaches on the anterior tonsillar pillar ➡ of the oropharynx.* **(Right)** *Axial T2 FS MR in a patient with a poorly healing socket following tooth extraction shows a mildly hyperintense soft tissue mass ➡ from the retromolar trigone, which infiltrates to the medial pterygoid ➡ (T4b disease). SCCa also infiltrates laterally to masseter & cheek ➡ along the buccinator.*

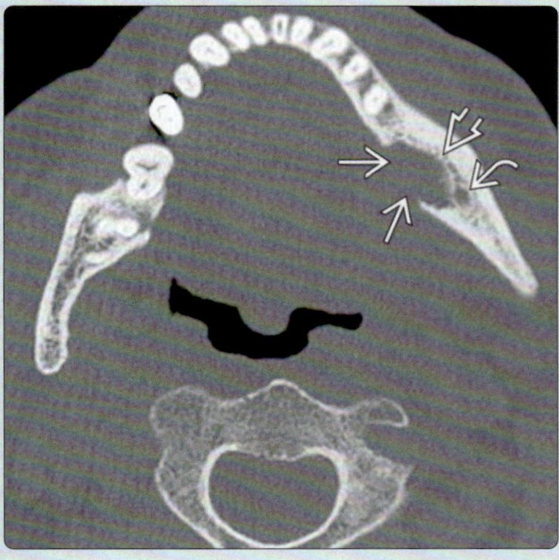

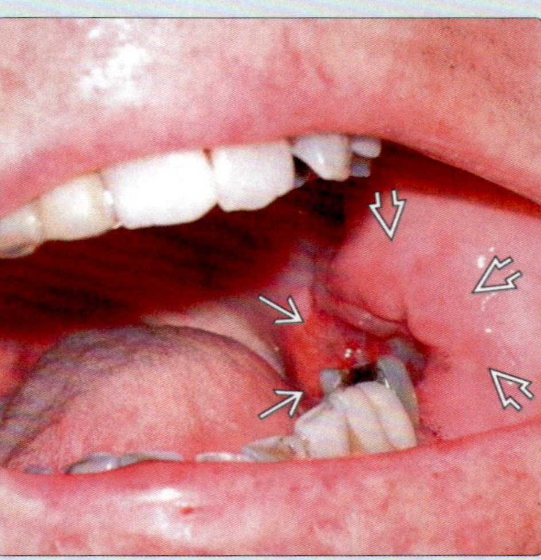

(Left) *Axial bone CT in the same patient shows a large lytic defect ➡ in the left mandible with an ill-defined lateral margin ➡. Note the proximity of the defect to the inferior alveolar canal ➡. Imaging features stage this as T4b.* **(Right)** *Clinical photograph in the same patient shows mucosal well-differentiated SCCa ➡ in the retromolar trigone. Note fullness of the left cheek ➡, indicating submucosal infiltration of the tumor & correlating with MR findings.*

KEY FACTS

TERMINOLOGY

- Buccal mucosa squamous cell carcinoma
- Oral cavity mucosal malignancy arising from inner lining of cheek and lips

IMAGING

- Typically difficult to identify with routine imaging
- Mild to moderately enhancing irregular lesion
- Look for asymmetrically infiltrated buccal fat
- 1st-order node drainage: Buccal and level I, II nodes
- CECT: "Puffed cheek" method works well to separate mucosal surfaces and see site of origin
- MR: Hypointense gauze padding works similarly and often better tolerated with long MR sequences
- FDG avid (reserved for advanced nodal disease)
    - Nodes are important prognostic factor

TOP DIFFERENTIAL DIAGNOSES

- Oral cavity infection
- Oral cavity minor salivary gland malignancy

PATHOLOGY

- Same prognosis as cancers in other oral cavity sites once age, tumor stage, treatment, and race considered
- Strong association with tobacco, alcohol, betel nut, & paan
- Imaging important to determine deep extent
    - Identifying buccal space invasion and T4 features
    - **T4a**: Tumor invades skin of face, through cortical bone, into extrinsic tongue muscles
    - **T4b**: Tumor invades masticator space, pterygoid plates, skull base, or encases carotid

CLINICAL ISSUES

- Clinical presentation: Pain, bleeding, nonhealing ulcer
    - Buccal mucosal lesion visible on direct exam
- Treatment options
    - Surgical: Resection ± reconstruction ± neck dissection
    - ± adjuvant radiation

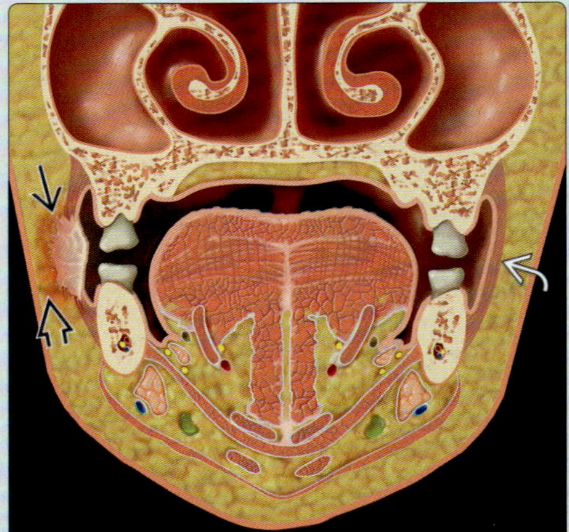

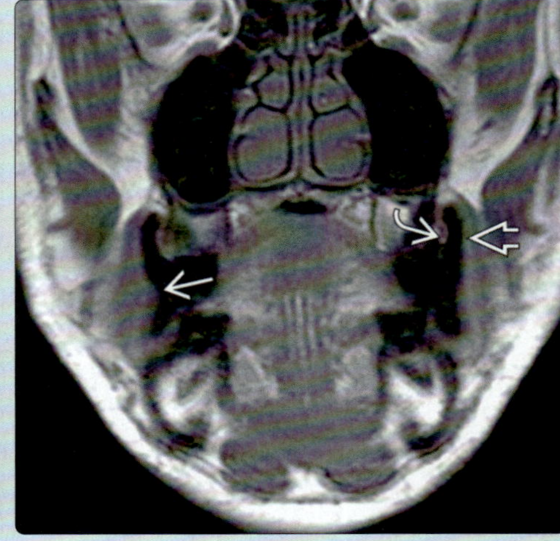

(Left) *Coronal graphic depicts a T2 (2-4 cm) buccal mucosal squamous cell carcinoma (SCCa) ⇨ that has invaded the underlying buccinator muscle and subcutaneous fat ⇨. If the lesion had involved the cheek skin, it would be staged as T4. Note the normal left buccinator ➡.* **(Right)** *Coronal T1WI MR performed with a patient using the "puffed cheek" method shows the cheek ➡ displaced from gingival mucosa ➡ and subtle nodularity of the right buccal mucosa ➡, representing SCCa. No evidence of deep infiltration is seen.*

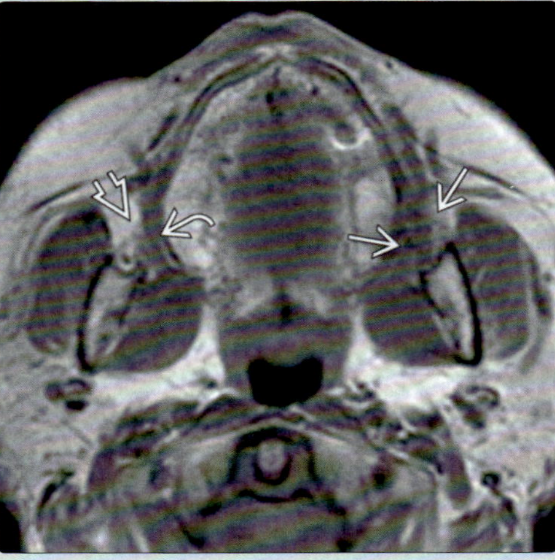

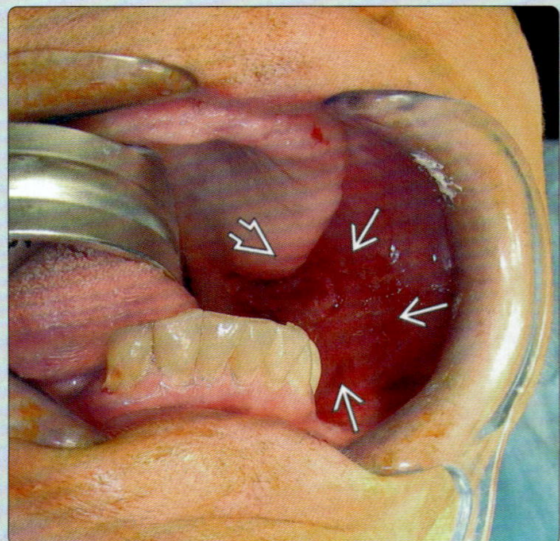

(Left) *Axial T1WI MR demonstrates an ill-defined tissue filling the buccal fat pad ➡ from deep infiltration of buccal mucosal malignancy. Note the smooth contours on the contralateral side ➡ and the clean buccal fat ➡. Without a clear history of the primary site, buccal fat infiltration may only be a subtle imaging finding.* **(Right)** *Clinical photograph in the same patient shows buccal mucosal primary SCCa ➡ along the posterior aspect of the inner cheek, extending to the posterior margin maxillary (edentulous) alveolus ➡.*

KEY FACTS

TERMINOLOGY

- Hard palate squamous cell carcinoma (SCCa)
- Oral cavity subsite: Mucosal malignancy of roof of mouth

IMAGING

- Often extremely subtle, may be occult to imaging
- Variable size from several mm to several cm
- **Coronal plane** imaging **key** for either CT or MR
- CECT: Mild to moderately enhancing ill-defined lesion with associated bone erosion
  - Both soft tissue and bone algorithm important
- MR: Low T1 tumor signal contrasts against hyperintense palate marrow and mucosa
  - T1 C+ FS and T2 FS aid tumor delineation
  - Look at **greater palatine canal** and **pterygopalatine fossa** for CNV2 perineural tumor (PNT)

TOP DIFFERENTIAL DIAGNOSES

- Hard palate minor salivary gland carcinoma
- Palate benign mixed tumor
- Invasive sinonasal SCCa

CLINICAL ISSUES

- Ulcer ± mass on roof of mouth; often painful
- Clinically obvious lesion may be subtle on CT or MR
- Rare tumor; least common oral cavity site
- In this location, SCCa is less common than minor salivary malignancies
- Overall 5-year survival: ~ 60%
- Treatment: Surgical resection ± neck dissection ± XRT
  - Elective neck dissection associated with lower recurrence rate, better overall survival

DIAGNOSTIC CHECKLIST

- Must evaluate bone for erosion ± infiltration
- MR better evaluates **greater palatine canal and pterygopalatine fossa** for CNV2 PNT
- Evaluate carefully for nodal metastases

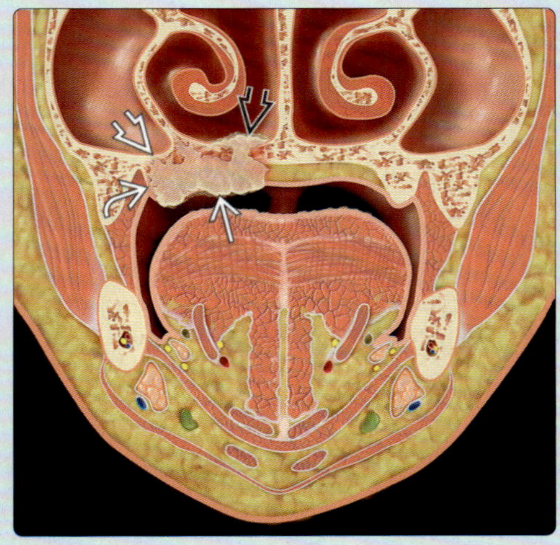

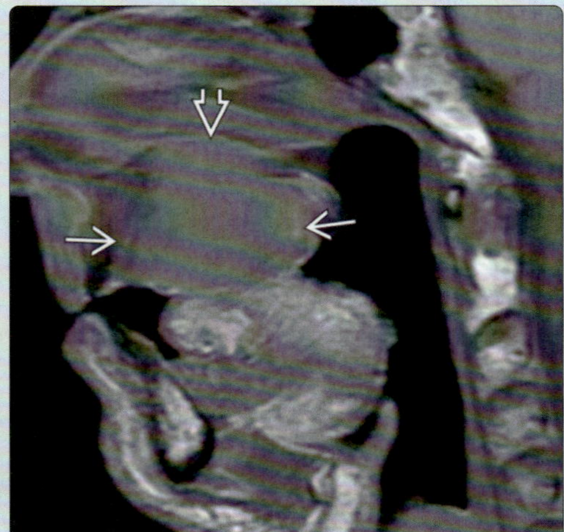

(Left) *Coronal graphic illustrates oral cavity SCCa ➡ arising from mucosa of the hard palate and infiltrating underlying bone. The tumor may extend through palatine portion of maxilla ⇨ to floor of the nasal cavity, or through the alveolar bone ➡, or to the maxillary sinus ➡. Perineural tumor spread may occur along the 2nd division of trigeminal nerve, V2.* **(Right)** *Sagittal T1WI MR shows a patient with prior retromolar trigone SCCa and a new large oral cavity SCCa ➡ that destroys the hard palate and extends into the nasal cavity ➡.*

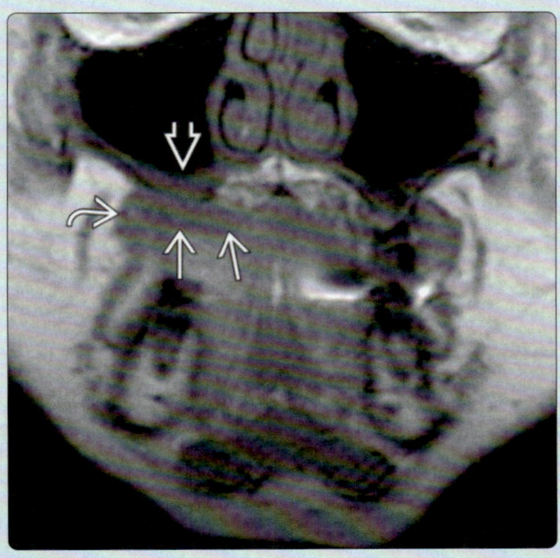

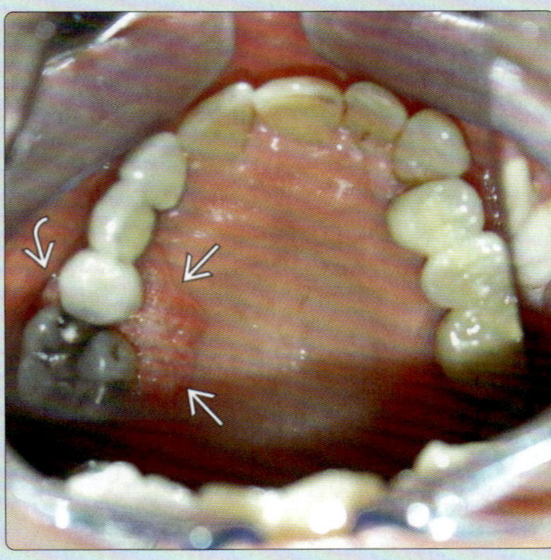

(Left) *Coronal T1 MR demonstrates a subtle mucosal lesion ➡ of hard palate that extends through maxillary alveolus to both buccal mucosa ➡ & maxillary sinus floor ➡. The tumor is T4aN0, stage IVA disease. Palatal lesions are often best seen on T1 precontrast and in coronal plane.* **(Right)** *Clinical photograph taken with an oral mirror demonstrates a clinically obvious maxillary mass involving the palatal mucosa ➡. The tumor was extremely subtle on imaging. Extension through to buccal surface is also evident ➡.*

T | Definition of Primary Tumor (T)

T Category	T Criteria
TX	Primary tumor cannot be assessed
Tis	Carcinoma in situ
T1	Tumor invades > 1 subsite of hypopharynx or adjacent site, or measures > 2 cm but ≤ 4 cm in greatest dimension without fixation of hemilarynx
T2	Tumor limited to 1 subsite of hypopharynx &/or ≤ 2 cm in greatest dimension
T3	Tumor > 4 cm in greatest dimension or with fixation of hemilarynx or extension to esophagus
T4a	Moderately advanced local disease: Tumor invades thyroid/cricoid cartilage, hyoid bone, thyroid gland, or central compartment soft tissue[1]
T4b	Very advanced local disease: Tumor invades prevertebral fascia, encases carotid artery, or involves mediastinal structures

[1]Central compartment soft tissue includes prelaryngeal strap muscles and subcutaneous fat.

All tables adapted with permission from AJCC Cancer Staging Manual 8th ed., 2017.

N | Definition of Regional Lymph Node (N[1]): Clinical N (cN)

N Category	N Criteria
NX	Regional lymph nodes cannot be assessed
N0	No regional lymph node metastasis
N1	Extranodal extension (ENE)(-)[2] metastasis in single ipsilateral lymph node, ≤ 3 cm
N2a N2b N2c	ENE(-) metastasis, single ipsilateral node > 3 cm but ≤ 6 cm ENE(-) metastasis in multiple ipsilateral lymph nodes, none > 6 cm ENE(-) metastasis in bilateral or contralateral lymph nodes, none > 6 cm
N3a N3b	ENE(-) metastasis in lymph node > 6 cm Clinically overt ENE(+)[3] in any metastatic nodes

[1]Designation of "U" or "L" may be used for any N category to indicate metastasis above (U) or below (L) lower border of cricoid cartilage.
[2]ENE should be recorded as ENE(-) or ENE(+); however, clinically overt ENE(+) corresponds solely with cN3b.
[3]Clinically overt ENE(+) can be diagnosed by presence of "matted" nodal mass, overlying skin or adjacent soft tissue involvement, or clinical signs of cranial nerve, brachial plexus, sympathetic chain, or phrenic nerve invasion. CT/MR imaging signs of ENE are adjacent fat/muscle infiltration, indistinct nodal margin, or irregular nodal capsular enhancement. US, less accurate than CT/MR, suggests ENE by interrupted or undefined nodal contours.

N | Definition of Regional Lymph Nodes (N[1]): Pathological N (pN)

N Category	N Criteria
NX	Regional lymph nodes cannot be assessed
N0	No regional lymph node metastasis
N1	Extranodal extension (ENE)(-)[2] metastasis in single ipsilateral lymph node, ≤ 3 cm
N2a N2b N3a	ENE(+)[2] metastasis in single ipsilateral lymph node, ≤ 3 cm or ENE(-) metastasis in single ipsilateral lymph node, > 3 cm but ≤ 6 cm ENE(-) metastasis in multiple ipsilateral lymph nodes, none > 6 cm ENE(-) metastasis in bilateral or contralateral lymph nodes, none > 6 cm
N3a N3b	ENE(-) metastasis in lymph node > 6 cm ENE(+) metastasis in single ipsilateral lymph node, > 3 cm in greatest dimension; **or** multiple ipsilateral, single or multiple contralateral, or bilateral nodes with any ENE(+) nodes

[1]Designation of "U" or "L" may be used for any N category to indicate metastasis above (U) or below (L) lower border of cricoid cartilage.
[2]ENE should be recorded as ENE(-) or ENE(+). As above, pathological ENE (+) increases pN category by 1.

M | Definition of Distant Metastasis (M[1])

M Category	M Criteria
M0	No distant metastasis
M1	Distant metastasis

[1]Mediastinal lymph nodes are considered distant metastasis, except level VII nodes (anterior superior mediastinal nodes above inominate/brachiocephalic artery).

AJCC | Prognostic Stage Groups

When T is...	And N is...	And M is...	Then the stage group is...
Tis	N0	M0	0
T1	N0	M0	I
T2	N0	M0	II
T3	N0	M0	III
T1, T2, T3	N1	M0	III
T4a	N0, N1	M0	IVA
T1, T2, T3, T4a	N2	M0	IVA
Any T	N3	M0	IVB
T4b	Any N	M0	IVB
Any T	Any N	M1	IVC

G | Histologic Grade (G)

G	G Criteria
GX	Grade cannot be assessed
G1	Well differentiated
G2	Moderately differentiated
G3	Poorly differentiated
G4	Undifferentiated

T1/T2 Pyriform Sinus

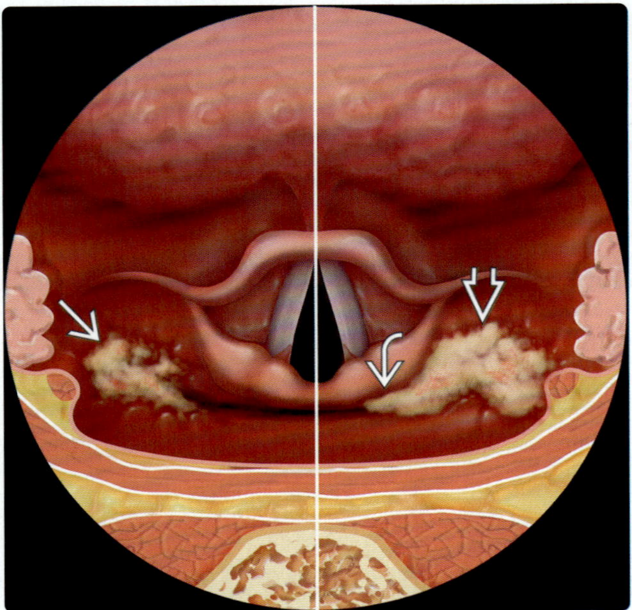

Graphic illustrates a small T1 squamous cell carcinoma (SCCa) → limited to the pyriform sinus and < 2 cm in greatest diameter. Another SCCa → is also shown, which is larger in size but < 4 cm. This tumor extends from the pyriform sinus to the postcricoid area →, which would also designate this as T2.

T3 Pyriform Sinus

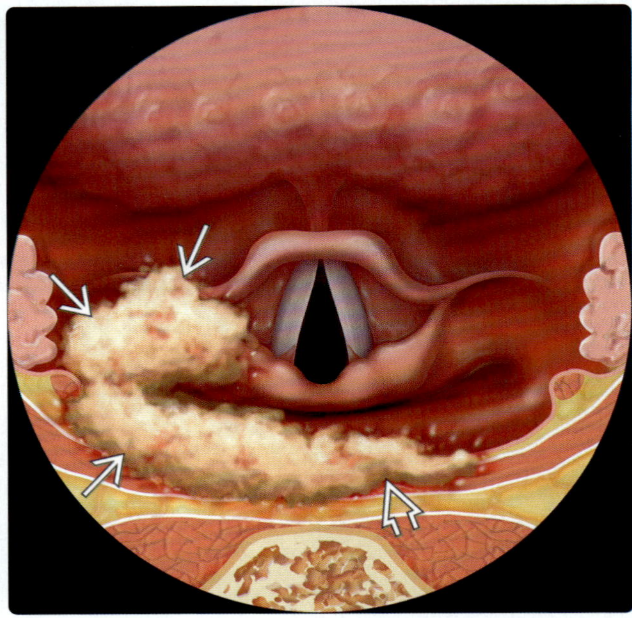

Graphic shows a large pyriform sinus SCCa → that is extending medially along the posterior hypopharyngeal wall →. A hypopharyngeal tumor > 4 cm or involving the esophagus is designated T3 disease. Hemilarynx fixation as determined by clinical examination also determines T3 disease.

T4a Pyriform Sinus

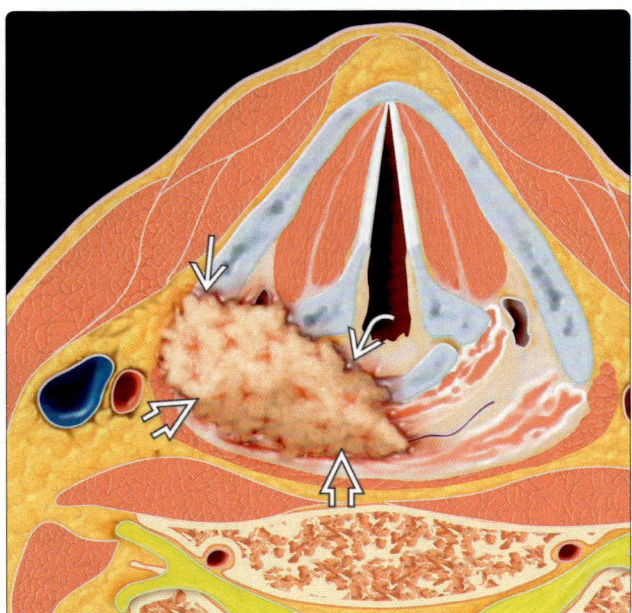

Axial graphic reveals a pyriform sinus SCCa → that, while not clearly > 4 cm, does show invasion of the cricoid → and thyroid → cartilages. Hyoid or cartilage invasion determines T4a disease as does invasion of the thyroid gland, the prelaryngeal strap muscles, &/or paralaryngeal fat.

T4b Pyriform Sinus

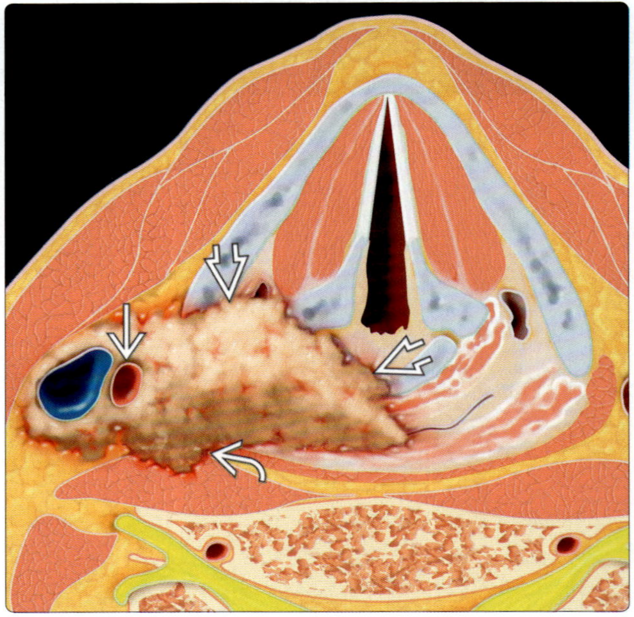

Axial graphic depicts a more extensive pyriform sinus SCCa → that is invading laterally into the soft tissues so that it encases the carotid artery →. Additionally, it penetrates the prevertebral fascia → to involve the prevertebral muscle. Either of these features determines T4b status.

T4a Postcricoid Region

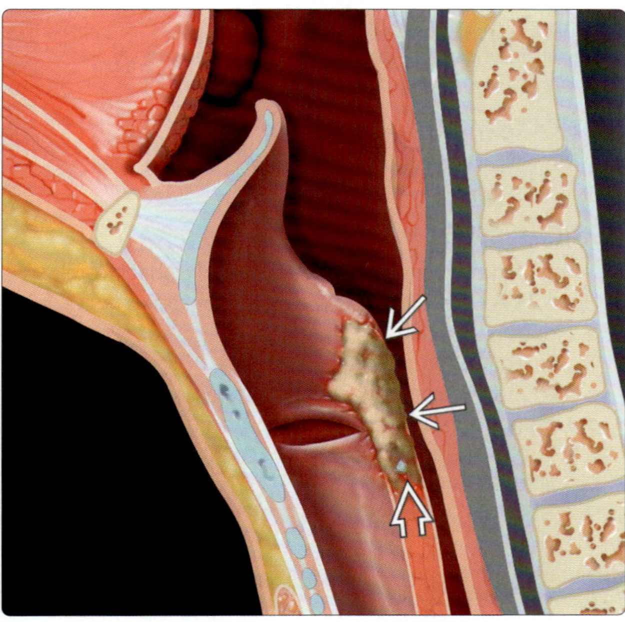

Graphic illustrates a moderately advanced hypopharyngeal tumor arising from postcricoid mucosa ➡ and invading anteriorly through the cricoid cartilage ⇨.

T4b Posterior Hypopharyngeal Wall

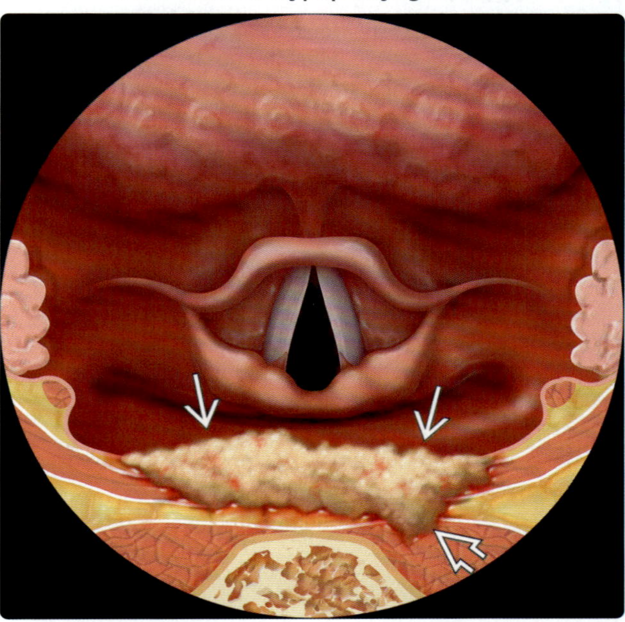

Graphic illustrates a sessile posterior hypopharyngeal wall SCCa ➡. This tumor has extended through the pharyngeal wall, then the prevertebral fascia to the left prevertebral muscle ⇨. This is T4b disease.

Metastases, Organ Frequency

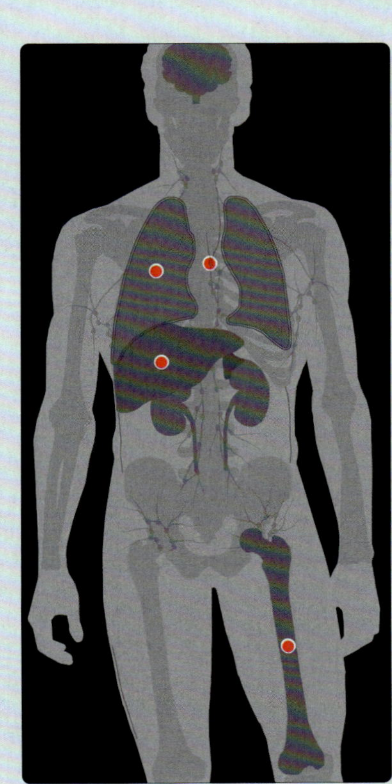

Lung
Liver
Bone
Mediastinal nodes

Overall incidence of distant metastases is 17% and more often seen with T4 stage primary tumors &/or nodal metastases. Distant metastases are most frequent with pyriform sinus carcinoma. No statistics regarding relative frequency of metastases sites are available.

Pyriform Sinus Squamous Cell Carcinoma

KEY FACTS

TERMINOLOGY

- Definition: Mucosal squamous cell carcinoma (SCCa) of pyriform sinus (PyrS) hypopharynx subsite
  - 2/3 of all hypopharyngeal SCCa are in PyrS

IMAGING

- General imaging features & comments
  - Variable tumor size/appearance at presentation
    - May present as small unknown primary with metastatic nodes
      - Or presents as large T3-4 tumor, minimal symptoms, metastatic adenopathy
  - Nota bene: Aryepiglottic fold SCCa = supraglottic laryngeal SCCa, with different staging
- CECT/enhanced T1 MR findings
  - Mild to moderately enhancing PyrS irregular mass
  - Arises from PyrS apex, anterior, posterior, or lateral wall
  - May fill PyrS ± circumferentially involve walls
- PET/CECT: Stages primary, nodes, and metastatic disease

TOP DIFFERENTIAL DIAGNOSES

- Supraglottic (aryepiglottic fold) SCCa
- Hypopharyngeal minor salivary gland malignancy
- Cervical esophageal carcinoma

PATHOLOGY

- Strong association with tobacco & alcohol use
- Overall **5-year survival**: ~ **40%**

CLINICAL ISSUES

- Often minimal symptoms: Sore throat, dysphagia, otalgia
- Up to **75%** have adenopathy at presentation
  - Nodes frequently bilateral (N2c)
- Treatment options
  - T1-T2: Endoscopic partial laryngopharyngectomy or XRT
  - Large tumors: Laryngopharyngectomy ± chemo/radiation **or** organ preservation with chemoXRT ± salvage surgery
  - T4b tumors: Chemotherapy ± radiation for palliation

(Left) *Lateral graphic illustrates pyriform sinus squamous cell carcinoma (SCCa) ➡ arising from the anterior wall and extending toward paraglottic fat ➡. Tumor location does not result in airway or swallowing obstruction.* **(Right)** *Axial CECT in a 65-year-old man with extensive smoking history and sore throat demonstrates a mass filling the right pyriform sinus ➡. The mass appears superficially spreading, involving all walls of the sinus but not spreading anteriorly to paraglottic fat ➡ or laterally into thyroid cartilage ➡.*

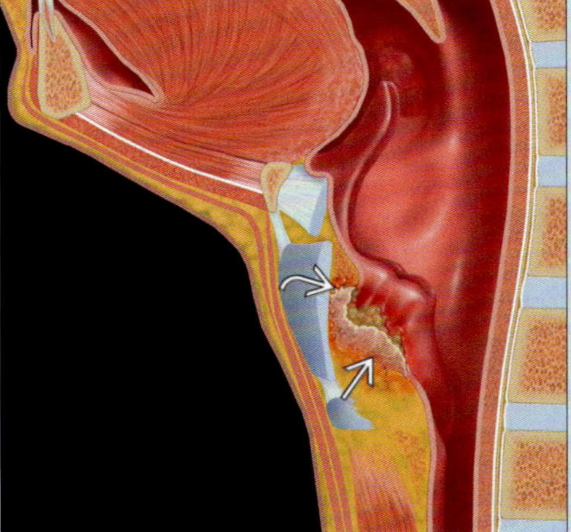

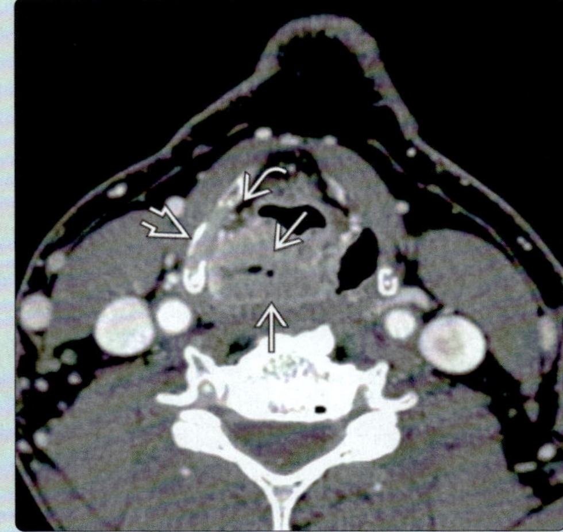

(Left) *Axial T1WI C+ FS MR in the same patient shows relatively less enhancement of SCCa ➡ than of mucosa of the larynx and hypopharynx. The right aryepiglottic fold is displaced anteriorly, but the laryngeal surface ➡ is normal.* **(Right)** *Coronal T1WI C+ FS MR in the same patient shows a lesion filling the pyriform sinus ➡ apex. Tumor abuts cartilage ➡ but does not invade or extend laterally to soft tissues. PET/CT obtained due to suspicious bone lesions on CT was negative. This was T2N1M0 SCCa treated with chemoradiation.*

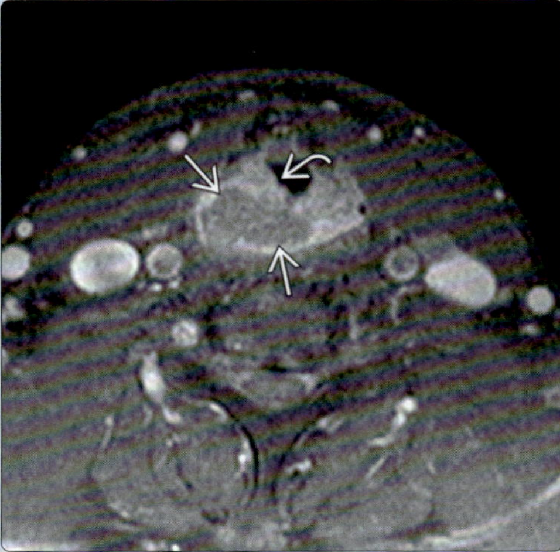

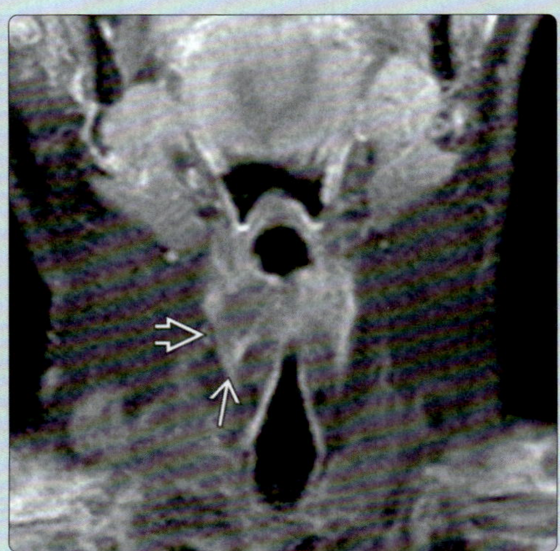

KEY FACTS

TERMINOLOGY

- Squamous cell carcinoma (SCCa) arising from mucosa overlying posterior cricoid cartilage
  - 1 of 3 subsites of hypopharynx (HP)

IMAGING

- General comments: Often difficult scans to read
  - Mass of lower HP with invasion anteriorly to larynx, superiorly and laterally in HP, or inferiorly to esophagus
- CECT: Mildly enhancing irregular mass
- MR: May better clarify cartilage invasion
- PET/CT: SCCa is reliably FDG avid

TOP DIFFERENTIAL DIAGNOSES

- Pharyngitis
- Posterior hypopharyngeal wall SCCa
- Cervical esophageal carcinoma

PATHOLOGY

- Strong association with tobacco and alcohol abuse
- Association with Plummer-Vinson syndrome
- Poorest prognosis of all H&N SCCa; 5-year survival = 30%

CLINICAL ISSUES

- Clinical presentation
  - Presents with sore throat, dysphagia
  - Often presents at late stage: T3 or T4 primary tumor
    - T3: > 4 cm or esophageal invasion
    - T4a: Cartilage or paralaryngeal invasion
    - T4b: ICA encasement, prevertebral fascia invasion
  - 60% have nodes at diagnosis; often bilateral
- Treatment options
  - T1-T2 (rare): Partial pharyngectomy or XRT
  - T3, T4a: Laryngopharyngectomy and neck dissection with adjuvant XRT
    - Organ preservation attempt: Chemoradiation
  - T4b: Chemoradiation

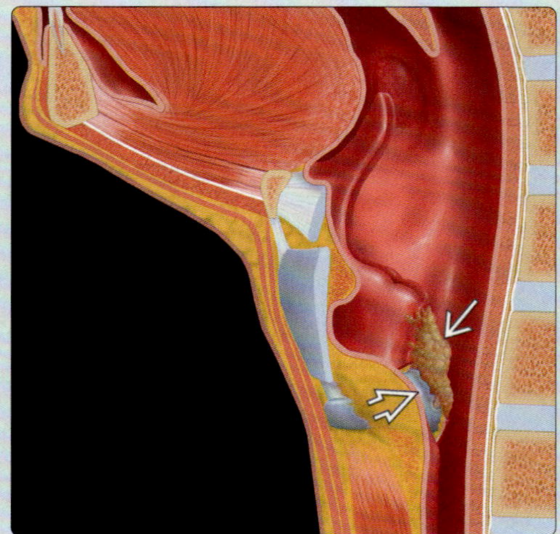

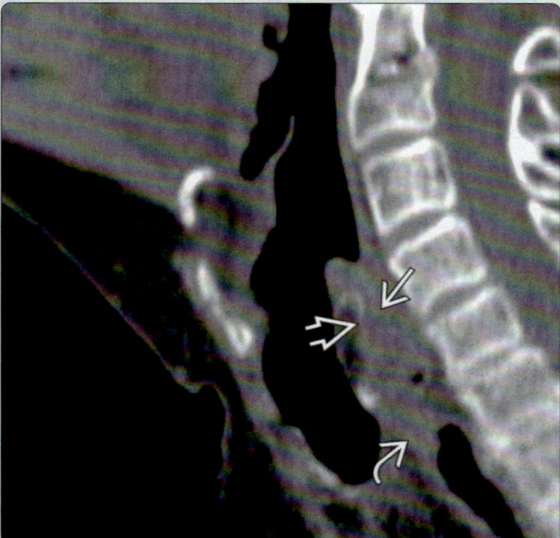

(Left) *Lateral graphic of the hypopharynx illustrates an irregular tumor ➡ arising from the mucosal surface covering the posterior cricoid ring ➡. Cartilage erosion is depicted here. Note the proximal cervical esophagus is just inferior to the postcricoid hypopharynx.* **(Right)** *Sagittal reformatted CECT shows an exophytic mass ➡ distending the lower hypopharynx, posterior to the cricoid ➡, without cartilage destruction. Note extension below the inferior cricoid cartilage to the cervical esophagus ➡. This is staged as T3N0 SCCa.*

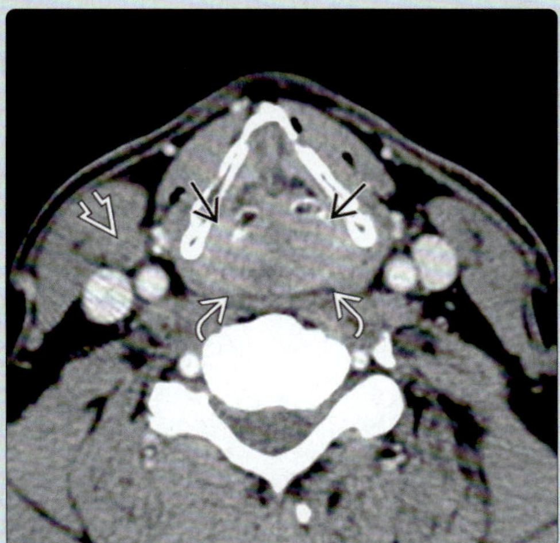

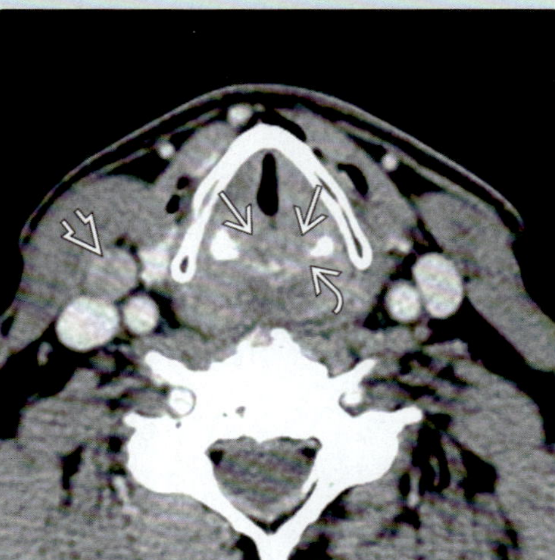

(Left) *Axial CECT in a different patient shows soft tissue fullness of the lower hypopharynx. A mildly enhancing tumor infiltrates around the arytenoid cartilages ➡, while the retropharyngeal fat is clear posteriorly ➡. This feature helps to distinguish it from a posterior hypopharyngeal wall tumor. Right adenopathy is present ➡.* **(Right)** *Axial CECT inferiorly shows fullness of the hypopharynx & irregular destruction of cricoid ➡ with tumor extension into posterior larynx ➡. Note the right neck node ➡. This is T4aN2c SCCa.*

Posterior Hypopharyngeal Wall Squamous Cell Carcinoma

KEY FACTS

TERMINOLOGY

- Definition: Squamous cell carcinoma (SCCa) arising from mucosa of posterior wall of hypopharynx (HP) from hyoid bone to esophageal inlet
  - 15% are hypopharyngeal SCCa

IMAGING

- General imaging features
  - Superficial spread superiorly to oropharynx or inferiorly to esophagus
  - Early invasion posteriorly into prevertebral muscles through prevertebral fascia
- CECT: Irregular, enhancing mass distending lower HP
  - Superior spread to oropharynx (T2)
  - Inferior spread to esophagus (T3)
  - Infiltrate prevertebral muscles (T4b)
    - Imaging not accurate for predicting invasion
    - Preservation of retropharyngeal fat excludes this
  - Carotid encasement or mediastinal invasion (T4b)
- PET/CT: SCCa is reliably FDG avid

TOP DIFFERENTIAL DIAGNOSES

- Postcricoid region SCCa
- Cervical esophageal carcinoma

PATHOLOGY

- Strong association with tobacco and alcohol abuse
- Poor prognosis; overall 5-year survival ~ 30%

CLINICAL ISSUES

- Clinical presentation: Posterior HP wall mucosal lesion
  - Asymptomatic until late, stages III-IV
  - ≤ **75%** have **nodes** at diagnosis; often bilateral
  - Up to 50% present with neck mass from nodes
- Treatment options
  - T1-T2 SCCa: Surgical resection ± radiation therapy (XRT)
  - T3-T4a: Laryngopharyngectomy ± XRT
    - Alternative treatment: Organ preservation chemoXRT
  - T4b: Palliative chemoXRT

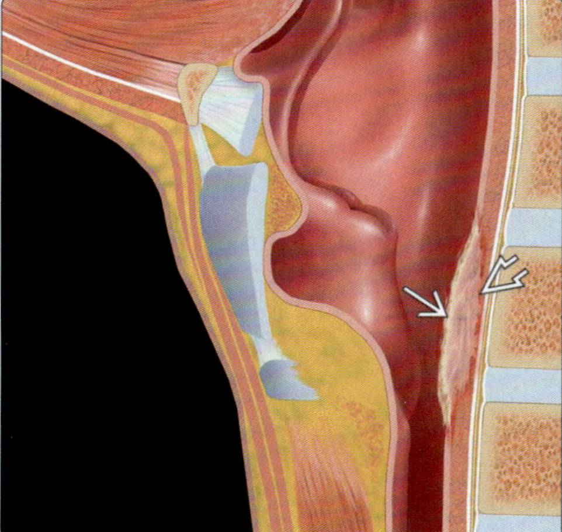

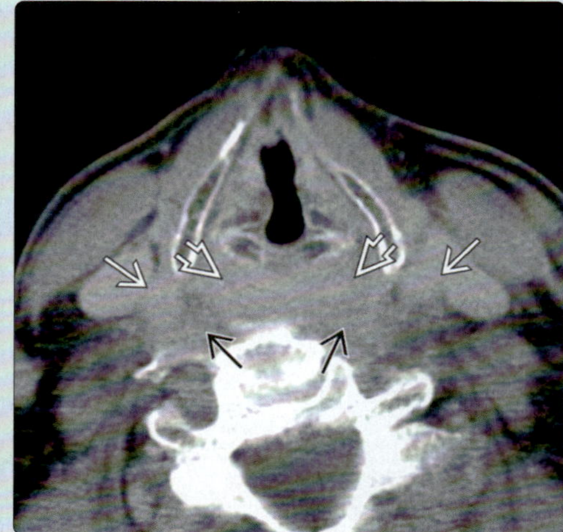

(Left) *Lateral graphic illustrates posterior hypopharyngeal wall SCCa ➡. These tumors often spread superiorly to the oropharynx or caudally to the esophagus. Invasion of the prevertebral muscles ➡ translates to T4b primary stage.* **(Right)** *Axial CECT at the level of the cricoarytenoid joints shows abnormal soft tissue ➡ with ill-defined margins posterior to the cricoid. Poor definition of the prevertebral muscles ➡ is highly suspicious for invasion, and a tumor abuts both common carotid arteries ➡. This is T4bN1 SCCa.*

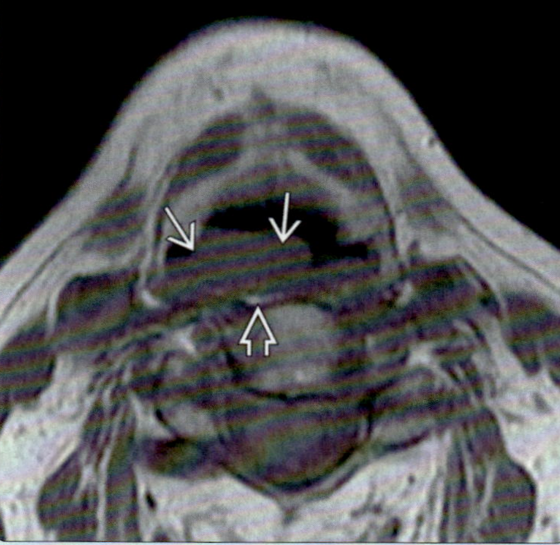

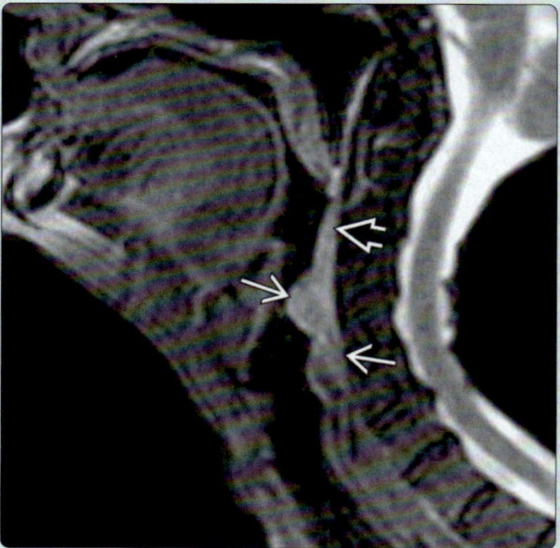

(Left) *Axial T1WI MR in an immunosuppressed woman with bilateral lung transplants shows a lobulated mass ➡ arising from the posterior pharyngeal wall. Retropharyngeal fat ➡ is not clearly defined; however, MR has limited accuracy in predicting prevertebral invasion.* **(Right)** *Sagittal T2WI FS MR in same patient shows superficial spreading nature of posterior hypopharyngeal wall SCCa ➡ extending superiorly to oropharynx ➡. Patient was asymptomatic; lesion was only found on clinical examination & was stage T2N1.*

Posterior Hypopharyngeal Wall Squamous Cell Carcinoma

TERMINOLOGY

Definitions

- Squamous cell carcinoma (SCCa) arising from posterior wall mucosa of pharynx from hyoid bone to esophageal inlet
  - Subsite of hypopharynx

IMAGING

General Features

- Best diagnostic clue
  - Irregular, moderately enhancing mass of posterior hypopharyngeal wall extending superiorly to oropharynx posterior wall
- Location
  - Posterior wall of hypopharynx from level of hyoid to inferior border of cricoid cartilage
    - Lateral limits are apex of pyriform sinuses
- Size
  - Variable; typically presents late
- Morphology
  - Irregular infiltrative mass

CT Findings

- CECT
  - Irregular, mildly enhancing mass distending lower hypopharynx
  - Tends to spread superiorly to oropharynx
  - May infiltrate posteriorly into prevertebral muscles

MR Findings

- T1 isointense to muscle, T2 moderately hyperintense
- Mild to moderate contrast enhancement

Nuclear Medicine Findings

- PET/CT
  - SCCa is reliably FDG avid

Imaging Recommendations

- Best imaging tool
  - CECT often best as patient may not tolerate long MR sequences
  - MR may be helpful if resection planned, to evaluate suspected prevertebral fascia invasion
- Protocol advice
  - T1 MR best for infiltration of retropharyngeal fat
  - T2 helpful for prevertebral muscle invasion

DIFFERENTIAL DIAGNOSIS

Postcricoid Region SCCa

- Arises from anterior wall lower hypopharynx

Cervical Esophageal Carcinoma

- Uncommon tumor but may spread superiorly to hypopharynx

Pharyngitis

- Infection/inflammation often in immunocompromised patients

PATHOLOGY

General Features

- Etiology
  - Strong association with tobacco and alcohol abuse
  - Association with Plummer-Vinson syndrome

Staging, Grading, & Classification

- Uses same American Joint Committee on Cancer TNM (2017) staging as for all hypopharyngeal SCCa

CLINICAL ISSUES

Presentation

- Most common signs/symptoms
  - Dysphagia, sore throat
- Other signs/symptoms
  - Up to 50% present with neck mass from nodes
  - Weight loss, otalgia

Demographics

- Age
  - Peak incidence in 7th decade
- Gender
  - M > > F
- Epidemiology
  - Least common hypopharyngeal site (15%)
    - Pyriform sinus (65%), postcricoid region (20%)

Natural History & Prognosis

- Tendency to present late, stages III-IV
- **≤ 75%** have **nodal metastases** at diagnosis
- Nodal drainage often bilateral
  - Levels III, IV, and VI
  - Superior spread to retropharyngeal nodes also
- Distant metastases develop in 20-40%
- **Hypopharyngeal SCCa has poorest prognosis of all H&N SCCa**
  - Overall 5-year survival ~ 30%

Treatment

- Small T1-T2 SCCa: Surgical resection ± radiation therapy (XRT)
- Some T2: ChemoXRT
- T3-T4a: Laryngopharyngectomy ± XRT or organ preservation chemoXRT
- T4b: Palliative chemoXRT

DIAGNOSTIC CHECKLIST

Image Interpretation Pearls

- May infiltrate posteriorly to prevertebral muscles (T4b)
  - Preservation of retropharyngeal fat excludes infiltration
  - Imaging not accurate for muscle invasion
- Look for carotid encasement, mediastinal invasion (both T4b)

SELECTED REFERENCES

1. Canis M et al: Oncologic results of transoral laser microsurgery for squamous cell carcinoma of the posterior pharyngeal wall. Head Neck. 37(2):156-61, 2015
2. Becker M et al: Imaging of the larynx and hypopharynx. Eur J Radiol. 66(3):460-79, 2008

T | Definition of Primary Tumor (T)

T Category	T Criteria
TX	Primary tumor cannot be assessed
Tis	Carcinoma in situ
Supraglottis	
T1	Tumor limited to 1 subsite of supraglottis with normal vocal cord mobility
T2	Tumor invades mucosa of > 1 adjacent subsite of supraglottis or glottis or region outside supraglottis (e.g., mucosa of base of tongue, vallecula, medial wall of pyriform sinus) without fixation of larynx
T3	Tumor limited to larynx with vocal cord fixation &/or invades any of following: Postcricoid area, preepiglottic space, paraglottic space, &/or inner cortex of thyroid cartilage
T4a	Moderately advanced local disease: Tumor invades through thyroid cartilage &/or invades tissues beyond larynx (e.g., trachea, soft tissues of neck, including deep extrinsic muscle of tongue, strap muscles, thyroid, or esophagus)
T4b	Very advanced local disease: Tumor invades prevertebral space, encases carotid artery, or invades mediastinal structures
Glottis	
T1	Tumor limited to vocal cord(s) (may involve anterior or posterior commissure) with normal mobility
T1a	Tumor limited to 1 vocal cord
T2b	Tumor involves both vocal cords
T2	Tumor extends to supraglottis &/or subglottis &/or with impaired vocal cord mobility
T3	Tumor limited to larynx with vocal cord fixation &/or invasion of paraglottic space &/or inner cortex of thyroid cartilage
T4a	Moderately advanced local disease: Tumor invades through outer cortex of thyroid cartilage &/or invades tissues beyond larynx (e.g., trachea, soft tissues of neck, including deep extrinsic muscle of tongue, strap muscles, thyroid, or esophagus)
T4b	Very advanced local disease: Tumor invades prevertebral space, encases carotid artery, or invades mediastinal structures
Subglottis	
T1	Tumor limited to subglottis
T2	Tumor extends to vocal cord(s) with normal or impaired mobility
T3	Tumor limited to larynx with vocal cord fixation
T4a	Moderately advanced local disease: Tumor invades cricoid or thyroid cartilage &/or invades tissues beyond larynx (e.g., trachea, soft tissues of neck, including deep extrinsic muscles of tongue, strap muscles, thyroid, or esophagus)
T4b	Very advanced local disease: Tumor invades prevertebral space, encases carotid artery, or invades mediastinal structures

All tables adapted with permission from AJCC Cancer Staging Manual 8th ed., 2017.

N | Definition of Regional Lymph Node (N[1]): Clinical N (cN)

N Category	N Criteria
NX	Regional lymph nodes cannot be assessed
N0	No regional lymph node metastasis
N1	Extranodal extension (ENE)(-)[2] metastasis in single ipsilateral lymph node, ≤ 3 cm
N2a N2b N2c	ENE(-) metastasis, single ipsilateral node > 3 cm but ≤ 6 cm ENE(-) metastasis in multiple ipsilateral lymph nodes, none > 6 cm ENE(-) metastasis in bilateral or contralateral lymph nodes, none > 6 cm
N3a N3b	ENE(-) metastasis in lymph node > 6 cm Clinically overt ENE(+)[3] in any metastatic nodes

[1]Designation of "U" or "L" may be used for any N category to indicate metastasis above (U) or below (L) lower border of cricoid cartilage.
[2]ENE should be recorded as ENE(-) or ENE(+); however, clinically overt ENE (+) corresponds solely with cN3b.
[3]Clinically overt ENE(+) can be diagnosed by presence of "matted" nodal mass, overlying skin or adjacent soft tissue involvement, or clinical signs of cranial nerve, brachial plexus, sympathetic chain, or phrenic nerve invasion. CT/MR imaging signs of ENE are adjacent fat/muscle infiltration, indistinct nodal margin, or irregular nodal capsular enhancement. US, less accurate than CT/MR, suggests ENE by interrupted or undefined nodal contours.

N | Definition of Regional Lymph Node (N[1]): Pathological N (pN)

N Category	N Criteria
NX	No regional lymph node metastasis
N0	ENE(-)[2] metastasis in single ipsilateral lymph node, ≤ 3 cm
N2a N2b N2c	ENE(+)[2] metastasis in single ipsilateral lymph node, ≤ 3 cm **or** ENE(-) metastasis in single ipsilateral lymph node, > 3 cm but ≤ 6 cm ENE(-) metastasis in multiple ipsilateral lymph nodes, none > 6 cm ENE(-) metastasis in bilateral or contralateral lymph nodes, none > 6 cm
N3a N3b	ENE(-) metastasis in lymph node > 6 cm ENE(+) metastasis in single ipsilateral lymph node, > 3 cm in greatest dimension; **or** multiple ipsilateral, single or multiple contralateral, or bilateral nodes with any ENE(+) nodes

[1]Designation of "U" or "L" may be used for any N category to indicate metastasis above (U) or below (L) lower border of cricoid cartilage.
[2]ENE should be recorded as ENE(-) or ENE(+). As above, pathological ENE(+) increases pN category by 1.

G | Histologic Grade (G)

G	G Definition
GX	Grade cannot be assessed
G1	Well differentiated
G2	Moderately differentiated
G3	Poorly differentiated

M | Definition of Distant Metastasis

M Category	M Criteria
M0	No distant metastasis
M1	Distant metastasis[1]

[1]Mediastinal lymph nodes are considered distant metastasis, except level VII nodes (anterior superior mediastinal nodes above the innominate/brachiocephalic artery).

AJCC | Prognostic Stage Groups

When T is...	And N is...	And M is...	Then the stage group is...
Tis	N0	M0	0
T1	N0	M0	I
T2	N0	M0	II
T3	N0	M0	III
T1, T2, T3	N1	M0	III
T4a	N0, N1	M0	IVA
T1, T2, T3, T4a	N2	M0	IVA
Any T	N3	M0	IVB
T4b	Any N	M0	IVB
Any T	Any N	M1	IVC

T1a/T1b Glottic

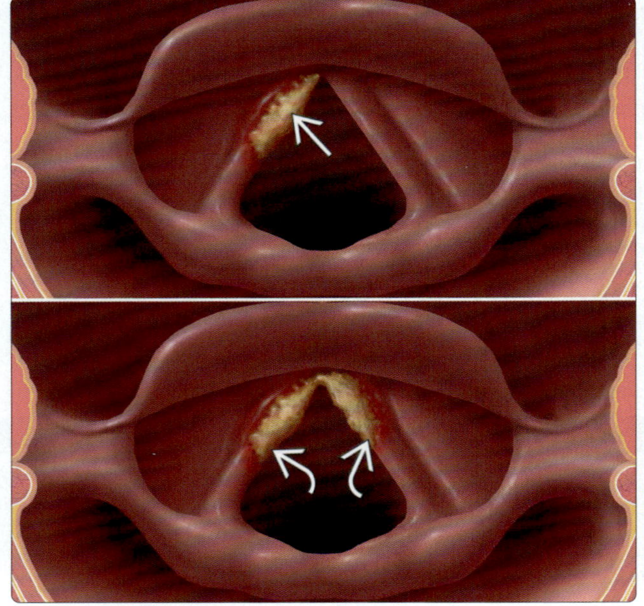

Graphic depicts endoscopic view of a T1a glottic tumor ➡ confined to 1 vocal cord and a T1b tumor ↪ that involves both vocal cords.

T2/T3 Glottic

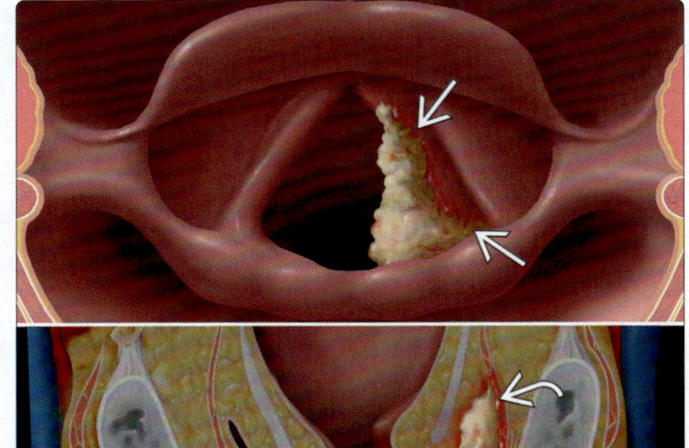

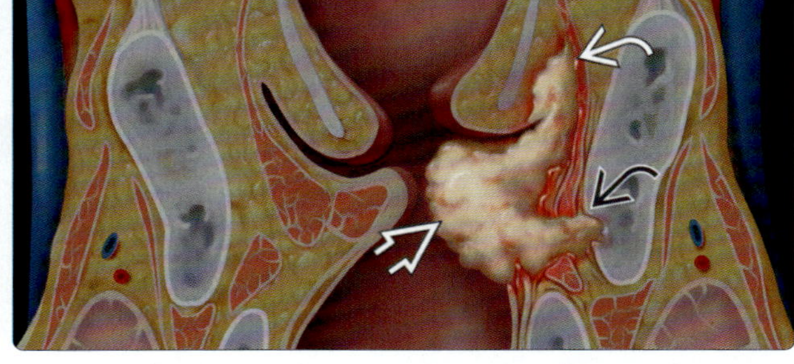

Upper graphic depicts a larger T2 glottic SCCa ➡ extending to supraglottic tissues. Impaired vocal cord mobility would also stage as T2. Lower graphic shows a glottic SCCa ➡ invading paraglottic fat ↪ and inner aspect of thyroid cartilage ⇨. Either feature &/or fixation of the vocal cord would also be stage T3.

T4a Glottic

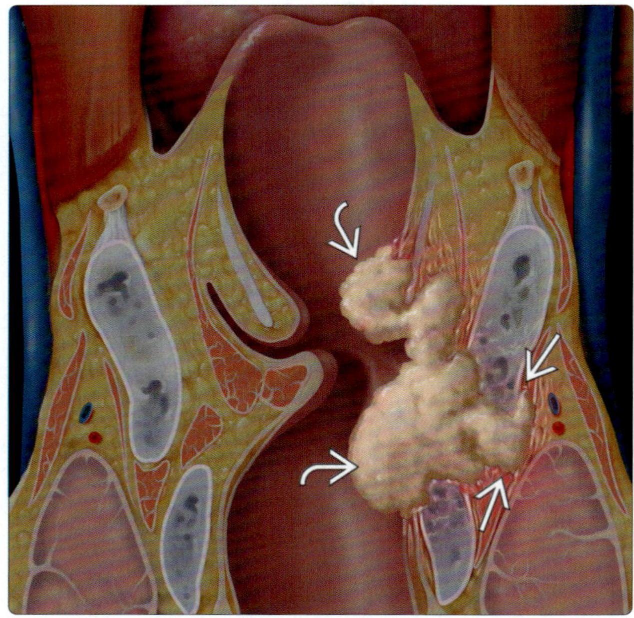

Coronal graphic illustrates a moderately advanced T4a glottic SCCa ↪ that is penetrating through thyroid cartilage ➡. Another feature that might be seen and denotes T4a is paralaryngeal extension, such as to the trachea or soft tissues of the neck, the strap muscles, thyroid, or esophagus.

T4b Glottic

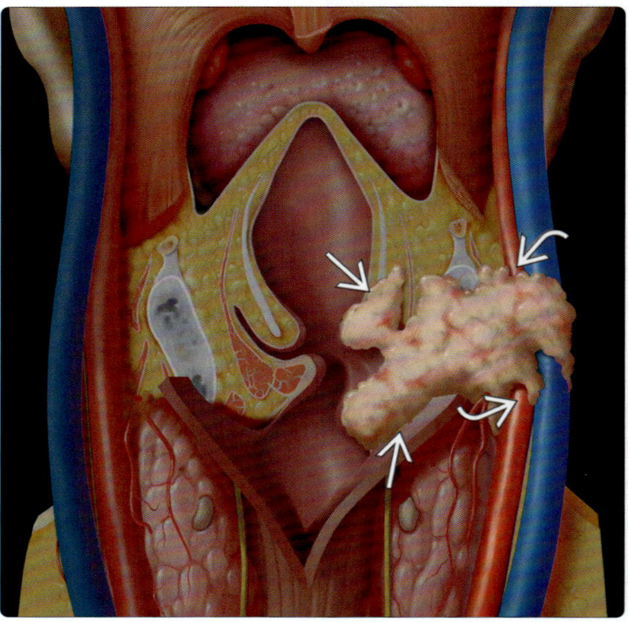

Coronal graphic demonstrates T4b glottic SCCa ➡, which is also known as very advanced local disease. This is determined when there is encasement of the carotid artery ↪ or prevertebral or mediastinal invasion. Definition of T4b tumor is the same for all laryngeal SCCa.

T1/T2 Supraglottic

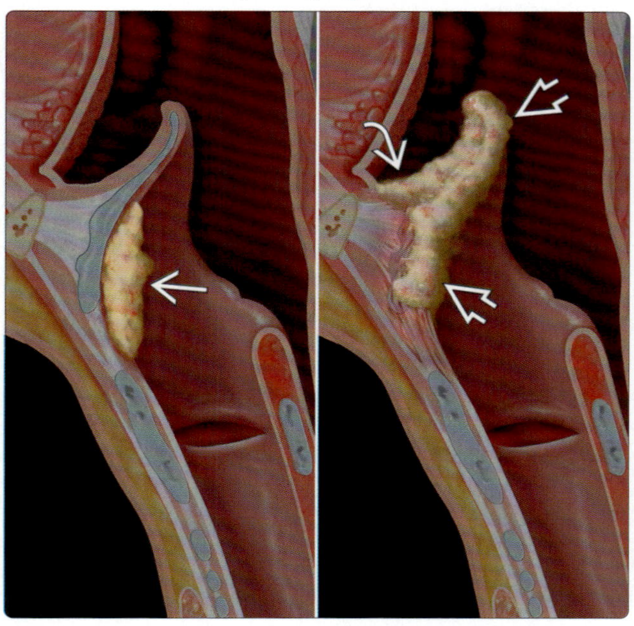

Sagittal graphic illustrates supraglottic SCCa. T1 SCCa ➡ is limited to 1 subsite (suprahyoid epiglottis, infrahyoid epiglottis, AE folds, arytenoids, false cords). T2 supraglottic SCCa ⇨ invades more than 1 adjacent subsite or region outside of the supraglottis, such as the vallecula ⇨.

T3 Supraglottic

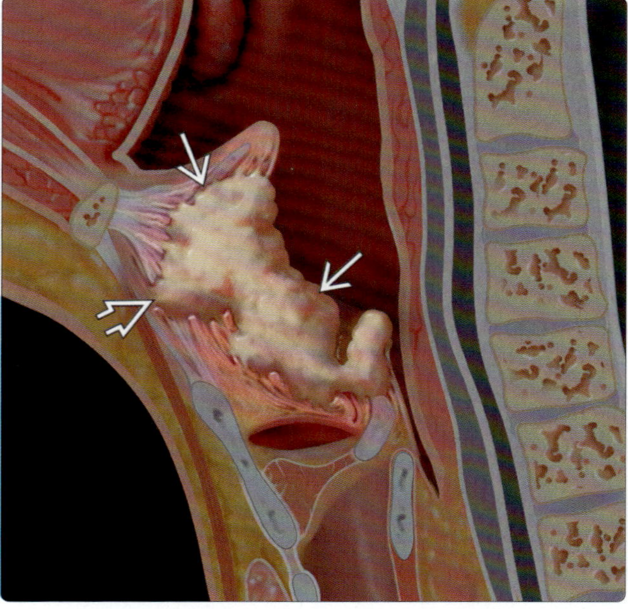

Sagittal graphic illustrates a T3 supraglottic SCCa ➡ as it invades preepiglottic space ⇨. T3 is also determined by vocal cord fixation &/or invasion of one of the following: Postcricoid area, paraglottic space, &/or inner cortex of thyroid cartilage.

T4a Supraglottic

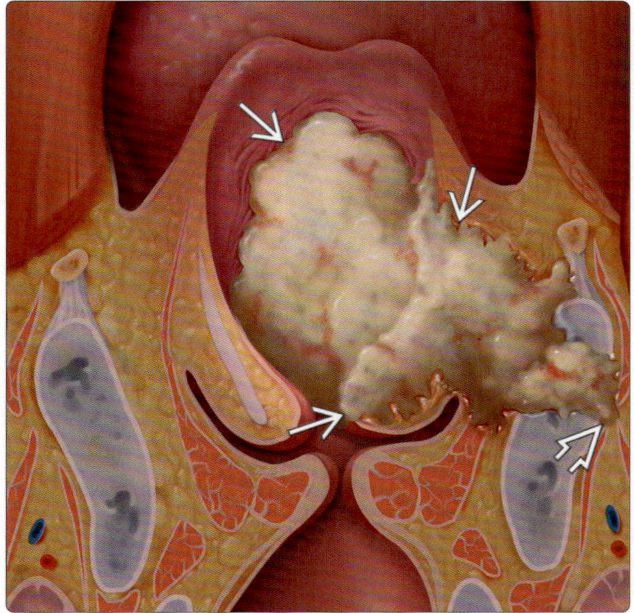

Coronal graphic shows a T4a supraglottic SCCa ➡ extending laterally from supraglottis through paraglottic fat to invade through the left thyroid cartilage ⇨. Extension to paralaryngeal tissues, such as trachea, thyroid, esophagus, or strap muscles, would also denote T4a.

T1/T2 Subglottic

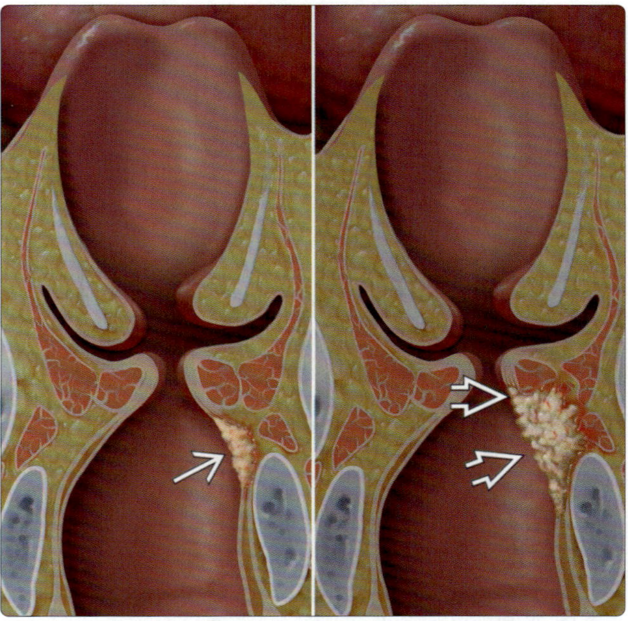

Coronal graphic images depict early-stage subglottic tumors. On the left, a small T1 SCCa ➡ is limited only to the subglottis, from the lower aspect of cord and above inferior cricoid. On the right, a T2 SCCa ⇨ is shown, extending to the vocal cord.

T3 Subglottic

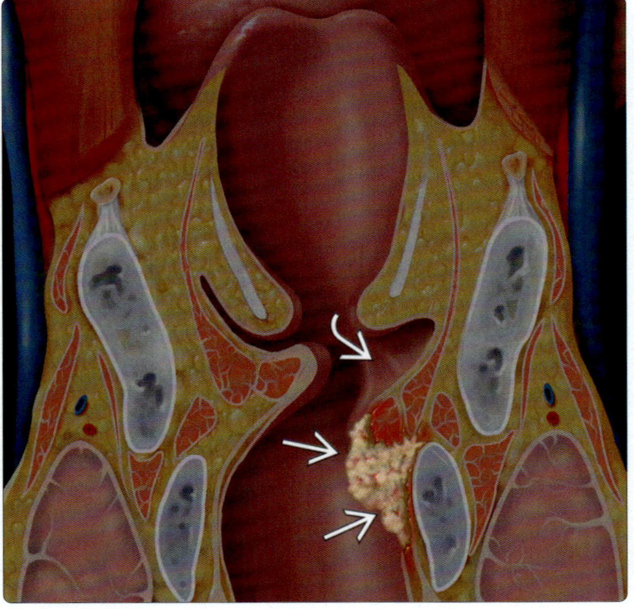

Coronal graphic reveals a subglottic T3 SCCa ➡ that is still limited to the larynx but now results in vocal cord fixation, demonstrated by dilation of the ipsilateral lateral ventricle ➡ and medialization of the cord.

T4a Subglottic

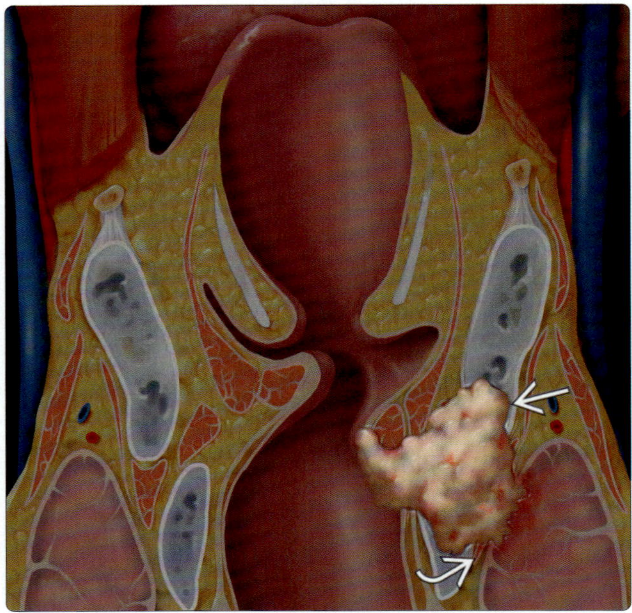

Coronal graphic illustrates moderately advanced local disease, or subglottic T4a SCCa, where tumor has invaded thyroid ➡ or cricoid ➡ cartilage &/or has spread to extralaryngeal soft tissues. Definition of T4b tumor is the same for all laryngeal SCCa (see Glottic T4b).

Metastases, Organ Frequency

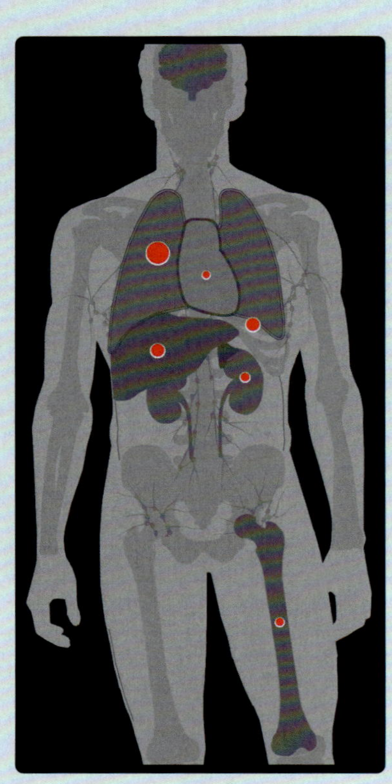

Lung	*43%*
Liver	*18%*
Diaphragm/pleura	*18%*
Kidney	*9%*
Bone	*7%*
Heart	*5%*
Spleen, nostril, small intestine	*2%*

Distant metastases for cancers of all laryngeal sites in autopsy series.

KEY FACTS

TERMINOLOGY

- Definition: Mucosal squamous cell carcinoma (SCCa) arising in supraglottic (SG) larynx

IMAGING

- CECT defines deep tissue extent; nodal involvement
- CECT: Enhancing mass arising from mucosa of supraglottis subsite (epiglottis, aryepiglottic fold, or false vocal cord)
  - Look for preepiglottic and paraglottic space involvement with tumor = **T3 disease**
  - Evaluate cartilage erosion for staging: Inner cortex (**T3**) or through cartilage (**T4**)
  - Look for extralaryngeal extension to surrounding soft tissues (**T4**)
  - Cartilage sclerosis is nonspecific: May be perichondritis from adjacent tumor or early tumor invasion
  - **Nodes frequent**; 1st nodal station is level II; can be **bilateral** due to embryologic lack of midline fusion plane

TOP DIFFERENTIAL DIAGNOSES

- Gastroesophageal reflux
- Rheumatoid larynx
- Laryngeal sarcoidosis
- Laryngeal adenoid cystic carcinoma

PATHOLOGY

- Secondary to long-term tobacco and alcohol use
- 5-year survival rate = 75% for all SG-SCCa

CLINICAL ISSUES

- Typical clinical presentation: > 50 years old, M:F = 9:1
  - Sore throat, dysphagia, hoarseness, referred ear pain
- Treatment options
  - **T1/T2** (smaller tumors): Laser surgery or XRT only
  - **T3/T4a** (larger tumors): XRT and chemotherapy
  - **T4a** with extralaryngeal or transcartilaginous extension: Total laryngectomy
  - Salvage treatment for XRT failure: Total laryngectomy

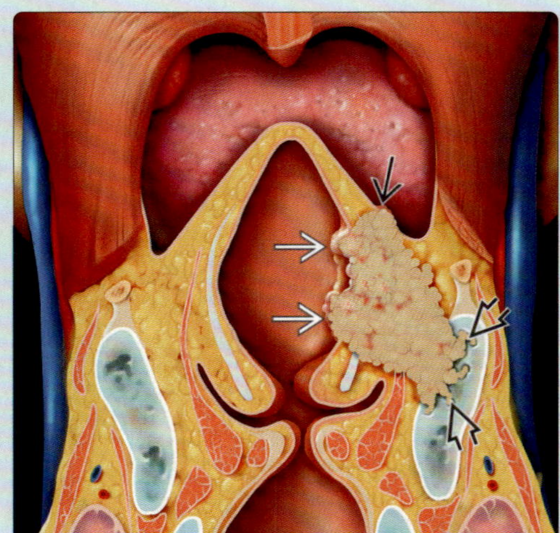

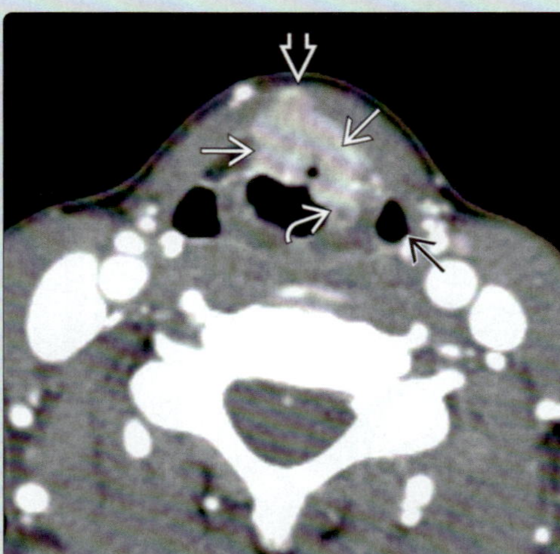

(Left) *Coronal graphic shows T4 supraglottic squamous cell carcinoma (SCCa) involving the left false vocal cord and aryepiglottic (AE) fold ➙ with invasion of thyroid cartilage ➙. Only the mucosal portion ➙ of the tumor is visible on endoscopy. The submucosal extent and cartilage invasion, which are only seen on imaging, are key to staging.* **(Right)** *Axial CECT shows similar findings with invasion of bilateral paraglottic fat ➙ and left AE fold ➙. Tumor bulges through the thyroid cartilage notch ➙. The pyriform sinus ➙ is normal.*

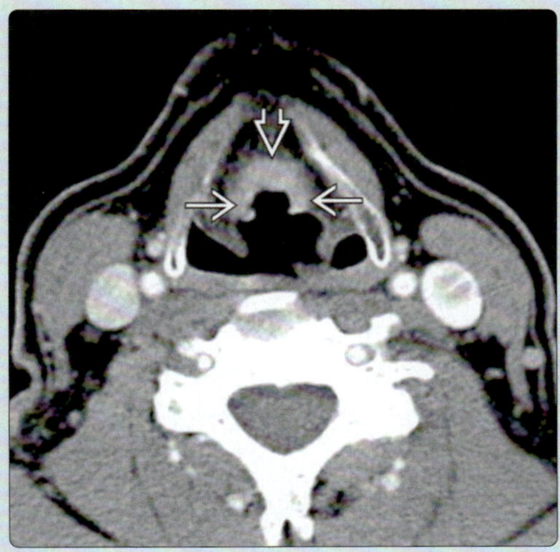

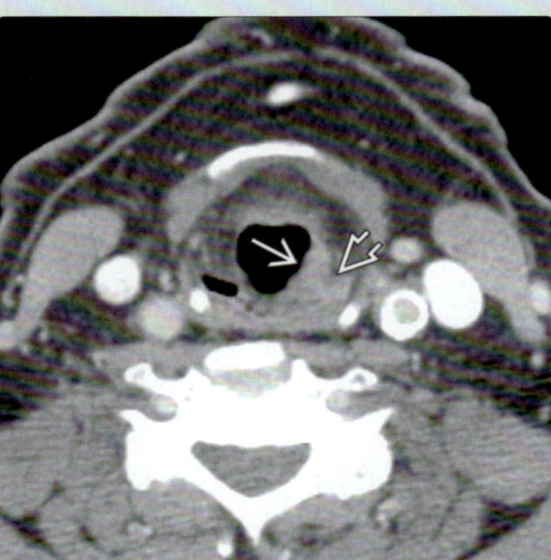

(Left) *Axial CECT shows a small epiglottic mass ➙, staged as T3 due to preepiglottic space invasion ➙. Mass is symmetric, making it hard to appreciate; however, epiglottis should never be this thick or enhancing. No nodes are evident but the search must be bilateral, especially with epiglottic tumors.* **(Right)** *Axial CECT shows a small T1 posterior laryngeal SCCa with a mass on the left AE fold ➙. Left pyriform sinus is collapsed ➙ but no tumor is present in the hypopharynx. Endoscopy is critical to confirm lack of tumor in the pyriform sinus.*

Glottic Laryngeal Squamous Cell Carcinoma

KEY FACTS

TERMINOLOGY

- Squamous cell carcinoma (SCCa) arising on mucosal surface of glottic larynx
- Glottis = vocal cord + anterior & posterior commissures

IMAGING

- Imaging issues
  - Typically, diagnosis known at time of imaging following clinical exam
    - Imaging important to assess supra- or subglottic extension, cartilage invasion, nodes
  - CECT/MR findings may be subtle if small tumor
  - CECT has fewer motion artifacts than MR
- CECT findings
  - Enhancing infiltrative or exophytic glottic mass
  - Location: Anterior true vocal cord ± anterior commissure
  - Metastatic nodes uncommon, typically late
- MR: Adjunctive role for **cartilage invasion** if CECT unsure
- FDG avid on PET; reserved for late-stage tumors only

TOP DIFFERENTIAL DIAGNOSES

- Gastroesophageal reflux disease
- Laryngeal chondrosarcoma
- Rheumatoid larynx
- Laryngeal adenoid cystic carcinoma

PATHOLOGY

- Strongly associated with tobacco & alcohol use
- Keratinizing well- to moderately differentiated SCCa

CLINICAL ISSUES

- Clinical presentation
  - Much more common in male patients; > 50 years
  - Often presents at low stage because of early presentation of persistent hoarseness or change in voice
- Treatment options
  - T1: XRT or laser surgery; > 90% 5-year survival
  - T4: Laryngectomy + XRT vs. chemoradiation therapy; 30-60% 5-year survival rate

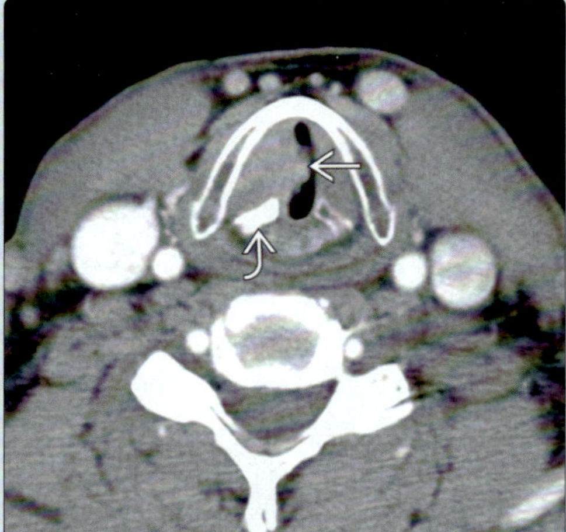

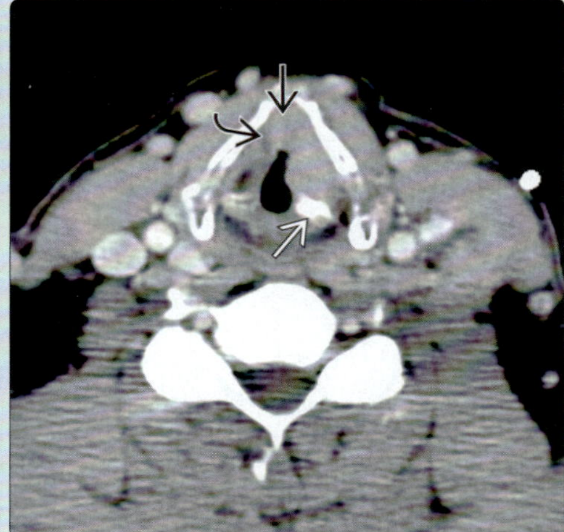

(Left) *Axial CECT shows an enhancing right true vocal card (TVC) exophytic mass ➡. Anterior and posterior commissures are normal. The right arytenoid cartilage sclerosis ➡ is nonspecific and may be either perichondritis from edema or tumor invasion. Diagnosis was T1a tumor.* **(Right)** *Axial CECT reveals SCCa involving the entire left true TVC, anterior commissure ➡, and anterior 1/3 of right cord ➡. Left arytenoid ➡ and thyroid cartilages are sclerotic but without destruction or cartilage penetration. This is T1b tumor by imaging.*

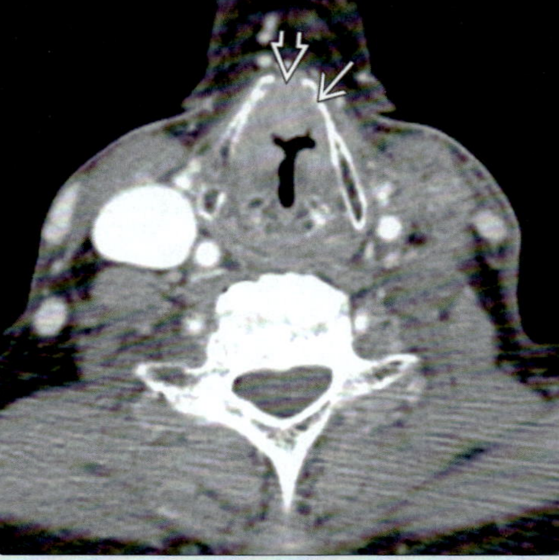

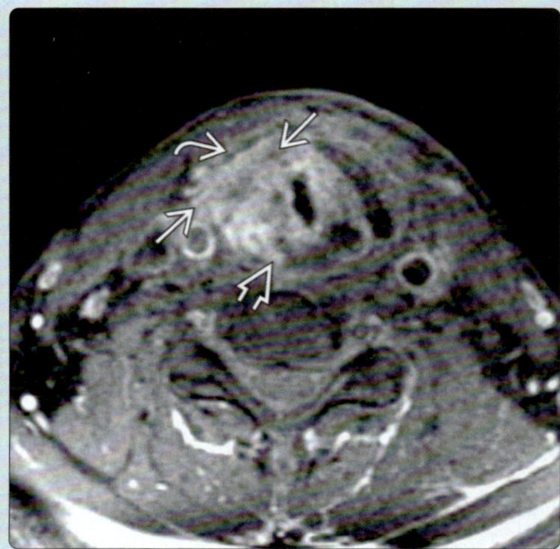

(Left) *Axial CECT shows bulky, ulcerated anterior SCCa involving both vocal cords and anterior commissure ➡. Both anterior thyroid cartilages are sclerotic with erosion of the inner cortex ➡, upstaging the tumor to T3.* **(Right)** *Axial T1WI C+ FS MR in a patient previously treated for right TVC SCCa and biopsy-proven recurrence shows an enhancing tumor involving the right cricoid cartilage ➡, penetrating through thyroid cartilage ➡ to the right strap muscles ➡. Diagnosis was T4a tumor.*

Glottic Laryngeal Squamous Cell Carcinoma

TERMINOLOGY

Abbreviations

- Glottic squamous cell carcinoma (G-SCCa)

Definitions

- SCCa arising on mucosal surface of glottic larynx
  - Glottis = vocal cord + anterior & posterior commissures

IMAGING

General Features

- Best diagnostic clue
  - Enhancing irregular true vocal cord (TVC)
- Location
  - Most often anterior TVC & anterior commissure

CT Findings

- CECT
  - Enhancing infiltrative or exophytic TVC mass
  - Imaging findings may be very subtle if small tumor
  - Metastatic nodes uncommon, typically late with large tumor

MR Findings

- T1WI
  - Low- to intermediate-intensity TVC mass
- T2WI
  - Intermediate-intensity TVC mass
- T1WI C+
  - Homogeneous enhancement

Nuclear Medicine Findings

- PET
  - Rarely obtained for G-SCCa, as nodal metastases unusual

Imaging Recommendations

- Best imaging tool
  - CECT obtained with quiet breathing has fewer motion artifacts than MR
  - MR has adjunctive role for cartilage invasion
- Protocol advice
  - CECT should be obtained during quiet respiration
  - < 1-mm slices allow coronal reformations
    - Supraglottic spread: Across laryngeal ventricle
    - Subglottic spread: > 1 cm below TVC

DIFFERENTIAL DIAGNOSIS

Gastroesophageal Reflux Disease

- Vocal cords edematous with mucosal enhancement

Rheumatoid Larynx

- Cricoarytenoid joint swelling

Laryngeal Chondrosarcoma

- T2-hyperintense submucosal mass of thyroid or cricoid cartilage

Laryngeal Adenoid Cystic Carcinoma

- Typically, submucosal & more hyperintense on T2

PATHOLOGY

General Features

- Etiology
  - Strongly associated with tobacco & alcohol abuse

Staging, Grading, & Classification

- American Joint Committee on Cancer (AJCC) **2017**
  - **T1**: Tumor limited to vocal cord(s) (may involve anterior or posterior commissure) with normal mobility
    - **T1a**: Tumor limited to 1 cord; **T1b**: Tumor involves both cords
  - **T2**: Tumor extends to supraglottis &/or subglottis &/or with impaired vocal cord mobility
  - **T3**: Tumor limited to larynx with vocal cord fixation &/or invasion of paraglottic space &/or inner cortex of thyroid cartilage
  - **T4a**: Tumor invades through outer cortex of thyroid cartilage &/or invades tissues beyond larynx
    - Involvement of trachea, soft tissues of neck, including deep extrinsic muscle of tongue, strap muscles, thyroid, or esophagus
  - **T4b**: Invades prevertebral muscles, encases carotid artery, or invades mediastinal soft tissues

CLINICAL ISSUES

Presentation

- Most common signs/symptoms
  - Typically presents with hoarseness, change in voice

Demographics

- Age
  - Patients typically > 50 years old
- Gender
  - M:F = 9:1
- Epidemiology
  - 60% of laryngeal SCCa are glottic tumors

Natural History & Prognosis

- Anterior cords are dense, avascular fibroelastic tissue without lymphatics
  - **Therefore nodal spread uncommon, late**
- Prognosis generally good for early tumors
  - T1: > 90% 5-year survival rate
  - T4: 30-60% 5-year survival rate

Treatment

- Small T1 tumors: Laser surgery or XRT alone
- Higher stage, larger tumor: Combination of XRT & partial or total laryngectomy

DIAGNOSTIC CHECKLIST

Consider

- Typically, diagnosis is known at time of imaging
- CECT to assess for supra- or subglottic extension, cartilage involvement, or nodal spread
- MR helpful to clarify cartilage penetration

Image Interpretation Pearls

- If anterior commissure > 1-mm thick, then likely involved with tumor

Subglottic Laryngeal Squamous Cell Carcinoma

KEY FACTS

TERMINOLOGY

- Definition: Mucosal squamous cell carcinoma (SCCa) originating from subglottic larynx
  - Subglottic larynx definition: Inferior aspect of true vocal cord (TVC) to inferior cricoid cartilage

IMAGING

- CECT findings: Enhancing mass internal to cricoid ring that fills lumen or invades extralaryngeal tissues
  - Local tumor spread patterns
    - May spread superiorly to TVC(s)
    - Cricoid cartilage invasion common (T4)
  - Nodal metastases: Uncommon (20%) except for advanced stage
- Thin-section CECT: Best to show tumor extent
  - Coronal reformats helpful for craniocaudal tumor
- MR: Intermediate T2, enhances with gadolinium
  - If cartilage signal = tumor signal, suggests invasion
- PET/CT: FDG-avid tumor and nodes

TOP DIFFERENTIAL DIAGNOSES

- Glottic larynx SCCa
- Larynx adenoid cystic carcinoma or chondrosarcoma

PATHOLOGY

- 50% present as T4 tumor
- < 5% of laryngeal SCCa are subglottic
- Overall 5-year survival: 50%

CLINICAL ISSUES

- Clinical presentation
  - > 50-year-old male smoker &/or drinker
  - Stridor, dyspnea, hoarseness if TVC involved
  - Subglottic SCCa has long asymptomatic period
  - **Imaging critical**: Clinical and endoscopic staging more difficult than glottic or supraglottic SCCa
- Treatment options
  - T4 tumors require total laryngectomy + adjuvant XRT
  - Primary XRT or chemoXRT for laryngeal conservation

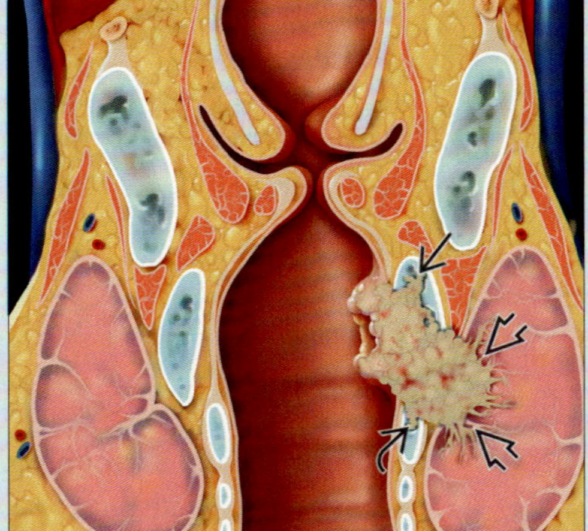

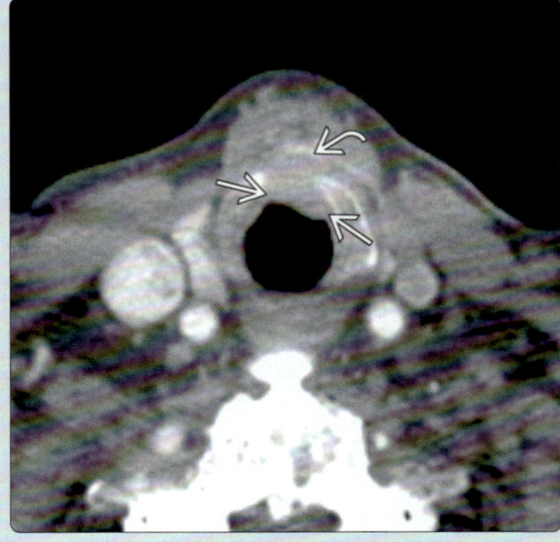

(Left) *Coronal graphic depicts a left subglottic squamous cell carcinoma (SCCa) tumor invading the cricoid ➔, 1st tracheal ring ➔, & thyroid gland ➔. This is an AJCC stage T4a SCCa tumor.* **(Right)** *Axial CECT demonstrates typical subglottic SCCa ➔ in the anterior subglottis. Note midline cricoid cartilage destruction with definite extralaryngeal extension into infrahyoid strap muscles ➔, designating T4a tumor. This is the most common pattern of extension. No soft tissue should be present between cartilage inner table & airway.*

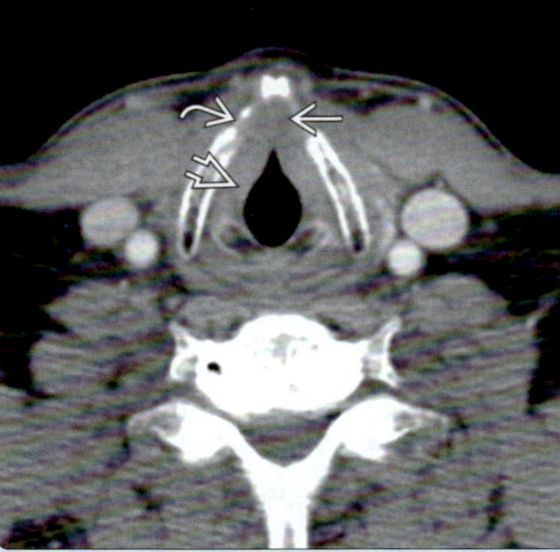

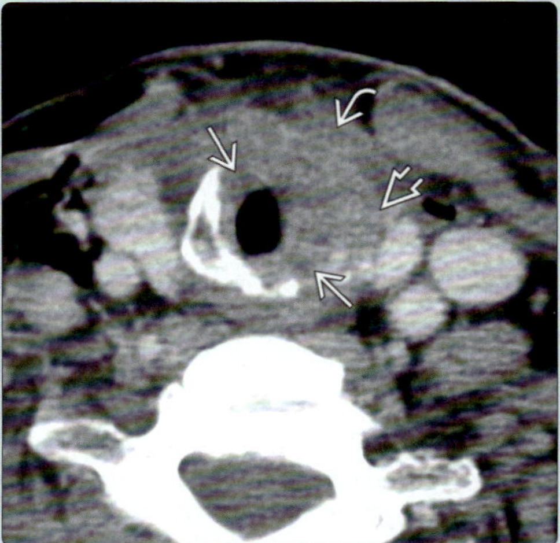

(Left) *Axial CECT immediately below the true vocal cord (TVC) ➔ reveals extremely subtle, symmetric, minimally enhancing subglottic SCCa ➔ in the anterior airway. The image level is below the TVC, as arytenoid cartilages are not present. There is subtle erosion and sclerosis of the right thyroid cartilage ➔. One must know if TVC mobility is normal to stage this tumor.* **(Right)** *Axial CECT of a T4a tumor shows a large mass destroying much of the cricoid cartilage ➔ with extralaryngeal spread ➔ and thyroid gland invasion ➔.*

Laryngeal Squamous Cell Carcinoma With Secondary Laryngocele

KEY FACTS

TERMINOLOGY

- Secondary laryngocele: Lesion obstructs laryngeal ventricle causing internal or mixed laryngocele
- Squamous cell carcinoma (SCCa) is most common cause of secondary laryngocele

IMAGING

- CECT with coronal reformats
  - Thin-walled air- or fluid-filled internal or mixed laryngocele with glottic &/or supraglottic soft tissue mass
  - Obstructing SCCa: Enhancing, infiltrative glottic or low supraglottic mass in area of ventricle
  - Paraglottic laryngocele extends to margin of SCCa
  - Internal laryngocele: Thin-walled fluid or air density paraglottic space cyst
  - Mixed laryngocele: Paraglottic cyst passes through thyrohyoid membrane into submandibular space

TOP DIFFERENTIAL DIAGNOSES

- Primary laryngocele
- 2nd branchial cleft cyst
- Thyroglossal duct cyst

PATHOLOGY

- Lesion obstructs laryngeal ventricle with consequent internal or mixed laryngocele
  - Laryngeal SCCa > > inflammation > trauma
  - 15% of all laryngoceles

CLINICAL ISSUES

- SCCa: Hoarseness, stridor from fixation of vocal cord
- Treatment: Single modality surgery or XRT for early stage, chemoXRT for advanced stage

DIAGNOSTIC CHECKLIST

- In smoker, search for laryngeal SCCa in area of ventricle
- Stage primary SCCa as if laryngocele not present

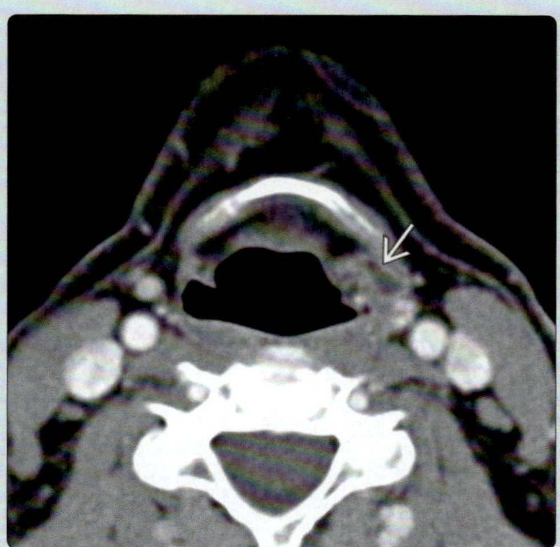

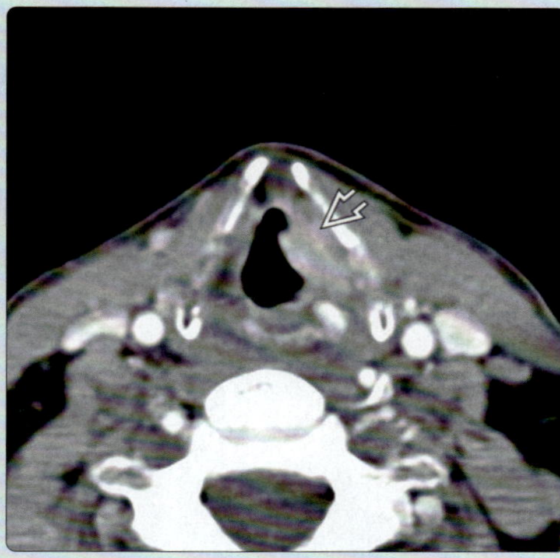

(Left) *Axial CECT reveals a small, left-sided, secondary internal laryngocele ➡ in the high left paraglottic space.* **(Right)** *Axial CECT at the level of the glottis in the same patient reveals an enhancing, infiltrative squamous cell carcinoma (SCCa) involving the left true vocal cord ➡. The endoscopic assessment suggests the tumor involves the superior false vocal cord, but the CECT demonstrated that a secondary internal laryngocele caused the submucosal mass effect in this area.*

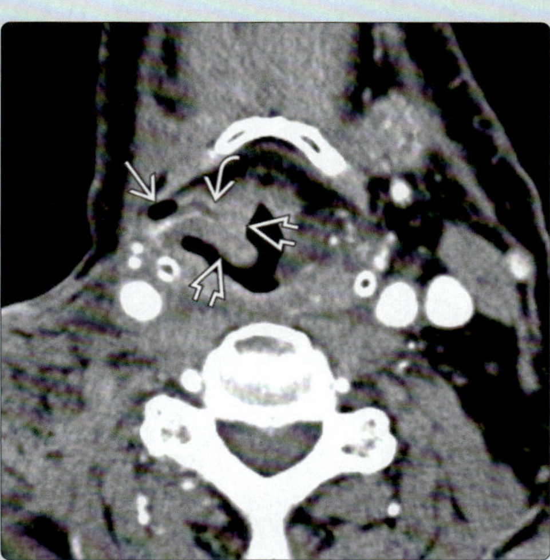

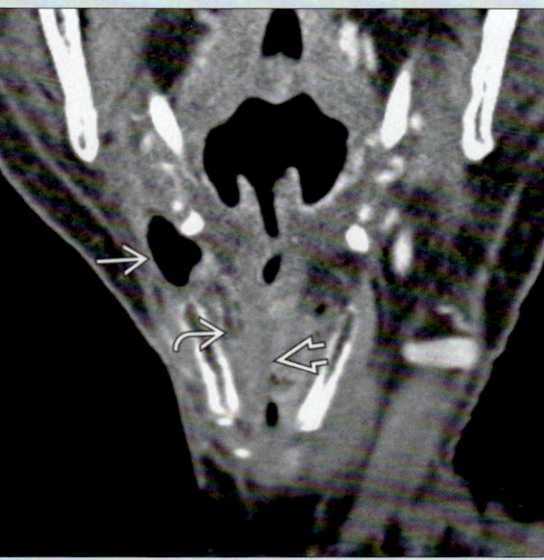

(Left) *Axial CECT shows an air-filled mixed secondary laryngocele ➡ with a fluid-filled stalk ➡ obstructed by a supraglottic enhancing SCCa ➡. The SCCa in this image involves the false cord and enlarges the aryepiglottic fold.* **(Right)** *Coronal CECT in the same patient reveals the air-filled external secondary laryngocele ➡, the fluid-filled tubular saccule ➡, and supraglottic and glottic SCCa ➡. Remember to search for a laryngeal SCCa in all adults where CECT reveals a laryngocele.*

Perineural Tumor Spread

KEY FACTS

TERMINOLOGY

- Definition: Malignant tumor spread along sheath of cranial nerves distant from 1° site

IMAGING

- General imaging findings and issues
  - Most often found along **CNV** and **CNVII** branches
  - MR more sensitive than CECT for perineural tumor spread (PNT)
  - Examine nerve(s) at risk from end organ to nucleus
  - PNT may spread anterograde and retrograde, may have skip lesions, and may cross between nerves
- CECT: May be extremely subtle
  - Enlarged nerve, ± mild enhancement
  - Smoothly widened bony foramina or canals
  - Muscular denervation atrophy (typically masticator from CNV3 PNT)
- MR: Nerve enlarged and enhancing, loss of normal fat signal along course of nerves
  - T1WI with fat saturation is mainstay of diagnosis

TOP DIFFERENTIAL DIAGNOSES

- Schwannoma, neurofibroma, lymphoma

PATHOLOGY

- Neurotropic tumors
  - **Adenoid cystic, squamous cell carcinoma, melanoma, lymphoma**
  - **Skin, parotid, palate, nasopharynx**

CLINICAL ISSUES

- Clinical presentation
  - Deep facial mass + facial numbness (CNV branches)
  - Parotid mass + peripheral facial nerve paralysis (CNVII)
- Treatment options
  - Surgery combined with postoperative radiation therapy ± chemo
  - With PNT, entire course of nerve must be treated

(Left) *Sagittal graphic illustrates the classic appearance of perineural tumor spread from cheek skin malignancy. Tumor gains access to the infraorbital nerve ➩ & spreads retrograde to the terygopalatine fossa ➩, foramen rotundum, & into the Meckel cave, involving the gasserian ganglion ➩.* **(Right)** *Coronal T1WI C+ FS MR in patient with left maxillary squamous cell carcinoma shows dramatic enlargement & enhancement of left CNV2 within the foramen rotundum ➩. A normal right CNV2 is shown for comparison ➩.*

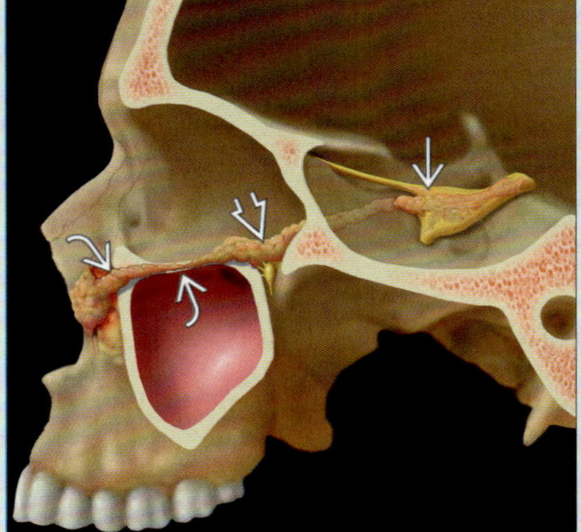

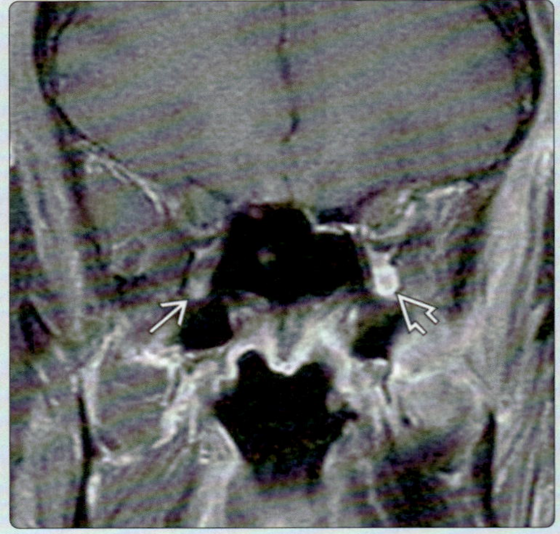

(Left) *Coronal graphic of the mandibular division of the trigeminal nerve (CNV3) shows a malignant lesion of the masticator space ➩ that follows the CNV3 ➩ superiorly and through the foramen ovale ➩ intracranially. Malignancy of the chin skin, mandible, and masticator space all can spread in a perineural fashion on CNV3.* **(Right)** *Coronal T1 FS C+ MR reveals a thickened CNV3 ➩ from perineural squamous cell carcinoma from the mandibular alveolar ridge spreading superiorly to the foramen ovale ➩.*

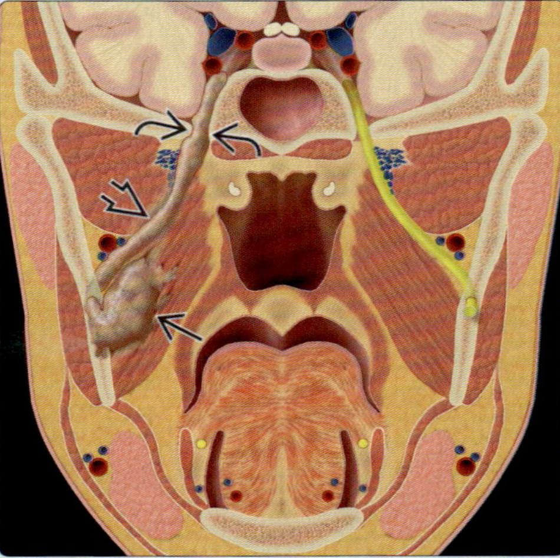

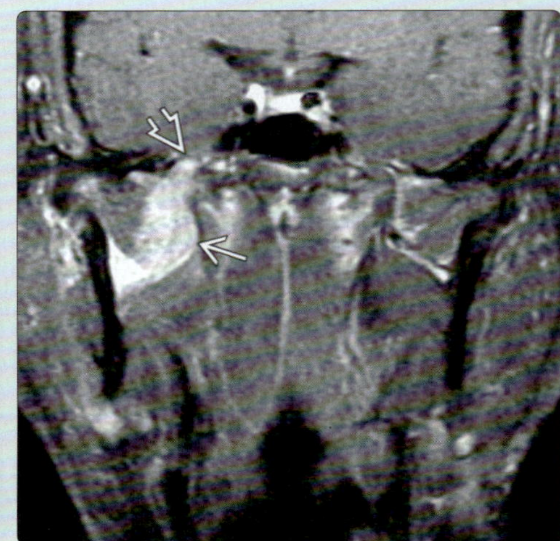

Nodal Squamous Cell Carcinoma

KEY FACTS

TERMINOLOGY

- Metastatic spread of primary H&N SCCa to nodes

IMAGING

- Change in morphology key to detecting nodal metastasis
- "**Malignant nodal criteria**" best used in combination
  - Nodal enlargement, typically > 10-mm long axis
  - Round node shape rather than oval
  - Clustered nodes: ≥ 3 nodes 8-9 mm
  - Focal nodal defect/necrosis
  - Extranodal extension
- Ultrasound can help
  - Shows **loss of hilar echogenicity**
  - Color Doppler: Chaotic intranodal vascularity, hilar and peripheral

TOP DIFFERENTIAL DIAGNOSES

- Reactive or suppurative nodes
- 2nd branchial cleft cyst
- Differentiated thyroid carcinoma or NHL nodes

PATHOLOGY

- Lymphatic spread of H&N SCCa follows expected pattern

CLINICAL ISSUES

- Nodal metastasis is **most important prognostic factor** for H&N SCCa
  - Unilateral node ↓ prognosis of survival 50%
  - Bilateral nodes ↓ prognosis of survival 75%
- Patient presenting with neck mass from metastatic SCCa + normal clinical & radiographic exam = "**unknown primary**"
- Classification of neck dissection
  - Radical neck dissection (RND): Resection of levels I-V + sternocleidomastoid (SCM), internal jugular vein (IJV), and spinal accessory nerve (CN11)
  - Modified radical neck dissection: RND with preservation of SCM, IJV, ± CN11
  - Selective neck dissection: One or more of nodal groups I-V preserved

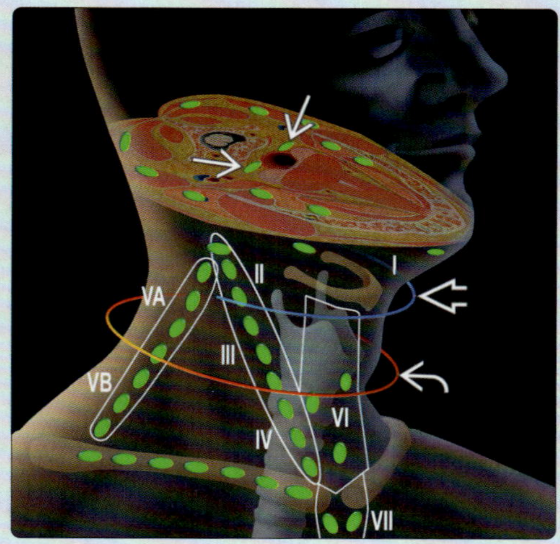

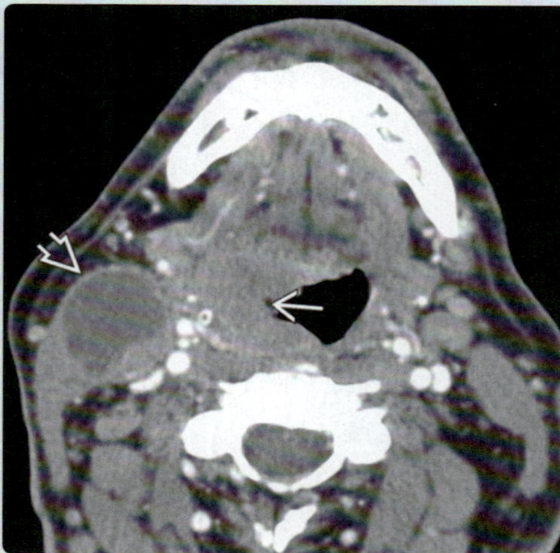

(Left) *Graphic of the cervical neck a depicts nodal network to which squamous cell carcinoma (SCCa) may metastasize. Superior axial slice shows retropharyngeal nodes ➡. The hyoid bone ➡ & cricoid cartilage ➡ planes subdivide the internal jugular & spinal accessory nodal group levels. Level II is most common site of SCCa nodal metastasis.* **(Right)** *Axial CECT in a patient with right oropharyngeal SCCa ➡ & level IIa metastatic node ➡ is shown. The round shape, cystic necrotic changes, & size allow the imager to label this node as malignant.*

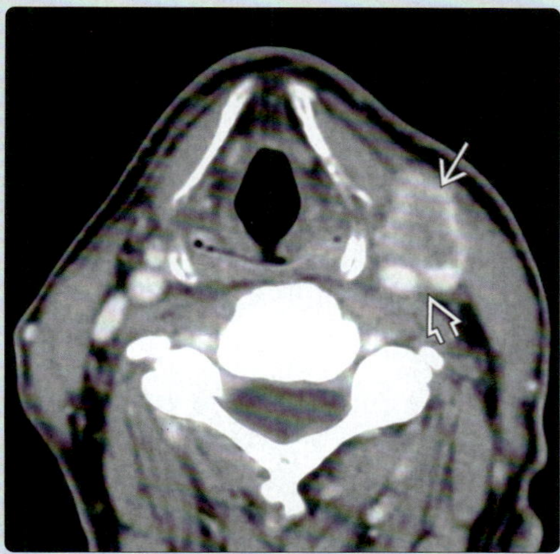

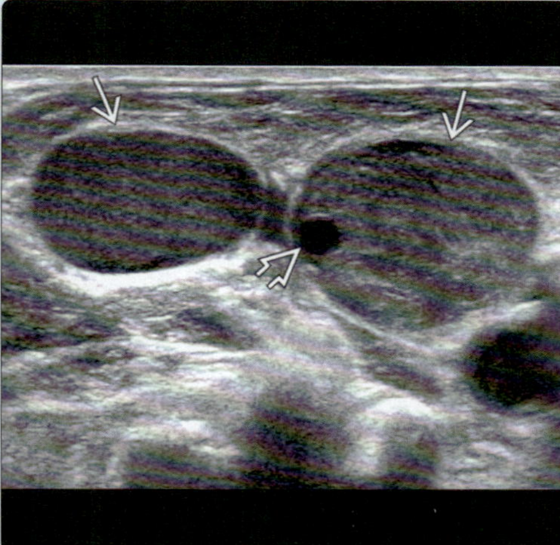

(Left) *Axial CECT through the level of the supraglottis reveals a left level II metastatic SCCa node ➡. The amorphous shape, irregular margins, and extension into the carotid space ➡ indicate extracapsular spread has occurred.* **(Right)** *Transverse grayscale US shows typical metastatic SCCa nodes ➡. They are round, predominantly solid, well defined, and hypoechoic with loss of normal hilar architecture. A small area of cystic necrosis is seen in 1 node ➡.*

Nodal Dissection in Neck

KEY FACTS

TERMINOLOGY

- Neck dissection (ND) performed to treat or accurately stage H&N cancer
- Nodal dissection definitions
  - **Selective ND (SND)**: Resection of known or potential nodal levels while preserving nonlymphatic structures
  - **SND (I-III)**: Resection of nodes in levels I, II, III
  - **SND (II-IV)**: Resection of nodes in levels II-IV
  - **SND (II-V)**: Resection of nodes in levels II-V
  - **SND (VI)**: Resection of nodes in level VI only
- **Modified (radical) ND (MND)**: Nodal resection levels I-V + preservation ≥ 1 nonlymphatic structure (IJV, SCM, or CNXI)
- **Radical ND (RND)**: Nodal resection levels I-V + IJV, SCM, & CNXI; SMG resected with level I nodes
- **Extended neck dissection**: RND + removal of additional structures

IMAGING

- Fibroadipose tissue resected with all NDs
- Imaging findings reflect different tissues resected
  - SND: Loss of fat around CS & beneath SCM; SCM "draped" over CS; IJV & SCM remain
  - MND: Loss of fat around CS; IJV or SCM resected
  - RND: Fibroadipose tissue removed around CS; IJV & SCM resected
- Atrophy of trapezius muscle seen in RND; may be present in MND or SND
- Levator scapulae hypertrophy in RND may mimic tumor
- If level I resected during ND, SMG will be absent

CLINICAL ISSUES

- "Elective" ND may be surgical standard of care to treat micrometastasis, even if diagnostic imaging studies do not show nodal metastases
- Physical exam for recurrent adenopathy after ND difficult due to scarring
- Imaging often only way to detect nodal recurrence after ND; PET/CECT has role in difficult cases

(Left) *Graphic illustrates nodal levels that may be removed in different combinations as part of neck nodal dissections. e.g., radical neck dissection involves removal of all groups; selective neck dissection (SND) is removal of levels I through III only.* **(Right)** *Axial CECT shows typical selective neck dissection findings at level II on the right. Note loss of fat beneath sternocleidomastoid muscle (SCM) ➡ and around carotid space (CS) ➡ (compared to normal left side). Right submandibular gland has been resected. Note normal flow in right IJV ➡.*

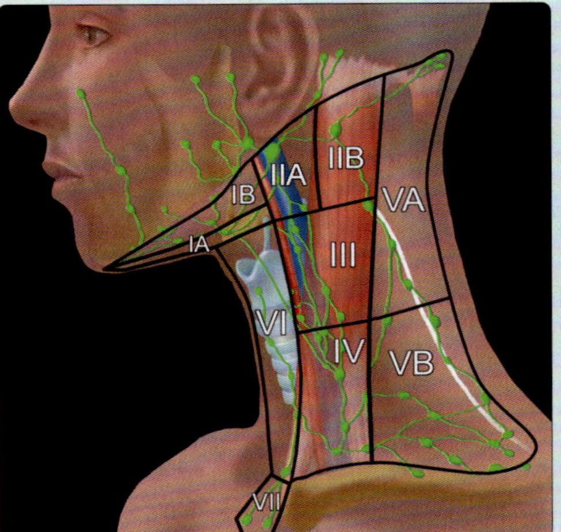

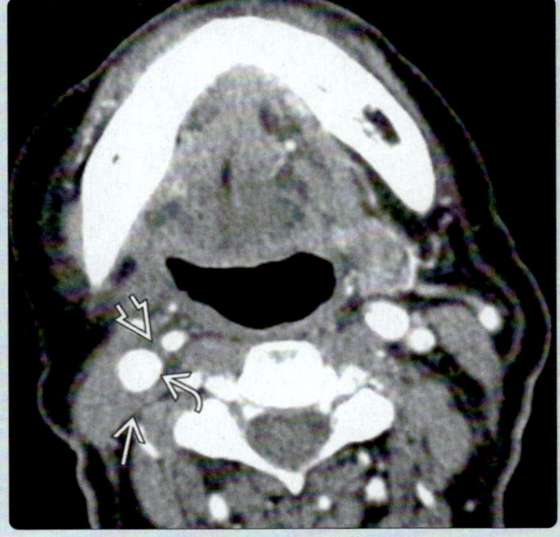

(Left) *Axial CECT shows subtle but definite loss of fat around right CS structures ➡, which is the typical appearance following selective neck dissection. Note the hypertrophy of contralateral trapezius muscle ➡, a common finding after neck dissection.* **(Right)** *Axial T1 MR shows subtle pericarotid changes ➡ of the right SND as compared to left. Note also loss of fat beneath the SCM. Right IJV, SCM ➡, and trapezius muscle ➡ appear normal, as expected with SND.*

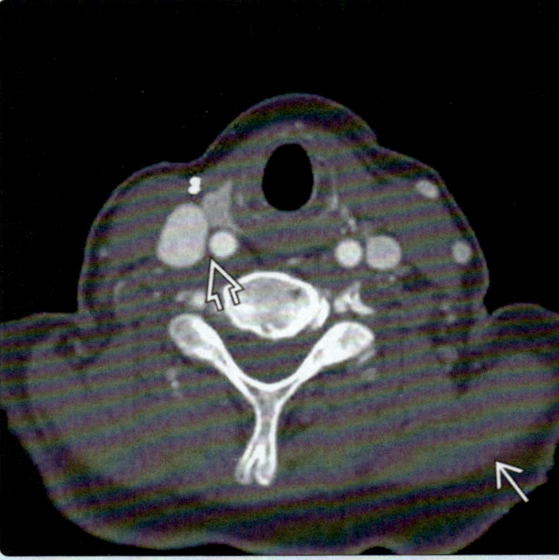

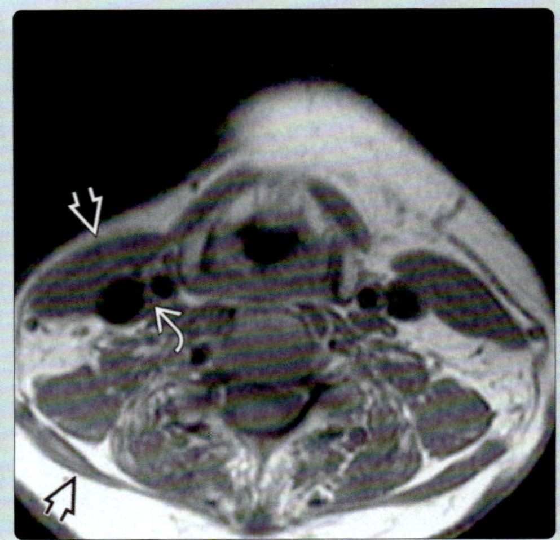

KEY FACTS

TERMINOLOGY

- Soft tissue or autologous bone used to reconstruct postoperative resection defect in H&N
- **Fasciocutaneous flap**
  - Deep muscle fascia, arterial perforators, & overlying skin
  - Used for smaller surgical reconstructions
  - Donor site is radial forearm or anterolateral thigh
- **Myocutaneous flap**
  - Muscle, soft tissue, & skin
  - Used when large surgical defect requires greater tissue volume to fill
  - Donor site is usually pectoralis major muscle or submental flap
- **Osteocutaneous flap**
  - Bone, soft tissue, & overlying skin ± muscle
  - Used when surgical reconstruction requires bone replacement (mandible, maxilla, face)
  - Donor site usually fibula or scapula

IMAGING

- General feature: Soft tissue or bone present in reconstruction site with **nonanatomic** appearance
- CECT/MR
  - Fasciocutaneous, small myocutaneous flaps: May look like normal soft tissue at surgical defect
  - Myocutaneous flap: Denervated at time of transfer to surgical defect; muscle in flap variable depending on time of imaging
  - Osteocutaneous flap: Bone contoured to approximate shape of excised bone

DIAGNOSTIC CHECKLIST

- Essential that history of flap reconstruction available when interpreting complex follow-up scans
  - Flap may be misinterpreted as recurrent tumor
- Look for new enhancing mass (CECT/MR) or hypermetabolic focus (PET) at deep aspect of flap
- Look for splayed/displaced surgical clips

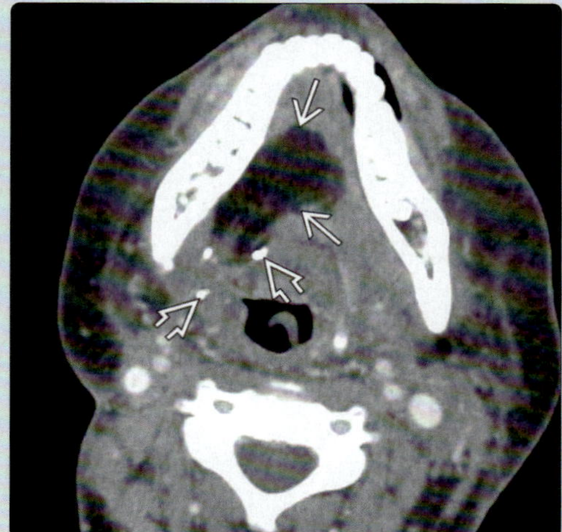

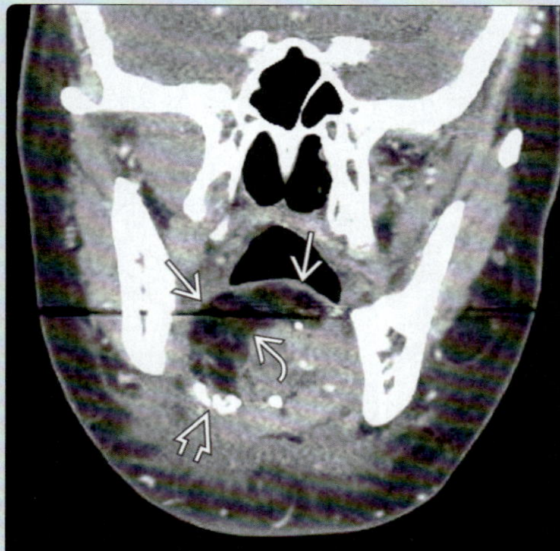

(Left) *Axial CECT of the fasciocutaneous radial forearm free flap shows a well-defined, rounded fatty component of the flap ➡ that provides volume to fill the surgical defect. Multiple surgical clips ➡ in the floor of mouth provide additional evidence that the flap has been placed.* **(Right)** *Coronal CECT in the same patient reveals a fatty flap ➡ filling the oral cavity surgical defect, providing soft tissue to reform a smooth contour to the tongue surface ➡. Surgical clips ➡ are again visible.*

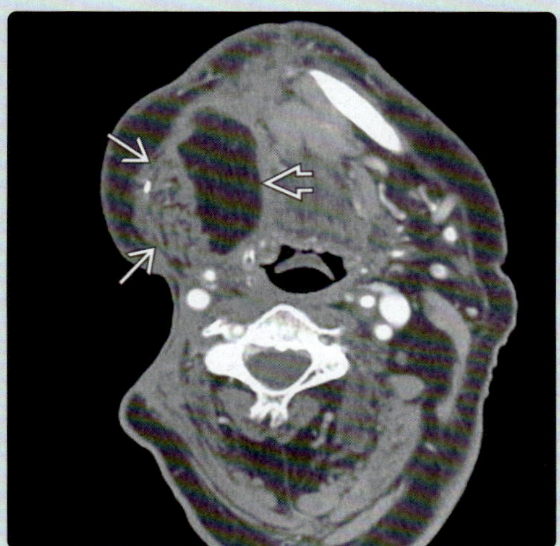

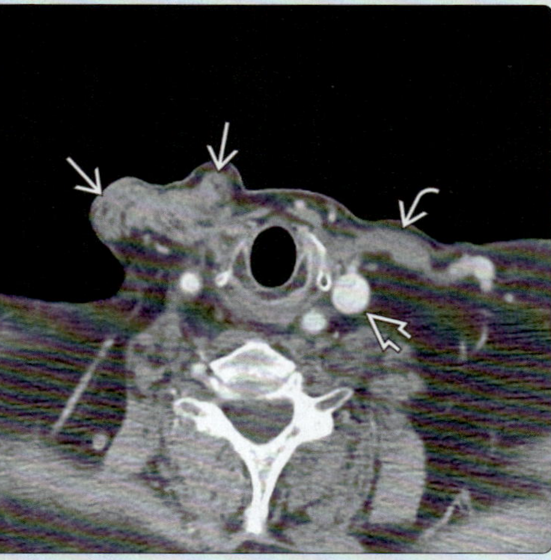

(Left) *Axial CECT in a patient with a pectoralis rotational myocutaneous flap following resection of a large retromolar trigone SCCa shows a medial hypodense fat component of the flap ➡ and a lateral striated pectoralis muscle component of the flap ➡.* **(Right)** *Axial CECT in the low neck (same patient) shows the flap ➡ coming up from the chest. The normal left internal jugular vein ➡ and sternocleidomastoid muscle ➡ are not seen on the right, as the right radical neck dissection was performed as part of the surgical procedure.*

Expected Changes of Neck Radiation Therapy

KEY FACTS

IMAGING

- **Early (1-4 months)**: Diffuse edema of all tissues
  - Reticulation of subcutaneous and deep fat planes
  - Thickening & enhancement of mucosa
  - Swollen, ill-defined enhancing parotid & submandibular glands
  - Subtly swollen muscles, especially pterygoids
- **Late (≥ 12 months)**: Diffuse fibrosis of all tissues
  - Edema and reticulation of fat resolves
  - Mucosal thickening and enhancement may resolve
  - Glandular tissues atrophy; often maintain increased enhancement
  - Lymph nodes and lymphoid tissues atrophy
- **MR**: T2 & T1 C+ accentuate changes seen on CECT
  - Marked T2 intensity & enhancement
- **PET/CT**: No focal uptake unless complication or residual/recurrent tumor

TOP DIFFERENTIAL DIAGNOSES

- Retropharyngeal space edema
- Retropharyngeal space abscess
- Acute parotitis
- Submandibular gland sialadenitis

PATHOLOGY

- XRT destroys endothelial cells lining small vessels
  - **Early**: Results in ischemia, edema, inflammation
  - **Late**: Results in tissue fibrosis

DIAGNOSTIC CHECKLIST

- 1st post-XRT imaging should be 10-12 weeks after end of treatment
- Careful, systematic imaging evaluation is key
- Radiation changes are generally readily identifiable
- Severe XRT changes make evaluating scan difficult
  - Residual or recurrent tumor may be easily missed
  - Focal tissue thickening/mass suggests tumor

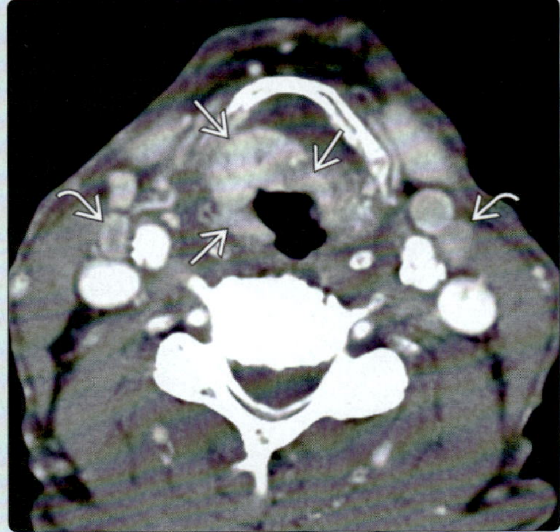

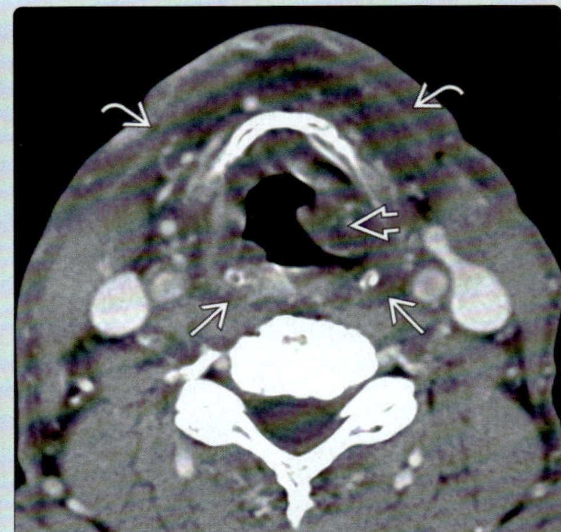

(Left) *CECT shows T3 N2c supraglottic squamous cell carcinoma with an enhancing mass ➔ at the base of the epiglottis, aryepiglottic (AE) fold, & pre- & paraglottic fat. Note bilateral nodes ➔.* **(Right)** *Axial CECT in the same patient 3 months following chemoXRT shows no residual enhancing tumor or nodes. All fat planes & submucosal tissues, including left AE fold ➔, are edematous with hazy density. Note retropharyngeal ➔ edema as well as thickened skin & platysma muscles ➔. These are expected posttreatment changes.*

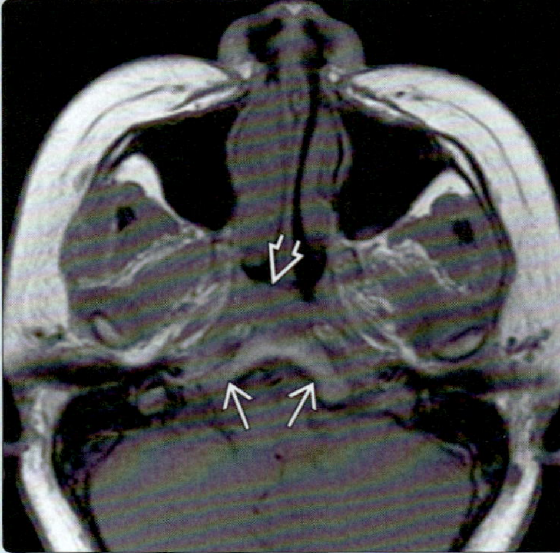

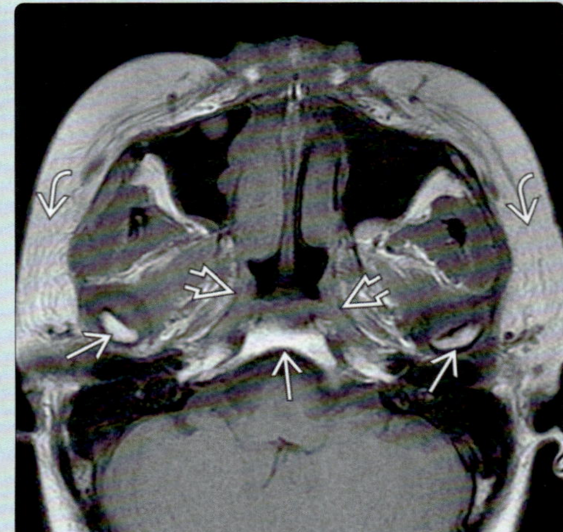

(Left) *Axial T1WI MR demonstrates small T1 primary nasopharyngeal carcinoma ➔, which was confined to nasopharynx. There is normal signal intensity in the clivus ➔, suggesting no infiltration by tumor.* **(Right)** *Axial T1WI MR after chemoXRT shows resolution of the small nasopharyngeal mass but symmetric, smooth, mild mucosal thickening ➔. Note new marked hyperintensity of the skull base & mandibular condylar marrow ➔. Only minimal facial fat reticulation is evident ➔.*

KEY FACTS

TERMINOLOGY

- Uncommon, unintended side effects from radiation therapy (XRT) seen in small proportion of patients

IMAGING

- Potentially involves any radiated neck tissue
  - Excessive inflammation, tissue necrosis, or tumor induction
- CT or MR may be complementary for detection and characterization of abnormality
- CECT typically 1st-order examination; evaluates soft tissues and bones
  - Mucosal ulceration and fistulae, myositis, osteoradionecrosis, chondronecrosis
- MR best for nervous system complications
  - Cerebral radionecrosis, myelopathy, brachial plexitis, cranial neuropathy
- PET may be misleading; intense focal FDG uptake common

TOP DIFFERENTIAL DIAGNOSES

- Recurrent tumor
- Skull base or mandible-maxilla osteomyelitis

PATHOLOGY

- XRT results in obstructive arteriopathy
- Tissues less able to withstand additional stress
- Infection, tumor recurrence, or biopsy may precipitate necrosis

CLINICAL ISSUES

- Uncommon; ~ 1% of patients receiving neck XRT
- Most complications occur ≤ 2 years after XRT
- May occur up to 5-8 years post XRT
- Treatment is largely conservative

DIAGNOSTIC CHECKLIST

- Key differential is always residual/recurrent tumor
- Look for solid enhancing mass

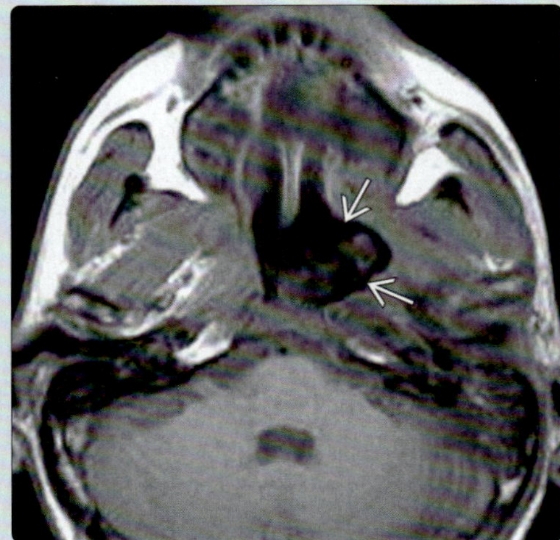

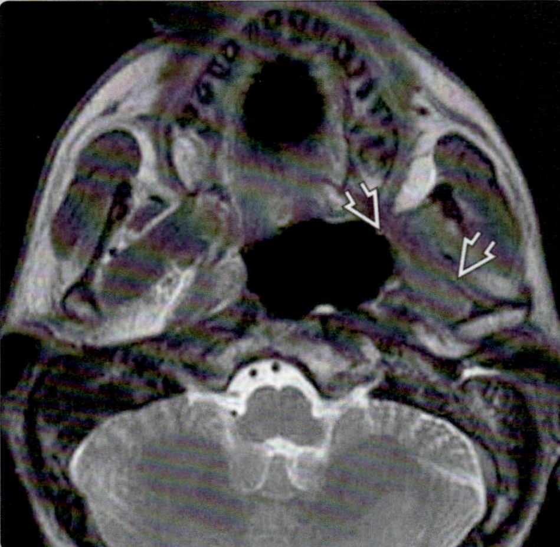

(Left) *Axial T1 MR in a patient treated the decade prior for nasopharyngeal carcinoma with chemoradiation demonstrates an enlarged nasopharyngeal airway following necrosis of the left lateral nasopharyngeal wall tissues ➡.* **(Right)** *Axial T2 MR in the same patient, slightly more inferiorly at the oropharynx, shows the left medial pterygoid muscle ➡ slightly hyperintense & smaller than the contralateral side, suggesting radiation-induced myositis & fibrosis. There are no mass or other imaging features of tumor recurrence.*

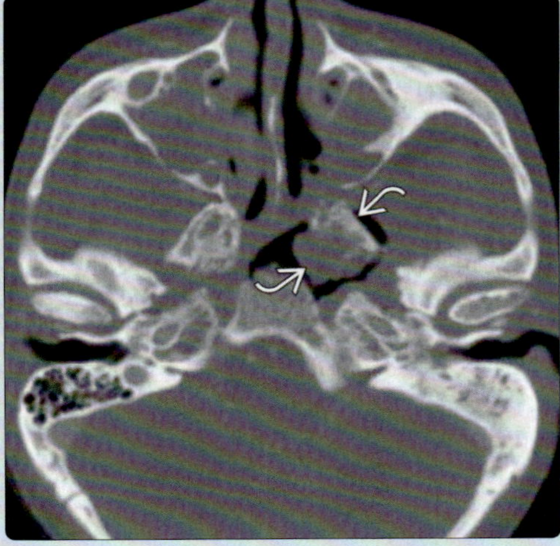

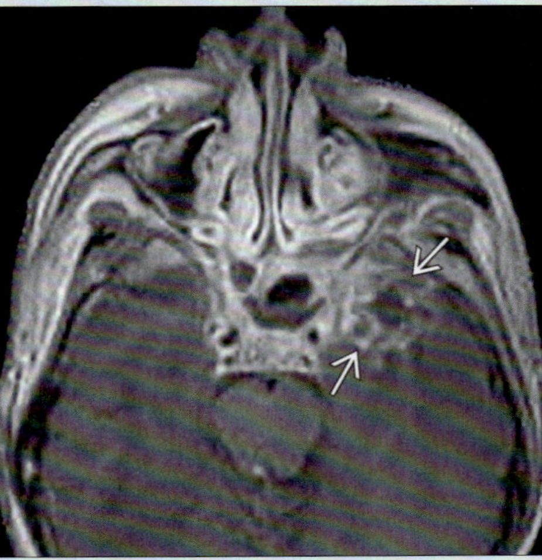

(Left) *Axial bone CT in the same patient shows frank destruction and "crumbling" of the lateral aspect of sphenoid body, creating a sequestrum ➡. This is osteoradionecrosis of sphenoid bone.* **(Right)** *Axial T1 C+ FS MR in the same patient reveals abnormal irregular enhancement of anteromedial left temporal lobe ➡, indicating cerebral radionecrosis. This case illustrates the potential for radiation-induced complications involving multiple tissues in the same field.*

KEY FACTS

TERMINOLOGY

- Imaging findings following resection of whole larynx or part of larynx
- Resection most often performed for malignancy
- **Total laryngectomy (TL)**: Larynx completely resected and neopharynx created
  - Neopharynx connects oropharynx to esophagus
  - Trachea no longer communicates with pharynx
  - Need tracheal stoma to breathe, tracheal-esophageal prosthesis to speak
- **Partial laryngectomy (PL)**: Conservative surgery
  - Aim is to preserve voice and breathing, swallowing without aspiration
  - Cordectomy → vertical or horizontal partial laryngectomy → near-total laryngectomy
  - Imaging varies from near-normal to complex reconstruction and deformity
  - Permanent tracheostomy often required with near total laryngectomy

TOP DIFFERENTIAL DIAGNOSES

- Larynx trauma
- Radiated larynx

CLINICAL ISSUES

- **Declining use of both PL and TL** with ↑ use of organ preservation chemoradiation
- Declining use of open surgery in favor of endoscopic transoral laser surgery
- Laryngectomy also used for cartilaginous laryngeal tumors, invasive thyroid tumors, salvage after failed chemoradiation, chondronecrosis, nonfunctioning larynx posttreatment

DIAGNOSTIC CHECKLIST

- Imaging confusion occurs most often with complex appearance of partial laryngectomy
- 1st determine type of procedure
- Look for recurrent mass and lymphadenopathy

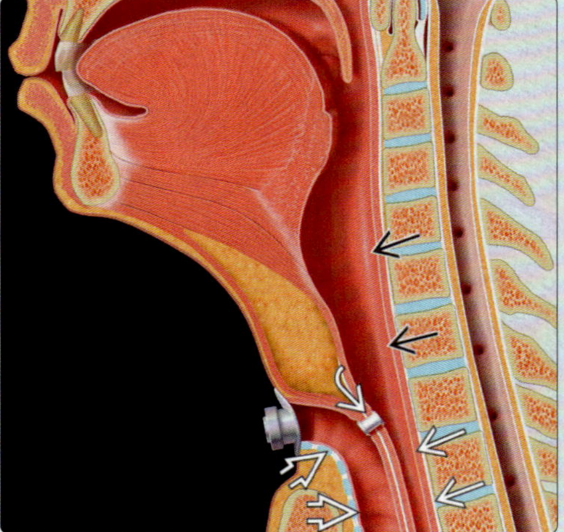
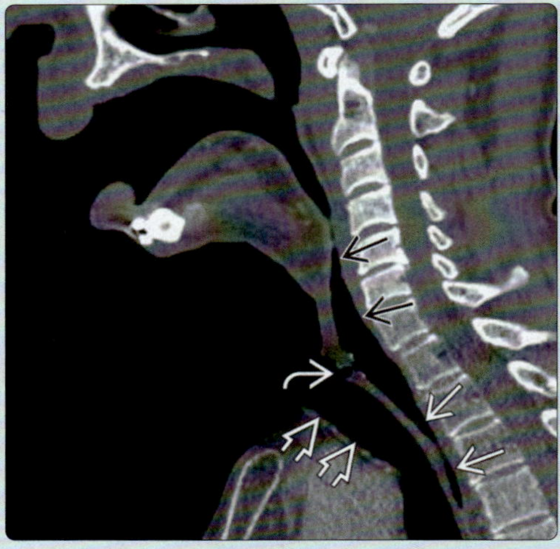

(Left) *Sagittal graphic after total laryngectomy shows the neopharynx ⇨ connects the oral cavity to the esophagus ➡. The trachea ➡ is brought to the skin surface with a tracheal stoma. There is a tracheoesophageal (TE) prosthesis ➡.* **(Right)** *Sagittal CECT reformation in a patient with total laryngectomy & total glossectomy shows deformity with absence of tongue plus absence of hyoid bone. Neopharynx ⇨ connects oral cavity to esophagus ➡ & trachea comes to skin surface with tracheal stoma ➡. Note the TE voice prosthesis ➡.*

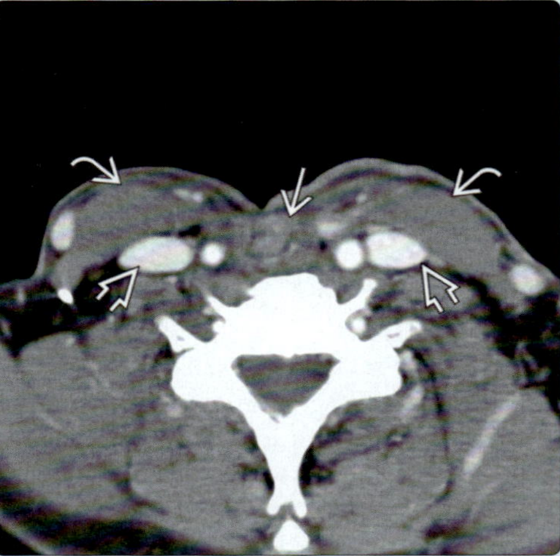
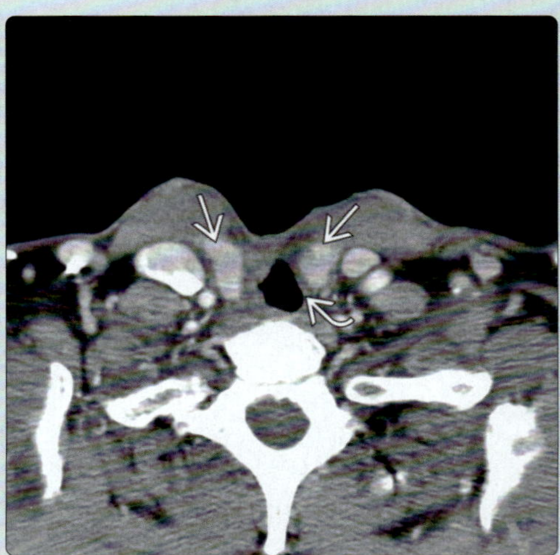

(Left) *Axial CECT in patient following total laryngectomy, right modified neck dissection, & gastric pull-up demonstrates neopharynx as a multilayered midline tubular structure ➡. Both sternocleidomastoid muscles ➡ and jugular veins ➡ are preserved.* **(Right)** *Axial CECT shows a new contour of thyroid lobes ➡ after midline splitting of the thyroid capsule. If 1 lobe is resected, the remaining lobe may be mistaken for a node, recurrent mass, or even pseudoaneurysm. Distal anastomosis ➡ often has slightly irregular contour.*

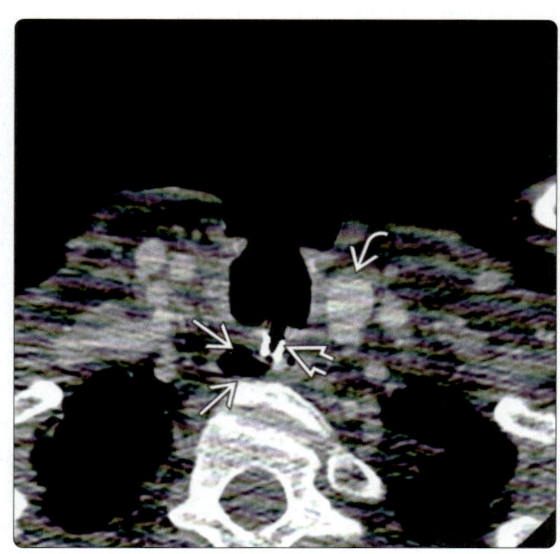

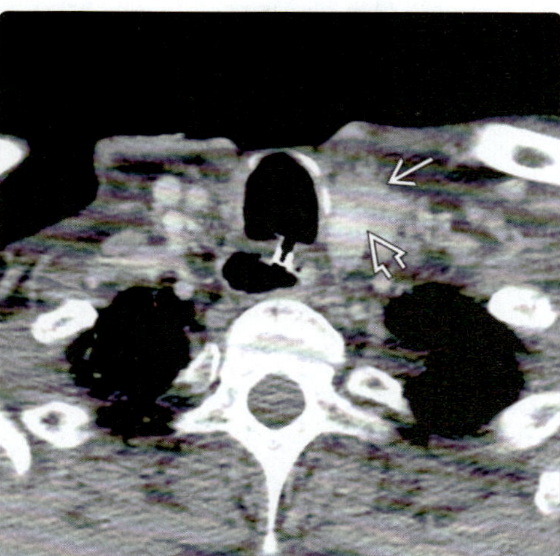

(Left) *Axial CECT 6 months following total laryngectomy and bilateral selective neck dissections in a patient with distal recurrence shows TE voice prosthesis ➡ connecting the trachea and proximal esophagus ➡. The left thyroid lobe is evident ➡.* **(Right)** *Axial CECT in the same patient 14 months following total laryngectomy and bilateral selective neck dissections shows new soft tissue mass ➡ involving the left sternocleidomastoid muscle & thyroid lobe ➡. Recurrent disease is most often nodal or occurs at anastomoses.*

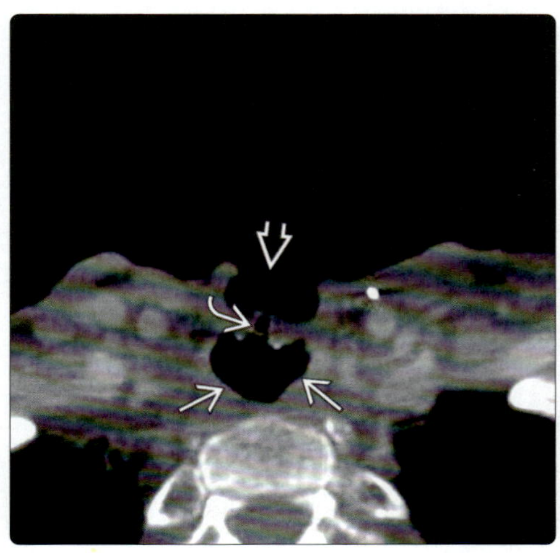

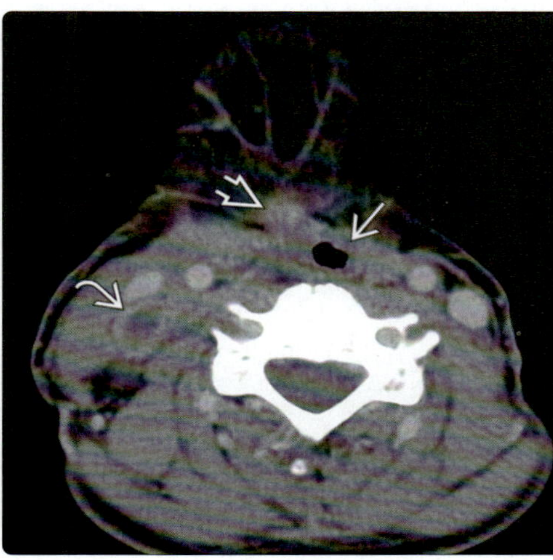

(Left) *Axial CECT in a patient status post total laryngectomy shows TE voice prosthesis ➡ connecting the trachea ➡ and proximal esophagus ➡. This 1-way valve allows the patient to speak when manually occluding the stoma.* **(Right)** *Axial CECT through the upper neck in a patient status post total laryngectomy reveals the neopharynx ➡ with an upper anastomosis recurrence ➡ along with simultaneous nodal recurrence ➡.*

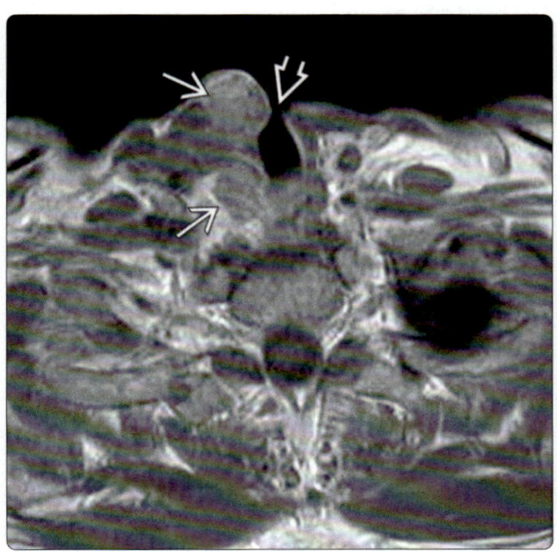

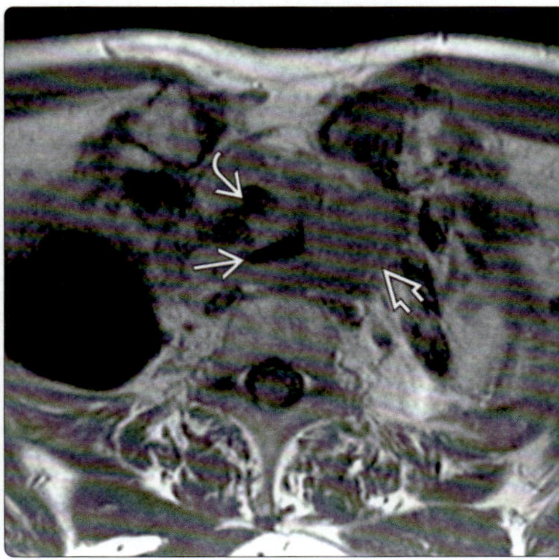

(Left) *Axial T1WI C+ MR through the lower neck in a patient with previous total laryngectomy shows 2 soft tissue enhancing masses ➡ in the lower neck at the level of the tracheostomy ➡ that proved to be distal recurrences.* **(Right)** *Axial T1 MR following total laryngectomy shows a soft tissue mass ➡ lateral to the proximal esophagus ➡ and posterolateral to the cervical trachea ➡. This is a paratracheal nodal recurrence.*

SECTION 3

Pediatric and Syndromic Diseases

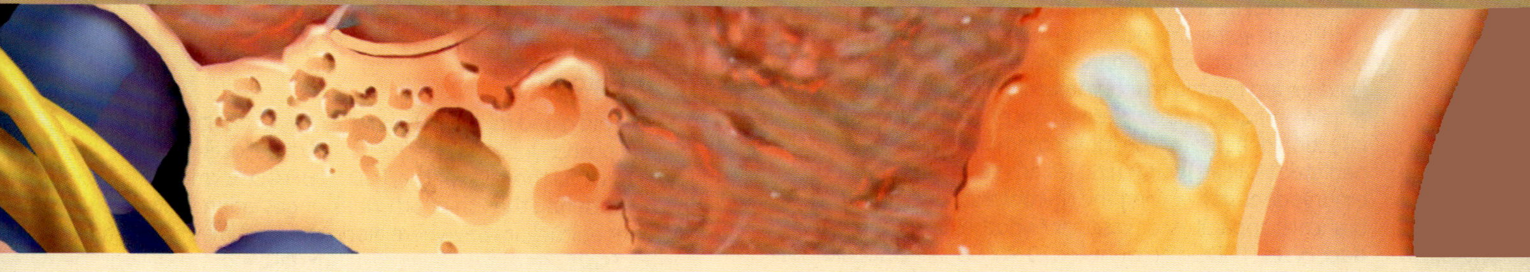

Pediatric Lesions

Syndromic Diseases

Summary Thoughts: Congenital Lesions of Head and Neck

Neck masses are a common indication for imaging the pediatric H&N. The majority of neck masses in children are either congenital or inflammatory in origin, with only 5% of childhood neoplasms occurring in the H&N. The most common extrathyroid, nonneoplastic solid neck masses in children are related to inflammatory disease and do not require imaging unless there is concern for deep neck infection or abscess. The most common cystic masses in the pediatric H&N are congenital lesions secondary to abnormal embryogenesis involving the thyroglossal duct (TGD), branchial apparatus, or vascular endothelium. **Thyroglossal duct cysts** (TGDCs) account for 70-90% of all congenital neck abnormalities in children. The most common **branchial apparatus lesion** is the 2nd branchial cleft cyst (BCC), and **lymphatic malformations** are the most common vascular malformations in the H&N.

Whenever a cystic neck mass in a child is encountered on an imaging study, a very reasonable differential diagnosis can be made based on location (midline, paramidline, or lateral, as well as location relative to carotid sheath), imaging appearance (simple cyst, complicated cyst, enhancement, ± solid component), and clinical presentation (present since birth or acute onset, ± clinical evidence of infection).

Terminology

TGDC or tract is an anomalous remnant of the TGD, which, during normal development, completely involutes. Cysts are located anywhere from the midline posterior tongue at the foramen cecum to the thyroid bed in the lower neck.

Branchial apparatus anomalies may be in the form of cysts, sinus tracts, or fistulae. **Cysts** are fluid-filled with well-defined walls secondary to the failure of obliteration of a branchial cleft or pouch. **Sinus tracts** are congenital tracts with **1 opening**, either externally to the skin surface (or external auditory canal) or internally to the pharynx or tonsillar fossa (2nd branchial cleft), superolateral hypopharynx (3rd branchial cleft), or pyriform sinus (4th or 3rd branchial pouch). **Fistulae** are congenital tracts with **2 openings**, 1 internally and 1 externally, secondary to failure of obliteration of the branchial cleft and pouch.

Imaging Techniques & Indications

US, CT, and MR are all reasonable options for initial imaging of neck masses in children. Modality choice depends on the clinical presentation, the referring clinical service, and the imaging modalities available at the time of imaging. For instance, if there is concern that a child with cellulitis and cervical adenitis has a drainable abscess deep to a palpable neck mass, US may be very helpful in determining the presence of underlying suppurative adenitis or frank abscess. Likewise, if a child is thought to have a TGDC, US is the imaging modality of choice to evaluate the suspected TGDC and prove the presence of a normal-appearing thyroid gland in the lower neck. Furthermore, US is the imaging modality of choice in patients with suspected infantile hemangioma, and color Doppler findings can be quite characteristic. However, CT is the initial imaging modality of choice to evaluate the total extent of disease in children with suspected deep neck infection and to assess for possible underlying pyriform sinus tract in children with left-sided neck abscesses that involve the left thyroid lobe.

In children who are not presenting with signs and symptoms of infection, CT or MR may be used as the initial imaging modality. The choice of which modality to use may depend on the need for sedation/anesthesia, which is usually required for MR in children under the age of 5 or 6 years. MR is the preferred imaging modality in children with suspected vascular malformations.

Embryology

The thyroid gland migrates from the foramen cecum at the midline posterior tongue to the paramidline location in the lower neck via the path of the **TGD**. The TGD normally involutes during the 5th or 6th week of gestation. However, remnant epithelium anywhere along the tract may persist and form a **TGDC**. As the TGD diverticulum descends caudally, it passes along the anterior surface of the developing hyoid bone, and therefore, remnants may be found anterior to the preepiglottic space of the larynx.

Branchial apparatus structures develop between the 4th and 6th week of gestation and consist of 6 pairs of mesodermal arches separated by 5 paired endodermal pouches internally and 5 paired ectodermal clefts externally. During the 6th week of gestation, the 2nd branchial arch overgrows the 3rd and 4th branchial arches, resulting in a combined 2nd, 3rd, and 4th branchial cleft, termed the "cervical sinus of His." Anomalies of the branchial apparatus include **cysts, sinus tracts, and fistulae**. The most common lesions for which imaging is indicated are **branchial apparatus cysts**, and most of these are related to anomalous development of a branchial cleft. However, a few are related to anomalous development of a branchial pouch.

Location of the lesion is the single most important determinant of the origin of a branchial apparatus anomaly. The **1st BCCs** account for ~ 8% of all branchial anomalies and are located in or around the external auditory canal, ear lobe, or parotid gland and may extend inferiorly to the angle of the mandible. The **2nd BCCs** account for up to 95% of all branchial apparatus anomalies and are subclassified by location using the Bailey classification: Type 1 cysts are located deep to the platysma muscle/anterior to the sternocleidomastoid muscle (SCM), type 2 cysts are posterior to the submandibular gland/anterior to the SCM and are the most common, type 3 cysts protrude between the external and internal carotid arteries, and type 4 cysts are directly adjacent to the pharyngeal wall (thought to be remnant of the 2nd pouch). Fistulas are rare; however, a 2nd branchial apparatus fistula is occasionally identified with an internal opening at the level of the pharynx and an external skin opening anterior to the lower aspect of the SCM.

Third BCCs are rare, located in the posterior compartment of the upper neck or anterior compartment of the lower neck. The 3rd pharyngeal pouch remnants are more common than cleft remnants and are related to descent of the thymic primordium from the lateral margins of the pharynx to the upper anterior mediastinum (via the thymopharyngeal duct) during the 6th to 9th week of gestation. If the duct does not undergo normal involution, a cervical thymic cyst may form that is usually in close association with the anterior margin of the carotid sheath. Formation is from interactions between the endodermal primordia and neural crest cells during normal thymic development and migration. Histologically, Hassall corpuscles will be identifiable within the cyst wall.

Differential Diagnosis of Congenital Lesions

Differential Diagnosis of Congenital Lesions
Thyroglossal Duct Lesions
Thyroglossal duct cyst (TGDC): Tongue base to thyroid bed; embedded in strap muscles when infrahyoid
Ectopic thyroid tissue: Lingual location most common
Branchial Apparatus Lesions
1st branchial cleft cyst (type 1): Located anterior, inferior, or posterior to EAC
1st branchial cleft cyst (type 2): Located in or adjacent to parotid gland; may extend inferiorly to angle of mandible
2nd branchial cleft cyst: Most common location posterior to submandibular gland, lateral to carotid space, & anteromedial to sternocleidomastoid muscle
3rd branchial cleft cyst: Posterior cervical space upper neck, anterior to SCM lower neck
3rd branchial pouch remnant → thymopharyngeal duct cyst or ectopic thymus: Along course from pharynx to upper mediastinum
4th branchial pouch remnant → pyriform sinus tract: Patients present with left-sided abscess involving thyroid gland
Vascular Malformations
Venous malformation: Slow-flow enhancing lesion, phleboliths common
Lymphatic malformation: Nonenhancing unilocular or multilocular ± fluid-fluid levels
Venolymphatic malformation: Mixed enhancing venous and nonenhancing lymphatic components

Ectopic foci of solid thymic tissue may also be deposited along the remnant duct.

Pyriform sinus tracts, or, rarely, fistulae represent a unique congenital anomaly of the 4th (or 3rd) pharyngeal pouch. This lesion should be suspected in any child presenting with neck infection involving the left thyroid lobe. The inflammation can frequently be traced superiorly to an asymmetric pyriform sinus apex. Post barium swallow CT study is frequently helpful to define the barium-filled tract extending from the pyriform sinus to the anterior lower neck.

Vascular malformations are congenital malformations of endothelial development that can be divided into capillary, lymphatic, venous, venolymphatic, and arteriovenous malformations based on the predominant endothelial characteristics of the lesion. The most common vascular malformations identified in the H&N are lymphatic malformations, venous malformations, and combined venolymphatic lesions.

Imaging Anatomy

Recognizing the defined location of a congenital abnormality, particularly congenital cysts, is key to arriving at the correct diagnosis or differential diagnosis. **Thyroglossal duct** remnants may be in the form of cysts or solid ectopic thyroid tissue anywhere from the midline tongue base to infrahyoid paramidline thyroid bed. The **1st BCCs** are in or around the EAC or parotid gland. The **2nd BCCs** are most commonly posteromedial to the submandibular gland and anteromedial to the SCM. Cysts in the posterior triangle of the upper neck may be **3rd BCCs or lymphatic malformations**. Cysts along the lower anterior margin of the SCM may be from the 2nd or 3rd branchial cleft or be lymphatic malformations. Cysts or solid masses in close association with the carotid sheath along the tract of the thymopharyngeal duct, from the angle of the mandible to the upper mediastinum, should raise the question of **cervical thymic cyst or ectopic thymus**.

Differential Diagnosis

Thyroglossal Duct Lesions

- Thyroglossal duct lesions are seen anywhere from the tongue base to the thyroid bed.
- The lingual thyroid is the most common ectopic thyroid lesion.

Branchial Apparatus Lesions

- First BCCs include type I and type II cysts. Type 1 cysts are located anterior, inferior, or posterior to the EAC. Type II cysts occur in the superficial, parotid, or parapharyngeal space, and may extend as low as the posterior submandibular space.
- Second BCCs most commonly occur posterolateral to the submandibular gland, lateral to the carotid space, and anteromedial to the SCM.
- Third BCCs are seen in the posterior cervical space of the upper neck or along the anterior border of the SCM in the mid and lower neck.
- Third branchial pouch remnants present as thymopharyngeal duct cysts or ectopic thymus.
- Fourth branchial pouch remnants present as a pyriform sinus tract with recurrent thyroiditis or thyroid abscess, usually left-sided. More recent literature suggests that this may be a 3rd branchial pouch remnant.

Vascular Malformations

- Venous malformations are slow-flow lesions with moderate postcontrast enhancement and phleboliths.
- Lymphatic malformations may be uni- or multilocular, may involve a single or multiple spaces, and most often present as nonenhancing multiseptated cystic masses with fluid-fluid levels.
- Mixed venolymphatic malformations have nonenhancing lymphatic and enhancing venous elements. Characteristic phleboliths may be present.

Selected References

1. Stern JS et al: Imaging of pediatric head and neck masses. Otolaryngol Clin North Am. 48(1):225-46, 2015
2. Wassef M et al: Vascular anomalies classification: recommendations from the international society for the study of vascular anomalies. Pediatrics. 136(1):e203-14, 2015
3. Friedman ER et al: Imaging of pediatric neck masses. Radiol Clin North Am. 49(4):617-32, v, 2011
4. Ibrahim M et al: Congenital cystic lesions of the head and neck. Neuroimaging Clin N Am. 21(3):621-39, viii, 2011

(Left) *Anteroposterior graphic of a 6-week fetus shows the 2nd branchial arch → growing inferiorly over the 3rd & 4th arches, resulting in the cervical sinus of His → that combines the 2nd, 3rd, and 4th branchial clefts (BCs). Notice the thymopharyngeal duct is a remnant of the 3rd branchial pouch →.* **(Right)** *Oblique graphic shows tract of type 1, 1st BC anomaly →, from medial bony EAC toward the retroauricular area. Tract of type 2, 1st BC anomaly →, connects the EAC to the angle of the mandible.*

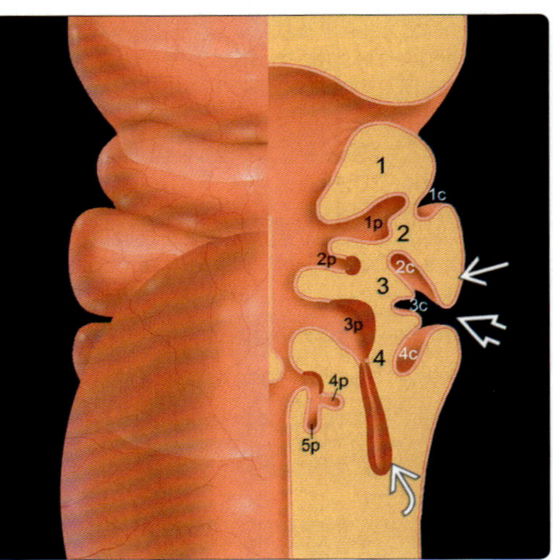

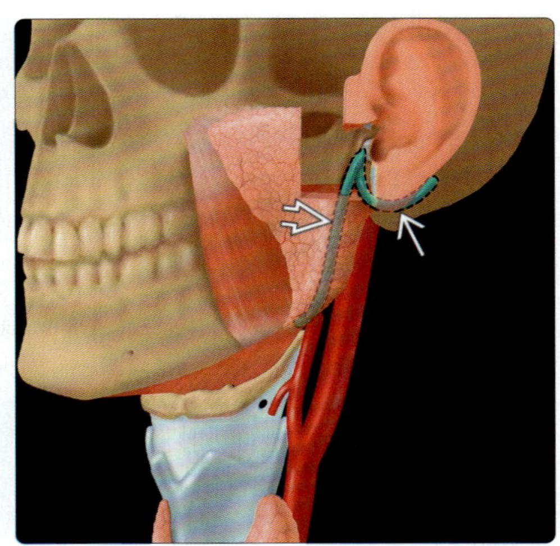

(Left) *Oblique graphic of tract of a 2nd BC cleft fistula → shows a proximal opening → in the faucial tonsil & a distal opening in the anterior supraclavicular neck →. Note the relationship to the carotid artery.* **(Right)** *Oblique graphic of neck illustrates tract of 3rd BC anomaly → extending from the cephalad aspect of the lateral hypopharynx → to the supraclavicular anterior neck skin →. Note the relationship to the carotid artery.*

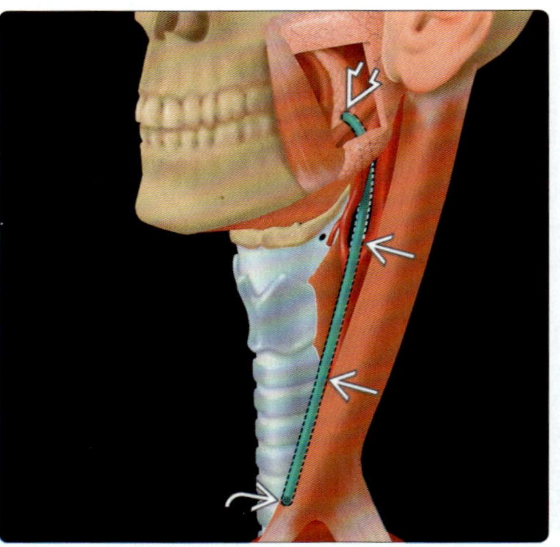

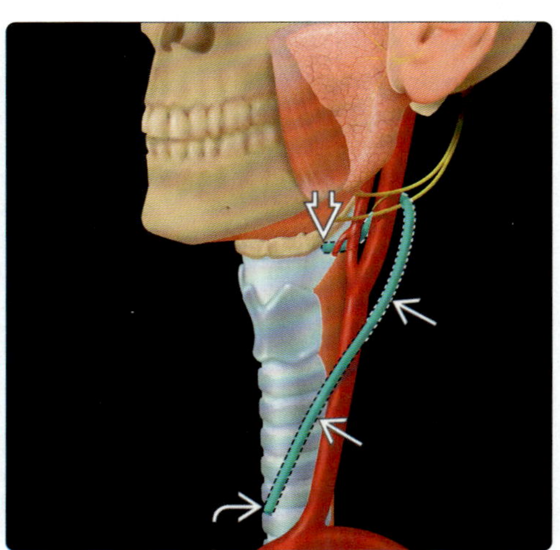

(Left) *Anteroposterior graphic shows both thymopharyngeal duct tracts → extending from the lateral hypopharyngeal area → to the location of the normal lobes of the thymus → in the superior mediastinum.* **(Right)** *Oblique graphic of the neck shows tract of 4th BC anomaly → extending from the hypopharynx → to the location of the left thyroid lobe →. This explains why this lesion often presents with thyroiditis.*

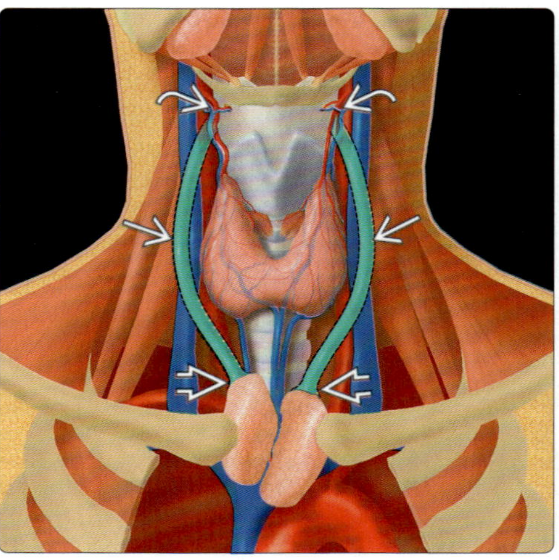

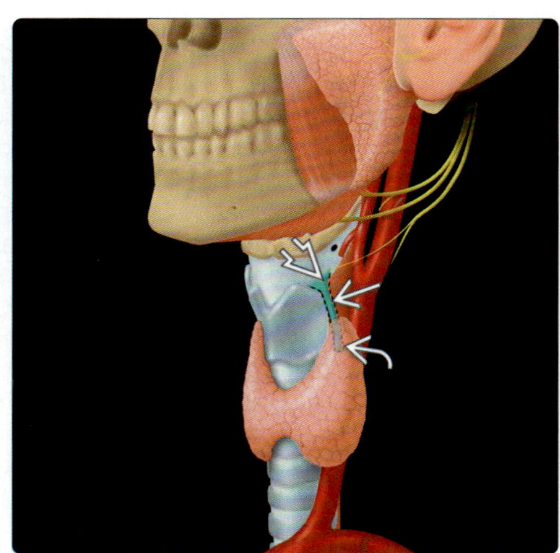

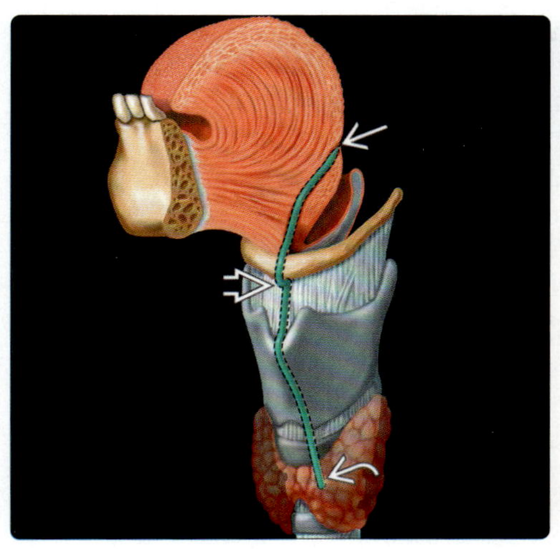

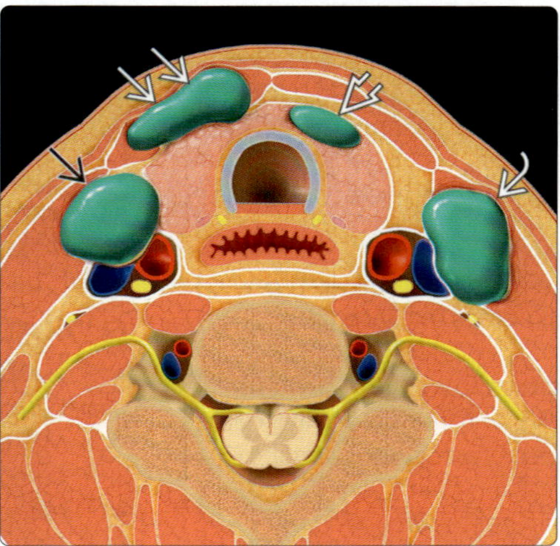

(Left) *Oblique graphic illustrates the tract of the thyroglossal duct descending from the foramen cecum ➡ at the tongue base, under the midline hyoid bone ➡, then tracking off midline to the thyroid lobe ➡.* **(Right)** *Axial graphic demonstrates the locations of 4 major congenital cystic lesions of the H&N. Shown here are the infrahyoid 2nd & 3rd BC cysts ➡, infrahyoid thyroglossal duct cyst ➡, cervical thymic cysts ➡, and 4th branchial apparatus sinus tracts ➡.*

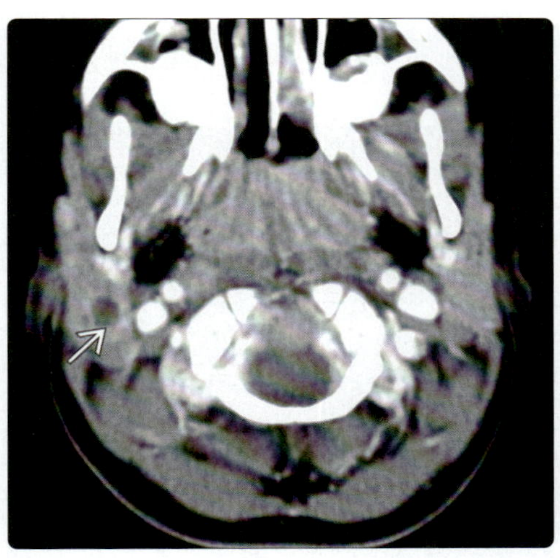

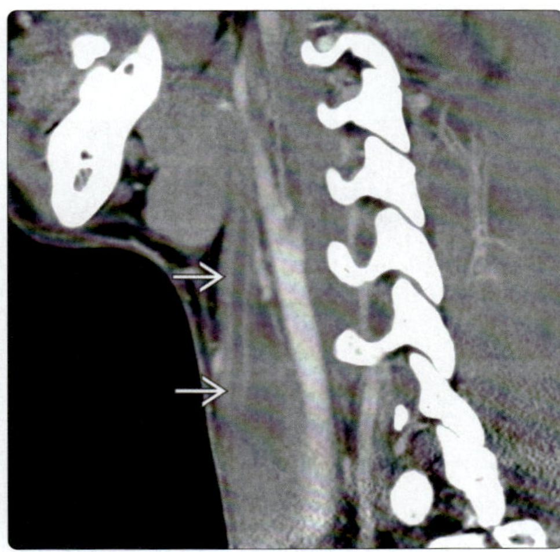

(Left) *Axial CECT in a 2-year-old boy shows intraparotid 1st BC cyst ➡ with mild peripheral enhancement and associated mild enlargement of the ipsilateral parotid gland consistent with parotitis.* **(Right)** *Sagittal reformatted CECT shows the typical location of a 2nd branchial apparatus fistula ➡ extending from the anterior lower neck skin opening (not included) toward the pharynx in a teenager with intermittent purulent drainage from the skin opening.*

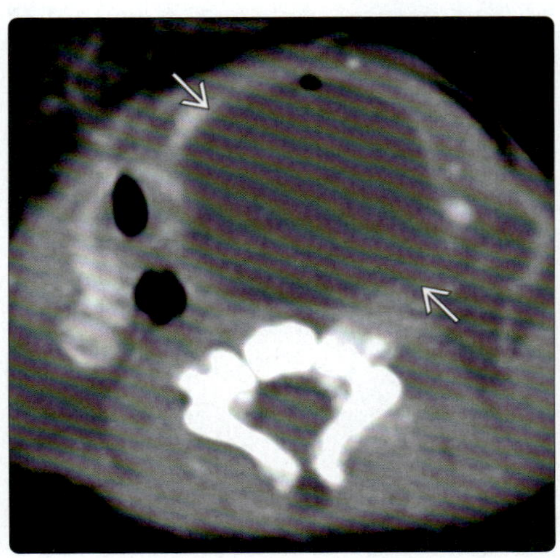

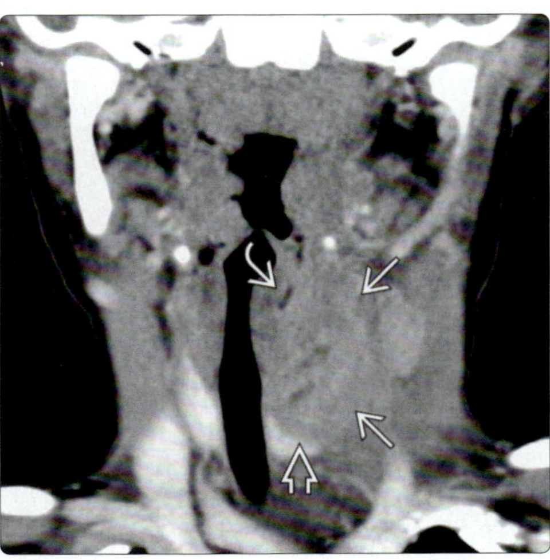

(Left) *Axial CECT in an infant shows a large, well-defined cystic mass ➡ in the left neck that displaces the airway and extends into the mediastinum, typical of a cervical thymic cyst. The bubble of gas is concerning for infection.* **(Right)** *Coronal CECT in a 4-year-old boy shows a phlegmonous mass ➡ in the left neck involving the left thyroid lobe ➡ and a tract of inflammation ➡ coursing toward the left pyriform sinus, consistent with inflamed pyriform sinus tract (remnant of 4th or 3rd branchial pouch).*

Lymphatic Malformation

KEY FACTS

TERMINOLOGY

- Subtype of congenital slow-/low-flow vascular malformation due to error in lymphatic vessel formation
- Results in well-defined, cyst-like (macrocystic), ± infiltrative, solid-appearing (microcystic) mass of abnormal lymphatic channels
  - Individual cyst size: Macrocyst > 1 cm, microcyst < 1 cm

IMAGING

- Macrocystic lymphatic malformation (LM): Lobulated, well-defined, **cystic** lesion with numerous thin **internal septations**
  - ± multiple **fluid-fluid levels**, typically due to hemorrhage
  - Soft and compressible by US with internal swirling debris
  - Protein, blood products, chyle/fat may cause bright T1 signal intensity on MR
  - Enhancement limited to rim, septations
- Microcystic LM: More poorly defined and solid-appearing
  - ± diffuse enhancement
- Locations: **Face, neck, chest, axilla** > > abdomen, pelvis, extremities
  - Frequently extend across tissue planes/compartments

TOP DIFFERENTIAL DIAGNOSES

- Infantile hemangioma
- Venous malformation
- Arteriovenous malformation
- Soft tissue sarcoma
- Soft tissue infection

CLINICAL ISSUES

- Soft and pliable mass, often apparent at birth
  - Can compress airway or other vital structures
  - May present later with pain and rapid enlargement due hemorrhage, inflammation, or hormonal stimulation
- Primary treatment: Percutaneous sclerotherapy (OK-432, ethanol, doxycycline, bleomycin,) ± surgical resection
  - Reports of successful medical therapy with sirolimus

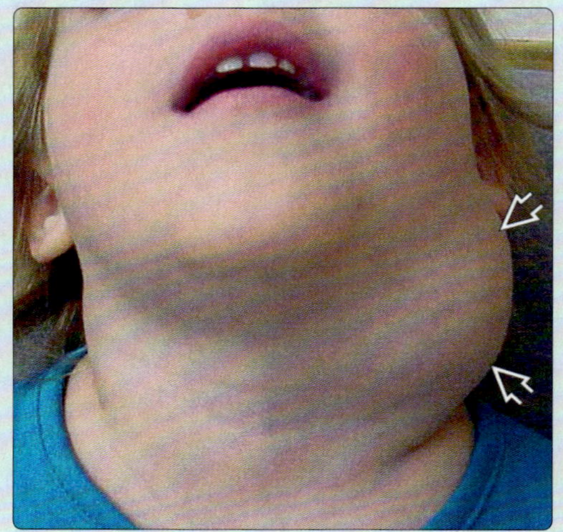

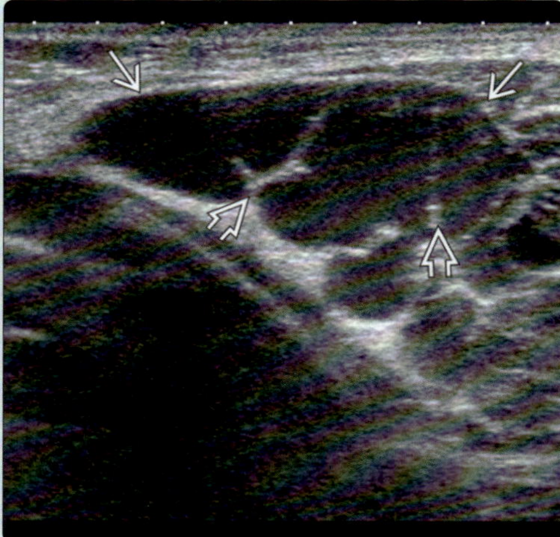

(Left) *Clinical photograph of a young girl shows a soft, pliable soft tissue mass ➡ in the left neck. No other symptoms were present. Note absence of skin vascular hue. Clinical impression of probable lymphatic malformation (LM) was confirmed on final path.* **(Right)** *Ultrasound in a 2-year-old patient with a soft, pliable mass shows a well-defined, lobulated, multicystic lesion ➡ with thin internal septations ➡, typical of a macrocystic LM.*

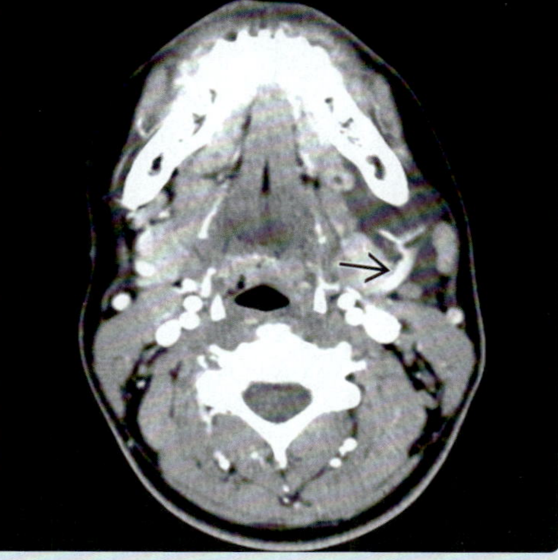

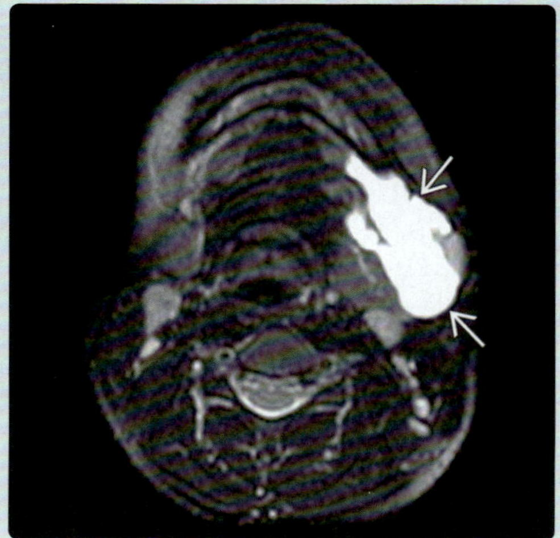

(Left) *Axial CECT in a 22-year-old woman with an angle of a mandible mass reveals a low-density submandibular space (SMS) LM ➡ with venous structures passing through it. The mass conforms to the shape of the SMS.* **(Right)** *Axial T2 FS MR in the same patient shows the high fluid signal ➡ of the LM with its lobular margins. In this case, no fluid-fluid levels are seen.*

KEY FACTS

TERMINOLOGY

- Venous malformation (VM)

IMAGING

- In child, use MR & US when possible
- General imaging findings
  - Lobulated soft tissue "mass" with **phleboliths**
  - **Solitary or multiple**
  - May be **circumscribed** or **transspatial**, infiltrating adjacent soft tissue compartments
  - ± combined lymphatic malformation (LM), i.e., mixed venolymphatic malformation (VLM)
- CT findings
  - **Rounded calcifications (phleboliths)**
  - Osseous remodeling in adjacent bone
  - Fat hypertrophy in adjacent soft tissues
- Enhancement features
  - **Variable enhancement** pattern reflects sluggish vascular flow to & through lesion
  - Patchy & delayed or homogeneous & intense enhancement

TOP DIFFERENTIAL DIAGNOSES

- Lymphatic malformation
- Infantile hemangioma
- Dermoid & epidermoid
- Arteriovenous malformation

PATHOLOGY

- Congenital venous vascular rest
- 70% of patients with periorbital LM or VLM have intracranial vascular & parenchymal anomalies
  - DVA, cerebral cavernous malformation, dural arteriovenous malformation (AVM), pial AVM, sinus pericranii

CLINICAL ISSUES

- Presents as spongy head & neck mass that grows proportionately with patient

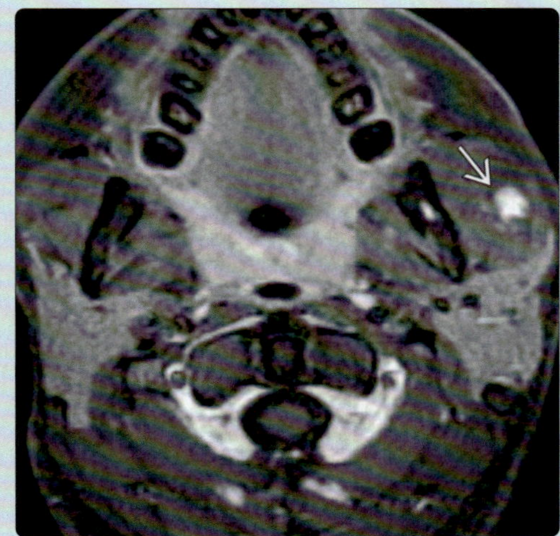

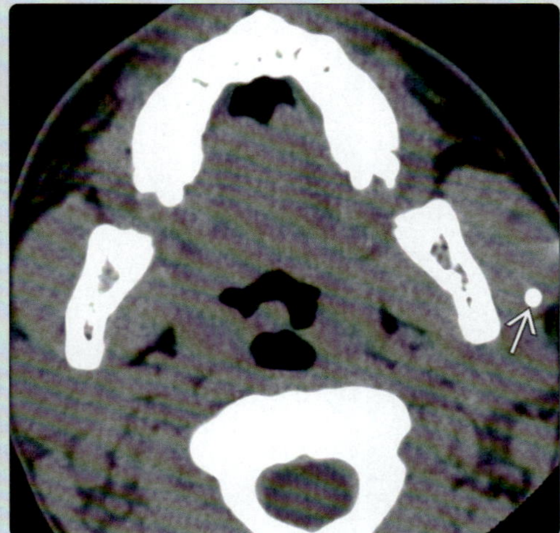

(Left) *Axial T1WI C+ FS MR in a 14-year-old boy demonstrates a small focal area of enhancement ➡ in an otherwise nonspecific lesion within the left masseter muscle within the masticator space.* **(Right)** *Axial NECT in the same patient shows an ill-defined intramuscular mass with small phlebolith ➡, consistent with venous malformation (VM).*

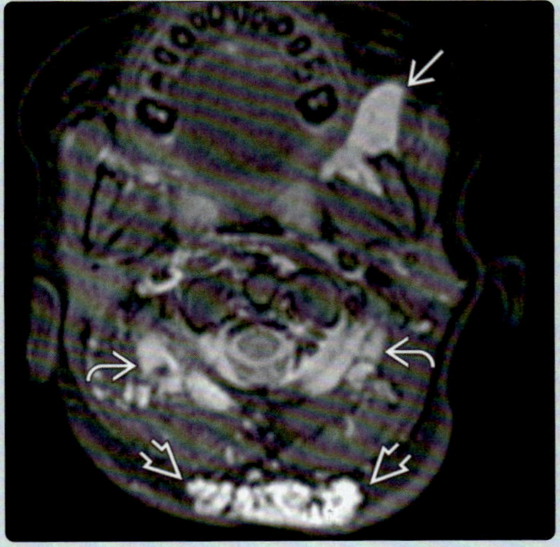

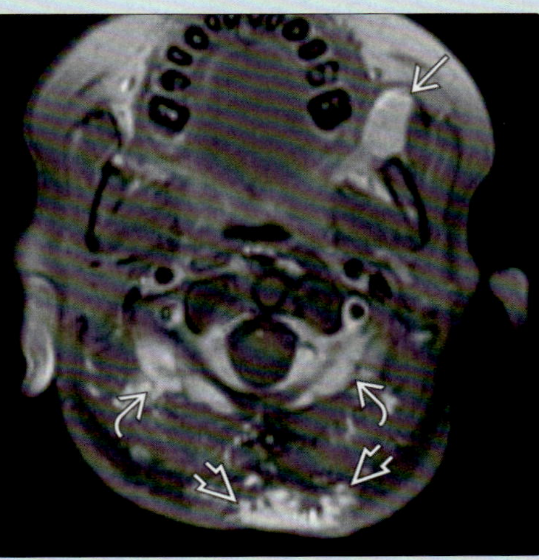

(Left) *Axial STIR MR in a 10-year-old girl with multiple VMs demonstrates hyperintense lesions in the left buccal space ➡, the midline posterior subcutaneous neck ➡, and the bilateral paraspinal soft tissues ➡.* **(Right)** *Axial T1WI C+ FS MR in the same patient shows variable enhancement of the VM in the left buccal space ➡, the midline posterior subcutaneous neck ➡, and the bilateral paraspinal soft tissues ➡.*

Congenital Vallecular Cyst

KEY FACTS

TERMINOLOGY

- Epiglottic cyst, base of tongue cyst, ductal cyst, saccular cyst
- Congenital cyst arising in vallecula

IMAGING

- Cystic mass in vallecula of child with inspiratory stridor
- Most diagnosed with direct laryngoscopy

TOP DIFFERENTIAL DIAGNOSES

- **Thyroglossal duct cyst**
  - When midline tongue base cyst (near foramen cecum), may be indistinguishable from congenital vallecular cyst
- **Retention cyst in pharyngeal mucosal space**
  - Benign postinflammatory retention cyst in nasopharynx or oropharynx
- **Lingual thyroid**
  - Midline, solid mass near foramen cecum
  - Increased attenuation on CT
  - Variable signal intensity on MR
- **Lingual hamartoma**
  - Midline posterior tongue mass near foramen cecum
- **Lymphatic malformation**
  - Cystic, usually transspatial congenital lesion
  - Rarely involves vallecula

CLINICAL ISSUES

- Most common signs/symptoms
  - **Inspiratory stridor with supraglottic lesion**
  - Airway obstruction: May lead to life-threatening airway obstruction if left untreated
  - Apnea
- Other signs/symptoms
  - Laryngomalacia
  - Feeding difficulties
  - Failure to thrive
- Treatment
  - Surgical excision, laser-assisted resection, marsupialization, radiofrequency ablation

(Left) *Lateral radiograph in an infant with stridor shows a well-defined soft tissue mass ➡ at the base of the tongue protruding into the vallecula.* **(Right)** *Axial CECT shows a well-defined, low-attenuation, nonenhancing cyst in the midline base of the tongue ➡. Based on CECT findings alone, this lesion cannot be distinguished from thyroglossal duct cyst in the location of the foramen cecum.*

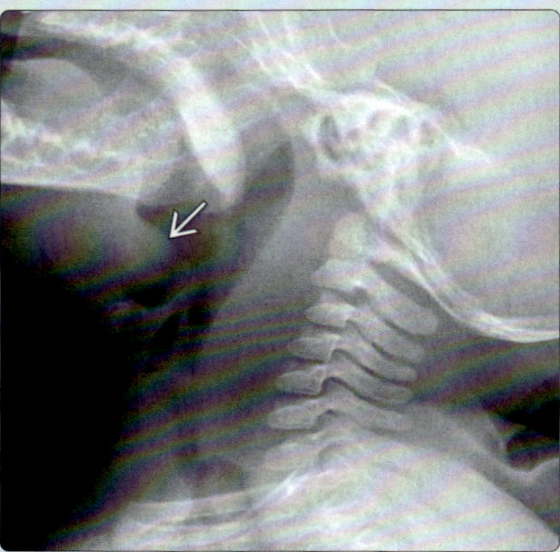

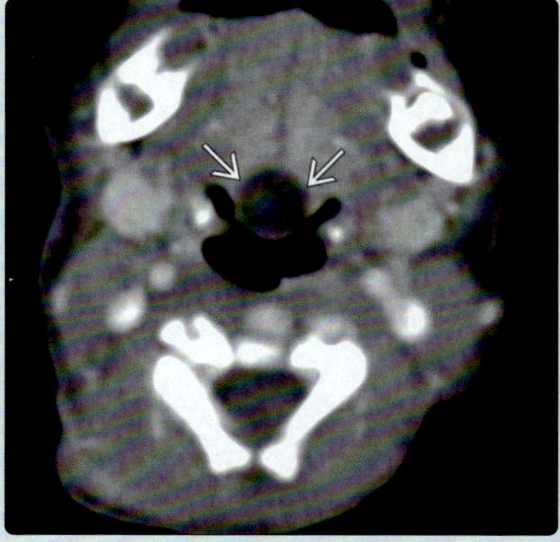

(Left) *Sagittal T1WI MR shows an incidentally noted, well-defined, fluid signal intensity congenital vallecular cyst at the base of the tongue ➡ in the anterior oropharynx.* **(Right)** *Coronal T2WI MR in the same patient shows a fluid signal intensity vallecular cyst to be somewhat lobulated in contour ➡ and located in the ventral aspect of the oropharynx.*

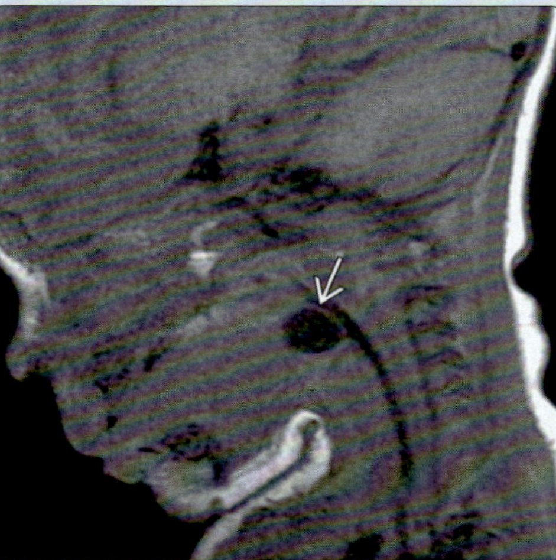

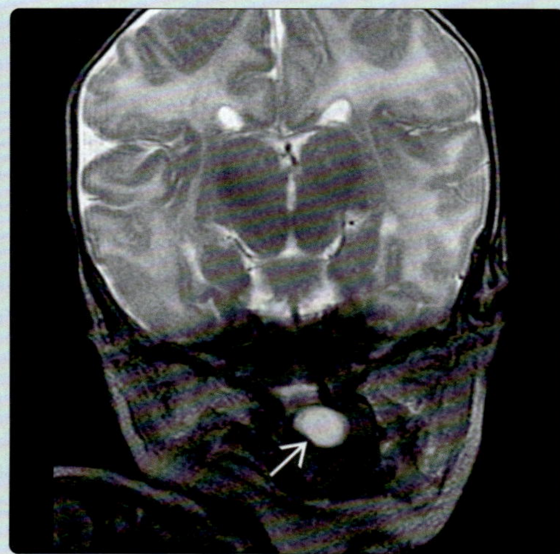

KEY FACTS

TERMINOLOGY

- Thyroglossal duct cyst (TGDC) is developmental anomaly derived from thyroglossal duct (TDG) remnant

IMAGING

- Best diagnostic clue: Midline perihyoid bone cyst
- Imaging findings
  - Nonenhancing, thin-walled cystic mass
    - Wall may enhance if infected
  - Embedded in strap muscles
  - May project into preepiglottic space
- Located between foramen cecum and thyroid bed
  - 60% in midline around hyoid bone
  - 20% midline hyoid bone to foramen cecum
  - 20% in infrahyoid neck

TOP DIFFERENTIAL DIAGNOSES

- Lymphatic malformation
- 2nd branchial cleft cyst
- Lingual thyroid
- Level VI (Delphian chain) necrotic node

PATHOLOGY

- Failure of involution of TGD & persistent secretion of epithelial cells lining duct → TGDC
- 90% of nonodontogenic congenital cysts
- Macroscopic features: Smooth-walled cystic mass
- Microscopic features
  - Wall lined with **respiratory epithelium**
  - Wall may contain thyroid follicles
  - Rarely papillary thyroid carcinoma arises in cyst

CLINICAL ISSUES

- Midline neck lesion in child
  - 90% < 19 years of age
  - Recurrent, intermittent swelling of mass following upper respiratory infection or trauma
- Excise cyst & midline hyoid bone (**Sistrunk procedure**)

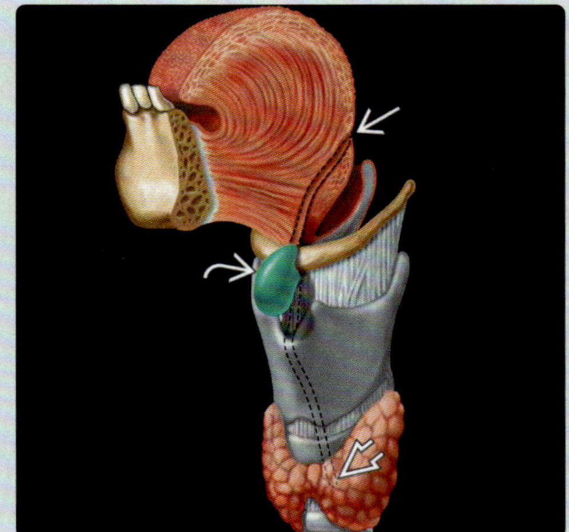

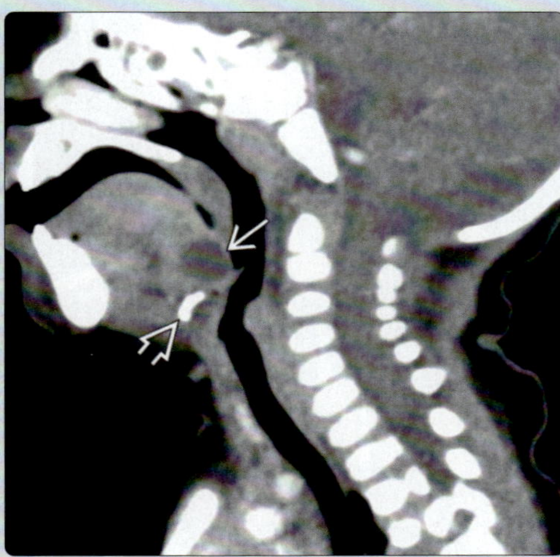

(Left) *Sagittal oblique graphic shows the course of the thyroglossal duct (dotted lines) from the foramen cecum ➡ to the thyroid bed ➡. Note the close relationship to the midportion of hyoid bone ➡.* **(Right)** *Sagittal CECT reformation shows a well-defined cystic TGDC ➡ above the hyoid bone ➡ at the midline base of the tongue in the location of the foramen cecum. This TGDC was incidentally found on a CT performed to evaluate the extent of deep neck infection (not shown).*

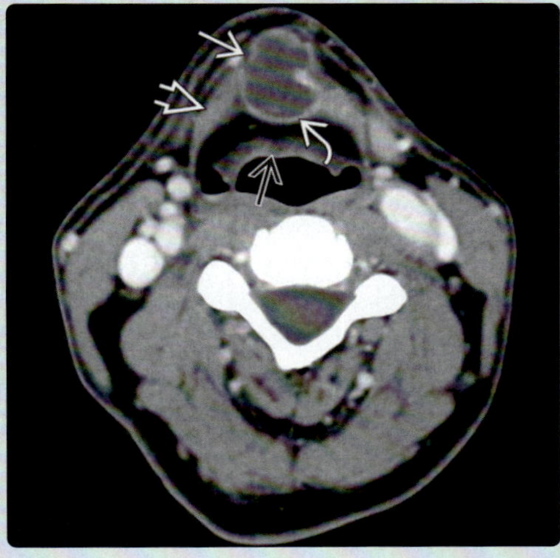

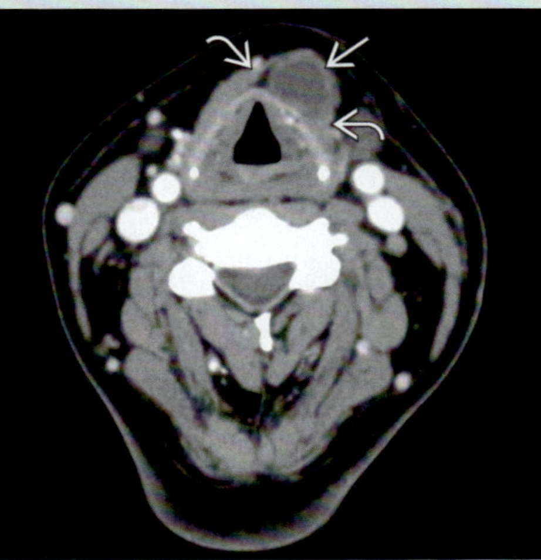

(Left) *Axial CECT just inferior to the hyoid bone reveals a lobulated TGDC ➡ in the midline, embedded in the strap muscles ➡ and bulging into the preepiglottic space ➡. Note the epiglottis ➡.* **(Right)** *Axial CECT shows an ovoid low-density TGDC ➡ superficial to the thyroid cartilage embedded in the strap muscles ➡ at the level of the low supraglottis. The more inferior the TGDC, the more paramedian in location.*

KEY FACTS

TERMINOLOGY

- Definition: Cystic remnant of **thymopharyngeal duct**
  - Derivative of **3rd pharyngeal pouch**

IMAGING

- General imaging findings: CECT/ultrasound
  - Cystic mass closely associated with carotid sheath
  - Found anywhere along thymopharyngeal duct from pyriform sinus to anterior mediastinum
  - **Usually lateral infrahyoid neck**
  - **Left > > right side of neck**
  - May splay carotid artery and jugular vein
  - Cystic component nonenhancing
  - Cyst wall or solid nodules may enhance slightly

TOP DIFFERENTIAL DIAGNOSES

- 2nd branchial cleft cyst
- 4th branchial anomaly
- Lymphatic malformation
- Abscess

PATHOLOGY

- **Hassall corpuscles** in cyst wall confirm diagnosis
- Cyst wall may contain lymphoid follicles, thymic or thyroid or parathyroid tissue, cholesterol crystals

CLINICAL ISSUES

- Clinical presentation
  - Smaller lesions asymptomatic
    - Gradually enlarging, soft, compressible
  - If large, may present with **dysphagia, respiratory distress**, ± vocal cord paralysis
  - Most present between **2-15 years** of age
- Treatment options
  - Complete surgical resection
  - Large cervicothoracic thymic cyst may require H&N and thoracic surgery

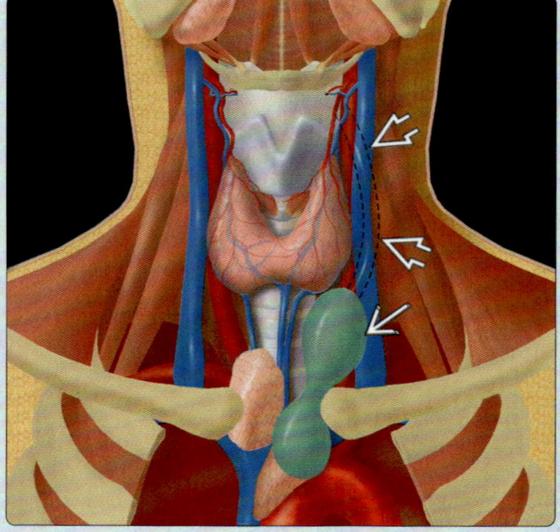

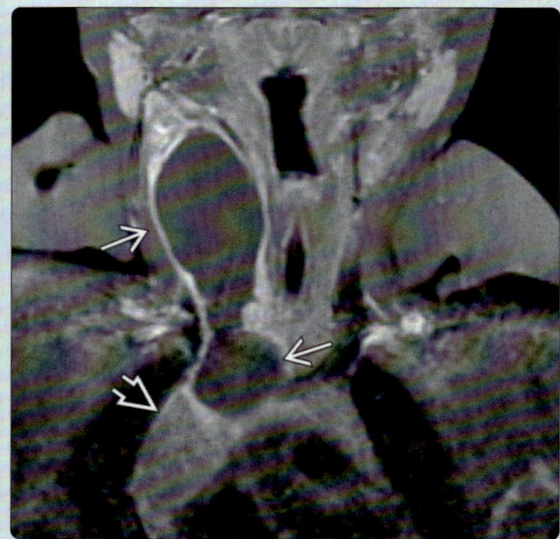

(Left) *Coronal graphic shows typical bilobed cervical thymic cyst ➡ extending from the anterior mediastinum into the lower neck along the course of the thymopharyngeal duct ➡. Notice the close association with the carotid space.* **(Right)** *Coronal T1 C+ FS MR in a 16 month old shows a thymic cyst in the right neck ➡ causing mild airway compression. The cyst extends to the otherwise normal-appearing thymus ➡. Mild diffuse wall enhancement is consistent with chronic inflammation identified histologically.*

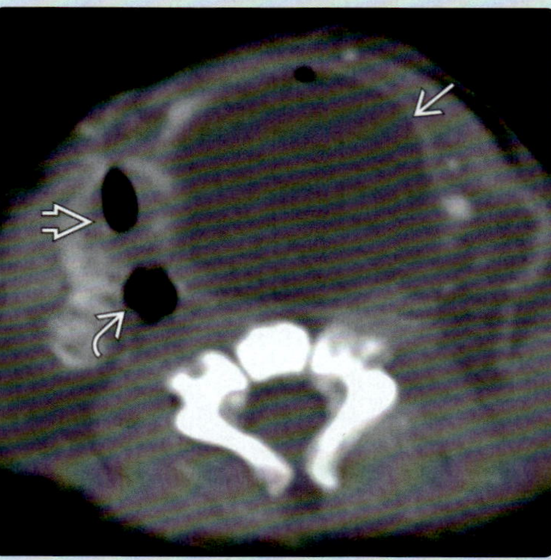

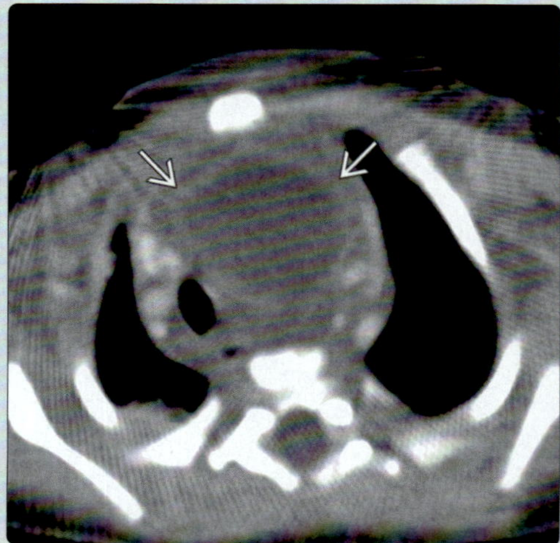

(Left) *Axial CECT in an infant with an infected thymic cyst demonstrates a small bubble of gas anteriorly within a large left-sided cystic neck mass ➡ that causes significant deviation of the airway ➡ and esophagus ➡ to the right.* **(Right)** *Axial CECT in the same infant shows the thymic cyst ➡ extending into the anterior mediastinum. Most thymic cysts are left-sided and may occur anywhere along the embryologic course of the thymopharyngeal duct from the angle of the mandible to the mediastinum.*

KEY FACTS

TERMINOLOGY

- Most common 1st branchial cleft (BC) anomalies are branchial cleft cysts (BCCs) or sinus tracts
- Work classification
  - Type I, cyst runs parallel to external auditory canal (EAC)
  - Type II (more common), angle of mandible to BC junction

IMAGING

- Best diagnostic clue: **Cystic mass near pinna & EAC or extending from EAC to angle of mandible**
- CECT: Well-circumscribed, nonenhancing or rim-enhancing, low-density mass
  - If infected, may have thickened, enhancing rim
  - Lesion may point toward bony-cartilaginous EAC junction

TOP DIFFERENTIAL DIAGNOSES

- Cholesteatoma, EAC
  - Submucosal mass with bone erosion
- Parotitis complicated by abscess (rare)
  - Parotitis with thick-walled, ring-enhancing cystic mass
  - Cellulitis extends to EAC and angle of mandible
- Lymphatic malformation
  - No contrast enhancement, ± fluid-fluid levels

PATHOLOGY

- **Remnant of 1st branchial apparatus**
  - Cysts > > sinus or fistula
- Most common location for 1st BCC to terminate is in EAC between cartilaginous & bony portions

CLINICAL ISSUES

- Clinical presentation
  - < 10 years old with periauricular painless mass
    - EAC or skin sinus tract possible, may cause otorrhea
    - May present as periauricular or intraparotid infection
  - Treatment options
    - Complete surgical resection of tract
    - Proximity to CNVII puts nerve at risk during surgery

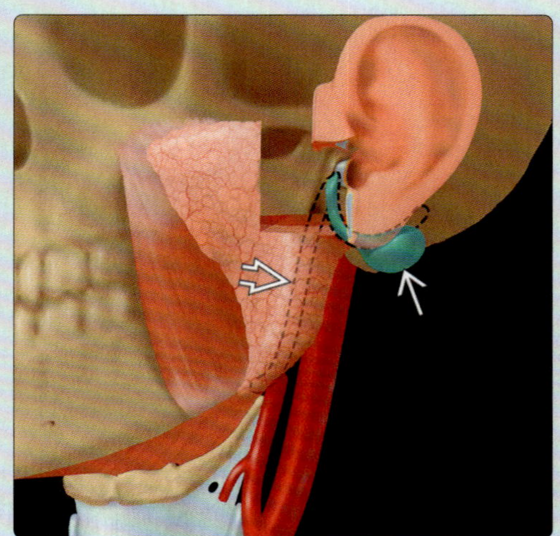

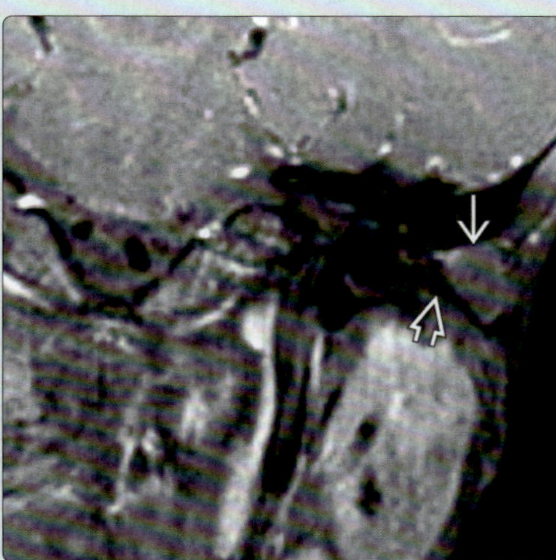

(Left) *Oblique graphic of the ear and cheek reveals a type I 1st branchial cleft cyst (BCC) ➡ along the tract from the bony-cartilaginous junction of the external auditory canal (EAC) situated just posteroinferior to auricle. The tract of the Work type II BCC ➡ would project inferiorly to the angle of the mandible.* **(Right)** *Coronal T1WI C+ FS MR shows an intermediate signal intensity, nonenhancing, type I 1st BCC ➡ causing near-complete obstruction of the left membranous EAC ➡.*

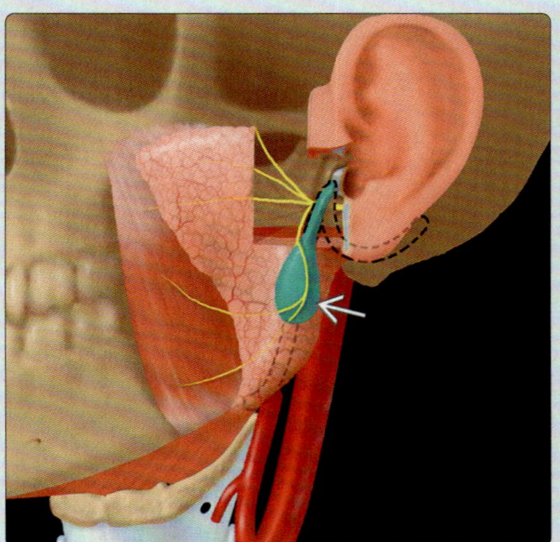

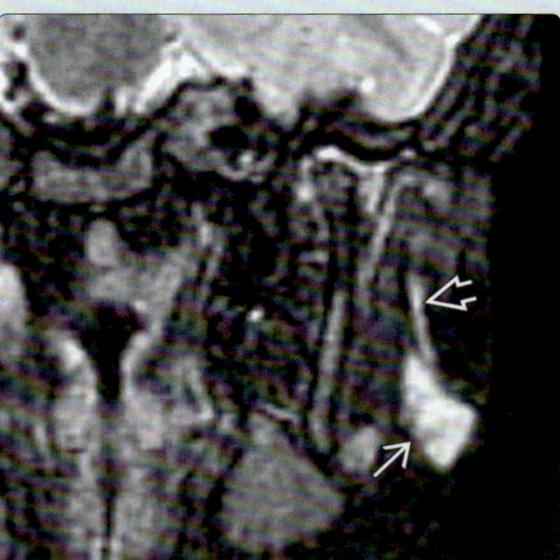

(Left) *Oblique graphic of the ear and cheek shows an example of a type II 1st BCC ➡ along the course of the tract from the bony-cartilaginous EAC to the angle of the mandible. Note the intimate relationship of the BCC to the facial nerve branches.* **(Right)** *Coronal T2WI FS MR demonstrates the cystic inferior component of a type II 1st branchial apparatus cyst ➡ and the sinus tract ➡ extending superiorly toward the EAC.*

2nd Branchial Cleft Cyst

KEY FACTS

TERMINOLOGY

- Cervical sinus of His cystic remnant: 2nd, 3rd, & 4th branchial clefts & 2nd branchial arch derivative
- Synonyms
  - 2nd branchial cleft cyst (BCC) or anomaly, 2nd branchial apparatus cyst or anomaly

IMAGING

- CECT or enhanced T1 MR findings
  - **Location key**: Mass posterolateral to submandibular gland, lateral to carotid space, anterior to sternocleidomastoid
  - Ovoid or round fluid density/intensity mass
  - Thin, minimally enhancing wall
- Infected 2nd branchial cleft cyst: Thick enhancing wall + surrounding soft tissue cellulitis

TOP DIFFERENTIAL DIAGNOSES

- Lymphatic malformation: Multilocular, transspatial
- Cervical thymic cyst: Cervical thoracic junction
- Lymphadenopathy/abscess
- Cystic squamous cell carcinoma or differentiated thyroid nodes

PATHOLOGY

- 2nd branchial apparatus cyst, sinus or fistulae
- Epidemiology: 2nd branchial apparatus anomalies (BAA) account for up to **95%** of all BAAs

CLINICAL ISSUES

- Clinical presentation
  - Angle of mandible mass; often after URI; can drain in track anterior to sternomastoid muscle, tonsillar fossa
  - If infected, heat, pain, redness and swelling
  - Caveat: In adult, "2nd BCC" diagnosis = nodal metastasis until proven otherwise
- Treatment options: Complete surgical resection; must resect associated sinus or fistula tract

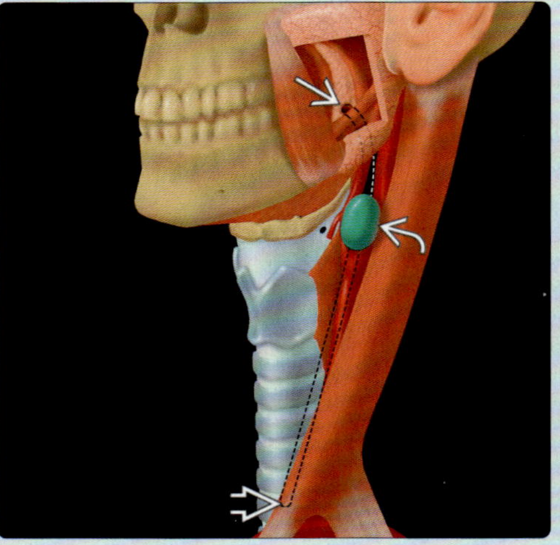

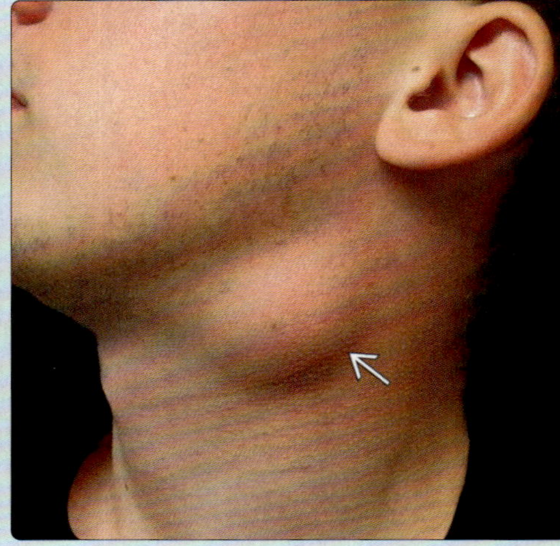

(Left) *Sagittal oblique graphic shows a 2nd branchial cleft cyst ➙ in its most common location: Anterior to the sternomastoid muscle (SCM) & anterolateral to the carotid space. The full tract may extend from the faucial tonsil ➙ to low anterior neck ➙.* **(Right)** *Clinical photograph shows a compressible lateral neck mass in a young adult male ➙, characteristic for a 2nd branchial cleft cyst. The patient came to clinical attention after an upper respiratory tract viral infection.*

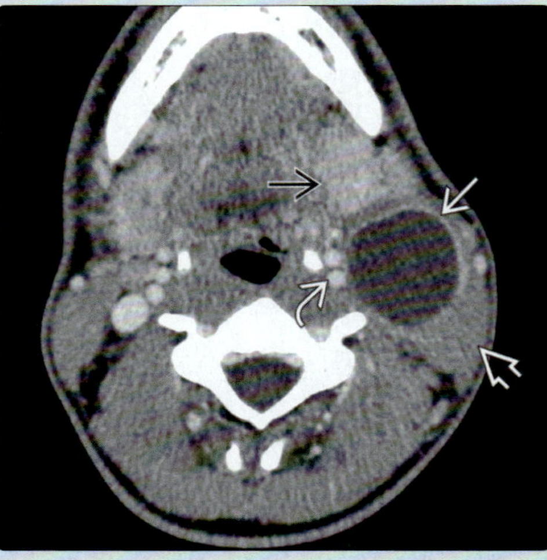

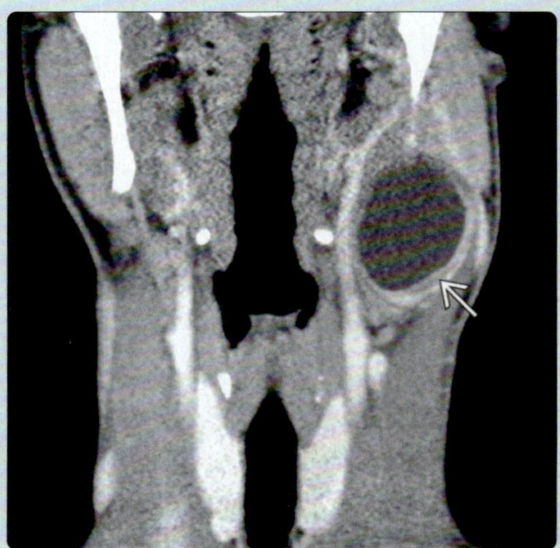

(Left) *Axial CECT in a 17-year-old boy shows a well-defined, low-attenuation mass ➙ in the typical location of a Bailey type II 2nd branchial cleft cyst: Anterior to the SCM ➙, lateral to the carotid sheath vessels ➙, and posterior to the submandibular gland ➙.* **(Right)** *Coronal CECT in the same patient demonstrates a thicker wall inferiorly ➙, which histologically represented lymphoid follicles in the wall of the cyst.*

KEY FACTS

TERMINOLOGY

- 3rd branchial cleft cyst (BCC)
  - Epithelial-lined **remnant 3rd branchial cleft**

IMAGING

- CT/MR/US
  - Unilocular thin-walled cyst in **upper posterior cervical space or lower anterior neck**
  - If infected, cyst wall thickens and enhances
  - ± adjacent cellulitis or myositis
- Barium or water-soluble contrast swallow may outline **associated sinus or fistula**

TOP DIFFERENTIAL DIAGNOSES

- 2nd branchial cleft cyst: Most common BCC
- Lymphatic malformation: Uni- or multilocular
- Abscess: Signs and symptoms of infection
- Cervical thymic cyst: Cervical-thoracic junction
- 4th branchial apparatus anomaly: Pyriform sinus tract and left thyroid abscess
- Infrahyoid thyroglossal duct cyst: Midline; embedded in strap muscles
- Cystic-necrotic metastatic lymph node: Usually known primary H&N squamous cell carcinoma or systemic non-Hodgkin lymphoma

CLINICAL ISSUES

- Clinical presentation
  - Fluctuant mass in posterolateral upper neck
  - Frequently presents in **adulthood**
  - Purulent drainage from skin ostium if fistula
    - Posterior triangle/posterior cervical space
- Treatment option: Surgical resection
  - Surgery includes resection of cyst and any associated sinus or fistula
  - If infected, treat with antibiotics prior to surgical resection

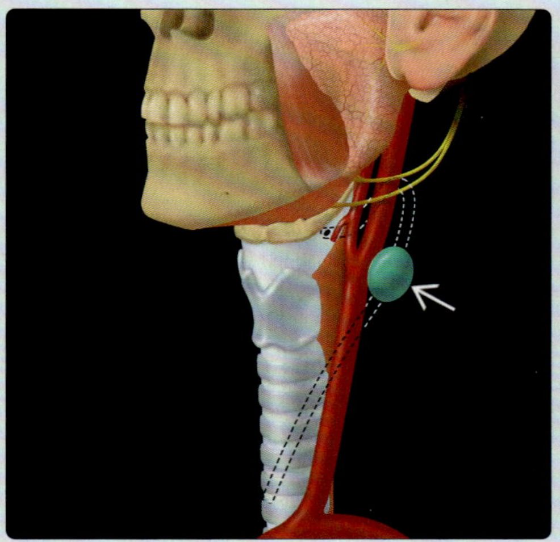

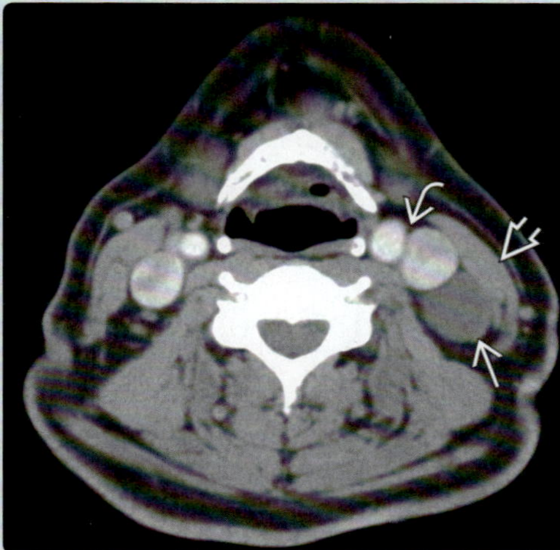

(Left) *Lateral graphic illustrates the course of a 3rd branchial anomaly (dashes), along which 3rd branchial cleft cysts arise, most commonly in the upper posterior triangle ➡.* **(Right)** *Axial CECT in this adult male patient with a posterior left neck mass demonstrates a well-defined, thin-walled, unilocular cyst ➡ in the posterior cervical space, deep to the sternocleidomastoid muscle ➡ and posterolateral to the carotid space ➡. Note that the cyst wall is imperceptible, indicating the lesion has not been infected.*

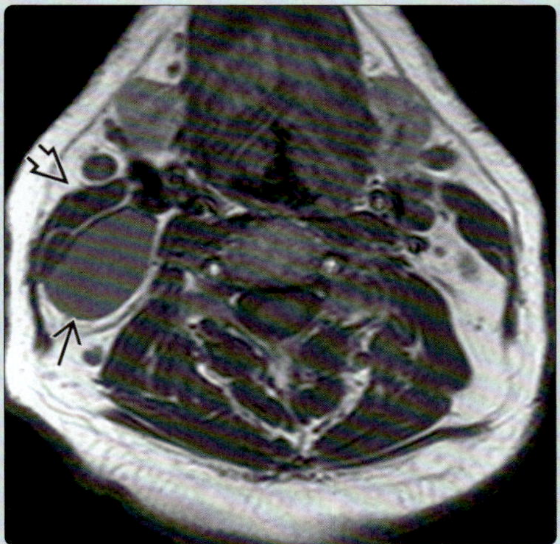

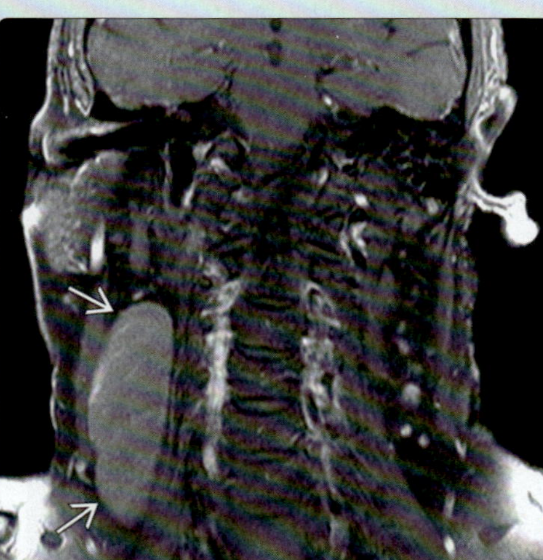

(Left) *Axial T1 MR in a 60-year-old man (imaged for other reasons) shows an incidental 3rd branchial cleft cyst in the right posterior triangle ➡ deep to the sternocleidomastoid muscle ➡.* **(Right)** *Coronal T1 C+ FS MR in the same patient shows the cyst ➡ deep to the sternocleidomastoid muscle, without significant internal or perilesional enhancement; this is typical of an uncomplicated 3rd branchial cleft cyst.*

4th Branchial Apparatus Anomaly

KEY FACTS

TERMINOLOGY

- Pyriform sinus "fistula" or 4th branchial apparatus anomaly
  - **Most** anomalies are actually **sinus tracts (not cysts) from 4th pharyngeal pouch remnant**
  - Course from apex of pyriform sinus to upper aspect of **left** thyroid lobe

IMAGING

- Sinus tract extending from **apex of pyriform sinus to lower anterior neck** after barium swallow
- CECT best demonstrates phlegmon or abscess
  - Abscess in or adjacent to anterior **left** thyroid lobe
  - CT after barium swallow best identifies sinus tract
- Direct injection of fistula best demonstrates course of fistulous tract

TOP DIFFERENTIAL DIAGNOSES

- Cervical thymic cyst
- Lymphatic malformation
- Thyroglossal duct cyst
- 3rd branchial cleft cyst

CLINICAL ISSUES

- Clinical presentation
  - Infant or young child presents with
    - **Recurrent neck abscesses**
    - **Recurrent suppurative thyroiditis or thyroid abscess**
- Treatment options
  - Initial treatment is antibiotics ± I&D of abscess
  - Next treatment is complete resection of sinus tract or fistula
    - Simultaneous obliterate opening in pyriform sinus
  - Thyroid lobectomy for lesions in thyroid lobe

DIAGNOSTIC CHECKLIST

- Suspect sinus tract from pyriform sinus in any child with abscess in or anterior to left thyroid lobe

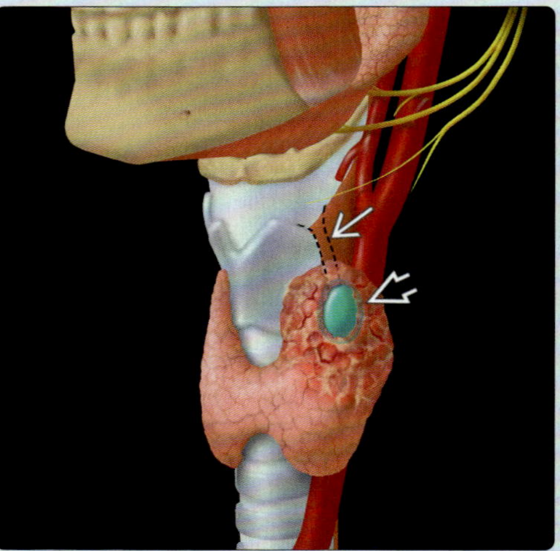

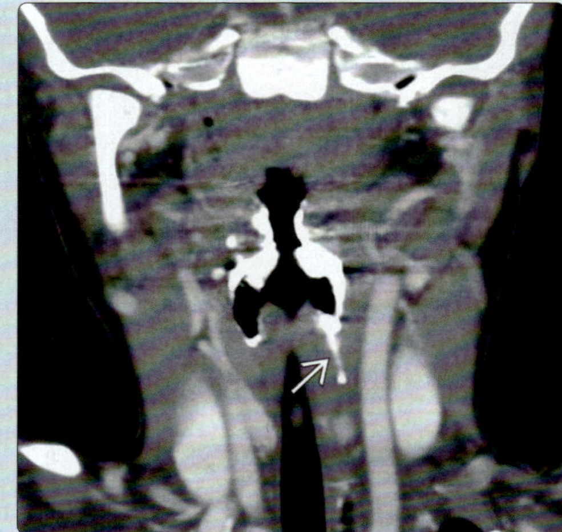

(Left) *Sagittal oblique graphic shows a sinus tract ➡ from the pyriform sinus to the left thyroid lobe with associated abscess ➡ and thyroiditis secondary to a 4th pharyngeal pouch remnant.* **(Right)** *Coronal CECT obtained after barium swallow defines a tract ➡ extending from the apex of the left pyriform sinus to the lower anterior left neck in a patient with prior history of left-sided thyroiditis.*

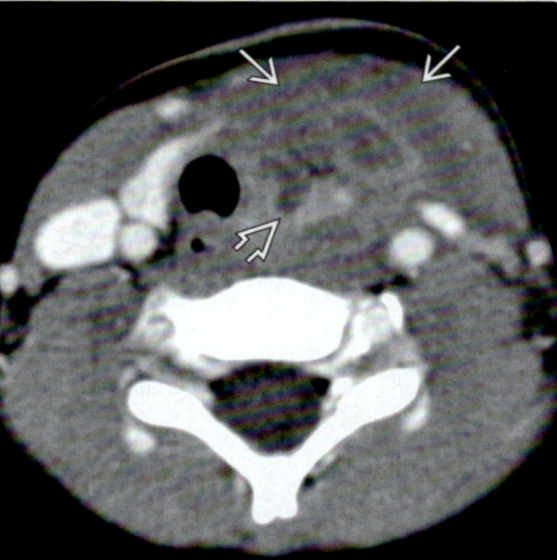

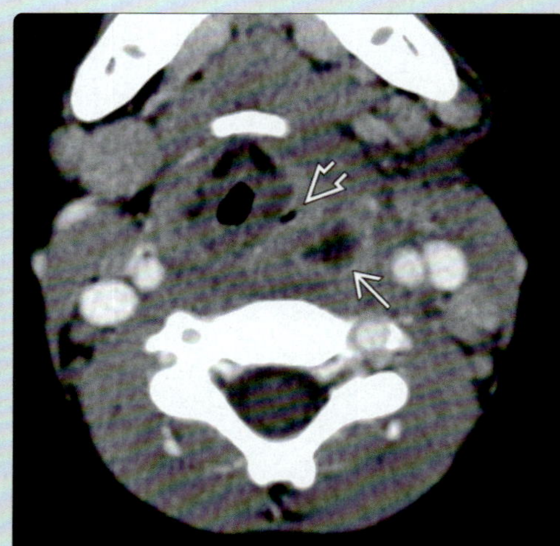

(Left) *Axial CECT in a child presenting with acute signs of infection demonstrates a phlegmonous mass ➡ in the anterior left neck, involving the left thyroid lobe ➡ and causing deviation of the airway to the right of midline.* **(Right)** *Axial CECT in the same patient shows a rim-enhancing early abscess ➡ deviating an air-filled sinus tract ➡ forward. This constellation of findings should alert the clinician to search for an opening at the apex of the pyriform sinus.*

KEY FACTS

TERMINOLOGY

- Definition: Cystic mass resulting from **congenital** epithelial inclusion or rest
  - Epidermoid: Epithelial elements only
  - Dermoid: Epithelial elements + dermal substructure, including dermal appendages

IMAGING

- Epidermoid: Cystic mass with **fluid contents** only
- Dermoid: Cystic mass with **fatty, fluid, or mixed contents**
- Location
  - Oral cavity: Submandibular space, sublingual space, or root of tongue
  - Anterior neck, usually midline
  - Orbit: Adjacent to frontozygomatic suture > frontolacrimal suture
  - Nasal cyst in association with nasal dermal sinus (NDS) ± intracranial extension
- Scalloping or remodeling of bone common
- Subtle rim enhancement of wall sometimes seen
- Dermoid & epidermoid cysts may see **restricted diffusion**
- Protocol advice
  - Routine CECT of cervical soft tissues
  - MR: T1 precontrast & use fat saturation postcontrast for orbit, neck, & oral cavity lesions
  - High-resolution anterior skull base MR in NDS; image from tip of nose to posterior to crista galli
  - Sagittal to define tract: Nose → anterior skull base

CLINICAL ISSUES

- Treatment: Complete surgical excision
- Congenital nasal mass requires imaging to evaluate intracranial extension before biopsy

DIAGNOSTIC CHECKLIST

- Complex lesion with fat, consider dermoid cyst
- Simple lesion (may be proteinaceous fluid) = epidermoid or dermoid cyst

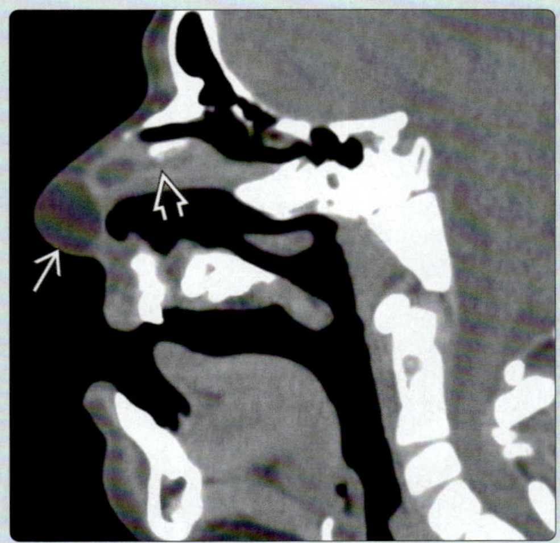

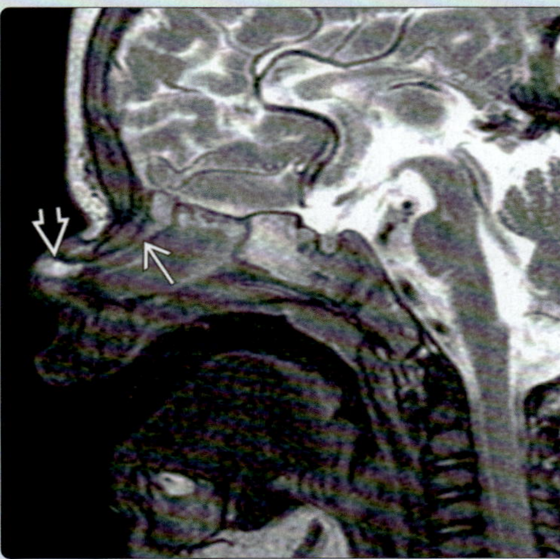

(Left) *Sagittal CT reconstruction in a 10-year-old child following cleft palate repair shows a large nasal dermoid ➡ with nasal dermal sinus tract ➡ extending toward the cribriform plate.* **(Right)** *Sagittal T2WI MR in an 8-month-old girl shows a hyperintense sinus tract ➡ extending from the dermoid at the tip of the nose ➡ toward the cribriform plate. Notice there is no evidence for intracranial dermoid or epidermoid.*

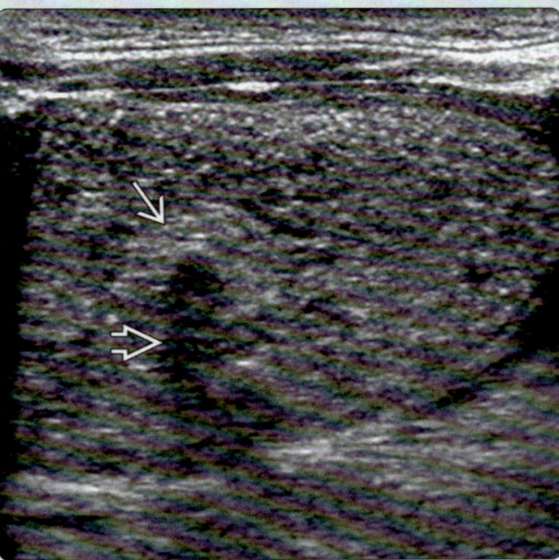

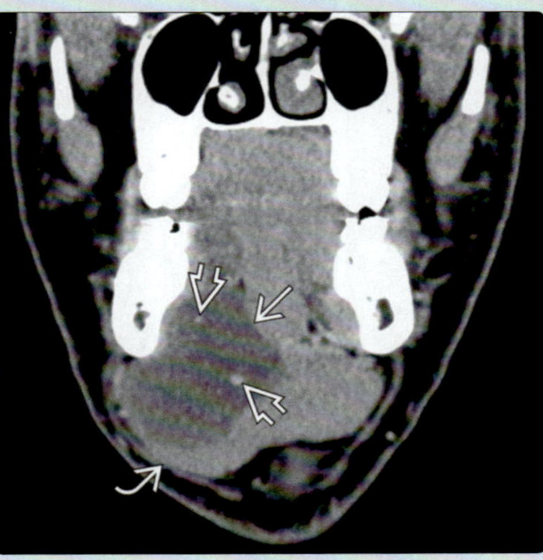

(Left) *Longitudinal ultrasound in a 14-year-old boy shows a submental mass with heterogeneous echotexture and minimal increase through transmission. One hyperechoic focus ➡ has posterior acoustical shadowing ➡, consistent with calcification in a dermoid.* **(Right)** *Coronal CECT in the same patient shows a low-density mass ➡ with a few calcifications ➡ within the oral cavity. Inferior displacement of the mylohyoid muscle ➡ indicates this dermoid is in the sublingual space.*

Fibromatosis Colli

KEY FACTS

TERMINOLOGY

- **Sternocleidomastoid (SCM) tumor of infancy**
- Nonneoplastic SCM muscle enlargement in early infancy

IMAGING

- General imaging findings and issues
  - **Nontender** SCM muscle **enlargement** in infant
  - No adjacent inflammation or significant adenopathy
  - Location: Right > left; rarely bilateral
- US: Modality of choice when imaging required
  - Variable echogenicity in enlarged SCM muscle
- CT: Enlarged muscle has similar attenuation to normal muscle pre- and postcontrast
- MR: Variable signal, diffuse enhancement

TOP DIFFERENTIAL DIAGNOSES

- Myositis related to neck infection
  - Tenderness, cellulitis evident clinically
  - Adenopathy conspicuous
- Systemic nodal metastases
  - Nodes deep to normal SCM muscle
- Primary cervical neuroblastoma
  - Close association with carotid sheath
- Rhabdomyosarcoma
  - More discrete mass with "aggressive" margins
- Teratoma
  - Often with fat, calcifications

CLINICAL ISSUES

- Clinical presentation
  - SCM muscle mass appears within 2 weeks of delivery
  - Usually **regresses by 8 months** of age
  - **Unilateral** longitudinal cervical neck mass
  - Torticollis in up to 30%
  - ↑ in breech presentation & forceps delivery
  - Occasionally with developmental dysplasia of hip
- Treatment: Physical therapy/stretching exercises to ↑ range of motion

(Left) *Longitudinal ultrasound in a 2-week-old infant shows typical fusiform enlargement of the left sternocleidomastoid (SCM) muscle with mildly increased echogenicity ➔ relative to the uninvolved portion of the muscle ➔.* **(Right)** *Axial T2 MR in the same child shows heterogeneous hyperintensity in the enlarged left SCM muscle ➔, relative to the contralateral normal right SCM muscle ➔.*

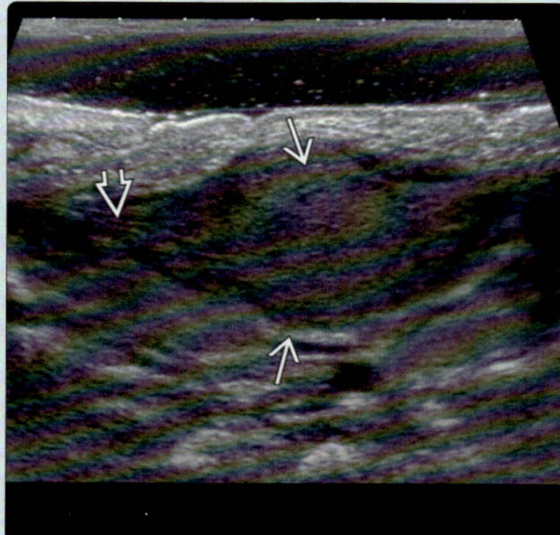

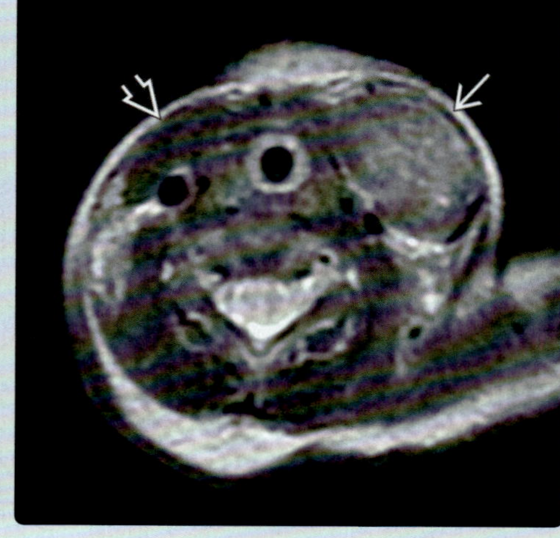

(Left) *Axial CECT demonstrates diffuse enlargement of the right SCM muscle ➔, isodense to the normal contralateral SCM muscle ➔, in a 1-month-old girl with fibromatosis colli.* **(Right)** *Posterior 3D surface-rendered soft tissue image in a child evaluated for bilateral cephalohematomas ➔ demonstrates incidental torticollis secondary to left SCM tumor of infancy (large left SCM not included).*

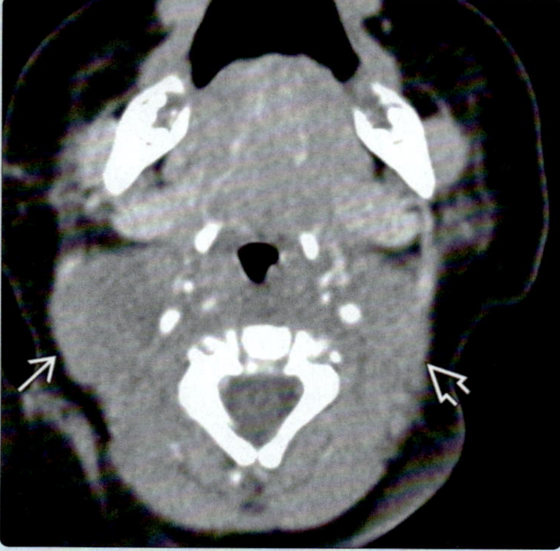

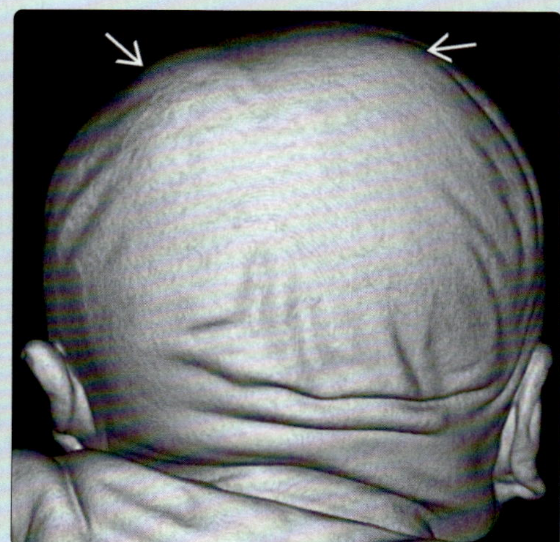

KEY FACTS

TERMINOLOGY

- Infantile hemangioma (IH): Benign **vascular neoplasm**; **not** vascular malformation

IMAGING

- Doppler will document characteristic flow
- Well-defined mass with **diffuse enhancement**
- **High-flow vessels** in/adjacent during proliferative phase
- ↓ size with **fatty replacement** during **involuting phase**

TOP DIFFERENTIAL DIAGNOSES

- **Congenital hemangioma**
  - Present at birth or on prenatal imaging; GLUT1(-)
- **Venous malformation**
  - Congenital vascular malformation, venous lakes
  - ↑ T2, ↓ T1, diffuse enhancement ± phleboliths
- **Soft tissue sarcoma**
  - Rhabdomyosarcoma, extraosseous Ewing sarcoma, undifferentiated sarcoma
- **Plexiform neurofibroma**
  - Ill-defined margins, transspatial involvement
- **Arteriovenous malformation**
  - Congenital vascular malformation
  - High-flow arteries, arteriovenous shunting

PATHOLOGY

- **GLUT1** immunohistochemical marker **positive** in all phases of growth & regression

CLINICAL ISSUES

- Typically **inapparent at birth**, appears in 1st weeks of life
- "Beard" distribution of IH with **PHACES association**
- Majority do not require treatment; treatment often required when causing vision issues or airway obstruction
- Propranolol (β-blocker) used if treatment needed; cardiology co-management can be helpful
- Rarely, intralesional steroids, laser, surgical excision or embolization

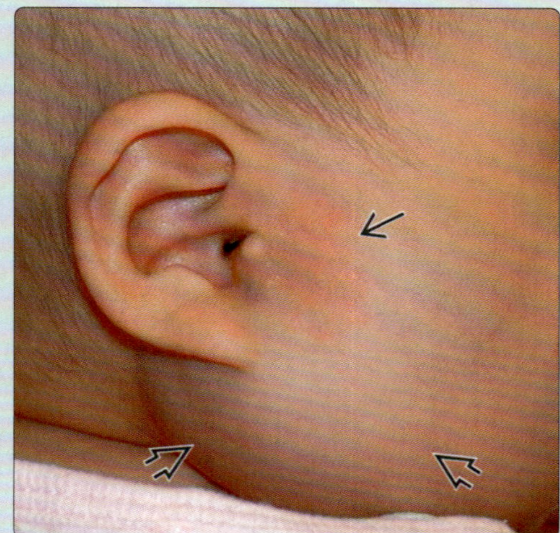

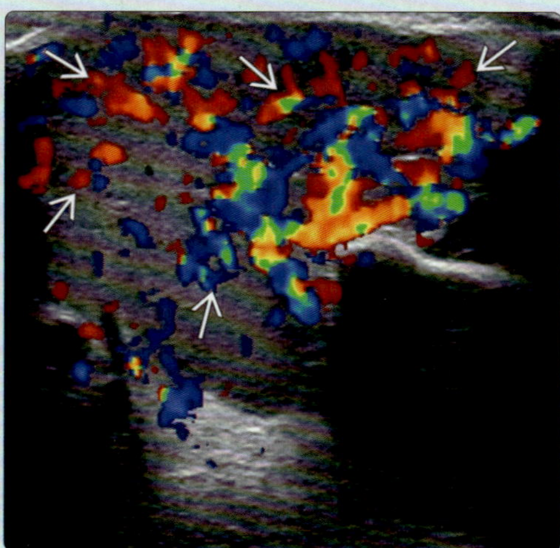

(Left) *Clinical photograph shows an infant with a large right parotid infantile hemangioma (IH). There is a large mass centered at the angle of the mandible ⇨ with reddish strawberry tinges of the overlying skin ⇨.* **(Right)** *Transverse color Doppler ultrasound in a 1-month-old child shows a lobular lesion replacing the parotid gland with high vessel density ➡ that is typical of a proliferating IH.*

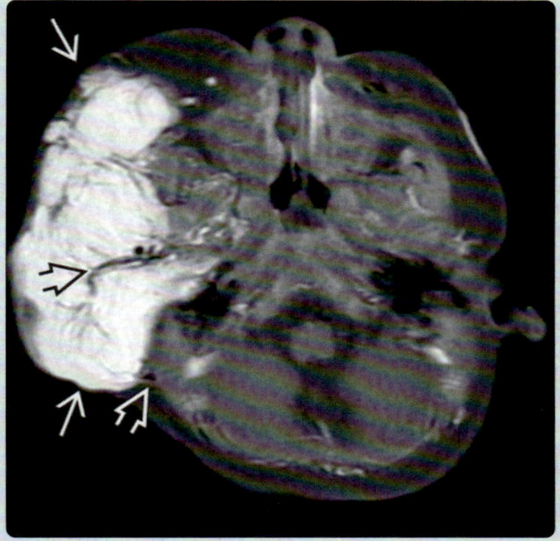

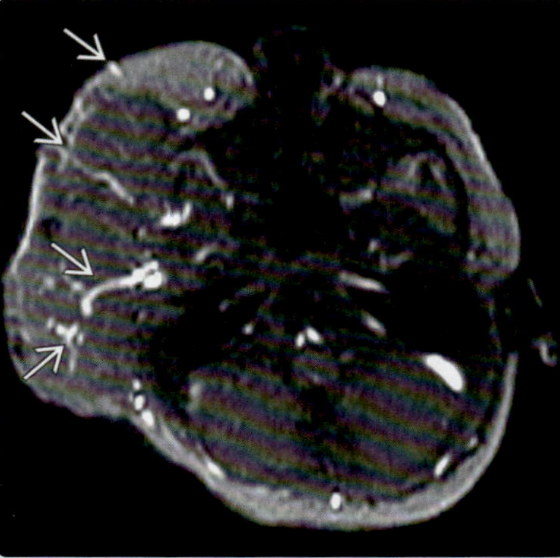

(Left) *Axial T1 C+ FS MR in a 5 month old shows a large, lobulated, intensely enhancing mass ➡ infiltrating the massively enlarged right parotid gland. Notice the prominent intralesional ⇨ and perilesional ➡ flow voids typical of IH.* **(Right)** *Axial SPGR flow-sensitive sequence in the same patient shows to better advantage the high-flow nature of the lesion typical of IH. Multiple high-flow vessels are noted within and adjacent to the primary parotid IH ➡.*

Rhabdomyosarcoma

KEY FACTS

TERMINOLOGY

- Abbreviation: Rhabdomyosarcoma (**RMS**)
  - Most common childhood soft tissue sarcoma

IMAGING

- General imaging findings & issues
  - Soft tissue mass with variable contrast enhancement
  - **Bone destruction** or **remodeling** possible
  - Up to **40%** occur in H&N
    - Orbit, parameningeal sites, & all other H&N sites
- Bone CT: Best to evaluate osseous erosion
- Enhanced MR: Best to evaluate intracranial spread
- Always include neck to look for metastatic adenopathy

TOP DIFFERENTIAL DIAGNOSES

- Juvenile angiofibroma
- Langerhans cell histiocytosis
- Plexiform neurofibroma
- Non-Hodgkin & Hodgkin lymphoma; leukemia

PATHOLOGY

- Originates from primitive mesenchymal cells (rhabdomyoblasts) committed to skeletal muscle differentiation
- 3 histologic subtypes
  - **Embryonal RMS**: Most common; younger children
  - **Alveolar RMS**: 2nd most common; patients 15-25 years
  - **Pleomorphic RMS**: Least common; adults 40-60 years

CLINICAL ISSUES

- Clinical presentation
  - Age: 70% under 12 years; 40% under 5 years
  - Symptoms location-dependent: Mass
    - Cranial neuropathy: Orbit (CNII), sinonasal (CNV), T-bone (CNVII)
- Treatment options
  - Surgical debulking, chemotherapy, ± radiation therapy
  - Research effort in proton therapy, immunotherapy, and vaccination

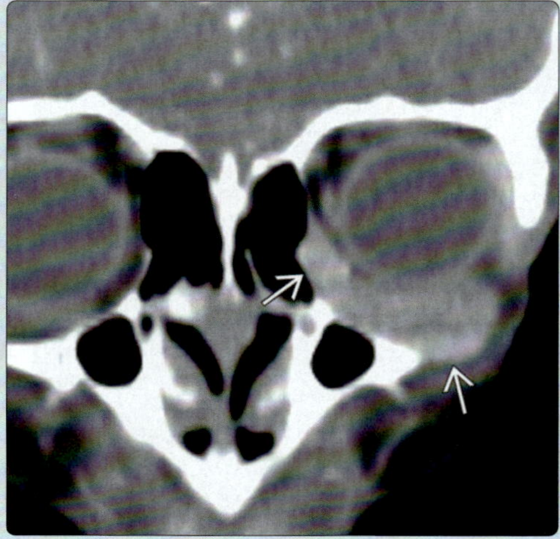

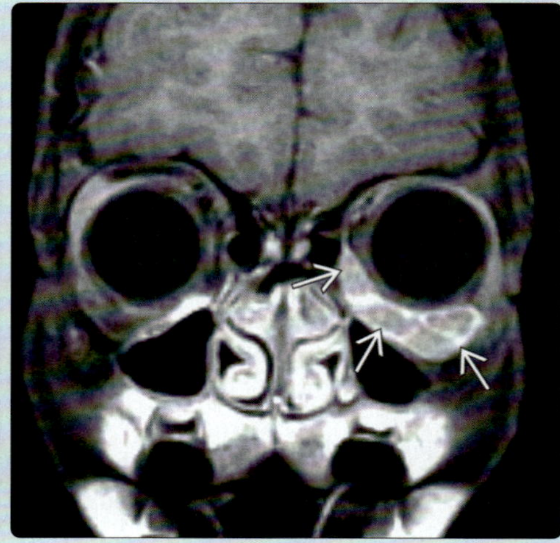

(Left) *Coronal CECT in an 8 year old shows a nonspecific, mildly heterogeneous extraconal mass ➡ in the inferior and inferomedial left orbit, without bone destruction.* **(Right)** *Coronal T1 C+ FS MR in the same child shows a heterogeneously enhancing mass ➡, atypical appearance for hematoma, hemangioma, and vascular malformation, histologically proven to be embryonal rhabdomyosarcoma (RMS). The absence of bone destruction does not exclude RMS.*

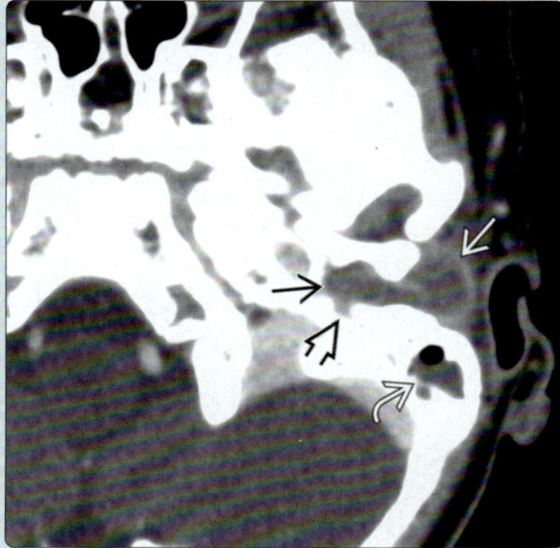

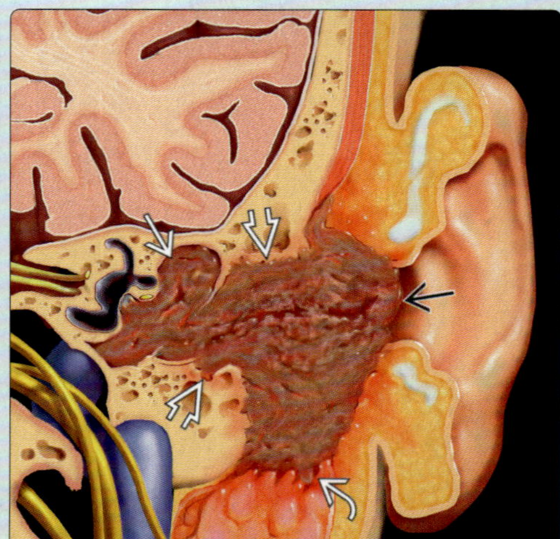

(Left) *Axial CECT in a 2-year-old boy presenting with few-day history of left external auditory canal (EAC) mass (rhabdomyosarcoma) ➡ shows minimal osseous irregularity ⇨ and postobstructive mastoid opacification ➡. Note middle ear involvement ⇨.* **(Right)** *Coronal graphic in a teenager with left ear rhabdomyosarcoma illustrates middle ➡ and external ear ➡ invasion with associated bone erosion and parotid involvement ➡. A patient would present with an EAC polyp ⇨.*

KEY FACTS

TERMINOLOGY

- Neurofibromatosis 1 (**NF1**); defect on chromosome 17
- **Neurofibromas**: Multiple localized neurofibromas & plexiform neurofibromas (PNF) in NF1

IMAGING

- MR shows hyperintense T2 signal
  - **Target** = ↓ signal center, ↑ signal periphery PNF
- Postcontrast CT or MR
  - Localized NF: Homogeneous or patchy enhancement, well-circumscribed fusiform mass
  - PNF: Heterogeneously enhancing, lobulated mass along course of peripheral nerve
- Most conspicuous on STIR & T2WI FS MR
- Other extracranial H&N manifestations of NF1
  - Orbit: **Optic pathway glioma (OPG)**, optic nerve sheath ectasia, Lisch nodules, buphthalmos, large foramina with PNFs
  - Skull & skull base: **Sphenoid dysplasia**, smooth bony foramina with PNF infiltration of cranial nerves, lambdoid suture defect
  - Vascular dysplasia: Internal carotid artery stenosis/occlusion & moyamoya; aneurysms & arteriovenous fistula rare

TOP DIFFERENTIAL DIAGNOSES

- Venous and lymphatic malformations
- Rhabdomyosarcoma

CLINICAL ISSUES

- Most commonly seen in late childhood to early adulthood
- Changes in skin coloring (pigmentation), tumors in peripheral nerves
- Patient with PNF or multiple localized neurofibromas, consider NF1
- Look for brain lesions, OPG, sphenoid wing dysplasia
- Treatment: Resection of neurofibromas that press on vital structures

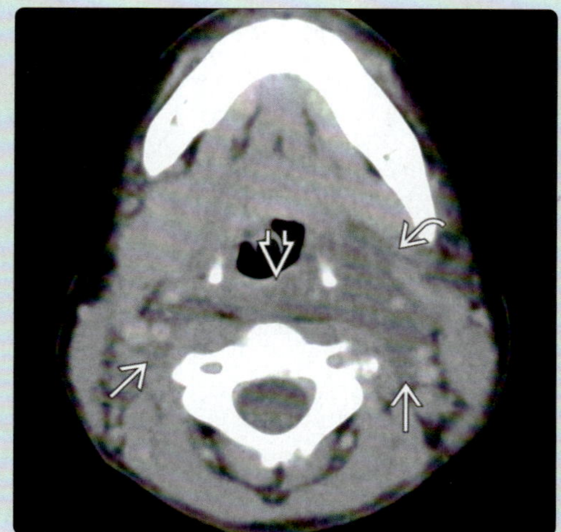

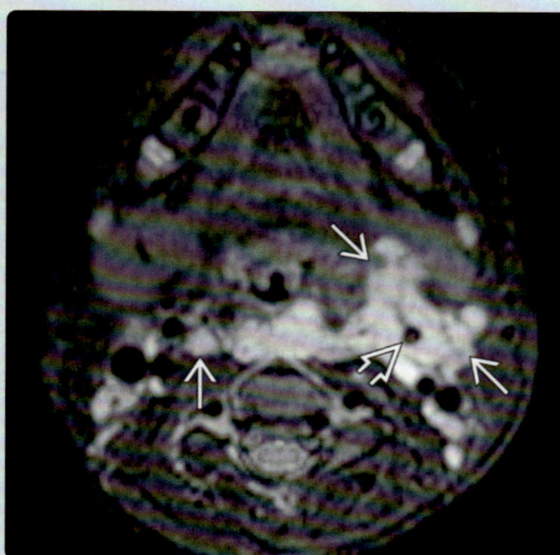

(Left) *Axial CECT in a child with neurofibromatosis type 1 (NF1) shows an ill-defined infiltrative transspatial plexiform neurofibroma (PNF) involving the bilateral carotid ➡, retropharyngeal ➡, and left submandibular ➡ spaces.* **(Right)** *Axial STIR MR in the same child better defines the margins of the PNF ➡. Notice the infiltrative pattern, with circumferential involvement of the left carotid artery ➡, typical of plexiform lesions.*

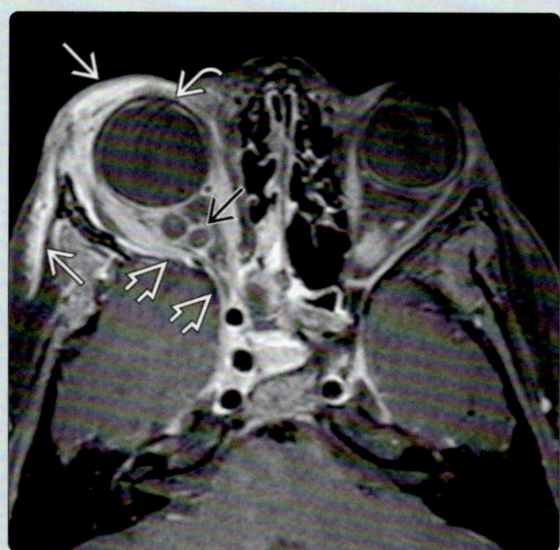

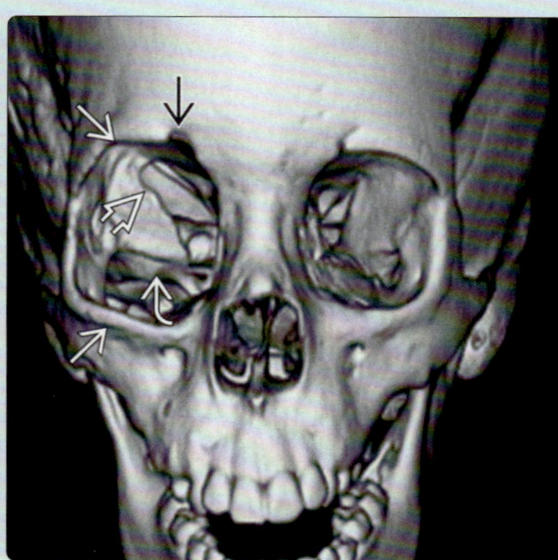

(Left) *Axial T1WI C+ FS MR shows diffusely enhancing neurofibroma ➡ involving the right pre- and postseptal orbit and temporalis scalp. There is also sphenoid wing hypoplasia ➡, buphthalmos ➡, and a tortuous optic nerve ➡.* **(Right)** *Frontal 3D reformation in the same patient shows diffuse right orbital expansion ➡. There is also enlargement of the superior ➡ and inferior ➡ orbital fissures and supraorbital foramen ➡ related to sphenoid dysplasia and adjacent PNF.*

Neurofibromatosis Type 2

KEY FACTS

TERMINOLOGY

- Neurofibromatosis type 2 (**NF2**): Inherited syndrome with multiple **schwannomas, meningiomas, & ependymomas**

IMAGING

- Bilateral **enhancing CPA-IAC masses**
  - Ovoid when small; "ice cream on cone" when large enough to fill IAC & CPA
- Brain: MR annually for surveillance
  - Calcifications: Choroid plexus, cerebellar hemispheres, & cerebral cortex
  - Other meningiomas & schwannoma (CNIII-XII)
  - Ependymomas > > gliomas
- Spine: MR every 3 years for surveillance
  - Meningiomas, schwannomas, & ependymomas

TOP DIFFERENTIAL DIAGNOSES

- CPA-IAC metastases
  - Bilateral IAC enhancing masses in older patient
- Facial nerve schwannoma, CPA-IAC
  - CPA-IAC mass with labyrinthine canal tail of enhancement
- Meningioma, CPA-IAC
  - Dural-based, eccentric CPA mass with dural tail of enhancement projecting into IAC

PATHOLOGY

- Autosomal dominant disorder
  - Mutation of *NF2* gene chromosome 22, protein Merlin
  - **50%** result from **new** dominant gene **mutation**

CLINICAL ISSUES

- Unilateral, then bilateral, **sensorineural hearing loss**
- Other symptoms: Tinnitus, vertigo, CNVII paralysis
- Mean age at diagnosis: ~ 25 years

DIAGNOSTIC CHECKLIST

- If diagnosis of NF2 made in adult, consider alternative diagnosis of metastases to CPA-IAC

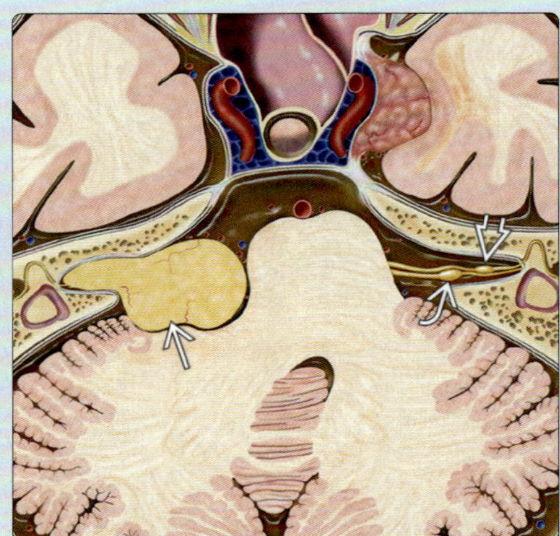

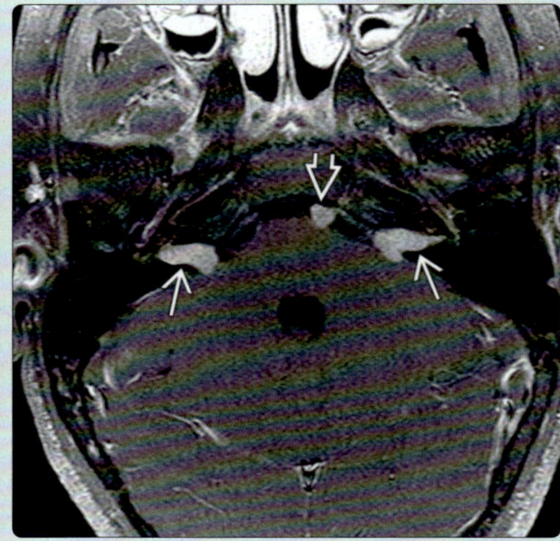

(Left) *Axial graphic depicts bilateral cerebellopontine angle-internal auditory canal masses in neurofibromatosis type 2 (NF2). Note the large right vestibular schwannoma ➡. On the left, there is a facial nerve schwannoma ➡ and a vestibular schwannoma ➡. Differentiating facial from vestibular schwannoma is important to assess therapy options.* **(Right)** *Axial T1 C+ FS MR in a 12-year-old child shows diffuse enhancement of the bilateral vestibular schwannomas ➡ and the left CNVI schwannoma ➡.*

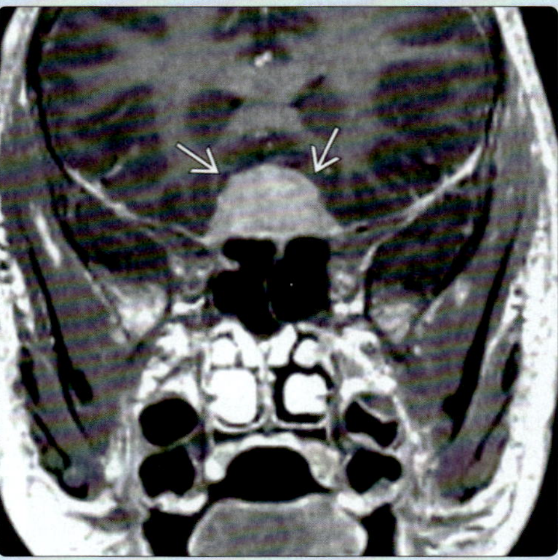

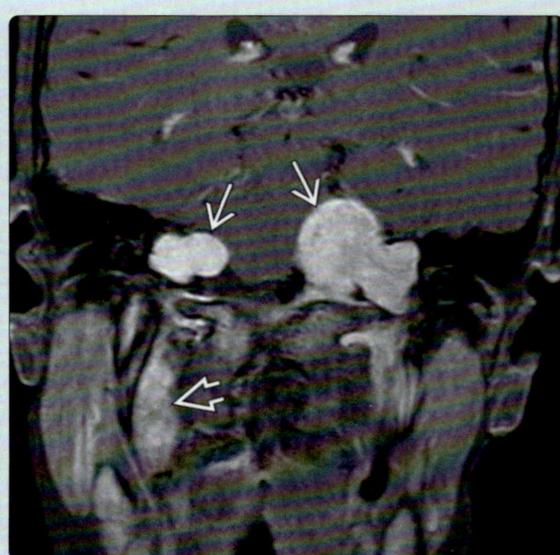

(Left) *Coronal T1 C+ MR in the same child reveals a broad-based, extraaxial sphenoidale mass ➡, proven to represent meningioma. This patient had a very high tumor burden at a young age, including multiple other intracranial and extracranial cranial nerve schwannomas as well as spinal lesions (not shown).* **(Right)** *Coronal T1 C+ FS MR in an 11-year-old child with severe phenotype of NF2 shows bilateral large vestibular schwannomas ➡ and right carotid space schwannoma ➡.*

KEY FACTS

TERMINOLOGY

- Abbreviation: Basal cell nevus syndrome (**BCNS**)
- Synonyms: Gorlin syndrome, **Gorlin-Goltz syndrome**
- **Autosomal dominant** disorder: Multiple keratocystic odontogenic tumors (KOTs), basal cell carcinoma, **medulloblastoma**, **intracranial dural Ca^{++}**, bifid ribs

IMAGING

- Multiple expansile, lucent lesions of **mandible and maxilla**
- May **displace developing teeth** ± **resorption of roots** of erupted teeth and tooth extrusion
- Variable attenuation/signal intensity depends on protein content &/or hemorrhage

TOP DIFFERENTIAL DIAGNOSES

- Periapical (radicular) cyst
- Dentigerous (follicular) cyst
- KOT (nonsyndromic)
- Ameloblastoma

PATHOLOGY

- Etiology: Arise from dental lamina remnants
- Autosomal dominant; 1/3 are new mutations
- Associated abnormalities
  - High incidence of **medulloblastomas**
  - Marked calcification of falx (80%), dura
  - Multiple skin **basal cell carcinoma**
  - Bifid ribs and scoliosis

CLINICAL ISSUES

- Clinical presentation
  - Syndrome apparent by **5-10 years**
  - Patients present by 3rd decade with multiple nevoid basal cell carcinomas; mean age = 19 years
  - Multiple enlarging jaw masses; asymptomatic or painful
    - Multiple KOTs seen in 80% of cases of BCNS
- Treatment options for KOTs
  - Surgical methods: Marsupialization, decompression, enucleation, curettage, en bloc resection

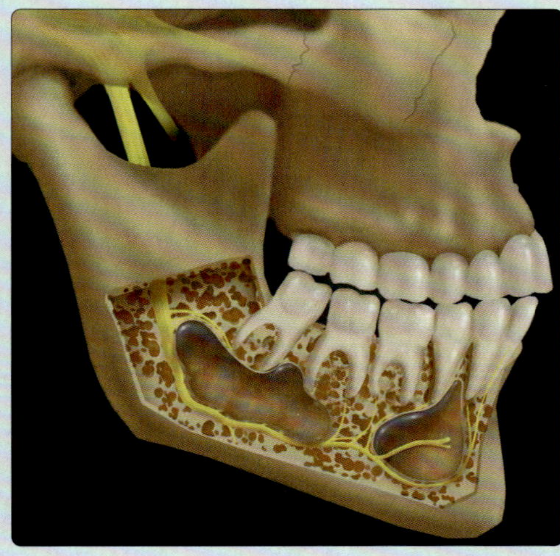

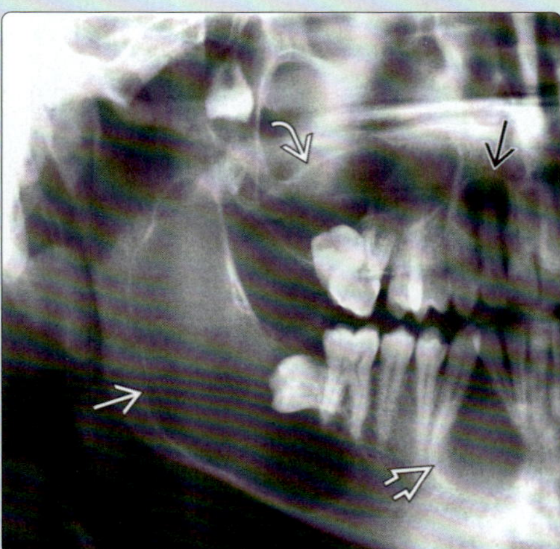

(Left) *Lateral graphic with the mandibular cortex removed shows the classic appearance of multiple keratocystic odontogenic tumors in basal cell nevus syndrome; lesions tend to splay tooth roots and displace nerves.* **(Right)** *Cropped panoramic radiograph shows at least 4 cystic jaw lesions: One in the posterior body and ramus ➡, 1 in the symphysis ➡, 1 in the posterior ➡, and 1 in midline ➡ maxilla. Multiple expansile lesions in the jaws raise suspicion of basal cell nevus syndrome.*

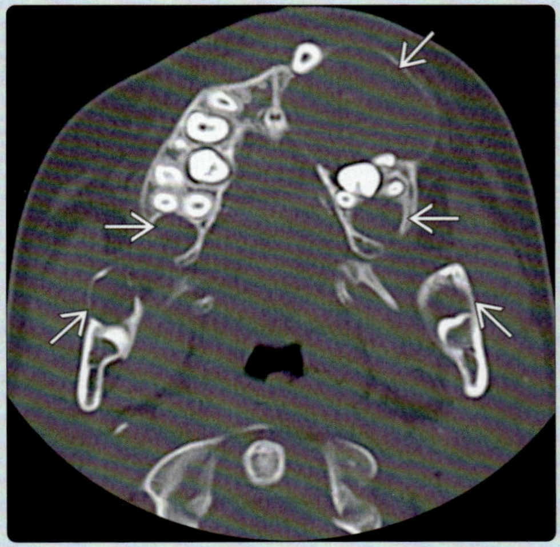

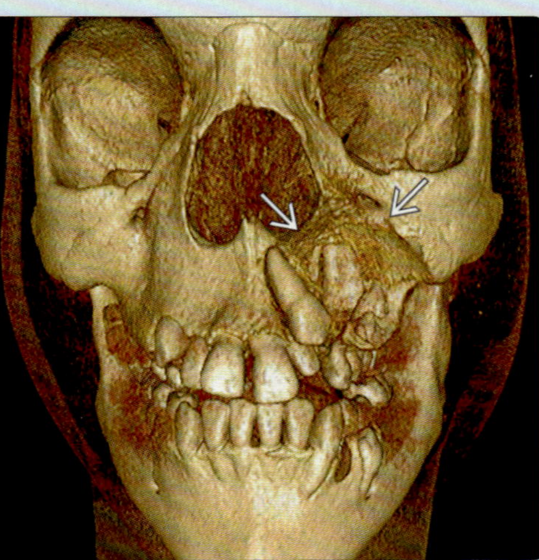

(Left) *Axial bone CT in a 9-year-old boy with basal cell nevus syndrome demonstrates multiple bilateral lytic lesions ➡ in the maxilla and mandible that are typical of keratocystic odontogenic tumors.* **(Right)** *Anteroposterior 3D reformation in a 9-year-old boy with basal cell nevus syndrome shows to better advantage the effect of the largest lesion ➡ on the adjacent teeth.*

KEY FACTS

TERMINOLOGY

- Branchiootorenal syndrome (BOR)
- Autosomal dominant syndrome
  - Deafness and ear anomalies
  - Branchial anomalies/preauricular pits
  - Renal abnormalities

IMAGING

- Neck: Branchial cleft cyst/fistula
- Temporal bone CT findings
  - Dilated eustachian tubes
  - External ear: Variable stenosis/atresia
  - Middle ear: Dysmorphic; fused, malformed ossicles
  - Cochlea: Tapered basal turn, hypoplastic and offset middle/apical turns
  - Semicircular canal anomaly
  - Dilated, bulbous vestibular aqueduct
  - Flared IAC; anomalous CNVII canal
- Abdominal CT findings: Renal cysts, dysplasia, agenesis
- Variable, asymmetric micrognathia

TOP DIFFERENTIAL DIAGNOSES

- Branchiootic syndrome
  - Normal kidneys; BOR genetic overlap
- Otofaciocervical syndrome: BOR genetic overlap
- Congenital nonsyndromic external ear and middle ear malformation

PATHOLOGY

- BOR1: 8q13.3 locus, *EYA1* gene mutation
- BOR2: 19q13.3 locus, *SIX5* mutation

CLINICAL ISSUES

- Clinical presentation
  - Hearing loss (sensorineural hearing loss, conductive hearing loss, mixed) (~ 98%)
  - Preauricular tag, pit (~ 84%)
  - Branchial anomalies (~ 70%)
  - Renal anomalies (~ 40%)

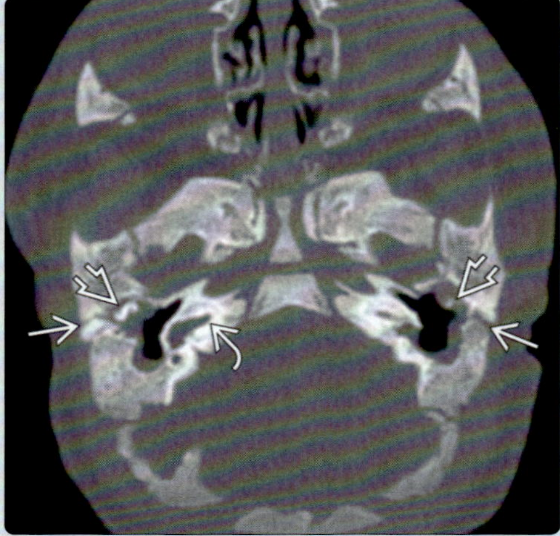

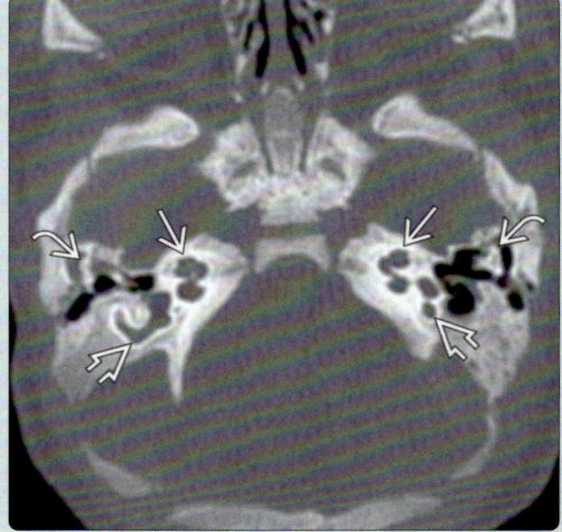

(Left) *Axial bone CT imaged at 10 days of age to evaluate microtia shows bilateral external auditory canal (EAC) atresia ➡. Ossicles are malformed, fused, & laterally located ➡. Note tapered basal turn of right cochlea ➡.* **(Right)** *Axial bone CT (same patient) shows "unwound" or offset, hypoplastic middle & apical cochlear turns ➡ & deficiency of the right cochlear modiolus. Posterior semicircular canals ➡ & ossicles ➡ are malformed. CT findings are characteristic of branchiootorenal syndrome (BOR).*

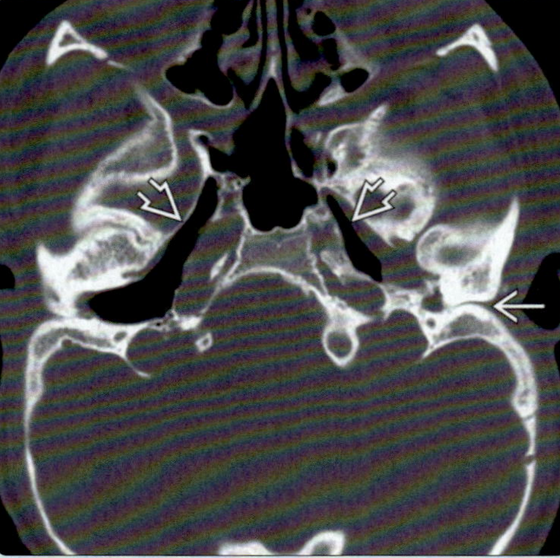

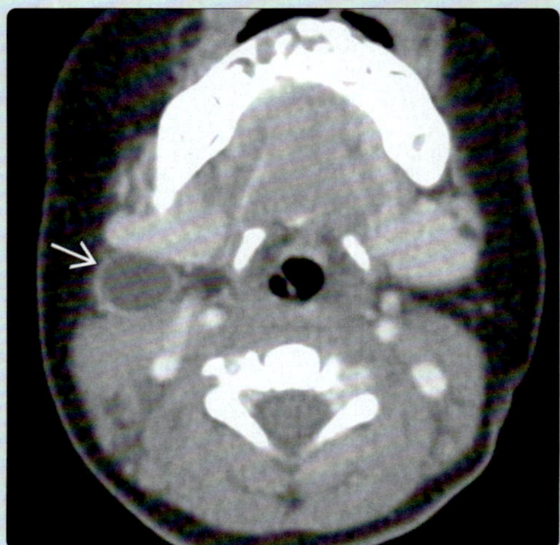

(Left) *Axial bone CT in a 12 year old with microtia and left EAC atresia ➡ shows marked dilatation of the eustachian tubes ➡, which terminate anomalously at the inferior aspect of the sphenoid bone. Dilatation of the eustachian tubes suggests BOR syndrome.* **(Right)** *Axial CECT in a 5-month-old boy with preauricular pits and a family history of pits and renal and ear anomalies shows a hypodense lesion ➡ consistent with a 2nd branchial cleft cyst. The patient also had ear anomalies of BOR syndrome.*

KEY FACTS

TERMINOLOGY

- **CHARGE**: **C**oloboma, **h**eart anomaly, **a**tresia choanae, **r**etardation (mental & somatic development), **g**enital hypoplasia, **e**ar abnormalities
- Major signs: Coloboma, choanal atresia, semicircular canal (SCC) hypoplasia/aplasia, cranial nerve (CN) involvement
- Minor signs: Hindbrain, external/middle ear, cardiac/esophageal malformations, hypothalamo-hypophyseal dysfunction, intellectual disability

IMAGING

- **Temporal bone CT**: Defines ear & facial nerve anatomy
- **High-resolution T2 MR** brain: Sagittal view of IAC
- Choanal atresia, coloboma (variable), cleft lip/palate
- Hypoplastic vestibule & hypoplastic/absent SCC
- Mildly flattened apical ± middle turns + thickened modiolus or single cochlear turn/hypoplasia
- Stenotic/atretic cochlear nerve canal, oval window & overlying anomalous tympanic segment of CNVII
- Large emissary veins, hypoplasia basiocciput, basilar invagination, & vertebral anomalies
- Hypoplastic pons, uplifted vermis ± cerebellar malformation
- CN hypoplasia/aplasia (mainly CNI, VII, & VIII)

TOP DIFFERENTIAL DIAGNOSES

- Kallmann syndrome: Allelic, less severe
- VACTERL association
- Branchiootorenal syndrome

PATHOLOGY

- *CHD7* mutation 60%; *SEMA3E* mutation
- Highly predictive of CHARGE: Cup-shaped pinna, agenesis/hypoplasia SCC, arrhinencephaly

CLINICAL ISSUES

- May require airway support for obligate nasal breathers
- If candidate for cochlear implantation, evaluate presence & location of CNVII/VIII

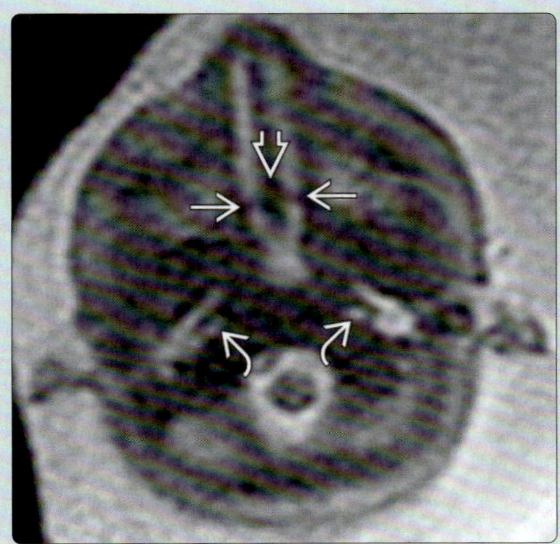

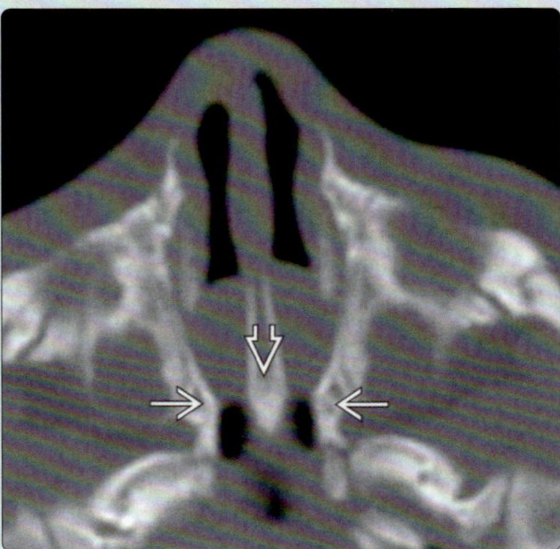

(Left) *Axial FSE T2-weighted fetal MR at 32-weeks gestation shows bilateral choanal atresia with linear hypointensity ➡ extending from the thickened vomer ⇨ to the lateral nasal walls, outlined by amniotic fluid. A single cochlear turn is seen bilaterally ↪, and the cochleae appeared isolated from the internal auditory canals.* **(Right)** *Axial bone CT in the same infant at 6 days of age shows lateral nasal wall medial deviation ➡ and a thickened vomer ⇨ with bilateral bony and membranous choanal atresia.*

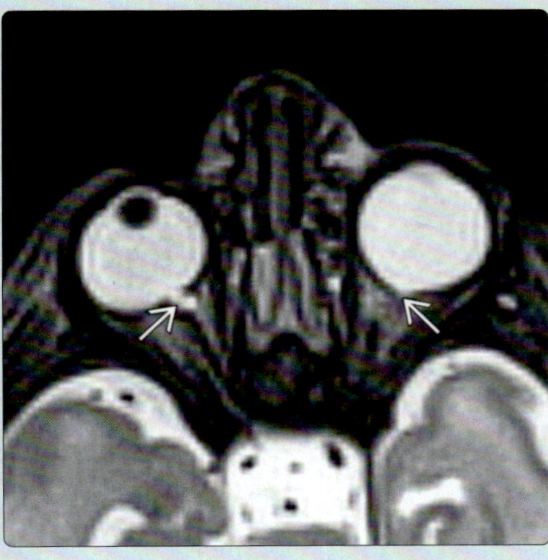

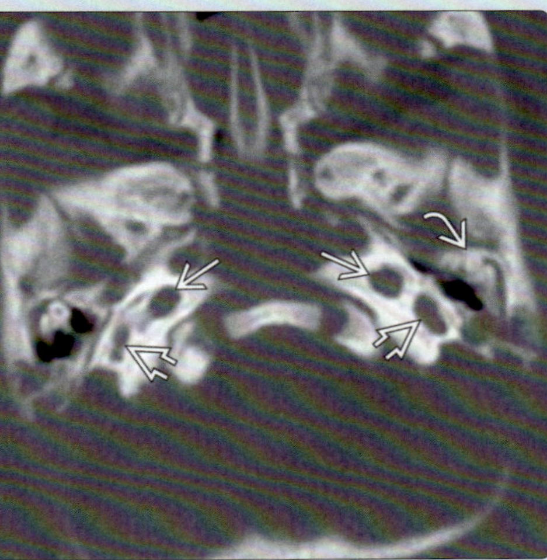

(Left) *Axial FSE T2-weighted MR in 4-day-old boy reveals right microphthalmia and bilateral colobomas ➡. A CHD7 mutation was found, confirming CHARGE syndrome.* **(Right)** *Axial bone CT in the same child confirms incomplete cochlear partitioning ➡, hypoplastic vestibules ⇨, and absent semicircular canals. The ossicles are dysmorphic, and the left malleus is fused to the attic ↪. It is unusual to see the ocular, ear, and nasal findings of CHARGE all in the same patient.*

Hemifacial Microsomia

KEY FACTS

TERMINOLOGY

- Oculoauriculovertebral spectrum, Goldenhar syndrome, facioauriculovertebral sequence
- Defect of 1st & 2nd pharyngeal arch derivatives ± neural crest cells

IMAGING

- Mandibular hypoplasia
  - Unilateral; rarely bilateral & asymmetric
- Zygomatic arch hypoplasia
- Hypoplasia muscles of mastication, facial muscles, & parotid gland
- EAC atresia/stenosis
- Middle ear hypoplasia & ossicular malformation/fusion
- Oval window atresia & CNVII anomaly/hypoplasia
- Cervical spine fusion/segmentation anomalies (Klippel-Feil anomaly)
- CNS (variable): Ventriculomegaly, brainstem cleft, cerebellar hypoplasia, cephalocele

TOP DIFFERENTIAL DIAGNOSES

- Teratogenic embryopathy (e.g., diabetes)
- Townes-Brocks syndrome
- Branchiootorenal syndrome
- Treacher Collins syndrome

CLINICAL ISSUES

- Common disorder, prevalence ~ 1 in 3,500 births
- Microtia/anotia, preauricular skin tags
- Hearing loss (~ 85%; conductive hearing loss > > SNHL)
- Facial asymmetry; unilateral micrognathia
- Facial nerve weakness (~ 50%)
- Variable facial clefts
- Epibulbar lipodermoid, coloboma
- TEF, cardiac, genitourinary, pulmonary abnormalities

DIAGNOSTIC CHECKLIST

- HFM as cause of facial asymmetry & external ear anomalies
- Facial weakness due to CNVII anomaly/hypoplasia

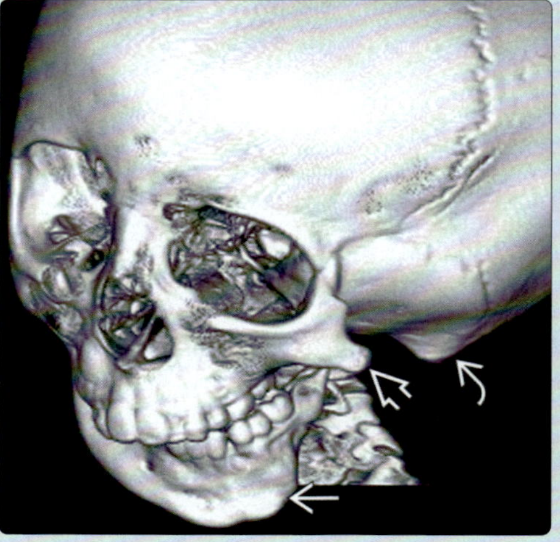

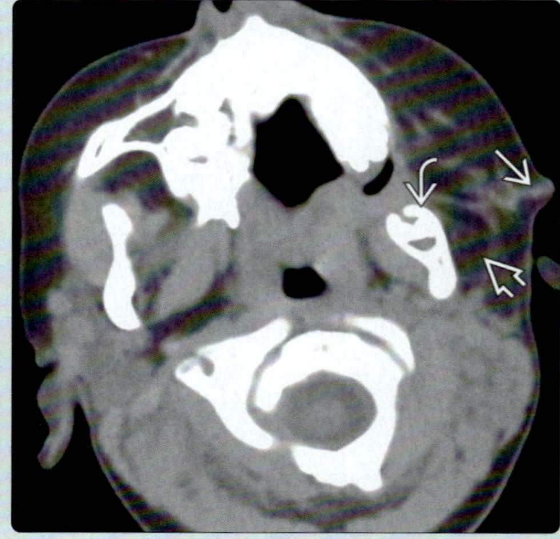

(Left) *3D NECT in a 7-year-old girl with hemifacial microsomia (HFM) reveals a smaller left hemimandible ➡, hypoplasia of the zygomatic arch ➡, underdevelopment of the mastoid process ➡, and external auditory canal atresia.* **(Right)** *Axial NECT in a 4-year-old girl with HFM demonstrates a smaller left mandibular ramus ➡, a preauricular sinus tract, and skin tag ➡. The left muscles of mastication are underdeveloped, and the masticator muscle and parotid tissue are not seen in their expected location ➡.*

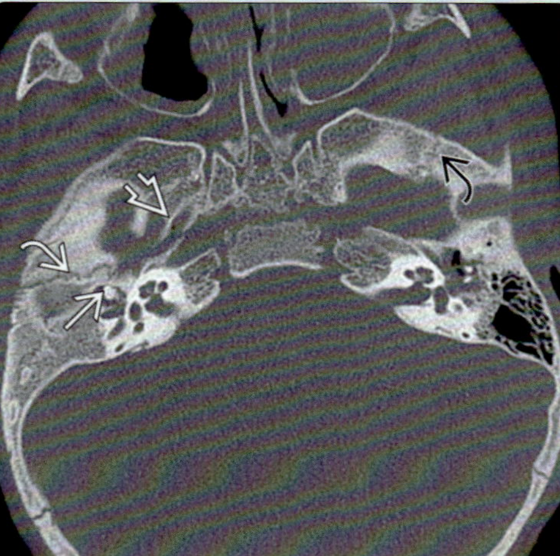

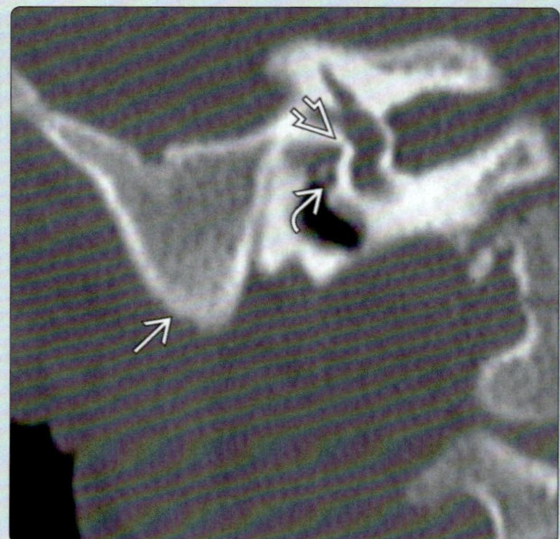

(Left) *Axial bone CT in a 23-month-old boy with HFM shows that the right middle ear cavity is hypoplastic and opacified. The ossicles ➡ are dysmorphic. The right eustachian tube is dilated and anomalous ➡. The right sphenosquamosal suture ➡ is rotated laterally compared with the left ➡.* **(Right)** *Reformatted coronal bone CT in the same patient shows absent mastoid pneumatization ➡, oval window atresia ➡, and an anomalous inferior course of CNVII tympanic segment ➡, running over the promontory.*

KEY FACTS

TERMINOLOGY

- Treacher Collins syndrome (TCS)
- Nager syndrome (NS): TCS + limb anomalies
- Craniofacial malformation: Down-slanting palpebral fissures, micrognathia, zygomatic and malar hypoplasia, microtia/anotia, ± limb defects

IMAGING

- Temporal bone findings
  - External auditory canal: Stenosis/atresia
  - Decreased/absent mastoid pneumatization
  - Hypoplastic/atretic middle ear space
  - Malformed or absent ossicles ± fixation
  - Oval window stenosis/atresia
  - Facial nerve canal anomalies/dehiscence
  - Normal or malformed cochlea (flattened turns)
  - Normal or malformed lateral semicircular canal ± vestibule
- Symmetric micrognathia, zygomatic/malar hypoplasia
- Coloboma

TOP DIFFERENTIAL DIAGNOSES

- Bilateral facial microsomia
- Nonsyndromic congenital external and middle ear malformation
- Branchiootorenal syndrome

PATHOLOGY

- Autosomal dominant > > recessive, phenotypic variability and genetic heterogeneity, "ribosomopathy"
- TCS: *TCOF1*, *POLR1D*, and *POLR1C* gene mutations
- NS: *SF3B4* gene mutation

CLINICAL ISSUES

- Airway obstruction, deafness
- Severity of atresia may preclude successful atresiaplasty; bone anchored hearing options may be best
- Treatment: Airway support, reconstructive surgery, hearing aids, developmental support

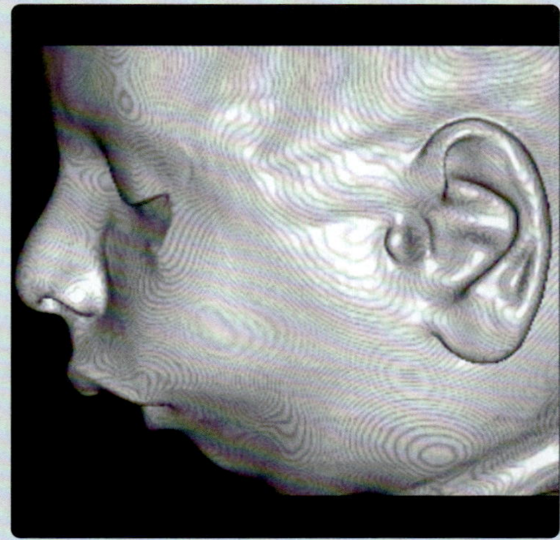

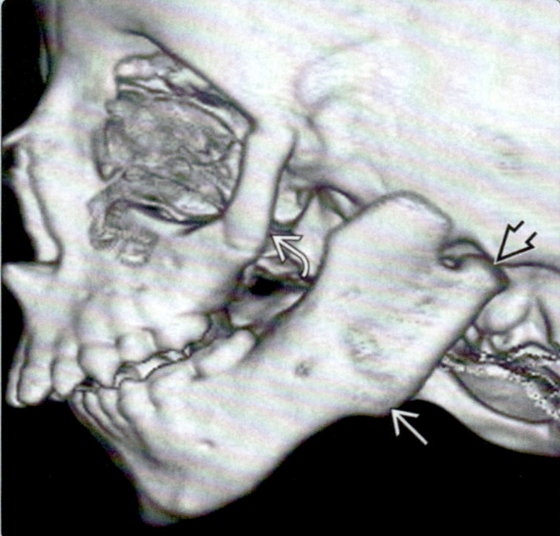

(Left) *Lateral 3D soft tissue surface-rendered reformation CT in an infant with Nager syndrome (NS) shows micrognathia, malar flattening, mildly low-set ears, & external auditory meatus atresia.* **(Right)** *Lateral 3D bone CT in the same infant with NS shows micrognathia with an obtuse mandibular angle ➡ & marked hypoplasia of the neck & condyle of the mandible ⇨. There is hypoplasia of the midface & zygomatic complex ➡ with absence of the zygomatic arch. There is external auditory canal (EAC) atresia.*

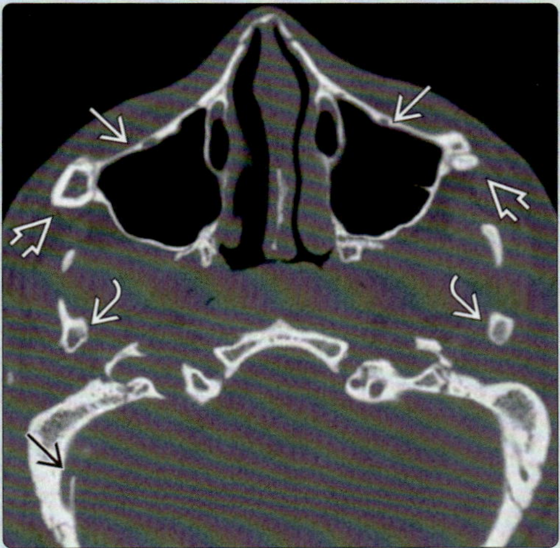

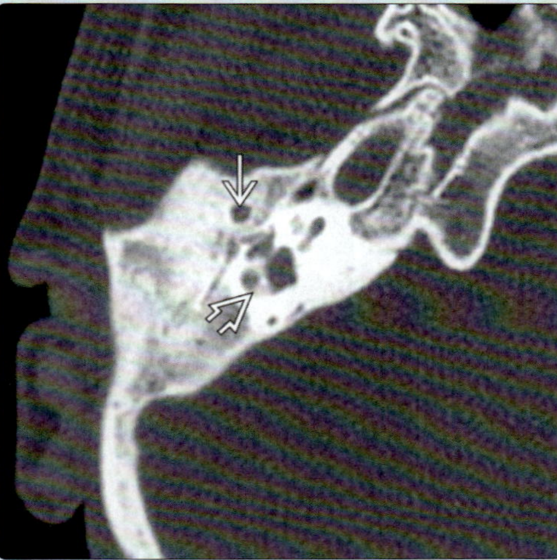

(Left) *Axial bone CT in a 13-year-old girl with Treacher Collins syndrome (TCS) shows zygomatic complex hypoplasia with posteriorly slanted maxillae ➡, absent zygomatic arches ➡, & hypoplastic mandibular condyles ➡. Note EAC atresia, absent mastoid pneumatization, & an enlarged mastoid emissary vein ⇨.* **(Right)** *Axial bone CT in a 16-year-old girl with TCS shows EAC atresia, absent middle ear space and ossicles, ventrally placed descending facial nerve canal ➡, and malformed lateral semicircular canal ➡ with small bone island.*

Pierre Robin Sequence

KEY FACTS

TERMINOLOGY

- Pierre Robin sequence (PRS)
- PRS triad: Micrognathia, glossoptosis, cleft palate

IMAGING

- Bilateral, usually symmetric **micrognathia**
- **Glossoptosis**: Elevated, posteriorly displaced tongue
- Posterior **U-shaped cleft palate**
- Additional features depend on syndromic etiology
- Temporal bone
  - EAC: Normal, stenotic, or atretic [e.g., Treacher Collins syndrome (TCS)]
  - Middle ear & mastoid: Normal or hypoplastic ± opacification
  - Ossicles: Normal, mildly malformed [e.g., stapes in velocardiofacial syndrome (VCFS)], or severely malformed ± fixation (e.g., TCS)
  - Inner ear: Normal or malformed (e.g., small semicircular canal bone island/anlage anomaly in VCFS & TCS)

TOP DIFFERENTIAL DIAGNOSES

- Stickler & related syndromes (18% of PRS)
- VCFS (~ 7% of PRS)
- TCS (~ 5% of PRS)

PATHOLOGY

- Primary micrognathia → glossoptosis → failure of palatal shelf elevation & fusion
- Collagen gene mutations: Stickler syndromes
- 22q11.2 deletion: Velocardiofacial syndrome

CLINICAL ISSUES

- Feeding & breathing difficulties, failure to thrive
- Stickler: Progressive myopia, joint degeneration
- VCFS: Cardiac anomalies, adenoidal hypoplasia, velopharyngeal insufficiency, medial deviation of cervical internal carotid arteries, learning difficulties
- TCS: Malar flattening, downslanting palpebral fissures, coloboma

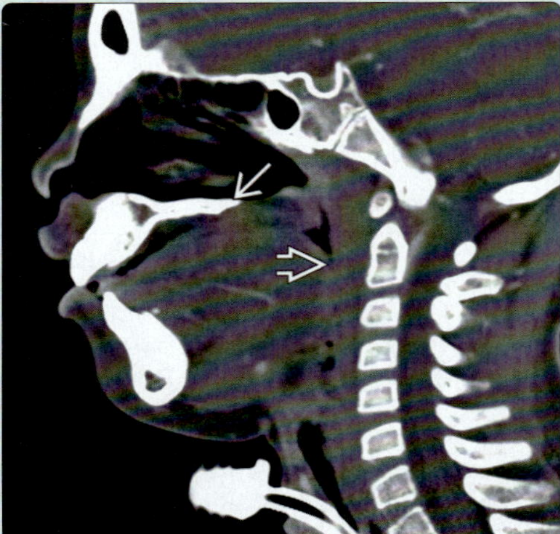

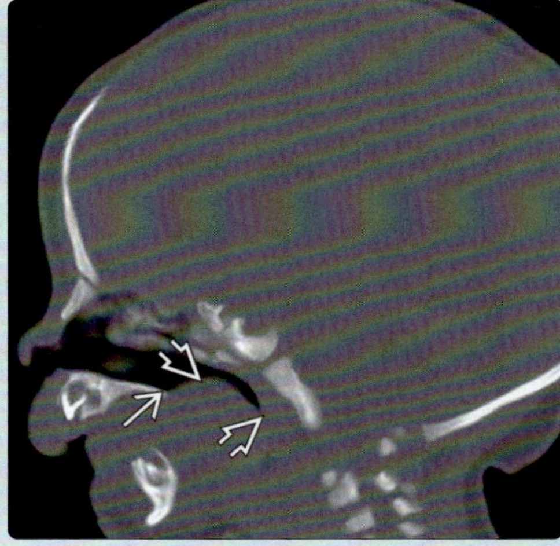

(Left) *Lateral CECT in 22q11 deletion patient reveals glossoptosis, deficiency of the hard palate ➡, and an absent uvula. Note the elevation and posterior displacement of the tongue ➡, resulting in obstruction of the airway. The patient has a tracheostomy tube in place.* **(Right)** *Sagittal CT reconstruction in a Pierre Robin sequence patient shows a shortened hard palate ➡ and abnormal downward or backward displacement of the tongue ➡. The tongue obstructs the oropharynx, resulting in difficulty with breathing and feeding.*

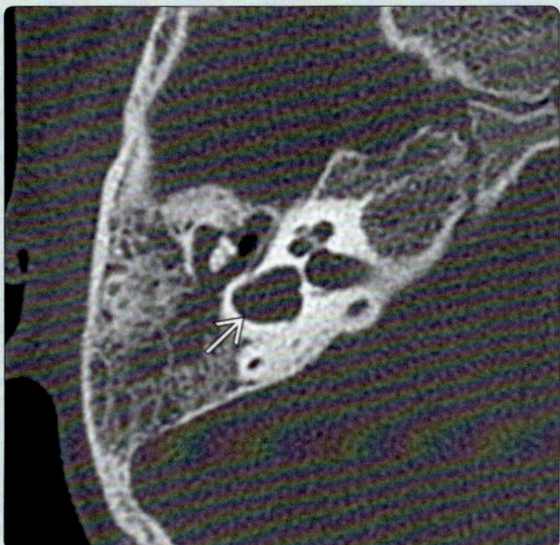

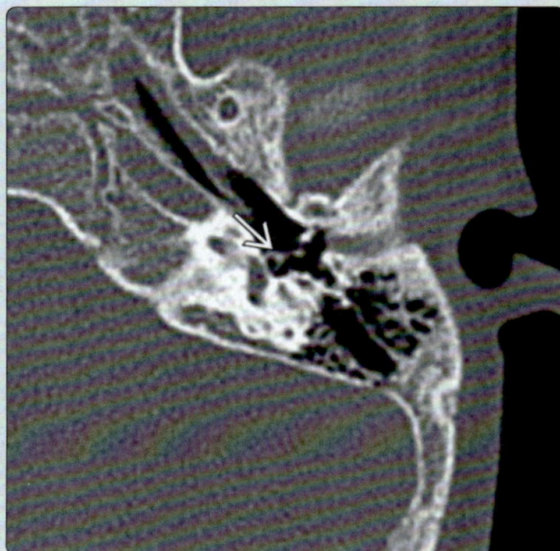

(Left) *Axial bone CT in a 5-year-old boy with velocardiofacial syndrome (VCFS) shows anlage anomaly where the lateral semicircular canal (SCC) & vestibule form a single globular space without a bone island ➡. There is diffuse opacification of the middle ear space & mastoid air cells.* **(Right)** *Axial bone CT in a 7-year-old girl with VCFS & hearing loss shows mild thickening of anterior crus of the stapes ➡ & mildly reduced mastoid pneumatization. More cephalad image (not shown) demonstrated slightly small lateral SCC bone island.*

X-Linked Stapes Gusher (DFNX2)

KEY FACTS

TERMINOLOGY

- **X-linked mixed hearing loss**; conductive hearing loss (CHL) with stapes fixation (DFN3)
- Mixed deafness with **perilymph gusher**
- Profound sensorineural hearing loss (SNHL) ± CHL + bilateral unique inner ear anomaly

IMAGING

- Cochlea: Deficient interscalar septa & osseous spiral lamina, absent modiolus → **corkscrew** appearance
- IAC: Bulbous dilatation laterally + deficient lamina cribrosa
- Vestibule & semicircular canals: ± slightly dilated, ± superior bulge protruding from vestibule ± semicircular canal ossification
- Vestibular aqueduct: ± large; CNVII canal: Wide labyrinthine & proximal tympanic segments

TOP DIFFERENTIAL DIAGNOSES

- Cochlear incomplete partition type I (IP-I)
- Large vestibular aqueduct + cochlear incomplete partition type II (IP-II)

PATHOLOGY

- X-linked recessive: **Males** affected, female carriers
- Molecular cause: *POU3F4* gene mutation
- Absent lamina cribrosa → communication between CSF & cochlear perilymph → perilymph hydrops

CLINICAL ISSUES

- Bilateral profound SNHL (may be progressive) ± CHL secondary to stapes fixation
  - CHL may be masked by severe SNHL
- Surgical perilymph fistula + perilymph/CSF gusher (e.g., during stapedectomy or cochleostomy) → dead ear postop
- Most common cause of X-linked hearing loss

DIAGNOSTIC CHECKLIST

- Essential imaging feature: Widened IAC, deficient lamina cribrosa, cochlear IP-III anomaly (corkscrew cochlea)

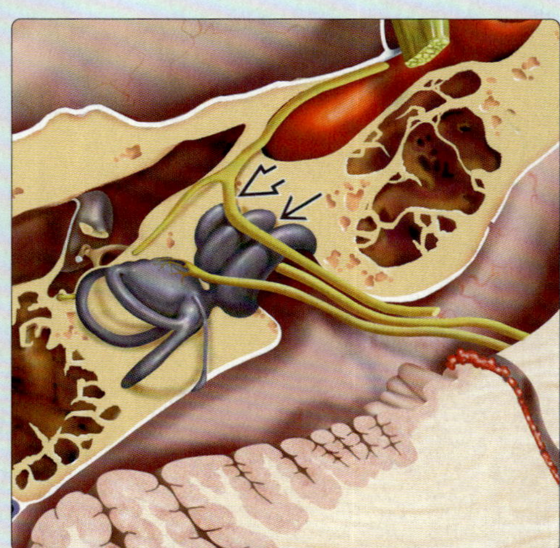

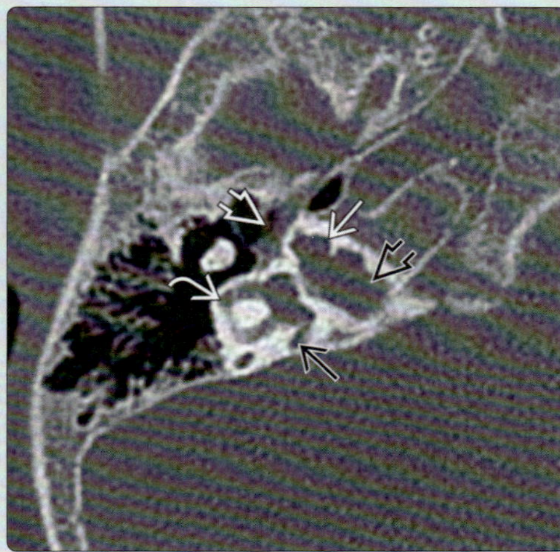

(Left) *Axial graphic of X-linked stapes gusher reveals corkscrew cochlea ⇨ with no modiolus. The IAC is foreshortened & widened. The labyrinthine CNVII segment is enlarged ⇨.* **(Right)** *Axial bone CT in a 2-year-old boy with profound sensorineural hearing loss shows internal osseous structures of the cochlea are essentially absent ➡. IAC is widened ⇨ & merges with cochlea. The lateral semicircular canal is mildly dilated ➡, vestibular aqueduct is slightly large ⇨, & the proximal tympanic CNVII canal is slightly widened ➡.*

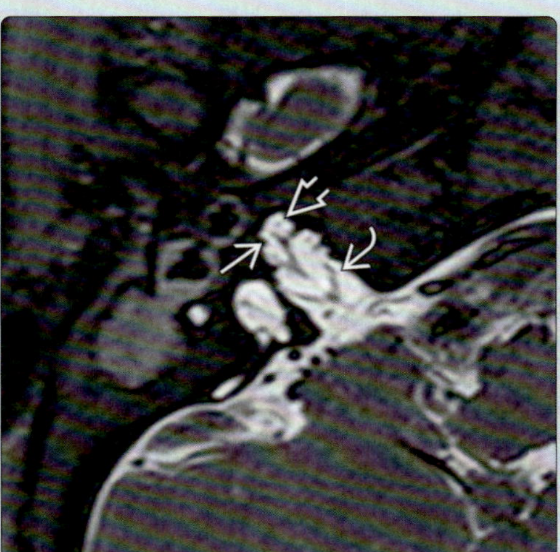

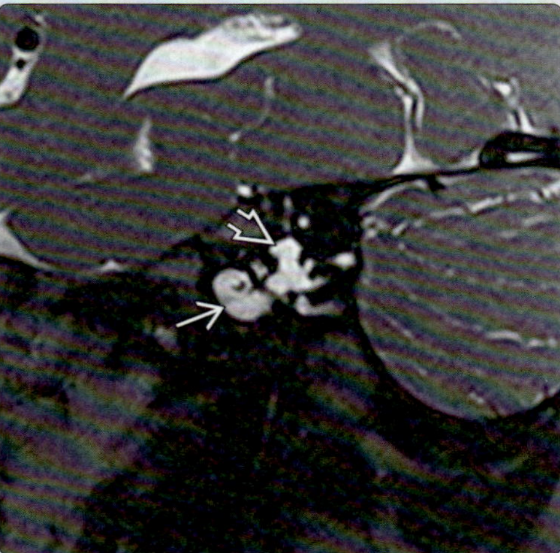

(Left) *Axial T2 SPACE MR in a 1-year-old boy with profound hearing loss shows a corkscrew morphology of the cochlea with deficiency of the interscalar septum ➡ and osseous spiral lamina (partially visualized) ➡ and absence of the modiolus. The IAC is widened and merges with the cochlear turns ➡.* **(Right)** *Sagittal oblique T2 SPACE MR in a 2-year-old boy with DFNX2 demonstrates the deficient internal structure of the cochlea ➡, which is dilated. There is a globular protrusion off the superior aspect of the vestibule ➡.*

McCune-Albright Syndrome

KEY FACTS

TERMINOLOGY

- McCune-Albright syndrome (MAS)
  - Subtype of **polyostotic fibrous dysplasia (FD)**
- **Classic triad**: Polyostotic FD, endocrine dysfunction with precocious puberty, and cutaneous hyperpigmentation

IMAGING

- Best diagnostic clues: Expanded ground-glass bone in child with precocious puberty and skin lesions
- Locations in H&N: Skull, skull base, or facial bones
  - Bilateral and asymmetric common
- CT: Imaging appearance depends on degree of fibrous vs. osseous components
  - **Ground glass**: Sclerotic
  - **Mixed** (pagetoid): Radiodensity and radiolucency
  - **Cystic**: Central lucency with thin sclerotic margins
  - Variable enhancement of fibrous component
- MR: Majority ↓ T1, intermediate or ↓ signal T2
  - Rim ↓ signal T2 and central ↑ T2 in cystic lesions
  - Fibrous component may enhance intensely

TOP DIFFERENTIAL DIAGNOSES

- Monostotic FD or polyostotic FD without MAS
- Jaffe-Campanacci syndrome
- Caffey disease
- Cherubism
- Garré sclerosing osteomyelitis

PATHOLOGY

- FD: Normal medullary bone replaced by mixture of fibrous tissue and immature, weak, woven bone
  - Defect in osteoblastic differentiation and maturation
- MAS represents 3-5% of FD cases

CLINICAL ISSUES

- FD < 10 years (~ 60%), > 10 years (40%); M > > F
- Treatment: Bisphosphonates decrease pain and fractures
- Surgical resection if severe deformity or vision loss
- Treat precocious puberty and renal phosphate wasting PRN

(Left) *Axial bone CT in a 7-year-old girl with McCune-Albright syndrome shows multiple areas of fibrous dysplasia ➡ with the typical expanded ground-glass appearance of lesions in the sclerotic stage.* **(Right)** *Coronal bone CT in the same child shows more extensive involvement of the skull base and typical narrowing of skull base foramina. Despite significant narrowing of both optic canals ➡, the child had only mild left-sided optic neuropathy with decreased vision and intermittent diplopia.*

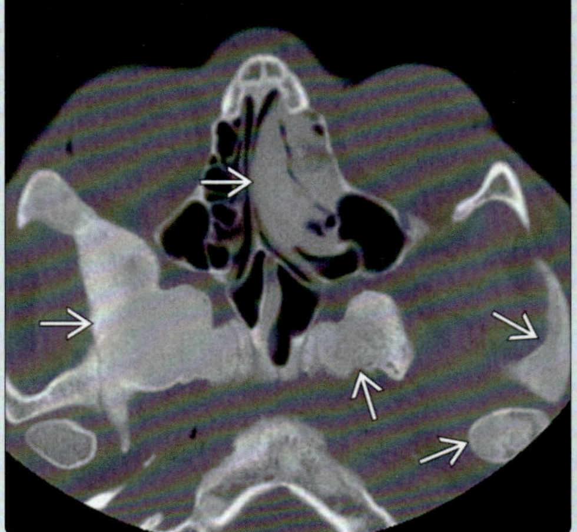

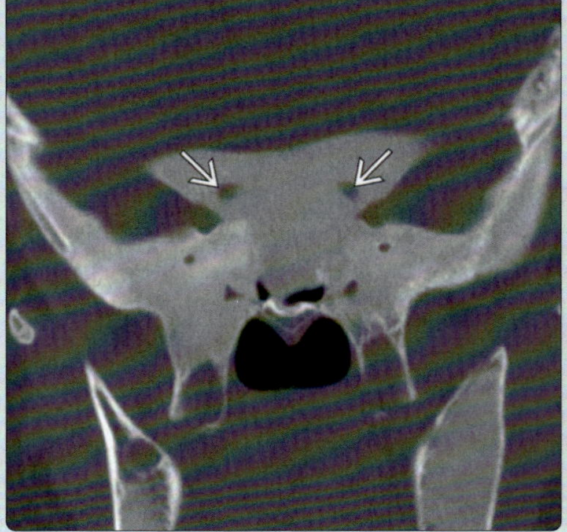

(Left) *Axial T2WI MR in a teenager with a frontal bone fibrous dysplasia lesion shows marked hypointensity within the majority of the expansile, sclerotic frontal bones ➡ with patchy hyperintensity that is typical of a small area of more active fibrous matrix ➡.* **(Right)** *Axial T1WI C+ FS MR in the same patient shows heterogeneous enhancement ➡ in the more active, fibrous component of fibrous dysplasia. This area was more lucent on CT (not shown).*

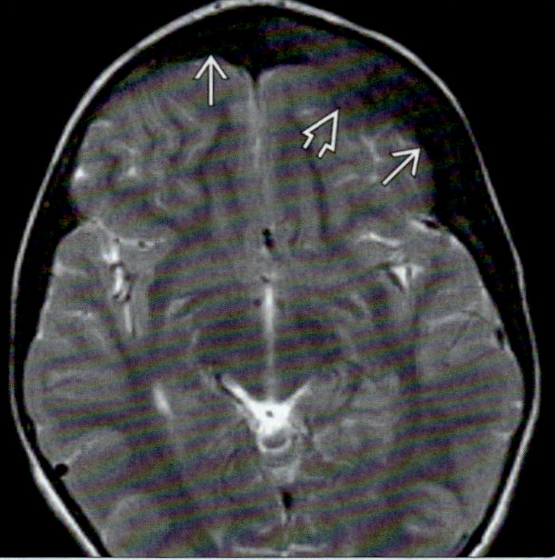

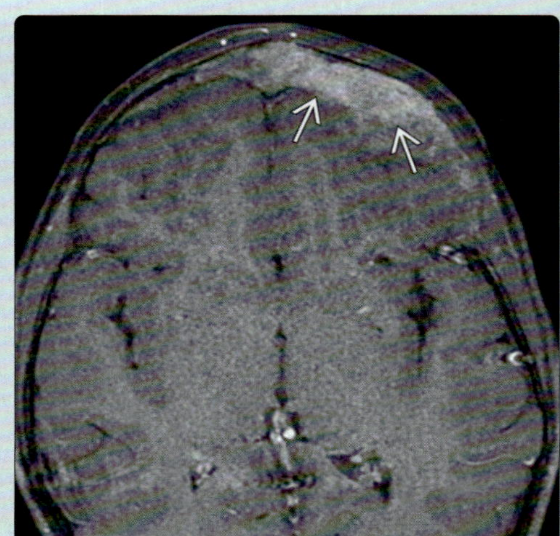

KEY FACTS

TERMINOLOGY

- Familial, bilateral fibroosseous jaw lesions
  - Genetically distinct from fibrous dysplasia (FD)

IMAGING

- **Bilateral** multilocular, **expansile** lucent lesions in **mandible**, displacing teeth
- ± submandibular lymph node enlargement

TOP DIFFERENTIAL DIAGNOSES

- FD
  - Ground glass, mixed cystic and sclerotic, or cystic
- Central giant cell granuloma
  - Expansile lesion with variable septations
  - Anterior midline mandible or ramus > maxilla
- McCune-Albright syndrome
  - Subtype of **polyostotic** FD
  - Classic triad of polyostotic FD, precocious puberty, and cutaneous hyperpigmentation

PATHOLOGY

- Autosomal dominant
  - Heterozygous mutation in *SH3BP2* gene, gene map locus 4p16.3
- Cherubism also reported in patients with Ramon syndrome, Noonan syndrome, and neurofibromatosis type 1

CLINICAL ISSUES

- **Painless** symmetric swelling of lower face
- Round face and lower eyelid retraction → eyes raised to heaven or cherub-like appearance
- Begins 14 months to 4 years of age
  - Progresses through puberty, then stabilizes
  - May regress in adulthood
  - Clinical swelling usually abates by 3rd decade
  - Radiographic changes seen until 4th decade
- Treatment: Conservative in most, curettage may improve chances of normal dentition and aesthetics

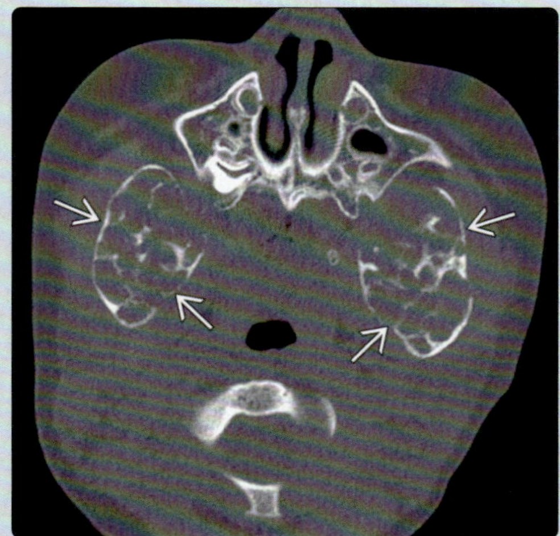

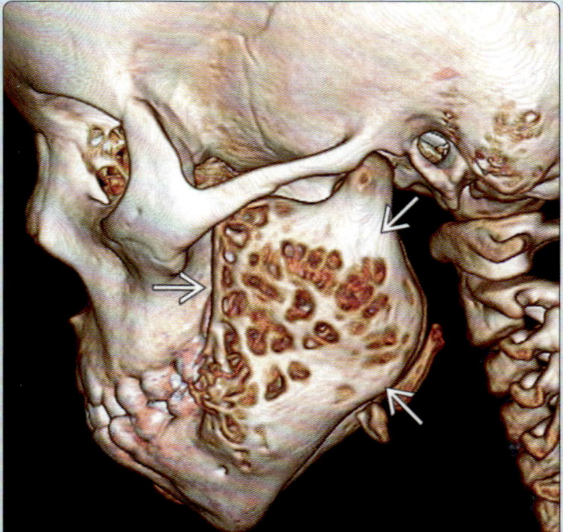

(Left) *Axial bone CT in a 17-year-old boy shows bilateral bubbly, expansile lesions ➡ confined to the mandible, a typical appearance of cherubism. Notice there are areas where the cortex appears to disappear without aggressive bone destruction or periosteal reaction.* **(Right)** *Lateral 3D reconstruction shows the diffuse expansion of the left mandible ➡ secondary to the multiple bone cysts. (Courtesy J. Cure, MD.)*

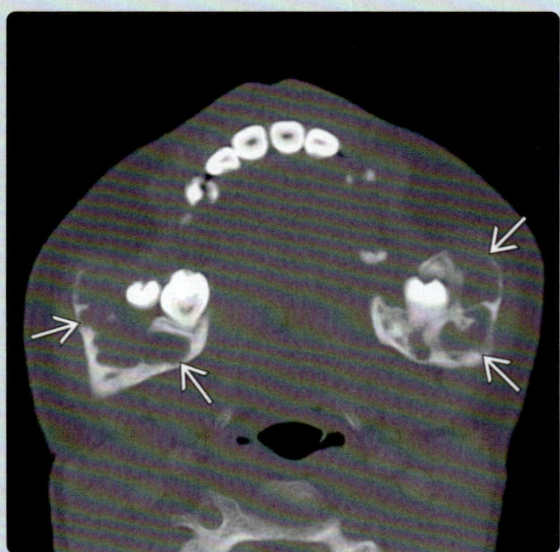

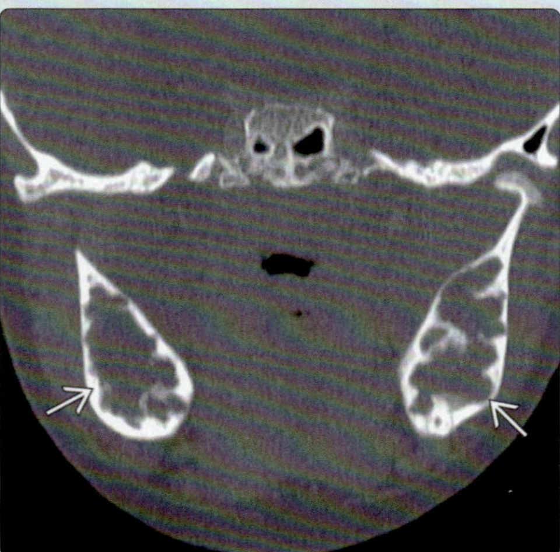

(Left) *Axial bone CT in a 4-year-old boy who presented with gradual increase in facial swelling shows bilateral cystic lesions in the mandible ➡ with several areas of diffuse cortical thinning, without aggressive bone destruction or periosteal reaction, typical of cherubism.* **(Right)** *Coronal bone CT in the same patient shows the multiloculated cystic, symmetric bilateral mandible lesions ➡ causing expansion of both sides of the mandible.*

SECTION 4

Sinonasal Cavities and Orbit

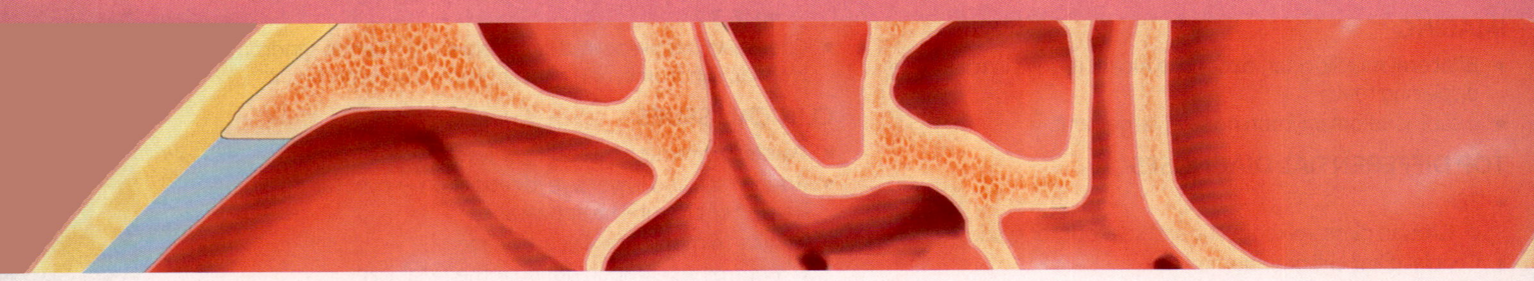

Nose and Sinus

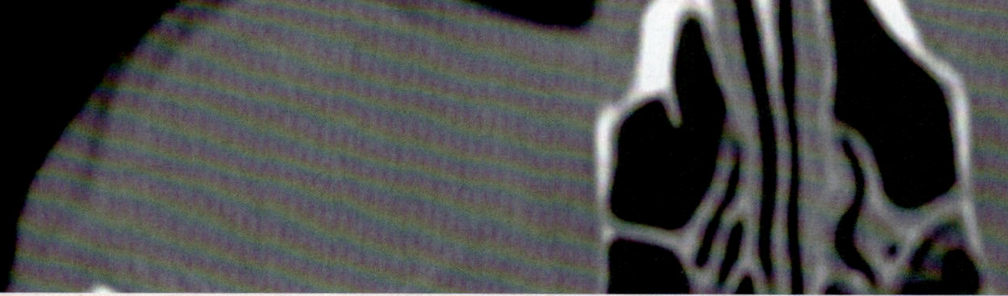

Orbit

Summary Thoughts: Sinus and Nose

Conditions related to the nose, nasal cavities (NC), and paranasal sinuses (PS) are some of the most common cases encountered by clinicians, prompting 25 million medical visits and costing $2 billion annually. Imaging is required when patients fail 1st-line treatments for inflammatory conditions, invasive disease or neoplasm is suspected, or presurgical planning becomes necessary. Given the complex bony architecture and the intervening air-filled spaces, **CT is the most common modality** for evaluating the sinonasal (SN) region. CT determines the extent of disease and is also helpful for surgical planning and intraoperative guidance. MR can be complementary in the evaluation of advanced infectious or inflammatory disease, and in the evaluation of neoplasms. As in all regions of the head and neck, information such as patient demographics, presenting symptoms, and clinical exam findings are critical for interpreting imaging studies of this area.

The NC is centrally located and is surrounded by the PS. It is important to understand the drainage pathways of the PS as one can then predict **patterns of disease** based upon the site of an obstructing lesion. However, this can be challenging due to limitless anatomic variation. Infectious/inflammatory diseases are by far the most common pathologies. Neoplasms, both benign and malignant, are relatively rare. They tend to present at an advanced stage and encroach upon vital structures (orbit, skull base, and cranial nerves). These tumors are difficult to completely resect and are associated with high surgical morbidity. Presurgical tumor mapping in such cases is best accomplished with multiplanar MR.

Imaging Approaches and Indications

CT is the preferred modality to evaluate inflammatory disease, depicting mucosal thickening, opacification, air-fluid levels, and soft tissue masses. CT easily depicts osseous changes such as remodeling, scalloping, hyperostosis, or erosion, and is sensitive for detecting Ca^{++} or bone in lesions such as osteomas, chronic fungal disease, fibroosseous lesions, chondrosarcoma, or inverted papilloma. **Coronal images** best demonstrate the anatomy of the **ostiomeatal unit** (OMU). CECT is usually reserved for complicated cases in which soft tissue abscess, neoplasm, or vascular complication (cavernous sinus thrombosis) is suspected.

MR is indicated for evaluation of **complex inflammatory disease and neoplasms**. It is optimal for assessing extension or invasion of disease beyond the SN cavities, evaluating perineural tumor spread, and differentiating tumor from postobstructive secretions.

Imaging Protocols

Historically, direct coronal images were obtained with patient in prone position and ≤ 3-mm slices angled perpendicular to the palate. With multidetector CT, coronal reformatted images can be generated from a thin-slice axial data set acquired in the supine position. This is preferred as images are less degraded by motion artifact and dental amalgam can be avoided. Axial source images can be used in image-guidance systems, obviating additional radiation for "treatment planning" CT prior to surgery. **Sagittal reformatted** images are helpful for delineating **frontal recess** (FR) and the sphenoethmoid region anatomy.

MR imaging protocols generally include axial and coronal T1, STIR, and T1 C+ images, typically with fat suppression.

Imaging Anatomy

The sinonasal region is composed of the NC and the surrounding PS. There are important anatomic relationships with adjacent structures including orbit, oral cavity, pterygopalatine fossa, and both the anterior and central skull base.

The SN cavities are pneumatized spaces within the maxillary, frontal, sphenoid, and ethmoid bones. Superiorly, the frontal sinuses border the anterior margin of the anterior cranial fossa. The cribriform plate (CP) and fovea ethmoidalis form the roof of the superior NC and ethmoid sinuses, respectively. The hard palate separates the NC from the oral cavity. The NC communicates posteriorly with the nasopharynx via the choanae. The orbits are separated from the ethmoid sinuses by the thin lamina papyracea and are separated from the maxillary sinuses by the orbital floors. Posterior to the maxillary sinuses are the pterygopalatine fossae, which communicate superiorly with the orbital apices, laterally with the masticator space, and posteriorly with central skull base.

The **NC is centrally located** and divided in the midline by the nasal septum. The posterior septum is bony and formed by the perpendicular plate of the ethmoid superiorly and vomer bone inferiorly. Anteriorly, the septum is cartilaginous. The bony superior, middle, and inferior turbinates project into the NC and divide the NC into inferior, middle, and superior meatuses. The middle turbinate is attached superiorly to the CP via the vertical lamella and posterolaterally to the lamina papyracea via the basal (ground) lamella.

The frontal sinuses are divided in the midline by an intersinus septum. Inferomedially, the frontal sinus narrows toward its ostium, which drains into its FR. The **FR is formed by the walls of surrounding structures**, best visualized on **sagittal reformations**. The drainage of the FR is determined by the insertion of the uncinate process. Most often, the uncinate inserts laterally onto the lamina papyracea and secretions drain into the middle meatus (MM). Less frequently, the uncinate inserts onto the anterior skull base or middle turbinate.

Paired groups of 13-18 air cells form the ethmoid sinuses. These cells are divided into anterior and posterior groups by the **basal lamella**. The anterior air cells drain into the anterior recess of the hiatus semilunaris and MM via the ethmoid bulla. The posterior air cells drain into the superior meatus and sphenoethmoidal recess (SER).

The maxillary sinuses lie lateral to the NC and inferior to the orbits. Each drains via its maxillary ostium into the infundibulum, then via the hiatus semilunaris into the MM.

The sphenoid sinuses are asymmetric air cells in the body of the sphenoid bone. Important surrounding structures include the maxillary division of CNV in the foramen rotundum laterally, the vidian nerve and artery in the vidian canal inferiorly, the optic nerves and sella superiorly, and the cavernous sinuses laterally. The sphenoid sinuses drain via their ostia into the SER.

The **OMU is a critical intersection** for drainage of the sinuses most affected by inflammatory disease (anterior ethmoid, maxillary, and frontal). Important components of the OMU include the ethmoid infundibulum, uncinate process, hiatus semilunaris, ethmoid bulla, and MM.

Differential Diagnosis of Sinonasal Lesion

Congenital	Benign tumors and tumor-like lesions	Anatomic variations
Nasolacrimal duct mucocele	Osteoma	Sinus hypo- or hyperpneumatization
Choanal atresia	Fibrous dysplasia	Nasal septal deviation and spurs
Nasal glioma	Ossifying fibroma	Frontal cells (types I-IV)
Nasal dermal sinus	Juvenile nasopharyngeal angiofibroma	**Ethmoid region**
Frontoethmoidal cephalocele	Inverted papilloma	Agger nasi cell
Pyriform aperture stenosis	Hemangioma	Infraorbital (Haller) cell
Infectious and inflammatory	Nerve sheath tumor	Supraorbital ethmoid cell
Acute rhinosinusitis	Benign mixed tumor	Large ethmoid bulla
Chronic rhinosinusitis	**Malignant tumors**	Sphenoethmoidal (Onodi) cell
Complications of rhinosinusitis	Squamous cell carcinoma	Asymmetric fovea ethmoidalis
Allergic fungal sinusitis	Esthesioneuroblastoma	Medial or dehiscent lamina papyracea
Mycetoma (fungal ball)	Adenocarcinoma	**Middle turbinate**
Invasive fungal sinusitis	Melanoma	Concha bullosa
Sinonasal polyposis	Non-Hodgkin lymphoma	Paradoxical curvature
Solitary sinonasal polyp	Sinonasal undifferentiated sarcoma	Hypoplasia
Mucocele	Adenoid cystic carcinoma	**Uncinate process**
Silent sinus syndrome	Chondrosarcoma	Pneumatized
Wegener granulomatosis	Osteosarcoma	Deviated
Sarcoidosis	Rhabdomyosarcoma	Fusion to middle turbinate or skull base
Nasal cocaine necrosis	Metastasis	Atelectatic (approximates orbital floor)

Approaches to Imaging Issues of Sinus and Nose

Congenital lesions can be classified as those presenting with **nasal obstruction vs. nasal mass**. Pyriform aperture stenosis and choanal atresia, for example, cause nasal obstruction without a mass. Frontonasal cephaloceles, dermoids, and extranasal gliomas present as extranasal masses. Frontoethmoidal cephaloceles, intranasal gliomas, and nasolacrimal duct mucoceles present with an intranasal mass. MR imaging can be very helpful for evaluating any connection to the intracranial space.

Rhinosinusitis (RS) is the **most common pathology** of the SN region. Acute RS is usually diagnosed clinically and may not require imaging. Because of the anatomy of the PS drainage pathways, predictable patterns of inflammatory disease exist based upon the point of obstruction. For example, obstruction of the MM would lead to disease in the ipsilateral frontal, anterior ethmoid, and maxillary sinuses. SER obstruction might lead to ipsilateral posterior ethmoid and sphenoid disease. Although uncommon, there are several forms of SN fungal disease. Mycetoma and allergic fungal sinusitis occur in immunocompetent patients and invasive fungal sinusitis (IFS) occurs in the immunocompromised or poorly controlled diabetics. It is important to note that **IFS may appear mass-like** or as **subtle infiltration of fat planes** adjacent to the PS at imaging. Granulomatous disease has a predilection for involving the nasal septum and turbinates.

There are a wide variety of SN neoplasms. Well-marginated tumors that cause bony remodeling suggest benign tumors, while infiltrative masses with osseous destruction suggest malignant lesions. The site of origin may also be predictive of histology. For instance, osteomas most often arise in the frontal and ethmoid sinuses, juvenile nasopharyngeal angiofibromas (JNA) arise in the posterior NC at the sphenopalatine foramen, inverted papillomas often arise along the lateral nasal wall, and esthesioneuroblastoma (ENB) typically arises near the CP. Squamous cell carcinoma is by far the **most common SN malignancy** and most often arises in the maxillary antrum. The imaging features of adenocarcinomas can be nonspecific, but they have a predilection for the ethmoid region. Three malignant neoplasms with a **predilection for the NC** include ENB, lymphoma, and melanoma.

Clinical Implications

It is important to note that studies have shown a poor correlation between symptoms of RS and CT findings. The diagnosis of RS is ultimately a clinical one. Lesions located within the NC can be evaluated with endoscopy. Lesions involving the PS are difficult to evaluate with scopes, so imaging is important for full evaluation.

Disease of the SN cavities often presents with nonspecific symptoms, such as nasal obstruction, discharge, and craniofacial pain. Additional symptoms, such as epistaxis, may be indicative of a vascular lesion (JNA or ENB). Pain may also be caused by mucoceles or neoplasms, while paresthesias can be linked to malignancies such as adenoid cystic carcinoma.

Selected References

1. Amine MA et al: Anatomy and complications: safe sinus. Otolaryngol Clin North Am. 48(5):739-48, 2015
2. Charles Burke M et al: A practical approach to the imaging interpretation of sphenoid sinus pathology. Curr Probl Diagn Radiol. 44(4):360-70, 2015
3. Vaid S et al: An imaging checklist for pre-FESS CT: framing a surgically relevant report. Clin Radiol. 66(5):459-70, 2011
4. Hoang JK et al: Multiplanar sinus CT: a systematic approach to imaging before functional endoscopic sinus surgery. AJR Am J Roentgenol. 194(6):W527-36, 2010

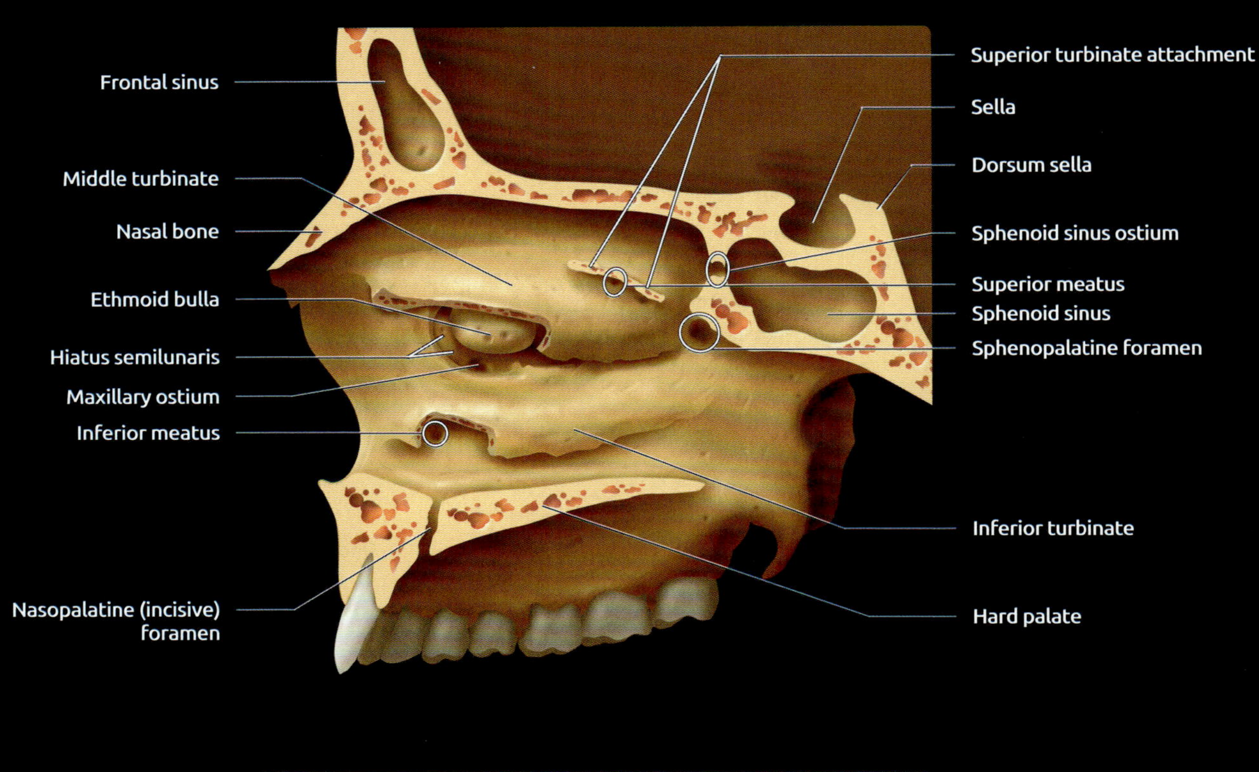

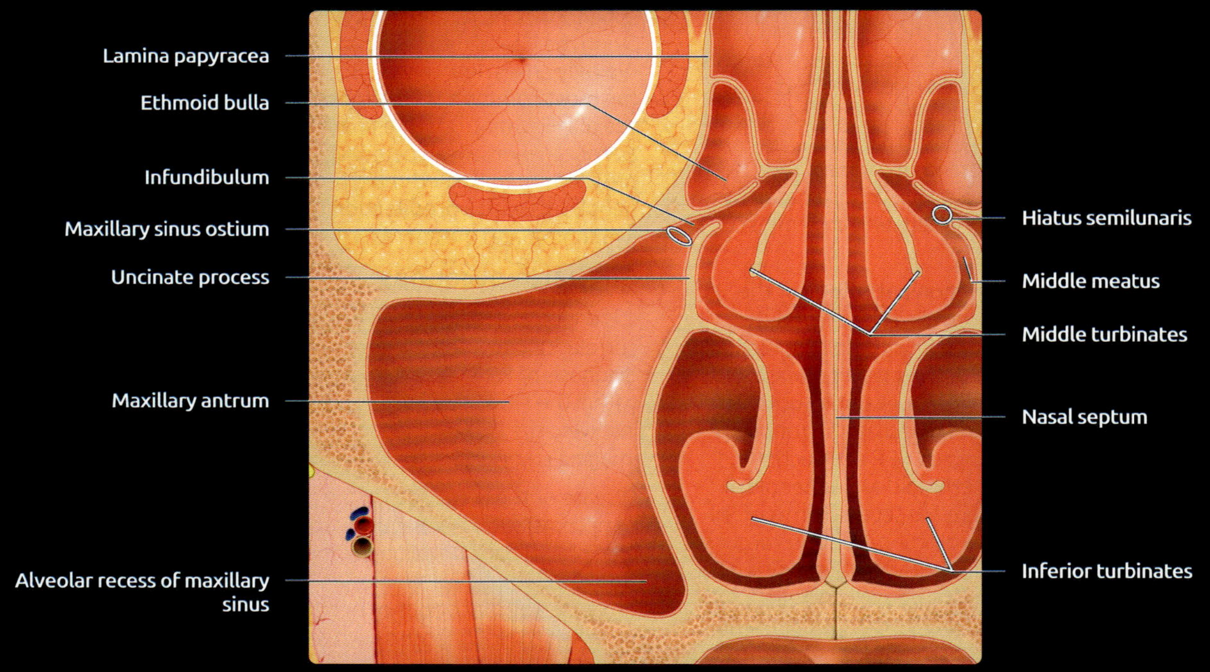

(Top) *Sagittal graphic demonstrates the osseous anatomy of the lateral nasal wall. The superior turbinate and portions of the middle and inferior turbinates have been resected. The superior, middle, and inferior meatuses drain inferior to their respective turbinates. The ipsilateral frontal, anterior ethmoid, and maxillary sinuses ultimately drain into the middle meatus. The nasolacrimal duct drains into the inferior meatus. The sphenoid ostium is located along the anterior sphenoid sinus wall and drains into the sphenoethmoidal recess.* **(Bottom)** *Coronal graphic of magnified right sinonasal region shows the important structures around the ostiomeatal unit. The vertically oriented uncinate process is bounded laterally by the ethmoid infundibulum, superiorly by the hiatus semilunaris, and medially by the middle meatus. The ethmoid bulla is the dominant anterior ethmoid cell located superior to the uncinate. The middle meatus drains beneath the middle turbinate.*

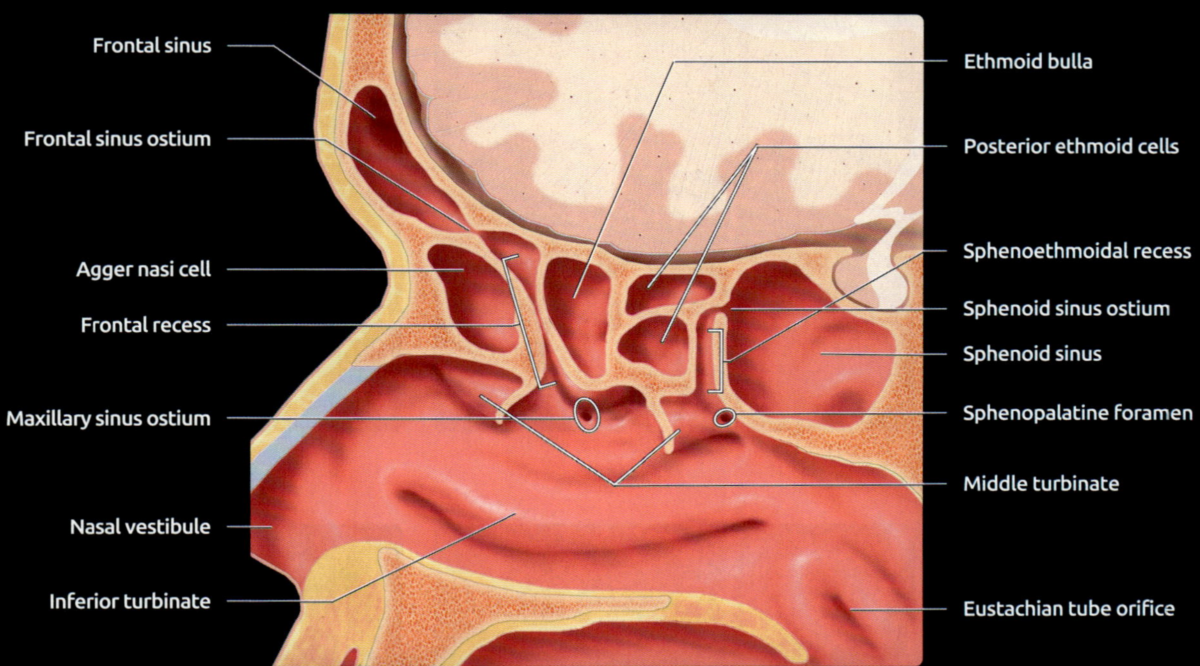

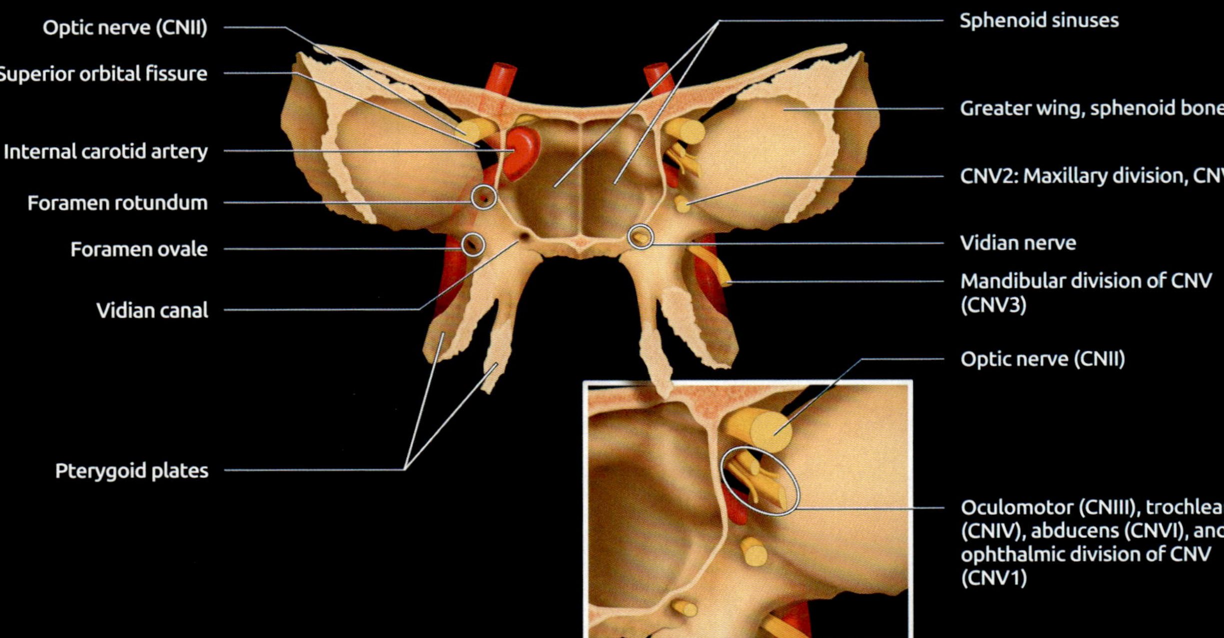

(Top) *Sagittal graphic shows the frontal sinus drainage pathway. The frontal sinus narrows inferiorly to its ostium. Secretions drain through the ostium into the frontal recess (FR). The FR is not a true duct in that its walls are composed of adjacent anatomy. In the graphic, the FR is bounded anteriorly by an agger nasi cell & posteriorly by the ethmoid bulla. Note that FR drainage may vary based upon the point of insertion of the uncinate process.* **(Bottom)** *Coronal graphic shows the important anatomy surrounding the sphenoid sinuses. The cavernous portions of the internal carotid arteries lie lateral and posterior to the sinuses. At the orbital apex, the optic nerve can be seen traversing the optic canal. The maxillary division of CNV in the foramen rotundum and the vidian nerve are positioned lateral and inferior to the sinus, respectively. Multiple cranial nerves pass through the superior orbital fissure (see inset) into the orbit, including CNs III, IV, and VI as well as the ophthalmic division on CNV.*

(Left) *Coronal bone CT shows the paired frontal sinuses separated by the intersinus septum. The most anterior ethmoid-type cells, the agger nasi, can be seen. Notice the air-filled lacrimal sac on the left.* **(Right)** *Coronal bone CT shows the medial and lateral lamellae of the cribriform plate forming the roof of the nasal cavity. The fovea ethmoidalis forms the ethmoid sinus roof. Note the patent frontal recesses leading to the middle meatuses.*

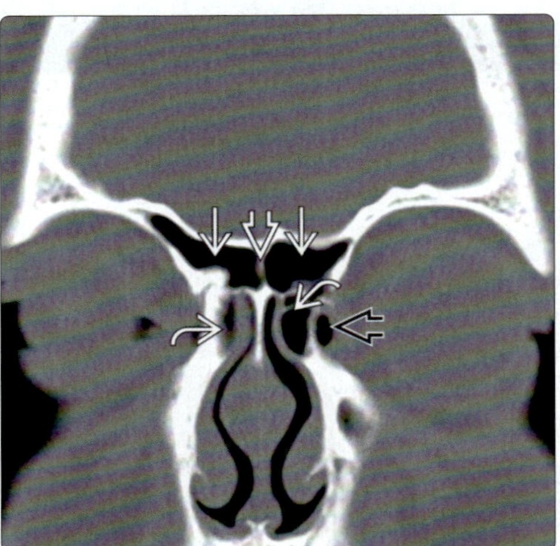

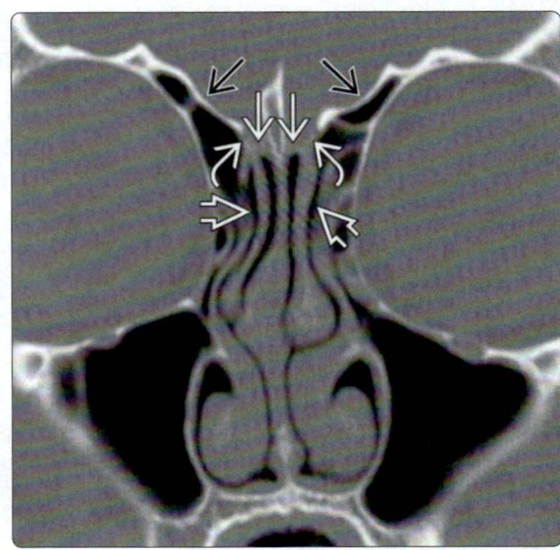

(Left) *Sagittal CT reconstruction shows the frontal sinus drainage pathway. The sinus drains inferiorly into the frontal recess. A frontal cell is anterior to the recess and the ethmoid bulla is posterior. Note the middle and inferior turbinates.* **(Right)** *Axial T1 MR shows the paired maxillary sinuses lateral to the nasal cavity. Note the inferior turbinates, midline nasal septum, and air-filled nasolacrimal ducts above the inferior meatuses.*

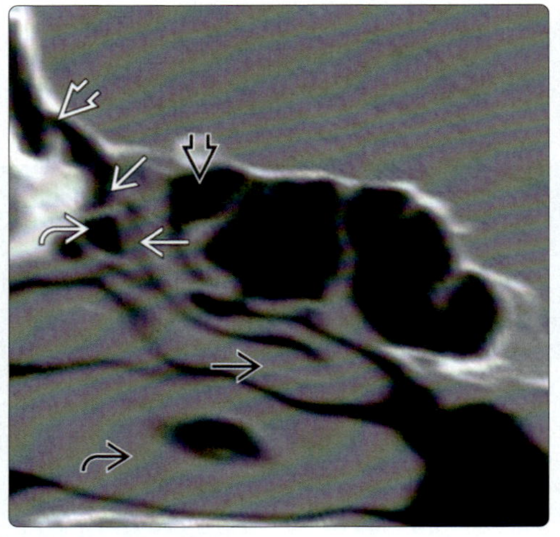

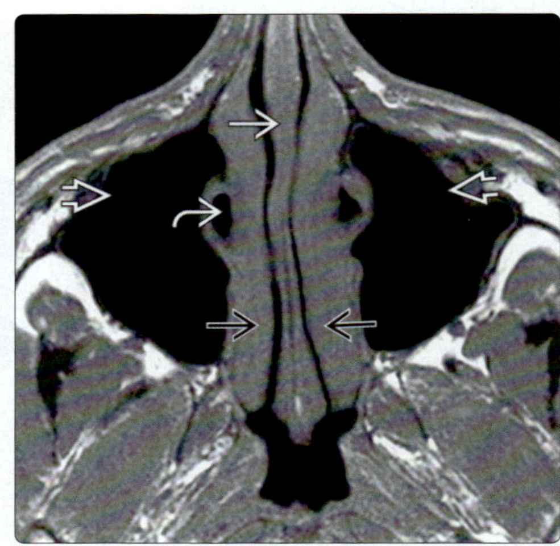

(Left) *Sagittal CT reconstruction shows the nasolacrimal duct draining into the inferior meatus. Note the pterygopalatine fossa (PPF) posterior to the maxillary sinus.* **(Right)** *Coronal bone CT at the level of the ostiomeatal units shows the uncinate processes, ethmoid bullae, and middle turbinates. They are pneumatized as is the right inferior turbinate. The middle meatus lies between the uncinate and middle turbinate. A retention cyst blocks the left maxillary ostium.*

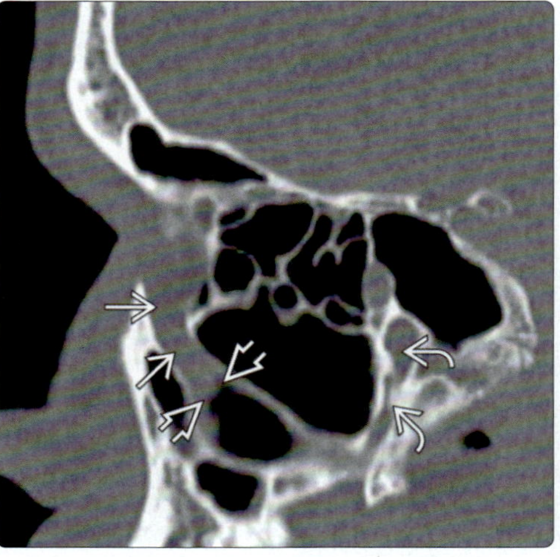

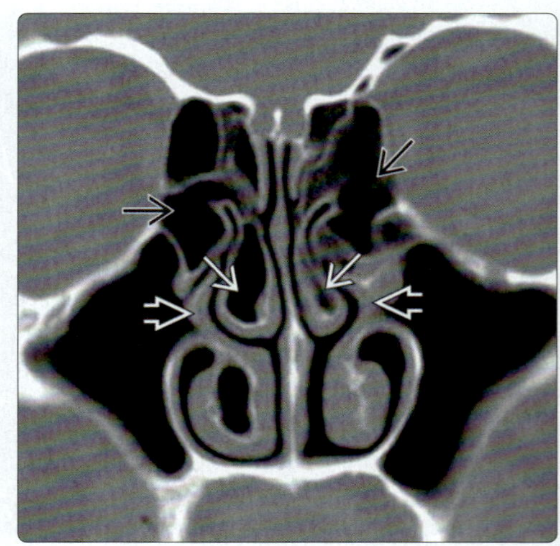

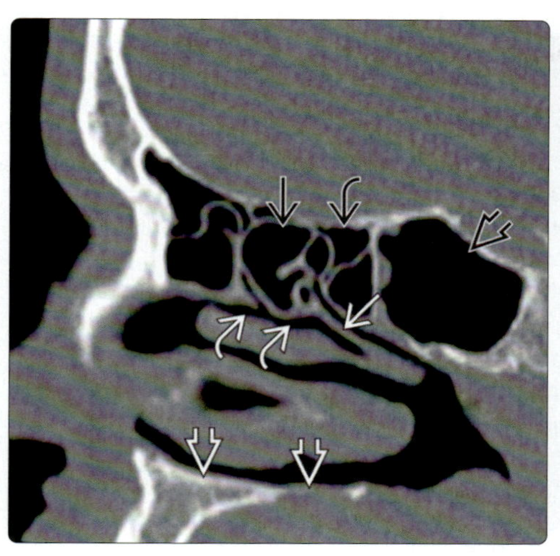

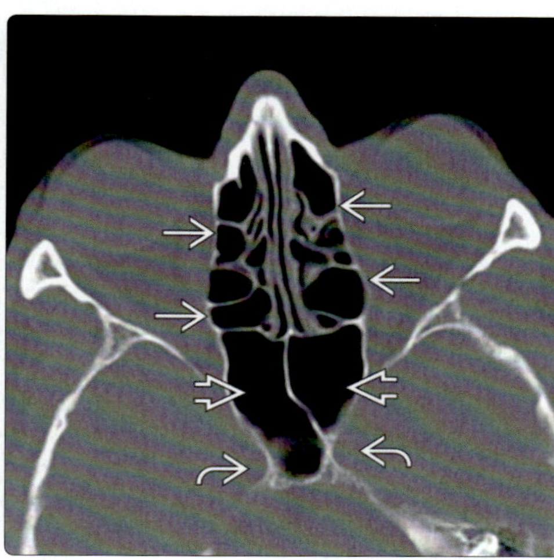

(Left) *Sagittal CT reconstruction shows anterior ➡ and posterior ➡ ethmoid cells and the sphenoid sinus ➡. The lateral attachment of the middle turbinate (basal lamella) is seen ➡. Note the hiatus semilunaris ➡. The palate is noted inferiorly ➡.* **(Right)** *Axial bone CT shows the thin lamina papyracea ➡ separating the ethmoid air cells from the orbits. The sphenoid sinuses ➡ are separated by an intersinus septum. The internal carotid arteries ➡ are immediately adjacent to the sinuses.*

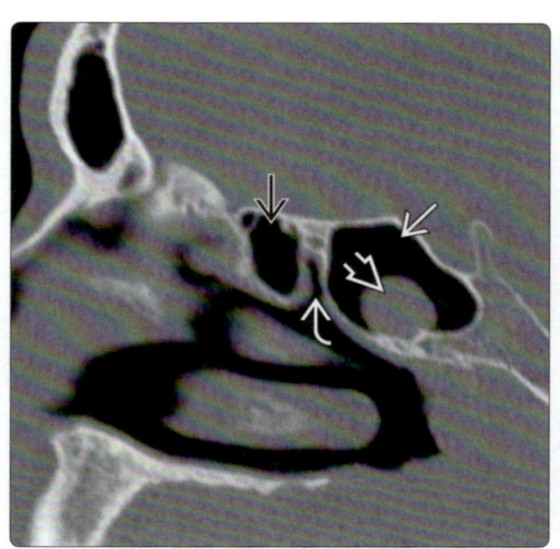

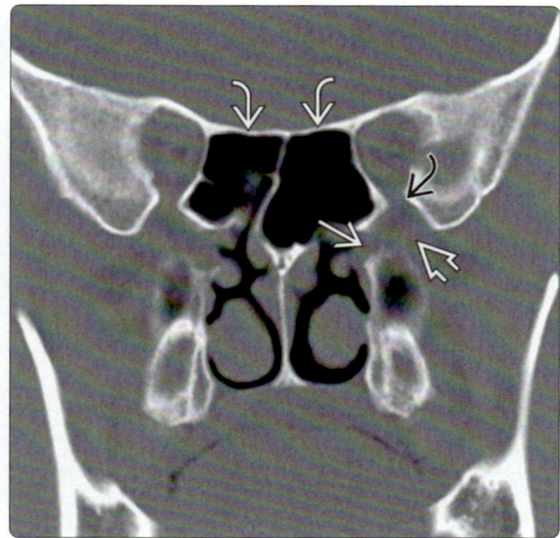

(Left) *Sagittal CT reconstruction shows the sphenoethmoidal recess ➡ bounded anteriorly by the most posterior ethmoid air cell ➡ and posteriorly by the sphenoid sinus ➡. A retention cyst is seen in the sphenoid sinus ➡.* **(Right)** *Coronal bone CT shows the sphenopalatine foramen ➡ connecting the nasal cavity to the PPF ➡. The inferior orbital fissure ➡ extends from the PPF to the orbital apex. Note the planum sphenoidale above the sphenoid sinuses ➡.*

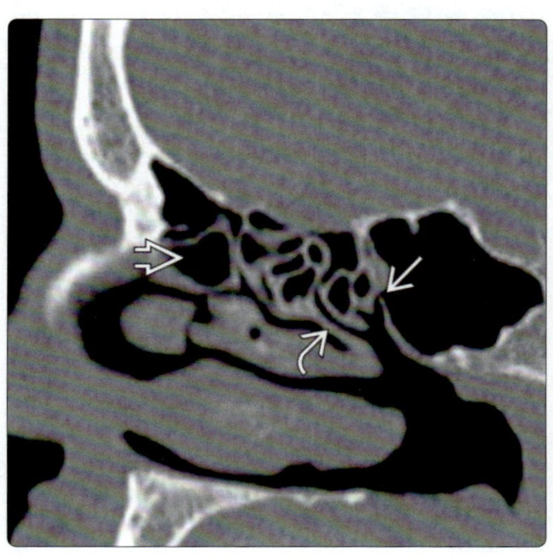

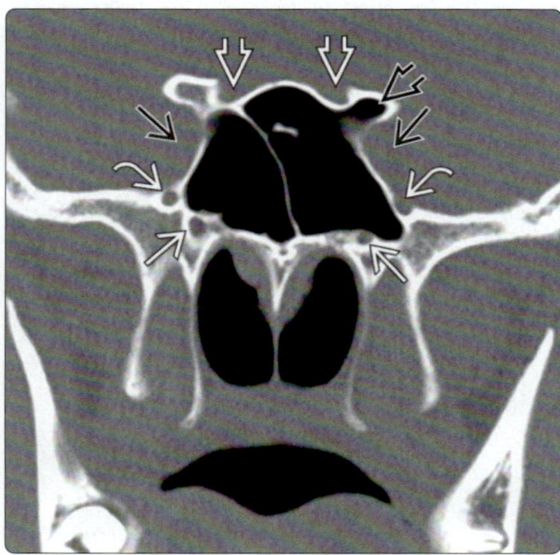

(Left) *Sagittal CT reconstruction shows the sphenoid sinus ostium ➡ along the anterior wall of the sphenoid sinus. An agger nasi cell ➡ & the basal lamella ➡ are also seen.* **(Right)** *Coronal bone CT shows the important structures around the sphenoid sinuses. The vidian canals ➡ are noted along the sphenoid sinus floors and the foramen rotundum ➡ is located laterally. The optic nerves lie medial to the anterior clinoids ➡ and the cavernous sinuses lie laterally ➡. Pneumatization of the clinoid ➡ is variant anatomy.*

KEY FACTS

TERMINOLOGY

- Synonym: Congenital dacryocystocele

IMAGING

- NECT: Well-defined, cystic, medial canthal mass in contiguity with enlarged nasolacrimal duct (NLD) in newborn
  - Unilateral or bilateral
- Absent or minimal wall enhancement (unless infected)
- Coronal/sagittal reformatted images show contiguity of cyst at lacrimal sac with NLD and inferior meatus cyst

TOP DIFFERENTIAL DIAGNOSES

- Orbital dermoid and epidermoid
  - Lateral > medial canthus
- Dacryocystocele, acquired lacrimal sac cyst
  - If dacryocystitis: Inflammatory changes in surrounding soft tissues and enhancing cyst rim around cyst

PATHOLOGY

- Tears and mucus accumulate in NLD with imperforate Hasner membrane (distal duct obstruction)

CLINICAL ISSUES

- Proximal lesion: Small, round, bluish, medial canthal mass identified at birth or shortly thereafter
- Distal lesion: Nasal airway obstruction with respiratory distress if bilateral
- Most common abnormality of infant lacrimal apparatus
- Treatment options
  - Daily **manual massage** ± prophylactic systemic/topical antibiotics
  - 10% require probing with irrigation ± Silastic stent placement
  - If endonasal component and no response to other options above → endoscopic resection with marsupialization

(Left) *Axial CECT in a 4 day old with bilateral lacrimal sac enlargement, bluish in color, and left-side draining purulent material demonstrates bilateral lacrimal sac enlargement ➔. Notice the bilateral enlargement of the lacrimal sac fossa ➔ on both sides.* **(Right)** *Coronal T2WI MR in an infant shows hyperintense signal in the mucoceles, not only at the inferior nasolacrimal ducts ➔, but also at the level of the lacrimal sacs ➔. Nasal obstruction results in difficulty breathing, as infants are obligate nose breathers.*

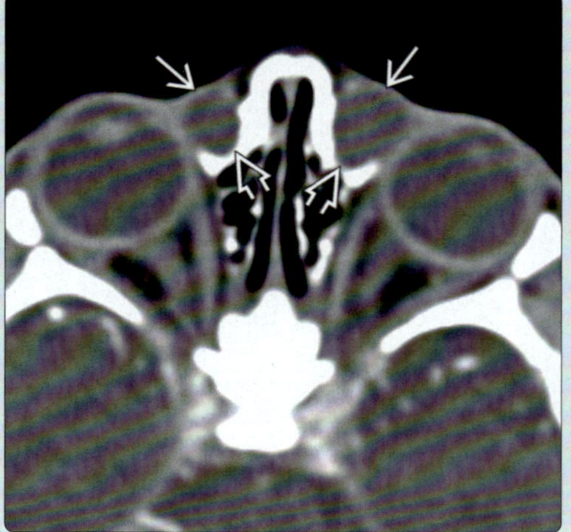

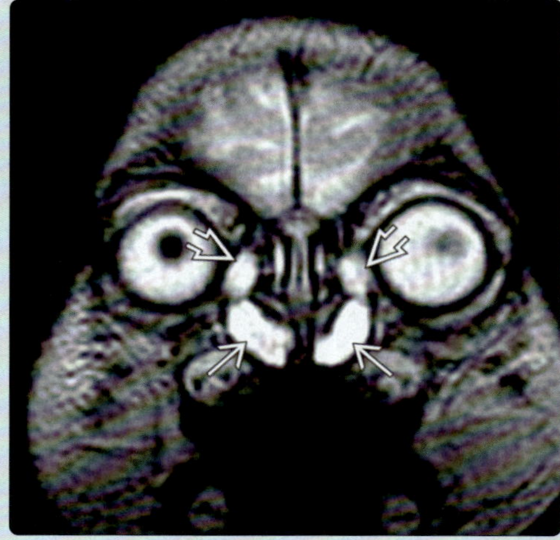

(Left) *Axial CECT in an infant demonstrates a cystic mass ➔ with an enhancing rim in the medial right orbit consistent with a mucocele. There is also enlargement of the right lacrimal sac fossa ➔. Note the normal left lacrimal sac fossa ➔. There is a mild amount of right preseptal periorbital soft tissue swelling ➔ consistent with secondary cellulitis.* **(Right)** *Axial CECT in the same patient shows extension of the mucocele inferiorly to the level of the inferior meatus ➔. The lesion obstructs the right nasal cavity at that level.*

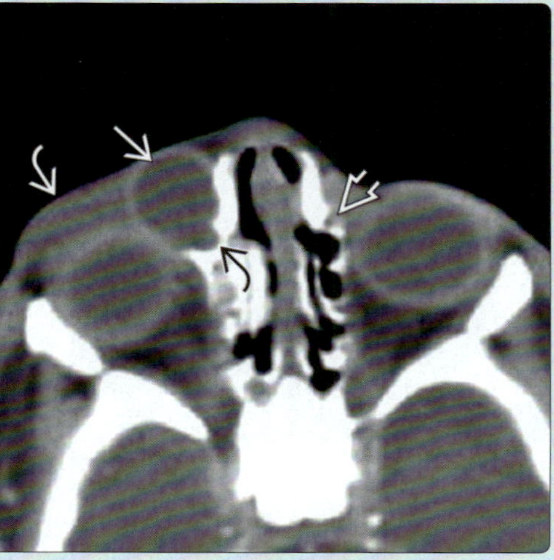

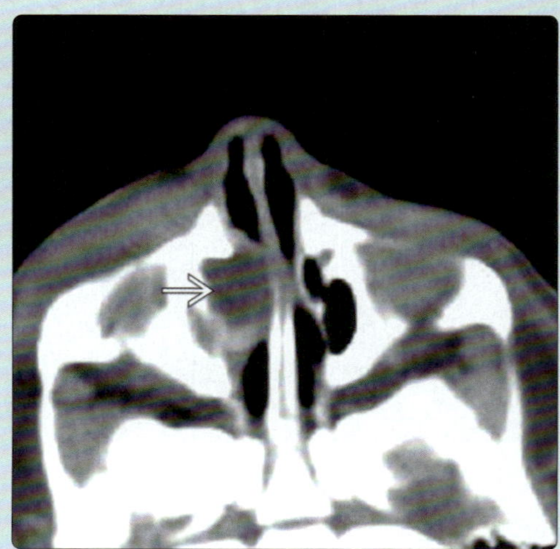

KEY FACTS

TERMINOLOGY

- Congenital obstruction of posterior nasal apertures

IMAGING

- NECT (bone CT) preferred imaging tool
  - Unilateral or bilateral narrowing of posterior nasal cavity with membranous or osseous obstruction of choana
- Bone CT findings
  - Thickening of vomer
  - Medial bowing of posterior maxilla
  - Unilateral in up to 75%: Right > left
  - Bilateral in up to 25%
    - 75% of bilateral have other anomalies

TOP DIFFERENTIAL DIAGNOSES

- Choanal stenosis
  - More common than true choanal atresia
- Pyriform aperture stenosis
  - Narrowed anterior nasal passage
- Nasolacrimal duct mucocele
  - Bilobed cysts in nasolacrimal fossae-inferior meatus
- Nasal foreign body

PATHOLOGY

- Choanal atresia types
  - Mixed bony and membranous atresia in up to 70%
  - Purely bony atresia in up to 30%

CLINICAL ISSUES

- Most common congenital intranasal lesion
- Bilateral choanal atresia → respiratory distress in newborn
- Unilateral choanal atresia: Chronic, purulent unilateral rhinorrhea with mild airway obstruction
- Treatment options
  - Membranous atresias: Perforated with nasogastric tube
  - Endoscopic/laser-assisted removal of blockage
  - Bilateral bony atresias require transpalatal resection of vomer with choanal reconstruction

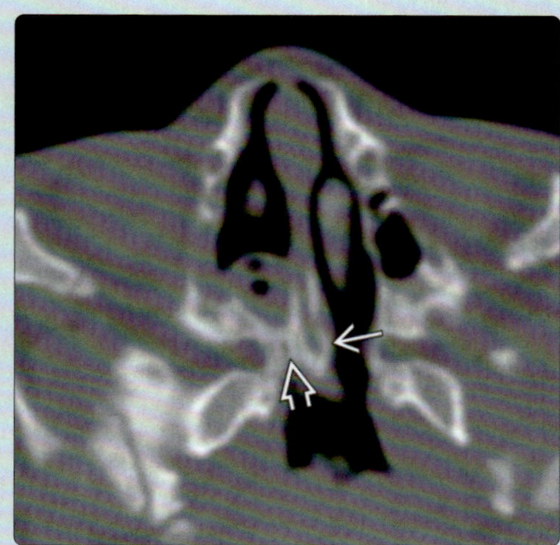

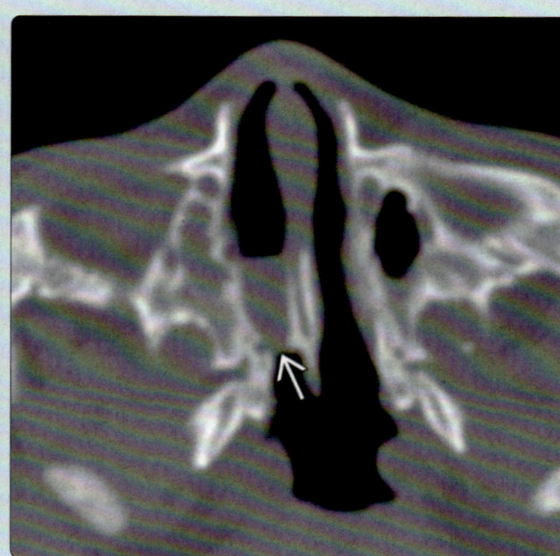

(Left) *Axial bone CT through the upper choana in a child with mixed bony/osseous choanal atresia shows osseous choanal obstruction secondary to an enlarged vomer ➡ fused to the thickened, medially positioned posterior maxilla ➡.* **(Right)** *Axial bone CT through the mid choana in the same patient shows membranous atresia ➡ bridging the narrowed inferior aspect of the choana. Notice also the retained nasal secretions on the right, secondary to obstruction of the choana.*

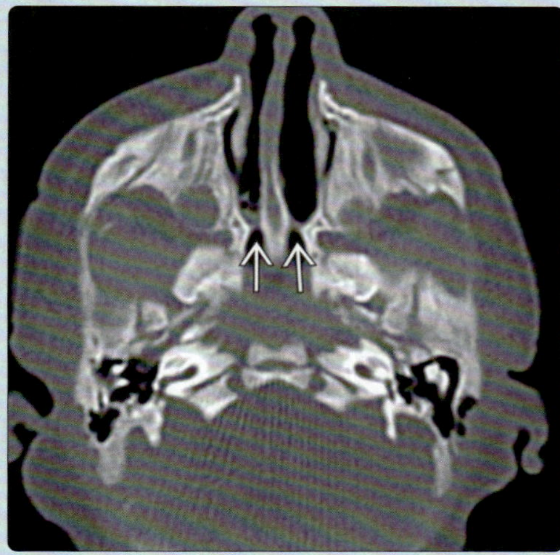

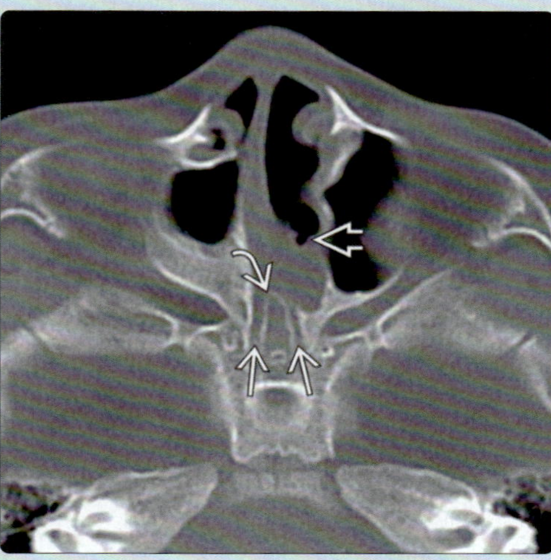

(Left) *Axial bone CT in a child with CHARGE syndrome demonstrates bilateral choanal obstruction secondary to linear membranes ➡ and mildly thickened and medially positioned posterior maxilla, typical of mixed choanal atresia.* **(Right)** *Axial bone CT in a newborn with complex nasal anomalies shows bilateral choanal atresia ➡, aplasia of the right nasal cavity, fluid layer in the left nasal cavity ➡, and thickened vomer ➡.*

KEY FACTS

TERMINOLOGY

- Developmental mass of **dysplastic neurogenic tissue** sequestered & isolated from subarachnoid space
  - "**Glioma**" is **misnomer** as is nonneoplastic tissue
    - Better term = **nasal glial heterotopia**
  - Extranasal glioma (ENG), intranasal glioma (ING)

IMAGING

- Well-circumscribed soft tissue mass at superior nasal dorsum (ENG) or within nasal cavity (ING) with no connection to brain
- Best imaging tool: Multiplanar MR; CT for skull base
  - May show pedicle of fibrous tissue (not brain parenchyma) between ING & intracranial cavity
  - MR better than CT for differentiating NG from cephalocele or dermoid
  - Gyral structure of gray matter rarely visible
  - Commonly shows hyperintensity related to gliosis

TOP DIFFERENTIAL DIAGNOSES

- Frontoethmoidal cephalocele
- Nasal dermal sinus
- Sinonasal solitary polyp

PATHOLOGY

- Similar spectrum of congenital anomalies as frontoethmoidal cephaloceles
  - Does **not** contain CSF contiguous with subarachnoid or intraventricular spaces
- **ENG: 60%**; **ING: 30%**; other sites: 10%
- Rarely associated with other brain or systemic anomalies

CLINICAL ISSUES

- Usually identified at birth
- Treatment of choice is complete surgical resection
  - ENG without intracranial connection removed via external incision with stalk dissection
  - ING, no intracranial connection: Remove endoscopically

(Left) *Sagittal graphic of a nasal glioma shows a mass of dysplastic glial tissue ➡ along the nasal dorsum. Notice the absence of a connection to the intracranial contents.* **(Right)** *Sagittal T2 MR in a 3 day old with a nasal mass demonstrates an intermediate signal intensity intranasal glioma ➡ without intracranial extension.*

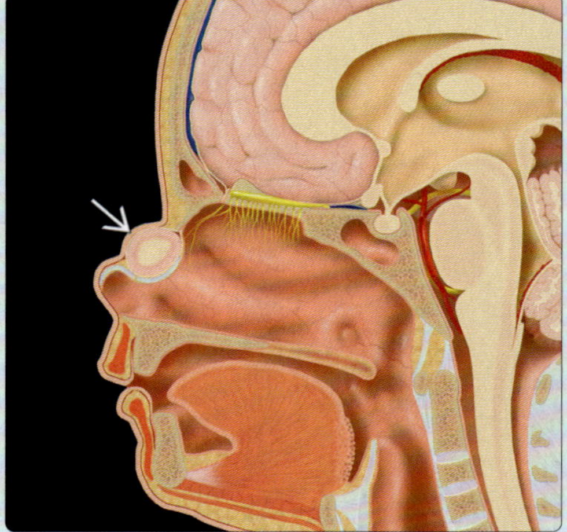

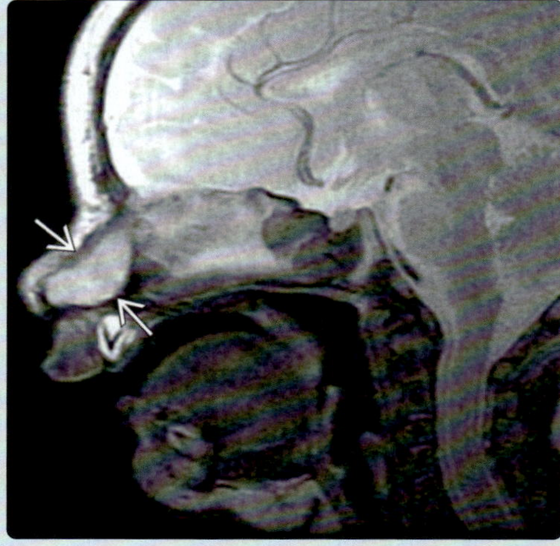

(Left) *Coronal NECT shows a well-defined, somewhat polypoid soft tissue mass ➡, consistent with an intranasal glioma, within the left nasal cavity. The nasal septum is slightly deviated toward the right. No definite connection to the frontal lobe parenchyma is appreciated.* **(Right)** *Axial CECT in same patient demonstrates a left-sided intranasal glioma ➡ widening the anterior nasal vault.*

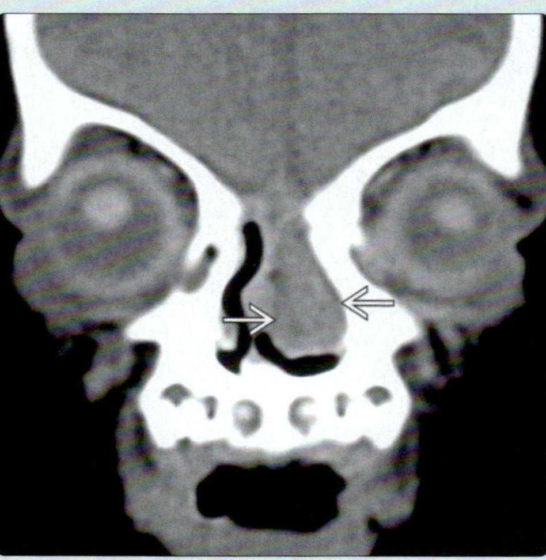

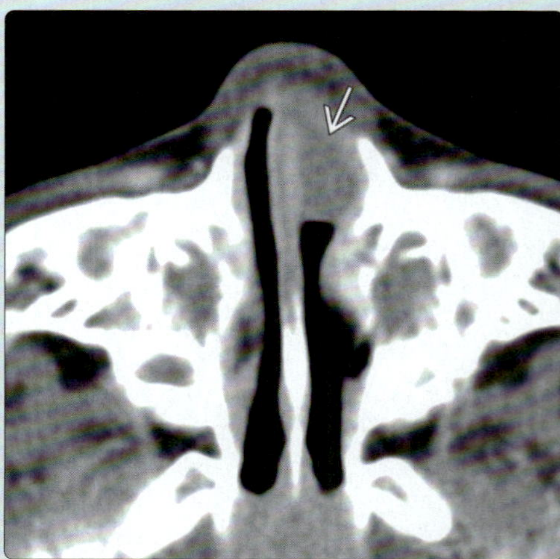

KEY FACTS

TERMINOLOGY

- Defective embryogenesis of anterior neuropore resulting any mixture of dermoid cyst, epidermoid cyst, &/or sinus tract in frontonasal region

IMAGING

- Midline location anywhere from nasal tip to anterior skull base at foramen cecum
- CT findings
  - Bifid crista galli with large foramen cecum
  - Fluid attenuation tract (sinus)/cyst or fat-containing mass (dermoid) from nasal dorsum to skull base within nasal septum
- MR findings
  - Fluid signal tract in septum from nasal dorsum to skull base (sinus)
  - Focal low-signal (epidermoid) or high-signal (dermoid) mass found between tip of nose and apex of crista galli

TOP DIFFERENTIAL DIAGNOSES

- Fatty marrow in crista galli
- Nonossified foramen cecum
- Frontoethmoidal cephalocele
- Nasal glioma (nasal glial heterotopia)

PATHOLOGY

- Intracranial extension of nasal dermal sinus (NDS) in 20%
- Associated craniofacial anomalies in 15%

CLINICAL ISSUES

- Nasoglabellar mass (30%); nasal bridge skin pit at osteocartilaginous nasal junction ± **protruding hair**
- Treatment options: Complete surgical excision required to prevent recurrence and distorted nasal growth
  - 80% require extracranial excision only
  - Local procedure to remove pit and epidermoid/dermoid
  - 20% combined extracranial & intracranial resection, craniofacial approach

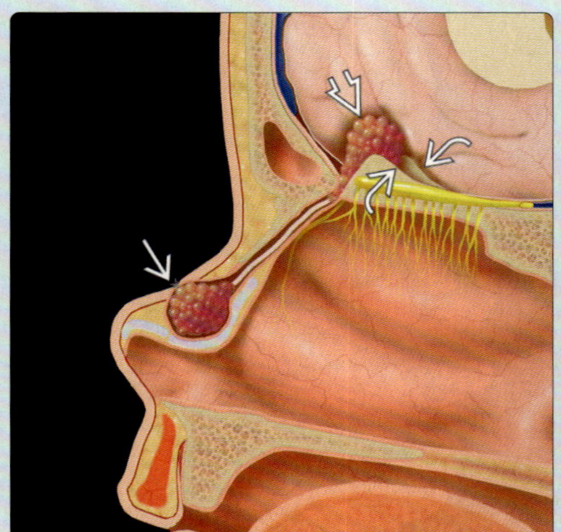

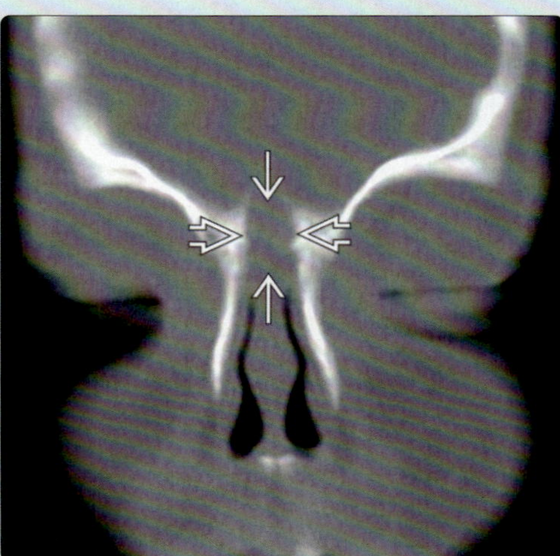

(Left) *Lateral graphic depicts a nasal dermal sinus with 2 dermoids. An extracranial dermoid is present just below a cutaneous nasal pit ➡. An intracranial dermoid ➡ splits a bifid crista galli ➡.* **(Right)** *Coronal bone CT demonstrates a nasal dermoid/epidermoid at the skull base. The low-attenuation midline mass ➡ causes remodeling of the adjacent bone ➡ at the margins of the foramen cecum.*

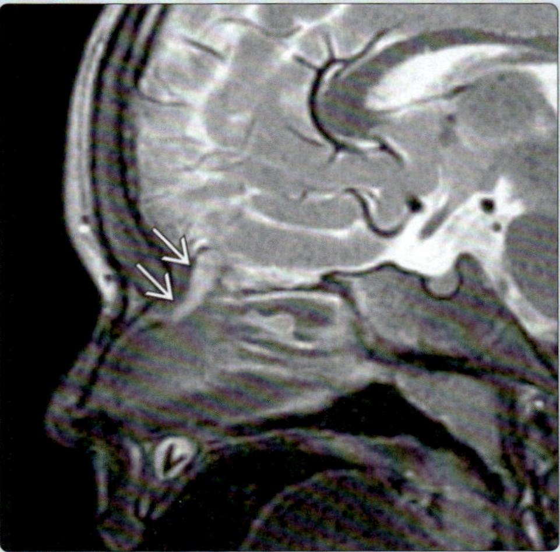

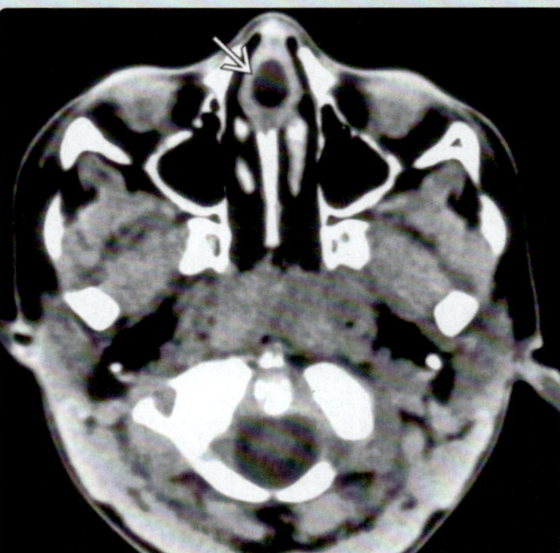

(Left) *Sagittal T2WI MR in a 3-year-old boy with a bump on the tip of the nose shows a hyperintense sinus tract ➡ extending from the anterior skull base into the nasal septum. The features are characteristic of a dermal sinus.* **(Right)** *Axial NECT demonstrates a low-attenuation dermoid ➡ centered in the cartilaginous portion of the nasal septum. The mass is slightly higher in attenuation than adjacent fat.*

KEY FACTS

TERMINOLOGY

- Congenital herniation of meninges, CSF ± brain tissue through mesodermal defect in anterior skull/skull base
- Synonym: Sincipital cephalocele

IMAGING

- Sagittal & coronal T1 & T2 MR optimal for showing contiguity of mass with intracranial contents
- NECT shows bony involvement details
- Heterogeneous, mixed-density mass (variable amounts CSF & parenchyma) extending through bony defect
  - Midline frontal: **Frontonasal** type (FNCeph)
  - Intranasal: **Nasoethmoidal** type (NECeph)
  - Inferomedial orbital: **Nasoorbital** type (NOCeph)

TOP DIFFERENTIAL DIAGNOSES

- Nasal glioma
- Orbital dermoid and epidermoid
- Nasal dermal sinus

PATHOLOGY

- **Frontonasal**
  - Protrudes through unobliterated **fonticulus frontalis**
- **Nasoethmoidal**
  - Protrudes through foramen cecum into **prenasal space**
- **Nasoorbital**
  - Protrudes into inferomedial orbit through defect in lacrimal/frontal process of maxillary bones

CLINICAL ISSUES

- Intracranial abnormalities in **~ 80%**
- F = 67%, M = 33%
- Treatment options
  - Biopsy contraindicated: CSF leak, seizures, meningitis
  - Complete surgical resection
    - Herniated brain tissue is dysfunctional (no neurological deficits result)
  - Meningeal & skull base defect repaired or CSF leak, meningitis, or recurrent herniation may result

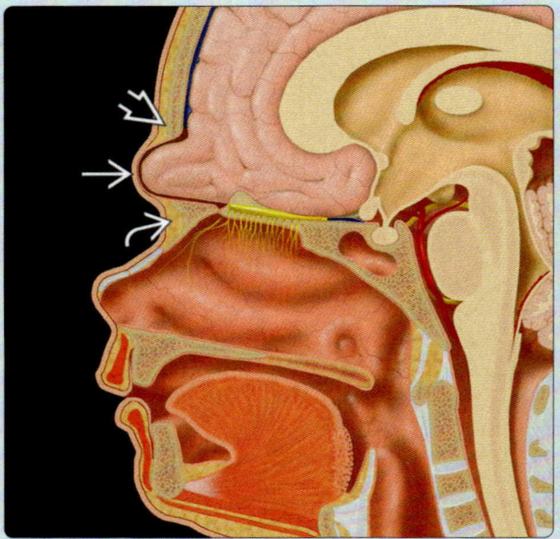

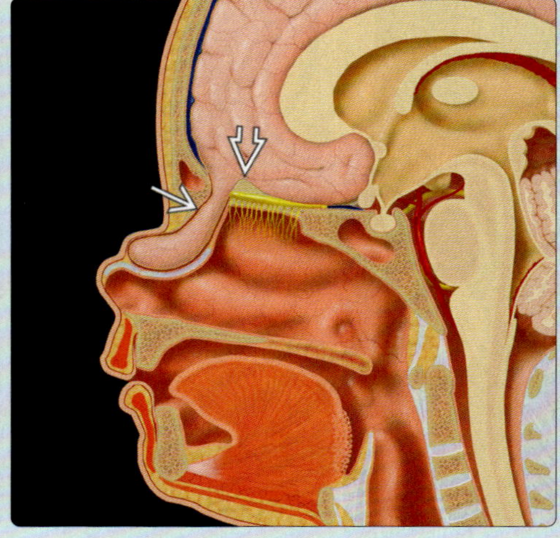

(Left) *Sagittal graphic of a frontonasal cephalocele shows herniation of the brain through a patent fonticulus frontalis ➡ between the frontal bones above ➡ and nasal bones below ➡.* **(Right)** *Nasoethmoidal cephalocele is depicted in this sagittal graphic. Notice the herniation of brain tissue ➡ into the nasal cavity through a patent foramen cecum. Also note the crista galli is positioned posterior to the skull base defect ➡.*

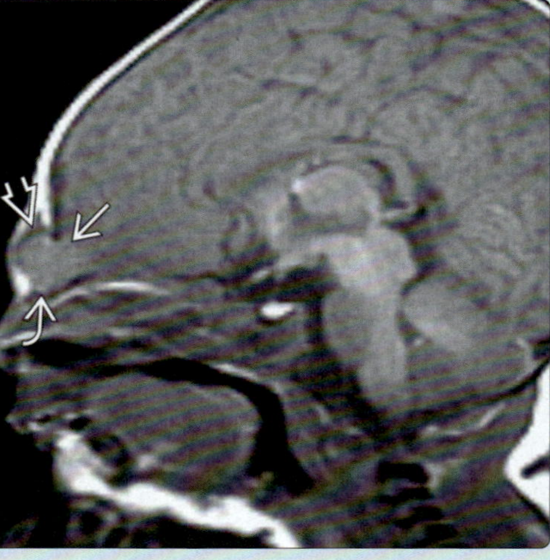

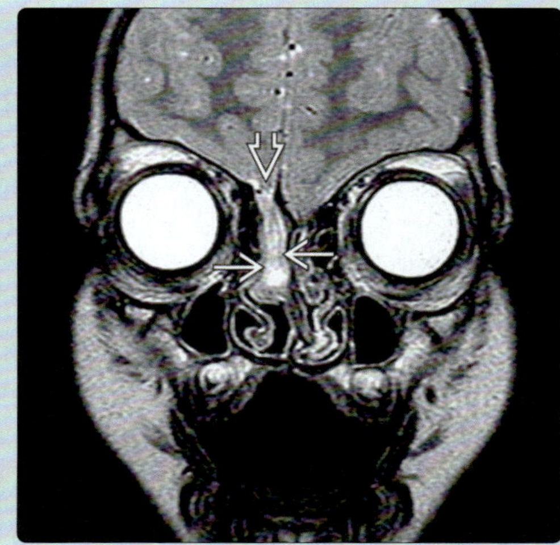

(Left) *Sagittal T1 MR in a 1 week old shows a frontonasal cephalocele ➡ with protrusion of the dysplastic-appearing inferior left frontal lobe through a patent fonticulus frontalis. The frontal bone ➡ is above and the nasal bone ➡ is below the cephalocele.* **(Right)** *Coronal T2 MR shows the typical appearance of a nasoethmoidal cephalocele. The gliotic brain parenchyma ➡ herniating into the nasal cavity is hyperintense. The cephalocele herniates through a skull base defect ➡ to the right of midline.*

KEY FACTS

TERMINOLOGY

- Congenital nasal pyriform aperture stenosis (CNPAS): Congenital narrowing of anterior bony nasal passageway

IMAGING

- Best tool: Bone CT in axial & coronal planes
  - Medial deviation of anterior maxillae ± thickening of nasal processes
  - Triangle-shaped palate
  - Abnormal maxillary dentition: **Solitary median maxillary central incisor (SMMCI)** (75%)
    - Add MR to exclude midline brain abnormalities

TOP DIFFERENTIAL DIAGNOSES

- Nasolacrimal duct mucoceles
  - Intranasal component narrows anterior nasal cavity
- Nasal choanal stenosis/atresia
  - Narrow posterior nasal passage by membrane or bone

PATHOLOGY

- CNPAS without SMMCI almost always isolated anomaly
- Solitary maxillary central incisor in 75% of cases
  - Associated with **holoprosencephaly**

CLINICAL ISSUES

- Respiratory distress in newborn/infant (obligate nasal breathers)
  - Can mimic choanal atresia/stenosis
  - Breathing problems may be triggered by URI
  - Symptoms may be more pronounced with feeding
- Narrow nasal inlet on clinical exam
- CNPAS 1/5 to 1/3 as common as choanal atresia
- Treated conservatively with special feeding techniques
- Surgery if persistent respiratory difficulty & poor weight gain
  - Resection of anteromedial maxilla ± anterior aspect of inferior turbinates & reconstruction of anterior nasal orifice

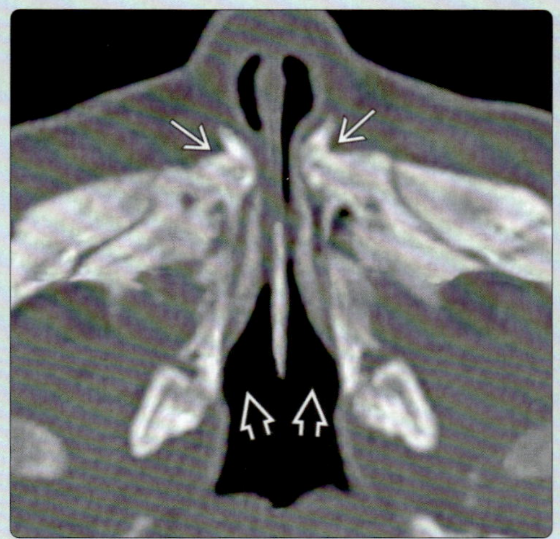

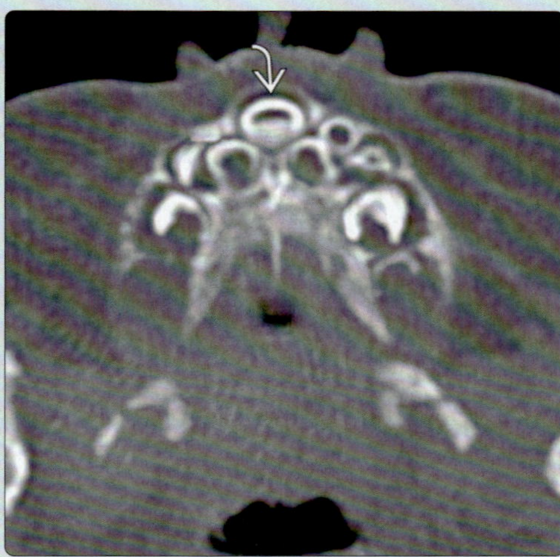

(Left) *Axial bone CT in a newborn shows the typical features of congenital nasal pyriform aperture stenosis. There is overgrowth of the anterior maxillae ➡ with marked narrowing of the anterior nasal passages. There is no associated choanal atresia ⇨.* **(Right)** *Axial bone CT at the level of the palate in the same patient shows a classic associated finding in patients with pyriform aperture stenosis, a solitary median maxillary central incisor or megaincisor ↪.*

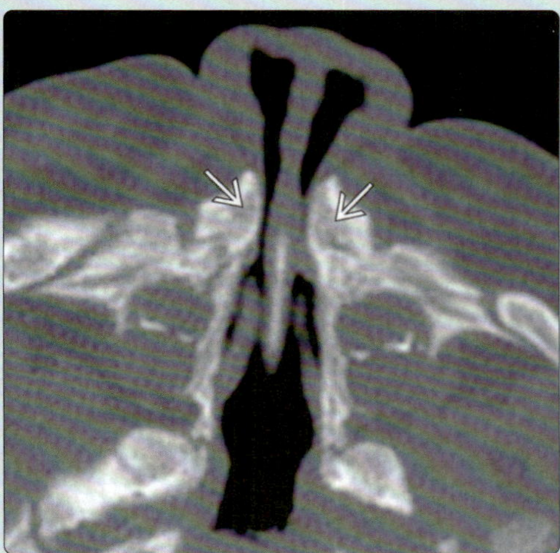

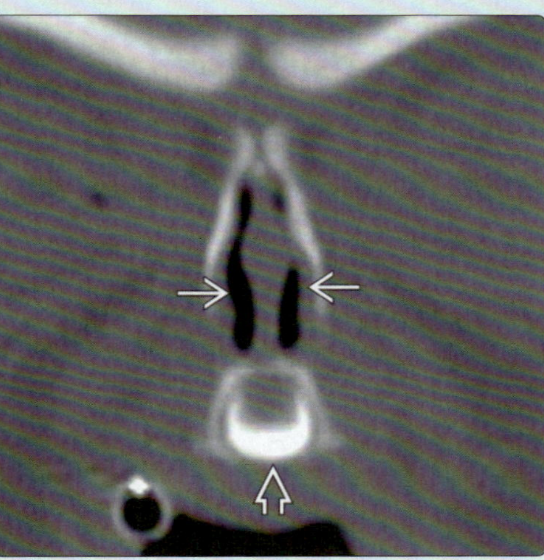

(Left) *Axial bone CT in a newborn with respiratory distress demonstrates bilateral congenital nasal pyriform aperture stenosis. The anterior and medial aspects of the maxillae are thickened ➡, causing narrowing of the anterior nasal airway.* **(Right)** *Coronal bone CT in the same patient demonstrates the narrowing of the anterior nasal airway ➡ bilaterally and the associated solitary maxillary central incisor ⇨.*

Acute Rhinosinusitis

KEY FACTS

TERMINOLOGY

- Acute inflammatory sinonasal process lasting ≤ 4 weeks
- Acute bacterial or rhinosinusitis (ARS), viral rhinosinusitis

IMAGING

- **ARS is clinical diagnosis** & imaging rarely necessary
- Radiography: Inaccurate & should be supplanted by CT
- NECT (bone CT): Confirms diagnosis, evaluates when medical therapy has failed, delineates anatomic variants, especially presurgical
  - CT technique: Axial ≤ 1-mm slice thickness + coronal & sagittal reconstructions
  - Best sign: **Air-fluid level** ± aerosolized secretions with mucosal thickening
  - Most common in ethmoid & maxillary sinuses; often asymmetric sinus involvement
- MR: Indicated for suspected complications; may overestimate clinical disease severity

TOP DIFFERENTIAL DIAGNOSES

- Noninfected secretions
- Pseudo fluid level from large maxillary polyp/cyst
- Posttraumatic blood level

PATHOLOGY

- Most cases follow viral URI; typically *Streptococcus pneumoniae, Moraxella catarrhalis, Haemophilus influenzae*

CLINICAL ISSUES

- **Clinical exam in ARS**: ≤ 4 weeks of **purulent** nasal drainage, nasal obstruction, & facial pain, pressure, fullness
- Viral rhinosinusitis usually self-limited; acute rhinosinusitis regional complications rare
- Treatment options
  - Medical: Saline nasal sprays & irrigants, mucolytics
  - Decongestants, antihistamines, antibiotics, nasal steroids
  - Drainage procedure in acute disease (frontal & sphenoid) to prevent regional complications

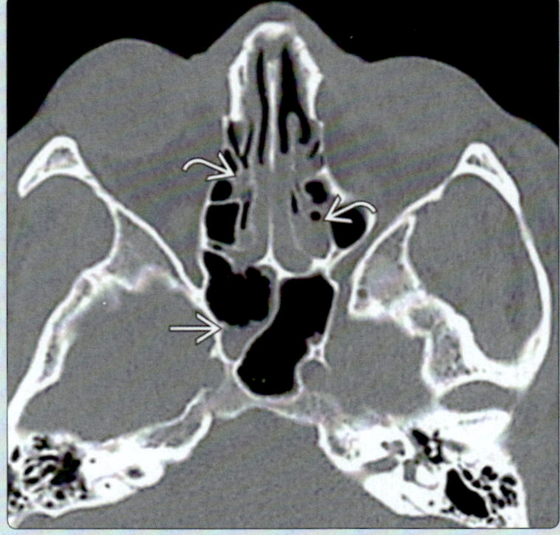

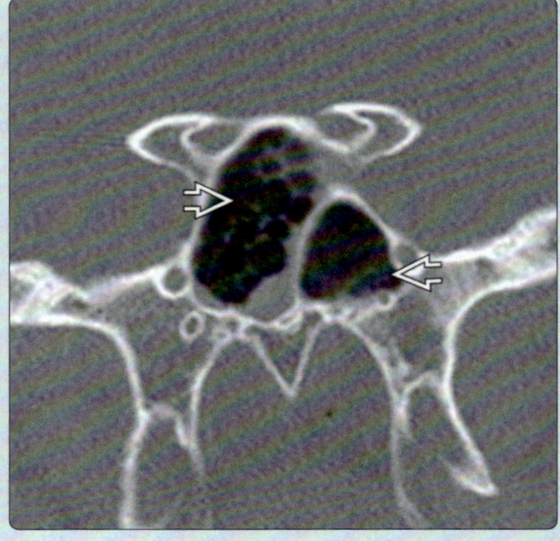

(Left) *Axial NECT in patient with purulent nasal discharge and headache shows patchy bilateral ethmoid sinus disease ➔ and an air-fluid level ➔ in the right sphenoid sinus corroborating the clinical history of acute bacterial rhinosinusitis (ABRS).* **(Right)** *NECT coronal reconstruction in the same patient demonstrates bubbly, frothy secretions in sphenoid sinuses ➔ in a patient with clinical diagnosis of ABRS.*

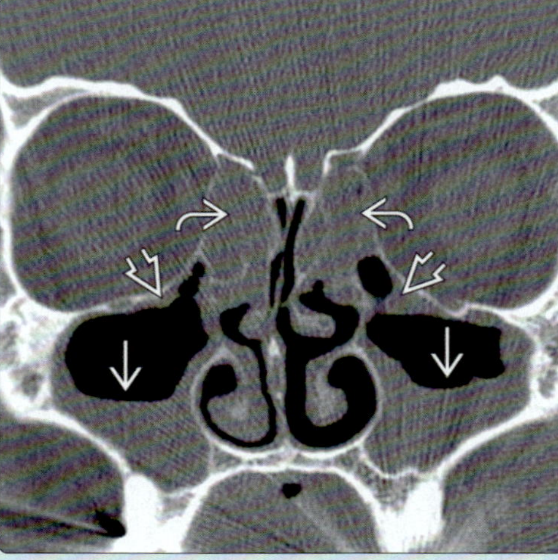

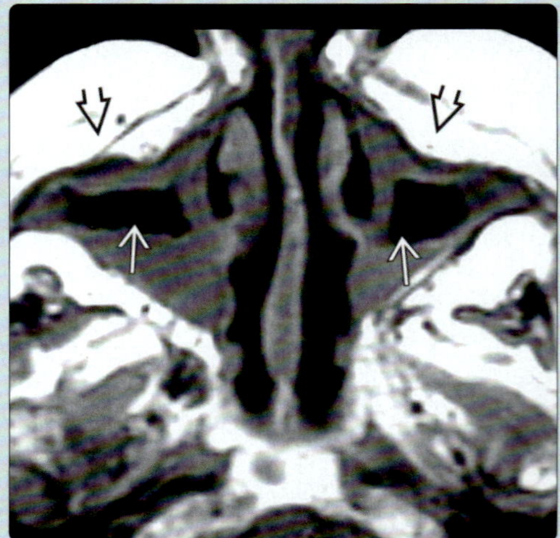

(Left) *Coronal bone CT shows bilateral maxillary and ethmoid sinusitis. Note air-fluid levels ➔ and mucosal thickening ➔ in maxillary sinuses and complete opacification of ethmoid sinuses ➔. Clinical findings drive the ABRS diagnosis as fluid may be just retained secretions as well.* **(Right)** *Axial T1WI MR in patient with clinical ABRS shows bilateral maxillary air-fluid levels ➔ and mucosal thickening ➔ on nondependent anterior sinus walls. The fluid is isointense to soft tissue on this T1 MR image.*

KEY FACTS

TERMINOLOGY

- Group of disorders characterized by inflammation of nose & paranasal sinuses ≥ 12 consecutive weeks' duration
- This broad definition is based on signs and symptoms and does not restrict to specific etiology

IMAGING

- Nonenhanced bone CT is gold standard for evaluation
  - Sinus mucosal thickening and opacification with thickening & sclerosis of bony walls
  - Involved sinus normal or decreased volume
  - Intrasinus hyperdensity or calcifications common
  - Mucus retention cysts and polyps are common
  - May show pattern of obstructive sinus disease

TOP DIFFERENTIAL DIAGNOSES

- Wegener granulomatosis, allergic fungal sinusitis, sinonasal polyposis, fungal mycetoma, sarcoidosis

PATHOLOGY

- Affects 12-14% of USA adult population
- Many factors & processes play role in etiology of chronic rhinosinusitis (CRS); causes are numerous, disparate, & frequently overlapping (i.e., allergy, anatomic variation)

CLINICAL ISSUES

- Chronic facial pain & pressure, headache, postnasal drip
  - Sinus CT shows finding of CRS
- Treatment options
  - Pharmacologic therapy: Antibiotics, decongestants, antihistamines, topical steroids (allergic cases)
  - Treatment of comorbid conditions (inhalant sensitivities, polyps, infections, immune deficiencies) critical for treatment success of CRS
  - Surgery in cases recalcitrant to medical therapy
    - Functional endoscopic sinus surgery to open natural sinus ostia

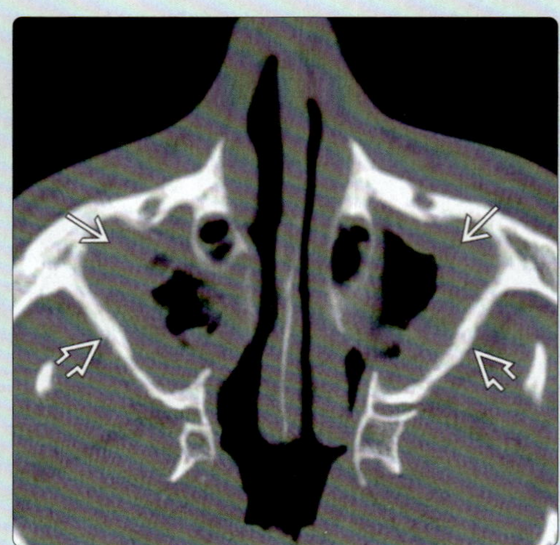

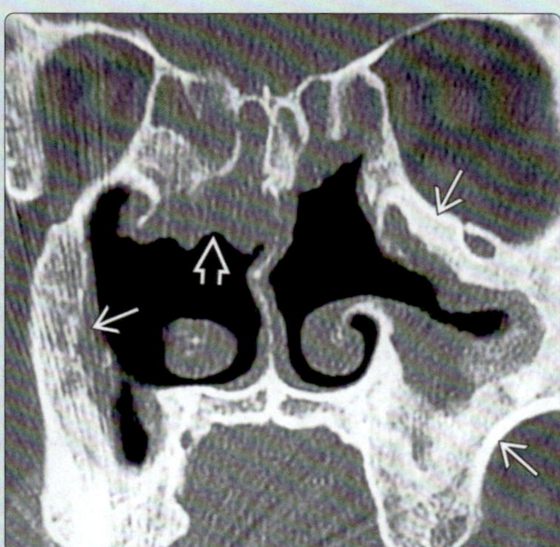

(Left) *Axial bone CT in a cystic fibrosis patient shows bilateral maxillary sinus mucosal thickening ➡ and thickening of the bony sinus walls (osteitis) ➡ consistent with chronic inflammatory disease.* **(Right)** *Coronal bone CT shows marked diffuse chronic osteitis of the sinus walls ➡ in a patient with chronic rhinosinusitis and sinonasal polyposis ➡. Extensive changes from prior endoscopic surgery are present.*

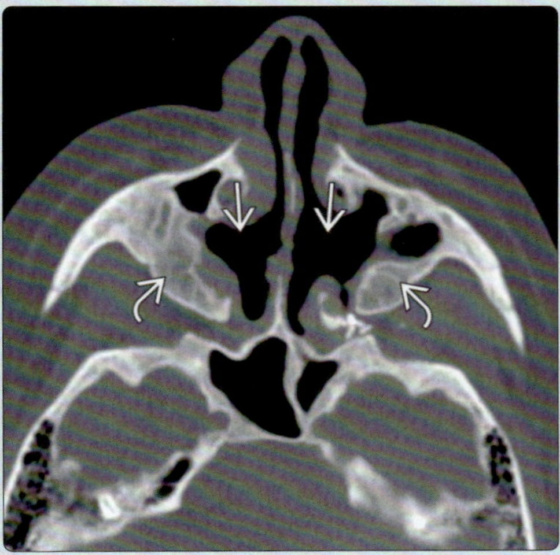

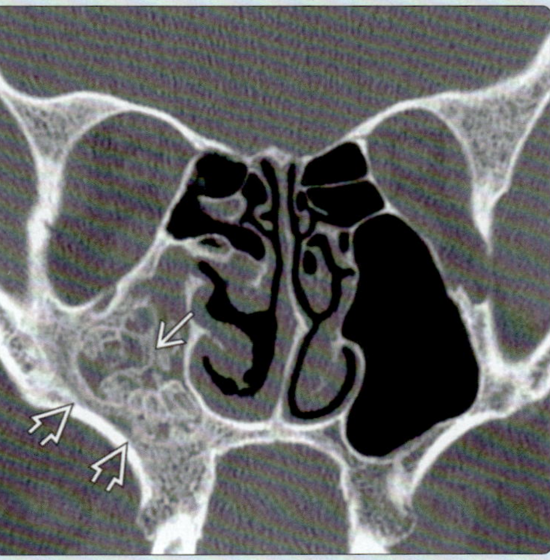

(Left) *Axial bone CT demonstrates marked chronic osteitis ➡ of the walls of both maxillary sinuses. The volume of the sinuses is diminished, and there is patchy mucosal thickening. Changes are noted from prior surgery with bilateral antrostomy defects ➡.* **(Right)** *Coronal bone CT in a patient with longstanding right maxillary inflammation shows prominent calcifications ➡ within the inspissated right maxillary sinus secretions. Osteitis of the walls of the sinus is also present ➡.*

KEY FACTS

TERMINOLOGY

- Superficial complications: Osteomyelitis, subgaleal abscess (Pott puffy tumor), septic thrombophlebitis
- Orbital complications: Preseptal cellulitis/abscess, subperiosteal postseptal abscess (SPA), myositis of extraocular muscles, optic neuritis, septic thrombophlebitis
- Intracranial complications: Meningitis, epidural abscess, subdural empyema (SDE), cerebritis, brain abscess, cavernous sinus thrombosis (CST)

IMAGING

- CECT for subperiosteal abscess
- All other complications: Contrast-enhanced MR
  - + diffusion-weighted images for intracranial issues

TOP DIFFERENTIAL DIAGNOSES

- SPA: Orbital pseudotumor, extraconal neoplasm
- CST: Pseudotumor of cavernous sinus (Tolosa-Hunt), cavernous sinus neoplasm
- SDE: Subdural hygroma/hematoma
- Cerebritis or cerebral abscess: Tumefactive MS, glioblastoma, solitary metastasis, radiation necrosis

PATHOLOGY

- Intraorbital/intracranial complications: ↑ in acute sinusitis
- Superficial complications with chronic rhinosinusitis
- Orbital complication most often from ethmoiditis
- Intracranial complications most often from frontal sinusitis

CLINICAL ISSUES

- Orbital complications more common in children
- Intracranial complications more common from adolescence to 2nd & 3rd decades
- Intracranial complications → 50-80% mortality if not diagnosed and treated early
- Treatment: Appropriate antibiotic therapy in all cases
  - Surgical intervention for SPA (functional endoscopic sinus surgery), some SDE, and cerebral abscesses

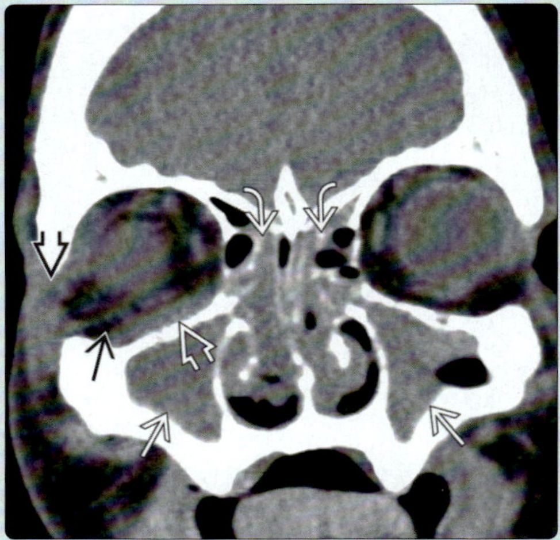

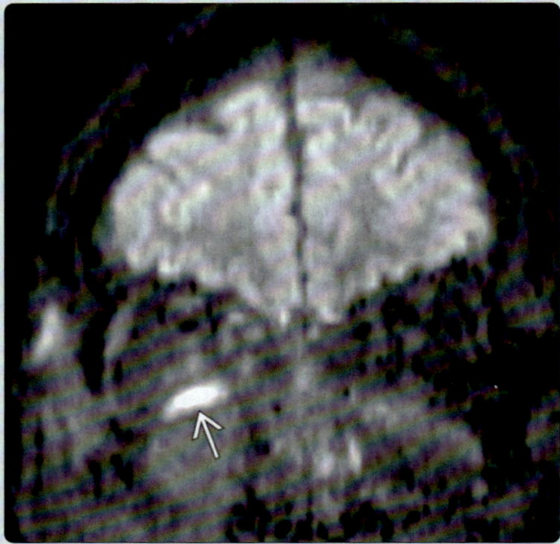

(Left) *Coronal NECT in a man with acute sinusitis complicated by orbital cellulitis and subperiosteal abscess shows extensive opacification of maxillary sinuses ➡ and ethmoid air cells ➡, plus retrobulbar, extraconal subperiosteal fluid collection ➡, retrobulbar edema/stranding ⇨, and preseptal edema ⇨. (Courtesy M. Sturgill, MD.)* **(Right)** *Coronal DTI trace in same patient shows diffusion restriction ➡, confirming subperiosteal abscess complicating acute sinusitis. (Courtesy M. Sturgill, MD.)*

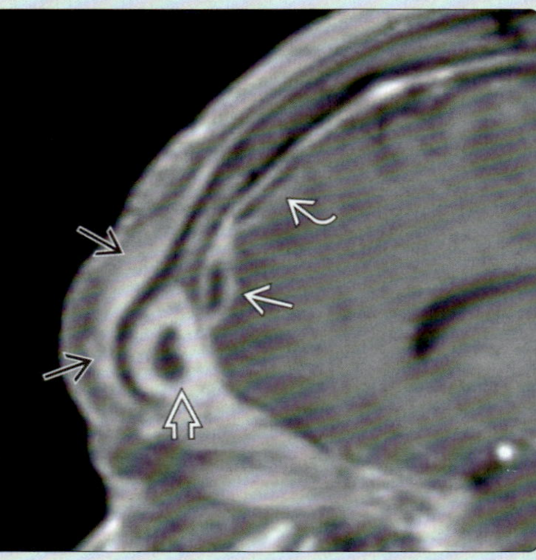

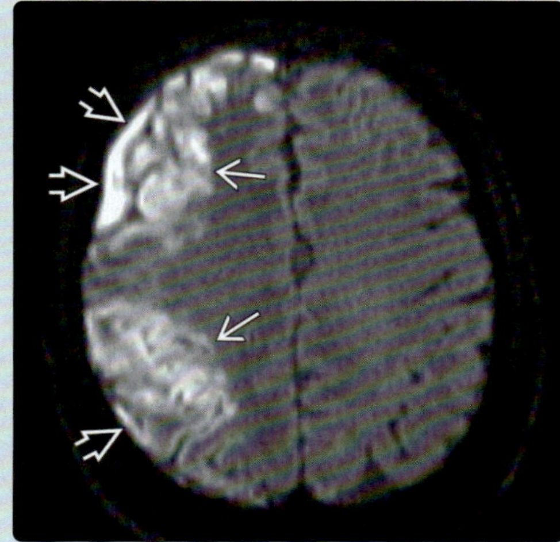

(Left) *Sagittal SPGR C+ in frontal sinusitis complicated by subdural empyema, meningitis, cerebritis, and subgaleal abscess shows frontal sinus mucosal thickening and opacification ➡ with rim-enhancing subdural collection ➡ and leptomeningeal enhancement ➡. Note overlying enhancing subgaleal collection ⇨.* **(Right)** *Axial DTI trace shows reduced diffusivity within a subdural empyema ➡, as well as diffuse cortical reduced diffusivity ➡ from cerebritis and associated acute infarcts complicating frontal sinusitis.*

KEY FACTS

TERMINOLOGY

- Severe form of chronic rhinosinusitis with polyposis
- Allergic response to fungi characterized by eosinophilic mucin with noninvasive fungal hyphae

IMAGING

- Opacification and expansion of multiple sinuses with inspissated material
- NECT: Centrally hyperdense & peripherally hypodense
  - Expansion of sinus with bony remodeling
- MR: Hypointense on T2WI; may mimic air

TOP DIFFERENTIAL DIAGNOSES

- Sinonasal polyposis
- Sinus fungal mycetoma
- Sinonasal solitary polyp
- Sinonasal mucocele
- Sinonasal non-Hodgkin lymphoma

PATHOLOGY

- **Type 1**, IgE-mediated hypersensitivity
- Immune response to fungal antigens
- Viscous, eosinophilic mucin with fungal hyphae
- **Absence** of tissue invasion

CLINICAL ISSUES

- Clinical presentation
  - Nasal obstruction due to **nasal polyposis**, rhinorrhea
  - Immunocompetent patient with longstanding chronic rhinosinusitis
  - Serum eosinophilia, elevated IgE
  - Cutaneous sensitivity to fungal antigens
- Treatment options
  - Topical steroids 1st-line medical therapy; allergy and immune therapy
  - Endoscopic surgical debridement + perioperative systemic steroids
  - Topical & systemic antifungal agents controversial

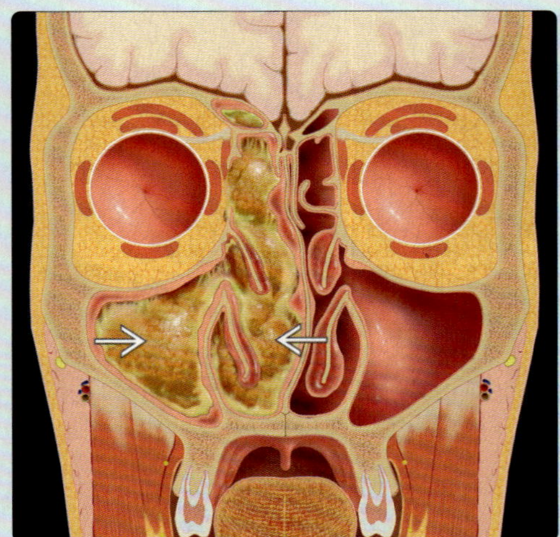

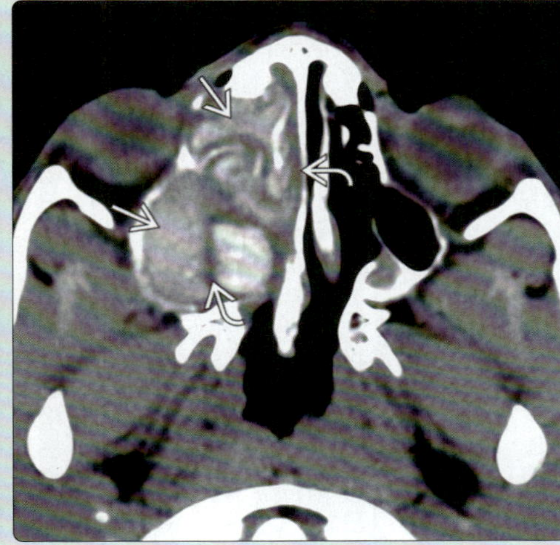

(Left) *Coronal graphic shows classic features of allergic fungal sinusitis (AFS), including opacification and expansion of multiple paranasal sinuses and the nasal cavity. Centrally inspissated material is present ➡, surrounded by peripheral edematous mucosa.* **(Right)** *Axial NECT shows unilateral involvement of AFS. The involved sinuses are expanded with centrally dense inspissated material ➡ and a peripheral rim of low attenuation ➡. Sinus involvement with AFS may be unilateral or bilateral.*

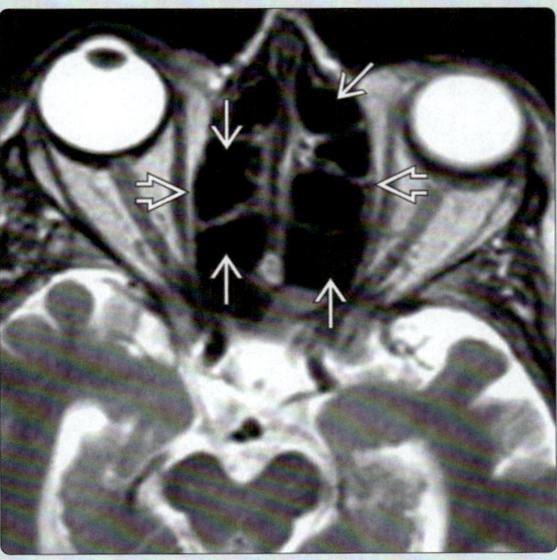

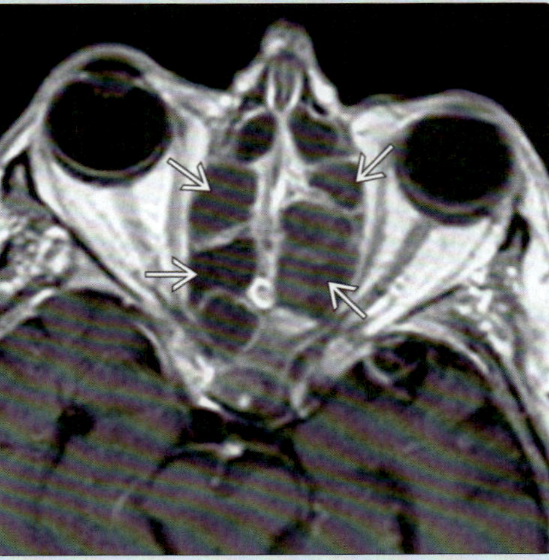

(Left) *Axial T2WI MR in a patient with bilateral AFS shows diffuse hypointense signal within the involved ethmoid air cells ➡. There is mild sinus expansion with lateral bowing of the lamina papyracea ➡. Note that the very low signal mimics normal sinus aeration.* **(Right)** *Axial T1WI C+ MR in the same patient confirms that the ethmoid sinuses are not aerated, but are in fact completely opacified ➡. The surrounding mucosa shows peripheral linear enhancement.*

KEY FACTS

TERMINOLOGY

- Synonyms: Fungus ball; aspergilloma
- Definition: Chronic, noninvasive fungal sinus infection
  - Fungal colonization of sinus cavity

IMAGING

- NECT: Single sinus containing high-density material
  - Fine, round-to-linear matrix **calcifications**
  - Maxillary > sphenoid > > frontal > ethmoid sinuses
    - Sinus often normal size and nonexpanded; may conform to sinus shape or be ball-shaped
- MR: Hypointense T1 signal in solid, mycetomatous mass
  - Hypointense T2 signal may be mistaken for air

TOP DIFFERENTIAL DIAGNOSES

- Chronic rhinosinusitis
- Allergic fungal sinusitis
- Sinonasal mucocele
- Invasive fungal sinusitis

PATHOLOGY

- Saprophytic fungal growth within paranasal sinus
  - Usually *Aspergillus fumigatus*
- No tissue invasion (mucosa, blood vessel, bone)
- Tightly packed fungal hyphae without allergic mucin

CLINICAL ISSUES

- Asymptomatic or mild pressure sensation overlying sinuses
- Immunocompetent, nonatopic, otherwise healthy patient
  - Most common in older female patients; indolent course for up to years
- Surgical curettage via functional endoscopic sinus surgery (FESS) is curative treatment of choice
- Antifungal therapy not effective

DIAGNOSTIC CHECKLIST

- Do not mistake low T2 signal for air
- Check for any signs of invasive disease
- May coexist with other forms of chronic rhinosinusitis

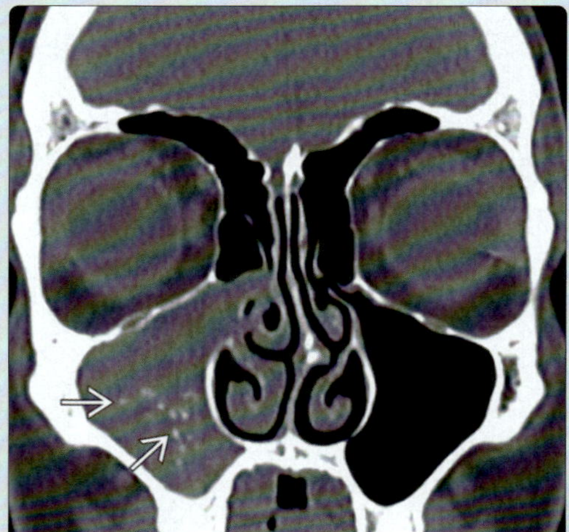

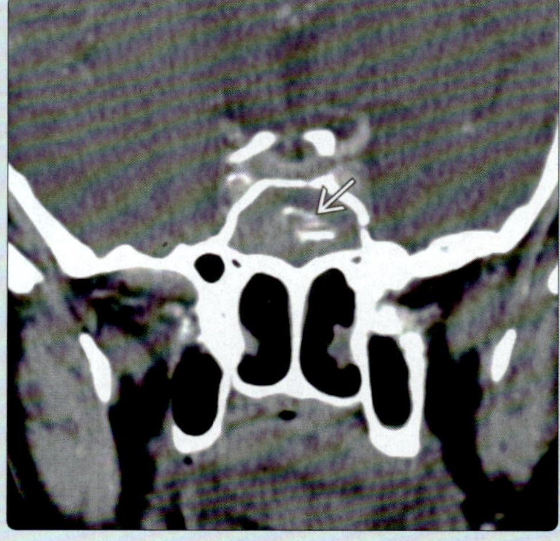

(Left) *Coronal bone CT shows the classic features of a mycetoma within the right maxillary sinus. The sinus is opacified but not expanded. Mixed-density material consistent with fungal elements and calcium deposits ➡ are present in the sinus.* **(Right)** *Coronal CECT in a patient with a sphenoid sinus mycetoma demonstrates multiple foci of calcification ➡ within the fungus ball. The sinus is opacified, and there is mild periosteal thickening, but it does not show expansion.*

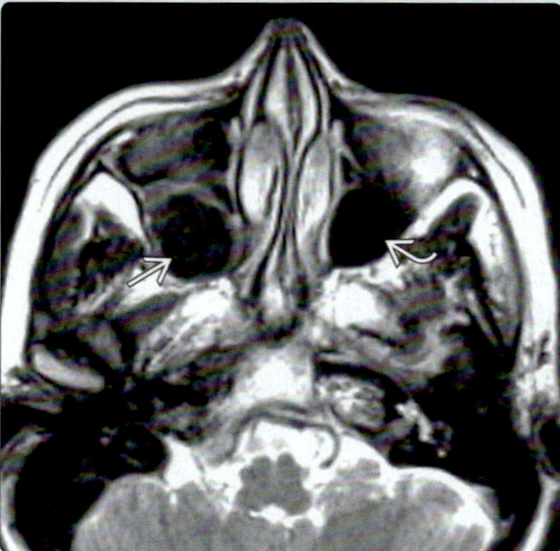

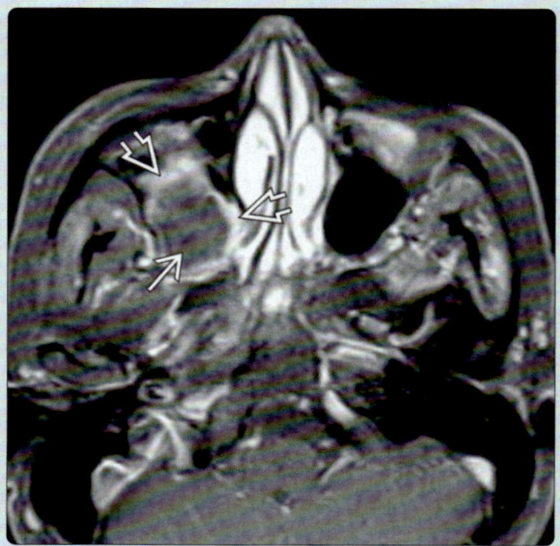

(Left) *Axial T2WI MR in a middle-aged woman with sensation of mild facial pressure shows a normally aerated left maxillary sinus ↪ and opacification of the right maxillary sinus ➡ with material that is nearly as dark in signal as air.* **(Right)** *Axial T1WI MR with fat suppression shows intermediate signal within the right maxillary sinus ➡, confirming that the cavity is opacified and not air-filled. The material within the sinus is nonenhancing, with rim enhancement evident in the surrounding mucosa ⇨.*

KEY FACTS

TERMINOLOGY

- Acute invasive fungal rhinosinusitis (AIFRS): Rapidly progressive (hours to days), transmucosal fungal sinus infection in immunocompromised patients with vascular, bone, soft tissues, orbit, & intracranial invasion resulting in "dry gangrene"; **mortality 50-80%**

IMAGING

- AIFRS: Commonly starts at middle turbinate, spreads to maxillary & ethmoid sinuses > sphenoid sinus
- Sinus opacification with focal bone erosion, adjacent soft tissue infiltration, & nonenhancing mucosa
- CT: Sinus opacification with focal bone erosion, adjacent soft tissue infiltration
- MR: Superior for evaluating intraorbital & intracranial extension; best defines foci of nonenhancing tissue

TOP DIFFERENTIAL DIAGNOSES

- Acute rhinosinusitis with complication
- Sinonasal granulomatosis with polyangiitis
- Sinonasal squamous cell carcinoma
- Sinonasal non-Hodgkin lymphoma

PATHOLOGY

- 3 distinct clinical/pathologic subgroups of IFRS
  - **Acute (fulminant) invasive** FRS
  - **Chronic** IFRS (CIFRS)
  - **Granulomatous** IFRS (GIFRS)

CLINICAL ISSUES

- AIFRS: Facial swelling (65%), fever (63%), nasal congestion (52%), orbital symptoms (50%), headache (46%), cranial nerve palsy (42%)
  - *Mucor* and *Aspergillus* species common
  - Treatment
    - Reverse underlying immunodeficiency when possible
    - Radical debridement until histopathologically normal tissue reached

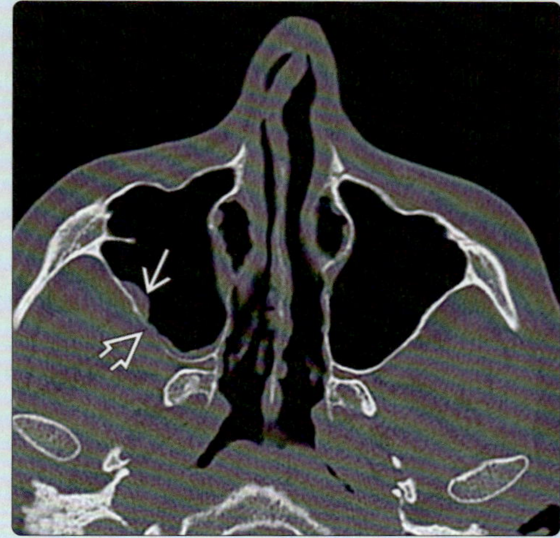

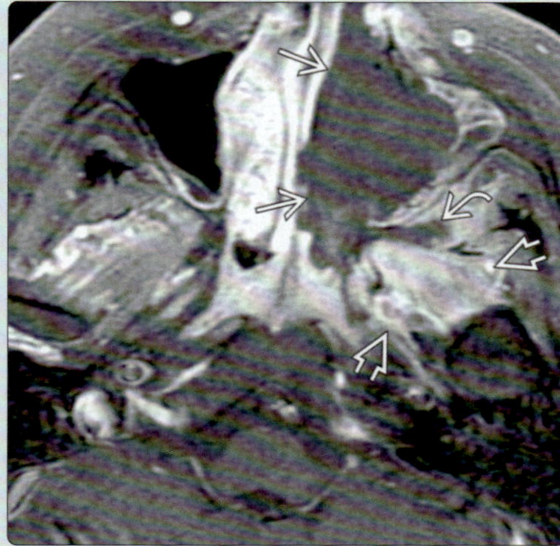

(Left) *Axial bone CT in an immunocompromised patient with facial pain shows findings of early invasive fungal sinusitis, including inflammatory soft tissue changes in the right maxillary sinus wall ➡ with significant thinning of underlying bone ⇨.* **(Right)** *Axial T1 C+ FS MR in a leukemic patient shows an area of nonenhancing necrotic tissue ➡ in the left maxillary sinus secondary to invasive fungal sinusitis. The IFS is seen advancing into the masticator space as a mixture of nonenhancing ⇨ and enhancing ⇨ components.*

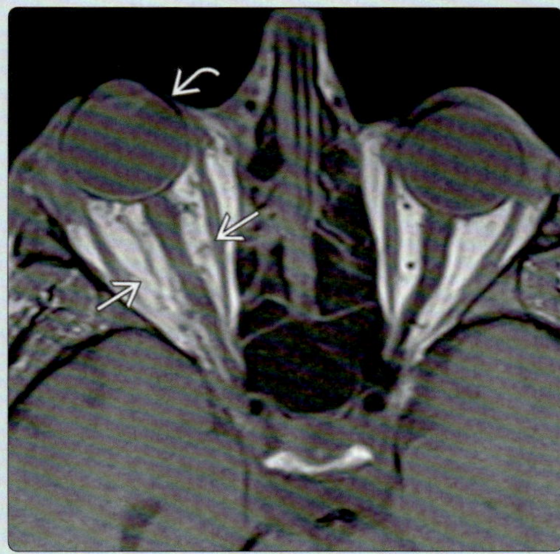

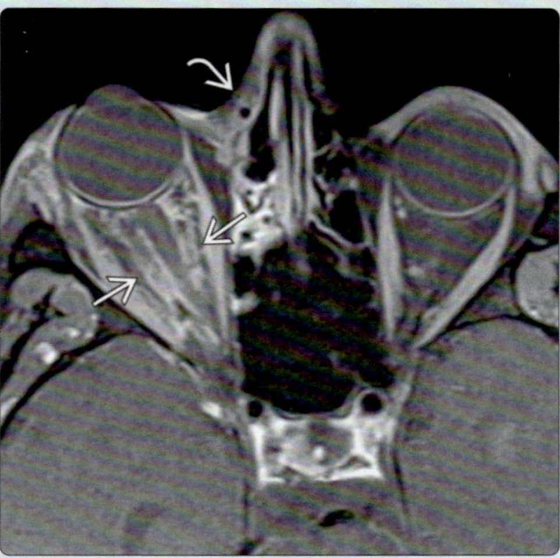

(Left) *Axial T1WI MR in a patient with chronic myelogenous leukemia complicated by Rhizopus acute invasive fungal rhinosinusitis shows ill-defined soft-tissue infiltration ➡ of the retrobulbar fat with associated proptosis ⇨.* **(Right)** *Axial T1 C+ FS MR better defines the extent of infiltrating retrobulbar soft tissue ➡ as well as early involvement of the soft tissues overlying the nasal bridge ⇨ in this patient who succumbed to disease.*

Sinonasal Polyposis

KEY FACTS

TERMINOLOGY

- Definition: Nonneoplastic, inflammatory swelling of sinonasal mucosa that buckles to form polyps

IMAGING

- NECT (bone CT) preferred imaging tool
- Involves nasal cavity and paranasal sinuses (vs. retention cysts mainly within sinuses)
  - Predominantly along lateral nasal wall and roof of nasal cavity
  - Commonly involves middle turbinate, sparing inferior turbinate
  - Anterior involvement > posterior
  - Primarily mucoid or soft tissue density
  - Remodeling of sinonasal bones common in severe cases
- MR may be complimentary to CT in assessing intraorbital and intracranial extension and differentiation of sinonasal polyposis (SNP) from neoplasm

TOP DIFFERENTIAL DIAGNOSES

- Allergic fungal sinusitis
- Cystic fibrosis
- Mucous retention cyst
- Solitary polyp
- Granulomatosis with polyangiitis

PATHOLOGY

- Formal pathogenesis of SNP has not been clarified
  - Chronic inflammation is major factor
  - Associated with allergy, asthma, primary ciliary dyskinesia, aspirin sensitivity, and cystic fibrosis

CLINICAL ISSUES

- Although not life threatening, chronic SNP unresponsive to therapy can be chronic, debilitating disease
- Medical therapy = maintenance treatment of choice
- Surgery reserved for symptomatic relief and correction of cosmetic deformities, orbital and intracranial involvement

(Left) *Coronal bone CT shows the classic appearance of sinonasal polyposis (SNP) with multiple lobular soft tissue masses involving the nasal cavity ➡ and paranasal sinuses ➡. In this case, the involvement is diffuse and bilateral, without expansion.* **(Right)** *Coronal bone CT in a patient with polyposis and new onset of acute sinusitis symptoms shows polyps ➡ in the nasal cavity occluding the middle meatuses. Fluid levels ➡ consistent with acute inflammation are present in the maxillary sinuses.*

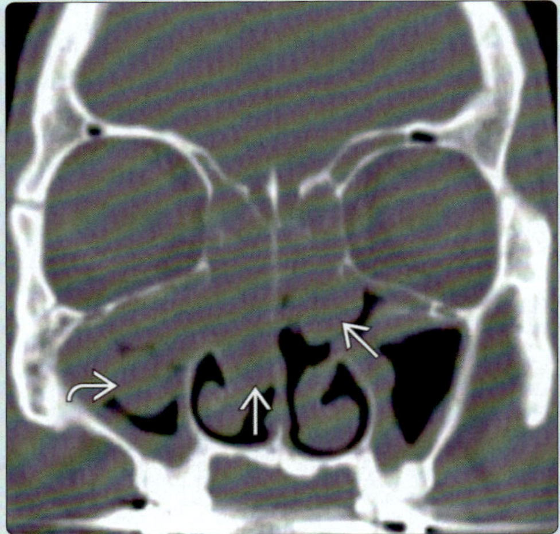

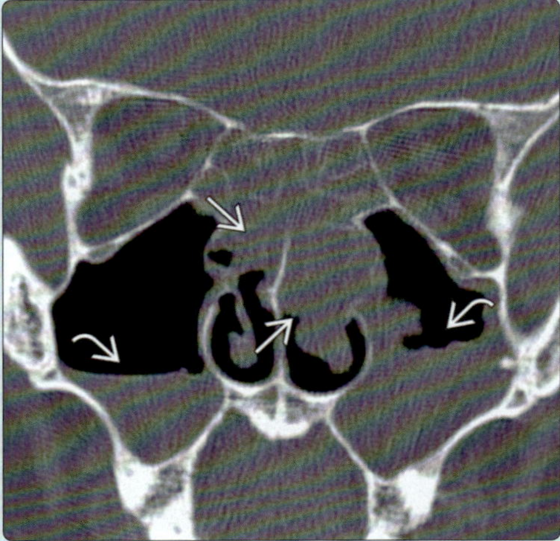

(Left) *Coronal T1WI MR shows multiple intermediate signal intensity polyps ➡ filling the nasal cavity maxillary and ethmoid sinuses. Trapped secretions with high protein content ➡ (T1 shortening) are also noted.* **(Right)** *Coronal T1WI C+ FS MR in the same patient shows enhancement of the inflamed mucosa ➡ at the periphery of the polyps. There is slight expansion of the right maxillary sinus with elevation of the orbital floor ➡.*

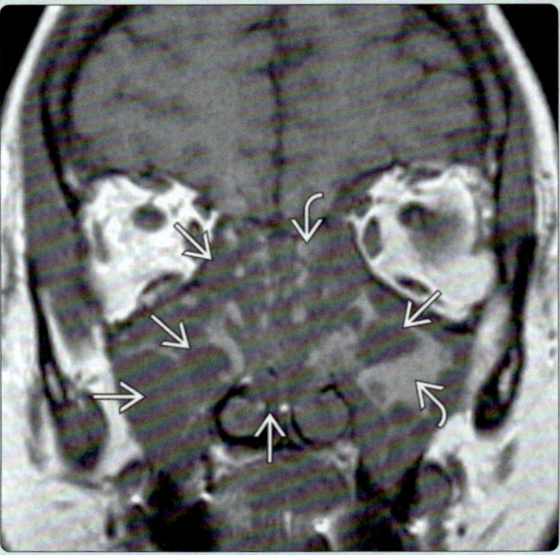

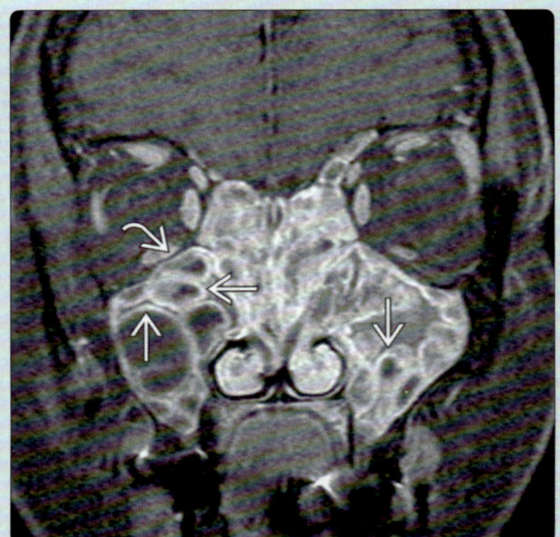

KEY FACTS

TERMINOLOGY

- **Solitary inflammatory polyp** resulting from edematous hypertrophy of respiratory epithelium

IMAGING

- Sinus CT 1st imaging exam
- Most common type is **antrochoanal**
  - Polyp extends from maxillary antrum → enlarged maxillary ostium or accessory ostium → nasal cavity
- Peripheral enhancement with **no** central enhancement
- Bone surrounding infundibulum/accessory ostium smoothly remodeled, not destroyed
- Large lesions extend into nasopharyngeal airway

TOP DIFFERENTIAL DIAGNOSES

- Intranasal glioma
- Nasoethmoidal cephalocele
- Juvenile angiofibroma
- Inverted papilloma
- Esthesioneuroblastoma

PATHOLOGY

- **Inflammatory polyp** resulting from edematous hypertrophy of respiratory epithelium
- Postobstructive inflammatory disease is often present
  - Greater when antrochoanal polyp exits antrum via accessory ostium > natural ostium
- Antrochoanal > > sphenochoanal > ethmochoanal polyp

CLINICAL ISSUES

- 4-6% of all sinonasal polyps
- Most common in **teenagers** & young adults
- Typical symptoms
  - Unilateral nasal obstruction, worse on expiration
  - Mouth breathing, snoring with sleep apnea
- Treatment options
  - Complete endoscopic surgical removal of nasal & antral components is treatment of choice

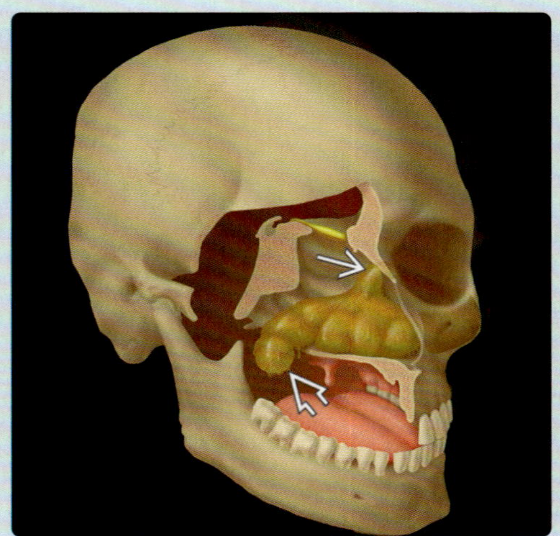

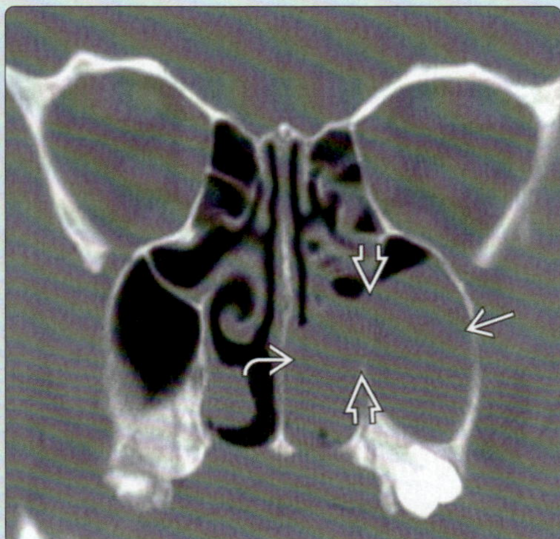

(Left) *Longitudinal oblique graphic shows an antrochoanal polyp (ACP) extending from maxillary antrum through a posterior fontanelle ➡ into the nasal cavity. Note the posterior extension of the polyp into the nasopharynx ➡.* **(Right)** *Coronal bone CT shows a typical ACP extending from the left maxillary antrum ➡ into the nasal cavity ➡ via a secondary ostium ➡ located posterior to the ostiomeatal complex.*

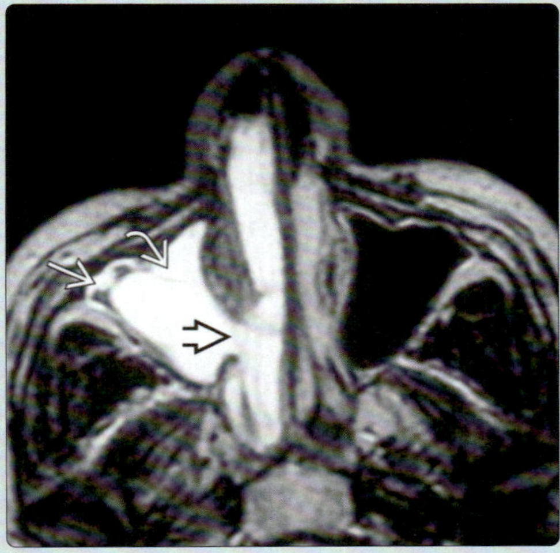

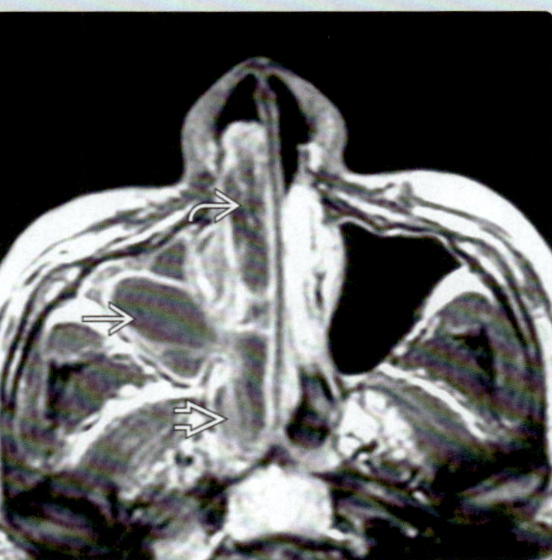

(Left) *Axial T2 MR shows diffuse, homogeneous, hyperintense signal ➡ within an ACP. The polyp extends into the nasal cavity via a secondary ostium ➡. A small amount of trapped secretions ➡ are noted lateral to the lesion.* **(Right)** *Axial T1 C+ MR shows the antral ➡, nasal ➡, and nasopharyngeal ➡ components of this ACP. Note that there is thin peripheral, but no central or nodular enhancement of the lesion, which helps to distinguish it from a neoplasm.*

KEY FACTS

TERMINOLOGY

- Mucocele: Cyst lined by normal respiratory epithelium and filled with mucus; will cause expanded, chronically obstructed sinus

IMAGING

- Opacified, **expanded** sinus with **smooth remodeled** walls
  - **Frontal (60%)** > **ethmoid (25%)** > maxillary (10%) > sphenoid (5%)
- Bone CT + coronal/sagittal reformats help surgical planning
  - Low-density opacified, expanded sinus
  - Bony sinus walls show benign remodeling
  - No central enhancement if mucocele only
    - Mild peripheral enhancement possible
- T1 C+ MR
  - Use if suspected obstructing nasal tumor or mucocele is projecting intracranially
  - High water content mucus typically ↓ T1, ↑ T2 signal
    - Signal varies with protein content (especially T1 signal)
      - Low signal, low protein; high signal, high protein

TOP DIFFERENTIAL DIAGNOSES

- Sinonasal polyposis
- Sinonasal solitary polyps
- Sinonasal neoplasia

PATHOLOGY

- Obstructed drainage pathway of affected sinus or air cell
- Most common expansile lesion of paranasal sinuses

CLINICAL ISSUES

- Symptoms & signs depend on affected sinus
  - Slowly progressive symptoms
  - > 90% have ophthalmic symptoms & signs
- Possible sequelae after sinonasal surgery or trauma
- Surgical issues
  - Creating patent sinus outflow tract key to prevent recurrence; endoscopic approach preferred to open when feasible

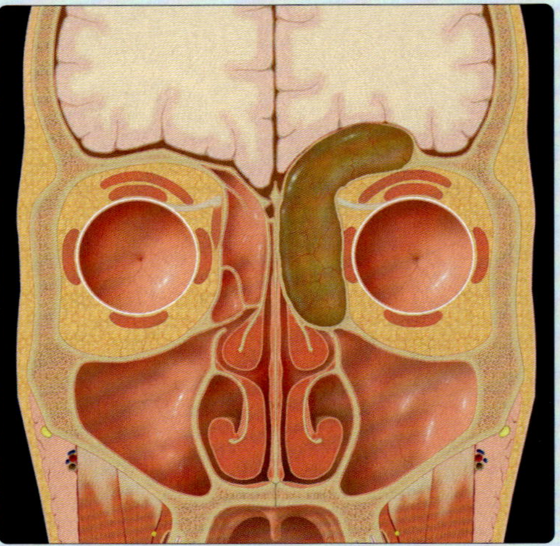

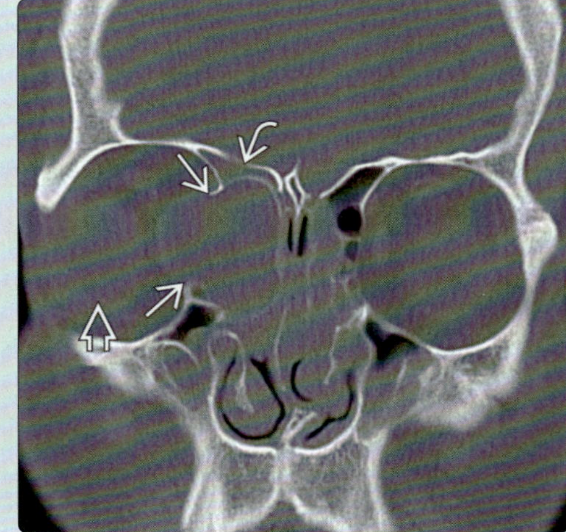

(Left) *Coronal graphic shows a large left anterior ethmoid mucocele extending into the left frontal sinus. The affected sinuses are expanded without evidence of aggressive bone destruction.* **(Right)** *Coronal bone CT shows the typical features of a right ethmoid mucocele. The sinus is opacified, and there is remodeling of the surrounding bony walls with erosion of the lamina papyracea ➡. Note the mass effect upon the orbit with lateralization of the globe ⇨ and frontal sinus obstruction with opacification ↗.*

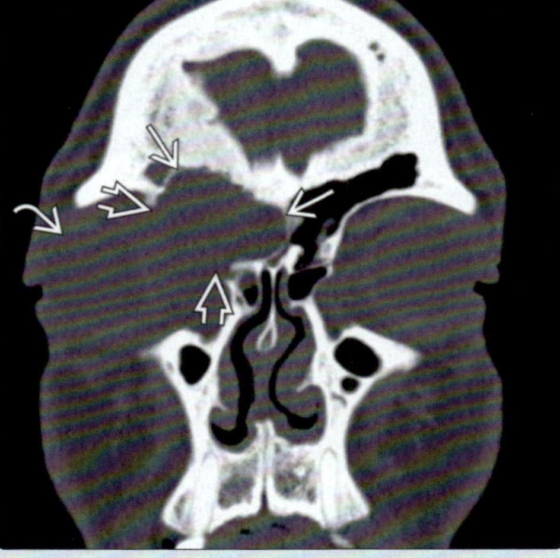

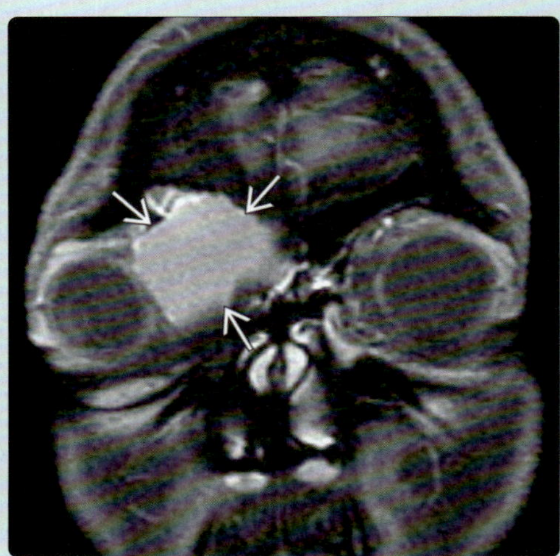

(Left) *Coronal bone CT demonstrates a right frontoethmoidal mucocele ➡ with smooth expansion medially and frank osseous dehiscence ➡ inferolaterally. The globe is laterally displaced ➡.* **(Right)** *Coronal T1 C+ FS MR in same patient reveals a lobulated, homogeneously hyperintense signal within a right frontoethmoidal mucocele ➡. The lesion extends into the right orbit, displacing the globe. Precontrast T1 MR (not shown) confirmed high signal was related to proteinaceous mucus and not enhancement.*

KEY FACTS

TERMINOLOGY

- Silent sinus syndrome (SSS): Acquired process with maxillary sinus walls retraction → reduced volume → depression of orbital floor → enophthalmos ± hypoglobus
- Synonym: Maxillary atelectasis with enophthalmos

IMAGING

- Axial NECT (bone CT) with coronal reformats
- NECT (bone CT) findings
  - Fully developed maxillary sinuses
  - Diminished maxillary antrum volume
  - Retraction (concavity) of all walls
    - With inferior position ("depression") of orbital floor
  - Lateralized uncinate and expanded middle meatus
  - Opacification of affected sinus

TOP DIFFERENTIAL DIAGNOSES

- Maxillary sinus hypoplasia
- Posttraumatic or postsurgical change

PATHOLOGY

- Occult chronic obstruction of maxillary ostium → negative pressure within sinus → stagnant mucus fills sinus → osteolysis thins/remodels bony walls → retraction of sinus walls including orbital floor

CLINICAL ISSUES

- Process is typically painless and asymptomatic ("silent")
- Adult with **unilateral enophthalmos** in absence of trauma
- **Diplopia** is most common visual symptom
- Hypoglobus (downward displacement of eye in orbit), malar depression, upper lid retraction, vague dental or facial pain
- Treatment options
  - Disease progress halted after restoration of sinus drainage
  - Functional endoscopic sinus surgery and transconjunctival reconstruction of orbital floor

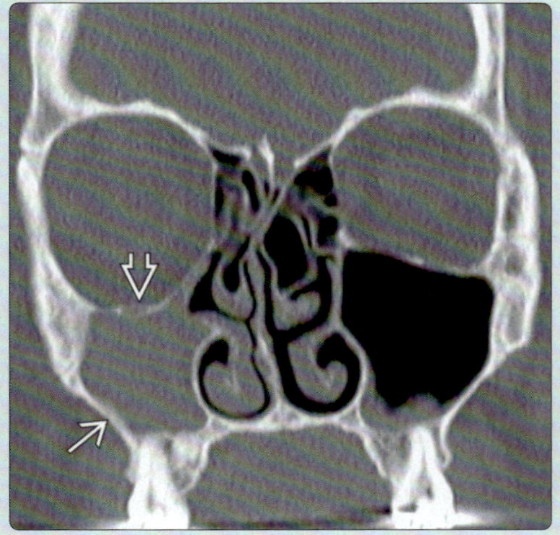

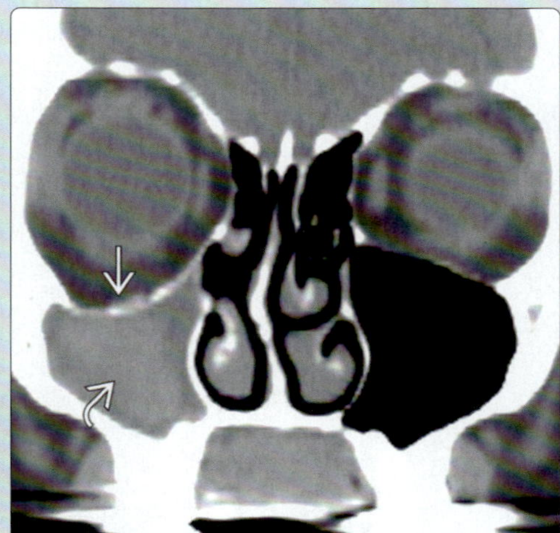

(Left) *Coronal bone CT in SSS shows opacification of the right maxillary sinus with slight thickening of the lateral wall ➡. The orbital floor is bowed inferiorly ➡ with increased orbital volume, which is characteristic of SSS. Enophthalmos is indicated by relative posterior position of globe.* **(Right)** *Coronal NECT shows typical features of SSS with decreased volume of right maxillary sinus, inferior position of the orbital floor ➡, and posterior position of ipsilateral globe. Increased density and chronic secretions ➡ are noted in the sinus.*

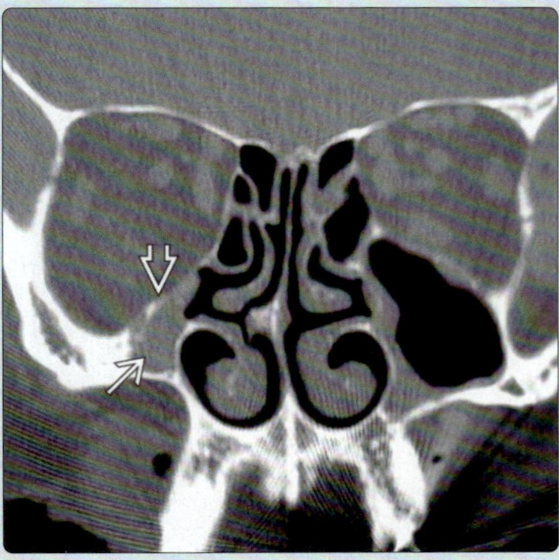

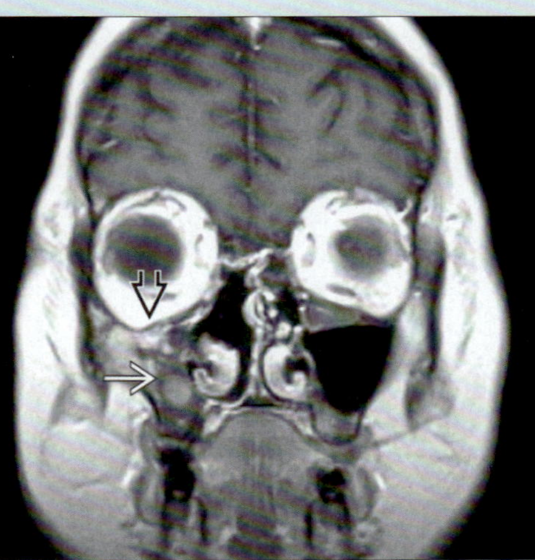

(Left) *Coronal bone CT shows the characteristic features of SSS. The volume of the opacified right maxillary antrum ➡ is diminished. The orbital floor is inferiorly positioned ➡ with increase in overall orbital volume.* **(Right)** *Coronal T1WI C+ MR in a patient with enophthalmos on the right side shows decreased volume of the maxillary sinus ➡, which is opacified with inspissated material. The ipsilateral orbital floor is depressed ➡.*

Granulomatosis With Polyangiitis (Wegener)

KEY FACTS

TERMINOLOGY

- Idiopathic, autoimmune **necrotizing granulomatous vasculitis** that preferentially involves upper and lower respiratory tracts, kidneys, skin, and joints

IMAGING

- Nodular soft tissue in nose with **septal and nonseptal cartilaginous and bone destruction**
  - **Orbital invasion** most common extrasinonasal H&N site
  - When severe, dura may be involved
- Multiplanar bone CT is best tool for initial evaluation
- Add enhanced MR best if extrasinonasal spread

TOP DIFFERENTIAL DIAGNOSES

- Sinonasal sarcoidosis
- Nasal cocaine necrosis
- Chronic rhinosinusitis
- Invasive fungal sinusitis
- Sinonasal non-Hodgkin lymphoma

CLINICAL ISSUES

- H&N involvement in 72-100% of granulomatosis with polyangiitis (GPA) patients
  - Rhinologic symptoms in > 80%
- Symptoms mimic chronic rhinosinusitis
  - Nasal obstruction and epistaxis
  - Diagnosis often delayed because symptoms mistaken for chronic rhinosinusitis
- Typically 40-60 years
- Generally indolent disease
  - May transition to fulminating disease
- Treatment options
  - Medical treatments: Immunosuppressive agents, cyclophosphamide, other cytotoxic drugs
    - Fulminant disease treated with high-dose prednisone followed by cyclophosphamide
  - Surgery reserved for selected H&N manifestations, such as saddle nose deformity and subglottic stenosis

(Left) *Coronal bone CT shows the classic features of sinonasal involvement by granulomatosis with polyangiitis (GPA). Nodular soft tissue ➡ is seen in the nasal cavity with an associated septal perforation ➡.* **(Right)** *Coronal bone CT shows sequelae of a severe chronic sinonasal inflammation in GPA with the combination of hyperostosis ➡ of the sinus walls and bony destruction of the turbinates ➡.*

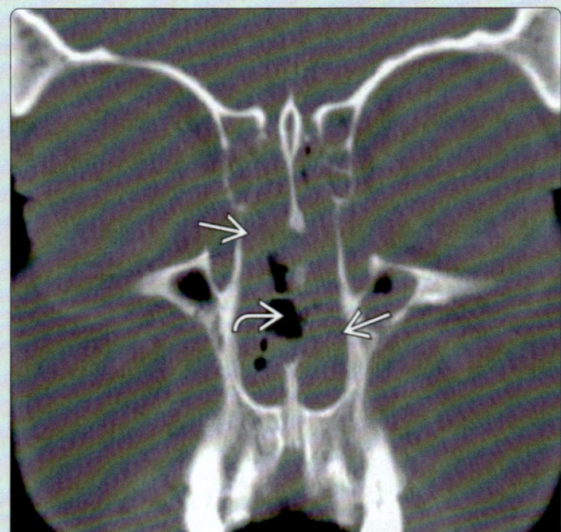

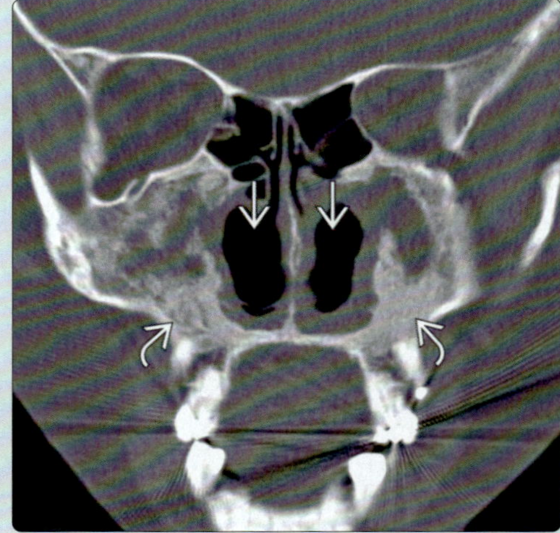

(Left) *Coronal bone CT in severe GPA shows extensive soft tissue thickening in the maxillary and ethmoid sinuses and nasal cavity. There is destruction of the nasal septum ➡ and bilateral inferior and middle turbinates ➡. Note diffuse soft tissue infiltration of the left orbit ➡ and milder disease right orbit ➡.* **(Right)** *Lateral clinical photo of the face reveals saddle nose deformity that can be seen in association with granulomatosis with polyangiitis secondary to nasal septal destruction.*

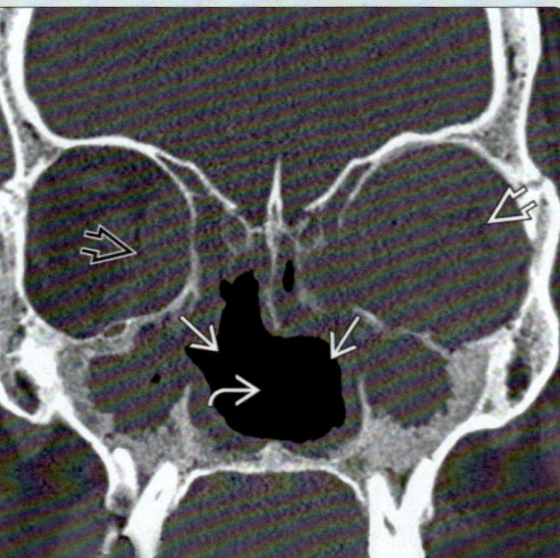

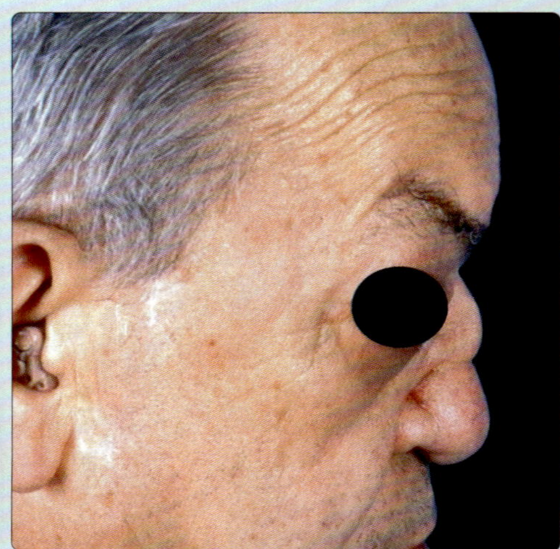

KEY FACTS

TERMINOLOGY

- Destruction of osteocartilaginous structures of nose, sinuses, and palate induced by chronic inhalation of cocaine

IMAGING

- Perforation of osteocartilaginous nasal septum ± turbinates/palate **without** soft tissue mass
    - 75% occur in quadrangular cartilage; 25% involve vomer-perpendicular ethmoidal lamina
- Thin-section CT with multiplanar reformat recommended to fully delineate extent of bone destruction

TOP DIFFERENTIAL DIAGNOSES

- Traumatic nasal septal perforation
- Granulomatosis with polyangiitis
- Sinonasal sarcoidosis
- Sinonasal non-Hodgkin lymphoma
- Other drug-related septal perforation

PATHOLOGY

- Nasal septal destruction results from combined effects of chemical irritation, ischemic necrosis from vasoconstriction, and direct trauma from autoinstrumentation
- Chemical agents (i.e., levamisole) added to cocaine to enhance its appearance, add weight, and produce additional psychoactive effects may contribute to necrosis

CLINICAL ISSUES

- Nasal obstruction and discharge are most common symptoms of acquired septal lesions
    - Extension to inferior (68%), middle (44%), and superior (16%) turbinates in 1 large study
- ~ 1.5 million Americans ≥ 12 years old (0.6% of population) are regular (at least 1x per month) cocaine users
    - Prevalence, cocaine sinonasal complications ~ 5%
    - Septal perforation = most common complication (5%)
- Treatment: Stop abuse; silicone buttons; surgical repair

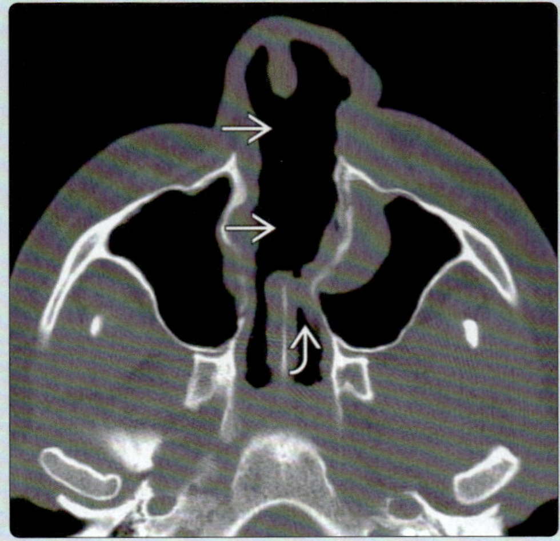

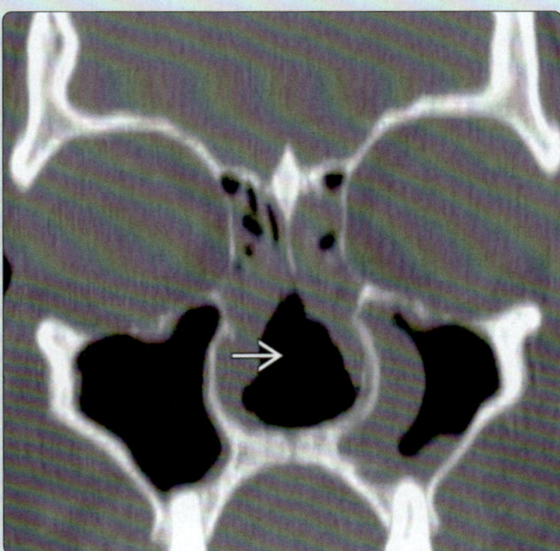

(Left) *Axial bone CT in a patient with a history of chronic cocaine inhalation shows a very large nasal septal perforation ➡. Scarring with adhesion formation ➡ is noted between the lateral nasal wall and septum posteriorly on the left.* **(Right)** *Coronal CT reconstruction demonstrates a large defect in the nasal septum ➡ related to cocaine necrosis. Note that the concha of the middle and inferior turbinates have been eroded and are absent.*

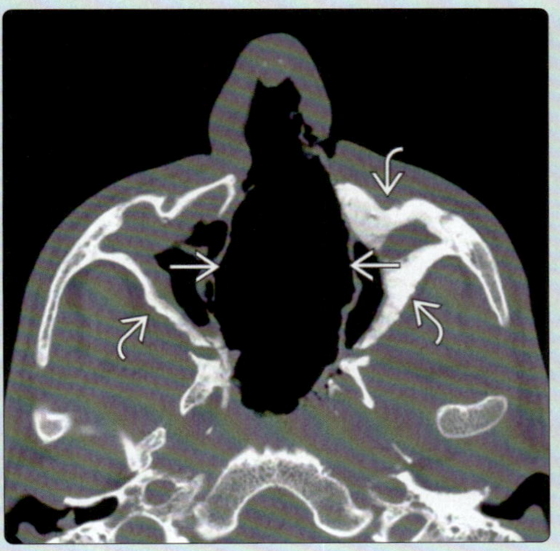

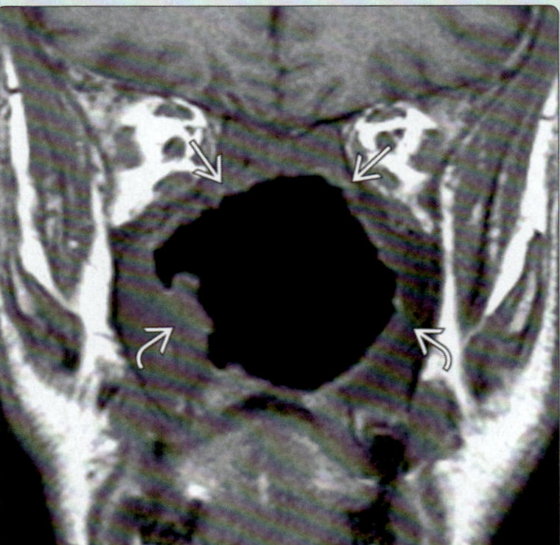

(Left) *Axial bone CT in a severe case of nasal cocaine necrosis shows complete erosion of the nasal septum. The lateral nasal walls ➡ are also involved. Extensive osteitis ➡ of the remaining antral walls is seen from chronic maxillary inflammation.* **(Right)** *Coronal T1WI MR demonstrates a large nasal septal perforation as well as ethmoid involvement ➡. Inflamed, thickened mucosa ➡ lines the walls of the sinuses.*

Sinonasal Fibrous Dysplasia

KEY FACTS

TERMINOLOGY

- Fibroosseous lesion in which normal medullary bone is replaced by weak osseous & fibrous tissue

IMAGING

- Classic appearance: **Ground-glass** density on NECT
  - Density varies with amount of fibrous tissue
  - Variable enhancement of fibrous component
  - Variable presence of lucent/lytic foci
- MR signal & enhancement are highly variable
  - **Expansion of diploic space** key feature of FD
  - **Low T2 signal** characteristic but often not present
  - When T2 hyperintense & enhancing: Neoplasm mimic
- Best imaging tool: Thin-section **bone algorithm NECT**

TOP DIFFERENTIAL DIAGNOSES

- Ossifying fibroma
- Osteoma
- Neo-osteogenesis

PATHOLOGY

- Etiology: Defective gene in bone-forming cells in early fetal life: ↑ osteogenesis in bone marrow
- Can obstruct sinus → recurrent infection, mucocele formation
- 3 forms of FD: Monostotic, polyostotic, & McCune-Albright syndrome

CLINICAL ISSUES

- Headache, pain, sinonasal obstruction & recurrent sinusitis
- Monostotic form most common, 25% in H&N
- Highest incidence: 3-15 years
  - Disease quiescent after cessation of skeletal growth

DIAGNOSTIC CHECKLIST

- MR appearance can be somewhat confusing: Fibrous component **enhances intensely**
  - **Mimics aggressive neoplasm** without comparison CT
  - **NECT critical** to establish correct diagnosis

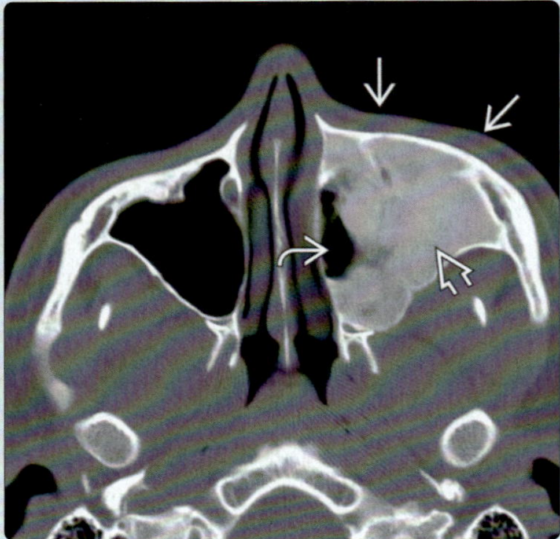

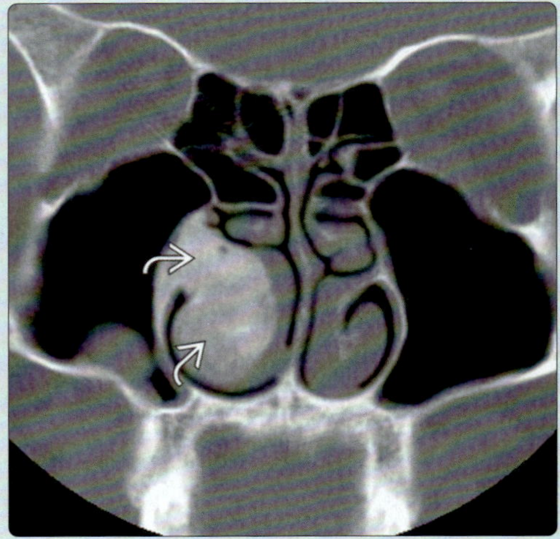

(Left) *Axial bone CT demonstrates the classic features of fibrous dysplasia. There is marked expansion of the left maxillary sinus walls with asymmetry of projection of the left cheek ➡. This case shows the typical ground-glass appearance ➡ of this entity. Note the markedly decreased antral volume ➡.* **(Right)** *Coronal bone CT shows fibrous dysplasia involving the concha of the right inferior turbinate ➡ and lateral nasal wall. The concha is markedly expanded with ground-glass density.*

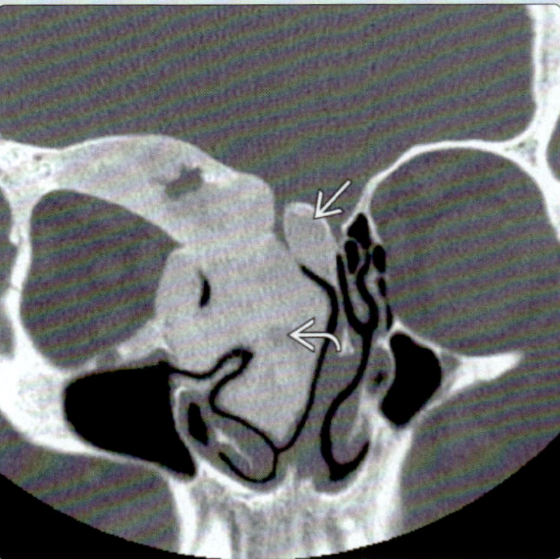

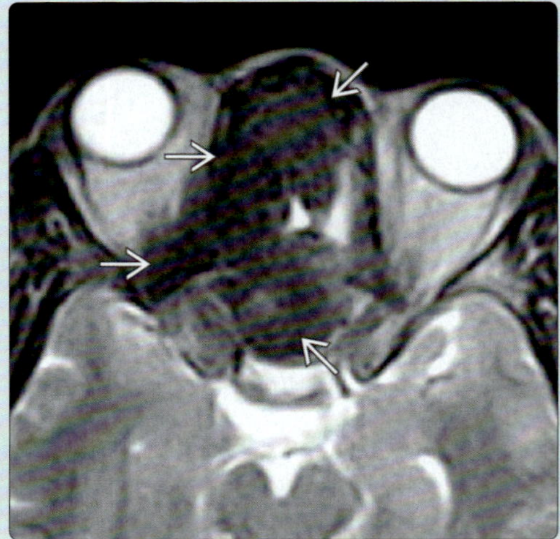

(Left) *Coronal bone CT shows extensive fibrous dysplasia involving the orbit, crista galli ➡, ethmoids, and middle turbinate ➡ on the right. The nasal septum is deviated to the left.* **(Right)** *Axial T2 MR shows characteristic marked hypointense signal in fibrous dysplasia ➡. These findings are typical when seen in conjunction with a ground-glass appearance on CT and are more diagnostic than when T2-hyperintense foci are present.*

KEY FACTS

TERMINOLOGY

- Benign, well-defined, slow-growing, bone-forming tumor

IMAGING

- Well-marginated bone density lesion that arises from wall of paranasal sinus & protrudes into sinus lumen
- Location: Frontal & ethmoid > > > maxillary & sphenoid
- Larger osteomas may be associated with
  - Sinus opacification or mucocele formation from ostial obstruction
  - Orbital mass effect from extraconal extension
  - Pneumocephalus or intraparenchymal tension pneumatocele
  - Brain abscess ± subdural empyema
- CT density depends on ivory vs. mature components

TOP DIFFERENTIAL DIAGNOSES

- Sinonasal fibrous dysplasia
- Sinonasal ossifying fibroma
- Sinonasal osteosarcoma

PATHOLOGY

- If multiple osteomas are discovered, consider Gardner syndrome
- Etiology not well established; theories include developmental, traumatic, and infectious causes
- Microscopic classifications in literature tend to distinguish between ivory, mature, and mixed types

CLINICAL ISSUES

- Most common benign tumor of paranasal sinuses
- Usually asymptomatic, incidental finding; M:F ~ 1.5-2.6:1.0
  - Found in 1% of patients on radiographs & 3% on CT done for sinonasal symptoms
  - < 5% of all osteomas are symptomatic
- Symptomatic lesions typically treated surgically
  - Small lesions: Endoscopic removal
  - Larger lesions: Open surgical procedure

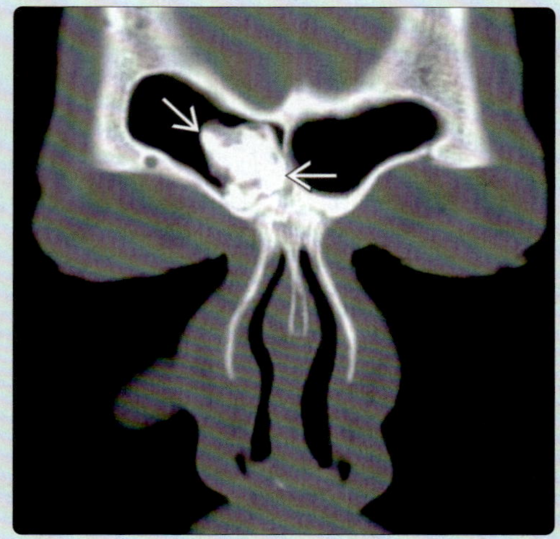

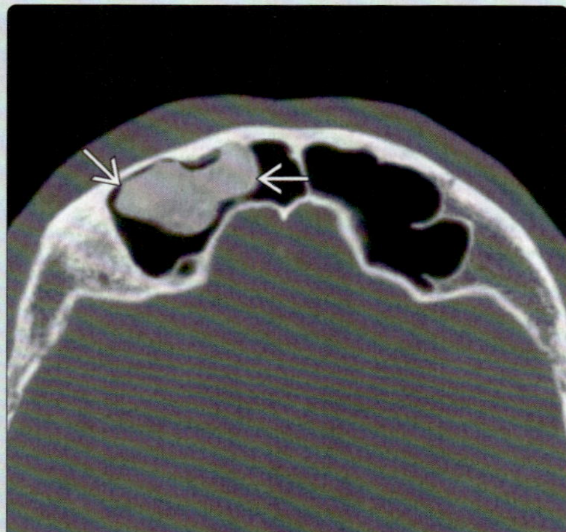

(Left) *Coronal bone CT demonstrates the classic appearance of an ivory osteoma ➡ of the right frontal sinus. The lesion is located medially but did not obstruct the frontal recess. The sinus is otherwise well aerated.* **(Right)** *Axial bone CT shows a well-defined, calcified mass within the right frontal sinus ➡, consistent with an osteoma. The ground-glass density is suggestive of a mature or mixed-type osteoma, rather than an ivory type.*

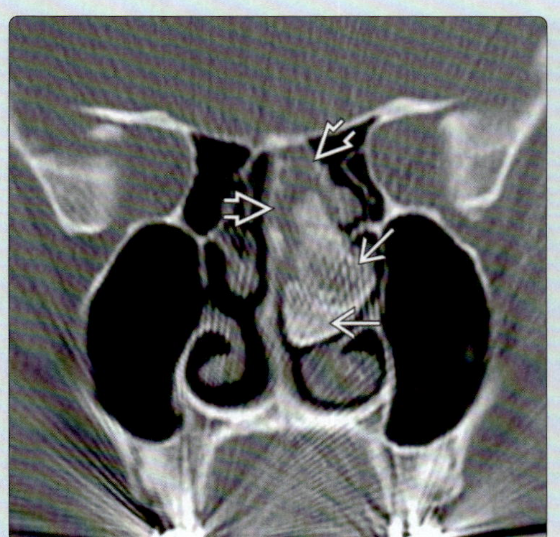

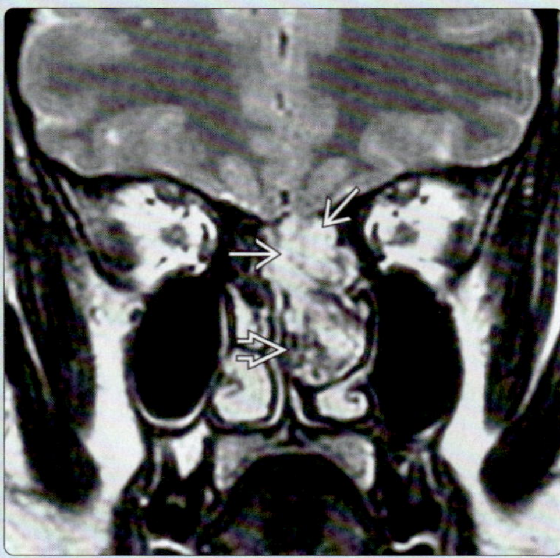

(Left) *Coronal bone CT shows a mixed calcified ➡ and soft tissue density ➡ mass involving the left ethmoid sinus and nasal cavity. Using imaging alone, it would be difficult to distinguish this osteoma from other fibroosseous lesions.* **(Right)** *Coronal T2WI MR shows high signal intensity ➡ in the superior component of an osteoma that appeared nonossified on CT and had low signal intensity ➡ in the inferior component that appeared densely ossified on CT.*

Sinonasal Ossifying Fibroma

KEY FACTS

TERMINOLOGY

- Rare, benign fibroosseous lesion composed of fibrous tissue & mature bone

IMAGING

- Imaging appearance depends on age (↑ ossified portions with age)
  - Classic appearance: Thick, bony peripheral rim surrounding fibrous center
- Location: **Sinus-nose** > orbit > mandible > temporal bone
- CT findings
  - **Expansile mass** with **soft tissue density** (fibrous) **central** area surrounded by **ossified rim**
  - May be indistinguishable from fibrous dysplasia & osteoma
- MR findings
  - T1: Intermediate to low signal throughout tumor
  - T2: Mixed low-signal (ossified) & high-signal (fibrous) areas
  - Inhomogeneous **enhancement of fibrous components**

TOP DIFFERENTIAL DIAGNOSES

- Fibrous dysplasia
- Osteoma
- Osteosarcoma

PATHOLOGY

- Thought to arise from mesenchyme of periodontal ligament

CLINICAL ISSUES

- Generally **asymptomatic** & found incidentally
- Age: 20-40 years most common
- Benign, but locally aggressive
  - May obstruct sinus drainage, cause cosmetic deformity & ocular dysfunction
- Complete surgical excision is treatment of choice
- High rate of recurrence with incomplete resection

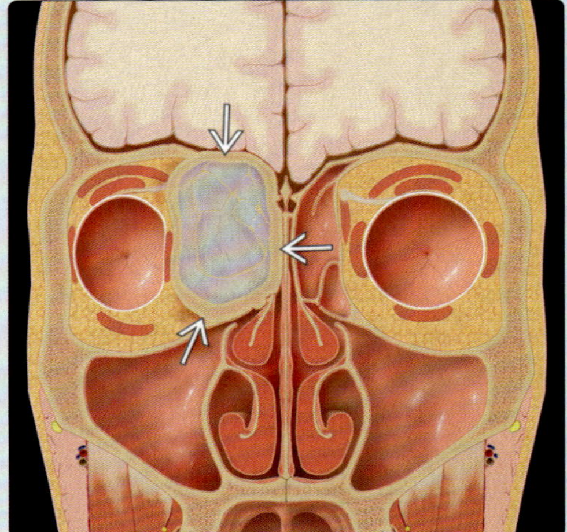

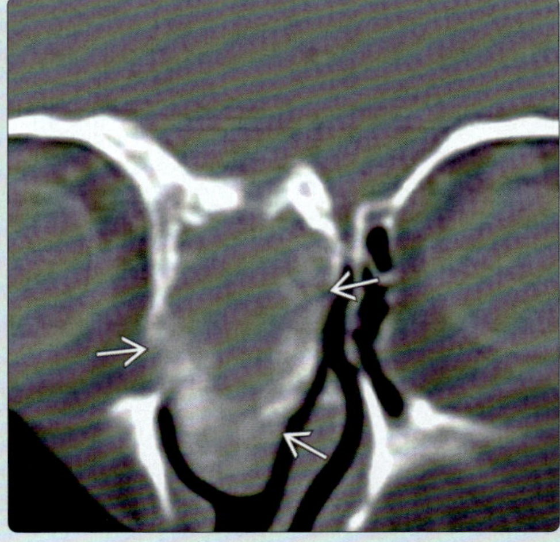

(Left) *Coronal graphic shows an ossifying fibroma (OsFib) of the ethmoid region with dense osseous material peripherally ➡ and a fibrous center. The margins are well defined. There is mass effect on the orbital contents.* **(Right)** *Coronal bone CT shows an OsFib of the anterior ethmoid sinus with an ossific outer margin ➡ surrounding a fibrous center. Unfortunately, not all OsFibs show this classic pattern.*

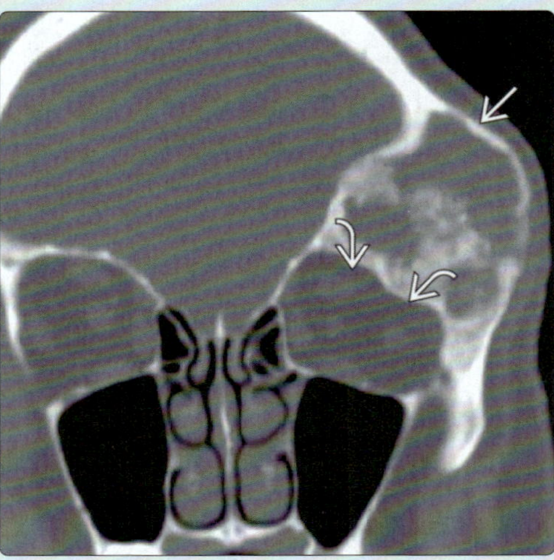

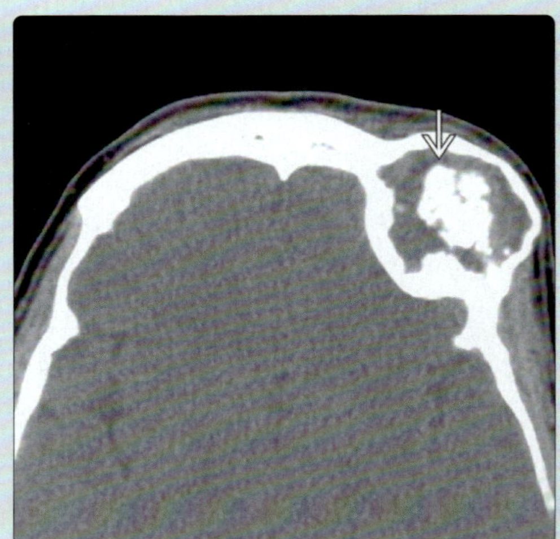

(Left) *Coronal bone CT shows a large OsFib of the orbital plate of the frontal bone. This OsFib shows a mixed ossified and fibrous density. It is expansile, and the patient presented with cosmetic deformity from forehead swelling ➡ and proptosis from orbital mass effect ➡.* **(Right)** *Axial NECT in the same patient shows that the dominant focus of ossification in this case is central ➡ with surrounding soft tissue density rather than the classic pattern with peripheral ossification.*

KEY FACTS

TERMINOLOGY

- Benign, vascular, locally invasive nasal cavity mass

IMAGING

- Location: Centered in posterior nasal cavity near **sphenopalatine foramen**
  - Extends into **pterygopalatine fossa**, nasopharynx, pterygoid plate, infratemporal fossa
- CT findings in juvenile nasopharyngeal angiofibroma (JNA)
  - Mass shows diffuse, avid enhancement
  - Posterior wall of maxillary sinus bowed anteriorly
  - Bone remodeling ± destruction
- MR findings in JNA
  - Signal voids represent flow in enlarged vessels
  - Intense enhancement ± flow voids
- Angiography typically performed at time of preoperative embolization shows tumor blush
  - Intense capillary blush characteristic
  - Internal maxillary artery most common feeding vessel

TOP DIFFERENTIAL DIAGNOSES

- Hypervascular polyp
- Antrochoanal polyp
- Rhabdomyosarcoma
- Esthesioneuroblastoma

CLINICAL ISSUES

- Symptoms
  - Unilateral nasal obstruction (90%); epistaxis (60%)
- Almost exclusively occurs in **male** patients
- Treatment: Complete endoscopic surgical resection
  - Radiation therapy may be used as adjuvant therapy after surgery or as primary treatment in some cases
  - Monitor intraoperative volume status; blood transfusions often necessary

DIAGNOSTIC CHECKLIST

- Look for JNA extension into surrounding structures, including orbit, infratemporal fossa, sphenoid sinus

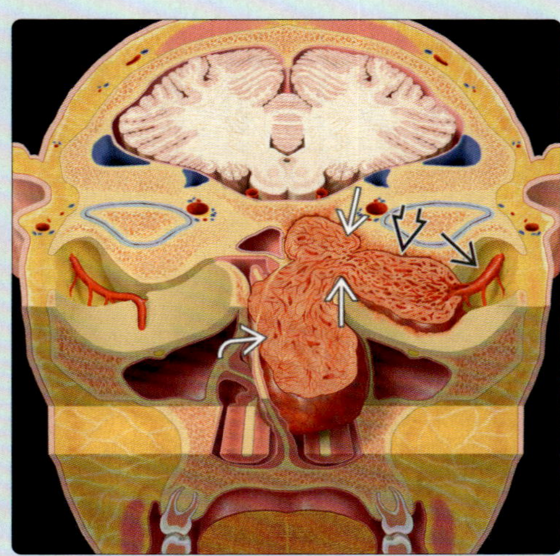

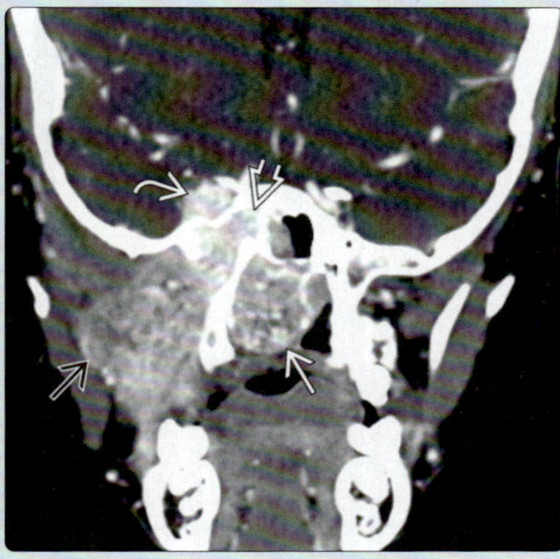

(Left) *Transverse oblique graphic shows classic features & location of a juvenile nasopharyngeal angiofibroma (JNA). Site of origin is in the sphenopalatine foramen ➡ with extension into the pterygopalatine fossa ➡ & nasal cavity ➡. Internal maxillary artery ➡ is the dominant feeding vessel of this vascular mass.* **(Right)** *Coronal CECT in a 13 year old shows typical growth pattern of a large, hypervascular JNA occluding nasopharynx ➡ & extending into right sphenoid ➡, middle cranial fossa ➡, & masticator space ➡.*

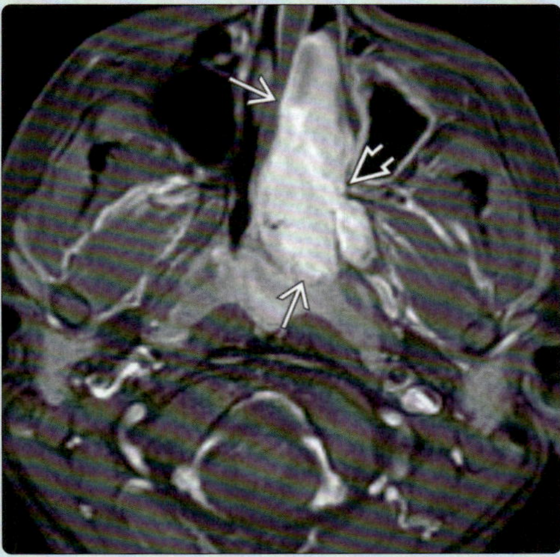

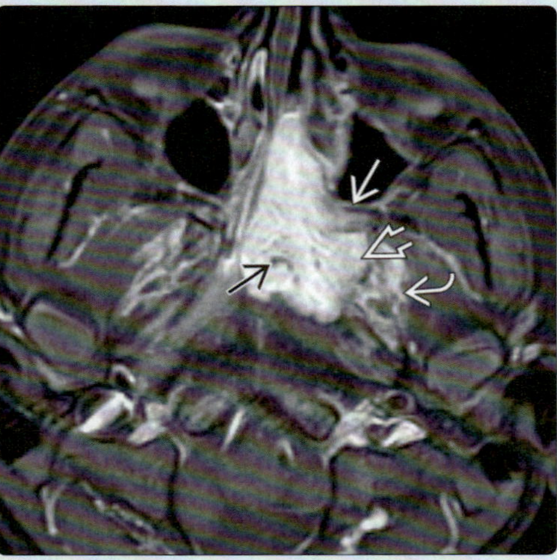

(Left) *Axial T1 C+ FS MR in a 15 year old with nasal obstruction shows enhancing angiofibroma ➡ filling the left nasal cavity and extending into the nasopharynx. The JNA presumed site of origin is the nasopalatine foramen ➡.* **(Right)** *Axial T1 C+ FS MR in the same patient shows a few intralesional high-flow vessels ➡ and extension of the angiofibroma into the widened pterygopalatine fossa ➡, destruction of the left pterygoid ➡, and extension into the masticator space ➡.*

KEY FACTS

TERMINOLOGY

- Inverted papilloma (IP): Benign nasal mucosa epithelial tumor with histology showing epithelium proliferating into underlying stroma

IMAGING

- Typical location: Along lateral nasal wall **centered at middle meatus** ± extension into antrum
- CT findings
  - 40% show entrapped bone
  - Focal bony hyperostosis suggests point of tumor origin
- MR findings
  - T2: Predominantly hyperintense to skeletal muscle
  - T2 & T1 C+ FS: Curvilinear striations or convoluted, **cerebriform pattern** is characteristic
  - If portion of tumor appears invasive or necrosis present → consider synchronous **SCCa**
- Multiplanar MR best maps tumor & differentiates tumor from obstructed secretions; CT complementary

TOP DIFFERENTIAL DIAGNOSES

- Solitary sinonasal (antrochoanal) polyp
- Sinonasal SCCa
- Sinonasal polyposis

PATHOLOGY

- Hyperplastic squamous epithelium replaces seromucinous ducts & glands in stroma with endophytic growth pattern
- **10%** either degenerate into or **coexist with SCCa**
  - SCCa may be synchronous (7%) or metachronous (4%)

CLINICAL ISSUES

- Typically 40-70 years
- M > F (4-5:1)
- Treatment options: Complete surgical removal = goal
  - Smaller tumors: Endoscopic resection effective
  - Larger tumors: Midfacial degloving
  - Medial maxillectomy through lateral rhinotomy + wide en bloc excision in more extensive IP

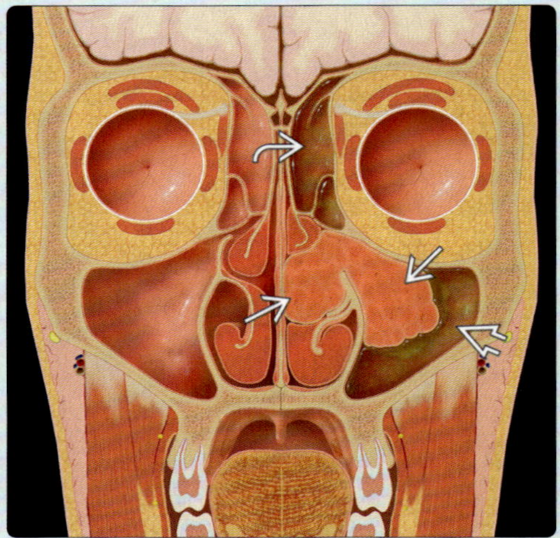

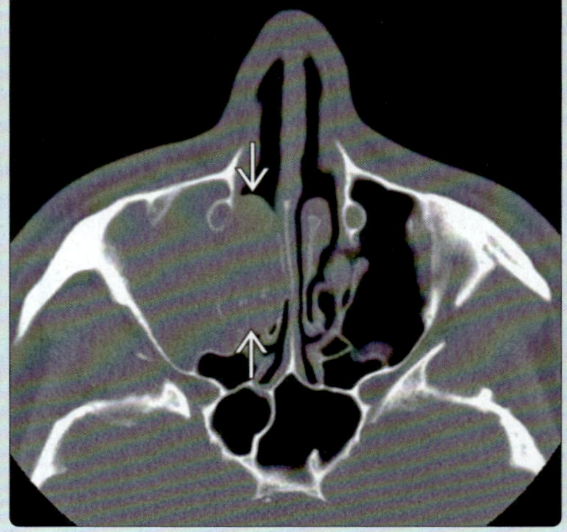

(Left) *Coronal graphic shows an inverted papilloma ➡ originating near the middle meatus and extending into the maxillary sinus. Blocked secretions are noted in the ethmoid ➡ and maxillary ➡ sinuses.* **(Right)** *Axial bone CT shows a mass in the nasal cavity ➡ along the lateral wall near the middle meatus. The maxillary sinus is opacified, but it is difficult to differentiate obstructed secretions from papilloma on the CT. MR in such a case would be helpful to delineate the margins of the mass.*

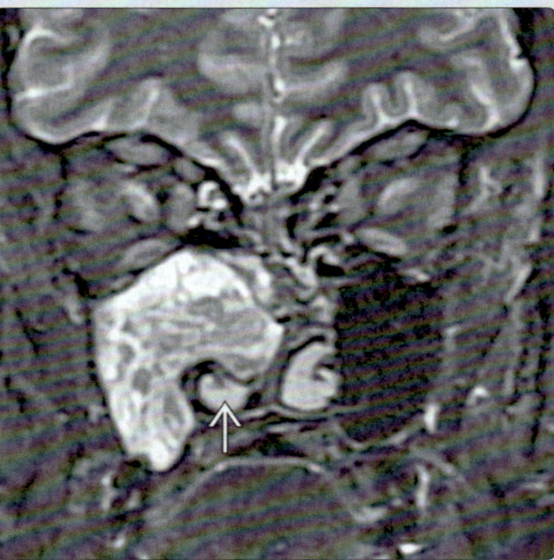

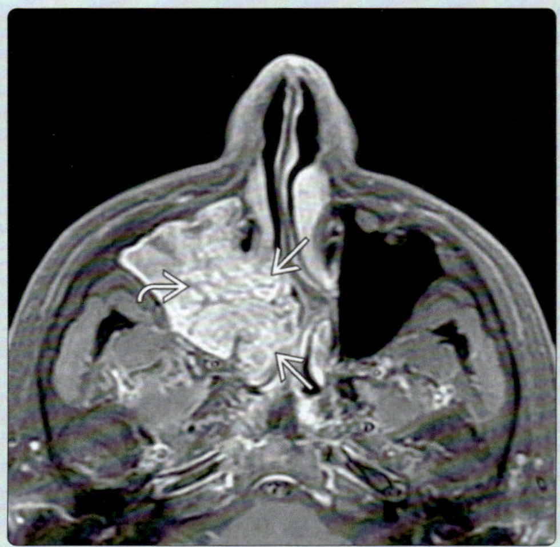

(Left) *Coronal T2 FS MR shows characteristic features of an inverted papilloma involving the right maxillary sinus and nasal cavity. The lesion has a convoluted, cerebriform architecture. Note the inferior displacement of the inferior turbinate ➡.* **(Right)** *Axial T1 C+ FS MR shows classic features of an inverted papilloma. The lesion is centered at the middle meatus with nasal cavity ➡ and antral ➡ components. This lesion shows characteristic convoluted, cerebriform architecture.*

KEY FACTS

TERMINOLOGY

- Lobular capillary hemangioma (LCH): Benign capillary proliferation with distinct lobular architecture
  - Old term: Pyogenic granuloma

IMAGING

- Location: Nasal septum (55%), particularly anteriorly (17%)
- Size: Typically ≤ 2 cm
- CT findings
  - Central areas of lobular enhancement surrounded by iso- to hypodense "cap" of variable thickness
  - May cause bone erosion or remodeling
- MR findings
  - Usually **T2 hyperintense**
  - Homogeneous, **avid enhancement ± flow voids**
- Lobular areas of capillary blush on angiography
  - Preoperative embolization ↓ intraoperative bleeding

TOP DIFFERENTIAL DIAGNOSES

- Venous malformation (old term: Cavernous hemangioma)
  - No central avid enhancement or flow voids
  - Centripetal pattern of enhancement with delayed filling
  - Variable T2 signal
- Sinonasal melanoma
- Juvenile angiofibroma
- Angiomatous polyp
- Hemangiopericytoma

PATHOLOGY

- Predisposing factors include trauma & hormonal influences

CLINICAL ISSUES

- Symptoms: Epistaxis & nasal obstruction
- Peak incidence in 5th decade with slight F > M
- Treatment options
  - Local surgical excision
  - Most can be done endoscopically under local anesthesia

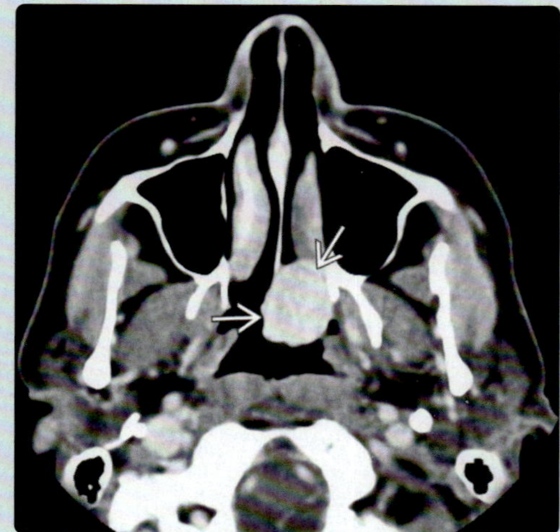

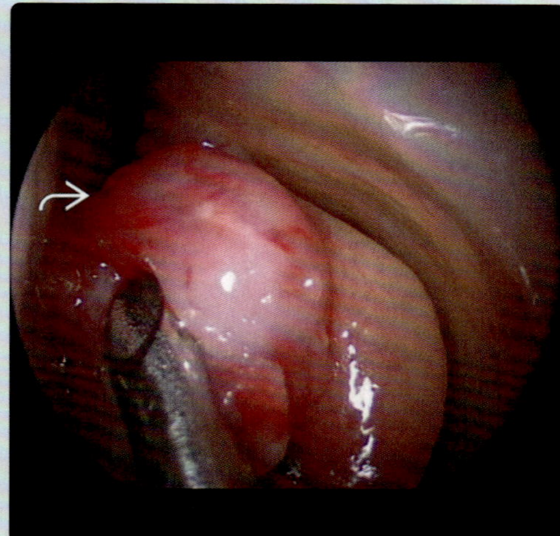

(Left) *Axial CECT demonstrates an avidly enhancing, well-circumscribed soft tissue mass ➡ in the posterior nasal cavity and protruding into the nasopharynx. No bony destructive changes were seen. This lobular hemangioma arose from the inferior turbinate; this patient presented with nasal bleeding.* **(Right)** *Endoscopic view of a lobular capillary hemangioma shows a lobulated, epithelial lined, red hypervascular mass ➡.*

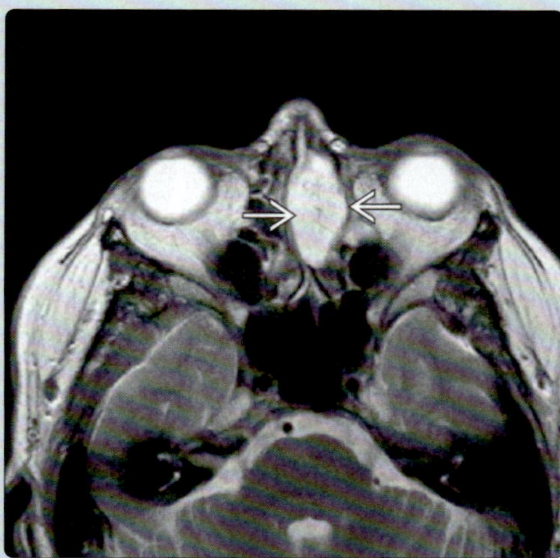

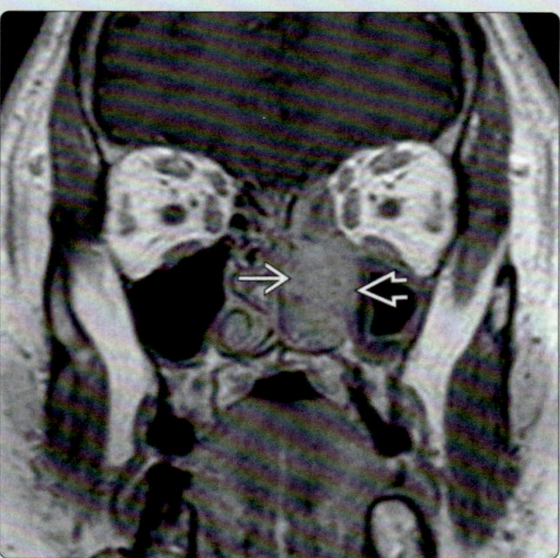

(Left) *Axial T2 MR demonstrates a well-defined, ovoid soft tissue mass ➡ in the superior aspect of the left nasal cavity in an adult patient with intermittent epistaxis. The lesion is homogeneously hyperintense on this sequence, typical of hemangioma. No orbital invasion is appreciated.* **(Right)** *Coronal T1 C+ MR shows homogeneous enhancement with a left nasal cavity hemangioma ➡. Note the mild expansion of the lateral nasal wall ➡ but no overtly invasive features.*

Sinonasal Squamous Cell Carcinoma

KEY FACTS

TERMINOLOGY

- Malignant epithelial tumor with squamous cell or epidermoid differentiation

IMAGING

- Location: Maxillary antrum involved in > 80%
- CT findings
  - Soft tissue density mass with irregular margins
  - Aggressive **bone destruction**
- MR findings
  - ↓ T2 signal due to ↑ nuclear:cytoplasmic ratio
  - Enhances to lesser degree than other sinonasal malignancies
- Multiplanar enhanced MR optimal for tumor mapping, detection of perineural tumor spread & nodes

TOP DIFFERENTIAL DIAGNOSES

- Sinonasal adenocarcinoma
- Sinonasal undifferentiated carcinoma
- Sinonasal non-Hodgkin lymphoma
- Adenoid cystic carcinoma
- Wegener granulomatosis

PATHOLOGY

- Risk factors: Inhaled wood dust, metallic particles (nickel & chromium), chemicals, HPV, inverted papilloma
  - Formaldehyde, arsenic & asbestos exposure may ↑ risk
  - HPV, pre- or coexisting inverted papilloma ↑ risk

CLINICAL ISSUES

- Symptoms mimic chronic sinusitis & delay diagnosis
- Age at presentation: 50-70 years old
- Most common malignancy of sinonasal area
- 15% maxillary sinus squamous cell carcinomas have malignant adenopathy
- Overall **5-year survival: 60%**
- Treatment options
  - Combined surgery & XRT most common

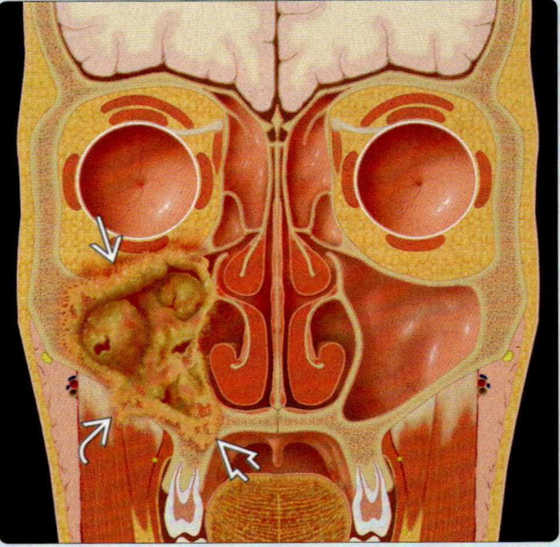
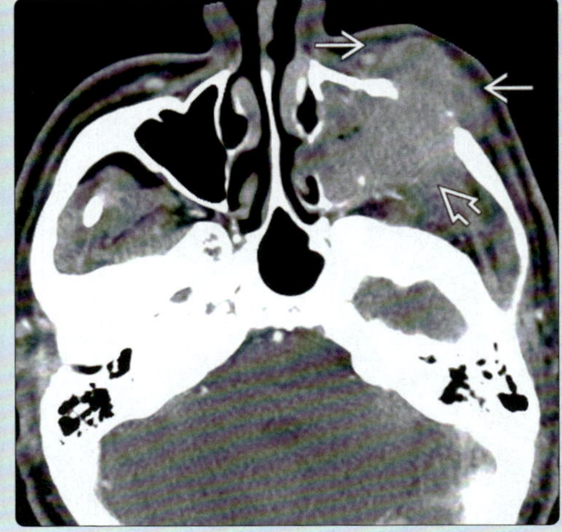

(Left) *Coronal graphic shows the typical features of an aggressive right maxillary squamous cell carcinoma (SCCa) with destruction of the maxillary sinus walls. Extension into the orbit ➡, maxillary alveolus ➡, and buccal space ➡ is noted.* **(Right)** *Axial CECT shows the typical location and appearance of an antral SCCa. There is extension into the premaxillary soft tissues anteriorly ➡ and through the posterior maxillary wall into the infratemporal fossa ➡.*

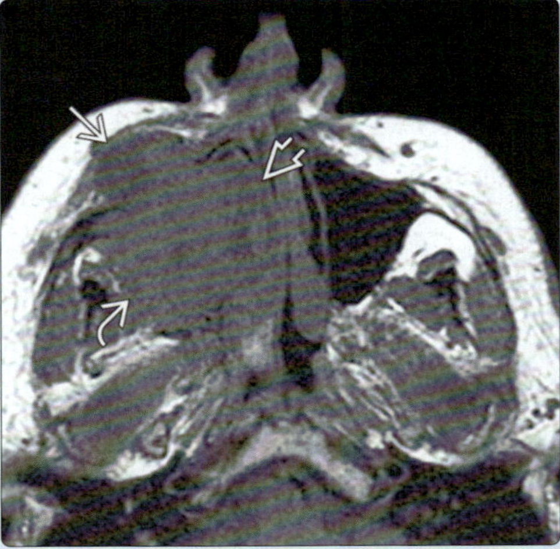
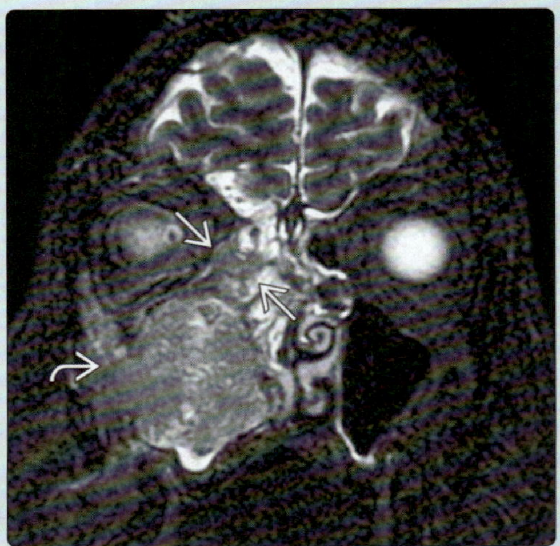

(Left) *Axial T1 MR shows a large antral SCCa. The signal of the mass is similar to other soft tissues. There is extension anteriorly into the premaxillary soft tissues ➡, medially into the nasal cavity ➡, and posteriorly into the masticator space ➡.* **(Right)** *Coronal T2 FS MR of SCCa demonstrates ethmoid sinus involvement ➡ and masticator space extension ➡. The low T2 signal of this mass is consistent with high cellularity and N:C ratio.*

KEY FACTS

TERMINOLOGY

- Malignant neuroectodermal tumor arising from **olfactory neuroepithelium** in superior nasal cavity

IMAGING

- Enhanced MR & bone CT best delineate esthesioneuroblastoma (ENB) for en bloc craniofacial surgery
- Shape & location
  - Large ENB: **Dumbbell-shaped**; "waist" at cribriform plate
  - Small ENB: Nasal polyp enlarges olfactory recess
- Bone CT: Bone destruction, especially of cribriform plate
- T1 C+ FS MR: Homogeneously enhancing mass
  - **Cysts** at intracranial tumor-brain margin
  - DWI MR: Mildly restricted diffusion
  - T2 best differentiate tumor from sinus secretions

TOP DIFFERENTIAL DIAGNOSES

- Sinonasal squamous cell carcinoma
- Sinonasal adenocarcinoma
- Sinonasal non-Hodgkin lymphoma
- Sinonasal undifferentiated carcinoma

PATHOLOGY

- No etiologic, genetic, or risk factors elucidated
- Staging: **Kadish classification**; good predictor of outcome
- Histologic grading: Hyams system
- Excellent prognosis vs. other sinonasal malignancies
  - 5-year survival rates: 75-77% overall; recurrence in ~ 30%; metastases in 10-30% of patients

CLINICAL ISSUES

- **Adolescent or middle-aged** patient with unilateral nasal obstruction & mild epistaxis
  - Bimodal distribution in 2nd & 6th decades
- Surgical resection & radiotherapy is best treatment
  - Chemotherapy reserved for advanced stage disease
- Smaller, intranasal tumors endoscopically resected

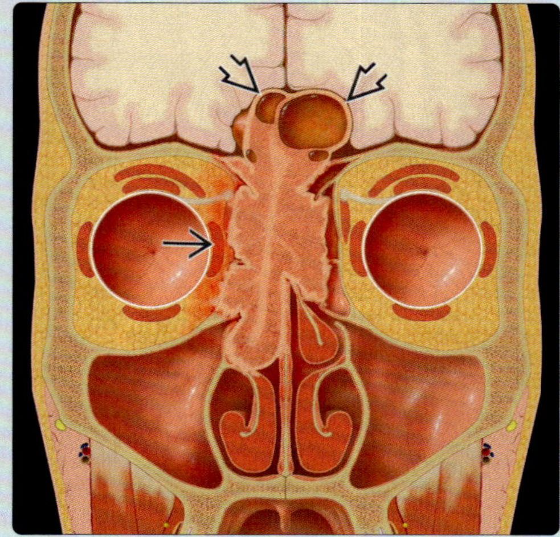

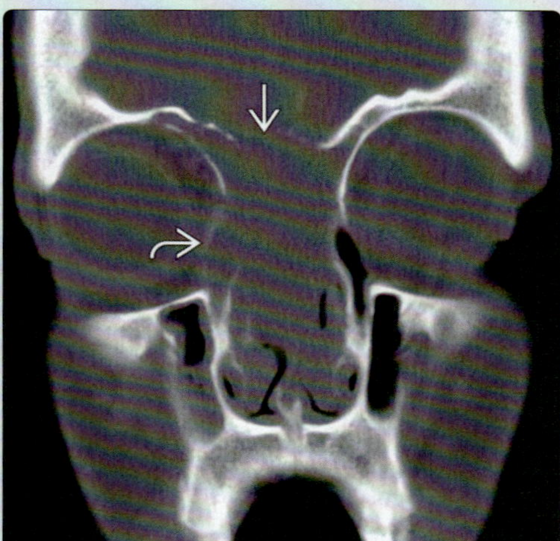

(Left) *Coronal graphic shows the classic features of esthesioneuroblastoma (ENB) centered below the cribriform plate and extending into the anterior cranial fossa and right orbit ➡. Cyst formation ➡ is noted at the tumor-brain interface.* **(Right)** *Coronal bone CT shows an ENB filling the upper nasal cavity and ethmoid sinuses. The lesion extends through the anterior skull base ➡. The lamina papyracea on the right is thinned and laterally displaced ➡.*

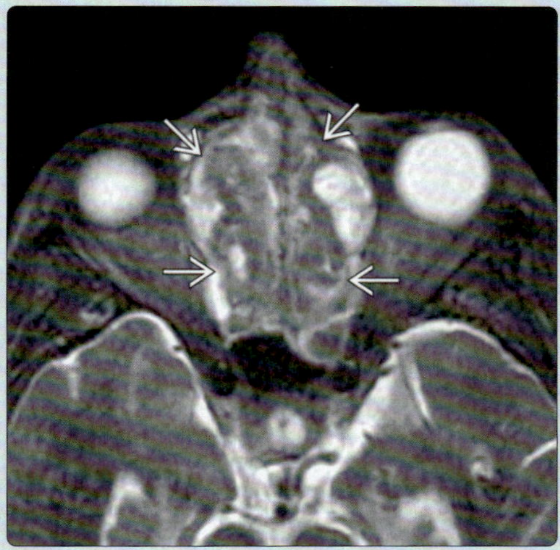

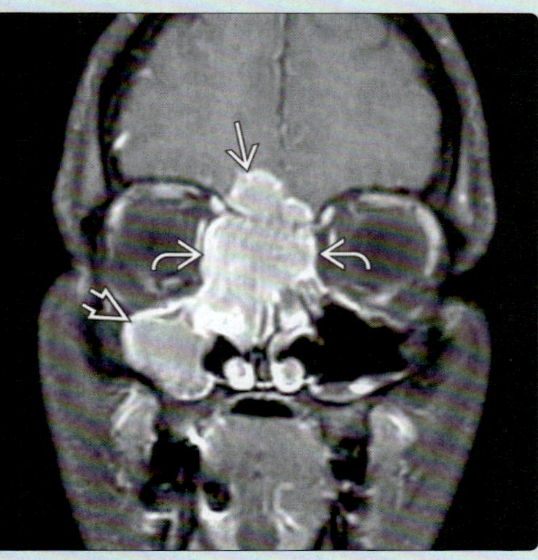

(Left) *Axial STIR MR demonstrates a large, heterogeneous ENB ➡ centered in the midline below the skull base and occupying the nasal cavity and ethmoid sinuses. The mass is predominantly hypointense in this case and causes hypertelorism.* **(Right)** *Coronal T1 C+ FS MR shows an avidly enhancing ENB with extension into anterior cranial fossa ➡ and both orbits ➡. Avid enhancement is characteristic of this highly vascular neoplasm. Note the trapped maxillary secretions ➡.*

KEY FACTS

TERMINOLOGY

- Malignant neoplasm with glandular differentiation arising from surface epithelium or minor salivary rests

IMAGING

- General imaging features
  - Predilection for nasal cavity & ethmoid sinuses
  - May reach large size due to delay in diagnosis
    - 75% with involvement of > 1 sinonasal (SN) region at diagnosis
- CT findings
  - Well- to poorly defined mass with bone destruction or remodeling
- MR findings
  - Typically intermediate to hyperintense T2 signal
  - Diffuse, heterogeneous enhancement

TOP DIFFERENTIAL DIAGNOSES

- Sinonasal squamous cell carcinoma; esthesioneuroblastoma
- Sinonasal undifferentiated carcinoma
- Sinonasal non-Hodgkin lymphoma

PATHOLOGY

- 2 major subtypes
  - Intestinal (related to **wood dust exposure**): Most frequent form colonic > solid > papillary > mucinous & mixed type
  - Nonintestinal: Unrelated to wood dust exposure
- Accounts for 15% of all SN cancers

CLINICAL ISSUES

- Clinical presentation
  - 6th decade most common; M > F (~ 3:1)
  - Poor prognosis with higher grades, incomplete resection, & intracranial involvement
  - 5-year survival rates generally poor (~ 50%)
- Treatment: Complete surgical excision for cure
  - Adjuvant postop radiation therapy & chemotherapy

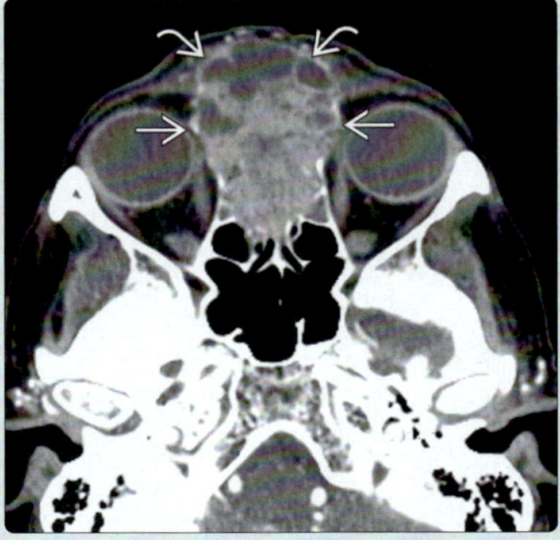

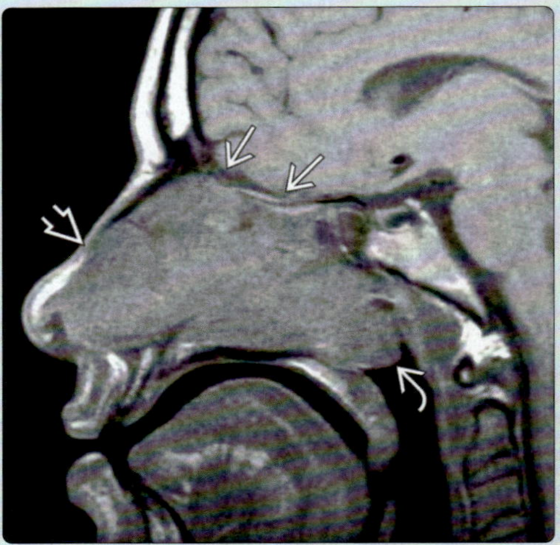

(Left) *Axial CECT shows a large, heterogeneously enhancing adenocarcinoma filling the upper nasal cavity and ethmoid sinuses. There is anterior extension into the soft tissues of the nasal dorsum → and destruction of bilateral lamina papyracea →.* **(Right)** *Sagittal T1WI MR shows a large adenocarcinoma filling the nasal cavity and extending into the nasopharynx →. No extension through the skull base → is seen. The lesion invades subcutaneous fat → of the dorsum of the nose.*

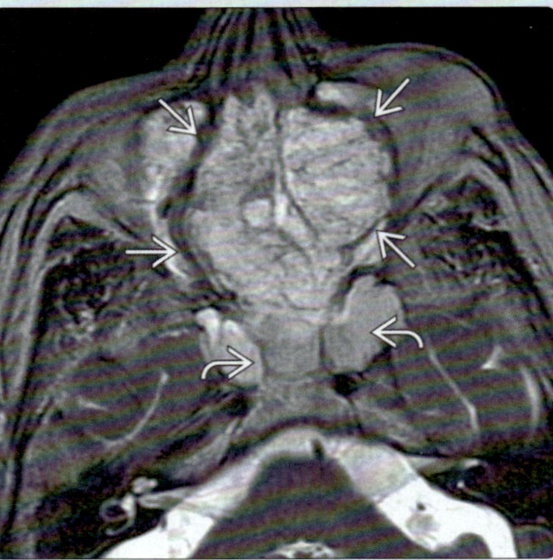

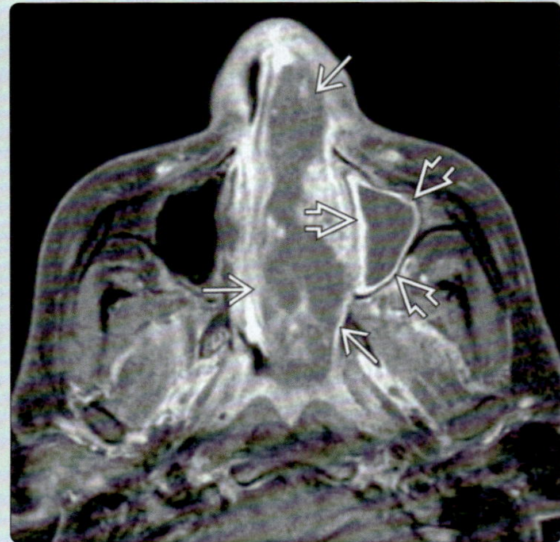

(Left) *Axial T2WI FS MR demonstrates a large, hyperintense, heterogeneous adenocarcinoma of ethmoids → filling the nasal cavity and causing mass effect on both orbits. Obstructed secretions → are present in the sphenoid sinuses.* **(Right)** *Axial T1WI C+ FS MR shows a left nasal cavity adenocarcinoma →, with heterogeneous enhancement. Note the left maxillary sinus is obstructed with peripheral (but no central) enhancement of retained secretions →.*

KEY FACTS

TERMINOLOGY

- Arises from melanocytes migrated from **neural crest origin** to sinonasal epithelium

IMAGING

- Soft tissue mass in nasal cavity > paranasal sinuses with bone destruction ± remodeling
  - Predilection for nasal septum, lateral nasal wall, and inferior turbinate
- MR (melanotic melanoma)
  - **↑ T1** & **↓ T2 signal** results from melanin, free radicals, metal ions, and hemorrhage
  - T2* GRE may show **blooming** when hemorrhage present in sinonasal melanoma (SNM)
  - Avidly enhances due to vascularity in SNM; enhancement may be difficult to appreciate if high precontrast T1 signal present

TOP DIFFERENTIAL DIAGNOSES

- Squamous cell carcinoma
- Non-Hodgkin lymphoma
- Esthesioneuroblastoma

CLINICAL ISSUES

- Adult with nasal stuffiness, epistaxis, and pigmented mass identified at nasal endoscopy
  - 5th-8th decades most common
  - > 90% occurs in whites, M > F
- Poor prognosis with 6-17% chance of 5-year survival
  - Mean survival ~ 24 months
  - Systemic metastatic disease typically precedes death
- Treatment options
  - Radical surgery with adjuvant radiotherapy
  - Chemotherapy, surgery, and XRT used for recurrences

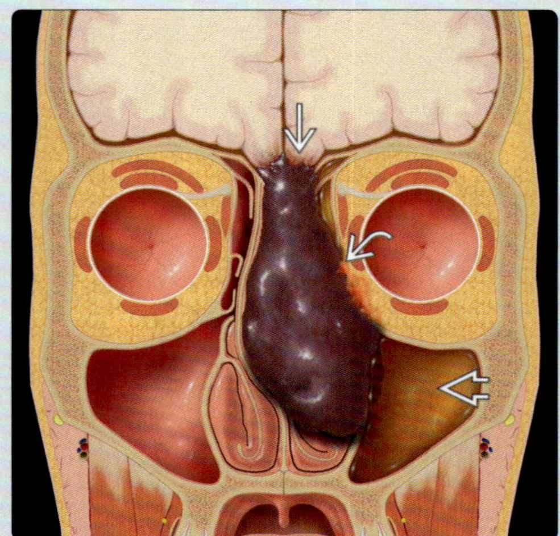

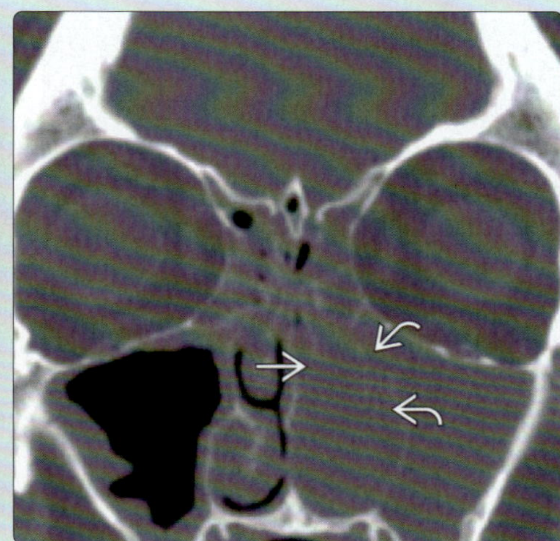

(Left) *Coronal graphic shows a darkly pigmented (highly melanotic) mass centered in the nasal cavity. Invasion of the skull base ➡, orbit ➡, and lateral nasal wall is seen, but the septum is deviated rather than invaded. Trapped secretions ➡ are noted in the left maxillary sinus.* **(Right)** *Coronal bone CT in a patient with left nasal obstruction and epistaxis shows a mass in the left nasal cavity with erosion of the left middle turbinate ➡ and portions of the lateral nasal wall ➡.*

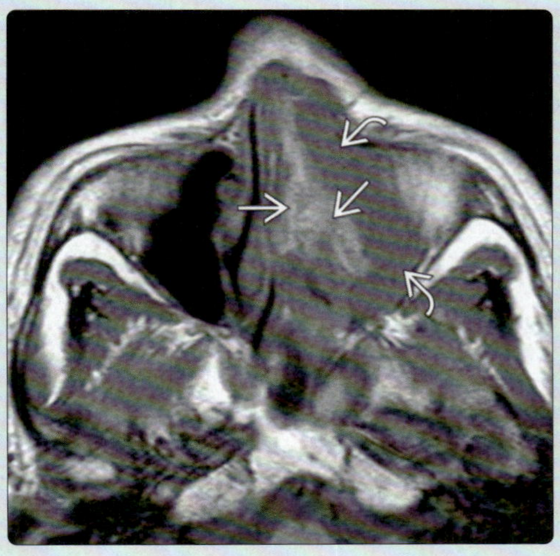

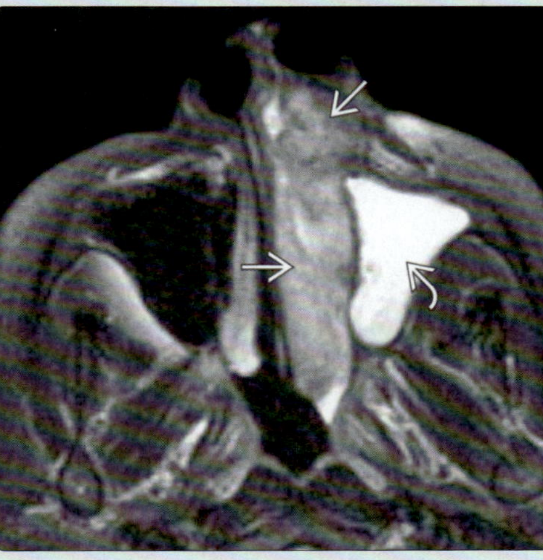

(Left) *Axial T1 MR demonstrates a mass in the left nasal cavity with maxillary sinus extension. The lesion is heterogeneous with areas of T1 shortening ➡ and intermediate signal ➡. T1 shortening on unenhanced images may indicate the presence of melanin or hemorrhage.* **(Right)** *Axial T2 FS MR shows a lobular melanoma ➡ within the left nasal cavity. It is somewhat hypointense and is readily distinguishable from the hyperintense obstructed secretions ➡ in the maxillary sinus.*

Sinonasal Non-Hodgkin Lymphoma

KEY FACTS

TERMINOLOGY

- Sinonasal non-Hodgkin lymphoma: Extranodal lymphoproliferative malignancy

IMAGING

- General imaging
  - Appearance can mimic variety of neoplasms & aggressive inflammatory disorders
  - Predilection for nasal cavity over sinuses
- CT: Homogeneous mass ± bone remodeling or destruction
  - May be hyperdense due to high N:C ratio
- MR: Imaging modality of choice; multiplanar, T1 C+ FS
  - MR: ↓ T2 signal
  - Restricted diffusion due to high cellularity
- PET: For initial staging & treatment response

TOP DIFFERENTIAL DIAGNOSES

- Wegener granulomatosis (with polyangiitis)
- Sinonasal adenocarcinoma
- Esthesioneuroblastoma
- Sinonasal squamous cell carcinoma

PATHOLOGY

- 3 pathologic subgroups
  - B-cell (Western) phenotype most common
  - T-cell (Asian) phenotype
  - Natural killer/T-cell lymphoma (Asian): Subtype of T cell

CLINICAL ISSUES

- Male patient in 6th decade with nonspecific symptoms of nasal obstruction & discharge
- Local radiotherapy = primary treatment
  - ± combination chemotherapy

DIAGNOSTIC CHECKLIST

- NHL could be included in DDx for almost any aggressive adult nasal soft tissue mass
- Imaging clue to diagnosis: Presence of enlarged cervical nodes & Waldeyer ring lymphatic mass

(Left) *Axial CECT shows a large non-Hodgkin lymphoma ➡ centered in the nasal cavity with slightly heterogeneous enhancement. There is gross destruction of the nasal septum ⇨. Obstructed secretions ↪ are noted in both maxillary sinuses.* **(Right)** *Axial STIR MR shows a large lymphoma involving the nasal cavity and ethmoid sinuses. Relatively hypointense signal is characteristic of this tumor with high nuclear:cytoplasmic ratio. Note the involvement of the right orbit ➡ with resulting proptosis.*

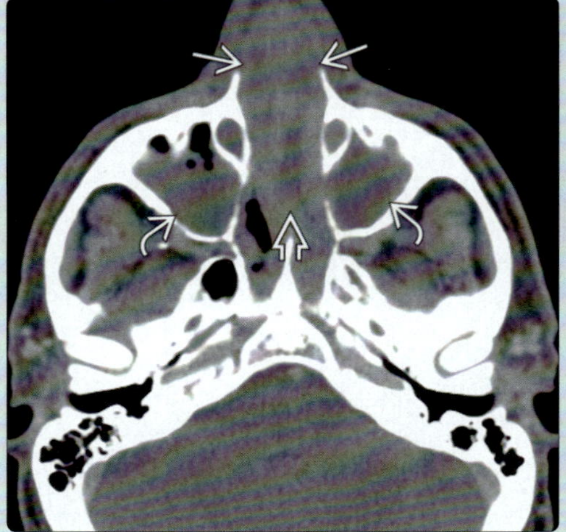

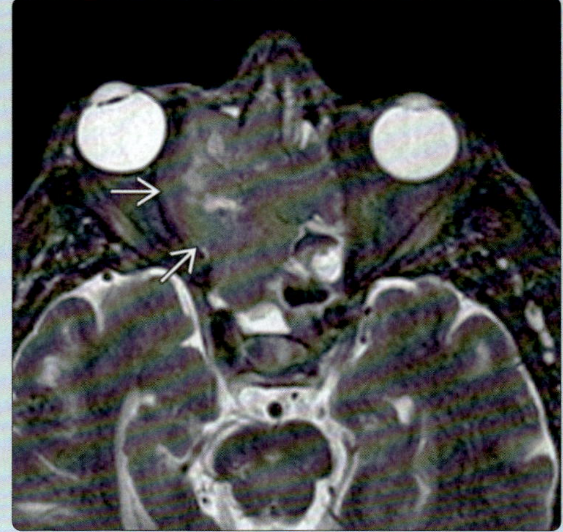

(Left) *Coronal bone CT shows the classic location of sinonasal non-Hodgkin lymphoma. The mass is centered around the nasal septum, and there is destruction of the septum ➡ as well as multiple ethmoid septations ↪.* **(Right)** *Axial T1 C+ FS MR demonstrates a large lymphoma filling the left nasal cavity. The septum is displaced ➡ but not eroded. Homogeneous mild enhancement is present. Trapped secretions ↪ are present in the left maxillary antrum.*

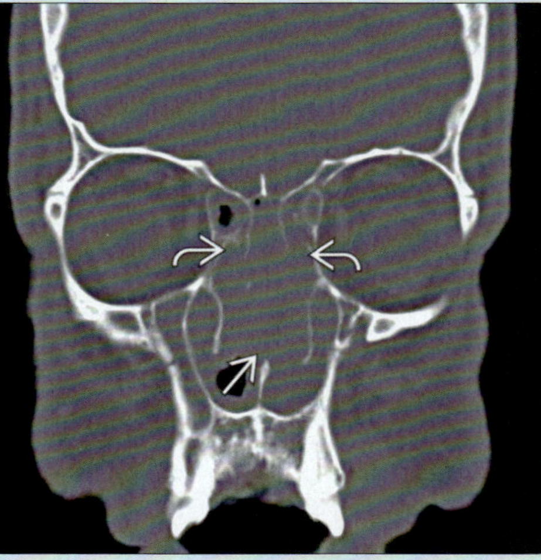

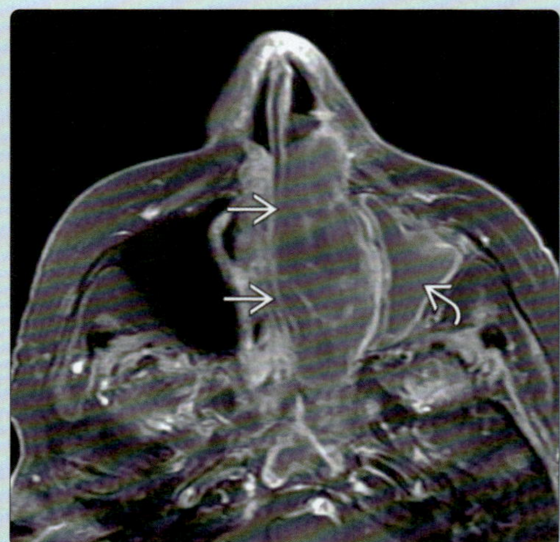

KEY FACTS

TERMINOLOGY

- Rare, aggressive, sinonasal nonsquamous cell epithelial or nonepithelial malignant neoplasm of varying histogenesis

IMAGING

- General imaging considerations
  - Sinonasal undifferentiated carcinoma (SNUC) imaging features are nonspecific
  - Consider extending coverage to evaluate for intracranial (particularly dural) & cervical nodal disease
  - Aggressive sinonasal mass with **bone destruction** & **rapid growth**
  - Large, typically > 4 cm at presentation
  - Origin mostly in nose with extension into sinuses
    - Ethmoid sinus origin more common than maxillary
- Bone CT findings
  - Poorly defined, soft tissue sinonasal mass with **aggressive bone destruction**
- MR findings
  - Isointense to muscle on T1
  - Low to intermediate T2 signal
  - Heterogeneous enhancement with necrosis

TOP DIFFERENTIAL DIAGNOSES

- Sinonasal squamous cell carcinoma
- Esthesioneuroblastoma
- Sinonasal non-Hodgkin lymphoma
- Sinonasal adenocarcinoma

CLINICAL ISSUES

- Nasal obstruction, epistaxis, proptosis, ± facial pain
  - Metastases common to neck nodes, bone, brain ± dura
- Treatment: Aggressive multimodality therapy
  - Craniofacial resection and adjuvant chemotherapy ± XRT

DIAGNOSTIC CHECKLIST

- Tumor growth rate & presence of nodes/distant metastases helpful for suggesting SNUC

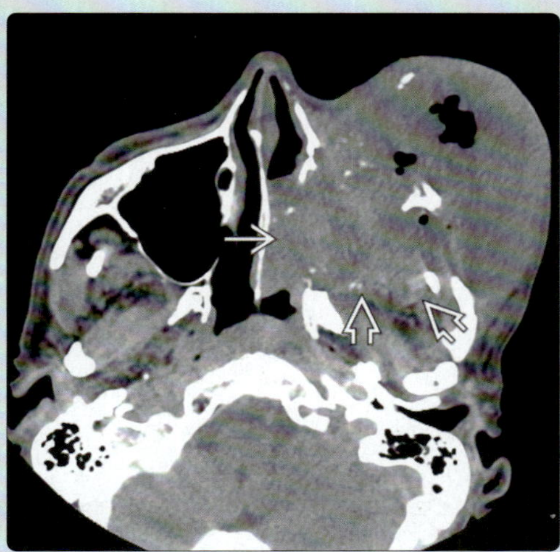

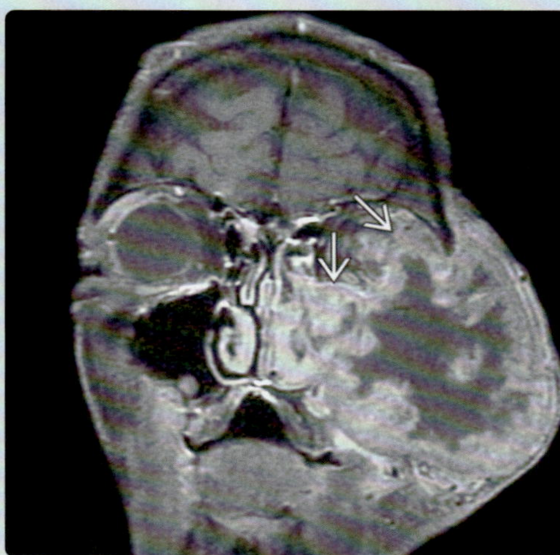

(Left) *Axial NECT demonstrates a large mass in the left maxillary antrum with marked bone destruction and extension into the nasal cavity ➡, masticator space ➡, and soft tissues of the cheek. Foci of air are seen within the necrotic portion of this rapidly growing lesion.* **(Right)** *Coronal T1WI C+ FS MR in the same patient shows a thick, nodular, enhancing rim at the periphery of the mass with central necrosis. There is aggressive invasion of the orbit ➡.*

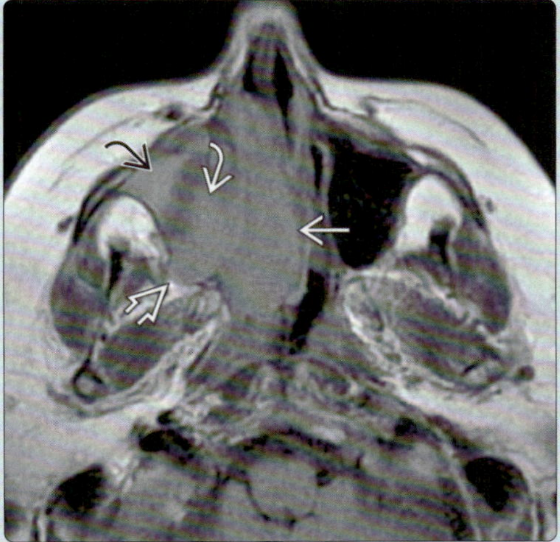

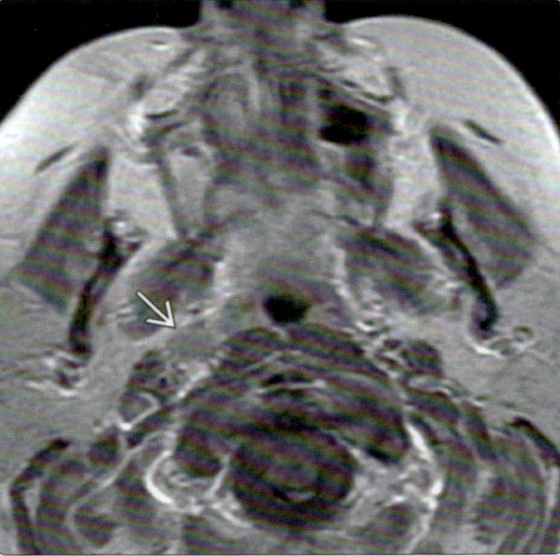

(Left) *Axial FLAIR MR demonstrates a large mass filling the right nasal cavity ➡ and extending into the right maxillary antrum ➡. There is extension into the retroantral fat ➡. Note the trapped secretions in the lateral aspect of the maxillary sinus ➡.* **(Right)** *Axial T1WI C+ MR in the same patient at the level of the nasopharynx shows a pathologic lateral retropharyngeal nodal metastasis ➡ from the patient's sinonasal undifferentiated carcinoma.*

Sinonasal Adenoid Cystic Carcinoma

KEY FACTS

TERMINOLOGY

- Malignant salivary type of adenocarcinoma

IMAGING

- Location: **Maxillary** > nasal cavity
- Low grade: Solidly enhancing, well-defined soft tissue mass
- High grade: Poorly defined, heterogeneous + bone destruction ± perineural tumor spread (PNTS)
- Multiplanar, **gadolinium-enhanced MR with fat suppression** recommended
  - Improves detection of PNTS

TOP DIFFERENTIAL DIAGNOSES

- Sinonasal squamous cell carcinoma
- Sinonasal adenocarcinoma (intestinal type)
- Esthesioneuroblastoma
- Sinonasal undifferentiated carcinoma

PATHOLOGY

- Not associated with inhalation exposures
- 3 histologic types
  - Cribriform (52%)
  - Tubular (20%)
  - Solid (29%); worst outcome; higher tendency for PNTS
- Most patients present with **T4 disease (65%)**

CLINICAL ISSUES

- Sinonasal adenoid cystic carcinoma (ACCa) accounts for 10-25% of H&N ACCa
  - Most common sinonasal salivary tumor
- Symptoms mimic sinusitis
  - **Facial pain ± numbness** (CNV2) → PNTS
- Treatment: Surgery followed by postop XRT
- Overall 5-year survival rate: > 50%
  - **Late recurrences** are common, even > 15 years after initial therapy; pulmonary metastasis

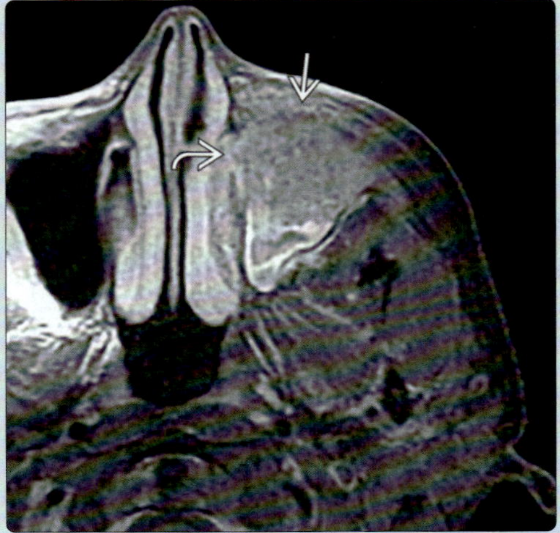

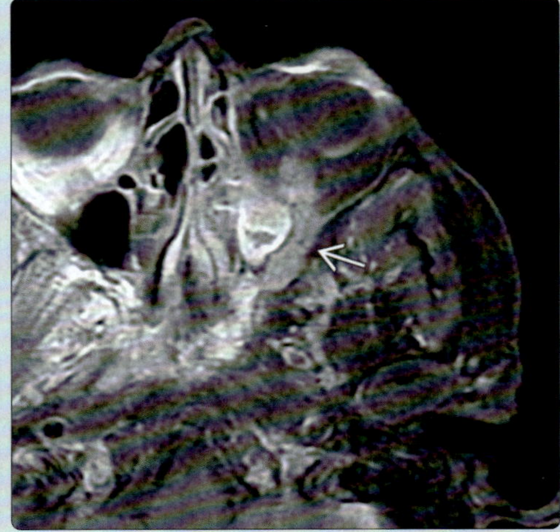

(Left) *Axial T1WI C+ FS MR demonstrates diffuse enhancement of a left maxillary sinus adenoid cystic carcinoma (ACCa). There is osseous destruction and extension through the anterior ➡ and medial ➡ maxillary sinus walls.* **(Right)** *Axial T1WI C+ FS MR in the same patient demonstrates linear enhancing soft tissue along CNV2 ➡ involving the left inferior orbital fissure extending toward foramen rotundum, compatible with perineural tumor spread.*

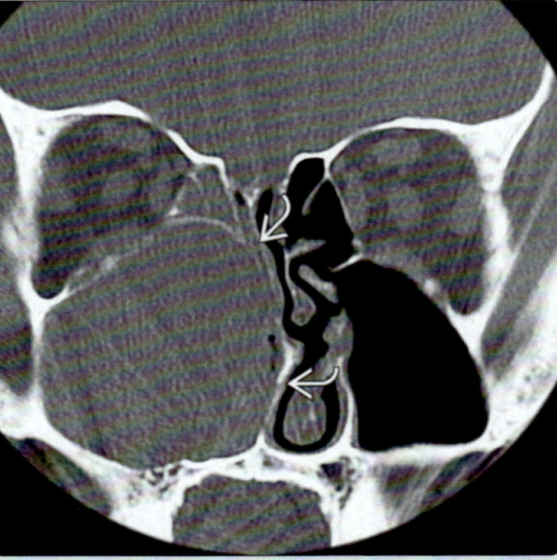

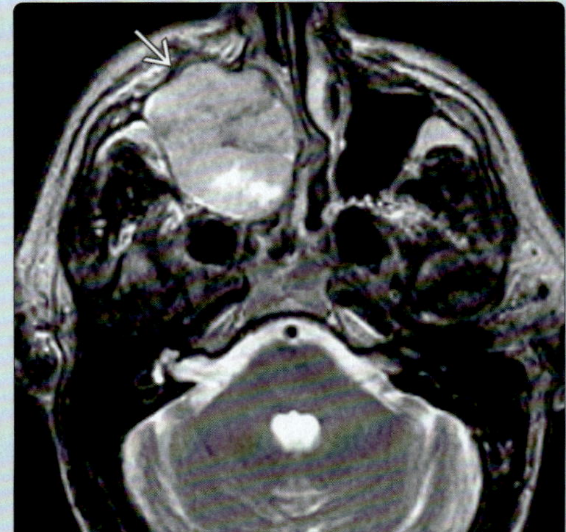

(Left) *Coronal bone CT shows opacification of the right maxillary sinus by a large, expansile ACCa. The medial maxillary wall is eroded, and the mass extends into the nasal cavity. Note the leftward deviation of the nasal septum ➡.* **(Right)** *Axial T2WI MR in the same patient shows slightly heterogeneous high signal throughout the mass. Slight extension into the premaxillary soft tissues is noted ➡. The relatively well-defined appearance of the ACCa may suggest a lower grade histology.*

KEY FACTS

IMAGING

- Arises from maxilla, nasal septum, and skull base
    - Nasal septum location: Posterosuperior vomer
- Bone CT: **Chondroid matrix calcification** and narrow bony transition zone
    - **50%** with chondroid matrix
- MR: Increased (high) signal on T2 images and heterogeneous enhancement

TOP DIFFERENTIAL DIAGNOSES

- Sinonasal osteosarcoma
- Skull base meningioma
- Sinonasal ossifying fibroma
- Sinonasal fibrous dysplasia
- Esthesioneuroblastoma

PATHOLOGY

- Malignant neoplasm arising from chondrocytes, embryonal rests, or mesenchymal cells
- May complicate Ollier and Maffucci syndromes

CLINICAL ISSUES

- Presents in 5th-7th decades
    - Duration from symptom onset to diagnosis: 3 months to 1 year
- Accounts for only 0.1% of H&N cancers
- Surgical resection is primary treatment modality
    - Difficult to achieve oncologic resection due to proximity of vital structures
    - Late recurrences after long disease-free periods are reported; long-term follow-up advised
- Overall 5-year survival: 50-80%

DIAGNOSTIC CHECKLIST

- **Arc-whorl** or **ring-like calcified matrix** on CT in lesion with ↑ T2 signal on MR may suggest diagnosis of sinonasal chondrosarcoma

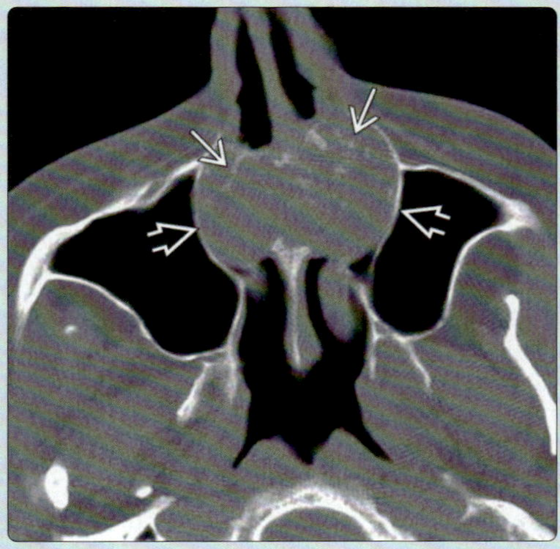

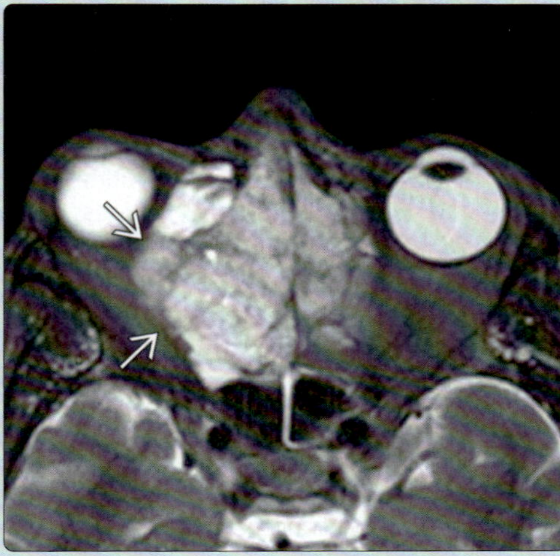

(Left) *Axial bone CT shows a bilobed chondrosarcoma centered around the nasal septum at the bone-cartilage junction. Note involvement of bilateral nasal cavities. Multiple chondroid calcifications* ➡ *are characteristic. The lateral nasal walls* ➡ *are remodeled but not destroyed.* **(Right)** *Axial STIR MR demonstrates a large chondrosarcoma involving the ethmoid sinuses bilaterally. There is extension into the right orbit* ➡*. High signal on T2-weighted images is a common feature of this histology.*

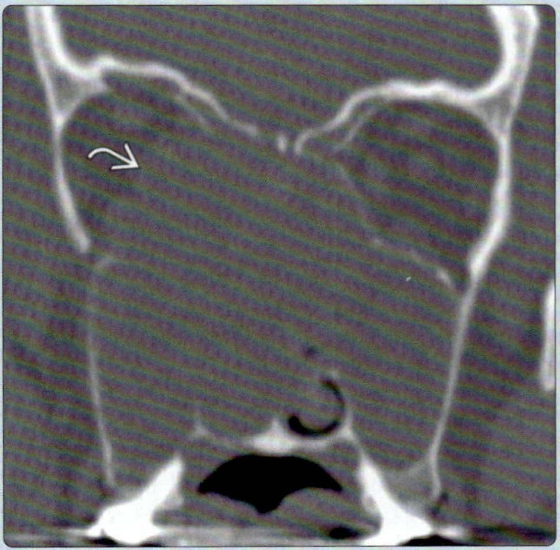

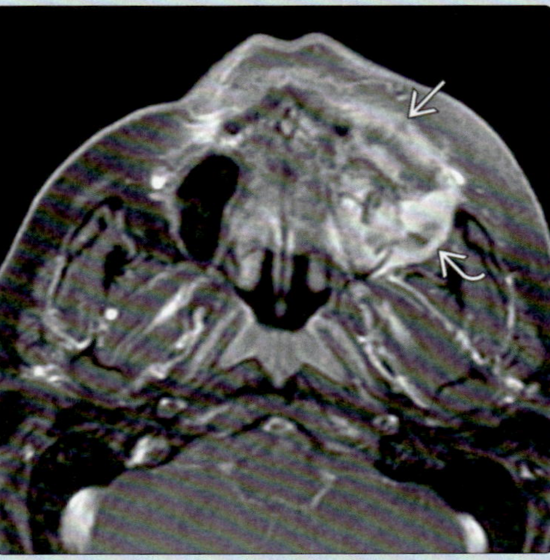

(Left) *Coronal CT reconstruction shows a large, aggressive mass filling the ethmoid sinuses and nasal cavity with bone destruction and extension into the right orbit* ➡*. There is no classic chondroid matrix but malignant features are present.* **(Right)** *Axial T1WI C+ FS MR shows a chondrosarcoma of the left maxilla with involvement of the maxillary antrum. The lesion enhances heterogeneously and extends into the premaxillary* ➡ *and retromaxillary* ➡ *soft tissues.*

Imaging Approach and Indications

General Approach

Imaging of the orbit encompasses 2 clinically distinct areas of ophthalmology.

- Eye (or globe)
- Bony orbit, soft tissues, and periorbita

Lesions in these 2 areas result in specific clinical profiles. When a patient is referred for imaging, it is usually clear to the clinician whether the problem involves the globe vs. some other structure of the orbit.

The term "orbital" refers to those bony structures and soft tissues that are extrinsic to the eye, as opposed to the term "ocular," which refers to the globe itself.

Most imaging referrals come from ophthalmologists, oculoplastic surgeons, neuro-ophthalmologists, neurosurgeons, and otolaryngologists. Imaging of the orbit and globe provides complementary information to the physical and ophthalmoscopic examination.

Ultrasound

Ultrasound of the eye is a readily available complement to funduscopic examination and is traditionally performed in the ophthalmology clinic. In addition to providing imaging of the globe, transocular ultrasound provides a limited, high-resolution assessment of other intraorbital soft tissues.

CT

Because of its superior bony characterization, CT has advantages over MR for orbital lesions that arise from or directly affect the bones, such as epithelial inclusions, osteocartilaginous tumors with matrix, osteodystrophic processes, benign masses that cause bony scalloping, and aggressive malignancies that cause bony destruction.

The presence of calcification is a specific differentiating feature in some lesions, and CT can provide essential diagnostic information, even after an MR has been obtained. For example, an indeterminate diagnosis of perioptic nerve meningioma on MR might be confirmed with identification of calcification on CT.

In some instances, CT can provide enough information to allow for a definitive diagnosis and guide therapy without the need for MR. Examples include thyroid ophthalmopathy, clinically benign lacrimal mass, orbital cavernous malformation, and orbital disease that is secondary to a sinonasal process.

MR

For evaluating complex orbital disease, MR is the preferred modality. Superior soft tissue differentiation and enhancement make MR ideal for characterizing the extent of complicated lesions, including extraocular tumors, vascular malformations, and complex infectious or inflammatory processes.

In particular, MR is the optimal modality for delineating the extent of malignant orbital disease. Important features visible on MR include optic nerve invasion, perineural extension of tumor to the orbit, intracranial extension of disease, and hematogeneous or CSF disseminated metastases.

Although ultrasound is usually the 1st line for imaging the globe, MR can provide a more accurate visualization of retrobulbar extension of intraocular malignancy, including retinoblastoma, ocular melanoma, and ocular metastases.

Additionally, MR provides exquisite characterization of the globe itself, which is particularly useful in circumstances wherein funduscopic evaluation is obscured, such as swollen or injured eye, retinal detachment, large intraocular mass, vitreal hemorrhage, or opaque media from any cause.

Imaging Anatomy

Bony Orbit

Major components of the bony orbital walls are the frontal bone superiorly, zygomatic bone laterally and inferiorly, maxillary bone inferiorly and medially, and ethmoid bone medially. Smaller contributions medially include the lacrimal bone, nasal bone, and a tiny portion of the palatine bone. The sphenoid bone makes up a large portion of the orbit posteriorly and laterally, forming the complex foramina at the orbital apex.

Globe

The aqueous-filled anterior segment includes anterior and posterior chambers, both anterior to the lens. The vitreous-filled posterior segment occupies the bulk of the globe posteriorly. The layers, or tunica, of the eye include the inner retina, vascular choroid, and outer structural sclera. The anterior refractive constructs include the iris and ciliary body, which are specialized portions of the uvea, as well as the lens.

Orbital Septum

The orbital septum is composed of fascia arising from the orbital periosteum that inserts onto the aponeurosis of the tarsal plates of the lids, providing a barrier between the anterior periorbita and the intraorbital contents. Although the septum itself is often not discernible as a discrete structure on routine imaging, its presence is readily evident when a disease process, especially preseptal infection, is contained on 1 side of the barrier.

Lacrimal Apparatus

The lacrimal gland lies in a bony fossa at the anterior aspect of the superolateral orbit. Lacrimal drainage occurs via the canaliculi and sac at the inferomedial orbit, and, from there, it passes through the nasolacrimal duct, which drains via the inferior meatus.

Extraocular Muscles

The 4 rectus muscles originate from the annulus of Zinn at the apex and insert on the corneoscleral surface. The superior oblique has similar origin and insertion but courses through the trochlea ("pulley") at the superomedial orbital rim. The inferior oblique has a short, more direct course originating from the anteroinferior orbital rim. The levator palpebrae superioris originates at the annulus, coursing just above the superior rectus, forming the superior muscle complex, and inserts at the upper eyelid.

Optic Nerve-Sheath Complex

The optic nerve (CNII) is actually a central nervous tract that traverses the optic canal and orbit to insert at the optic nerve head. The surrounding dural sheath is contiguous with the intracranial dura posteriorly and with the sclera anteriorly. A thin rim of CSF surrounding the nerve is typically visible on MR and is contiguous with CSF in the intracranial cisterns.

Peripheral Cranial Nerves

CNIII, CNIV, and CNVI supply motor innervation to the extraocular muscles (EOMs), as well as parasympathetics to the iris via CNIII. The individual branches of these nerves are not reliably distinguished within the orbit. However, knowledge of their course through the cavernous sinus and

Differential Diagnosis: Orbit

Congenital lesions (globe)	Infectious lesions (globe)	Benign tumors
Coloboma	Ocular toxocariasis	Lacrimal benign mixed tumor
Persistent hyperplastic primary vitreous	Acute endophthalmitis	Optic pathway glioma
Coats disease		Optic nerve sheath meningioma
Congenital lesions (orbit)	**Infectious lesions (orbit)**	**Malignant tumors (globe)**
Orbital dermoid and epidermoid	Orbital subperiosteal abscess	Retinoblastoma
Orbital neurofibromatosis, type 1	Orbital cellulitis	Uveal melanoma
Vascular malformations	**Inflammatory lesions**	**Malignant tumors (orbit)**
Orbital lymphatic malformation	Orbital idiopathic pseudotumor	Lacrimal epithelial carcinoma
Orbital varix	Orbital sarcoidosis	Lymphoproliferative lesions
Orbital cavernous malformation	Thyroid ophthalmopathy	Orbital Langerhans histiocytosis
Vascular neoplasms	Optic neuritis	Metastases
Orbital infantile hemangioma		

superior orbital fissure (SOF) allows localization of pathology that involves these nerves.

Two of the branches of CNV course through the orbit. V1 passes with other nerves through the SOF and exits the orbit through the supraorbital foramen. V2 passes through foramen rotundum and inferior orbital fissure and exits the orbit through the infraorbital foramen.

Vascular Structures

The ophthalmic artery enters the orbit alongside the optic nerve within the optic canal; it is frequently visible in the orbit, as it diverges from the nerve near the apex. High-resolution angiography, CT, and MR show the artery originating as the 1st intradural branch of the internal carotid artery. The superior ophthalmic vein is variable but typically found coursing between the superior rectus muscle and the optic nerve.

Orbital Fat

In addition to acting as a volume "filler" for the orbital cavity, orbital fat provides intrinsic imaging contrast, making other structures and disease processes more conspicuous.

Anatomy-based Imaging Issues

In approaching orbital lesions, it is useful to localize the process to a subregion of the orbit and ascertain relationship of the lesion to the critical structures.

- **Globe**: Is lesion entirely intraocular, or is there transscleral extension, particularly with regard to optic nerve head?
- **Optic nerve**: Does lesion arise within nerve proper or involve primarily dural sheath?
- **EOM**: Is lesion intraconal or extraconal, or does it arise from muscles themselves? Is muscle involvement symmetric or otherwise characteristic?
- **Lacrimal gland**: Is lesion unilateral, or is it bilateral, indicating systemic process?
- **Bone**: Does lesion arise from bone itself? If lesion is adjacent to bone, does bone show benign scalloped remodeling or aggressive destruction?
- **Focality**: Is lesion isolated or multiple, focal or diffuse and poorly defined? Does lesion extend beyond orbit?

Imaging Protocols

CT

Routine imaging of the orbit with CT does not require special discussion, except for 1 clinical circumstance: Intermittent proptosis due to orbital varix. This dynamic lesion enlarges with increases in venous pressures and is best demonstrated with provocation. After performing routine enhanced CT, the scan is repeated with the breath held in Valsalva maneuver, increasing venous pressures and dynamically enlarging the varix.

MR

Routine imaging of the orbit with MR is usually adequate for the majority of ophthalmologic indications. The protocol includes 3 sequence types, each of these performed in axial and coronal planes, at 3-mm slice thickness and 18-cm field of view. Whole-brain imaging is added when indicated.

- Precontrast T1WI (without fat suppression)
- T2WI with fat suppression (alternatively STIR)
- Postcontrast T1WI with fat suppression

Pathologic Issues: Vascular Malformations

Vascular malformations are congenital, nonneoplastic lesions, with classification that reflects their histologic and hemodynamic features.

Orbital cavernous malformation: This common mass is unique to the orbit. It is encapsulated with low-flow venous channels. The term "hemangioma" is commonly used to refer to this lesion but is actually a misnomer.

Venolymphatic malformation: Lesions may have no flow (type 1), venous flow (type 2), or may be mixed. There may be a distensible component, resulting in varix. Outdated terminology to be avoided includes "lymphangioma" and "cystic hygroma."

Arteriovenous malformations (AVM): True orbital AVMs are rare lesions, with high-flow arterial (type 3) hemodynamics.

Selected References

1. Yanoff M et al: Ophthalmology. Expert Consult. 4th ed. Saunders: Philadelphia: Saunders, 2013
2. Rootman J: Diseases of the Orbit: A Multidisciplinary Approach. Philadelphia: Lippincott, 2003

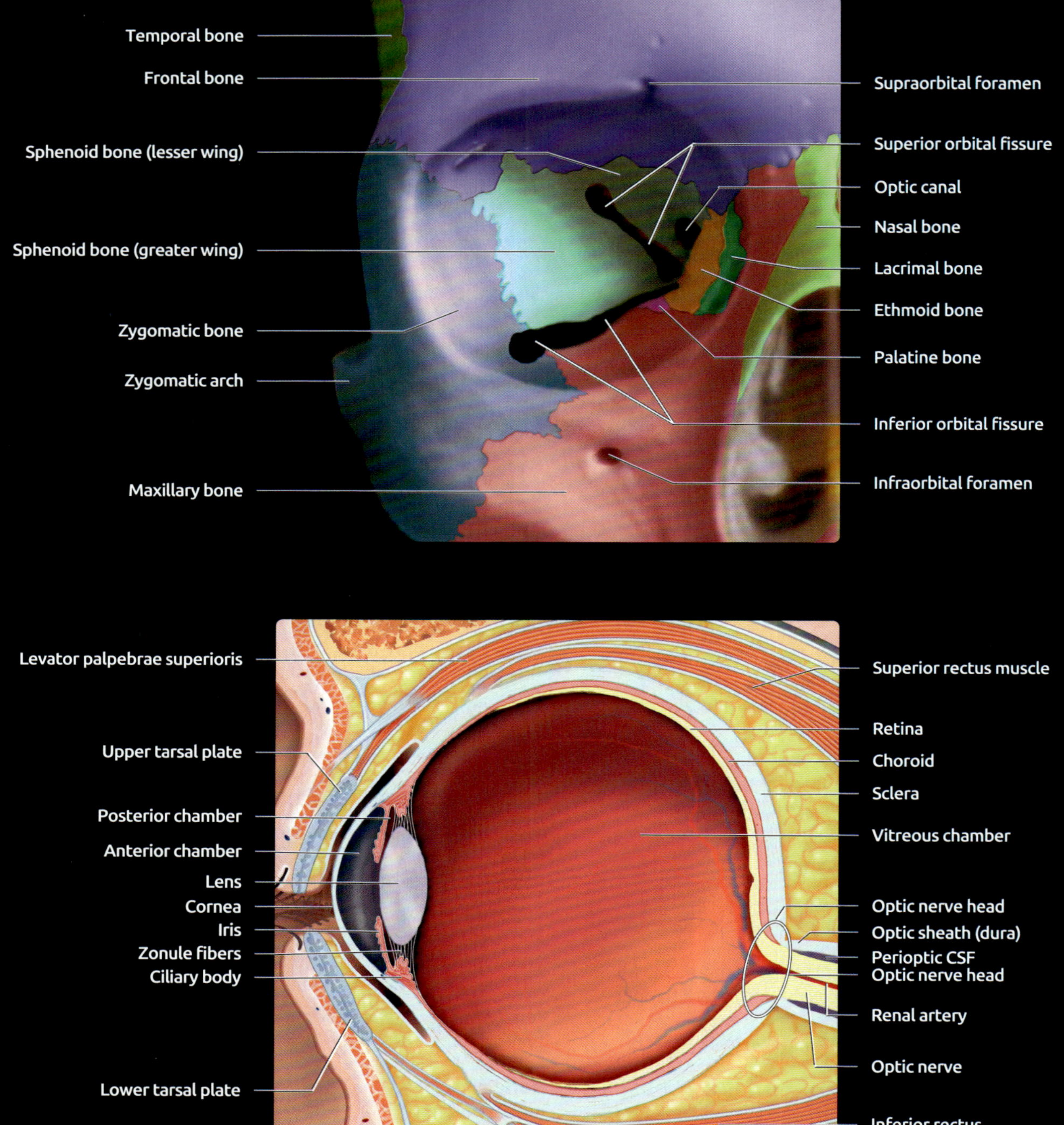

(Top) *Frontal graphic demonstrates the complex anatomy of the bony orbit. The walls of the orbital cavity receive contributions from 8 different bones of the skull. The complex foramina and fissures at the apex are located primarily within the greater and lesser wings of the sphenoid bone and its junctions with adjacent bones.* **(Bottom)** *Sagittal graphic demonstrates the anterior and posterior segments of the globe. The aqueous anterior segment is composed of the anterior chamber and very small posterior chamber. The much larger posterior segment is filled by the vitreous chamber. The layered tunicae of the retina, choroid, and sclera are demonstrated as well as the components of the optic nerve at its insertion. Some of the extraocular muscles and eyelid structures are also demonstrated.*

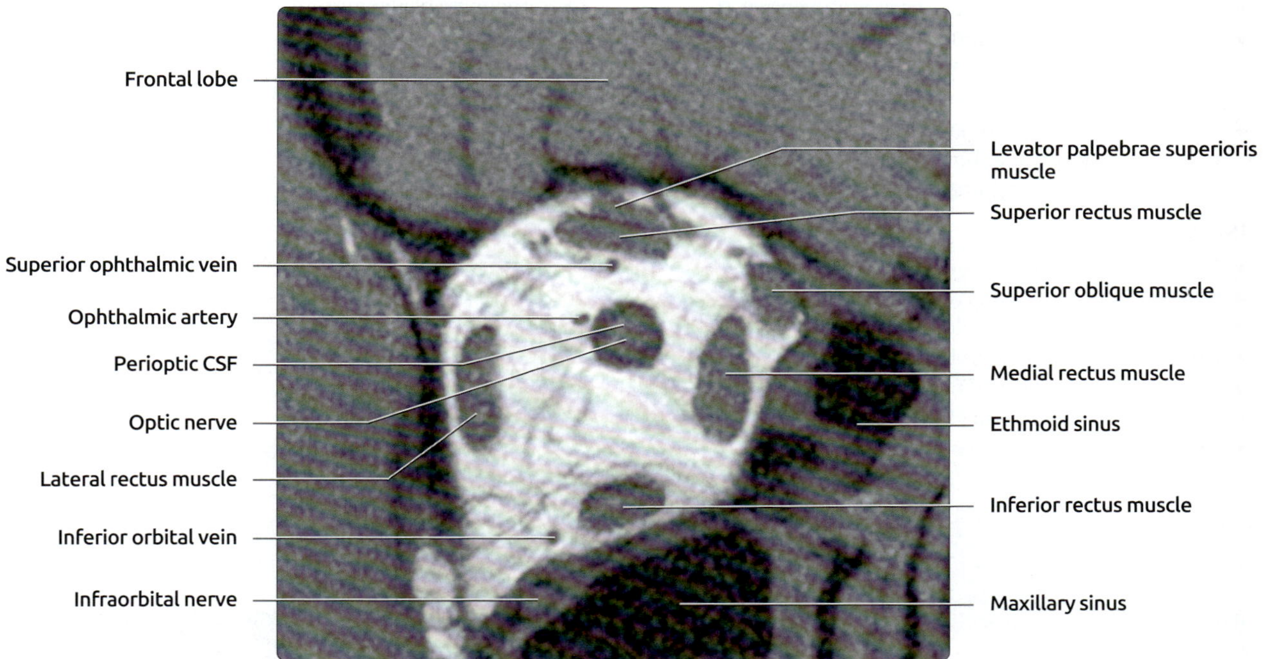

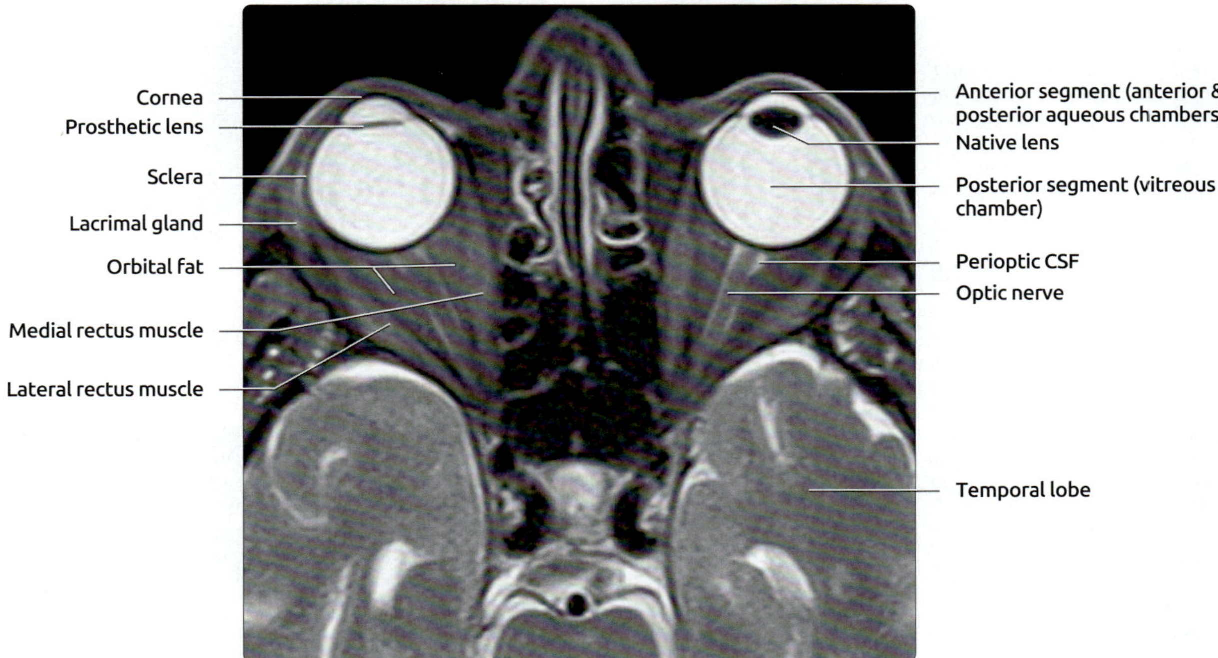

(Top) *Coronal T1WI MR demonstrates the peripherally located "cone" of extraocular muscles, the central optic nerve sheath complex, and the vascular structures of the orbit. The intrinsic T1 signal of the orbital fat provides excellent contrast for visualizing the intraorbital contents.* **(Bottom)** *Axial T2WI MR with fat suppression nearly eliminates the signal from orbital fat, allowing for conspicuity of fluid signal structures. A small amount of CSF surrounding the optic nerve is usually visible on T2WI. The normal extraocular muscles show intermediate to low signal. A small portion of the lacrimal gland is seen, but the majority of the gland is located further superiorly. The anterior segment of the eye shows water signal, primarily representing the anterior chamber; the posterior chamber is not separately discernible on routine MR. The posterior segment also shows water signal, composed of the vitreous chamber. Note that this patient has a prosthetic lens on the right.*

KEY FACTS

TERMINOLOGY

- Coloboma = gap or defect of ocular tissue
- May involve any or all structures of embryonic cleft
- Types of posterior coloboma
  - Optic disc coloboma
  - Choroidoretinal coloboma
- Related but distinct anomalies
  - Morning glory disc anomaly
  - Peripapillary staphyloma

IMAGING

- Focal defect at posterior pole of globe
- Outpouching contiguous with vitreous
- Oriented posteriorly with long axis of globe
- Microphthalmos and retrobulbar cysts often present
- Isodense to vitreous on CT
- Isointense to vitreous on MR
- Bulging of posterior globe on prenatal MR

TOP DIFFERENTIAL DIAGNOSES

- Congenital microphthalmos
- Congenital glaucoma
- Neurofibromatosis type 1
- Degenerative staphyloma
- Axial myopia

PATHOLOGY

- Failure of embryonic fissure fusion
- Isolated, sporadic, and syndromic genetic etiologies
- Bilateral when syndromic

CLINICAL ISSUES

- Decreased visual acuity; leukocoria
- Treatment to address refractive errors, strabismus, amblyopia, retinal detachment

DIAGNOSTIC CHECKLIST

- Look for syndromic and systemic associations

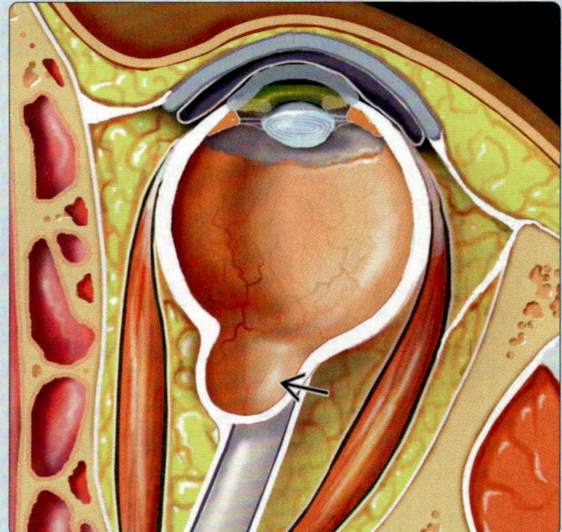

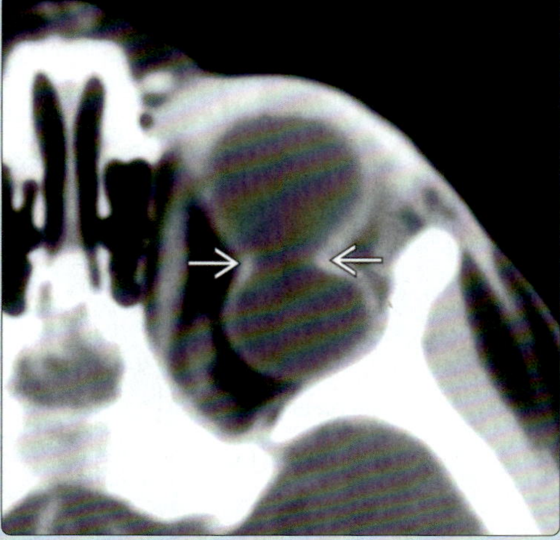

(Left) *Axial graphic of classic optic disc coloboma shows a focal defect in the posterior globe at the site of the optic nerve head insertion ⇒.* **(Right)** *Axial CECT demonstrates a broad colobomatous defect ➡ centered on the upper margin of the optic disc. Note that the vitreous appears contiguous to retrobulbar outpouching. Apart from the retrobulbar outpouching, the globe is small.*

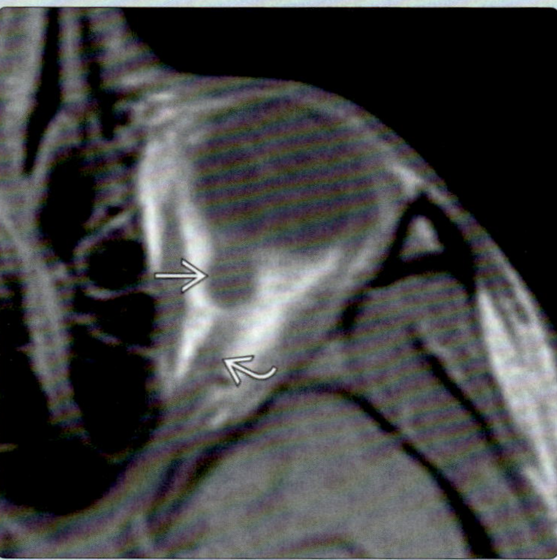

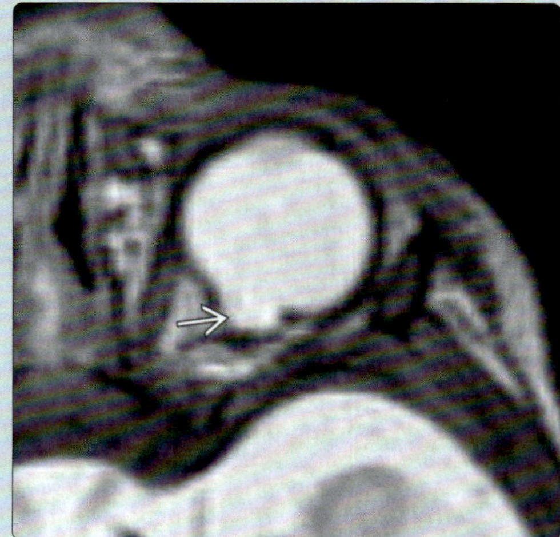

(Left) *Axial T1 MR of the orbit demonstrates a focal posterior pole outpouching of the globe ➡, located just above and medial to optic nerve head. Note posterior intraorbital optic nerve ➡.* **(Right)** *Axial T2 MR in the same patient demonstrates a focal globe defect near the optic nerve insertion ➡. Note fluid signal within the outpouching is identical to the intraocular vitreous.*

Orbital Dermoid and Epidermoid

KEY FACTS

TERMINOLOGY

- Congenital orbital **ectodermal inclusion lesion** resulting in choristomatous cyst
- **Dermoid**: Includes dermal appendages
- **Epidermoid**: Dermal adnexal structures absent

IMAGING

- CT without contrast often adequate for diagnosis
- Presence of **fat** is **pathognomonic**
- Cystic, well-demarcated, extraconal mass with lipid, fluid, or mixed contents
- Adjacent to orbital periosteum, near suture lines
- Osseous remodeling in majority of lesions with smooth scalloped margins and thinning or dehiscence
- Superolateral at frontozygomatic suture most common
- May contain debris or fluid levels
- Distinguishing features
  - Dermoid: Typically but not exclusively contains fat; more heterogeneous with **complex signal** on MR
  - Epidermoid: Density and intensity similar to fluid; more homogeneous; **diffusion restriction** on MR

TOP DIFFERENTIAL DIAGNOSES

- Dermolipoma
- Frontal or ethmoid sinus mucocele
- Lacrimal gland cyst

PATHOLOGY

- Congenital inclusion of trapped ectoderm at suture site
- Fibrous capsule lined by squamous epithelium

CLINICAL ISSUES

- Firm, nontender mass, fixed to underling bone
- Slowly progressive; may rupture with acute inflammation
- Presentation typically in childhood; deeper lesions in adults
- Surgical resection is curative
  - Steroids if lesion ruptures at surgery

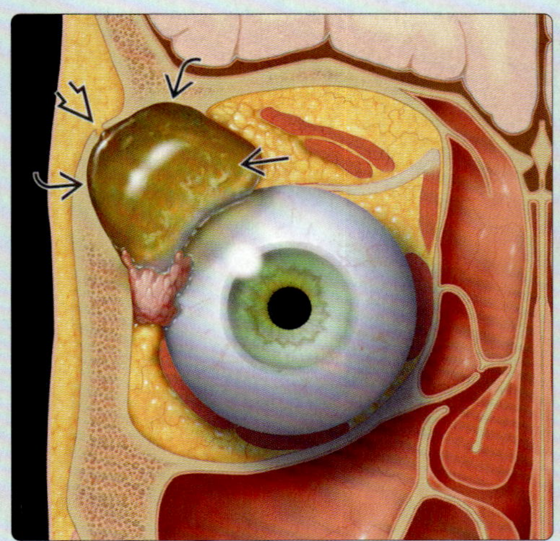

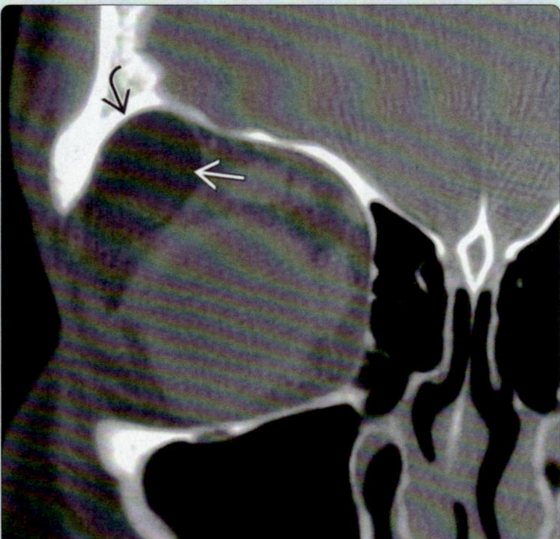

(Left) *Coronal graphic depicts a superotemporal dermoid cyst ➡ located adjacent to the frontozygomatic suture of the right orbit ➡. There is resultant mass effect on the globe with remodeling of the bony orbit ➡.* **(Right)** *Coronal CT demonstrates an ovoid, well-marginated cystic mass in the superotemporal quadrant of the right orbit ➡. Even on bone windows, the lipid density within the mass can be readily appreciated. Smooth remodeling of the adjacent bony orbit is evident ➡.*

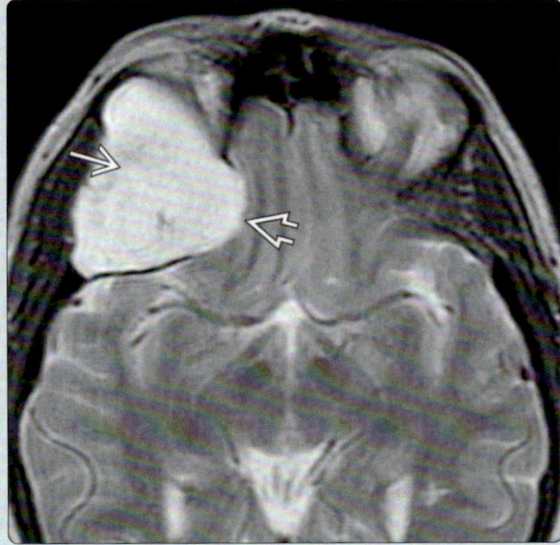

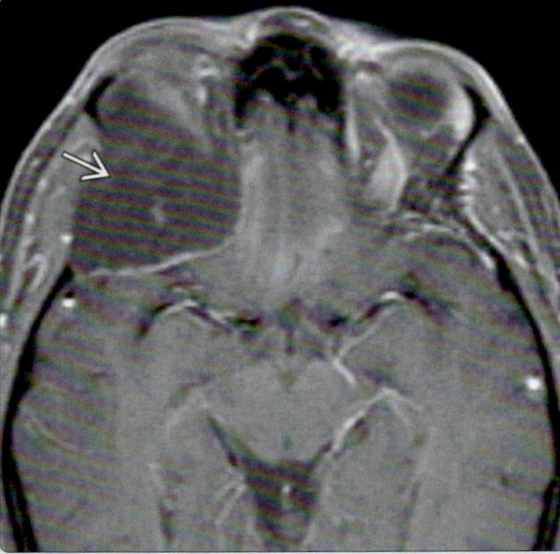

(Left) *Axial T2WI MR shows a very large, lobulated mass centered at the deep right orbit and sphenoid ➡. This epidermoid cyst shows fluid signal with some internal heterogeneity. Marked thinning of the adjacent bony orbit and skull base is evident ➡.* **(Right)** *Axial T1WI postcontrast MR in the same patient shows low signal with mild irregularity in the epidermoid cyst ➡ but no appreciable enhancement. The lesion showed no evidence of lipid signal on precontrast images.*

Orbital Lymphatic Malformation

KEY FACTS

TERMINOLOGY

- Definition: Congenital vascular malformation with variable lymphatic and venous vascular elements

IMAGING

- General imaging findings
  - Poorly marginated, lobulated, transspatial mass
  - Multiloculated cystic features with **fluid-fluid levels**, **blood products**, and variable irregular enhancement
  - Variants: Superficial vs. deep, macrocystic vs. microcystic
  - Variable C+ on margins, ↑ if prominent venous components
- CT: Irregular cystic hypodense mass with mixed hyperdense blood products
- MR: Variable signal resulting from mixed age hemorrhagic, lymphatic, or proteinaceous fluid
- US: Hypoechoic with heterogeneous internal echoes
- Best imaging tool
  - Dedicated enhanced orbital MR with fat suppression

TOP DIFFERENTIAL DIAGNOSES

- Orbital varix
- Orbital cavernous malformation
- Infantile hemangioma
- Plexiform neurofibroma

PATHOLOGY

- Congenital nonneoplastic vascular malformation
- Dilated dysplastic lymphatic ± venous channels

CLINICAL ISSUES

- Mass effect with proptosis in pediatric patient
- May rapidly ↑ in size due to acute hemorrhage
- Treatment options
  - Conservative therapy preferred due to surgical risk
  - Percutaneous sclerotherapy for suitable lesions
  - Difficult resection due to complex **insinuation** with normal orbital structures
    - **Recurrence** after surgery common (~ 50%)

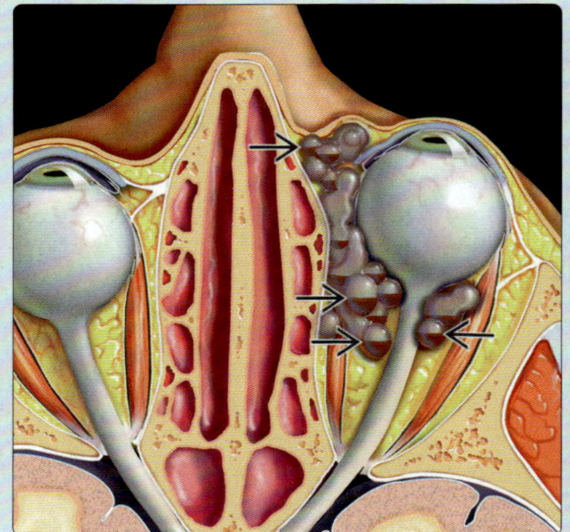

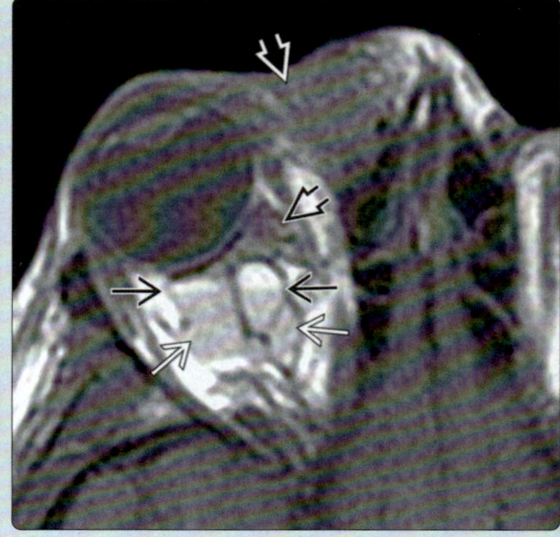

(Left) *Axial graphic depicts the typical features of orbital lymphatic malformation, including transspatial extension and characteristic fluid-fluid levels within loculations ➔.* **(Right)** *Axial T1-weighted MR shows an infiltrative, transspatial mass. The posterior intraconal component ➔ demonstrates fluid-blood levels ➔ within macrocystic loculations. The preseptal ➔ and anterior intraorbital ➔ components appear more homogeneously hypointense, suggesting microcystic or venous elements.*

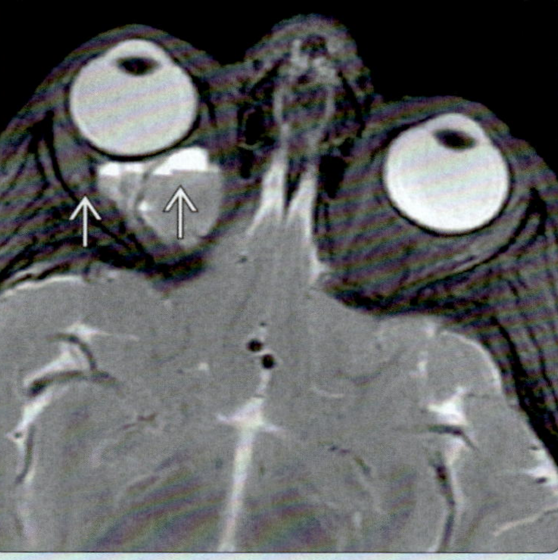

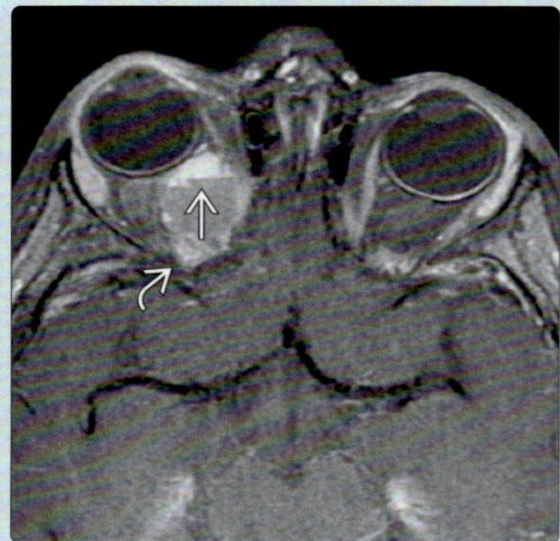

(Left) *Axial T2-weighted MR in an older child with acute worsening of longstanding right proptosis shows a large, lobulated retrobulbar mass with characteristic fluid-fluid levels ➔. The differing heights of levels are indicative of the multilocular nature of the lesion.* **(Right)** *Axial T1 C+ FS MR in the same patient demonstrates that the variable signal of contents again manifest as fluid-fluid levels ➔, indicating proteinaceous and hemorrhagic products. Mild venous enhancement is evident posteriorly ➔.*

Orbital Cavernous Venous Malformation (Hemangioma)

KEY FACTS

TERMINOLOGY

- Venous vascular malformation of orbit characterized by endothelial-lined cavernous spaces
- Pseudoencapsulated morphology distinguishes orbital cavernous venous malformation from venous malformations elsewhere in head & neck
- Synonymous with cavernous "hemangioma" (misnomer)

IMAGING

- Solid enhancing intraorbital mass
  - Most intraconal, usually lateral
  - Ovoid or round, sharply marginated
  - Pseudocapsule of compressed surrounding tissue
- CT
  - Benign remodeling of bone in larger lesions
- MR
  - T2 hyperintense; internal septations may be visible
  - Characteristic dynamic enhancement
    - Heterogeneous early patchy central enhancement
    - Fills in homogeneously on delayed images

PATHOLOGY

- Slowly growing vascular malformation
- ISSVA classification as slow-flow venous lesion
- Dilated vascular channels of thin-walled sinusoidal spaces, flattened endothelial cells, scant fibrous connective stroma
- Pseudocapsule with surrounding compressed tissue
- No evidence of cellular proliferation

CLINICAL ISSUES

- Slowly progressive painless proptosis
- Most common isolated orbital mass in adults
- Female predominance; faster growth during pregnancy
- Excellent prognosis; rare recurrence after surgery
- Treatment: Surgical resection, often via lateral orbitotomy

DIAGNOSTIC CHECKLIST

- Often discovered incidentally during brain MR
- Patchy dynamic enhancement is characteristic

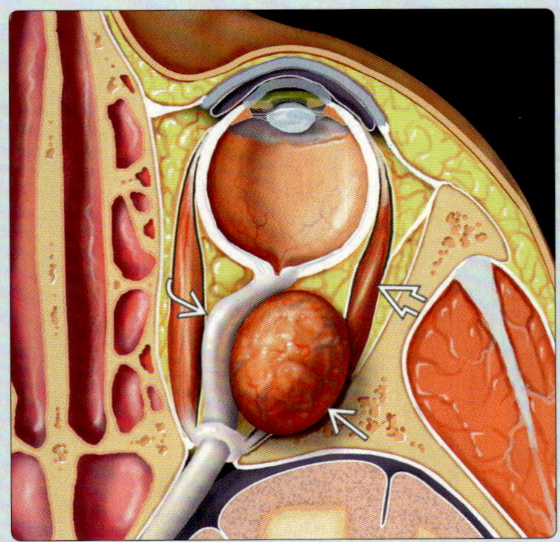

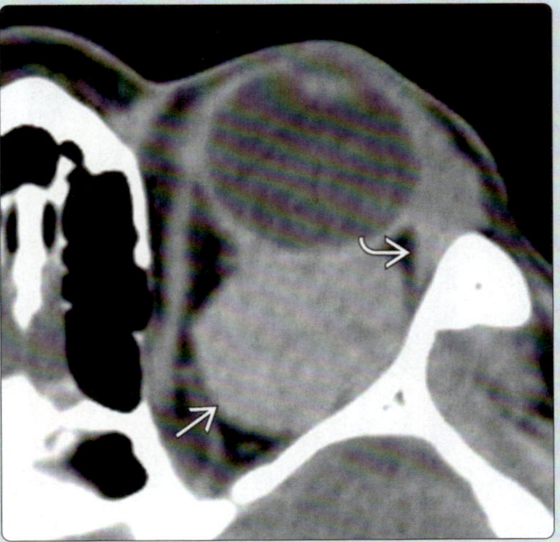

(Left) *Axial graphic through the orbit shows an ovoid, well-demarcated, intraconal mass ➡ that displaces the optic nerve ➡ and adjacent lateral rectus muscle ➡. Note the lack of adjacent structure invasion.* **(Right)** *Axial NECT shows a well-demarcated, ovoid, slightly hyperdense mass centered in the lateral aspect of the left orbit ➡. The lateral rectus muscle is seen draping around the lateral margin of this intraconal mass ➡.*

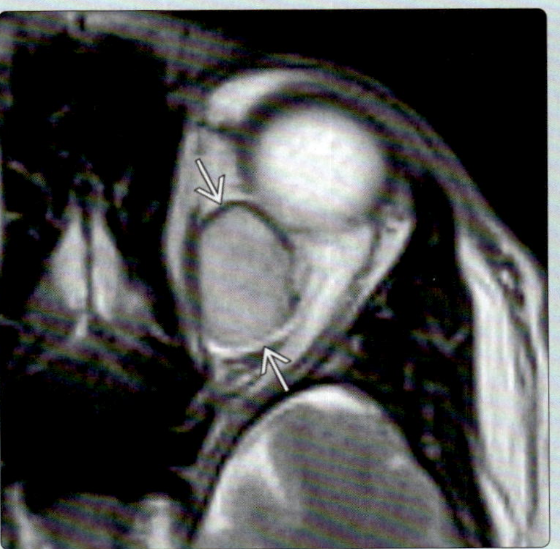

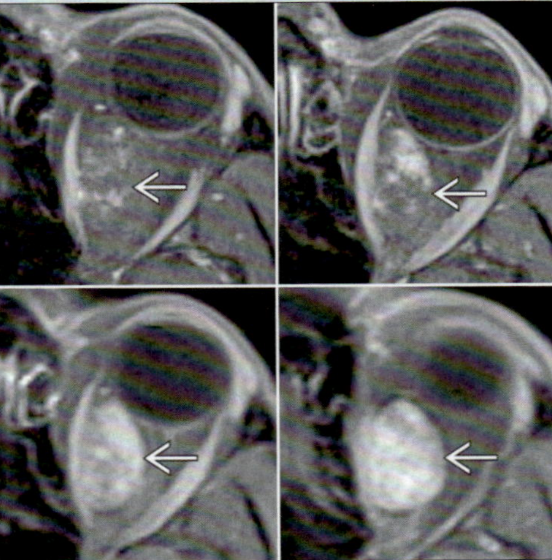

(Left) *Axial T2-weighted MR reveals a sharply marginated, ovoid, hyperintense intraconal mass. A thin rim of signal ➡ represents the pseudocapsule, accentuated by a chemical shift artifact.* **(Right)** *Axial T1 C+ FS MR demonstrates progressive enhancement of a vascular mass in the medial left orbit ➡. Serial scans were obtained over the course of several minutes, from earliest (top left) to latest (bottom right) following contrast injection.*

Orbital Subperiosteal Abscess

KEY FACTS

TERMINOLOGY

- Definition: **Purulent** accumulation between bony **orbital wall** & orbital **periosteum**

IMAGING

- **Imaging recommendations**
  - CT with contrast for diagnosis & monitoring
  - MR with contrast for complications or to avoid radiation
- Lentiform, rim-enhancing fluid collection along orbital wall
  - Loculated fluid density/signal on CT/MR
  - Adjacent ethmoid sinusitis
- Demineralization &/or dehiscence of orbital wall
- Diffusion restriction within abscess on MR

TOP DIFFERENTIAL DIAGNOSES

- Orbital cellulitis
- Idiopathic orbital inflammation
- Sinonasal mucocele
- Nasolacrimal duct mucocele ± infection

PATHOLOGY

- Secondary to adjacent sinusitis
- Upper respiratory microbes: Simple & aerobic in children
  - Polymicrobial & anaerobic in adults

CLINICAL ISSUES

- Presentation & natural history
  - Eye swelling, erythema, gaze restriction
  - Rapidly progressive, **potentially blinding disease**
  - Venous thrombosis, intracranial extension complications
- Treatment options
  - Targeted IV antibiotics
  - Surgical drainage via FESS &/or external approach
  - Factors that may indicate need for surgical drainage
    - > 10 years old, mass effect, or visual compromise
    - Large-volume abscess or frontal sinus origin

DIAGNOSTIC CHECKLIST

- Risk of blindness, which requires immediate attention

(Left) *Axial graphic depicts spread of infection from the left ethmoid sinuses ⇨ through the lamina papyracea into the medial orbit. Resultant subperiosteal abscess ⇨ causes mass effect, displacing the adjacent muscle cone and putting the optic nerve at risk.* **(Right)** *Axial CECT shows asymmetric opacification of the left ethmoid sinuses ⇨ with a large subperiosteal abscess extending into the medial extraconal orbit ➡. Displacement of the medial rectus ➡ is a typical finding.*

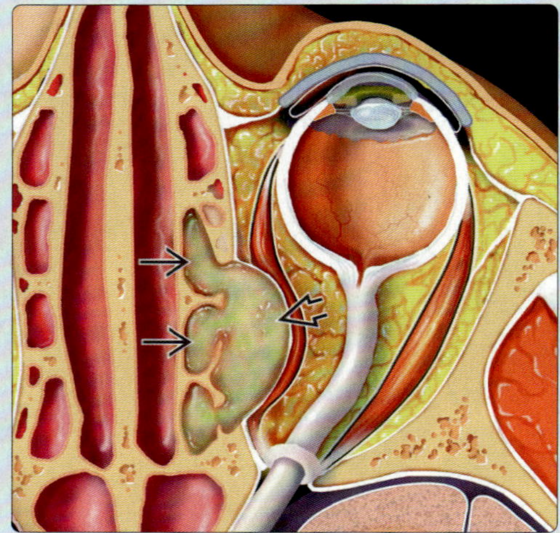

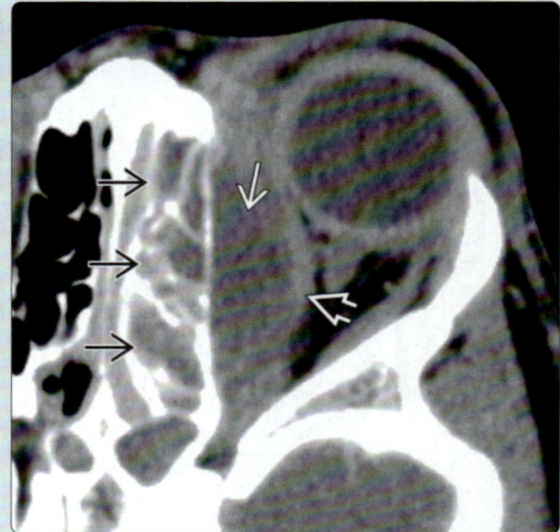

(Left) *Coronal T1WI C+ FS MR in a patient status post endoscopic sinus surgery shows phlegmonous enhancement in the medial right extraconal fat ➡ with a small abscess pocket forming centrally ➡.* **(Right)** *Axial T1WI C+ FS MR shows a large subperiosteal abscess ➡ extending through the lamina papyracea with findings of acute sinusitis ⇨ and extensive right orbital cellulitis ➡. Marked proptosis is evident ➡. Posterior extension of the abscess implies a higher risk of vision loss.*

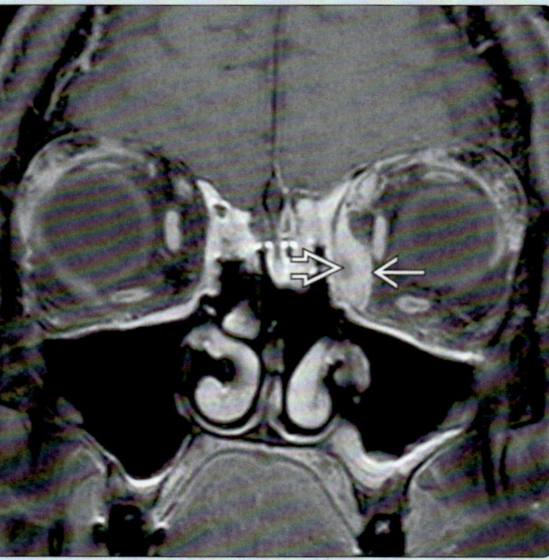

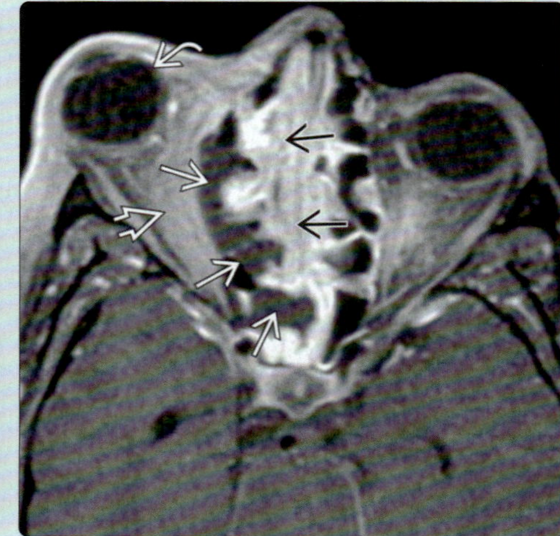

KEY FACTS

TERMINOLOGY

- Preseptal cellulitis
  - Infection limited to superficial periorbita
- Intraorbital (postseptal) cellulitis
  - Infection posterior to orbital septum
- Orbital septum
  - Connective tissue plane that acts as diaphragm

IMAGING

- Superficial periorbital or deep intraorbital soft tissue infiltration with mass effect & enhancement
- Enhanced CT adequate for uncomplicated cases
- MR shows diffusion restriction if abscess is present

TOP DIFFERENTIAL DIAGNOSES

- Orbital subperiosteal abscess
- Invasive fungal infection
- Idiopathic orbital inflammatory disease
- Orbital sarcoidosis

PATHOLOGY

- Etiology
  - Preseptal cellulitis: Trauma, insect bites common
  - Intraorbital cellulitis: Sinusitis most common
- Microbiology
  - Related to traumatic & sinogenic etiologies
  - Adults more likely polymicrobial & less responsive

CLINICAL ISSUES

- Presentation
  - Preseptal cellulitis
    - Periorbital edema & erythema
  - Intraorbital cellulitis
    - Axial (forward) displacement of globe
- Treatment
  - Targeted antimicrobials with cultures
  - Concomitant corticosteroids to reduce inflammation
  - Surgical drainage ± functional endoscopic sinus surgery may be required if abscess develops

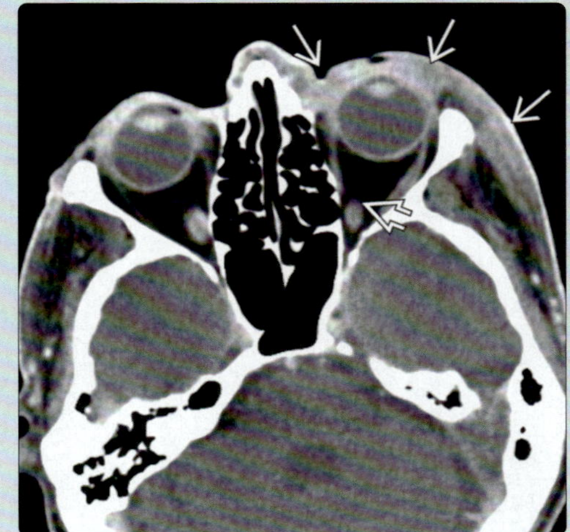

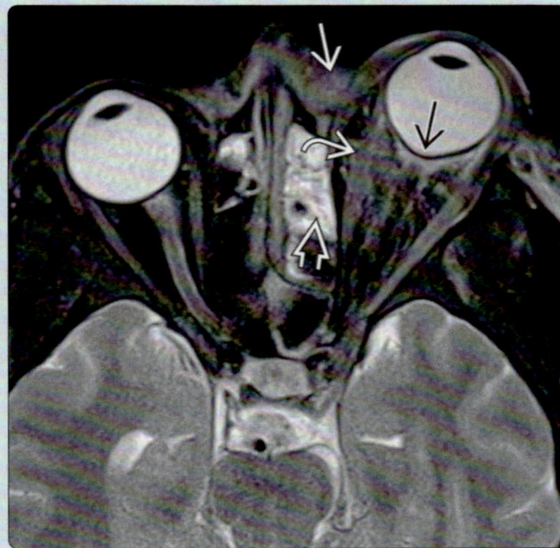

(Left) *Axial CECT in a patient with facial impetigo shows edema and enhancement of the preseptal soft tissues ➡ with normal appearance of the intraorbital fat ➡. Note that the adjacent sinuses are clear.* **(Right)** *Axial STIR MR in a teenage girl shows infiltrating signal representing both preseptal ➡ and postseptal ➡ cellulitis secondary to ethmoid sinusitis ➡. Although no abscess is present, there is significant proptosis with tenting of the posterior globe ➡.*

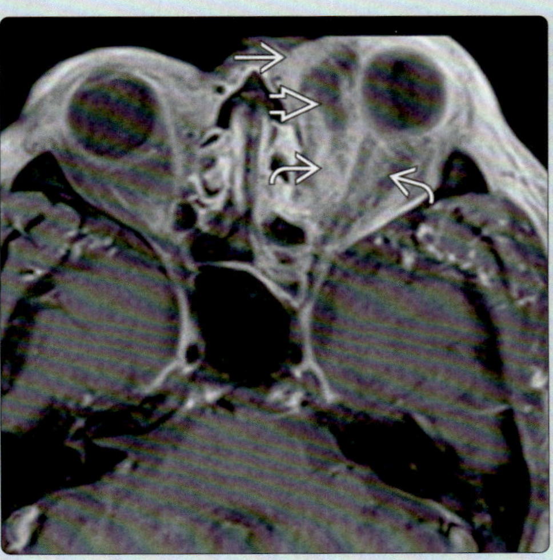

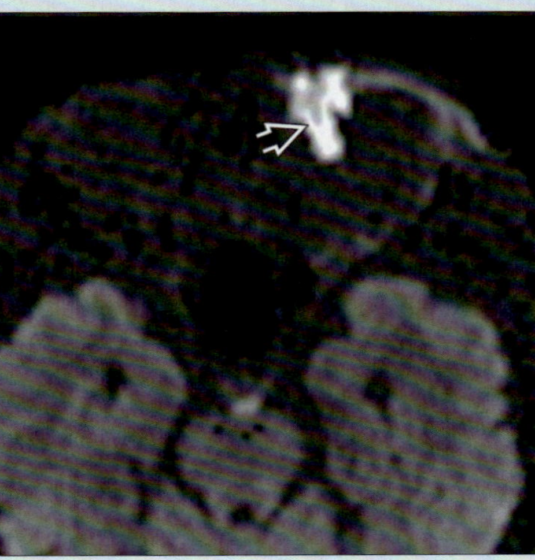

(Left) *Axial T1-weighted postcontrast MR in a patient with recent penetrating facial trauma shows extensive preseptal ➡ and intraorbital ➡ infiltration and enhancement. A rim-enhancing collection is seen extending along the trajectory of injury ➡.* **(Right)** *DWI MR in the same patient shows restriction within the collection ➡, indicating acute abscess. The abscess crosses the plane of the orbital septum, which was violated due to the trauma.*

Idiopathic Orbital Inflammation (Pseudotumor)

KEY FACTS

TERMINOLOGY

- Nonspecific orbital inflammation, not due to any known etiology or systemic illness

IMAGING

- Poorly marginated, mass-like, or infiltrative enhancing inflammatory tissue involving any area of orbit
  - **Myositic** (extraocular muscles)
  - **Lacrimal** (lacrimal gland)
  - **Anterior** (globe, retrobulbar orbit)
  - **Diffuse** (multifocal intraconal ± extraconal)
  - **Apical** (orbital apex, intracranial extension)
- Diffuse irregularity, muscle enlargement, and enhancement
- T2/STIR hypointense due to cellular infiltrate and fibrosis
- Best imaging tool: Contrast-enhanced MR with fat suppression
- Disease variants
  - Tolosa-Hunt: Through fissures into cavernous sinus
  - Sclerosing: More often bilateral, may extend into sinuses
  - IgG4: Predilection for lacrimal gland and nerves

TOP DIFFERENTIAL DIAGNOSES

- Lymphoproliferative lesions, especially lymphoma
- Thyroid ophthalmopathy
- Sarcoidosis
- Granulomatosis with polyangiitis (Wegener)
- Orbital cellulitis

PATHOLOGY

- Polymorphous chronic inflammation and fibrosis

CLINICAL ISSUES

- Acute to subacute orbital pain, swelling, restricted motion, diplopia, proptosis, and impaired vision
- Steroid treatment effective in most patients

DIAGNOSTIC CHECKLIST

- Idiopathic orbital inflammation (pseudotumor) is diagnosis of exclusion

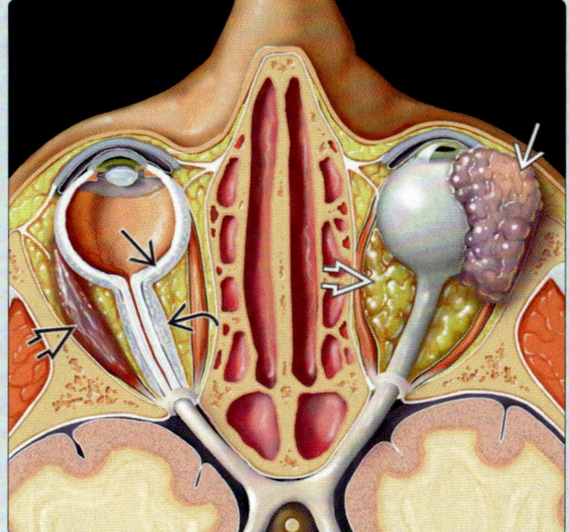

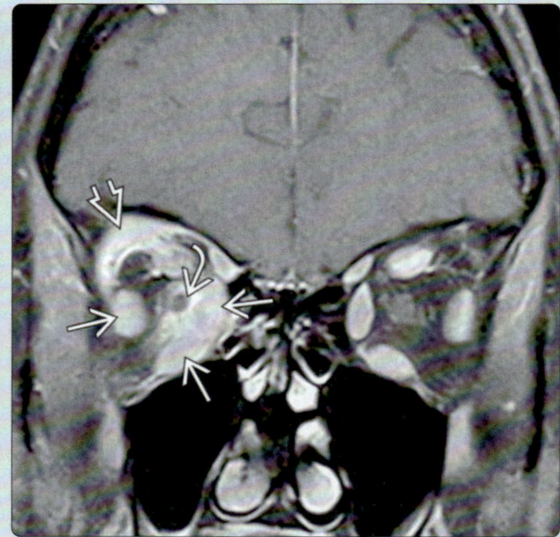

(Left) *Axial graphic depicts multifocal idiopathic orbital inflammation, including involvement of the extraocular muscles ⇨, orbital fat ➡, lacrimal gland ➡, sclera ⇨, and optic sheath ⇨.* **(Right)** *Coronal T1WI C+ FS MR demonstrates extensive orbital inflammation with ill-defined enlargement and enhancement of the rectus muscles ➡, extraconal infiltration extending to the lacrimal gland ➡, and intraconal enhancement partially surrounding the optic nerve ➡.*

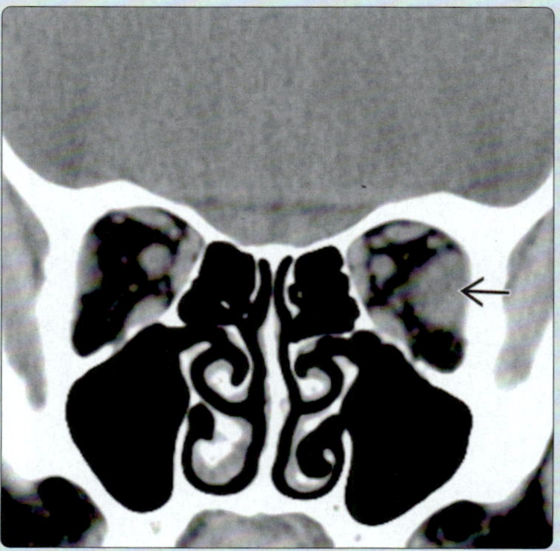

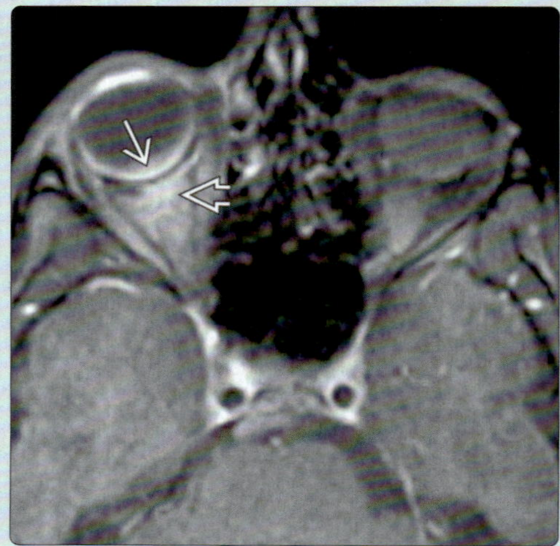

(Left) *Coronal NECT in a middle-aged woman with left eye pain and diplopia shows enlargement and hypodensity of the left lateral rectus muscle ⇨. Isolated lateral rectus myositis is a typical manifestation of idiopathic orbital inflammatory disease, rare in thyroid orbitopathy.* **(Right)** *Axial T1WI C+ FS MR in a patient with uveitis shows inflammatory changes of the anterior right orbit. Marked uveoscleral "shaggy" enhancement is evident ➡ as well as ill-defined enhancement of retrobulbar fat ➡.*

Thyroid-Associated Orbitopathy

KEY FACTS

TERMINOLOGY

- Synonyms: Graves ophthalmopathy, thyroid eye disease
- Definition: Autoimmune orbital inflammation associated with autoimmune thyroid dysfunction

IMAGING

- CT: Bilateral extraocular muscle (EOM) enlargement
  - Nonuniform, symmetric involvement
  - **I'M SLO** mnemonic for sites of predilection
    - Inferior ≥ medial ≥ superior > lateral ≥ oblique
  - Enlargement of muscle bellies; typically spares tendons
  - Heterogeneous areas of internal lower density
  - Exophthalmos and increased orbital fat
  - Decreased EOM enhancement compared to normal
- T2/STIR MR signal correlates with disease activity
  - ↑ in acute disease due to edema and inflammation
  - ↓ in chronic disease from involutional changes/fibrosis

TOP DIFFERENTIAL DIAGNOSES

- Idiopathic orbital inflammation
- Orbital sarcoidosis
- Orbital cellulitis
- Lymphoproliferative disease

PATHOLOGY

- **Autoimmune inflammation** due to thyrotropin receptor autoantigens present in both thyroid gland and orbit
- Orbital fibroblasts and adipocytes involved in T-cell lymphocyte cytokine-mediated inflammation
- Associated with other autoimmune diseases

CLINICAL ISSUES

- Typical patient is middle-aged woman with lid retraction, periorbital edema, proptosis, and restricted gaze
- Orbital disease may not be concordant with thyroid disease
- Corticosteroids 1st line of therapy in acute disease
- Surgery for decompression in severe cases

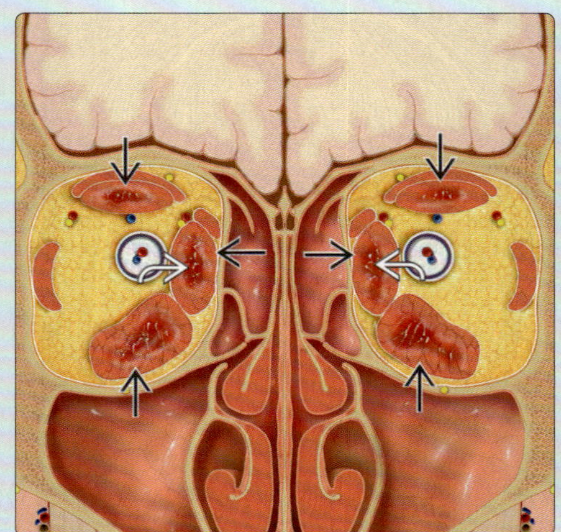

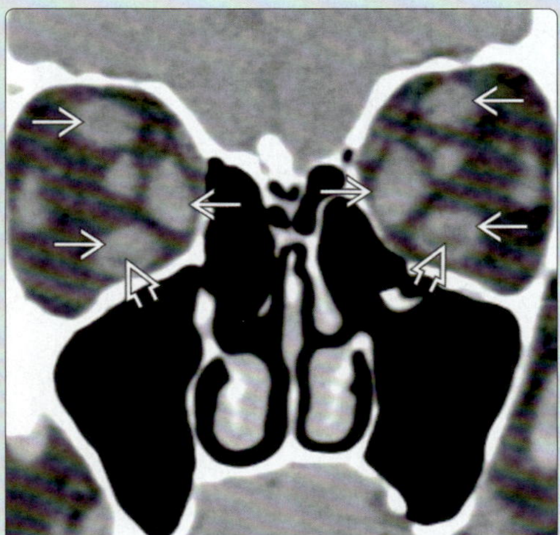

(Left) *Coronal graphic shows bilateral symmetric enlargement of extraocular muscles (EOMs) ➔. Irregularity within the muscles ➔ represents accumulation of lymphocytes and mucopolysaccharide deposition.* **(Right)** *Coronal NECT shows enlargement of the bilateral inferior, medial, and superior rectus muscles ➔ in a patient with thyroid eye disease. Mucopolysaccharide deposition manifests as areas of low density ➔ within the muscles, particularly the inferior recti.*

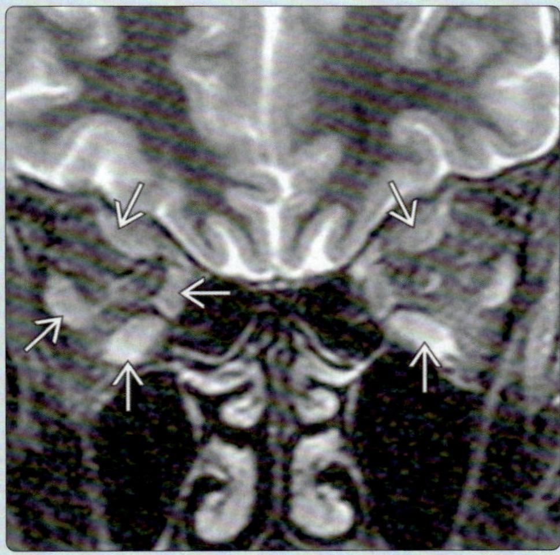

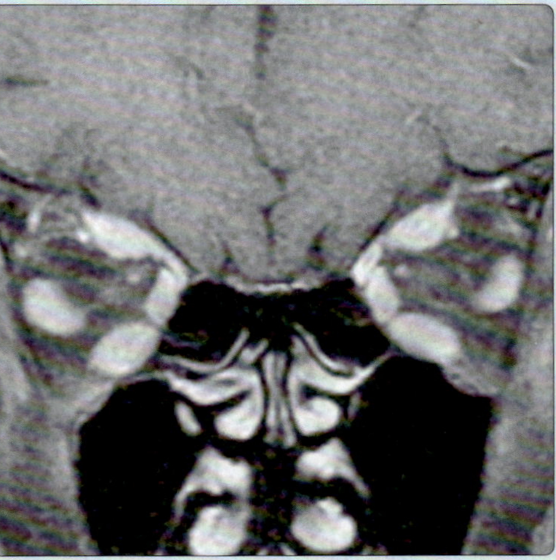

(Left) *Coronal STIR MR demonstrates bilateral diffuse enlargement of multiple rectus muscles ➔. Hyperintensity on STIR imaging correlates with acuity of disease as well as responsiveness to glucocorticoid therapy.* **(Right)** *Axial T1 C+ FS MR in the same patient with acute thyroid eye disease shows diffuse enlargement of essentially all of the rectus muscles. EOMs affected by acute thyroid orbitopathy typically enhance less intensely than normal muscles.*

KEY FACTS

IMAGING

- MR findings
  - Focal or segmental **T2 hyperintensity** of optic nerve
  - Central or diffuse **optic nerve enhancement**
  - Optic nerve diffusely & mildly enlarged
  - **Increased diffusivity** (diffusion restriction) on DWI sequence due to disruption of myelinated axons

TOP DIFFERENTIAL DIAGNOSES

- Ischemic optic neuropathy
- Infectious optic neuritis
- Idiopathic perineuritis (pseudotumor)
- Granulomatous optic neuropathy (sarcoid)
- Optic nerve sheath meningioma
- Optic nerve glioma

PATHOLOGY

- Autoimmune demyelination in susceptible patients
- Triggered by infection, systemic disease, or other stressor
- Nerve edema acutely, atrophy chronically

CLINICAL ISSUES

- Symptoms
  - Acute loss of visual acuity & color vision; eye pain
- Distinct clinical profiles
  - Acute multiple sclerosis-associated optic neuritis (ON)
  - Neuromyelitis optica (Devic syndrome)
  - Acute demyelinating encephalomyelitis (ADEM)
  - Pediatric ON
- Spontaneous recovery of vision is characteristic
- 2x or more as common in female patients

DIAGNOSTIC CHECKLIST

- Identification of demyelinating lesions in CNS is critical neuroimaging task in setting of ON
  - High incidence of MS in patients with ON
  - Findings on MR strongly predictive of MS
- Recommend brain & spinal cord imaging

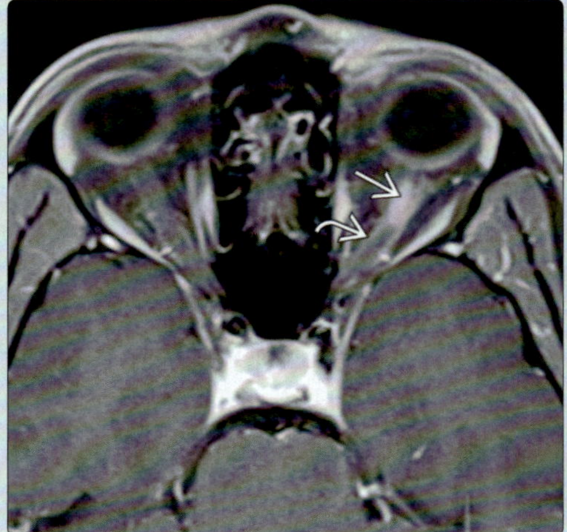

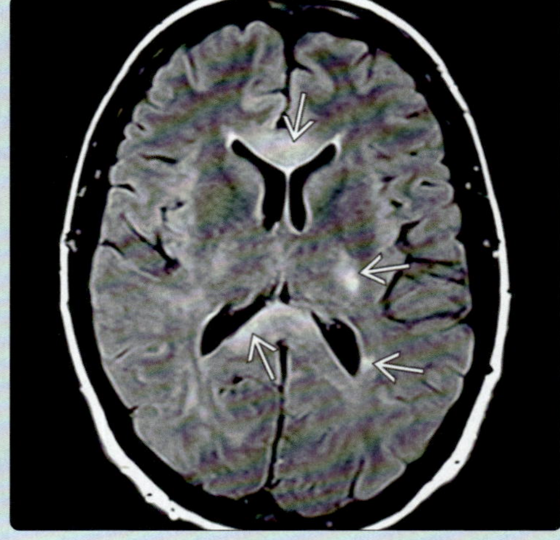

(Left) *Axial T1WI C+ FS MR in an adult woman with left eye pain and decreased color vision shows intense segmental enhancement of the left intraorbital optic nerve ➡. A component of peripheral nerve sheath enhancement is seen extending posteriorly ➡.* **(Right)** *Axial FLAIR MR of the brain in the same patient shows multiple periatrial, capsular, and callosal white matter lesions ➡. CSF analysis yielded oligoclonal bands, and the patient was diagnosed with multiple sclerosis.*

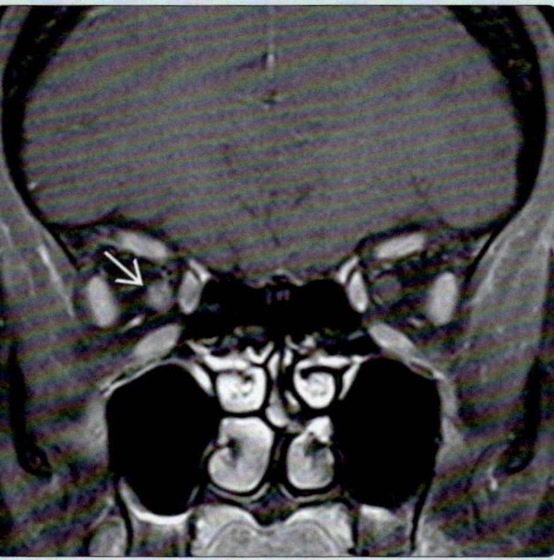

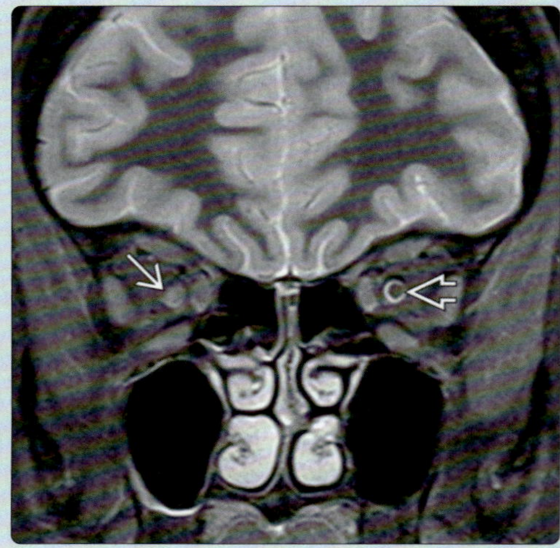

(Left) *Coronal T1WI C+ FS MR in a young adult woman with right eye vision loss, pain, & afferent pupillary defect shows moderate enhancement of the intraorbital optic nerve ➡. There are no other inflammatory changes in the orbit.* **(Right)** *Coronal STIR MR in the same patient shows increased signal in the right optic nerve ➡. Note that the hyperintense signal of the right nerve is similar to CSF in the optic nerve sheath, whereas the normal left nerve is distinct from the surrounding CSF ➡.*

Orbital Infantile Hemangioma

KEY FACTS

TERMINOLOGY

- Synonyms: Orbital capillary hemangioma, infantile periocular hemangioma
- Definition: **Benign vascular tumor** of infancy
- Distinct lesion from vascular malformation

IMAGING

- Location: Preseptal &/or postseptal orbit
  - Exclusively retrobulbar in 10%
- CT findings
  - Lobular, slightly hyperdense, homogeneous
  - Intense enhancement
- MR findings
  - T1 intermediate; prominent internal **flow voids**
  - Moderate T2 hyperintensity (high cellularity)
- US: High vessel density, absent arteriovenous shunting, high peak arterial Doppler shift
  - When superficial, US confirms clinical diagnosis
- MR best for mapping larger, deeper lesions

TOP DIFFERENTIAL DIAGNOSES

- Rhabdomyosarcoma
- Metastatic neuroblastoma
- Orbital Langerhans cell histiocytosis
- Orbital venous malformation
- Plexiform neurofibroma
- Orbital non-Hodgkin lymphoma

CLINICAL ISSUES

- Distinguish from vascular malformations
  - Present at birth; grow in monophasic fashion
- 3 distinct phases
  - **Proliferative phase**: Appears few weeks after birth and grows rapidly for 1st year or 2
  - **Involuting phase**: Regression over 3-5 years
  - **Involuted phase**: Usually complete regression by late childhood
- Treatment: Expectant observation unless complications
  - Propranolol ± corticosteroids; surgery if refractory

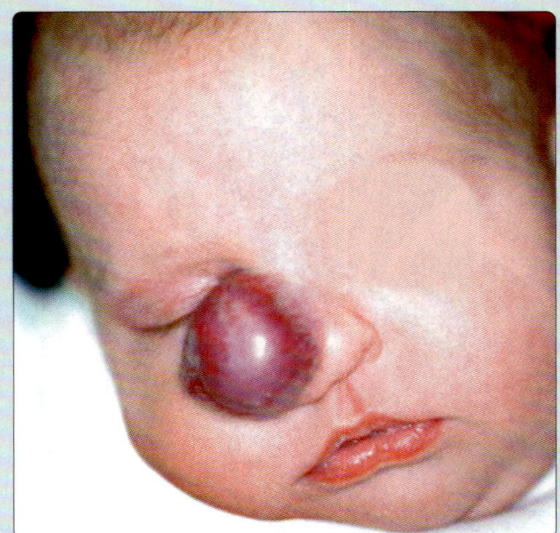

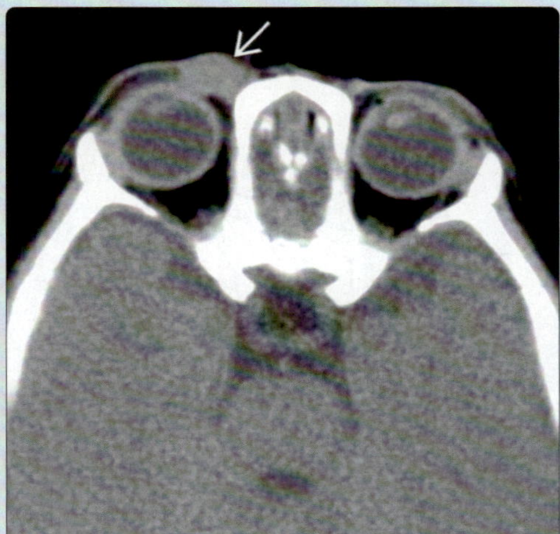

(Left) *Clinical photograph shows a superficial vascular mass centered at the medial orbit and nose with typical violaceous discoloration seen in infantile hemangioma.* **(Right)** *Axial CT without contrast demonstrates the most common location for orbital infantile hemangioma within the superior medial preseptal soft tissues ➡. There is no evidence of postseptal extension.*

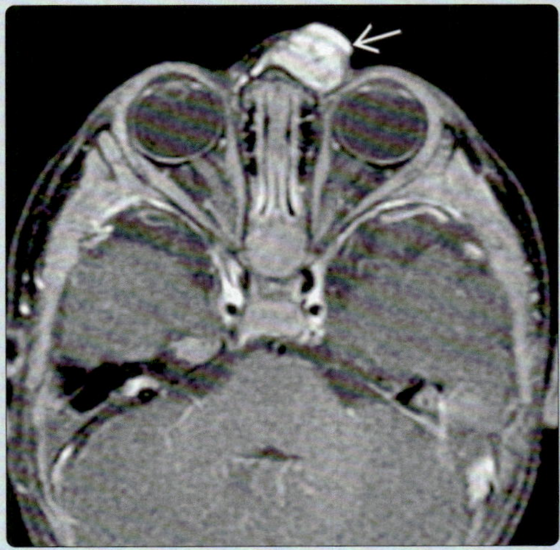

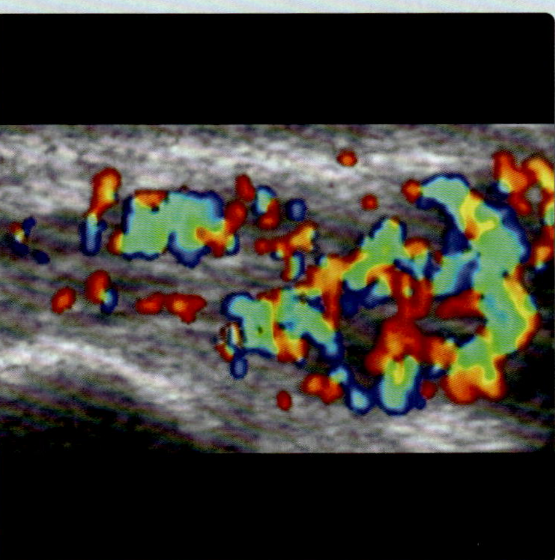

(Left) *Axial enhanced T1WI MR depicts a well-delineated, intensely enhancing infantile hemangioma ➡ with internal septations &/or flow voids in a typical periorbital location. Once again, postseptal extension is absent.* **(Right)** *Doppler US in the same patient shows striking internal flow, typical for phase I (proliferating) infantile hemangioma.*

KEY FACTS

TERMINOLOGY

- Optic nerve sheath meningioma
  - a.k.a. perioptic meningioma
- Benign, slow-growing tumor of optic nerve sheath
- Distinct entity from intracranial (sphenoorbital) meningioma that extends through orbital apex

IMAGING

- MR is preferred imaging modality
- Use CECT to look for Ca^{++} when diagnosis in doubt
- Imaging findings
  - Uniformly enhancing fusiform mass surrounding intraorbital optic nerve
    - With Ca^{++} around optic nerve in ~ 1/3 of cases (CT)
  - Tram-track pattern of enhancement (MR)
  - Variably hyperintense to hypointense on T2WI

TOP DIFFERENTIAL DIAGNOSES

- Optic nerve glioma
- Orbital pseudotumor
- Orbital sarcoidosis
- Metastasis
- Orbit lymphoproliferative lesions

PATHOLOGY

- Benign tumor **arising from arachnoid "cap" cells** within optic nerve sheath
- Histologic subtypes and degree of calcification affect signal intensity on T2WI MR

CLINICAL ISSUES

- Classic triad: Visual loss, optic atrophy, and optociliary venous shunting
  - Look for other findings of neurofibromatosis type 2, especially in younger patients
- Treatment options
  - Fractionated radiotherapy currently 1st-line therapy
    - Stereotactic radiation also being explored

(Left) *Axial graphic depicts a fusiform meningioma ➡ arising from the optic nerve sheath. Characteristic "perioptic cyst" ⇨ behind the globe represents trapped cerebrospinal fluid (CSF) within nerve sheath.* **(Right)** *Axial CECT shows enhancing optic nerve sheath meningioma (ONSM) ➡ with punctate and linear calcification surrounding the left optic nerve complex extending through the orbital apex. Note adjacent hyperostosis ⇨.*

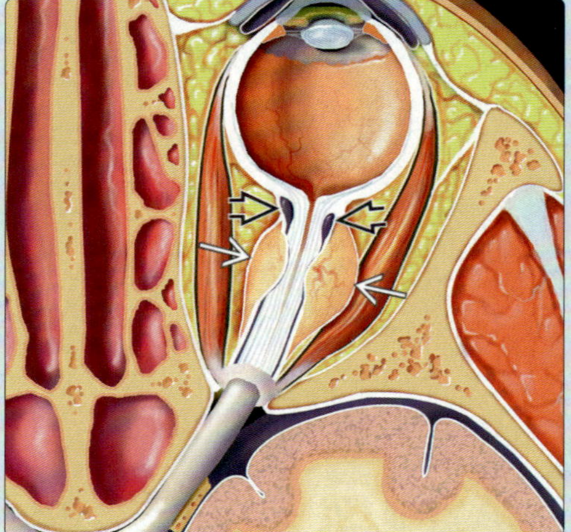

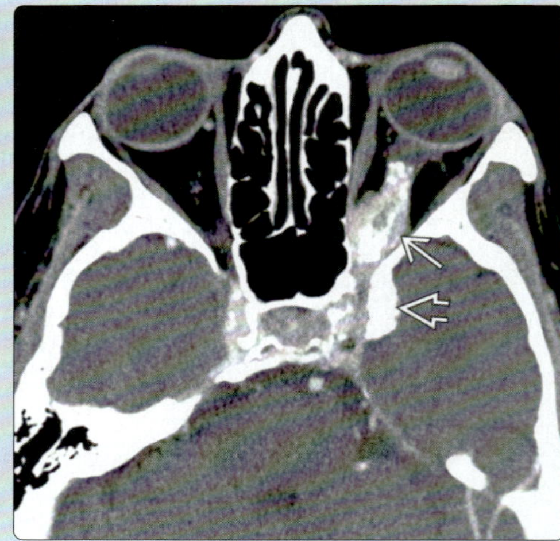

(Left) *Axial T2WI FS MR reveals a globular meningioma involving the intraorbital segment of the right optic nerve ⇨. Note T2 signal similar to brain parenchyma. Though signal intensity may be variable, ONSMs, like intracranial lesions, are often relatively hypointense on T2WI.* **(Right)** *Axial T1WI C+ FS MR demonstrates a globular configuration of avidly enhancing ONSM ➡ eccentrically surrounding orbital segment of right optic nerve. Note tumor spares optic nerve immediately posterior to globe ↩, a common pattern.*

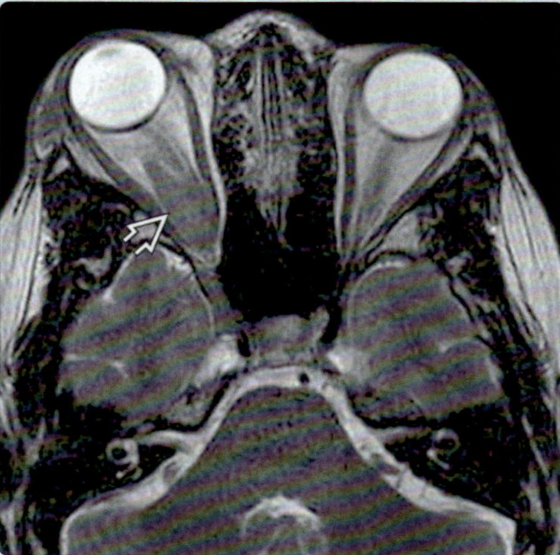

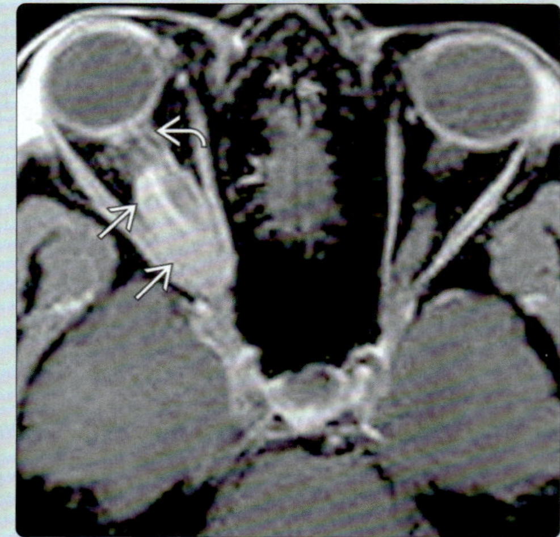

KEY FACTS

TERMINOLOGY

- Definition: Malignant primary retinal neoplasm
- Trilateral/quadrilateral retinoblastoma (RB): Bilateral ocular RB + pineal ± suprasellar tumors

IMAGING

- General imaging findings
  - Unilateral in 60%, bilateral in 40%
  - Trilateral or quadrilateral disease rare
  - **Extraocular extension** in **< 10%**
    - Indicates poor prognosis
- CT: **Calcification** in **> 90%**
- MR: Assess extent of intraocular tumor and presence of optic nerve, orbital, or intracranial involvement
  - T1: Mild hyperintensity
  - T2: Moderate to marked **hypointensity**
  - Moderate to marked heterogeneous enhancement

TOP DIFFERENTIAL DIAGNOSES

- Persistent hyperplastic primary vitreous
- Coats disease
- Retinopathy of prematurity
- Orbital toxocariasis

PATHOLOGY

- **Primitive neuroectodermal tumor**
- Inherited (germline): Multilateral > unilateral
- Requires "two-hit" mutation of both *Rb* tumor suppressor genes

CLINICAL ISSUES

- Most common intraocular tumor of childhood
- **Leukocoria** in 50%; 90-95% diagnosed by 5 years of age
- Treatment options
  - Many treatment approaches
  - Challenge is maintaining eye and vision
  - > 95% of RB (USA) cured with modern techniques

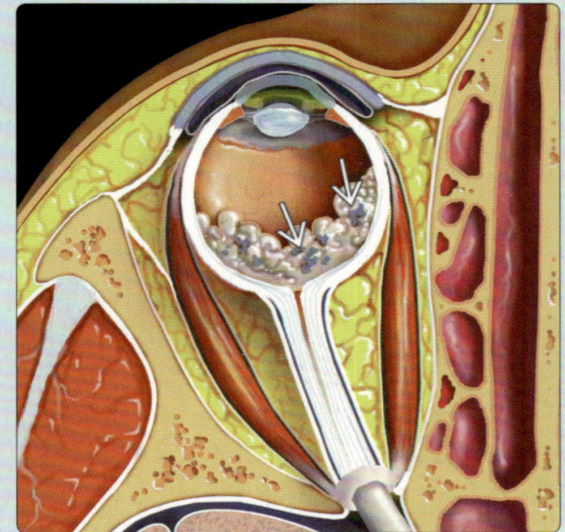

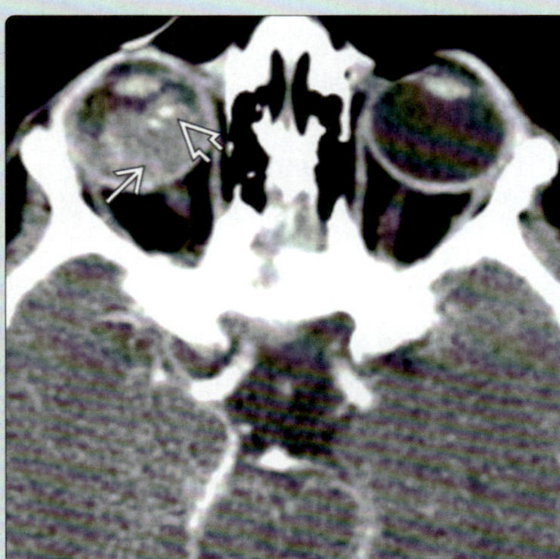

(Left) *Axial graphic depicts retinoblastoma with a lobulated tumor extending through the limiting membrane into the vitreous. Punctate calcifications ➡ are characteristic.* **(Right)** *Axial CECT demonstrates a lobular endophytic retinoblastoma ➡ containing small calcifications ➡ and filling much of the vitreous compartment. A calcified ocular mass in a child represents retinoblastoma until proven otherwise.*

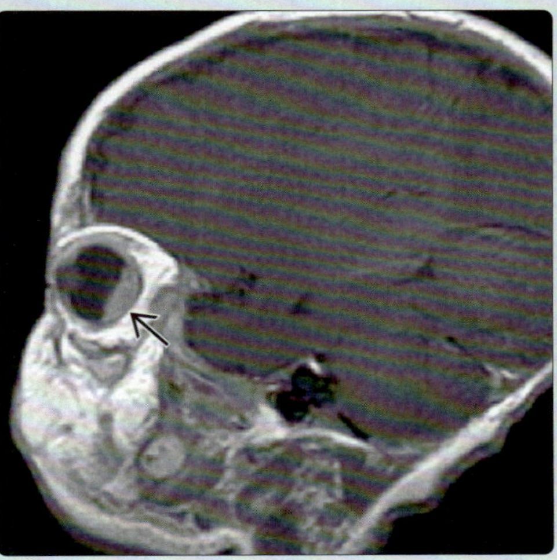

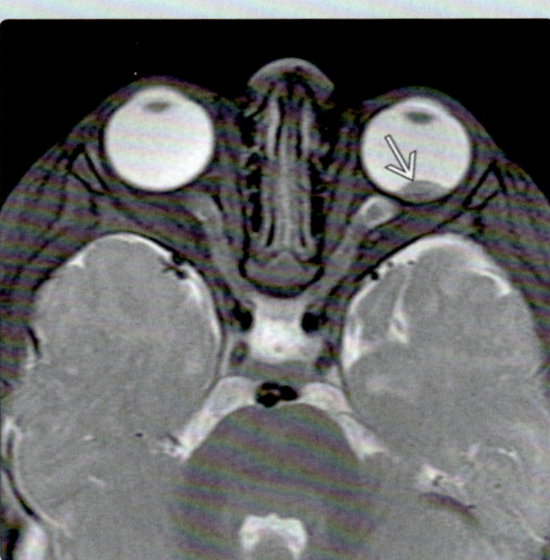

(Left) *Sagittal postcontrast T1WI MR through the orbit shows an enhancing intraocular mass ➡ without visible extraocular extension.* **(Right)** *Axial T2WI FS MR shows a mass at the margin of the left optic disc ➡. Virtually all retinoblastomas demonstrate hypointensity relative to vitreous on T2WI; the lenticular shape is typical for early lesions.*

SECTION 5

Skull Base

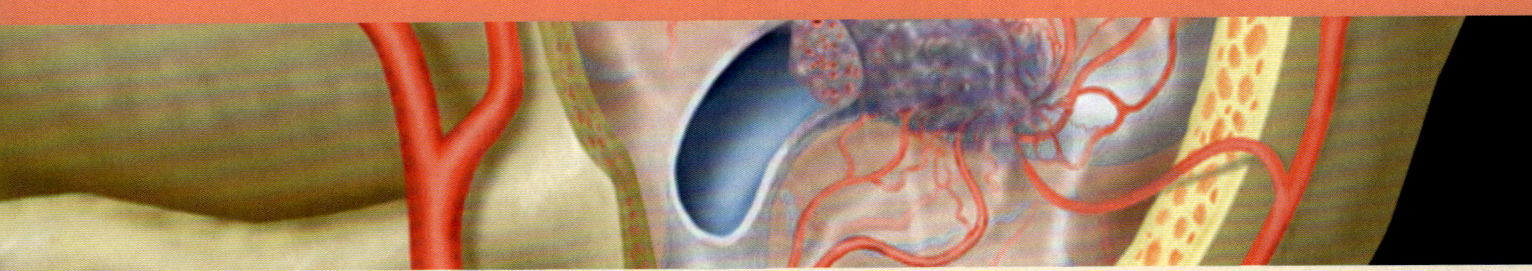

Skull Base Lesions

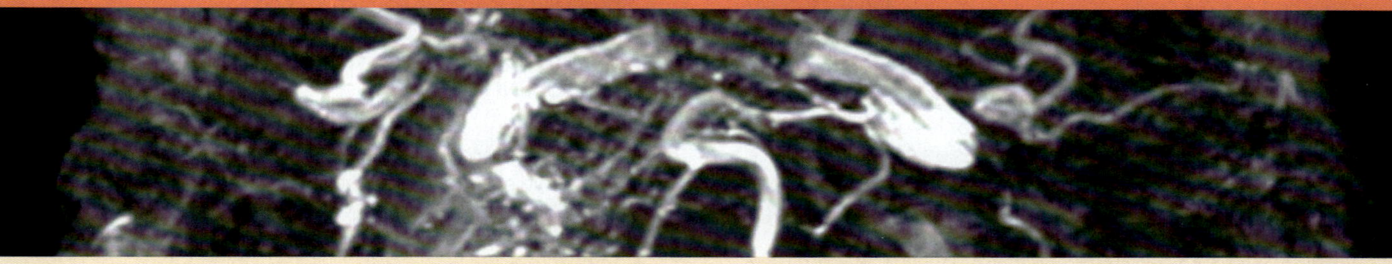

Imaging Approaches and Indications

CT is primary imaging tool for evaluating bony details of the skull base (SB). Multislice CT scanners allow thin slices (≤ 1 mm) & provide multiplanar reformatted images. These function as a mainstay for evaluating bony changes associated with SB diseases and providing evidence for calcific/bony matrices of these lesions.

MR is an essential partner to bone CT in evaluating SB lesions as it provides the best understanding of lesion soft tissue extent. T1 precontrast images show lesion margins against the contrast of skull base marrow fat. T1 also reveals high-signal subacute blood and intralesion high-velocity flow voids to best advantage. Enhanced, fat-saturated T1 sequences define enhancement characteristics of the lesion in question. GRE may show blooming if hemorrhage or venous sinus thrombosis is present. DWI hyperintensity in a focal SB lesion suggests the diagnosis of epidermoid. MRA and MRV are important sequences to acquire if internal carotid and vertebral artery or venous sinus involvement is suspected.

Imaging Anatomy

The SB is made up of five bones: The paired frontal and temporal bones and the unpaired ethmoid, sphenoid, and occipital bones. Two major surfaces of the SB can be described: The **endocranial surface**, which faces the brain, cisterns, cranial nerves (CN), and intracranial vessels, and the **exocranial surface**, which faces the extracranial H&N. The exocranial surface anteriorly interfaces with the sinus, nose, and orbits, centrally with the masticator (MS), parotid (PS), parapharyngeal, and anterior pharyngeal mucosal spaces (PMS), and posteriorly with the carotid (CS), retropharyngeal (RPS), perivertebral (PVS), and posterior PMS.

The **endocranial surface** can be further divided into three regions: The anterior, central, and posterior SB.

- **Anterior SB** (ASB): Floor of anterior cranial fossa, comprised of orbital plate of frontal bone, ethmoid bone cribriform plate and ethmoid sinus roof, and planum sphenoidale and lesser wing (LWS) of sphenoid bone; important ASB foramina include **foramen cecum** (FC) and **cribriform plate foramina**
- **Central SB** (CSB): Floor of middle cranial fossa, made up of **basisphenoid**, **greater wing** of sphenoid bone (GWS), and **temporal bone** (T-bone) anterior to petrous ridge; bony landmarks of CSB include sella turcica, tuberculum sellae, and posterior clinoid process; important CSB foramina and fissures are optic canal, superior orbital fissure (SOF), inferior orbital fissure (IOF), foramen rotundum, foramen ovale, foramen spinosum, vidian canal, carotid canal, and foramen lacerum
- **Posterior SB** (PSB): Bony bowl floor of posterior cranial fossa, made up of **posterior T-bone wall** & **occipital bone**; occipital bone has 3 parts: Basilar part (lower clivus/basiocciput), condylar part lateral to foramen magnum, including occipital condyles, & squamous part (large bony plate posterosuperior to foramen magnum); PSB foramina/fissures include internal auditory canal (IAC), jugular foramen, hypoglossal canal, stylomastoid foramen, & foramen magnum

Skull Base Foramina/Fissures and Contents

Anterior skull base

- **Foramen cecum**: Midline, anterior to crista galli; embryologic remnant of anterior neuropore, which normally involutes in early childhood
- **Cribriform plate foramina**: Roof of nasal cavity; transmits afferent fibers from nasal mucosa to olfactory bulbs of **CNI**

Central skull base

- **Optic canal**: Medial LWS; transmits **CNII** to **globe**, dura, arachnoid and pia, CSF, ophthalmic artery
- **SOF**: Between LWS and GWS; transmits **CNIII**, **CNIV**, **CNVI**, **CNV1**, and superior ophthalmic vein
- **IOF**: Cleft between maxilla body and GWS; transmits inferior orbital artery, vein, and nerve
- **Foramen rotundum**: Conduit to pterygopalatine fossa (PPF) within sphenoid bone superolateral to vidian canal; transmits **CNV2** to **PPF**, artery of foramen rotundum, emissary veins from cavernous sinus to pterygoid plexus
- **Foramen ovale**: Within GWS; conduit to masticator space; transmits **CNV3** into **masticator space**, lesser petrosal nerve, and accessory meningeal branch of internal maxillary artery
- **Foramen spinosum**: Within GWS posterolateral to foramen ovale; transmits middle meningeal artery and vein and recurrent branch of CNV3
- **Vidian canal**: Inferolateral to foramen rotundum within GWS; connects foramen lacerum to PPF; transmits vidian nerve and artery
- **Carotid canal**: In T-bone and GWS; transmits petrous (C2) and lacerum (C3) segments of internal carotid artery (ICA) and **sympathetic plexus**
- **Foramen lacerum**: Pseudoforamen; cartilaginous floor of lacerum ICA segment

Posterior skull base

- **IAC**: In posterior wall of T-bone; opening called porus acusticus; transmits **CNVII**, **CNVIII**, and labyrinthine artery
- **Jugular foramen** (JF): Cleft between temporal and occipital bones with 2 parts (pars nervosa and vascularis/venosa); pars nervosa transmits **CNXI** into **CS**, Jacobsen nerve, inferior petrosal vein; pars vascularis/venosa transmits **CNX**, **CNXI**, Arnold nerve, posterior meningeal artery, jugular bulb
- **Hypoglossal canal**: Found with condylar occipital bone inferomedial to JF; transmits **CNXII** into **CS**
- **Stylomastoid foramen**: Exocranial surface of T-bone between medial mastoid tip and styloid process; transmits **CNVII** into **parotid space**
- **Foramen magnum**: Occipital bone inferior ring; transmits medulla oblongata, vertebral arteries, and **CNXI** (ascending spinal component)

Embryology

ASB embryology is the key to understanding disease in this area (anterior neuropore anomaly, cephalocele, nasal glioma). Failure to close the space between the nasal and frontal bones, also known as the **fonticulus nasofrontalis**, can lead to these congenital conditions. The **prenasal space** is a transient prenatal region separating the nasal bones and cartilaginous nasal capsule. The anterior neuropore extends from the intracranial space to the prenasal space and briefly contacts

Skull Base Differential Diagnosis: Tumors & Tumor-Like Lesions by Site

Skull base, anterior, central, or posterior	Melanoma, N
Meningioma	Lacrimal gland carcinoma, O
Giant cell tumor	**Central skull base**
Hemangiopericytoma	Sella: Pituitary macroadenoma
Metastases	Clivus: Chordoma, ecchordosis physaliphora
Multiple myeloma	Petrooccipital fissure: Chondrosarcoma
Plasmacytoma	Meckel cave: Trigeminal schwannoma
Osteosarcoma	T-bone: Tumor
Rhabdomyosarcoma, parameningeal	Endolymphatic sac tumor
Langerhans cell histiocytosis	T-bone: Tumor-like lesions
Tumor-like lesions	Acquired cholesteatoma
Fibrous dysplasia	Congenital cholesteatoma
Paget disease	Cholesterol granuloma
Idiopathic extraorbital inflammation (pseudotumor)	**Posterior skull base**
Anterior skull base	Clivus (occipital bone): Chordoma
Mucocele, SN	Jugular foramen
Osteoma, SN	Glomus jugulare paraganglioma
Esthesioneuroblastoma, N	Jugular foramen schwannoma
Squamous cell carcinoma, SN	Jugular foramen meningioma
Non-Hodgkin lymphoma, SN or O	Hypoglossal canal: Hypoglossal schwannoma

SN = sinonasal; N = nasal; O = orbit.

skin at the bridge of the nose but involutes prior to birth. The prenasal space reduces to a small canal anterior to the crista galli called the **foramen cecum**. The newborn FC diameter is ~ 4 mm. The FC should be completely ossified by 2 years of age.

As the ASB originates largely from cartilaginous precursors, the process of ossification can be confusing on imaging. The ASB ossifies from posterior to anterior and lateral to medial. At birth the ASB is composed of cartilage, which progressively ossifies. Ossification of the crista galli and cribriform plate begins at 2 months and is nearly complete by 24 months. The crista galli contains fat at about 12 months (**do not** call it a dermoid). The area of the FC ossifies last, reaching its adult configuration by 2 years.

The CSB forms from ~ 24 ossifications centers. Major centers include the presphenoid (planum sphenoidale), postsphenoid (basisphenoid containing sella, dorsum, and sphenoid sinus), alisphenoid (GWS), and orbitosphenoid (LWS). The **sphenooccipital synchondrosis** lies between the basisphenoid and basiocciput. It is the site of most postnatal SB growth and the last sutures to fuse (completed by age 20 years). Persistence of the **craniopharyngeal canal** (remnant of Rathke pouch) may occur between the presphenoid & basisphenoid. Persistence of **median basal canal** may be seen between the basioccipital ossification centers.

Approaches to Skull Base Imaging Issues

Creating skull base lesion DDx can be difficult because some lesions can occur anywhere along the SB. Understanding the DDx list of the lesions that can occur anywhere in the SB is essential. Adding this group to a site-specific DDx can yield a near complete set of possible lesions to be considered. ASB, CSB, and PSB DDx lists can be constructed. The CSB can be further refined into shorter, site-specific DDx lists for the sella, clivus, petrooccipital fissure, and Meckel cave. The PSB has one important site-specific DDx for the jugular foramen.

Knowledge of SB lesions requires the clinician to understand the interface relationships between the SB and the extracranial H&N. The ASB sits atop the frontal and ethmoid sinuses, orbit, and nose. Many of the ASB lesions originate in these structures. The CSB resides superior to the MS, PS, and PMSs. Nasopharyngeal carcinoma directly accesses the intracranial compartment via the foramen lacerum (perivascular spread). MS and PS space malignancies may reach the intracranial compartment via perineural spread along CNV3 and CNVII, respectively. The PSB directly interacts with the CS, RPS, and PVSs. When JF lesions exit the skull base inferiorly, they plunge directly into the nasopharyngeal CS.

Without a clear understanding of perineural tumor (PNT) SB spread, the clinician may not identify this key imaging finding. PNT from PS malignancy enters the stylomastoid foramen and climbs the CNVII mastoid segment. MS malignancy at CNV3 PNT traverses the foramen ovale on its way to Meckel cave. Cheek skin, palate, sinus, or orbit carcinoma can access CNV2 via the infraorbital nerve or PPF, following CNV2 through the foramen rotundum into the middle cranial fossa. PPF malignancy may also show PNT spread via the vidian nerve to the foramen lacerum. PNT also connects between CNV and CNVII along the greater superficial petrosal nerve on the superior ridge of the petrous T-bone.

Selected References

1. Borges A: Skull base tumours part I. Imaging technique, anatomy and anterior skull base tumours. Eur J Radiol. 66(3):338-47, 2008
2. Borges A: Skull base tumours part II. Central skull base tumours and intrinsic tumours of the bony skull base. Eur J Radiol. 66(3):348-62, 2008

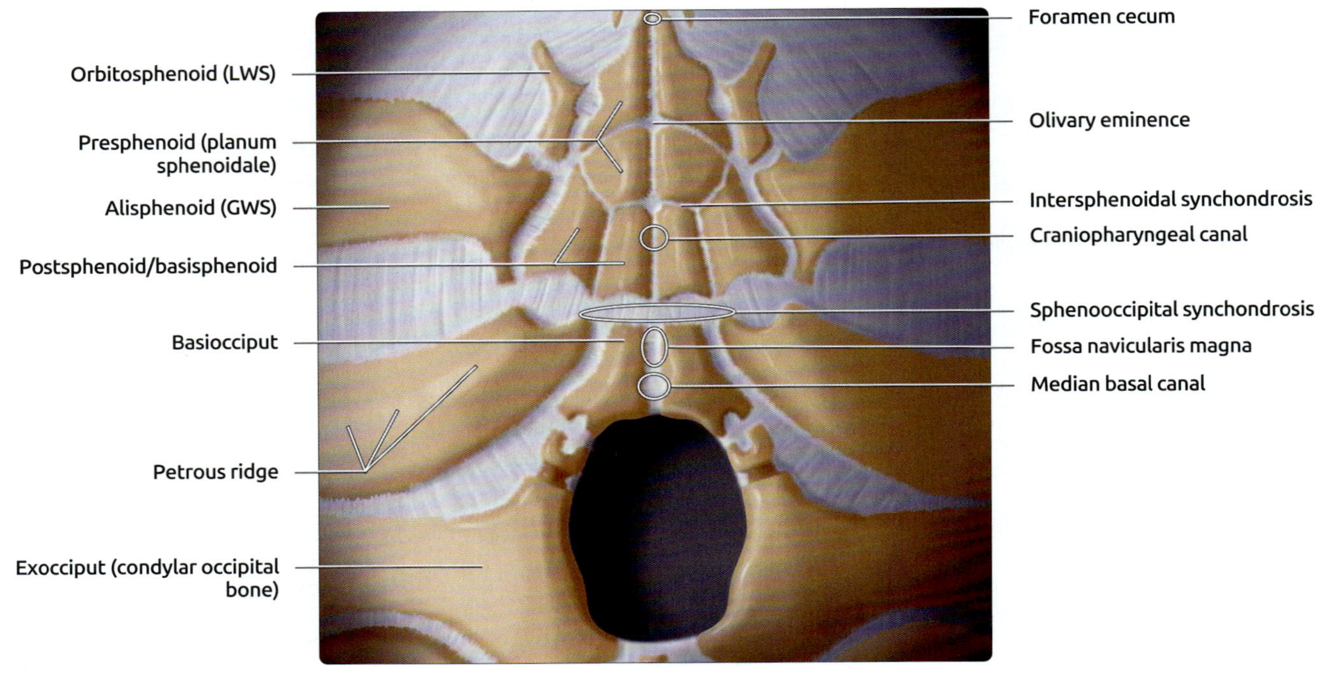

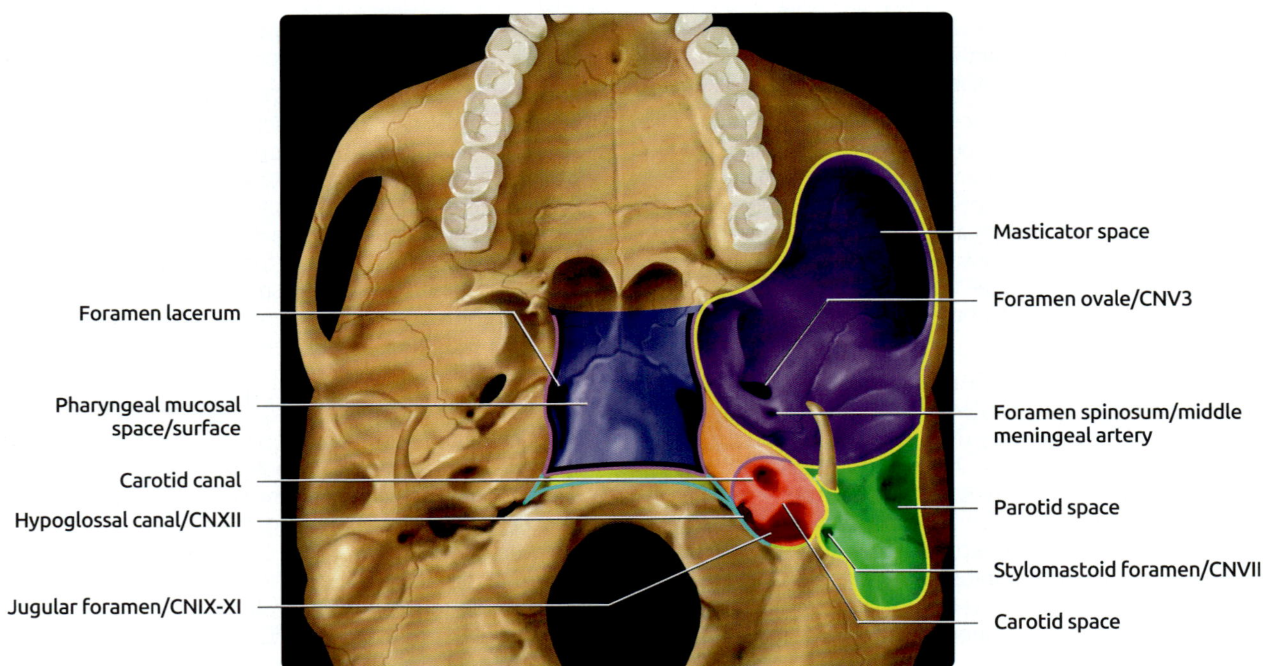

(Top) *Graphic of the skull base shows many ossification centers. Between the ossification centers of presphenoid is a cartilaginous gap called the olivary eminence, which is obliterated shortly after birth. In the midline, note the craniopharyngeal canal, sphenooccipital synchondrosis, fossa navicularis magna, and median basal canal. The sphenooccipital synchondrosis fuses over the first 20 years of life while the craniopharyngeal and median basal canals are rarely persistent into childhood. When persistent, these 2 canals can rarely be the source of meningitis.* **(Bottom)** *Graphic of the skull base viewed from below shows the relationship of spaces of the suprahyoid neck to the skull base. Four spaces have key interactions with the skull base: Masticator, parotid, carotid, and pharyngeal mucosal spaces. Parotid space (green) malignancy can follow CNVII into the stylomastoid foramen. The masticator space (purple) receives CNV3 while CNIX-XII enters the carotid space (red). The pharyngeal mucosal space abuts the foramen lacerum, which is covered by fibrocartilage in life.*

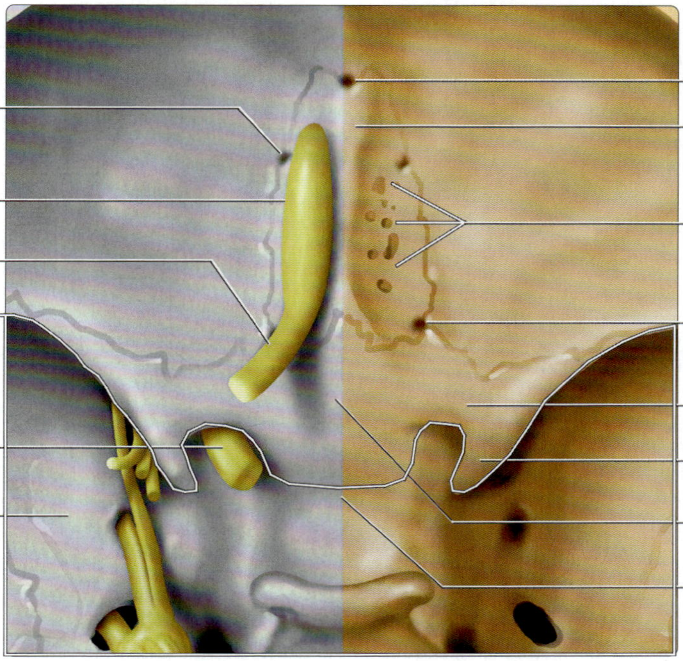

Anterior ethmoid foramen
Olfactory bulb
Olfactory nerve (CNI)
Line dividing anterior and central skull base
Optic nerve (CNII)
Central skull base
Foramen cecum
Crista galli
Cribriform plate of ethmoid
Posterior ethmoid foramen
Lesser wing, sphenoid bone
Anterior clinoid process
Planum sphenoidale
Tuberculum sellae

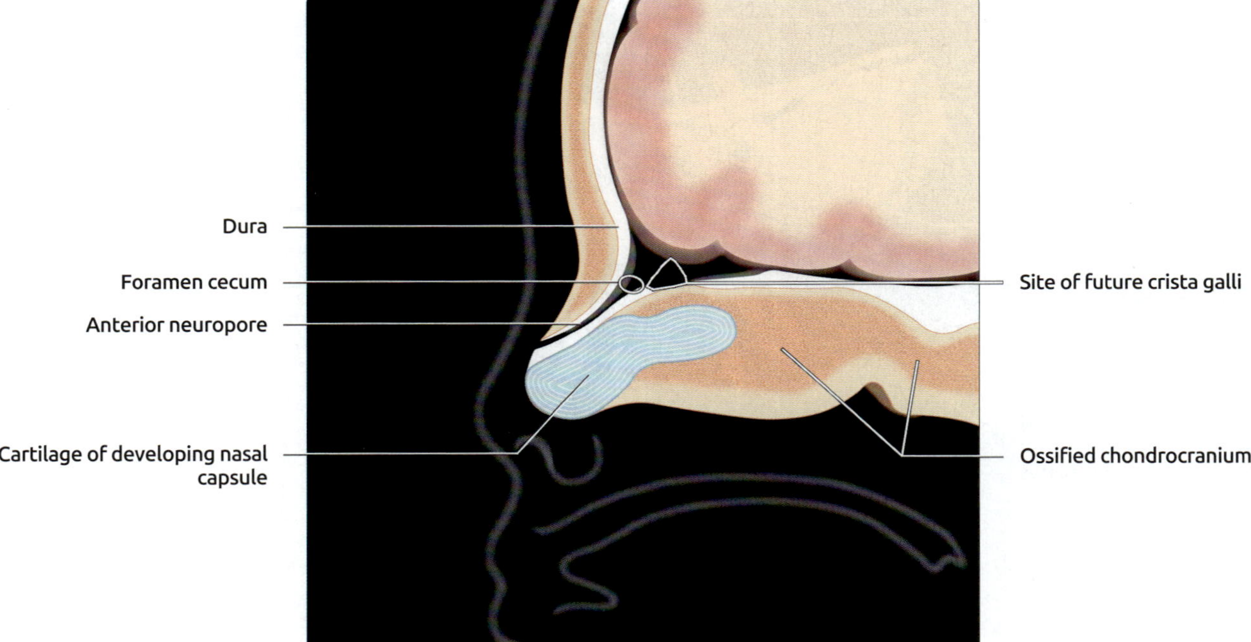

(Top) *Graphic of the anterior skull base seen from above shows the olfactory bulb of CNI lying on the cribriform plate. Neural structures have been removed on the right panel, allowing visualization of numerous perforations in the cribriform plate, through which afferent fibers from olfactory mucosa pass to form the olfactory bulb. The posterior margin of the anterior skull base is formed by the lesser wing of the sphenoid and planum sphenoidale. Note the foramen cecum, a small pit anterior to the crista galli, bounded anteriorly by the frontal bone and posteriorly by the ethmoid bone. If the anterior neuropore persists, an enlarged foramen cecum, bifid crista galli, and epidermoid along the neuropore tract are possible.* **(Bottom)** *Sagittal graphic of the anterior skull base during development shows ossification of the chondrocranium proceeding from posterior to anterior. The prenasal space is now encased in bone and has become the foramen cecum. A normal stalk of dura extends through the foramen cecum to skin (anterior neuropore).*

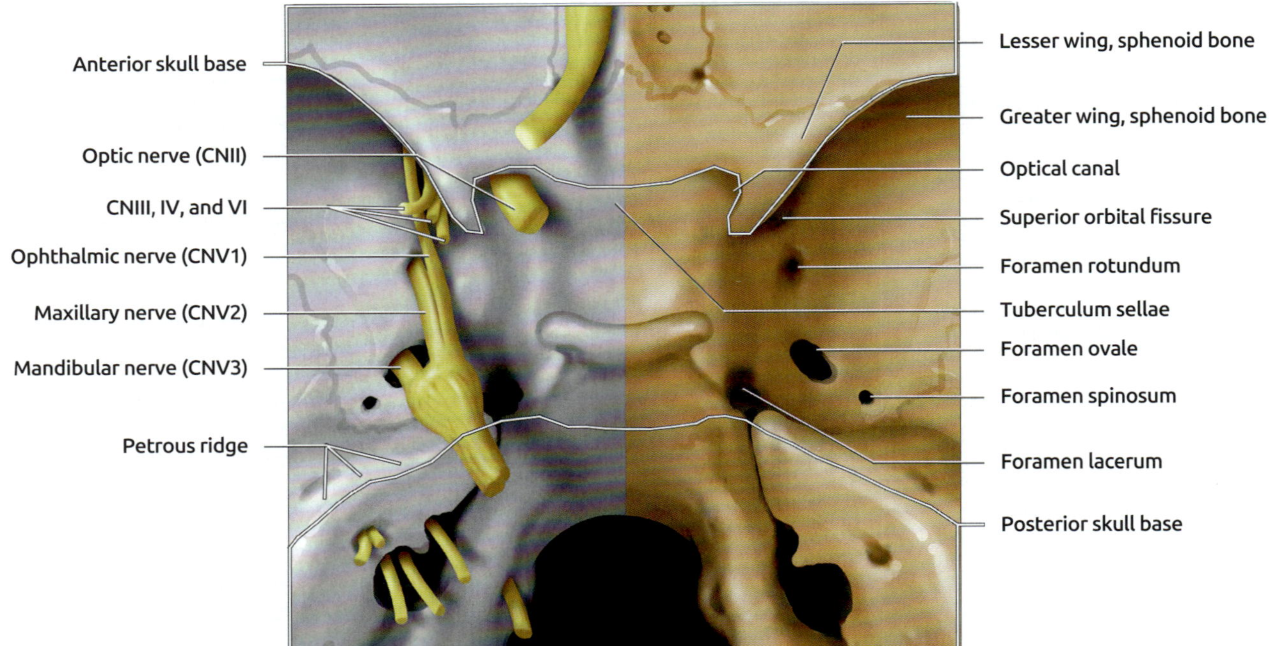

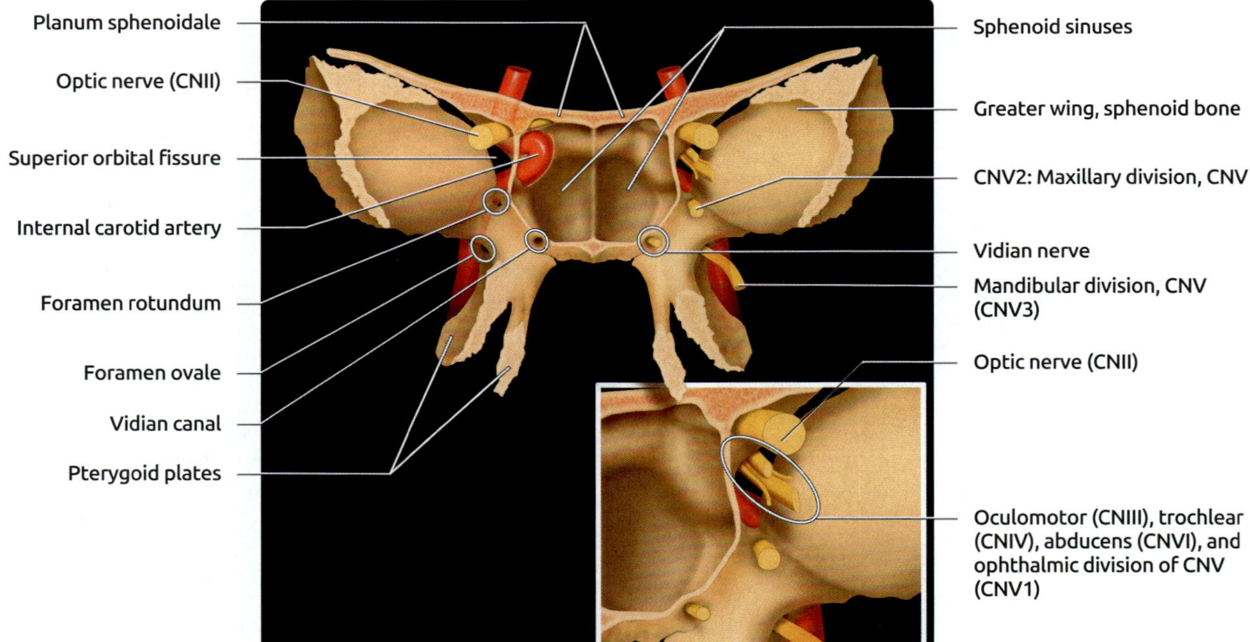

(Top) *Graphic of the central skull base seen from above shows the important nerves on the left and the numerous fissures and foramina on the right. The greater wing of the sphenoid bone forms the anterior wall of the middle cranial fossa. The posterior limit of the central skull base is the dorsum sella medially and the petrous ridge laterally.* **(Bottom)** *Coronal graphic shows the important anatomy of the central skull base/sphenoid bone. The cavernous portions of the internal carotid arteries lie lateral and posterior to the sinuses. At the orbital apex, the optic nerve can be seen traversing the optic canal. Multiple cranial nerves pass through the superior orbital fissure into the orbit, including CNs III, IV, and VI as well as the ophthalmic division on CNV. The maxillary division of CNV in foramen rotundum and the vidian nerve are positioned lateral and inferior to the sinus, respectively.*

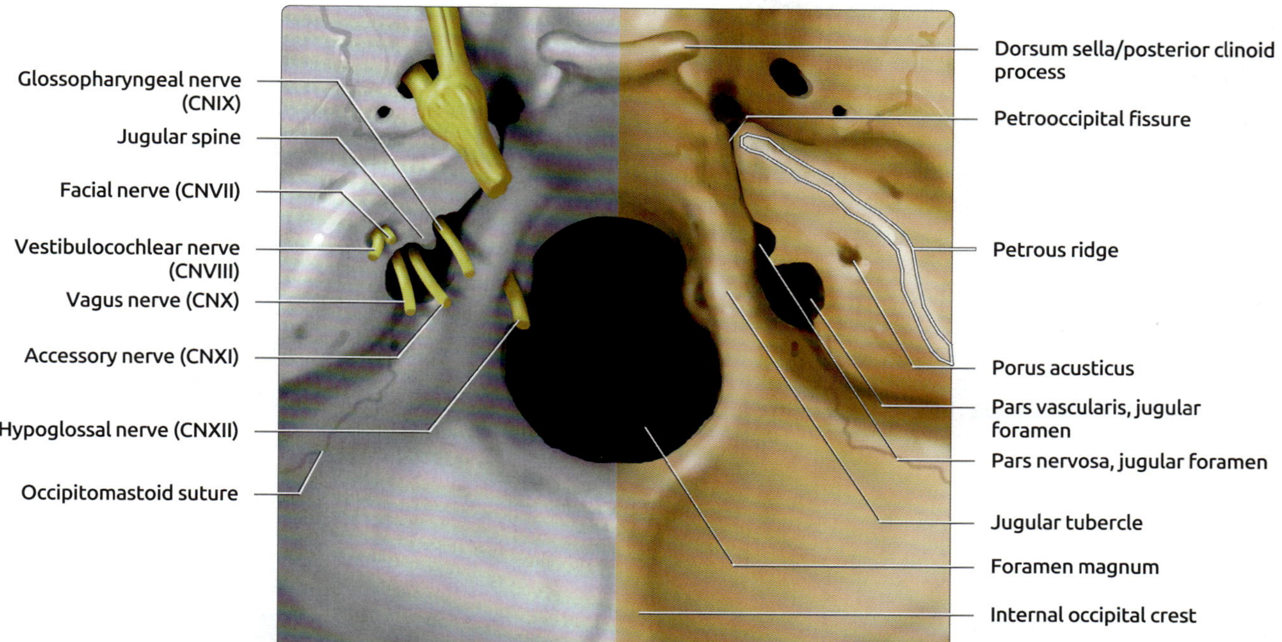

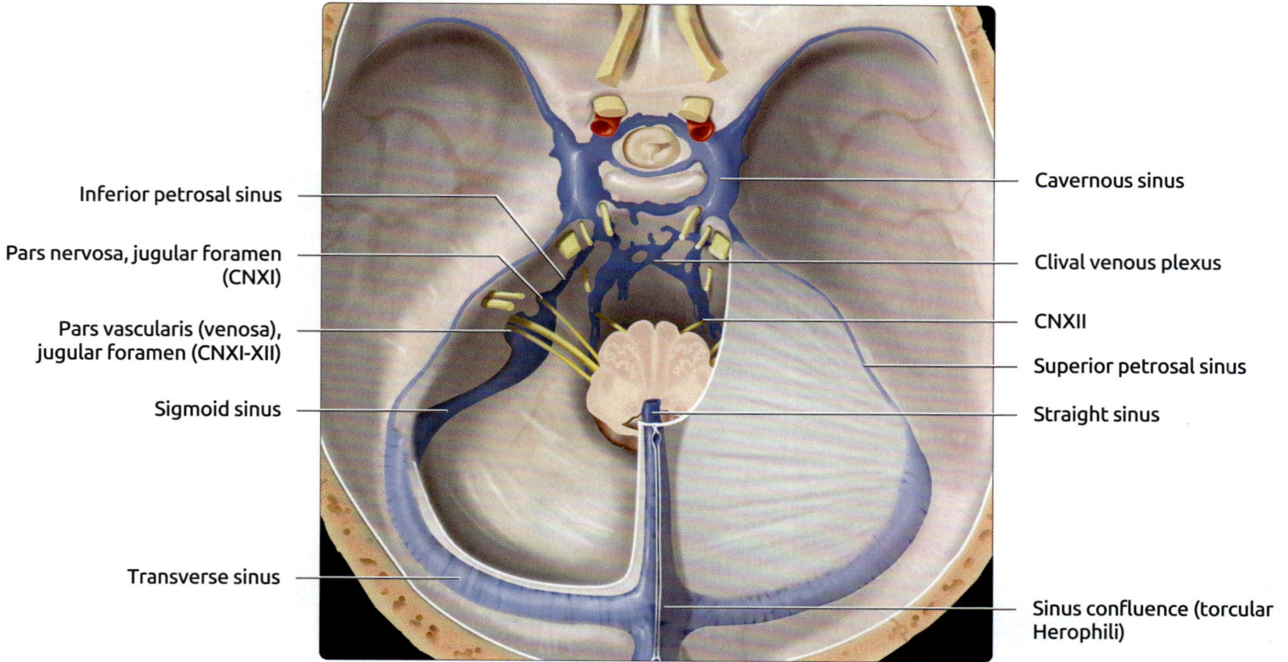

(Top) *Graphic shows the posterior skull base as seen from above. The neural structures are shown on the left while the bony landmarks are seen on the right. The anterior boundary of the posterior skull base is clivus medially and petrous ridge laterally. The major foramina are the foramen magnum, porus acusticus, jugular foramen, and hypoglossal canal. Notice that the jugular foramen connects anteriorly with the petrooccipital fissure.* **(Bottom)** *Graphic of the posterior skull base shows the major dural venous sinuses and jugular foramen from above. The midbrain and pons as well as the tentorium cerebelli have been removed on the left. Notice the transverse sinus is in the wall of the occipital bone while the sigmoid sinus is in the medial wall of the temporal bone. The 2 portions of the jugular foramen are also visible. The anterior pars nervosa receives the glossopharyngeal nerve (CNIX), while the pars vascularis (or venosa) has the vagus (CNX) and accessory (CNXI) nerves passing through it.*

Ecchordosis Physaliphora

KEY FACTS

TERMINOLOGY

- Definition: Benign **cystic mass arising dorsal to clivus with intradural component in prepontine cistern**
  - Considered to be ectopic notochordal remnant

IMAGING

- CT: Prepontine **intradural mass** connected by osseous stalk or pedicle to clivus
  - May have associated well-marginated, **scalloped clival lesion** with sclerotic margins
- MR: Provides best depiction of lesion, stalk, and intradural component
  - Uniformly **T2 hyperintense**
  - Clival component hypointense compared to normal bone marrow
  - Restricted diffusion often noted
  - **Lack of enhancement** differentiates from chordoma

TOP DIFFERENTIAL DIAGNOSES

- Chordoma
- Skull base metastasis
- Dermoid or epidermoid
- Arachnoid cyst

PATHOLOGY

- Few clear cells ("**physaliphorous cells**") surrounded by chondromyxoid stroma

CLINICAL ISSUES

- Asymptomatic incidental lesion found on head MR
  - Found in 2% of autopsies & 1.6% of MR studies
- Indolent lesion, which does not grow
- Not managed surgically in most cases
- Surgery indicated when atypical imaging findings, significant brainstem compression, or other symptoms

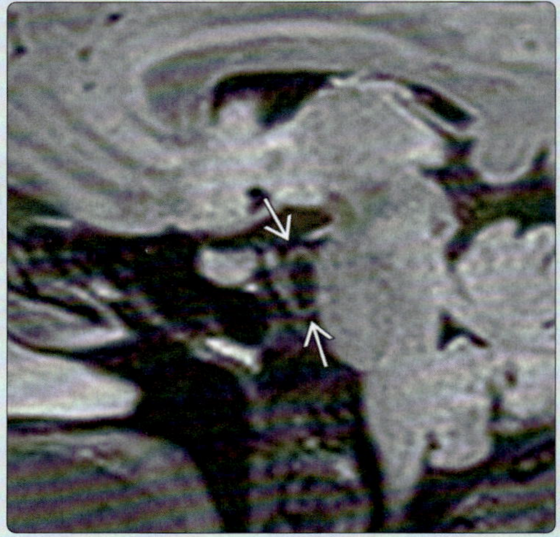

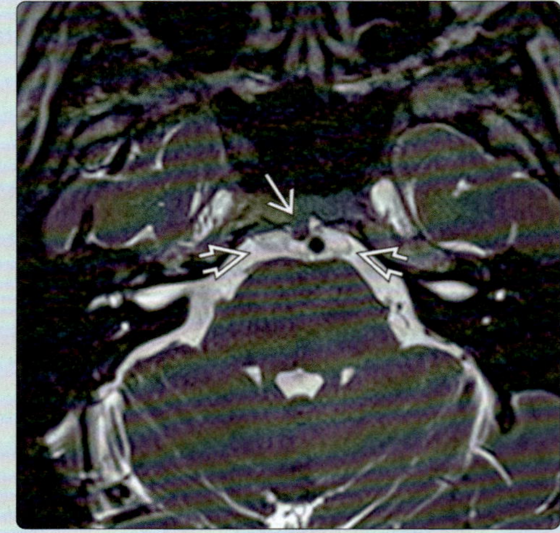

(Left) *Sagittal T2 FLAIR MR demonstrates the intradural component of a classic ecchordosis physaliphora with a notable thin-walled ➡ cyst, which is otherwise isointense with CSF. The clival portion of lesion is not well seen.* **(Right)** *Axial 3D T2 SSFSE MR demonstrates a small bony strut ➡ of classic ecchordosis physaliphora and the intradural cystic component of the lesion ➡, which is surrounding the basilar artery. Cystic lesion within the clivus is not apparent on this section.*

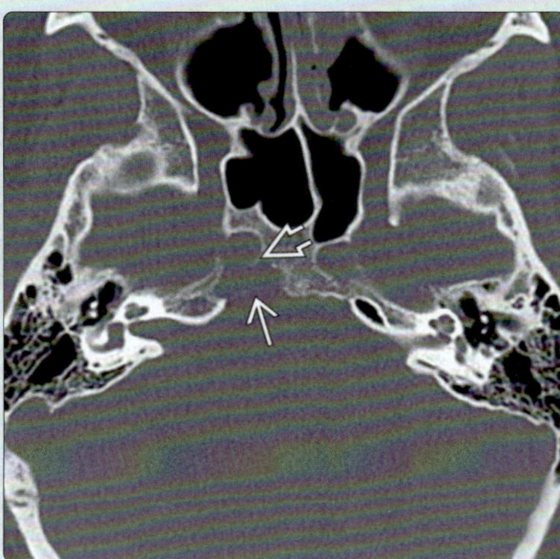

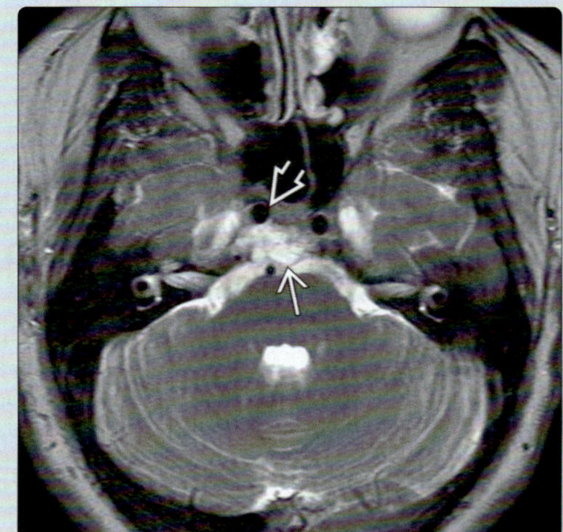

(Left) *Axial bone CT shows a well-marginated lytic lesion of the clivus with sclerotic borders ➡. This lesion extended to the carotid canal ➡, but the carotid artery was normal. No intradural component is appreciated on this bone window CT.* **(Right)** *Axial T2 MR in the same patient shows hyperintense T2 signal with internal septations within the clival portion of the lesion and demonstrates intradural extension into the prepontine cistern ➡, adjacent to the basilar artery. A normal internal carotid artery flow void is evident ➡.*

Invasive Pituitary Macroadenoma

KEY FACTS

TERMINOLOGY

- Definition: Invasive, benign pituitary adenoma with inferior extension into skull base

IMAGING

- Best imaging tool: Multiplanar gadolinium-enhanced MR
- MR findings
  - Mass invading central skull base **contiguous with and inseparable from soft tissue mass in sella**
  - Ill-defined soft tissue mass centered in sella with invasion of surrounding bone and soft tissue
  - Intense heterogeneous tumor enhancement
  - May **extend into cavernous sinus**
- CT findings: Sella floor dehiscent
  - Bone erosion of central skull base and dorsal clivus

TOP DIFFERENTIAL DIAGNOSES

- Clival chordoma
- Skull base meningioma
- Skull base metastasis
- Petrooccipital chondrosarcoma
- Skull base plasmacytoma

CLINICAL ISSUES

- Mean age at presentation: ~ 40 years
- If hormone secreting, symptoms depend on which hormone secreted
- 25% visual field defect or other cranial nerve palsy
- Treatment: Multimodality therapy required for best outcome
  - Surgery often indicated for decompression of optic apparatus; transsphenoidal endoscopic when possible
  - Resection often incomplete and leads to recurrences
  - ↑ morbidity due to proximity to vital structures

DIAGNOSTIC CHECKLIST

- Look for normal pituitary gland on sagittal images; if absent, invasive adenoma should be at top of DDx

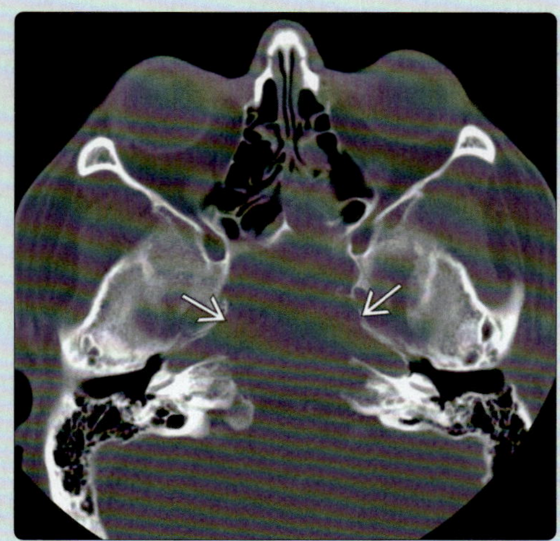

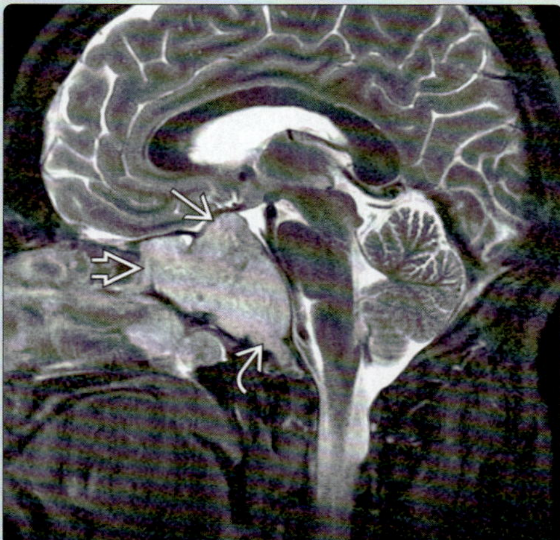

(Left) *Axial bone CT of invasive pituitary macroadenoma shows extensive bone erosion of the central skull base and dorsal clivus. The sella and basisphenoid are largely destroyed. Tumor extends to the medial aspects of the petrous internal carotid artery canals ➡.* **(Right)** *Sagittal T2WI MR shows extensive invasive pituitary tumor with suprasellar extension ➡ and invasion anteriorly into the basisphenoid ➡ and inferiorly into the clivus ➡. Tumor also extends anteroinferiorly into the nasopharynx and posterior nasal cavity.*

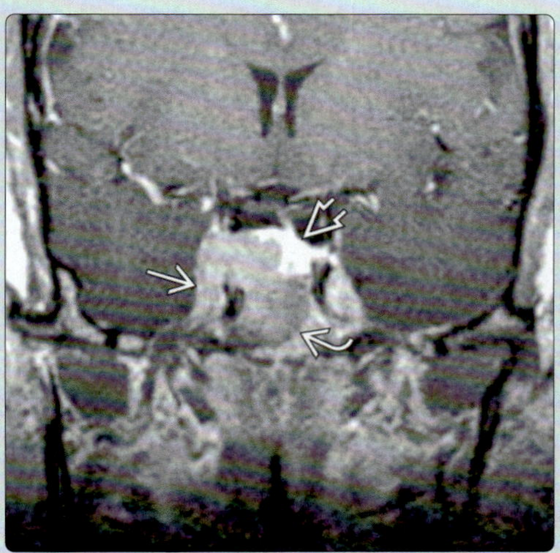

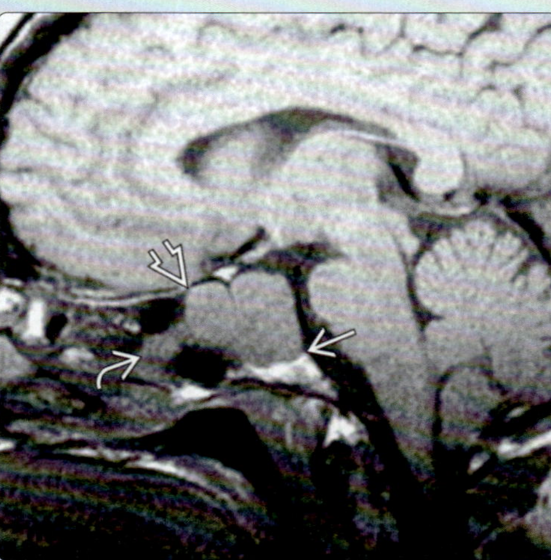

(Left) *Coronal T1WI C+ MR demonstrates pituitary adenoma with invasion of the right cavernous sinus ➡ and encasement of the carotid artery. Tumor extends inferiorly into skull base ➡. Residual normal enhancing pituitary gland is seen superior to invasive adenoma ➡.* **(Right)** *Sagittal T1WI MR shows an invasive pituitary adenoma extending inferiorly into the clivus and replacing normal clival fat ➡. The mass also invades the sphenoid sinus ➡ and posterior nasal cavity ➡. The normal pituitary gland is not visualized.*

KEY FACTS

TERMINOLOGY

- Definition: Rare, locally aggressive tumor of clivus arising from cranial end of primitive notochord remnant

IMAGING

- Location: **Clivus**; sphenooccipital synchondrosis
  - Can occur anywhere along primitive notochord
- CT findings
  - **Midline**, expansile, multilobulated, well circumscribed
  - Lytic underlying bone; intratumoral bone fragments
  - Variable enhancement due to variable myxoid content
- MR findings
  - T1: Intermediate to low signal ≈ brain
  - T2: Classically **hyperintense**
  - T1WI C+: Moderate to marked enhancement
    - Low-signal foci from ↑ myxoid content
  - DWI: Mean ADC value 1474 ± 117 x 10^{-6} mm^2/s, generally less than chondrosarcoma

TOP DIFFERENTIAL DIAGNOSES

- Ecchordosis physaliphora
- Invasive pituitary macroadenoma
- Skull base chondrosarcoma
- Skull base plasmacytoma or metastases
- Skull base meningioma

CLINICAL ISSUES

- **35%** of all chordomas arise in **skull base**
  - Sacrococcygeal (50%); vertebral (15%)
- Common symptoms: Headache & diplopia (CNVI)
- Most common age: 30-50 years
- Treatment
  - Managed by multidisciplinary skull base team
  - Surgical resection (conventional surgery vs. endonasal transclival resection)
  - Proton beam RT: Postop & unresectable tumors
- Brachyury: Molecular marker distinctive for chordoma

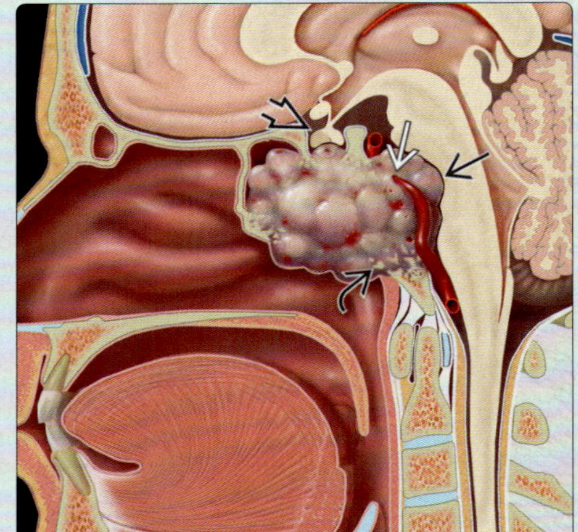

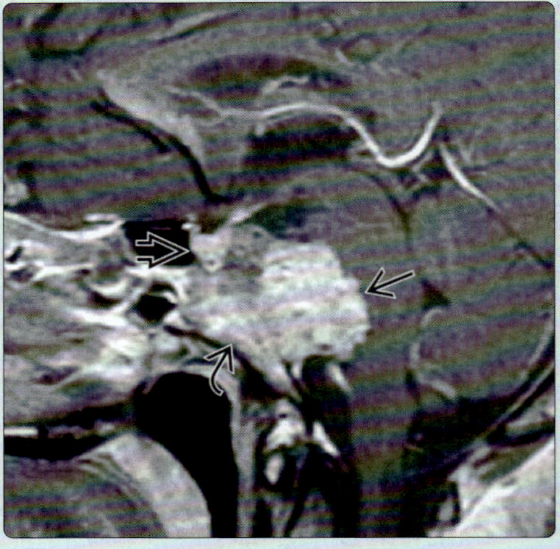

(Left) *Sagittal graphic shows an expansile, destructive mass originating from the clivus, "thumbing" the pons ➾, and elevating the pituitary gland ➾. Note bone fragments floating in the chordoma ➾ and tumor engulfing the basilar artery ➡.* **(Right)** *Sagittal T1 C+ MR demonstrates heterogeneous enhancement of chordoma. Note posterior extension into the prepontine cistern with resulting "thumbing" of the pons ➾. Note the peserved pituitary ➾ and clival invasion ➾.*

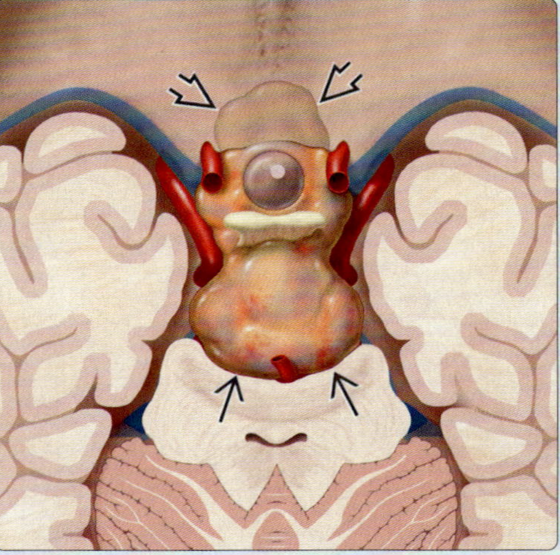

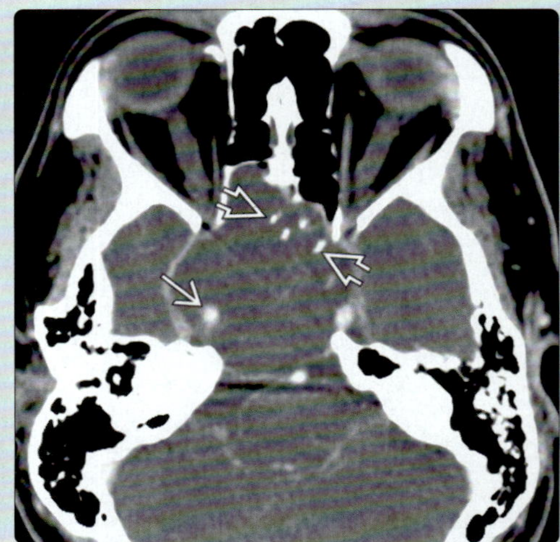

(Left) *Axial graphic illustrates a large clival chordoma pushing posteriorly to indent the low pons and basilar artery ➾. Basisphenoid invasion ➾ is also seen lifting the pituitary gland in the sella.* **(Right)** *Axial CECT shows an unenhancing chordoma with elevated myxoid content engulfing the right internal carotid artery ➡ without significant narrowing. Bone fragments ➡ in anterior tumor margin are typical.*

KEY FACTS

TERMINOLOGY

- Synonyms: Transsphenoidal canal, craniopharyngeal duct, hypophyseal canal, basipharyngeal canal
- Persistent craniopharyngeal canal: Developmental anomaly with persistent tract from nasopharynx to pituitary fossa
- Believed to be **persistent adenohypophyseal stalk**

IMAGING

- Skull base bone CT
  - **Midline**, well-marginated tract from sella to roof of nasopharynx
  - Anterior to sphenooccipital synchondrosis
  - When incidental, < 1.5 mm in diameter
- Multiplanar MR
  - Smoothly marginated cylindrical "canal" extending from sella to nasopharynx
  - Variable signal intensity in canal itself
  - Coronal sections reveal adenohypophysis perched on craniopharyngeal canal like **ball on tee**

TOP DIFFERENTIAL DIAGNOSES

- Skull base cephalocele
- Sphenobasilar synchondrosis
- Persistent medial basal canal

PATHOLOGY

- 3 types of persistent craniopharyngeal canal
  - Small caliber, incidental
  - Larger caliber with ectopic adenohypophysis
  - Larger caliber + cephalocele, ectopic pituitary, craniopharyngioma, dermoid, teratoma or glioma

CLINICAL ISSUES

- Incidental finding (~ 75%)
- Seen in 0.42% of population
- When large, MR needed to look for associated anomalies
- Treatment: **"Leave alone" lesion** when incidental
  - Larger lesions with associated anomaly: Treatment directed at associated lesion(s)

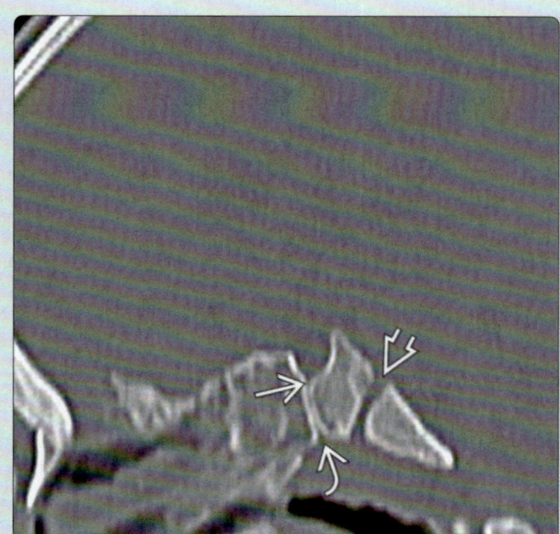

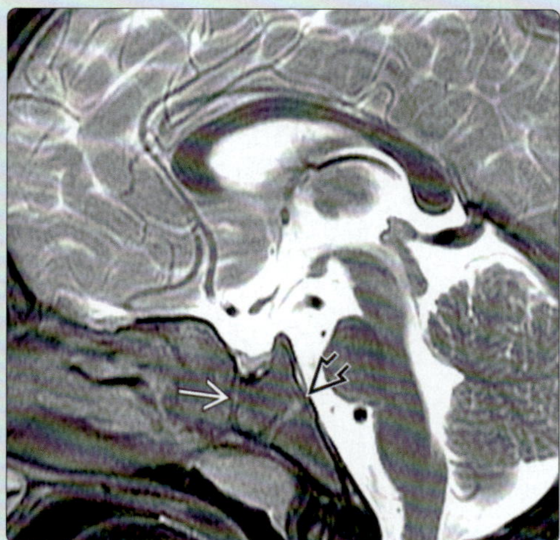

(Left) *Sagittal reformatted CT shows bony tract originating in the floor of the sella turcica ➡ and extending to the roof of the nasopharynx ➡. Note sphenooccipital synchondrosis ➡ posteriorly is unfused in this child.* **(Right)** *Sagittal T2 MR in the same patient shows a persistent craniopharyngeal canal ➡ evident as a small tract with central intermediate signal and hypointense margins extending from the pituitary fossa to the nasopharynx. A normal sphenooccipital synchondrosis ➡ is posterior to the craniopharyngeal canal.*

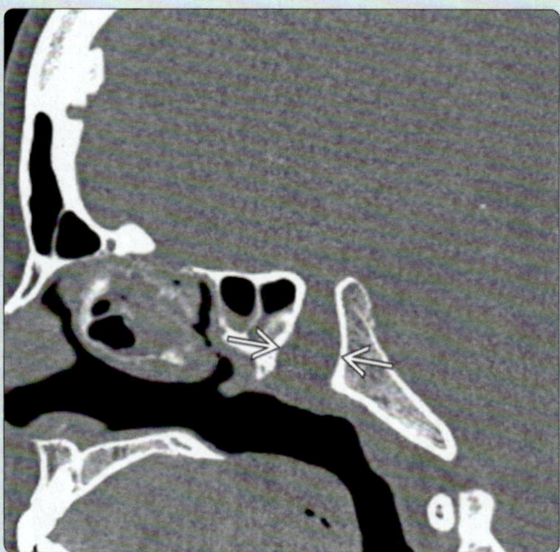

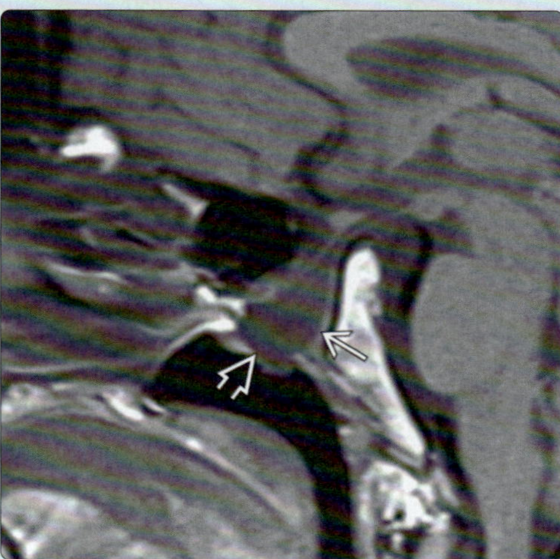

(Left) *Sagittal bone CT reformation of the skull base reveals a large persistent craniopharyngeal canal ➡. MR should be acquired to answer the question of what is in the canal.* **(Right)** *Sagittal T1 MR shows a transsphenoidal cephalocele ➡ filling the enlarged persistent craniopharyngeal canal, bulging into the roof of the nasopharynx ➡. No normal pituitary is visible. This patient is at risk to develop meningitis.*

Sphenoid Benign Fatty Lesion

KEY FACTS

TERMINOLOGY

- Synonym: Arrested pneumatization of sphenoid
- Definition: Well-corticated, fat-containing lesion of sphenoid bone
  - Occurs in regions where primary or accessory pneumatization known to occur
  - Usually adjacent to posterior sinus wall

IMAGING

- Bone CT findings
  - Thin-section axial images best for depicting uniform cortical bone rim
  - Well-defined, **low-attenuation** (fat density), nonexpansile lesion with **sclerotic rim**
  - May have occasional curvilinear calcification or soft tissue density
- MR findings
  - Can help delineate smaller lesions
  - **Central ↑ T1**, variable T2, & ↓ T1 signal post fat suppression
  - Hypointense rim
  - Minimal if any enhancement

TOP DIFFERENTIAL DIAGNOSES

- Fibrous dysplasia
- Hemangioma
- Chordoma
- Ossifying fibroma

CLINICAL ISSUES

- Common **incidental finding** on CT or MR depicting skull base identified by radiologists
- **"Leave alone"** lesion

DIAGNOSTIC CHECKLIST

- Identification of internal fat & sclerotic margin is essentially pathognomonic of benign fatty lesion of sphenoid bone

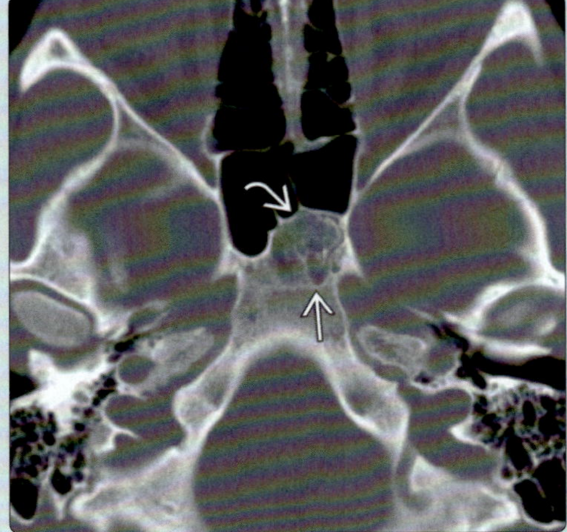

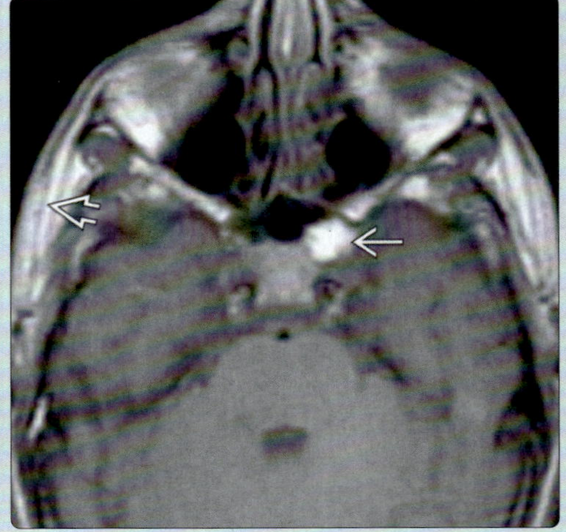

(Left) *Axial bone CT shows characteristic features of an incidentally discovered fatty lesion of the sphenoid. The lesion ➡ bulges into the left sphenoid sinus ➡ and has well-defined sclerotic margins and predominantly low density (fat) centrally. Note a normal trabeculae traverse lesion.* **(Right)** *Axial T1WI MR (same patient) demonstrates a homogeneously hyperintense, nonexpansile lesion ➡ in the left aspect of the basisphenoid similar that is similar in signal to subcutaneous fat ➡. MR may be useful to confirm internal fatty contents.*

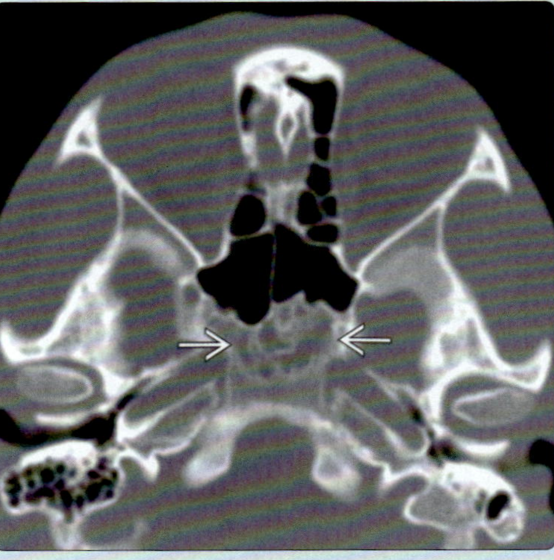

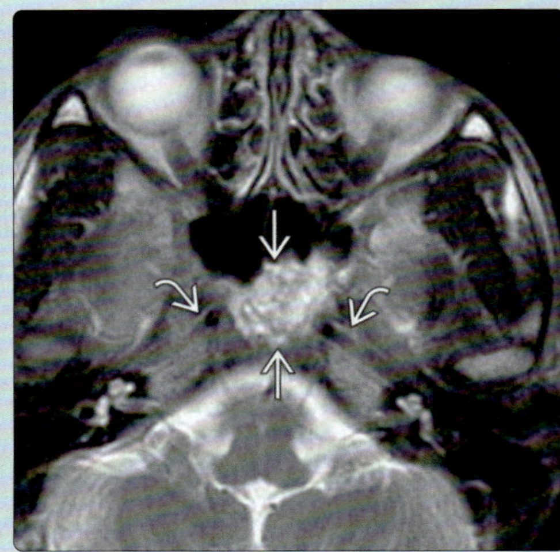

(Left) *Axial bone CT demonstrates a typical benign, fatty lesion of the sphenoid ➡ with well-defined margins and a low-density central component, confirmed on MR to represent fat.* **(Right)** *Axial T2WI MR in the same patient confirms predominantly hyperintense (paralleling fat) signal with a lobulated contour to the lesion ➡. There is no significant distortion of skull base foramina or normal structures, such as petrous segments of internal carotid arteries ➡.*

KEY FACTS

TERMINOLOGY

- Synonym: Giant trigeminal schwannoma (TS), "dumbbell" TS

IMAGING

- **Tubular mass** along course of trigeminal nerve
  - Can involve preganglionic (cisternal) segment, Meckel cave, CNV1 (superior orbital fissure), CNV2 (foramen rotundum), CNV3 (foramen ovale)
  - May extend extracranially via CNV exit foramina
- Size: Small to giant
- Morphology: **Dumbbell** shape secondary to constriction at porus trigeminus or skull base foramen
- CT: Soft tissue mass with smooth bony erosion of central skull base, ± foraminal widening
  - Bone CT best for identifying foraminal enlargement
- MR: T1 isointense to hypointense, T2 hyperintense, variable enhancement
  - **Cyst formation** is common
  - Enhanced MR best to identify intracranial and extracranial extent of lesion

TOP DIFFERENTIAL DIAGNOSES

- Meningioma
- CNV3 perineural tumor
- CNV2 perineural tumor
- Non-Hodgkin lymphoma

PATHOLOGY

- Benign nerve sheath tumor
  - 2nd most common intracranial schwannoma next to vestibular schwannoma
- May occur in setting of neurofibromatosis type 2; look for additional intracranial schwannomas

CLINICAL ISSUES

- Management options include microsurgical resection (may need combined intra- and extracranial approach), stereotactic radiation, or active surveillance

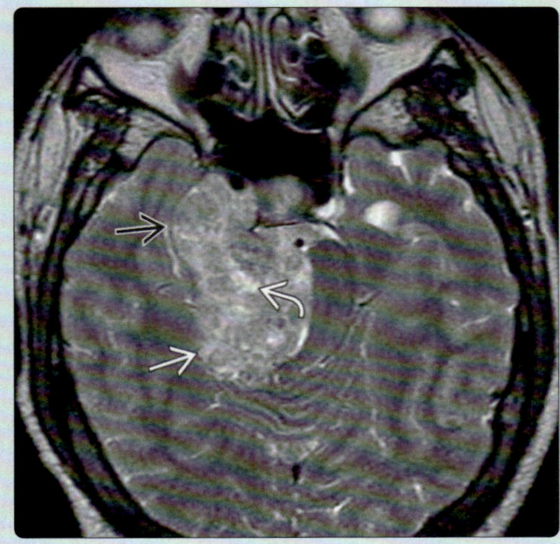

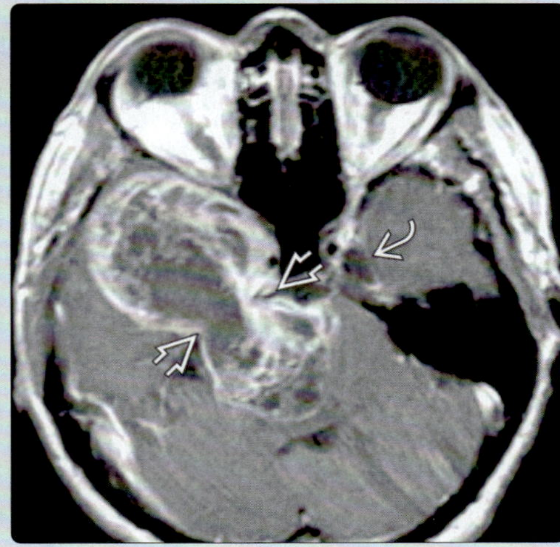

(Left) *Axial T2WI MR shows a mass in both the middle ⇨ and posterior ➡ cranial fossae, consistent with an extraaxial location. Internal areas of higher T2 signal intensity ➡ may indicate cystic degeneration.* **(Right)** *Axial T1WI C+ MR reveals a dumbbell-shaped giant trigeminal schwannoma (TS) with a waist formed at the level of the porus trigeminus ➡. Extensive cystic components are present. Note the normal left Meckel cave containing CSF signal ➡.*

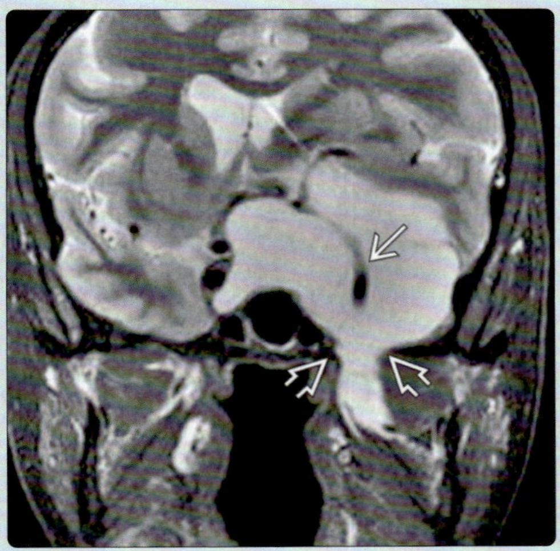

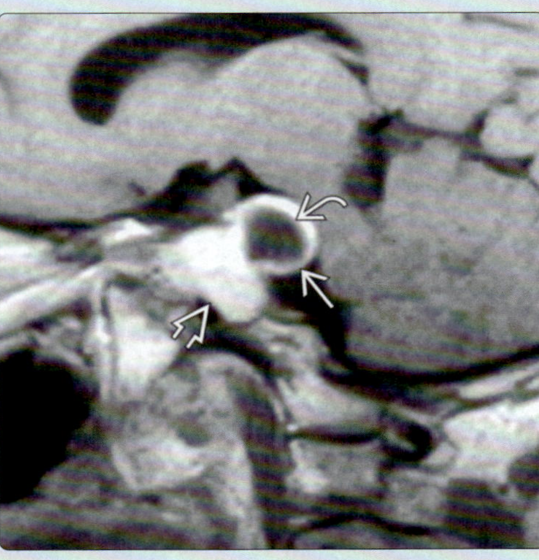

(Left) *Coronal T2WI FS MR demonstrates a well-demarcated, hyperintense, giant TS encasing, but not significantly compressing, the left internal carotid artery ➡. In this location, a waist is formed as the mass extends through the enlarged foramen ovale ➡.* **(Right)** *Sagittal T1WI C+ MR reveals a "dumbbell" TS affecting the preganglionic ➡ and Meckel cave ➡ segments of the trigeminal nerve. Notice the intramural cyst in the preganglionic segment ➡, common in schwannomas.*

Hypoglossal Nerve Schwannoma

KEY FACTS

TERMINOLOGY

- Benign tumor of differentiated Schwann cells surrounding CNXII

IMAGING

- Multiplanar contrast-enhanced MR with bone CT for delineation of bone margins
- CT findings
  - Sharply marginated, fusiform mass with enlarged hypoglossal canal (HC)
  - Coronal plane: Remodeling of undersurface of jugular tubercle
  - Tongue muscle atrophy with fatty replacement
- MR: Homogeneous, enhancing mass following course of CNXII
  - Cephalad growth toward preolivary sulcus
  - Caudal growth into nasopharyngeal carotid space
- Distal lesions may present in carotid space, submandibular space, or in tongue

TOP DIFFERENTIAL DIAGNOSES

- Asymmetric HC venous drainage
- Skull base metastasis
- Persistent hypoglossal artery
- Jugular foramen meningioma
- Glomus jugulare paraganglioma

PATHOLOGY

- Smooth, encapsulated mass arising eccentrically from CNXII

CLINICAL ISSUES

- Can result in unilateral tongue denervation
- Larger lesions may produce multiple lower cranial neuropathies
- Surgical removal in single operation is curative
  - Will often require far lateral approach
  - Staged procedure may be required if there is cisternal or nasopharyngeal carotid space extension
- Stereotactic radiation is option in select patients

(Left) *Axial T1 MR through the tongue demonstrates asymmetric signal of tongue. Right hemitongue is normal; left hemitongue has sharply marginated abnormally ↑ signal ➡. Increased signal signifies fatty infiltration and should direct attention to hypoglossal canal (HC).* **(Right)** *Axial T1 C+ MR at HC reveals lobulated mass ➡ on left extending into medullary cistern ➡. Note normal right hypoglossal canal ➡. Mass demonstrates uniform enhancement consistent with schwannoma. Cystic change is common with large tumors.*

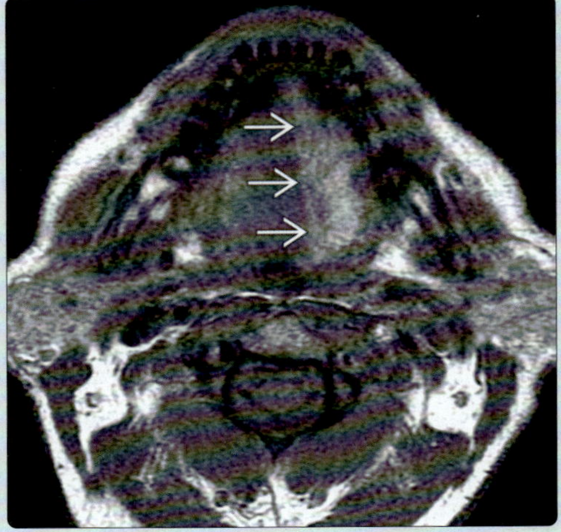

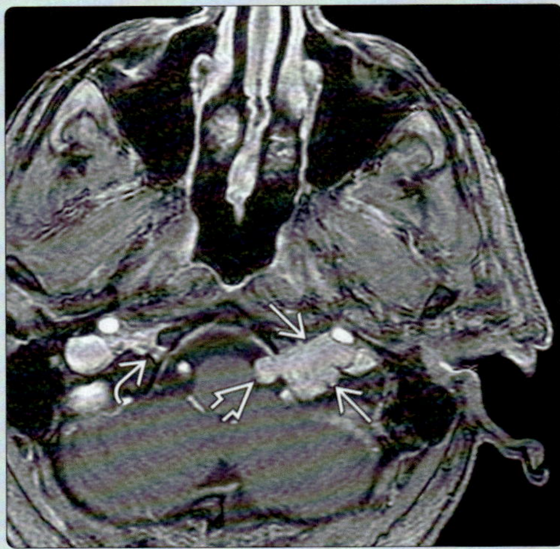

(Left) *Coronal bone CT shows a markedly expanded HC on the right ➡, eroding undersurface of "eagle's beak." Contrast this with the normal left HC ➡ and jugular tubercle ➡.* **(Right)** *Coronal T1 C+ FS MR in the same patient reveals heterogeneous enhancement of the schwannoma ➡ with marked scalloping of adjacent occipital bone & obliteration of normal "eagle's beak" as seen on CT. The normal hypoglossal canal ➡ & jugular tubercle ➡ are identified on left.*

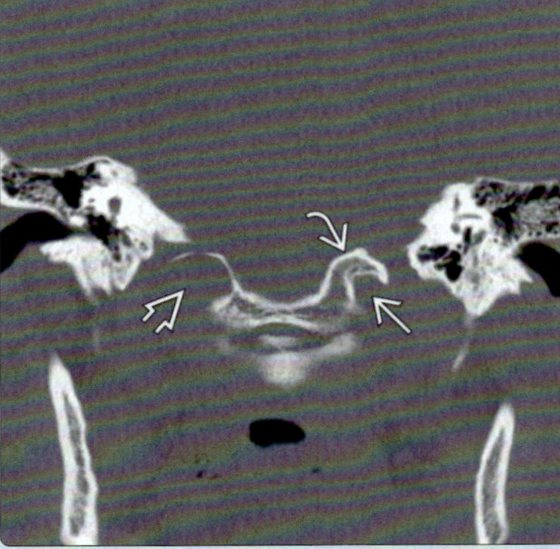

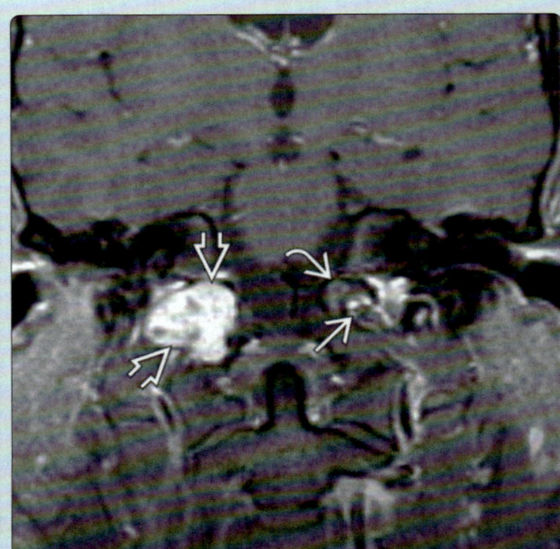

KEY FACTS

TERMINOLOGY

- Asymmetric, large jugular bulb flow phenomenon simulates neoplasm or thrombosis on MR sequences

IMAGING

- Best diagnostic clue: **Complex MR signal in jugular bulb** with normal jugular foramen (JF) cortex & jugular spine
  - Complex MR signal **does not persist** on all MR sequences
  - Normal bony margins of jugular bulb on T-bone CT

TOP DIFFERENTIAL DIAGNOSES

- High jugular bulb
- Jugular bulb diverticulum
- Dehiscent jugular bulb
- Sigmoid sinus-jugular bulb thrombosis
- Jugular foramen schwannoma
- Jugular foramen meningioma

CLINICAL ISSUES

- **Found incidentally on brain MR** during work-up for unrelated symptoms
- Surgical exploration must be avoided by clinician making correct diagnosis
- No treatment or follow-up required

DIAGNOSTIC CHECKLIST

- Jugular bulb pseudolesion is most common jugular bulb "lesion"
- Once abnormality is seen in JF on MR, 1st question to ask is, "Am I looking at jugular bulb pseudolesion?"
  - Do not mistake jugular bulb pseudolesion for schwannoma or venous sinus thrombosis
- If jugular bulb pseudolesion is observed while patient is in imaging center, add MRV to protocol to clarify
- Use bone CT to evaluate bony margins of jugular foramen if MR diagnosis uncertain

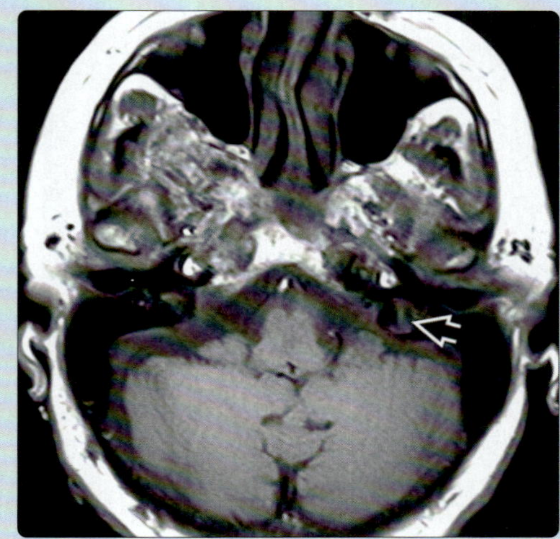

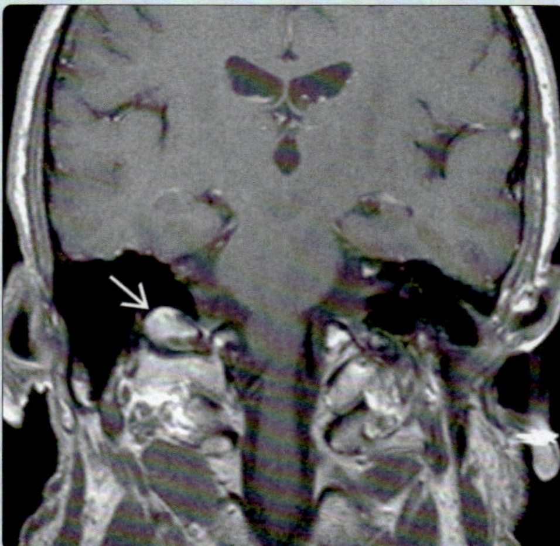

(Left) *Axial T1WI MR shows heterogeneous signal intensity within the left jugular foramen ➡, concerning for pathology. Other MR sequences proved this to be a jugular bulb pseudolesion, related to an asymmetric, large jugular bulb.* **(Right)** *Coronal T1WI C+ MR shows a jugular bulb pseudolesion ➡ related to turbulent flow in a mildly asymmetric right jugular bulb. This pseudolesion may be mistaken for a schwannoma or venous thrombosis. Other MR sequences confirmed this pseudolesion.*

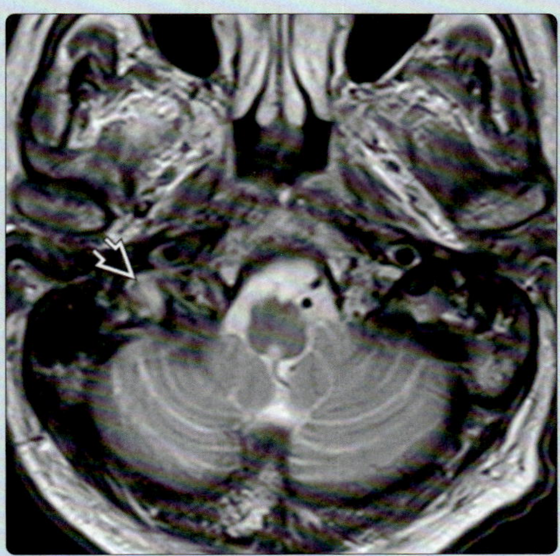

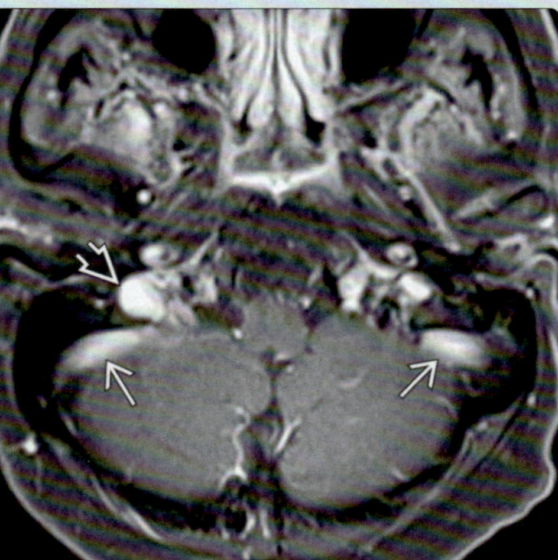

(Left) *Axial T2WI MR shows a hyperintense right jugular foramen "lesion" ➡, concerning for a jugular foramen schwannoma in this elderly patient with new-onset right-sided numbness.* **(Right)** *Axial T1WI C+ FS MR in the same patient shows normal enhancement of a mildly prominent right jugular bulb ➡. The enhancement is similar to the enhancement of the normal sigmoid sinuses ➡. Other sequences including an MRA/MRV confirmed this as a jugular bulb pseudolesion.*

High Jugular Bulb

KEY FACTS

TERMINOLOGY

- **High jugular bulb** (JB): Superior aspect of JB extends above floor of IAC with **no** middle ear connection
  - If dehiscence into middle ear present, use "dehiscent JB" not "high JB" to describe

IMAGING

- Most cephalad portion of JB extends superior to **floor of IAC** ± at level of basal turn of cochlea
  - Jugular foramen cortical margins intact
  - High JB occurs most commonly on **right**
- Best imaging tool: T-bone CT
  - Axial: JB at level of IAC or cochlea
  - Coronal: JB medial ± inferior to semicircular canals
- T1 C+ MR: High JB enhances same as jugular vein
- MRV: Same signal as surrounding venous structures

TOP DIFFERENTIAL DIAGNOSES

- JB pseudolesion (variant flow signal on MR)
- JB diverticulum
- Dehiscent JB
- Glomus jugulare paraganglioma
- Jugular foramen schwannoma
- Jugular foramen meningioma

PATHOLOGY

- High JB is more commonly seen with poorly aerated mastoid air cells
- JB diverticulum present in 35% of cases with high JB

CLINICAL ISSUES

- High JB is typically **incidental**; may increase risk of inadvertently entering JB during mastoidectomy
- Otoscopic exam: Normal
- Conservative management most common treatment
- Rarely reported to be associated with pulsatile tinnitus or Meniere disease; causality uncertain
- Do not confuse with IAC of CPA mass, especially on MR

(Left) *Axial T-bone CT of the right ear shows a high jugular bulb ➡ at the level of the cochlea ➡ with intact cortical margins. They are often incidental, but may be seen with pulsatile tinnitus, especially with diverticula.* **(Right)** *Coronal T1WI C+ FS MR shows a high jugular bulb ➡ connected inferiorly to a large internal jugular vein ➡. The top of the high jugular bulb reaches the level of the floor of the internal auditory canal ➡. On axial images, this may mimic an inner ear lesion if the connection to the jugular vein is not appreciated.*

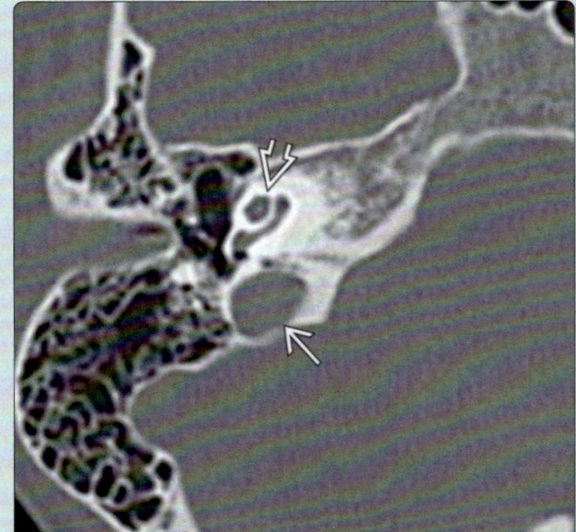

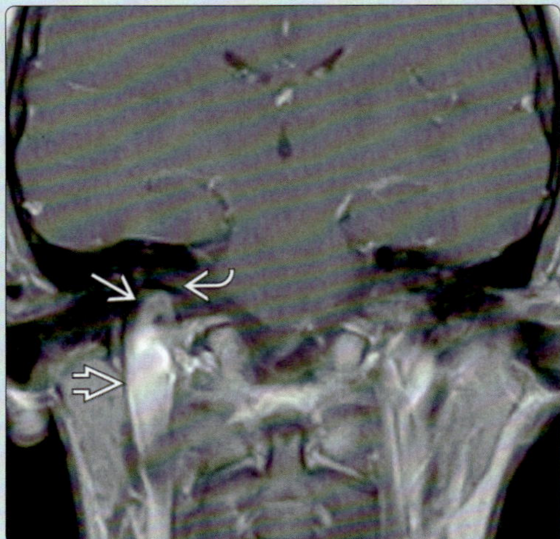

(Left) *Axial T-bone CT of the left ear shows a high jugular bulb ➡ present at the level of the internal auditory canal ➡. The high jugular bulb abuts the bony vestibular aqueduct ➡ on its posterior margin.* **(Right)** *Coronal T-bone CT in the same patient shows the high jugular bulb ➡ as a cephalad extension of the jugular foramen. A high jugular bulb occurs most commonly on the right side. This congenital lesion can be associated with jugular bulb dehiscence or a jugular bulb diverticulum.*

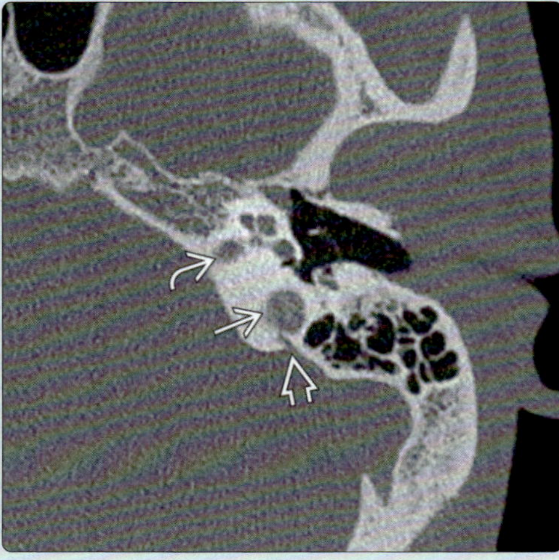

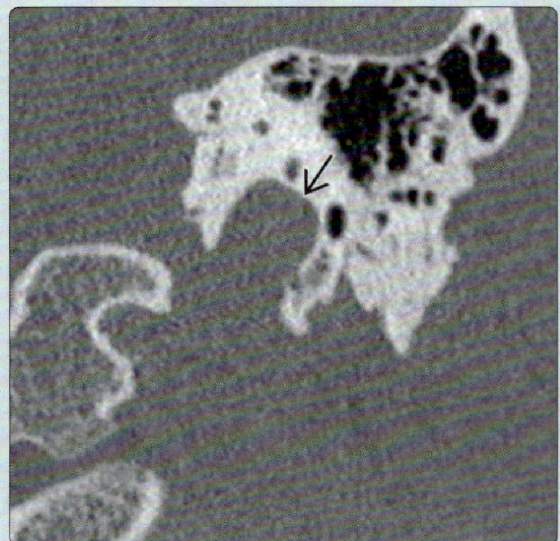

KEY FACTS

TERMINOLOGY

- Dehiscent jugular bulb (DJB): Normal venous variant with superior & lateral extension of jugular bulb (JB) into middle ear (ME) cavity through dehiscent sigmoid plate

IMAGING

- Soft tissue mass in ME contiguous with JB through **dehiscent sigmoid plate**
  - **Lateral outpouching** from JB best seen on coronal CT
  - Enhances to same degree as adjacent venous structures on C+ CT and MR
  - CTA or MRA may be performed in equivocal cases

TOP DIFFERENTIAL DIAGNOSES

- High-riding jugular bulb
- Jugular bulb diverticulum
- Glomus tympanicum paraganglioma
- Glomus jugulare paraganglioma
- Jugular foramen schwannoma
- Jugular foramen meningioma

CLINICAL ISSUES

- DJB has been reported as linked to many symptoms, though **causality** is **disputed**
  - Pulsatile tinnitus (due to turbulent flow), hearing loss, Ménière disease
- Otoscopy: **Vascular blue "mass"** behind intact tympanic membrane may prompt imaging
- Otoscopic + bone CT findings make correct diagnosis
  - Correct imaging diagnosis of DJB provides warning to surgeons when surgery occurring for other indications (i.e. pressure equalization tubes or middle ear surgery)
    - Helps avoid injury to jugular bulb

DIAGNOSTIC CHECKLIST

- DJB in differential diagnosis list of any vascular retrotympanic mass
- Coronal temporal bone CT will show direct continuity of middle ear mass with JB

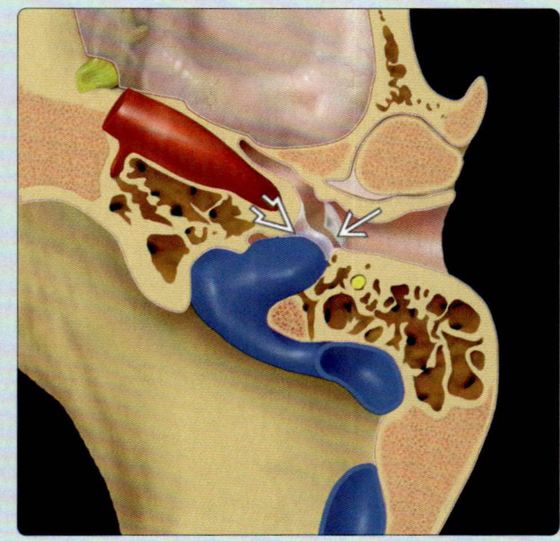

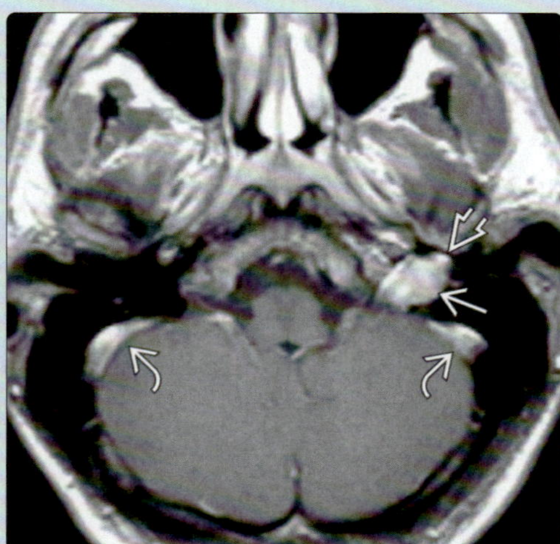

(Left) *Axial graphic depicts a dehiscent jugular bulb projecting superolaterally into the middle ear through the dehiscent sigmoid plate ➡. Typically, a blue-colored vascular "mass" is identified behind the posteroinferior quadrant of the intact tympanic membrane ➡.* **(Right)** *Axial T1WI C+ MR shows enhancement of the prominent jugular bulb ➡ contiguous with the dehiscent component in the middle ear ➡. Enhancement is identical to the sigmoid sinuses ➡.*

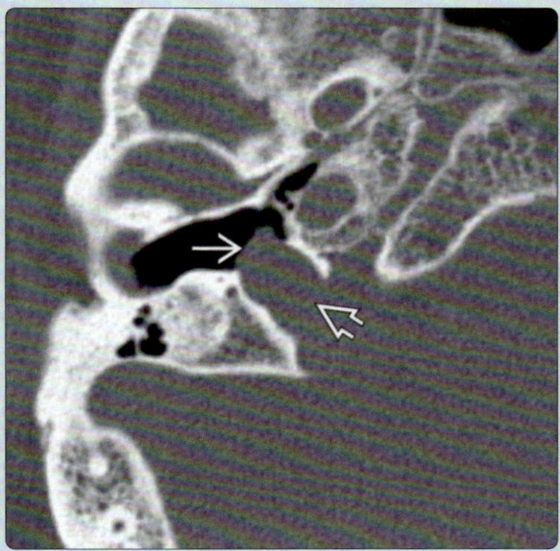

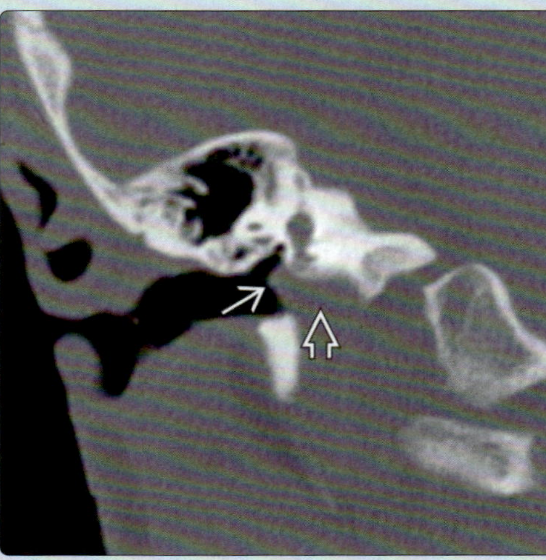

(Left) *Axial bone CT demonstrates the jugular bulb ➡ and soft tissue density mass ➡ within the inferior right middle ear cavity contiguous through the widely dehiscent jugular plate.* **(Right)** *Coronal bone CT shows a laterally lobulated extension ➡ of the dehiscent jugular bulb ➡ into the right middle ear. Dehiscent jugular bulb is the most common vascular variant of the temporal bone and is more frequent on the right.*

Jugular Bulb Diverticulum

KEY FACTS

TERMINOLOGY

- Definition: Congenital vascular anomaly of jugular bulb (JB) with **focal finger-like projection extending from JB** into surrounding skull base

IMAGING

- Best imaging tool: T-bone CT
- T-bone CT findings
  - Focal projection extending off JB margin **superiorly** in most cases into deep T-bone just behind IAC
  - Other directions of extension: **Medial, anterior, or posterior**
    - If lateral into middle ear = dehiscent jugular bulb
- Imaging protocol: Start with thin-section T-bone CT
  - If concern lingers, MR with contrast & MRV

TOP DIFFERENTIAL DIAGNOSES

- JB pseudolesion (variant flow phenomenon on MR)
- High JB; dehiscent JB
- Glomus jugulare paraganglioma
- Jugular foramen schwannoma or meningioma

PATHOLOGY

- JB diverticulum = expansion of high JB into surrounding bone
  - Hindered by dense otic capsule

CLINICAL ISSUES

- Often **asymptomatic**, incidental finding commonly; if symptomatic, consider eval for intracranial hypertension
- Pulsatile tinnitus may result from turbulent flow

DIAGNOSTIC CHECKLIST

- JB diverticulum in differential of medial T-bone mass with smooth margins on CT
- CT shows smooth bony remodeling + continuity with JB
- On axial T1 C+ MR, enhancing foci behind IAC may be mistaken for vestibular schwannoma or intralabyrinthine schwannoma

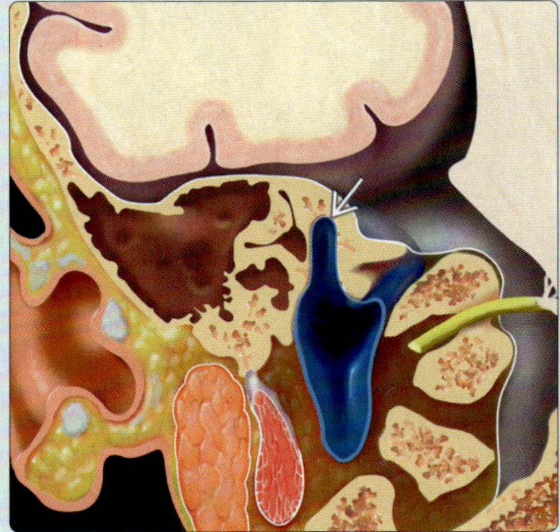

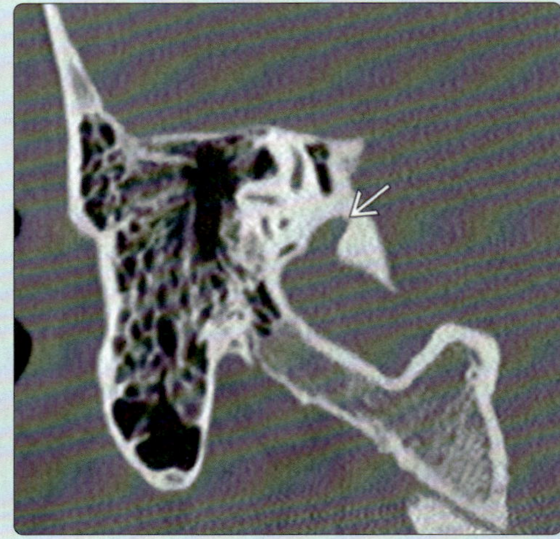

(Left) *Coronal graphic depicts a jugular bulb diverticulum (JBD) as a finger-like superior projection off the jugular bulb (JB) into the petrous T-bone ➡ without extension into the middle ear.* **(Right)** *Coronal right ear CT shows a JBD ➡ as a thumb-like projection arising from the superior JB margin. Continuity with the normal JB and smooth bony margins helps confirm the diagnosis. This JB lesion is more common on the left side. Patients are asymptomatic as a rule.*

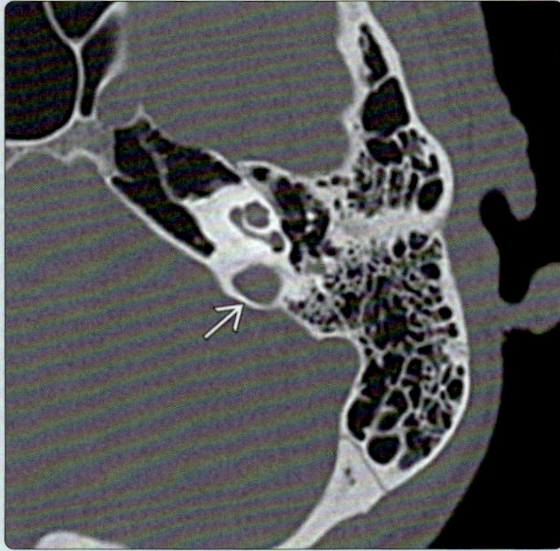

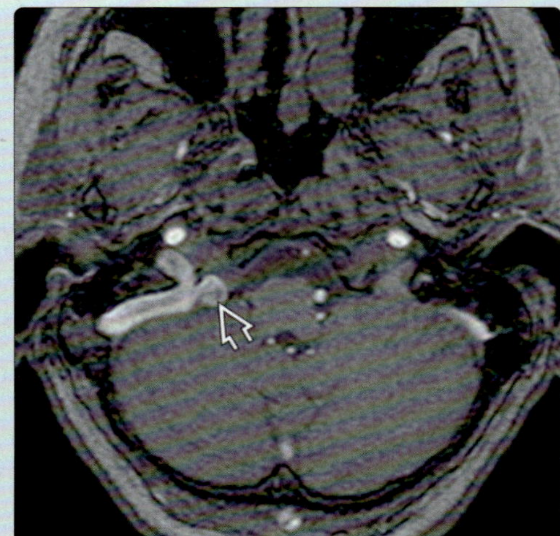

(Left) *Axial left T-bone CT shows a JBD ➡ projecting cephalad from the JB into the medial T-bone. These diverticula are typically located posterior to the internal auditory canal and have smooth bony margins.* **(Right)** *Axial MRV source image shows a medially projecting JBD ➡. This polypoid extension from the JB has similar enhancement characteristics as the JB and jugular vein. A JBD may be discovered at any age.*

Glomus Jugulare Paraganglioma

KEY FACTS

TERMINOLOGY

- Glomus jugulare paraganglioma (GJP): Benign tumor arising from **neural crest** progenitor crest cells (glomus bodies) located in & around jugular foramen

IMAGING

- Bone CT: **Permeative-destructive** bone changes
  - Jugular spine erosion is common
  - Floor of middle ear cavity dehisced
- MR: Lesions > 2 cm demonstrate characteristic **salt & pepper** appearance
- Vector of spread: **Superolateral spread** from JF through floor of middle ear into middle ear is typical
- CTA/angiography: Main arterial supply is typically from **ascending pharyngeal artery**
- **Paraganglia rests** occur in 3 distinct bodies around JF: Jugular bulb, along tympanic branch of CNIX (Jacobsen nerve), & along auricular branch of CNX (Arnold nerve)
- Caveat: Always check if multifocal paraganglioma present

TOP DIFFERENTIAL DIAGNOSES

- Glomus tympanicum paraganglioma
- Jugular foramen schwannoma
- Jugular foramen meningioma
- Dehiscent jugular bulb

CLINICAL ISSUES

- Presentation: Pulsatile tinnitus most common with **red, pulsatile** retrotympanic mass seen on otoscopy
  - CNVII or CNVIII neuropathy less often, though conductive ± sensorineural hearing loss common
  - Other symptoms: CNIX-XI ± CNXII cranial neuropathy
- 10% secreting, check urine for catecholamine metabolites
- GJP = most common jugular foramen tumor
- GJP & carotid body paraganglioma: 80% of H&N paragangliomas
- Treatment: Surgical resection ± radiation
  - Stereotactic radiation may be used as primary therapy
- Familial paraganglioma syndrome: High % multifocal

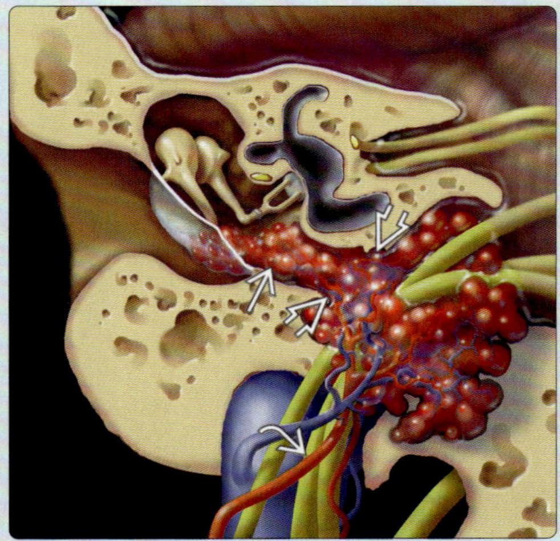

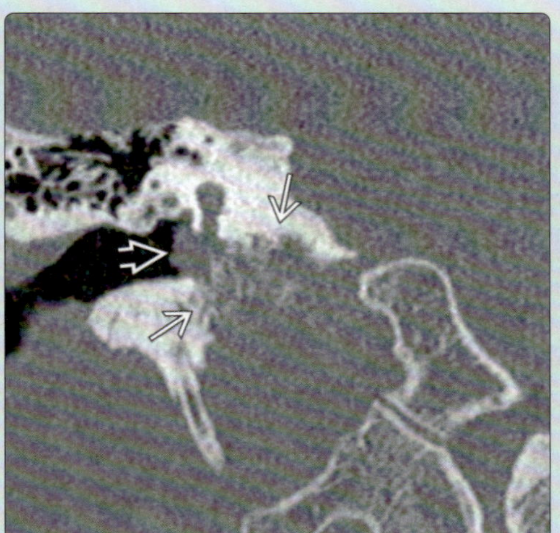

(Left) *Graphic shows a glomus jugulare paraganglioma (GJP) centered in jugular foramen (JF) dehiscing the middle ear floor ➡ to reach the middle ear cavity ➡. Main arterial supply for this vascular tumor is ascending pharyngeal artery ➡.* **(Right)** *T-bone CT (right ear) shows classic permeative-destructive margins ➡ of GJP. Note typical vector of spread superolateral into middle ear ➡. On otoscopy, it can be difficult to differentiate a retrotympanic mass as GJP vs. glomus tympanicum. Eroded jugular bulb on imaging favors GJP.*

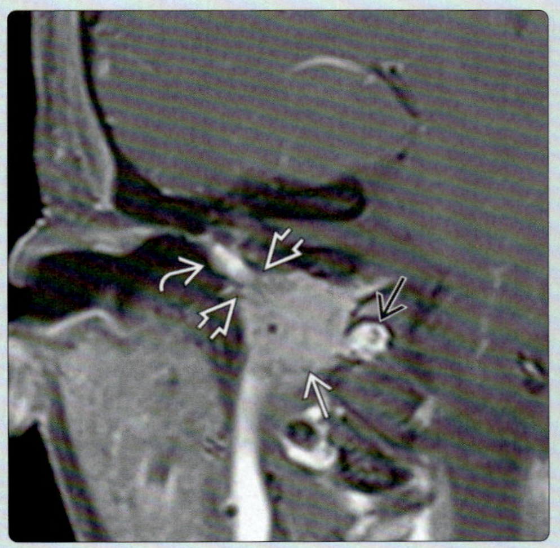

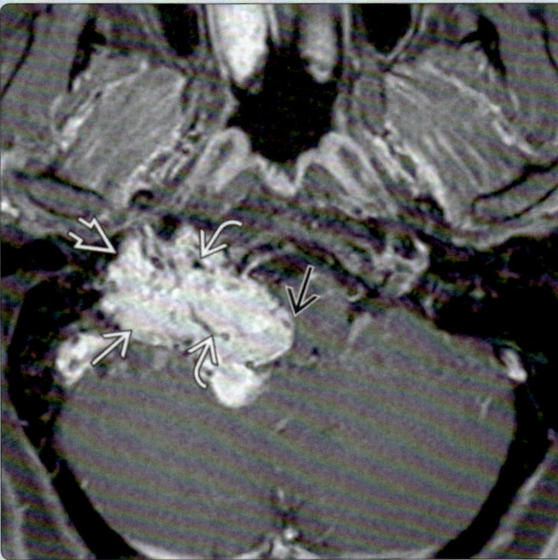

(Left) *Coronal T1 C+ FS MR shows a GJP ➡ filling the jugular foramen, passing through the middle ear floor ➡, and invading the middle ear ➡. Otoscopy reveals a pulsatile retrotympanic mass. The hypoglossal canal ➡ is spared.* **(Right)** *Axial T1 C+ FS MR shows the classic intense enhancement of this large GJP ➡. There is intracranial extension with mass effect on the adjacent medulla ➡. Flow voids from larger vessels are seen as curvilinear and punctate low-signal areas ➡ within the tumor ➡: GJP is in the middle ear.*

Jugular Foramen Schwannoma

KEY FACTS

TERMINOLOGY

- Benign tumor of differentiated Schwann cells wrapping around cranial nerves (CNs) IX, X, or XI within jugular foramen (JF)

IMAGING

- Bone CT: Sharply marginated, enlarged JF
- T1WI C+ MR
  - Tubular or dumbbell-shaped, uniformly enhancing
  - **No flow voids** ("pepper") (vs. paraganglioma)
  - Nonenhancing **cystic areas** in large lesions
- T2WI hyperintense
- Superomedial vector of tumor growth
  - Follows craniocaudal course of CNs IX-XI
  - Grows cephalad from JF through basal cistern toward retroolivary sulcus of lateral medulla
  - Grows inferiorly from JF into nasopharyngeal carotid space
- MRV: Dural sinus compressed, not occluded

TOP DIFFERENTIAL DIAGNOSES

- Jugular foramen pseudolesion (MR)
- Glomus jugulare paraganglioma
- Jugular foramen meningioma
- Skull base metastasis

CLINICAL ISSUES

- Mean age: 45 years old
- CNs IX-XI related symptoms possible
- Sensorineural hearing loss in 90% at presentation
  - May present clinically like vestibular schwannoma
- 2nd most common JF tumor
  - Glossopharyngeal nerve (CNIX) most common nerve of origin
- Complete surgical removal of tumor in single procedure is goal
  - May be complicated by lower cranial neuropathy
- Stereotactic radiation as primary or adjuvant therapy

(Left) *Coronal graphic depicts a classic jugular foramen (JF) schwannoma as a fusiform mass arising on one of the lower cranial nerves (IX-XI) within the JF. Note the vector of spread is superomedial. The JF ➡ is enlarged with an intact cortex.* **(Right)** *Coronal bone CT shows a sharply marginated, enlarged JF with amputation of the lateral jugular tubercle ➡. The smooth enlargement ➡ with sclerotic margins is characteristic of JF schwannoma.*

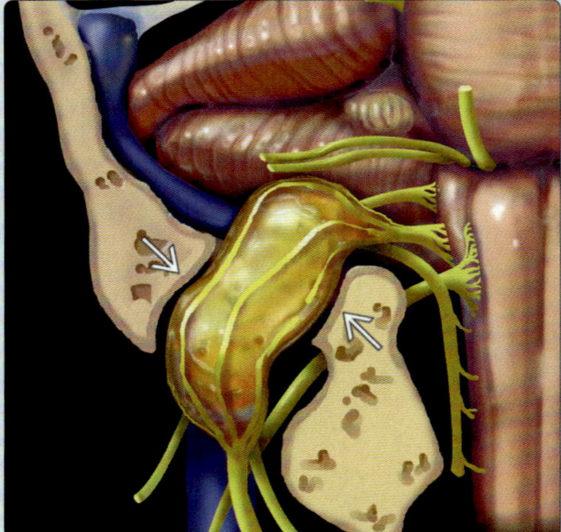

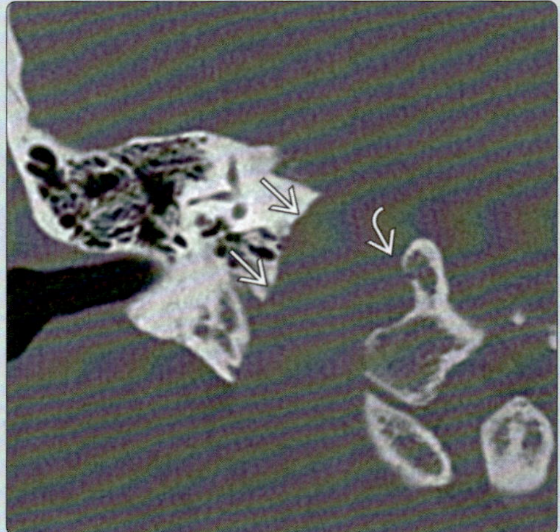

(Left) *Coronal T1 MR shows a JF schwannoma ➡ projecting superomedially from the JF toward the brainstem. Inferiorly, the schwannoma extends into the nasopharyngeal carotid space ➡. There is amputation of the lateral aspect of the jugular tubercle ➡. Lack of flow voids helps differentiate this schwannoma from the more common glomus jugulare paraganglioma.* **(Right)** *Coronal T1 C+ MR in the same patient shows enhancement of the JF schwannoma ➡.*

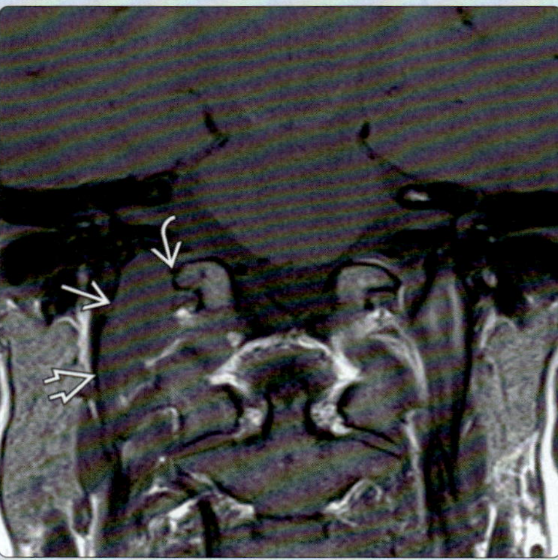

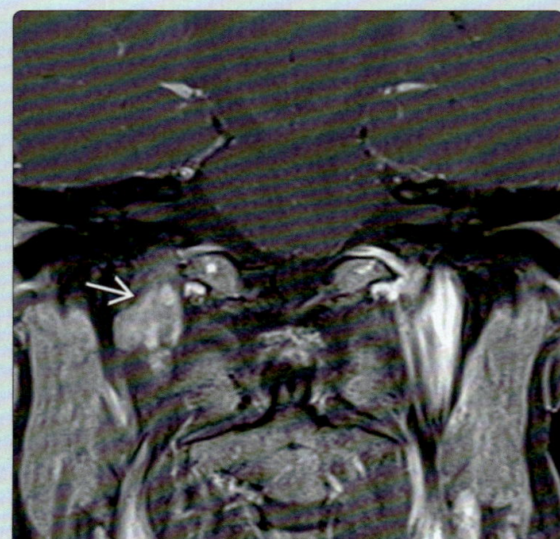

Jugular Foramen Meningioma

KEY FACTS

TERMINOLOGY

- Benign neoplasm arising from arachnoid cap cells found along cranial nerves within jugular foramen (JF)

IMAGING

- Bone CT: **Permeative-sclerotic** JF margins; may also see subjacent hyperostosis
- T1WI C+ MR: Enhancing JF mass spreading along dural surfaces
  - Enhancing **dural tails** may be seen
  - No high-velocity flow voids
- **Centrifugal** vector of spread: Extends in all directions from JF along dural surfaces and through surrounding bones
  - May protrude into basal cisterns or nasopharyngeal carotid space

TOP DIFFERENTIAL DIAGNOSES

- Glomus jugulare paraganglioma
- JF schwannoma
- JF metastasis
- JF pseudolesion
- Dehiscent jugular bulb

PATHOLOGY

- Proliferation of arachnoid meningothelial cap cells along CNs IX-XI in JF

CLINICAL ISSUES

- CNs IX-XI neuropathy most common presentation
- Risk factors: Prior nasopharynx, skull base, or brain radiation; neurofibromatosis type 2; female sex hormones
- Meningioma is 3rd most common JF mass
  - Paraganglioma > > schwannoma > meningioma
- Treatment: Complete surgical removal is goal
  - Surgical cure often results in multiple lower cranial neuropathies
  - Radiotherapy for growing tumor, elderly or poor surgical candidate, patient preference, subtotal resection

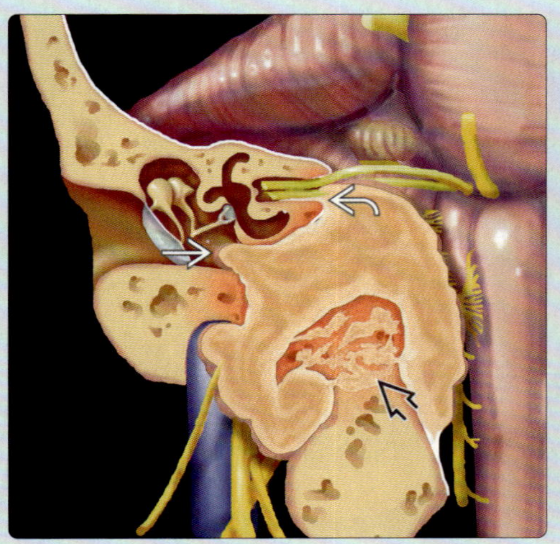

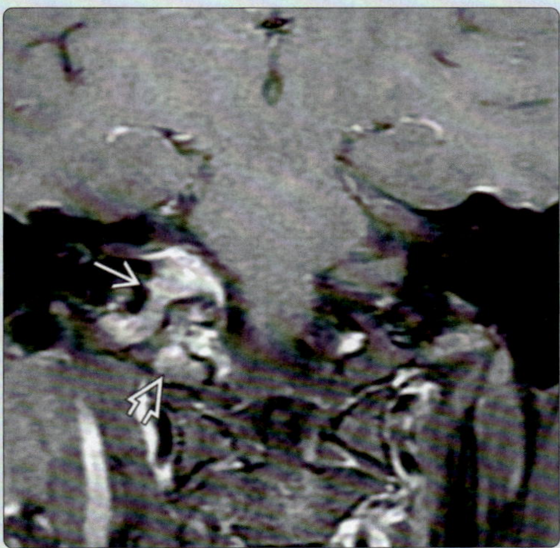

(Left) *Coronal graphic shows a large jugular foramen meningioma invading the middle ear ➡, skull base marrow ⇨, and internal auditory canal ⮌. Note the cranial nerves of the jugular foramen (CN IX-XI) are engulfed.* **(Right)** *Coronal T1WI C+ FS MR shows a large jugular foramen meningioma ➡ with invasion of the skull base marrow ⇨. Jugular foramen meningiomas have a centrifugal vector of spread and often extend along dural surfaces and through the surrounding bones.*

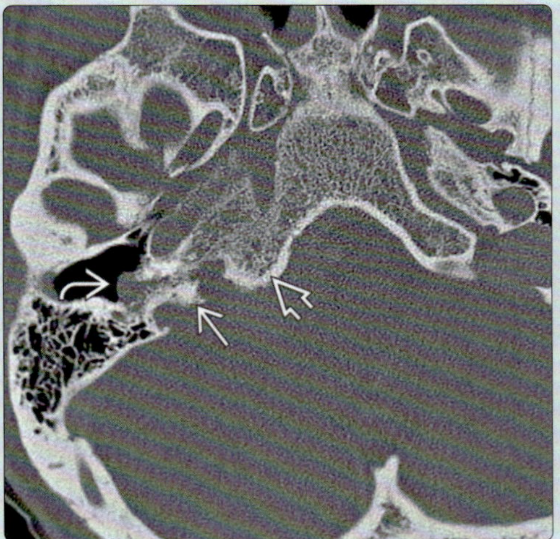

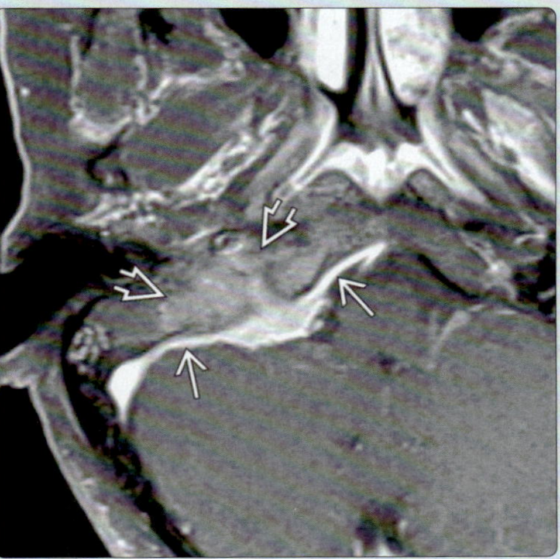

(Left) *Axial bone CT shows the characteristic permeative sclerotic changes along the jugular foramen ➡ and lateral clivus ⇨ of this jugular foramen meningioma. The meningioma extends into the middle ear ⮌ and may present clinically as a vascular retrotympanic mass on otoscopy.* **(Right)** *Axial T1WI C+ FS MR shows a jugular foramen meningioma with en plaque morphology and dural tails ➡. Note the lack of flow voids and the jugular foramen involvement with extensive adjacent skull base infiltration ⇨.*

Dural Sinus and Aberrant Arachnoid Granulations

KEY FACTS

TERMINOLOGY

- **Arachnoid granulation** (AG)
  - Defined as enlarged arachnoid villi projecting into major dural venous sinus lumen
- **Aberrant arachnoid granulation** (AbAG)
  - Defined as AG that penetrates dura, but fails to reach venous sinus, typically in sphenoid or T-bone

IMAGING

- Intrasinus AG: Well-circumscribed, discrete, filling defect in venous sinus ± inner calvarial table erosion
  - CECT: Nonenhancing; density like CSF
  - MR: T1/T2 intensity follows CSF; FLAIR often hyperintense
- AbAG: Multiple outpouches in sphenoid bone or T-bone
  - Sphenoid bone location: Greater wing
  - T-bone location: Posterior wall or tegmen
  - CT: Multiple smooth pits in sphenoid or T-bone
  - MR: T1 and T2 intensity follows CSF

TOP DIFFERENTIAL DIAGNOSES

- Dural sinus hypoplasia-aplasia
- Transverse-sigmoid sinus pseudolesion
- Dural sinus thrombosis
- Dural arteriovenous fistula

CLINICAL ISSUES

- Intrasinus AG: Asymptomatic with rare exception
- AbAG: Mostly asymptomatic
  - If large with rupture, **CSF leak** ± meningitis possible
  - Sphenoid bone: CSF leak → sphenoid fluid → rhinorrhea
  - T-bone: CSF leak → middle ear-mastoid fluid → otorrhea
    - Evaluate CT for superior semicircular canal dehiscence
  - Large AG may have associated **cephalocele** (± seizure)
  - **Meningitis** may complicate CSF leak
- Treatment
  - Intrasinus AG: No treatment required
  - AbAG: No treatment unless CSF leak present; treat surgically with multilayer repair

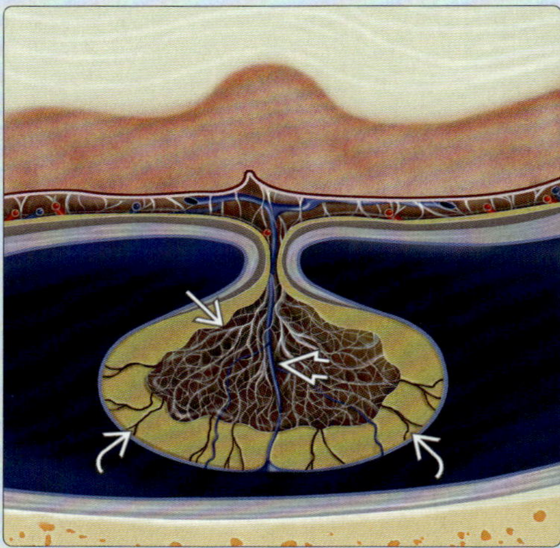

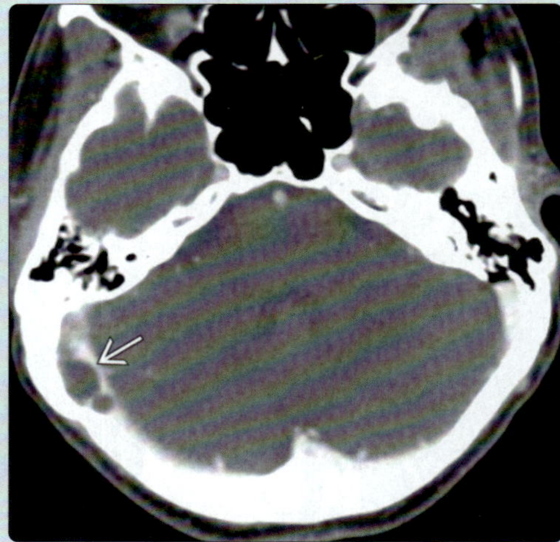

(Left) *Graphic shows a giant arachnoid granulation (AG) projecting from the subarachnoid space into the transverse sinus. CSF core ➡ extends into the AG and is separated by arachnoid cap cells from the venous sinus endothelium ➡. Giant AGs often contain prominent venous channels ➡ and septations.* **(Right)** *Axial CECT shows a giant AG cluster at the transverse-sigmoid venous sinus junction ➡. The 1st imaging interpretation of this finding mistakenly suggested venous sinus thrombosis.*

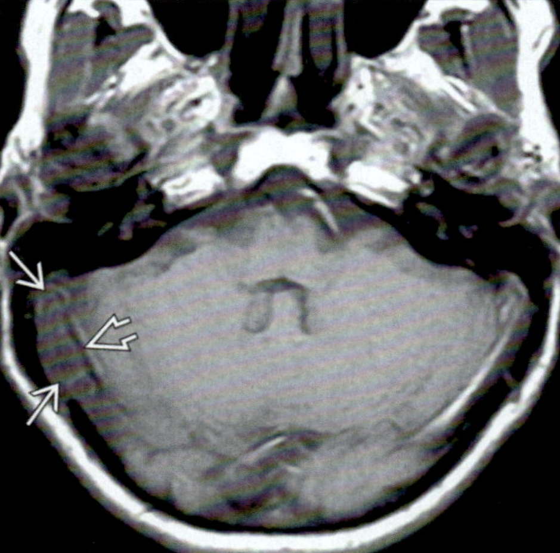

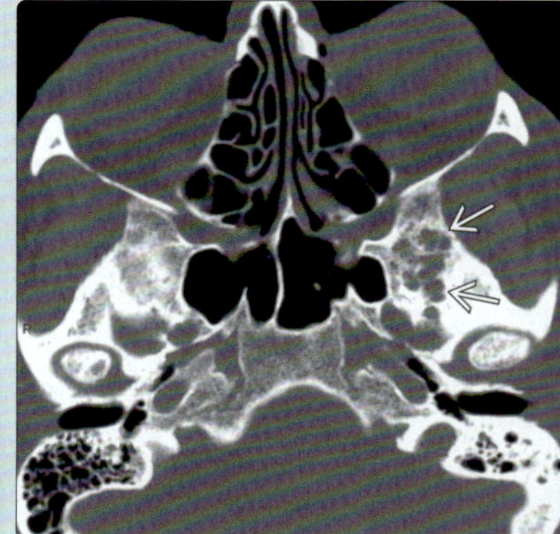

(Left) *Axial T1WI MR in the same patient reveals the multiple giant AGs ➡ as low signal within the transverse and proximal sigmoid sinuses. The medial low-signal line ➡ is the dura.* **(Right)** *Axial bone CT through the mid sphenoid sinus shows multiple ovoid bony defects in the greater wing of the sphenoid bone ➡ representing aberrant arachnoid granulations, also sometimes referred to as arachnoid pits. These AGs may enlarge from CSF pulsations.*

KEY FACTS

TERMINOLOGY

- Abbreviation: Dural sinus thrombosis (DST)

IMAGING

- MR with MRV is best single imaging exam for DST
  - CT venography close 2nd if MR contraindication
- CT findings
  - ↑ **density** thrombus in affected dural sinus
  - Conforms to shape of sinus; fusiform enlargement acutely
  - CECT shows enhancing dura surrounding less dense thrombus
- MR findings
  - ↓ **signal** (blooming) on **T2*** sequences in thrombus
  - Restricted diffusion in parenchymal venous infarction in temporal/occipital lobes or cerebellum
  - Parenchymal hemorrhage more common than arterial infarct
- Serial imaging to determine if thrombus is propagating

TOP DIFFERENTIAL DIAGNOSES

- Dural sinus asymmetric hypoplasia-aplasia
- Physiologic sinus flow asymmetry
- Large arachnoid granulation
- Subdural hematoma

PATHOLOGY

- Wide variety of causes (> 100 identified)
  - Otomastoiditis most common
  - Pregnancy & oral contraceptives
  - Trauma (temporal bone fracture) or postsurgical
  - Metabolic (dehydration, thyrotoxicosis, cirrhosis)

CLINICAL ISSUES

- Headache most common symptom (70-90%)
- Young female (autoimmune, oral contraceptives)
- **≤ 50%** of DSTs progress to venous **infarction**
- Treat inciting cause of thrombosis
- When indicated, anticoagulation is mainstay of therapy

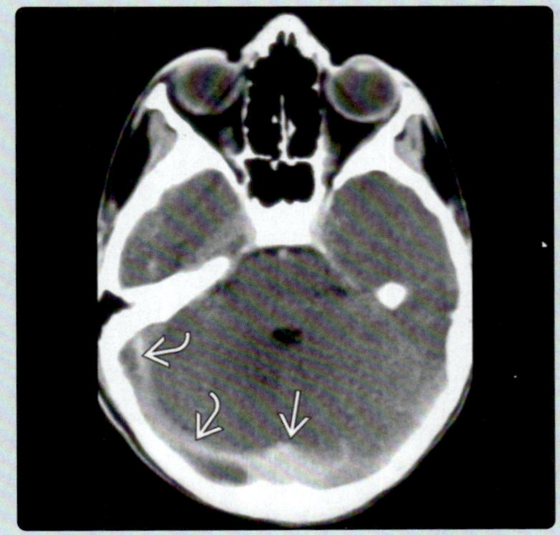

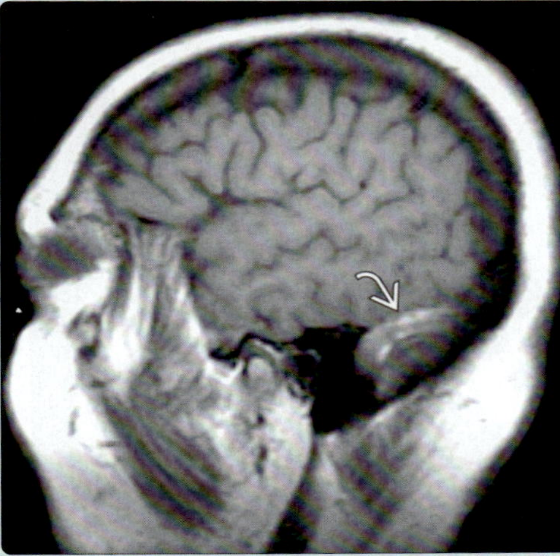

(Left) *Axial CECT shows sinus thrombosis secondary to oral contraceptive use. A tubular filling defect ➡ represents thrombus in the right transverse sinus with enhancement of the anterior dura of the sinus. The torcular enhances normally ➡.* **(Right)** *Sagittal T1WI MR demonstrates heterogeneous signal representing acute & subacute blood products within the transverse sinus clot extending into the sigmoid sinus ➡. No evidence of temporal lobe infarction is seen.*

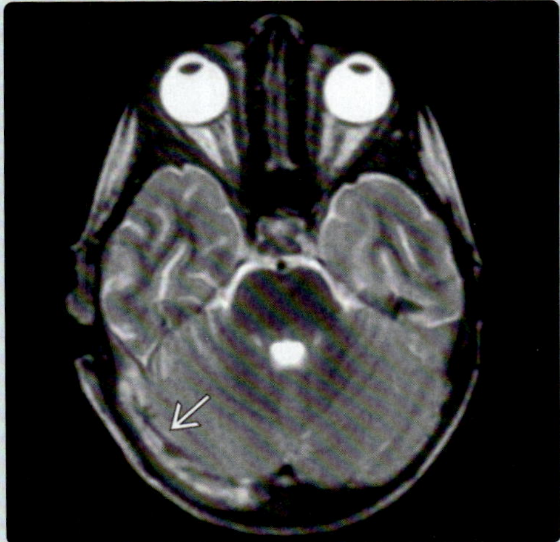

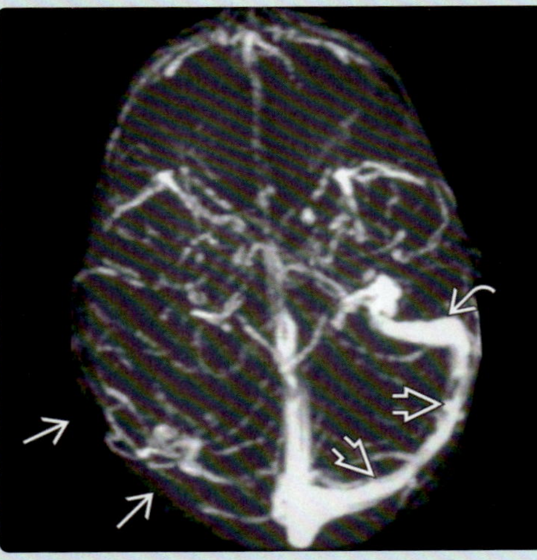

(Left) *Axial T2WI MR shows heterogeneous but largely high signal ➡ representing thrombus in the right transverse & sigmoid sinuses. No abnormal signal is identified in the right cerebellar hemisphere that would suggest venous infarction.* **(Right)** *Axial MRV in the same patient confirms the absence of flow-related signal in the thrombosed portions of the right transverse and sigmoid sinuses ➡ and confirms the patency of other dural sinuses and contralateral transverse ➡ and sigmoid ➡ sinuses.*

KEY FACTS

TERMINOLOGY

- Cavernous sinus (CS) thrombosis/thrombophlebitis (CST)
- CST: Blood clot in CS ± infection/thrombophlebitis

IMAGING

- Relevant anatomy
  - CS = trabeculated venous cavities
  - Receive blood from multiple valveless veins
  - Blood flows any direction (pressure gradient-dependent)
- CECT or MR
  - CT findings often subtle or negative in CST
  - Enlarged CS with convex margins, filling defect
  - Enlarged superior ophthalmic vein ± clot, proptosis
  - Enlarged extraocular muscles
  - Intracavernous carotid artery: Rarely stenosis, thrombosis, or pseudoaneurysm formation

TOP DIFFERENTIAL DIAGNOSES

- Cavernous sinus neoplasm
  - Meningioma, lymphoma, metastasis
- Cavernous carotid aneurysm, fistula
- Infection/inflammation
  - Idiopathic inflammatory extraorbital pseudotumor, sarcoidosis, Wegener granulomatosis

PATHOLOGY

- Often complication of sinusitis/orbital/midface infection
  - *Staphylococcus aureus* most common pathogen

CLINICAL ISSUES

- Headache most common early symptom
- Orbital pain, ophthalmoplegia, visual loss
- Treatment: Intravenous antibiotics; supportive care
- I&D of source infection if indicated (i.e., orbital abscess or functional endoscopic sinus surgery for sinusitis)

DIAGNOSTIC CHECKLIST

- Clinical setting + high index of suspicion

(Left) *Axial CECT of the head in a child with extensive sinusitis (not shown), demonstrates near-complete lack of cavernous sinus enhancement* ➡. **(Right)** *Coronal CECT shows classic laterally convex margins of the heterogeneously enhancing cavernous sinuses* ➡.

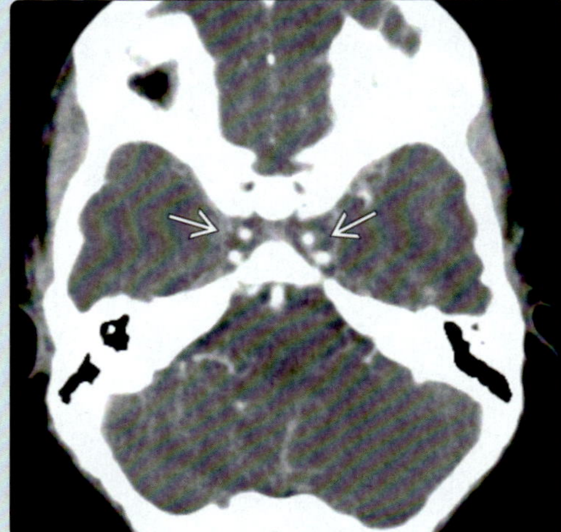

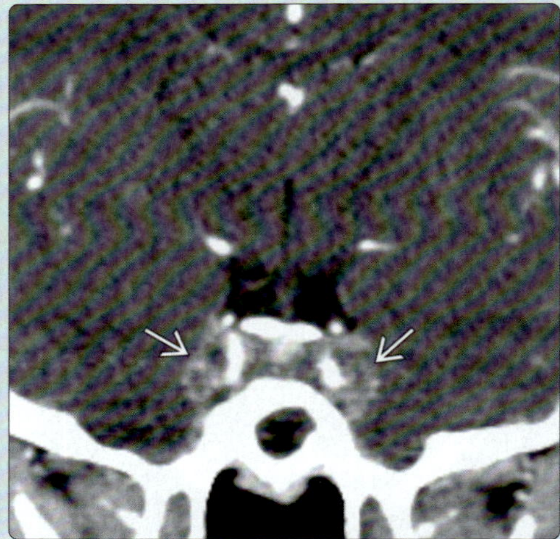

(Left) *Axial T1 C+ FS MR in the same patient demonstrates multiple filling defects in the cavernous sinuses* ➡, *right preseptal cellulitis, proptosis, lateral rectus muscle enlargement, and extensive sinus disease.* **(Right)** *Axial DWI MR in the same patient shows corresponding hyperintense signal within cavernous sinus clots* ➡ *and associated right superior ophthalmic vein thrombus* ➡.

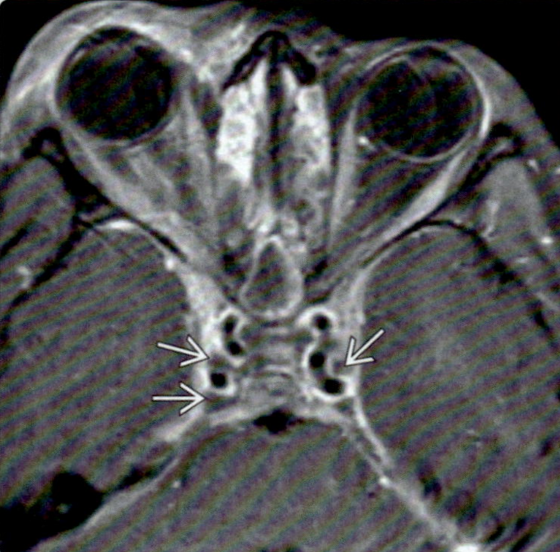

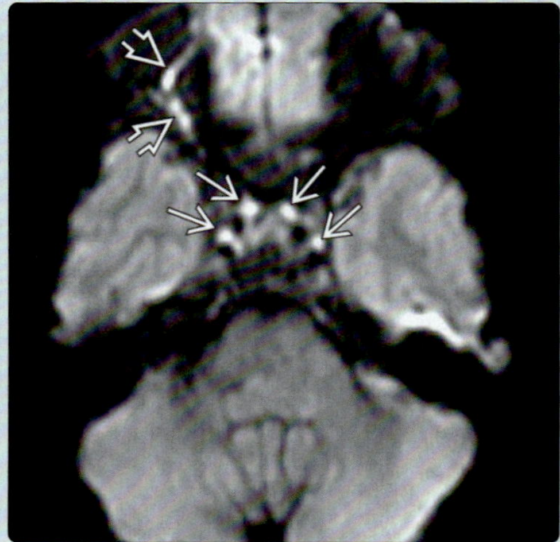

KEY FACTS

TERMINOLOGY

- Definition: Acquired direct shunt between dural artery and dural venous sinus or cortical vein

IMAGING

- Best imaging modality: Digital subtraction angio (DSA)
  - If objective pulsatile tinnitus + no other vascular lesion on CTA or MRA, DSA necessary to exclude dural arteriovenous fistula (DAVF)
  - Single pedicle DAVF often not seen on CTA or MRA
- Most common site: Transverse sinus (TS)
- CECT findings in DAVF
  - Tortuous, enhancing dural feeders with enlarged dural sinus
  - Enlarged cortical draining veins → aggressive DAVF
  - ± flow-related aneurysms
- MR findings in DAVF
  - Localized or generalized venous dilatation
  - Focal T2 hyperintensity in adjacent white matter (venous congestion)

TOP DIFFERENTIAL DIAGNOSES

- Hypoplastic TS-sigmoid sinus (TS-SS)
- Jugular bulb pseudolesion (MR artifact)
- Dural sinus thrombosis
- Pial arteriovenous malformation

CLINICAL ISSUES

- Presents in middle-aged to older patients
- Accounts for 35% of infratentorial vascular malformations
- TS-SS DAVF presents with **pulsatile tinnitus**
- Clinical options
  - Observe in selected cases (older patient ± small DAVF)
  - Treatment options if hemorrhage risk exists
    - Endovascular → embolization
    - Surgical resection → skeletonization sinus
    - Stereotactic radiotherapy

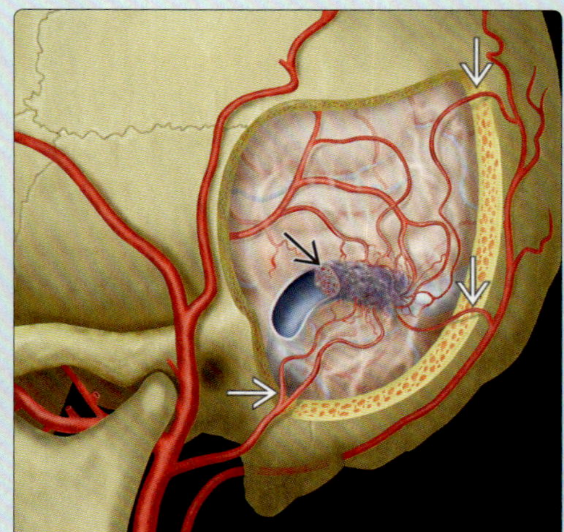

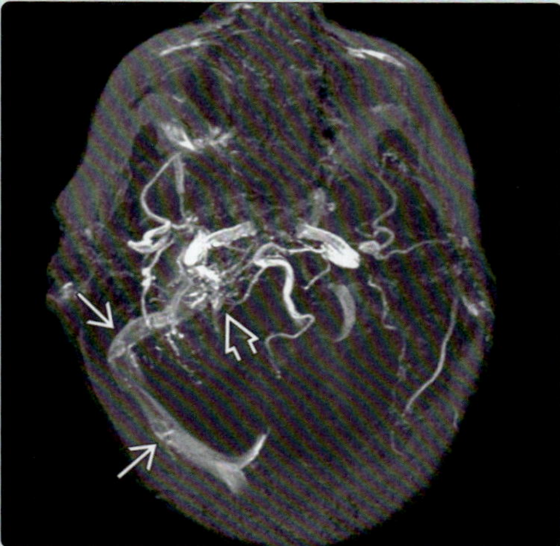

(Left) *A typical dural arteriovenous fistula (DAVF) with a short segment of thrombosed transverse sinus (TS) ⇨ shows DAVF consisting of multiple dural vessels in the wall of a thrombosed segment. Multiple dural & transosseous feeders arise from external ➡ & internal carotid arteries.* **(Right)** *MRA shows extensive prominent vascularity in the right skull base ➡ from DAVF. Source images from MRA should be reviewed for correlation with MIP images. Dural sinuses ➡ remain patent in this case. Thrombosis is often seen.*

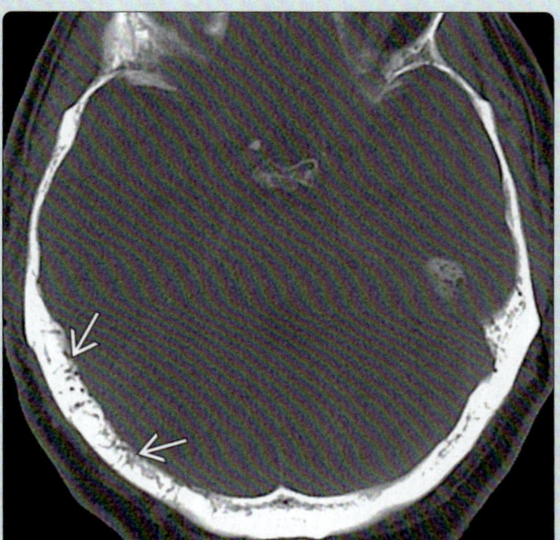

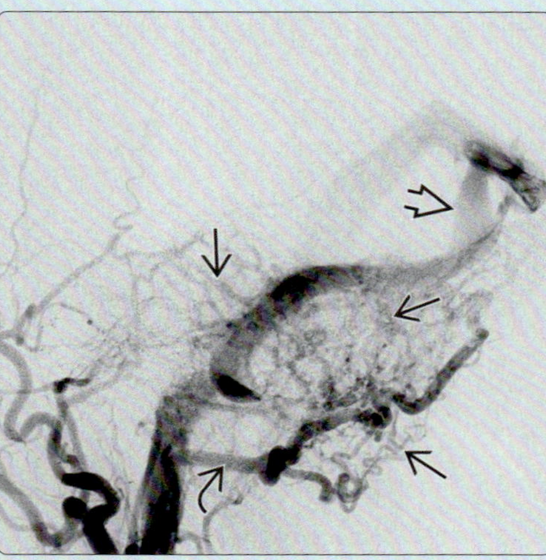

(Left) *Bone CT in a patient with DAVF shows innumerable enlarged transcalvarial vascular channels ➡. These particularly numerous vascular markings are usually noted but less impressive findings may go overlooked. Clinical suspicion may be helpful information.* **(Right)** *Selective right external carotid artery angiogram shows a large occipital artery ⇨ and auricular artery with prominent transosseous perforating vessels ⇨. Venous reflux into a large right TS ⇨ is present.*

Skull Base Cephalocele

KEY FACTS

TERMINOLOGY

- Basal cephalocele = congenital extracranial herniation of meninges, CSF, ± brain tissue through mesodermal defect in sphenoid, ethmoid, or basiocciput

IMAGING

- Nasopharyngeal
  - Transethmoid: Defect in cribriform plate
  - Sphenoethmoid: Bony defect junction of cribriform plate and planum sphenoidale
  - Sphenonasopharyngeal = transsphenoid: Defect in body of sphenoid bone is large craniopharyngeal canal
    - Most common
  - Basioccipital-nasopharyngeal (transbasioccipital): Bony defect parallel & inferior to sphenooccipital synchondrosis
    - Area of median basal canal
- Sphenoorbital
- Sphenomaxillary
- Best imaging tool
  - MR best identifies meninges, CSF, brain, pituitary, and optic nerves/chiasm position
  - Bone CT defines osseous defects prior to surgery

TOP DIFFERENTIAL DIAGNOSES

- Nasal glioma
- Nasal dermal sinus
- Teratoma

CLINICAL ISSUES

- Most common signs/symptoms
  - May be clinically occult
  - Hypertelorism, nasal mass, nasal stuffiness, endocrine dysfunction
  - Recurrent meningitis
- Combined craniofacial procedure may involve neurosurgery, otolaryngology, &/or plastic surgery

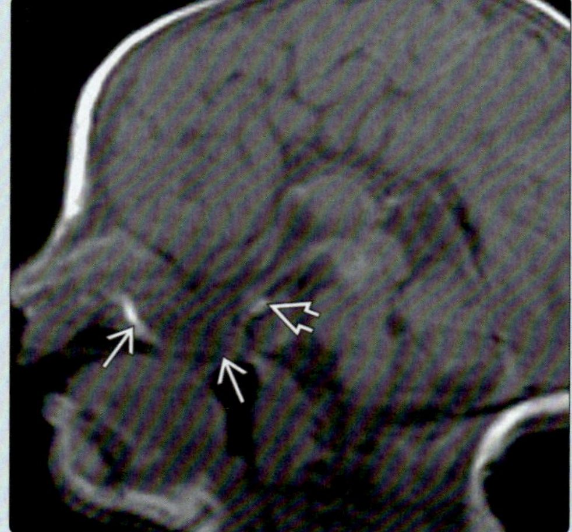
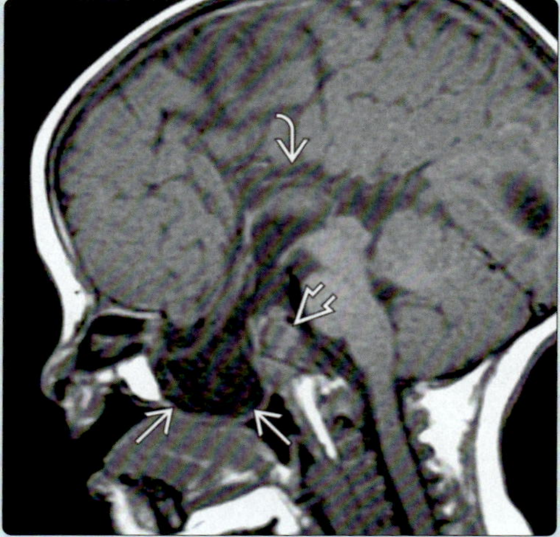

(Left) *Sagittal T1 MR in a 3-day-old boy with a nasal mass shows a CSF intensity transsphenoidal meningocele → protruding into the nasopharynx via a skull base defect in the floor of the sella (persistent craniopharyngeal canal). Note posterior pituitary hyperintensity in the dorsal aspect of the sella →.* **(Right)** *Sagittal T1 MR in the same child at 9 months of age shows an increase in the size of the cephalocele →, a defect anterior to the sphenooccipital synchondrosis →, and associated callosal agenesis →.*

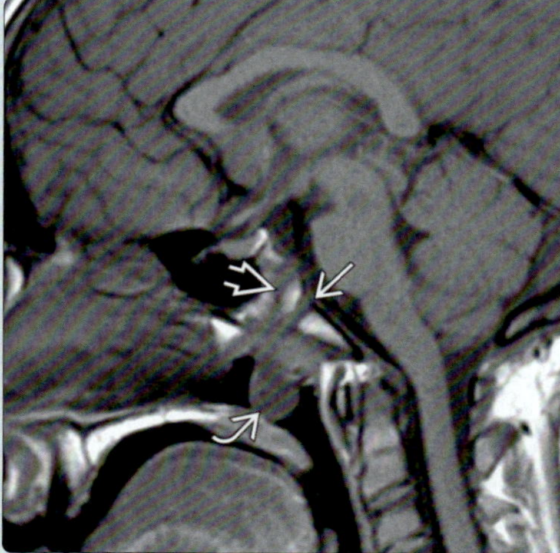
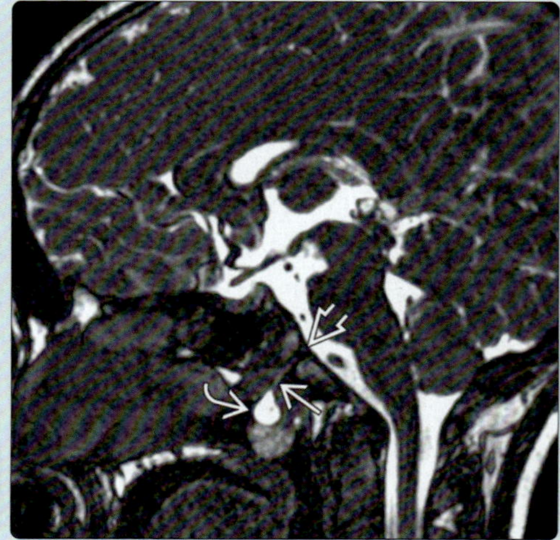

(Left) *Sagittal T1 MR in a 13 year old with meningitis shows a median basilar canal → inferior to residual sphenooccipital synchondrosis → and an associated nasopharyngeal mass →.* **(Right)** *Sagittal FIESTA in the same child shows the nasopharyngeal mass to be mixed signal intensity with a hyperintense linear tract → extending from the median basilar canal → to the cystic-appearing portion of the nasopharyngeal mass →. Histologically, the mass was thought to be an infarcted Thornwaldt cyst.*

KEY FACTS

IMAGING

- Best clue: Anterior or central **skull base (SB) defect** on bone CT with **positive β2-transferrin** test on nasal secretions
- Anterior skull base bone CT findings
  - Bone defect in cribriform plate, lateral lamella of middle turbinate or ethmoid roof
  - Other evidence for fracture, endoscopic sinus surgery, congenital cephalocele
- Central skull base bone CT findings
  - Bone defect in sella floor (transnasal pituitary surgery), lateral wall sphenoid (osseous dural defect)
- Multiple defects often present in obese patient with **idiopathic intracranial hypertension**
- MR used if cephalocele suspected

TOP DIFFERENTIAL DIAGNOSES

- Vasomotor rhinitis
- Skull base defect without CSF leak

PATHOLOGY

- Congenital CSF leak
  - Cribriform defect ± congenital cephalocele, persistent craniopharyngeal canal
- Acquired leak: Spontaneous leak from osseous dural defect
  - Lateral roof of sphenoid sinus
- Posttraumatic leak: Can occur with any facial or SB fx, or even closed head injury
  - Roof or lateral wall of sphenoid sinus, or cribriform plate/ethmoid roof
- Postoperative defect: Can occur after sinonasal or skull base surgery

CLINICAL ISSUES

- Rhinorrhea with Valsalva or head down maneuvers
- **β2-transferrin** is best test to confirm fluid from nose is CSF
- Treatment options
  - 1st try bed rest; lumbar drain
  - Persistent CSF leaks endoscopically repaired

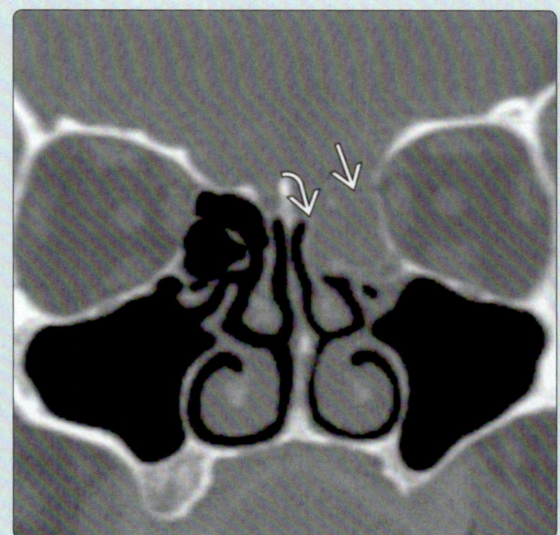

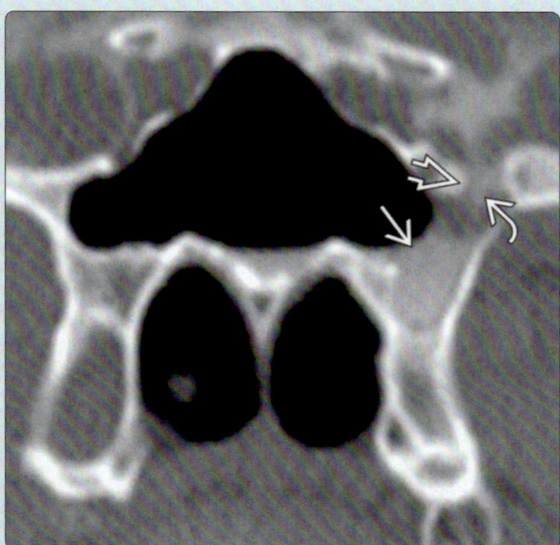

(Left) *Coronal bone CT shows a large bony defect ➡ in the left ethmoid roof, lateral to insertion of the middle turbinate ➡. Because there is complete opacification of the ethmoid cells, an MR was performed that showed meningoencephalocele.* **(Right)** *Coronal bone CT after intrathecal contrast shows CSF ➡ in the left sphenoid chamber, bone defect ➡, and contrast extending through the defect ➡. CT cisternography is rarely necessary when high-resolution bone CT and MR are performed 1st for CSF leak.*

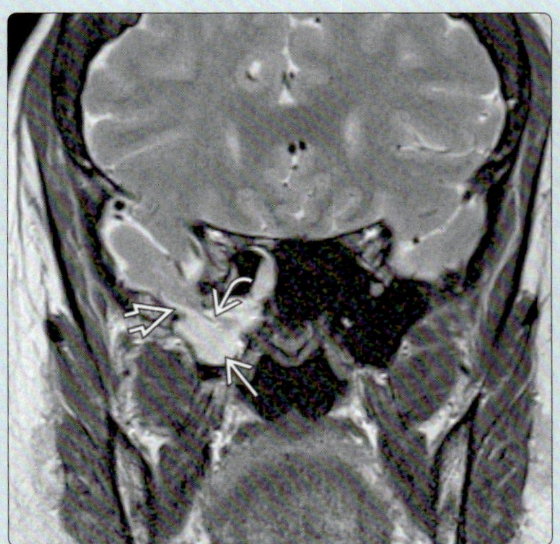

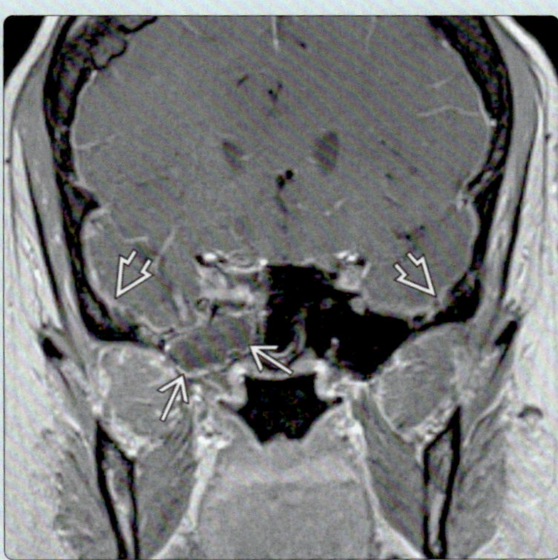

(Left) *Coronal T2 MR reveals a lateral sphenoid sinus filled with CSF ➡. Note the osseous defect in the lateral sphenoid roof ➡ & brain herniating through the defect ➡. This patient had a spontaneous CSF leak. Many such leaks are caused by large osseous dural defects.* **(Right)** *Coronal T1WI C+ MR (same patient) shows peripheral enhancement ➡ of the sphenoid meningoencephalocele. Note diffuse thin dural enhancement ➡, including at the defect site. Dural enhancement may be present without infection.*

KEY FACTS

TERMINOLOGY

- Definition: Congenital disorder with defect in osteoblastic differentiation and maturation, resulting in progressive replacement of normal cancellous bone by mixture of fibrous tissue and immature woven bone

IMAGING

- May affect calvarium, skull base, and facial bones
- Density (CT) and signal (MR) appearance highly variable
- CT findings
  - Expansile lesion centered in medullary space with variable attenuation
  - Sclerotic fibrous dysplasia (FD): Ground-glass density
  - Pagetoid FD: Mixed lucent and sclerotic areas
  - Cystic FD: Centrally lucent with thin sclerotic borders
- MR findings
  - Low signal in ossified ± fibrous portions of lesion
  - Variable enhancement depending on lesion pattern
- PET findings
  - Can be variably hypermetabolic on FDG PET

TOP DIFFERENTIAL DIAGNOSES

- Paget disease
- Ossifying fibroma
- Meningioma
- Skull base metastasis

PATHOLOGY

- Contains fibrous tissue with interspersed trabeculae of immature woven bone that resemble Chinese letters
- Sporadic mutation of *GNAS* gene; is not inherited
- Associated abnormalities include aneurysmal bone cyst, multiple endocrine disorders in McCune-Albright syndrome

CLINICAL ISSUES

- 3 presentations: Monostotic, polyostotic, and McCune-Albright syndrome
- Surgical resection when lesions symptomatic, resectable

(Left) *Coronal T2WI MR in a patient with fibrous dysplasia (FD) of the skull base shows expanded bone and marked hypointensity extending into the pterygoid processes ➡.* **(Right)** *Coronal CT in the same patient demonstrates expansion of the body and greater wing of the sphenoid with obliteration of the left sphenoid sinus lumen. The left foramen rotundum ➡ is narrowed and laterally displaced. Note the marked expansion of left pterygoid process and medial and lateral pterygoid plates ➡.*

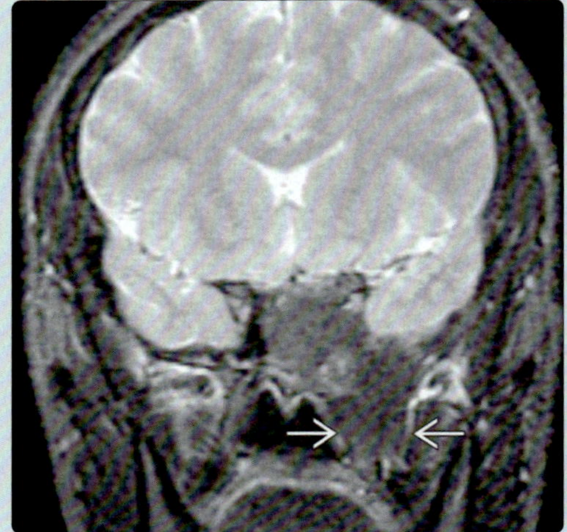

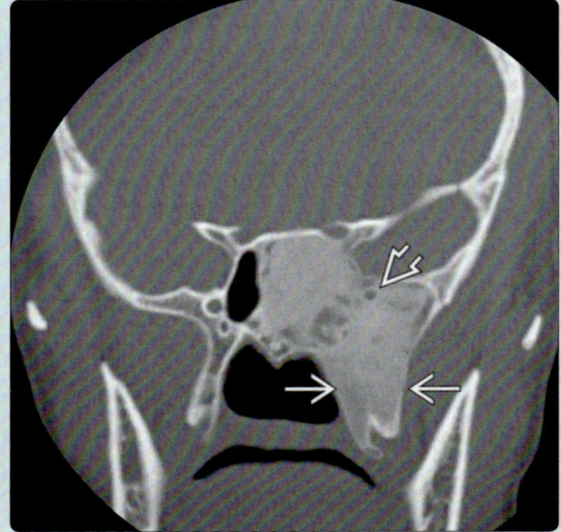

(Left) *Axial bone CT shows FD involving the temporal bone with smooth, expanded appearance of the bone ➡. The petrous temporal bone is extensively involved with sparing of the inner ear structures. The more posterior-lateral component ➡ shows classic ground-glass density.* **(Right)** *Axial T1WI C+ FS MR in the same patient demonstrates enhancement of the entire extent of the involved petrous bone ➡. In this case, enhancement is diffuse and homogeneous.*

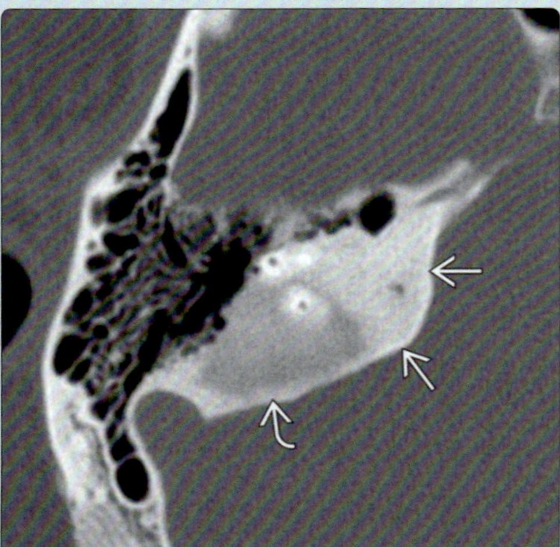

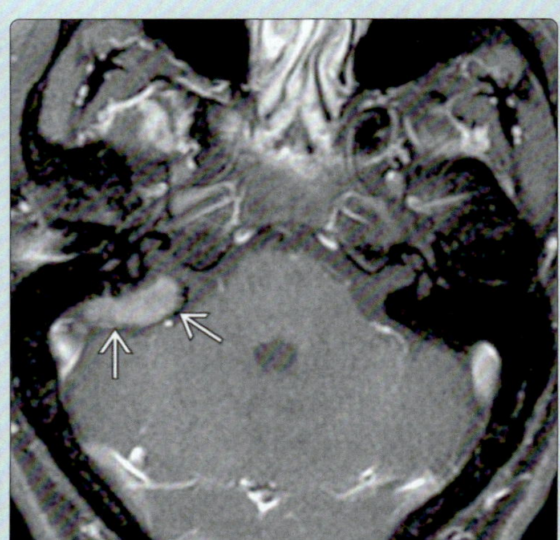

KEY FACTS

TERMINOLOGY

- Primary metabolic bony disease of unknown etiology

IMAGING

- CT findings: Diploic widening common
  - Bone CT most demonstrative of **mixed sclerosis & lysis**
  - Well-defined **lytic regions** with expansion of bone in **early-phase disease**
  - **Cotton-wool** appearance in later **lytic-sclerotic phase**
- MR findings
  - T1: Hypointense signal due to fibrovascular replacement of marrow space
  - T1 C+: Heterogeneous C+ from hypervascular new bone
- Basilar invagination from bone softening & expansion

TOP DIFFERENTIAL DIAGNOSES

- Fibrous dysplasia
- Skull base metastasis
- Osteopetrosis
- Osteogenesis imperfecta

PATHOLOGY

- Cases may have autosomal dominant transmission
  - Some consistent mutations identified in familial cases & some sporadic cases
- Both environmental and genetic causes likely
- Histologic mosaic bone pattern in final stage of disease

CLINICAL ISSUES

- Common presentation: Expansile, lytic, & sclerotic bony disease of axial skeleton and skull in elderly male patient
  - **Hearing loss** if temporal bone involvement
  - May be incidental finding
- Total serum alkaline phosphatase ↑ (85%)
- Malignant transformation in < 1% of cases
- Pagetic bone pain is uncommon (constant, boring)
- Treatment: Lasting response to **bisphosphonate agents**
  - Watch for osteonecrosis complication (mandible)

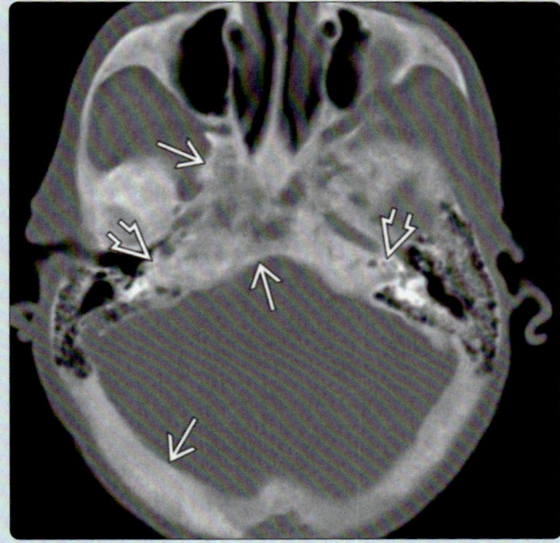

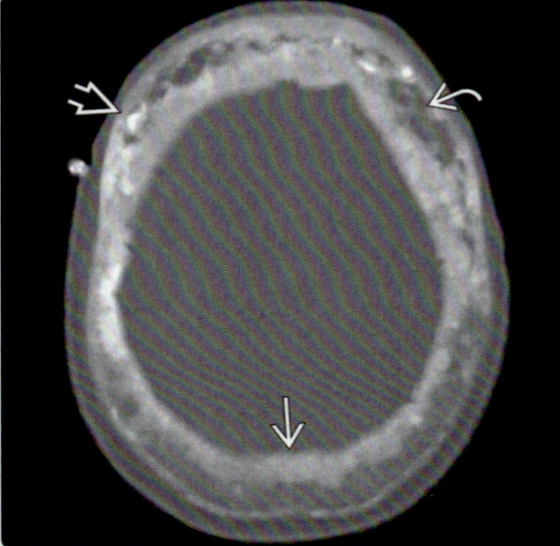

(Left) *Axial bone CT of the skull base shows Paget disease with diffuse expansion and hyperdensity of the skull base ➡ and a fluffy appearance of the abnormally thickened bone. This process also involves the temporal bones and otic capsules ➡.* **(Right)** *Axial bone CT in the same patient demonstrates the extensive nature of the disease with diffuse irregular calvarial cortical thickening ➡, patchy osteolysis ➡, and islands of sclerotic bone ➡ representing cotton-wool lesions.*

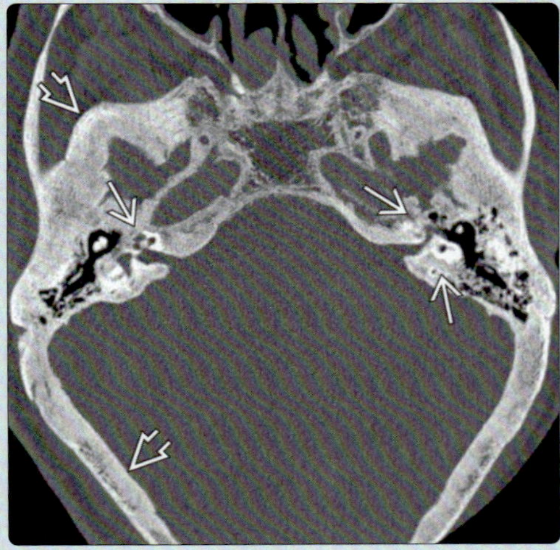

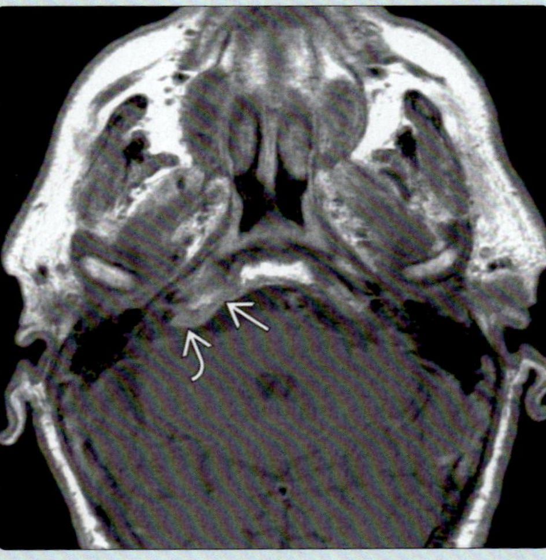

(Left) *Axial bone CT demonstrates diffuse skull base sclerosis with mild bony expansion, irregular cortical thickening ➡, and poor corticomedullary differentiation. There is demineralization of the otic capsules ➡ bilaterally. Temporal bone involvement may result in hearing loss.* **(Right)** *Axial T1WI C+ MR in the same patient demonstrates avid enhancement of the pagetoid focus ➡, which is mildly expanded and results in stenosis of the internal auditory canal ➡.*

Skull Base Langerhans Cell Histiocytosis

KEY FACTS

TERMINOLOGY

- **Langerhans cell histiocytosis**: Spectrum of disorders caused by neoplastic clonal proliferations of CD1a, CD207, S100 (+) dendritic cells
  - Single system (unifocal or multifocal) vs. multisystem disease
  - Bone and skin most frequently involved
  - High-risk organ involvement: Liver, spleen, marrow = worse prognosis
  - Other organs: Lymph nodes, pituitary, thymus, GI tract, central nervous system
  - **70%** have involvement of H&N: Skull base, T-bone, craniofacial

IMAGING

- CT findings
  - Geographic, lytic lesion of skull base/T-bone
  - Associated with enhancing soft tissue mass
- MR findings
  - Heterogeneous, strongly enhancing soft tissue mass ± intracranial/dural extension

TOP DIFFERENTIAL DIAGNOSES

- Acute coalescent otomastoiditis
- Rhabdomyosarcoma
- Acquired cholesteatoma

CLINICAL ISSUES

- Typical presentation: **Young male patient** with otalgia, otorrhea, & postauricular mass
  - Usually presents in 1st decade; M:F = 1.2-3:1
  - Otologic symptoms may be only initial sign of disease
  - More common among Caucasians
- 90% cure rate for unifocal disease of T-bone
- Usually responds well to medical management
- Surgical curettage or mastoidectomy for localized disease
  - Treatment can include surgery, radiation, chemo, or steroid injections

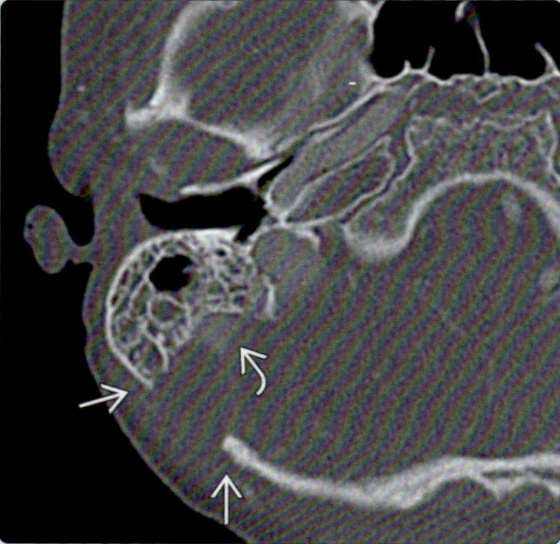
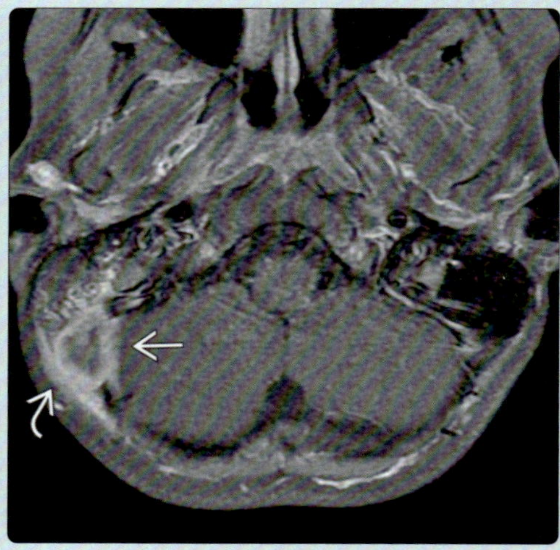

(Left) *Axial CECT in Langerhans cell histiocytosis (LCH) demonstrates involvement of the posterior mastoid with well-defined destruction ➡ displacing the adjacent sigmoid sinus ➡.* **(Right)** *Axial T1 C+ FS MR in the same patient demonstrates heterogeneous enhancement of LCH and depicts the extent of soft tissue disease ➡ contiguous with a bony lesion and involvement of contiguous dura ➡.*

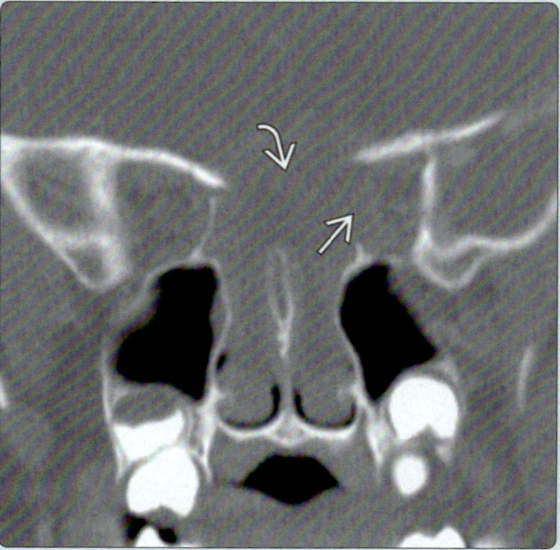
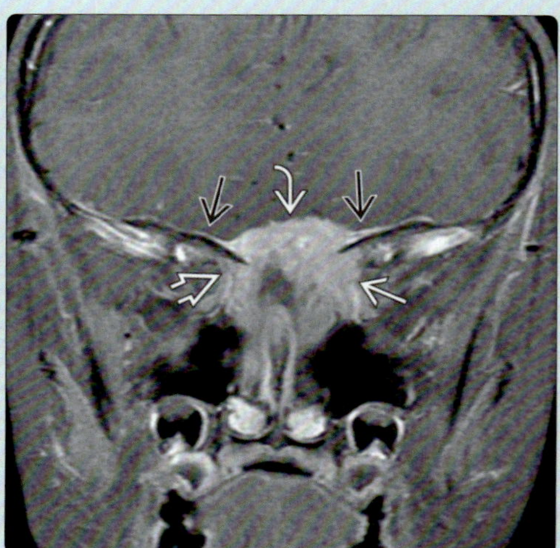

(Left) *Coronal bone CT shows LCH lesion centered in the basisphenoid and extending into the left ➡ orbital apex through the medial orbital wall. A large area of bone dehiscence involves the planum sphenoidale ➡.* **(Right)** *Coronal T1 C+ MR in the same patient shows involvement of the left orbit near apex ➡, right orbital apex ➡, and anterior cranial fossa ➡. Dural involvement is also noted with abnormal dural enhancement ➡ at the tumor margins.*

KEY FACTS

TERMINOLOGY

- Rare heritable metabolic bone disease with defective bone remodeling resulting in overproduction of immature bone
- **Autosomal recessive osteopetrosis** (AROP): Childhood severe form
- **Autosomal dominant osteopetrosis** (ADOP): Adult benign, less severe form

IMAGING

- **AROP**: CT findings seen in **infancy**
  - Diffuse increase in overall bone density
  - Temporal bone: Internal auditory canal (IAC) & internal carotid artery canal stenoses, middle ear encroachment
  - Skull base: Foraminal & dural sinus stenoses
- **ADOP type 1**: Adult CT findings
  - Universal otosclerosis
    - Spares spine
  - Dense sclerosis of calvarium
- **ADOP type 2** (Albers-Schönberg): Adult CT findings
  - Dense sclerosis of skull base, spine, pelvis
    - Spares calvarium
  - Generalized ↑ density of entire skull base
  - Endobones (unresorbed primary ossification centers)
  - Sclerotic otic capsule beyond normal bony labyrinth margins
  - IAC short & trumpet-shaped
  - Enlarged subarcuate fossa possible

TOP DIFFERENTIAL DIAGNOSES

- Skull base Paget disease
- Skull base fibrous dysplasia

PATHOLOGY

- Hereditary disorder: *CLCN7* gene mutation

CLINICAL ISSUES

- **AROP** is apparent in **infancy**
- ADOP manifests later in life

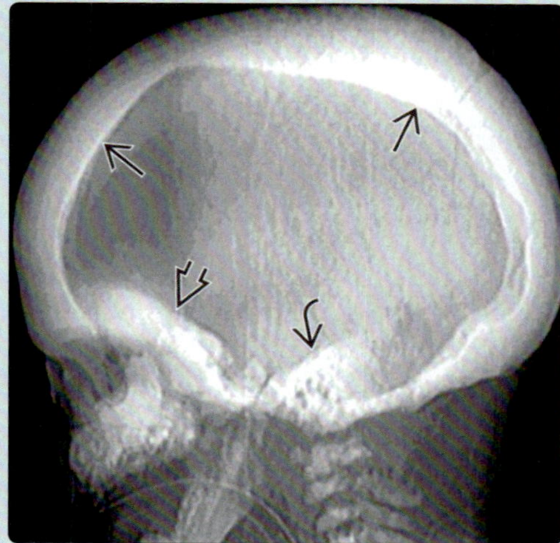

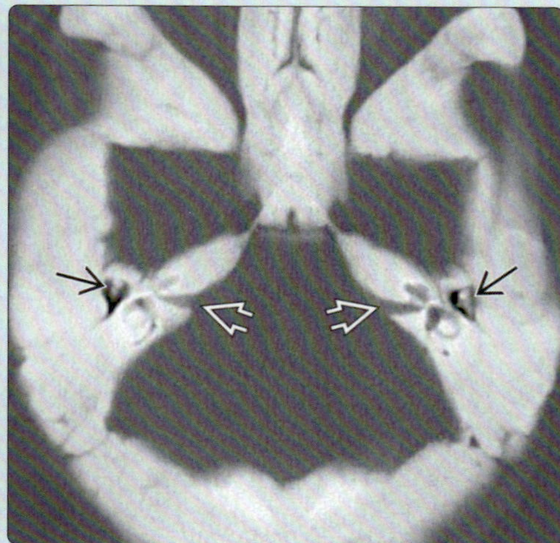

(Left) *Lateral radiograph shows diffuse thickening of the calvarium ➙, cranial base ➙, and temporal bone ➙, characteristic of the more severe form of osteopetrosis (autosomal recessive).* **(Right)** *Axial skull base bone CT shows diffuse sclerosis of the entire cranial base. There is narrowing of both middle ears ➙. Note also compromise of each internal auditory canal ➙. This child has autosomal recessive osteopetrosis.*

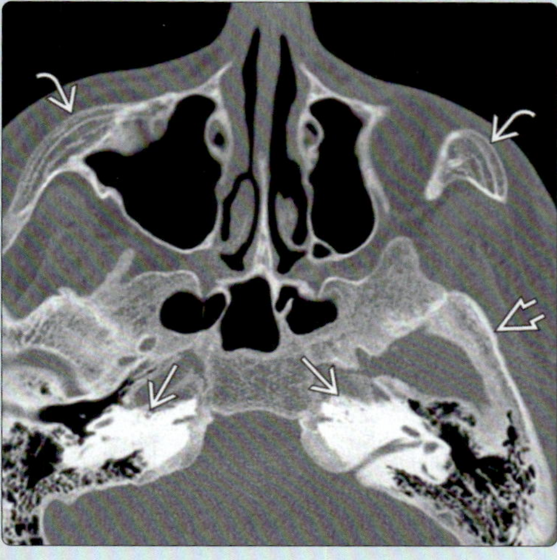

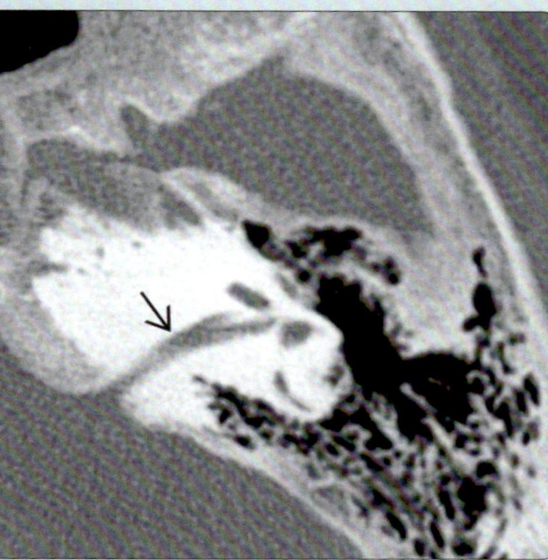

(Left) *Axial bone CT through the skull base in a young adult with type 2 autosomal dominant osteopetrosis shows bilateral dense sclerosis of the temporal bone ➙ with thickening of the calvarium ➙ without increased density. Notice the endobone appearance of both malar eminences ➙ from unresorbed primary ossification centers.* **(Right)** *Axial bone CT of the left temporal bone in the same patient reveals encroachment upon the internal auditory canal ➙ by osteopetrosis of the inner ear bone.*

KEY FACTS

TERMINOLOGY

- Definition: Nonspecific, nonneoplastic benign inflammatory lesion without identifiable local or systemic causes characterized by polymorphous lymphoplasmacytic infiltrate
- Idiopathic orbital inflammation (IOI)
  - May involve any part(s) of orbit
- Idiopathic extraorbital inflammation
  - **Intracranial involvement**: Spread through superior orbital fissure (SOF) or optic canal (OC)
    - Cavernous sinus, dura, Meckel cave
  - **Skull base-extracranial involvement**: Spreads from inferior orbital fissure (IOF) or through orbital wall
    - Anterior skull base, sinuses, nasopharyngeal spaces
- IgG4-related disease: Subgroup of idiopathic inflammation with systemic involvement
  - Intracranial noncontiguous sites: Pituitary, infundibulum
  - Extracranial noncontiguous H&N sites: Parotid, submandibular glands, thyroid

IMAGING

- T1WI C+ FS MR: Diffusely enhancing, infiltrating mass
  - Extends from orbit through SOF ± OC to cavernous sinus, dura, Meckel cave
  - Extends through IOF to pterygopalatine fossa, nose, deep nasopharyngeal spaces
- T2 MR: Iso- to **hypointense** lesion; ↑ fibrosis, ↓ intensity

TOP DIFFERENTIAL DIAGNOSES

- En plaque meningioma
- Meningeal non-Hodgkin lymphoma
- Nasopharyngeal carcinoma
- Neurosarcoid

CLINICAL ISSUES

- Symptoms: Painful proptosis ± headaches ± cranial neuropathies
- Diagnosis of exclusion; must be biopsied
- Treatment: High-dose systemic **steroids**

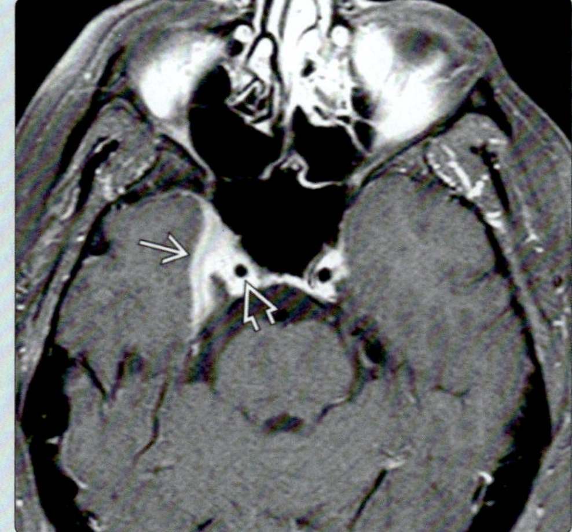

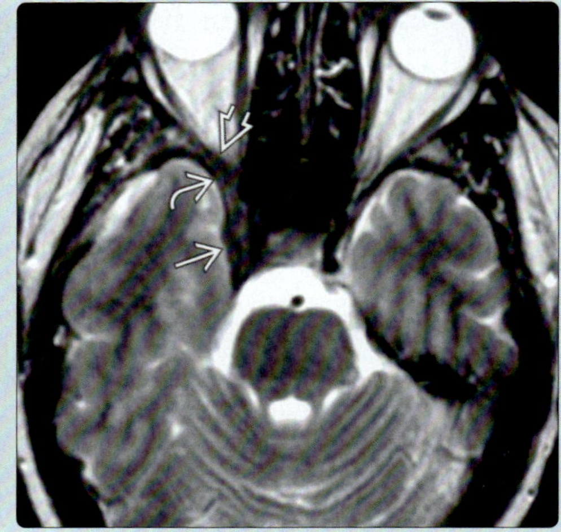

(Left) *Axial T1WI C+ FS MR shows a focus of enhancing idiopathic extraorbital inflammation (IEI) involving the right cavernous sinus ➡ with subtle narrowing ➡ of the intracavernous internal carotid artery.* **(Right)** *Axial T2WI MR in the same patient reveals an idiopathic orbital inflammation lesion ➡ that connects to the cavernous sinus IEI ➡ through the superior orbital fissure (SOF) ➡. Both areas of idiopathic inflammation are hypointense due to the fibrosis often found within this lesion.*

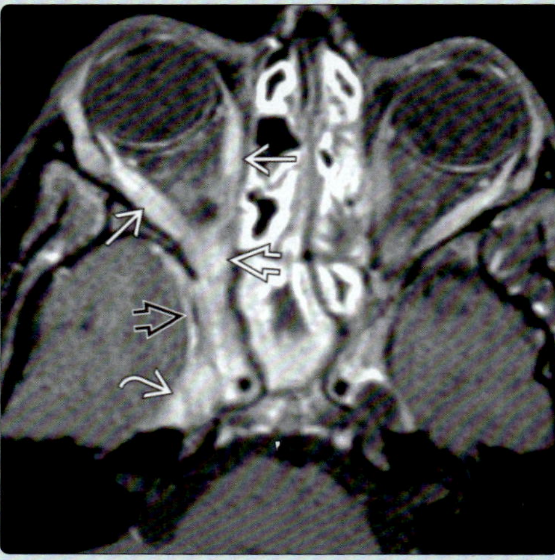

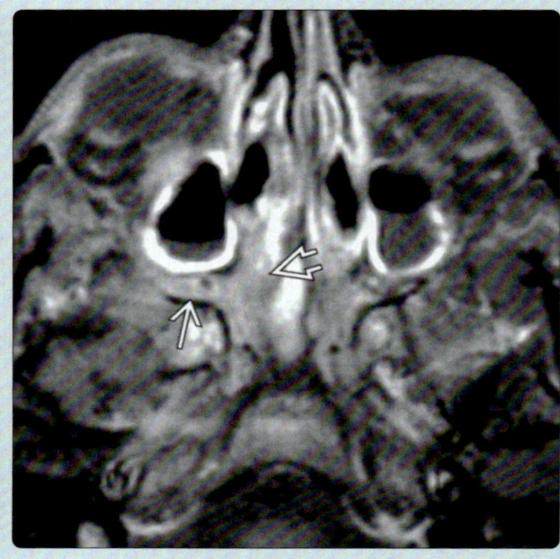

(Left) *Axial T1WI C+ FS MR through the orbits shows enlarged, enhancing orbital rectus muscles ➡ connecting through the SOF ➡ with the cavernous sinus ➡ and Meckel cave ➡. The initial impression of adenoid cystic carcinoma gave way to biopsy-proven idiopathic inflammation with both intraorbital and intracranial components.* **(Right)** *Axial T1WI C+ FS MR in the same patient shows the lesion invading inferiorly through the inferior orbital fissure into the pterygopalatine fossa ➡ and nose ➡.*

KEY FACTS

TERMINOLOGY

- Giant cell tumor (GCT): Benign intraosseous neoplasm arising from **multinucleated giant cells**

IMAGING

- CT: **Expansile** intraosseous soft tissue mass with thinned surrounding **cortical shell**
- MR: **Hypointense rim** & prominent internal enhancement
- Sphenoid bone > temporal bone > > frontal bone

TOP DIFFERENTIAL DIAGNOSES

- Aneurysmal bone cyst
- Chordoma
- Chondrosarcoma
- Fibrous dysplasia
- Plasmacytoma

PATHOLOGY

- Hemorrhage/hemosiderin deposition common
- Overlap with other giant cell containing tumors, such as giant cell lesion, aneurysmal bone cyst, brown tumor, pigmented villonodular synovitis
- Major neoplastic component of GCT comprised by stromal cells, not multinucleated giant cells

CLINICAL ISSUES

- Rare lesion: 2% of all GCT arise in skull base
- Peak incidence: 3rd-4th decade
- Metastases in 2% of cases
- Treatment: Preop embolization if needed, complete surgical resection with approach based on location of lesion
- Recurrence rate 40-60% after resection

DIAGNOSTIC CHECKLIST

- If in patient < 30 years of age, consider fibrous dysplasia
- If lesion centered in sella & normal pituitary not seen, consider invasive adenoma
- If patient has known malignancy, consider metastasis

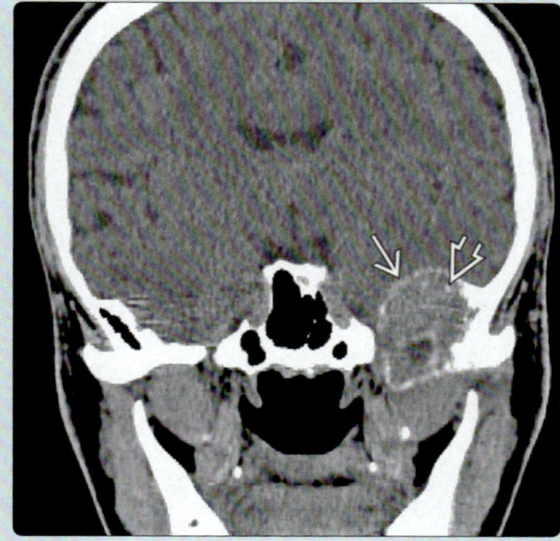
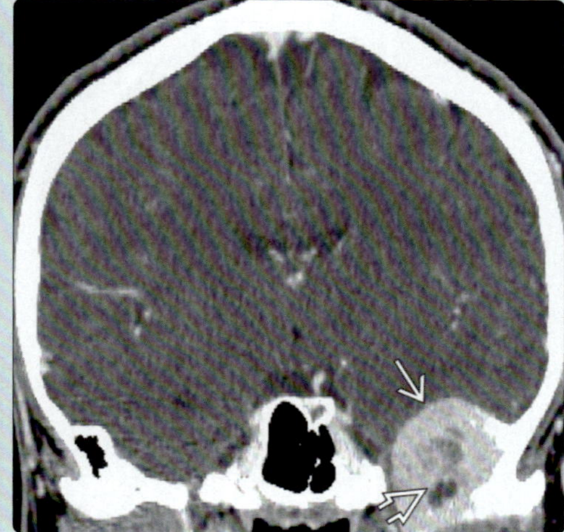

(Left) *Coronal NECT demonstrates an expansile mass centered in the floor of the left middle cranial fossa. There is thin peripheral (egg shell) calcification as well as specks of internal matrix calcification.* **(Right)** *Coronal CECT of the same patient shows the mass enhances intensely except for in areas of cystic change.*

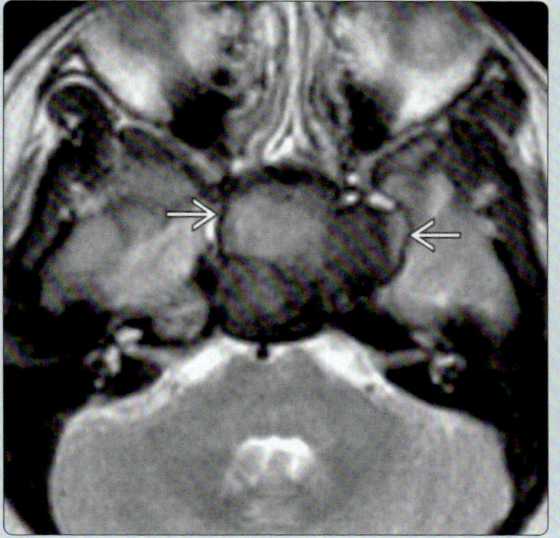
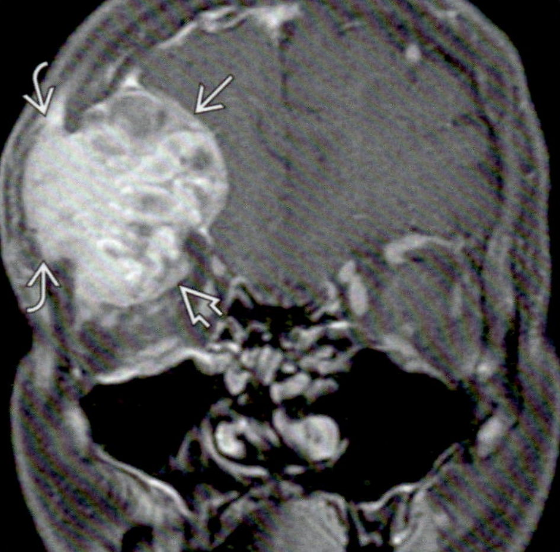

(Left) *Axial T2WI MR shows expansile sphenoid giant cell tumor with central heterogeneous hypointensity with a markedly hypointense rim. Fibrous dysplasia may mimic this appearance.* **(Right)** *Coronal T1 C+ FS MR demonstrates a giant cell tumor in its least common skull base location, the frontal bone. There is intracranial and extracranial extension, including involvement of the superior orbit.*

Skull Base Meningioma

KEY FACTS

TERMINOLOGY

- Benign extraaxial neoplasm arising from arachnoid cap cells

IMAGING

- Assess involvement of critical skull base structures
  - Optic canal, vessels, cavernous sinus, Meckel cave
- Anterior skull base: Olfactory groove, tuberculum sella, and sphenoid wing
- Central skull base: Petroclival and pericavernous
- Posterior skull base: Lower clival and foramen magnum
- Morphology: Sessile (en plaque)/lentiform > globose/spherical
- CT findings
  - Hyperdense, homogeneously enhancing mass
  - **25%** intramural calcification
  - Bone: **Hyperostosis** > **permeative sclerotic**
- MR findings
  - Isointense to gray matter with prominent enhancement
  - Enhancing reactive **dural tail** (60%)
  - **Cerebrospinal fluid-vascular cleft** between tumor and parenchyma

TOP DIFFERENTIAL DIAGNOSES

- Skull base schwannoma
- Giant pituitary macroadenoma
- Chordoma
- Skull base/dural metastasis
- Sarcoidosis

CLINICAL ISSUES

- 2nd most common primary intracranial tumor
- Middle-aged to elderly patients; M:F = 1:3
- Treatment options
  - Surgery curative; complexity and morbidity depend on location
  - Preoperative angiography/embolization as needed
  - Radiotherapy may be used primarily or adjunctive when resection is incomplete; high control rate

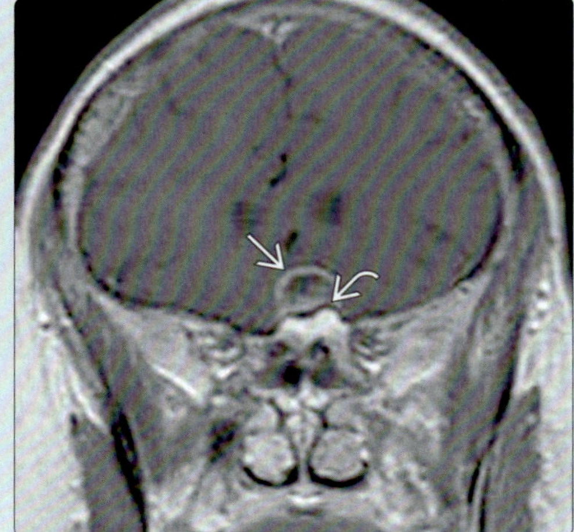

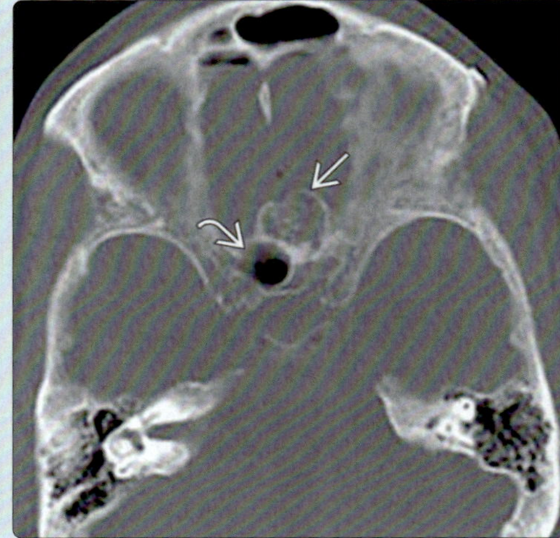

(Left) *Coronal T1WI C+ MR demonstrates a peripherally enhancing mass ➡ based along the floor of the anterior fossa. Although the central low signal is atypical (reflecting heavy calcification), the presence of hyperostosis and upward "blistering" ➡ of the planum sphenoidale is highly characteristic of meningioma.* **(Right)** *Axial bone CT in the same patient shows the calcified meningioma ➡ along the planum sphenoidale with accompanying pneumatosis dilatans of the adjacent sphenoid sinus ➡.*

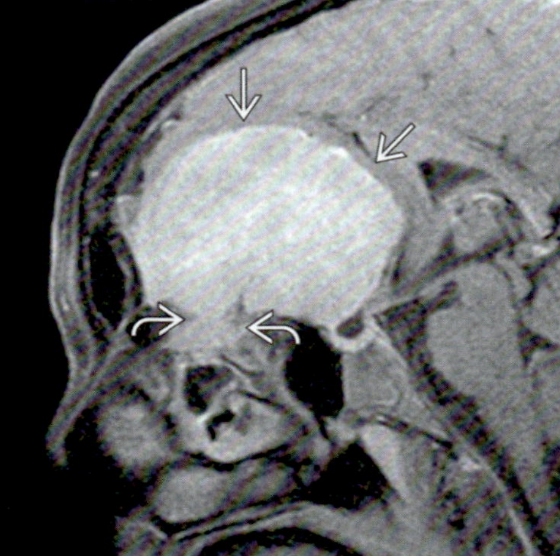

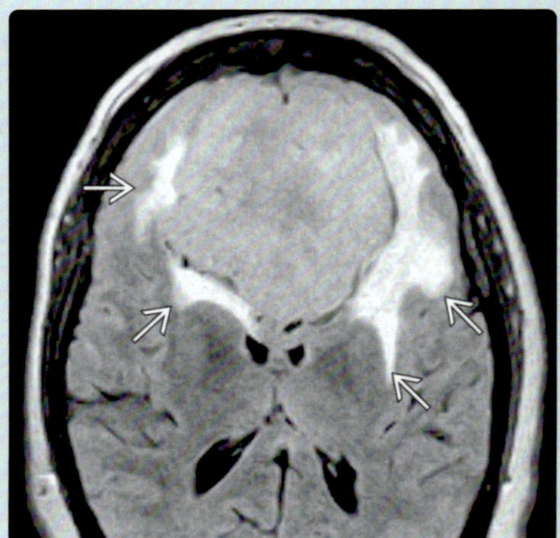

(Left) *Sagittal T1WI C+ FS MR shows a large, avidly enhancing anterior cranial fossa meningioma buckling the medial frontal lobe ➡. There is inferior extension through the cribriform plate into the olfactory recess of the nasal cavity ➡.* **(Right)** *Axial FLAIR MR in the same patient demonstrates signal intensity similar to gray matter with only mild heterogeneity. There is extensive peritumoral edema ➡, a finding that increases surgical morbidity and likelihood of recurrence.*

Skull Base Plasmacytoma

KEY FACTS

TERMINOLOGY

- Abbreviations: Solitary bone plasmacytoma (SBP), extramedullary plasmacytoma (EMP), multiple myeloma (MM)
- Definition: Isolated intramedullary or extramedullary neoplasm of plasma cells in absence of clinical or radiographic findings of MM

IMAGING

- CT findings
  - SBP: Solitary intraosseous, **lytic mass with nonsclerotic margins**
  - EMP: Sinonasal mass with secondary osseous invasion of skull base
- MR findings
  - Homogeneously enhancing intraosseous/extraosseous skull base mass
  - More sensitive for marrow space involvement and excluding additional small/early lesions
- Bone CT best defines trabecular and cortical destruction
- MR best defines marrow extent & extraosseous soft tissue

TOP DIFFERENTIAL DIAGNOSES

- Multiple myeloma
- Skull base metastasis
- Invasive pituitary macroadenoma
- Chordoma

PATHOLOGY

- Monoclonal proliferation of immunoglobulin-secreting plasma cells

CLINICAL ISSUES

- Symptoms: Local pain, headache, cranial nerve deficits
- M > F in 5th-9th decade
- SBP has higher rate of conversion to MM than EMP
- If skull base plasmacytoma diagnosed, complete clinical and radiologic work-up for MM required
- Treatment: Surgical resection and radiation therapy

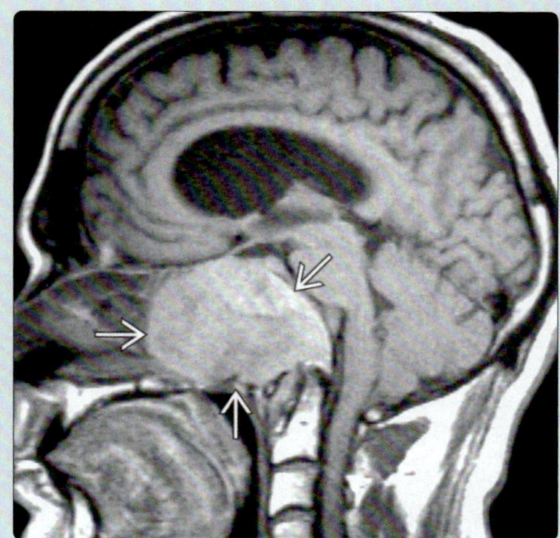

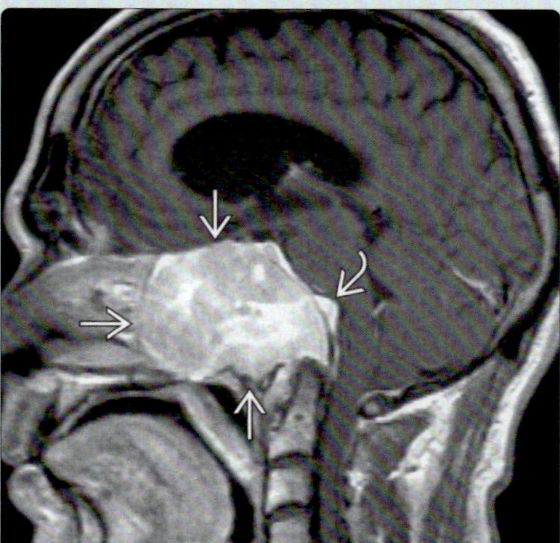

(Left) *Sagittal T1WI MR in a 61-year-old man demonstrates a large solitary mass ➡ expanding the clivus, obliterating the sphenoid sinus, and extending into the posterior nasal cavity and nasopharynx. The plasmacytoma is slightly hyperintense to brain parenchyma.* **(Right)** *Sagittal T1WI C+ MR shows heterogeneous enhancement of the lesion ➡ without necrosis. Dural thickening ➡ is noted posteriorly as epidural extension begins to compress the medulla.*

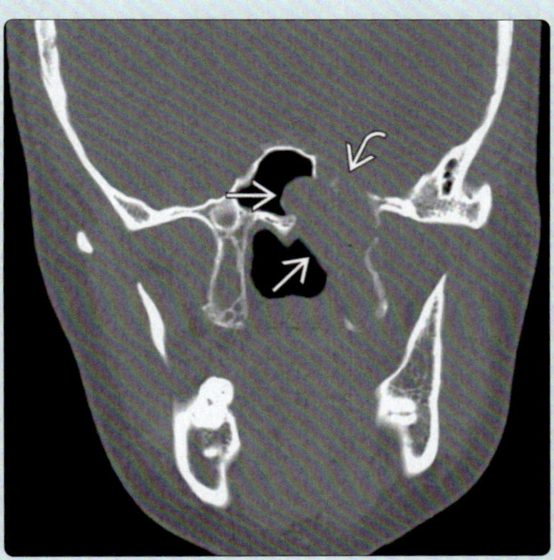

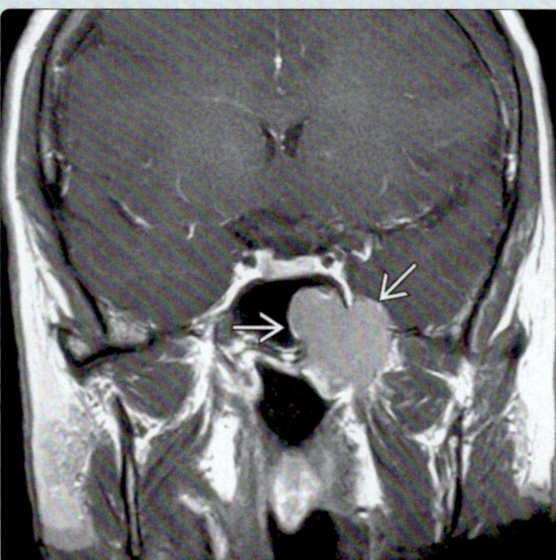

(Left) *Coronal bone CT in a 45-year-old woman with sinus pain demonstrates an expansile mass ➡ centered in the left sphenoid bone. The mass expands medially into the sphenoid sinus and erodes medial floor of the middle cranial fossa ➡. The margins of the tumor are relatively sharp, and in some areas there is preservation of thin eggshell margin of cortical bone.* **(Right)** *Coronal T1WI C+ MR demonstrates homogeneous enhancement of this skull base plasmacytoma ➡.*

Skull Base Multiple Myeloma

KEY FACTS

TERMINOLOGY

- Malignant monoclonal plasma cell proliferation

IMAGING

- CT shows osteolytic lesion(s) of skull base with additional skeletal lesions of calvarium, facial bones, cervical spine, etc.
- MR is most sensitive for evaluation of marrow involvement & assessing soft tissue characteristics
  - Homogeneous, isointense to gray matter on T1 & T2WI with moderate, diffuse enhancement

TOP DIFFERENTIAL DIAGNOSES

- Skull base metastases
- Non-Hodgkin lymphoma
- Chordoma
- Chondrosarcoma
- Invasive macroadenoma

CLINICAL ISSUES

- Most patients > 40 yr (average: 62 yr)
- 70% men
- Patients have localized pain and cranial neuropathy depending on lesion location
- Systemic symptoms related to anemia, renal failure, hypercalcemia
- Treatment options
  - Melphalan and prednisone primary treatment

DIAGNOSTIC CHECKLIST

- Key to imaging diagnosis is demonstrating multiple marrow replacing, **osteolytic lesions** on CT or plain films
- **Use T1 C+ FS MR** images to evaluate commonly overlooked regions of skull base & face
  - Clivus, petrous apex, occipital condyle, greater wing of sphenoid, mandibular condyle
- Whole-body imaging is recommended to evaluate for extracranial disease

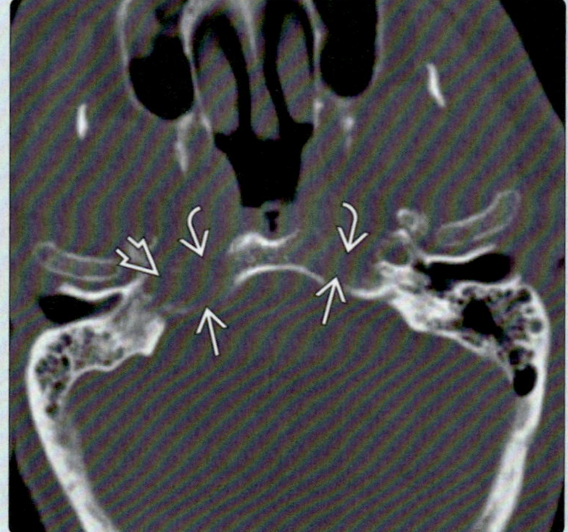

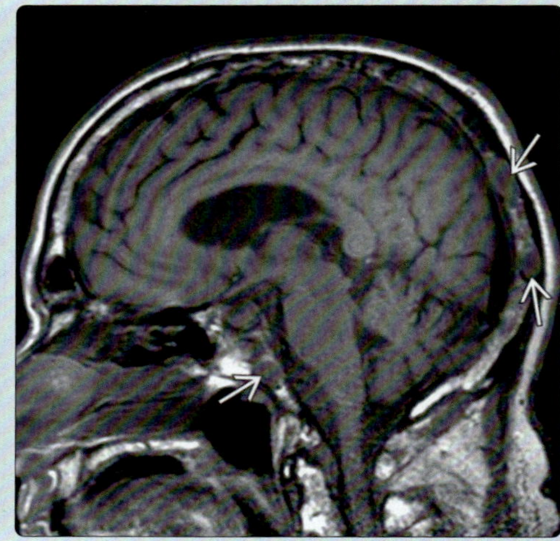

(Left) *Axial bone CT demonstrates nearly symmetric bilateral occipital bone lytic lesions ➡ of multiple myeloma. Symmetry can reduce conspicuity; however, loss of the expected outer white cortical line is clearly abnormal ➡. Note erosion into the right carotid canal ➡.* **(Right)** *Sagittal T1 MR shows multiple low-signal foci of multiple myeloma ➡. This is a relatively sensitive sequence (without FS) for osseous malignancy, particularly if the whole skull enhances &/or no FS is applied on the postcontrast sequence.*

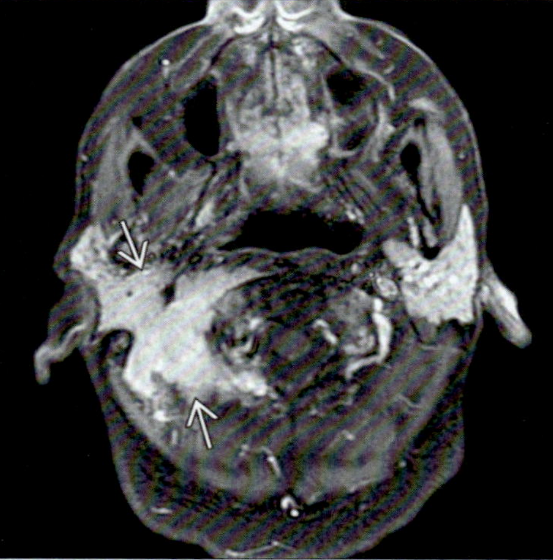

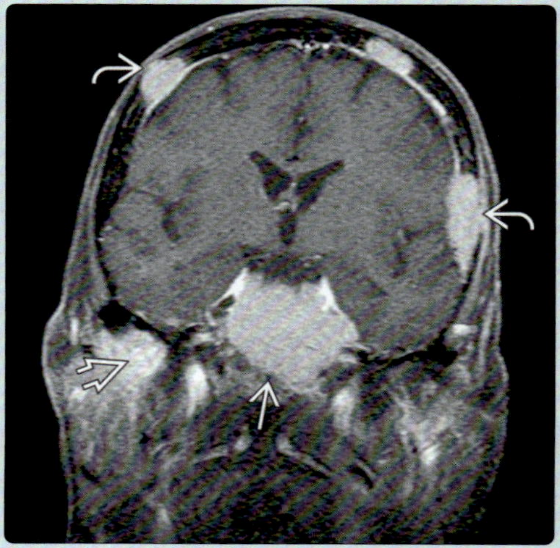

(Left) *Axial T1 C+ FS MR in a patient with right facial nerve palsy shows homogeneously enhancing osseous and extraosseous tumor ➡ destroying the mastoid segment of the right temporal bone and obliterating the stylomastoid foramen. T1 C+ FS MR is typically the most sensitive sequence to detect marrow involvement.* **(Right)** *Coronal T1 C+ FS MR shows a dominant enhancing mass in the clivus ➡ with additional smaller myelomatous lesions in the calvarium ➡ and right infratemporal fossa ➡.*

KEY FACTS

TERMINOLOGY

- Metastatic disease (mets) affecting osseous skull base &/or adjacent dura

IMAGING

- Enhancing, destructive mass of osseous skull base in patient with **known extracranial primary malignancy**
- Often dominant lesion seen in context of multiple additional skeletal lesions affecting skull base, calvarium, spine, etc.
- MR most sensitive modality
  - **Osseous metastasis**: Enhancing marrow space mass ± extraosseous extension
  - **Dural metastasis**: Enhancing, infiltrating, dural-based lesion
  - Noncontrast T1 & T1 C+ FS MR best sequences
- CT shows variable pattern of cortical and trabecular bone involvement: Lytic, permeative, sclerotic

TOP DIFFERENTIAL DIAGNOSES

- Multiple myeloma
- Non-Hodgkin lymphoma
- Skull base meningioma
- Solitary central skull base mass
  - Invasive pituitary adenoma, chordoma, chondrosarcoma

PATHOLOGY

- Cancer sources: Breast (40%) > lung (14%) > prostate (12%)

CLINICAL ISSUES

- Skull base mets from extracranial primaries occur in 4% of cancer patients
- Treatment: Radiotherapy is mainstay for focal/isolated disease; ± chemo; surgery for palliation/symptom control

DIAGNOSTIC CHECKLIST

- Consider metastatic disease if skull base lesion seen in patient with known malignancy who develops craniofacial pain or cranial neuropathy

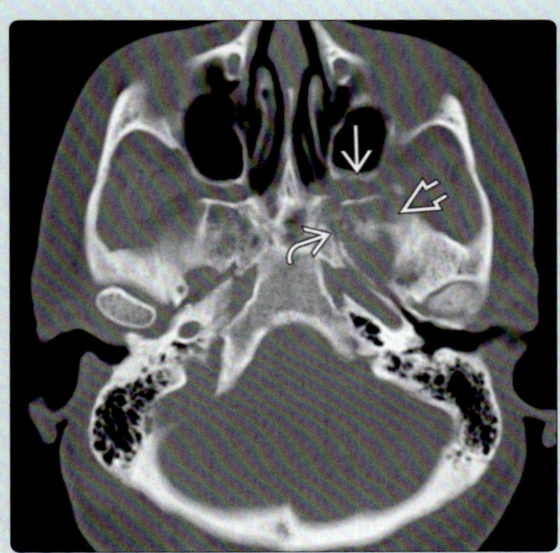

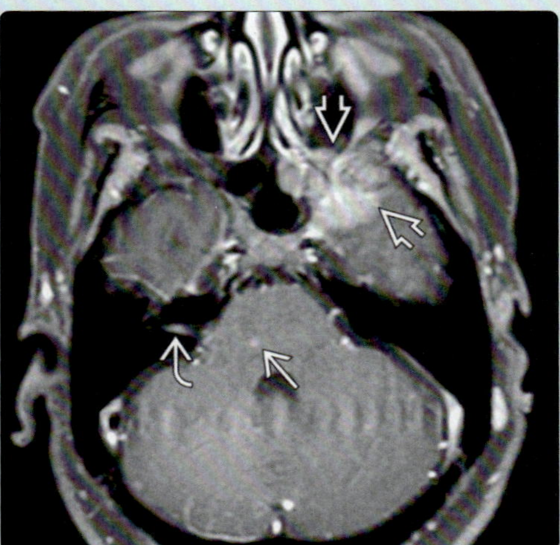

(Left) *Axial bone CT in a lung cancer patient with new left facial pain and dizziness shows a lytic lesion of the left sphenoid body ➡. Note erosion of the vidian canal ➡ and cortical irregularity of the margins of pterygopalatine fossa ➡ with associated soft tissue invasion.* **(Right)** *Axial T1 C+ FS MR reveals an enhancing mass ➡ of the sphenoid wing with dural invasion. Close inspection shows a leptomeningeal tumor in the right internal auditory canal ➡ and tiny pontine brain metastasis ➡.*

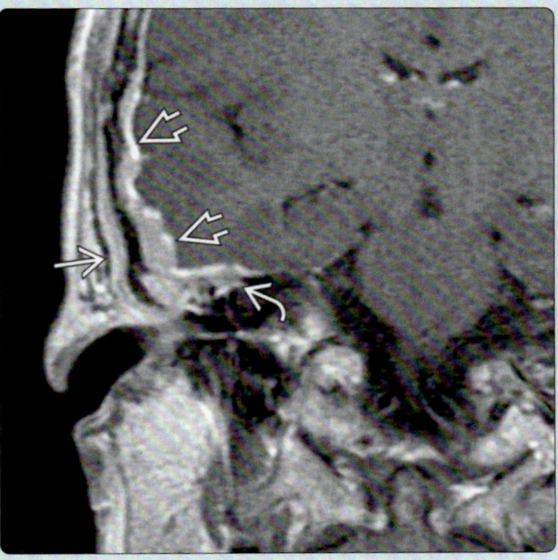

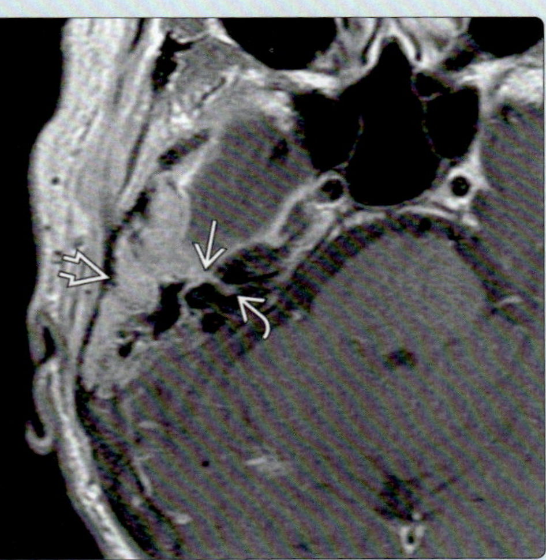

(Left) *Coronal T1 C+ MR in a 60 year old with breast cancer and right facial palsy shows a smooth, enhancing dural metastasis ➡ along the squamous temporal bone and petrous ridge. Tumor extends to the geniculate ganglion ➡. Note extracranial tumor lateral to the involved squamous temporal bone ➡.* **(Right)** *Axial T1 C+ MR shows thick dural tumor ➡ infiltrating the petrous ridge with perineural extension to CNVII geniculate ganglion ➡ to the fundus of the internal auditory canal ➡.*

Skull Base Chondrosarcoma

KEY FACTS

TERMINOLOGY

- Definition: Chondroid malignancy of skull base most commonly found in petrooccipital fissure

IMAGING

- Typical location **off-midline in petrooccipital fissure**
  - Off-midline location differentiates chondrosarcoma from midline chordoma in most cases
- CT findings
  - **Chondroid tumor matrix calcification** in **< 50%**
    - Arc or ring-like calcifications
    - Compared to chordoma fragmented destroyed bone
  - Sharp, narrow, nonsclerotic transition zone to adjacent normal bone
- MR findings
  - **High T2 signal** with scattered hypointense foci (calcifications)
  - Heterogeneously enhancing
  - Whorls of enhancing lines within tumor matrix often seen
- Consider MRA or CTA for preoperative characterization of vessel involvement

TOP DIFFERENTIAL DIAGNOSES

- Chordoma
- Skull base metastasis
- Plasmacytoma
- Nasopharyngeal carcinoma (invasive)
- Meningioma
- Benign petrous apex lesions

CLINICAL ISSUES

- Typically middle-aged patient with insidious onset of headache & cranial nerve palsies (especially CNVI)
- Treatment: Combined radical resection & postoperative, high-dose, fractionated precision conformal radiotherapy most often utilized

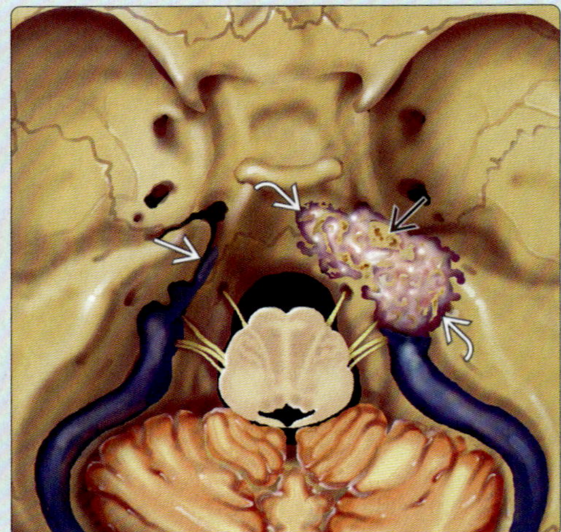
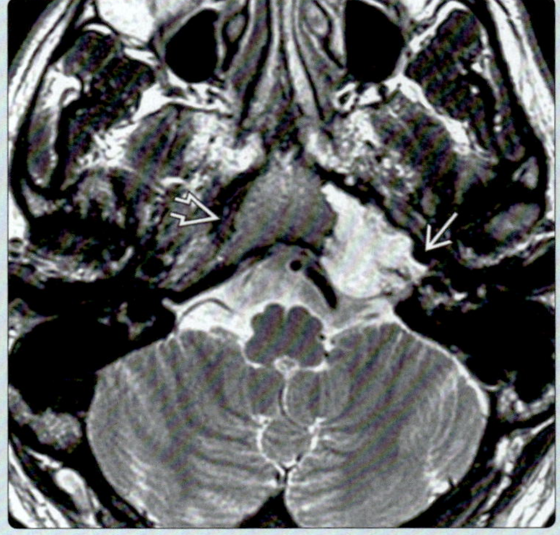

(Left) *Axial graphic depicts the classic location of a chondrosarcoma of the skull base centered in the left petrooccipital fissure* ➔. *Note the normal right petrooccipital fissure* ➔. *Chondroid calcifications, depicted in yellow, are present within the lesion* ➔. **(Right)** *Axial T2 MR reveals a large, high-signal chondrosarcoma of the left petrooccipital fissure. Note that the vertical segment of the petrous internal carotid artery is compressed* ➔. *Note the normal right petrooccipital fissure* ➔.

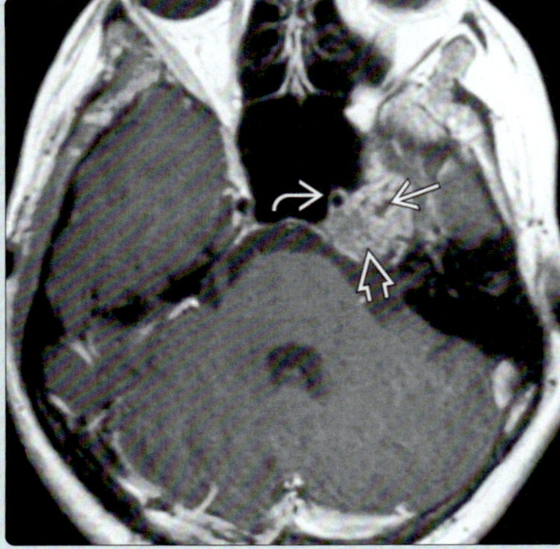
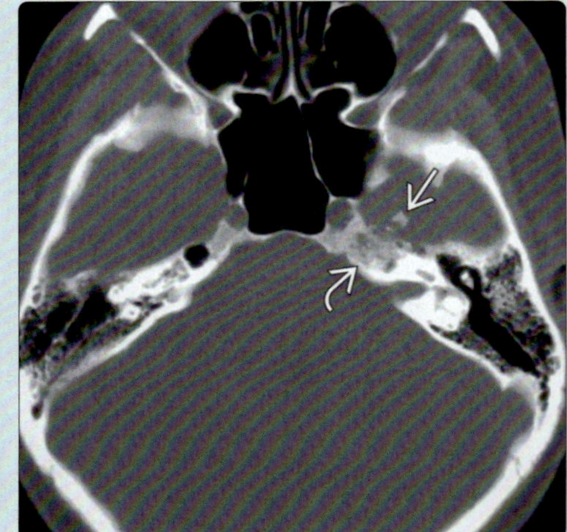

(Left) *Axial T1 C+ MR shows mottled enhancement* ➔ *within a chondrosarcoma centered at the left petrooccipital fissure. Calcified matrix is seen as a focal low signal intensity area* ➔ *within the otherwise enhancing tumor. The left internal carotid artery is patent* ➔. **(Right)** *Axial bone CT demonstrates typical chondroid calcification* ➔ *in a left petrooccipital fissure chondrosarcoma. In this case, no significant destruction of the adjacent petrous apex* ➔ *is appreciated.*

KEY FACTS

TERMINOLOGY

- Definition: Neoplasm composed of malignant cells producing osteoid matrix, or immature bone

IMAGING

- Very rare in skull base → clivus, parasellar, sphenoid wing, & anterior skull base
- CT findings
  - Often destructive & expansile
  - May be **lytic** or **blastic**
  - May show **tumor bone formation** & periosteal reaction
- MR findings
  - Heterogeneous low to intermediate T1 signal
  - Intermediate to high T2 signal; bone components ↓ T2 signal
  - Marrow/soft tissue enhancement

TOP DIFFERENTIAL DIAGNOSES

- Chordoma
- Chondrosarcoma
- Metastatic disease
- Plasmacytoma
- Non-Hodgkin lymphoma
- Invasive macroadenoma

PATHOLOGY

- May occur as late effect of previous irradiation
- Associated with Paget disease, fibrous dysplasia, giant cell tumor, Ollier disease, chronic osteomyelitis

CLINICAL ISSUES

- Nonspecific symptoms: Swelling, pain
- Present in 3rd-4th decade; M = F
- Difficult to completely resect due to proximity to critical structures within skull base
- Relatively resistant to radiation therapy
- Treatment: Maximal safe surgical resection with adjuvant radiation therapy

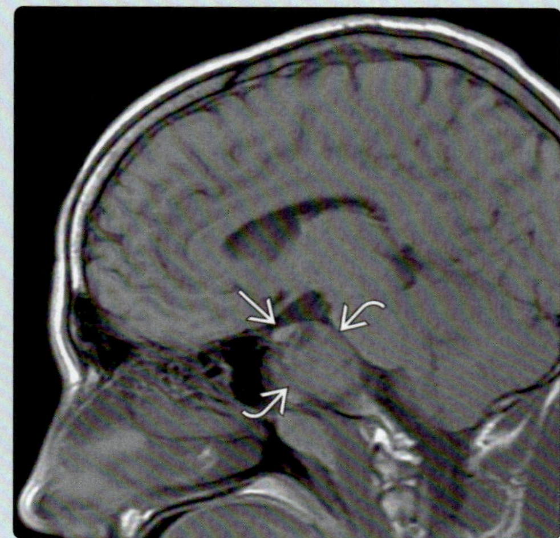

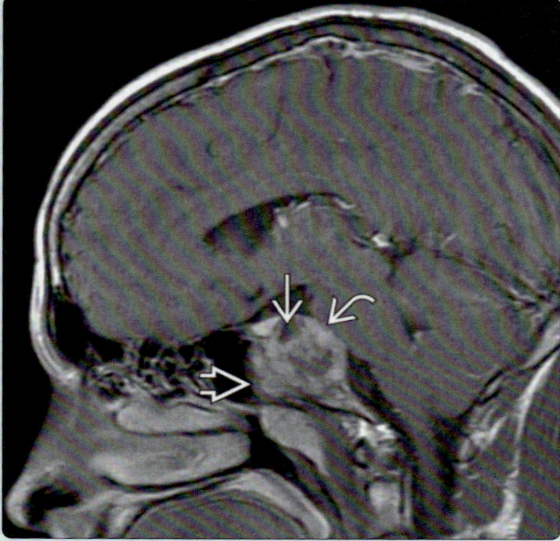

(Left) *Sagittal T1WI MR demonstrates an expansile, intermediate-signal clival osteosarcoma ➡. Normal pituitary parenchyma ➡ is seen at the superior aspect of the mass. This finding helps to exclude invasive pituitary adenoma from the differential diagnosis.* **(Right)** *Sagittal T1WI C+ MR in the same patient shows heterogeneous enhancement throughout the mass ➡. Note extension into the sphenoid sinus ➡. Nonenhancing foci with hypointense signal ➡ may represent areas of osteoid.*

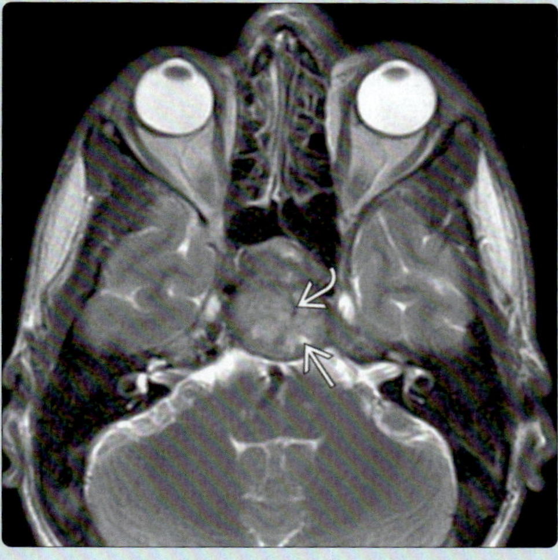

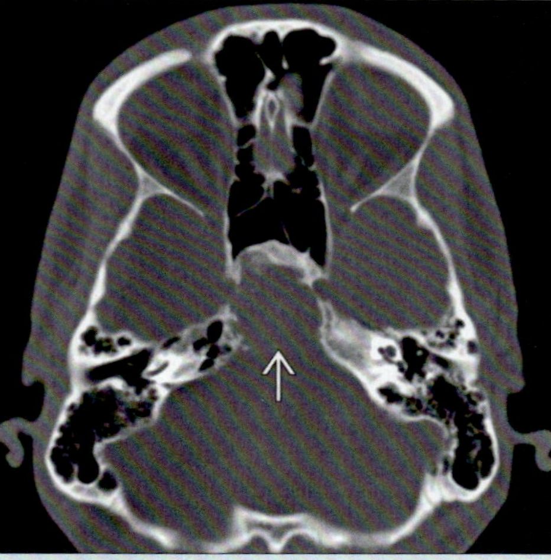

(Left) *Axial T2WI MR in the same patient shows heterogeneous, intermediate signal with areas of higher signal ➡, which may be due to focal necrosis. Curvilinear lower signal area may represent an area of internal calcification ➡.* **(Right)** *Axial bone CT in the same patient shows that this osteosarcoma is predominantly lytic. There is some expansion of the clivus with a large area of bone destruction posteriorly ➡. This lesion does not show osteoid matrix.*

Summary Thoughts: Skull Base & Facial Trauma

Skull base fractures (fxs) require considerable force & are often associated with other craniofacial injuries. Blunt trauma is responsible for over 90% of skull base & facial fxs & are frequently related to vehicular accidents. Injuries may range from a solitary linear fx to complex injuries involving the craniofacial skeleton. Associated intracranial injuries, such as cerebral contusion, intra-/extraaxial hemorrhage, dural tears, & vascular injuries, are common in these cases. The objective of imaging in these trauma patients is to depict the location & extent of fxs & to recognize associated injuries to vital structures. Accurate imaging interpretation also aids in surgical planning & in preventing complications.

Imaging Approaches & Indications

High-resolution bone algorithm CT is the modality of choice for imaging skull base & facial trauma. Thin-slice (0.6-1.0 mm) axial images extend from the skull vertex through the facial bones with coronal & sagittal reformatted images generated from the axial data set. Sagittal reformatted images are helpful for assessing injuries to the anterior & central skull base (ASB & CSB), particularly in patients with CSF leak. **3D-reformatted** images of facial fxs are beneficial for surgical planning as they provide a more anatomic representation of fx malalignment prior to reconstruction.

Patients with **CSF leak** or **recurrent meningitis** usually have visible defects in the ASB & CSB that are demonstrated with high-resolution bone CT. If a defect is not identified on bone CT or there are multiple fxs & it is unclear which is the source of the leak, CT cisternography may better delineate the leak site.

Arterial vascular injuries may be seen with CSB fxs that traverse the carotid canals. CTA can be performed in these patients to assess for **dissection**, traumatic **pseudoaneurysm**, or presence of **carotid-cavernous fistula**. Fxs of the petrous temporal bones & posterior fossa may extend into the major venous sinuses, resulting in posterior fossa epidural hematoma or posttraumatic venous thrombosis. CTV or MRV may be obtained in such cases. Conventional angiography is typically not necessary but used for treating vascular complications.

Cerebral injuries are often seen in high-impact trauma. Although MR is not performed initially, it is more sensitive for assessing the degree of parenchymal injury.

Approaches to Imaging Issues in Skull Base & Facial Trauma

Anterior Skull Base

ASB, or frontobasal, trauma is frequently associated with injury to the sinonasal cavities & orbits. The majority of these patients have facial injuries, including fxs of the frontal bone, orbital roofs, & cribriform plates (CP). Imaging analysis should address the following questions.

- Do fx lines involve CP or traverse anterior or posterior walls of frontal sinuses?
- Do fxs involve orbital apex or optic canals?

Central Skull Base

CSB (lateral basal) trauma may involve the sphenoid sinus walls, cavernous sinuses, & clivus & may present with carotid vascular injury or cranial nerves (CNs) III, IV, VI, or CNVI-III deficits. Imaging analysis should address the following questions.

- Are walls of sphenoid sinuses, carotid canals, & clivus intact?
- Do cavernous sinuses appear symmetric?

Temporal Bone

Petrous temporal fxs typically have a longitudinal or transverse trajectory. The longitudinal type more often spares the otic capsule traversing the mastoid & middle ear cavities & squamous portion & may result in ossicular chain disruption. Transverse fxs more often involve the otic capsule extending into the occipital bone after traversing the inner ear. Imaging analysis should address the following questions.

- Does main fx line involve or spare otic capsule?
- Is ossicular chain intact?
- Does fx traverse inner ear or CNVII canal?
- Does fx traverse tegmen?

Posterior Skull Base

Fxs of the occipital bones may be isolated or associated with transverse petrous ridge fxs. The fx may extend into a dural venous sinus, jugular foramen (CNIX-XI), or CNXII canal. Craniocervical junction injuries should also be suspected in these patients. Imaging analysis should address the following questions.

- Does fx extend into transverse sinus, sigmoid sinus, or jugular foramen?
- Does fx involve internal auditory canal or hypoglossal canal?

Orbital Trauma

Orbital fxs are classified as follows: (1) Those involving the orbital walls, frequently the inferior orbital rim & (2) the orbital "blowout" fx. Blowout fxs may involve the orbital floor or medial orbital wall, but the inferior orbital rim remains intact. Imaging analysis should address the following questions.

- Is there **entrapment** of inferior ± medial rectus muscles & fat; how large & displaced are fx fragments?
- Is fx isolated or are other orbital or facial fxs present [zygomaticomaxillary complex fx (ZMC), nasoorbitalethmoid fx (NOE), Le Fort]?

Transfacial Fracture (Le Fort)

There are 3 types of Le Fort fxs, & a consistent feature of all 3 types is the presence of bilateral pterygoid plate fxs. Le Fort I is a horizontal fx through the maxilla involving the piriform aperture. Le Fort II is a pyramidal fx involving the nasofrontal junction, infraorbital rims, medial orbital walls & orbital floors, & zygomaticomaxillary suture lines. Le Fort III (craniofacial separation) consists of fxs at the nasofrontal junction extending laterally through the lateral orbital walls & zygomatic arches. Le Fort fxs are rarely pure & are often seen in combination with other fxs. Imaging analysis should address the following questions.

- Which Le Fort types are involved; are fxs same on each side of face?
- Are other facial fx patterns present (ZMC, NOE)?

Zygomaticomaxillary Complex Fracture

The prominent position of the zygomatic arch makes it susceptible to trauma. This fx type was formerly referred to as the tripod fx; however, that is a misnomer as the zygoma has 4 involved articulations, & 5 distinct fxs are evident. Imaging analysis should address the following questions.

- How displaced & comminuted is ZMC fx?

Temporal Bone, Skull Base, & Facial Trauma Complications

Fracture Locations/Type	Potential Complications
Skull Base Trauma	
Anterior skull base	Posterior wall frontal sinus contaminated fx; cribriform plate fx: CSF leak/cephalocele/meningitis, CNI injury; orbital apex or optic canal fx: CNII injury
Central skull base	Internal carotid artery injury: Thrombosis, dissection, pseudoaneurysm, CCF; sphenoid sinus superior wall fx: CSF leak/cephalocele if dural tear; CNs at risk: CNIII, IV, VI, CNVI-III
Posterior skull base	Transvenous sinus fx: Venous sinus thrombosis, epidural hematoma; CNs at risk: CNVII-VIII (internal auditory canal); CNIX-XI (jugular foramen); CNXII (hypoglossal canal)
Temporal bone	Tegmen mastoideum/tympani fx: CSF leak/cephalocele if dural tear; conductive or sensorineural hearing loss; CNs at risk: CNVII (facial nerve canal fx), CNVIII (transcochlear fx)
Orbital Trauma	
Medial blowout	Medial rectus entrapment; diplopia, enophthalmos
Inferior blowout	Inferior rectus entrapment; infraorbital nerve injury, diplopia, enophthalmos
Foreign body	Globe rupture; CNII laceration/transection; infection
Facial Trauma	
Transfacial (Le Fort I-III), zygomaticomaxillary complex fx, complex midfacial, nasoorbitalethmoid fxs	Traumatic telecanthus, nasolacrimal apparatus injury, epiphora, inferior orbital nerve injury (CNV2), malocclusion, mucocele
Mandibular fx	Trismus, inferior alveolar nerve injury, infection, loss of teeth

- What is extent of involvement of orbital floor, orbital apex, & lamina papyracea?
- How is lateral orbital wall displaced, & is pterygoid plate fractured?

Complex Midfacial Fracture

The complex midfacial fx or "facial smash injury" consists of multiple facial fxs that cannot be classified as one of the named patterns (Le Fort, ZMC, NOE). Imaging analysis should address where the fxs are concentrated & the presence of associated orbital or skull base injuries.

Nasoorbitalethmoid Fracture

High-force trauma to the nasal bones is transmitted to the ethmoid sinuses & orbits in NOE fxs. The **medial canthal tendon** (MCT) may be disrupted in these cases & fxs may extend into the lacrimal apparatus. Imaging analysis should address the following questions.

- Is bone fragment to which MCT attaches displaced or comminuted?
- Is nasal bridge displaced posteriorly into ethmoids or superiorly into anterior fossa?
- Are there injuries to CP, frontal recess, or globes?

Mandible Fracture

Mandible fxs may occur within the alveolus (parasymphysis, body, or angle) or posterior to the teeth (ascending ramus, subcondylar region, condyle, or coronoid process). The mandible is essentially a ring of bone & multiple fxs are common, often bilaterally. Fx fragment displacement is affected by muscular attachments to the bone. Imaging analysis should address the following questions.

- Where are fxs located, & what is degree & direction of displacement?
- Is inferior alveolar foramen or canal involved?
- Are condyles subluxed or dislocated?
- Do fxs involve periodontal ligament space (tooth socket)?

Clinical Implications

Understanding the mechanisms & complications of injury is essential for managing skull base trauma. The objective of treatment in patients with facial trauma is to stabilize & restore facial anatomy & to provide skeletal support for the function of mastication. Treatment is also directed toward relief of early & prevention of late complications.

Clinical signs of ASB injury include epistaxis, proptosis, chemosis, rhinorrhea, anosmia, & visual deficits. In addition to CSF leak, patients with fxs of the posterior frontal sinus wall or CP are at risk for subsequent meningitis. Fxs at the orbital apex & optic canal may cause visual deficits. Signs of temporal bone trauma may include postauricular hematoma (Battle sign), hemotympanum, otorrhea, conductive or sensorineural hearing loss, vertigo, or facial weakness. Clinical signs of posterior skull base trauma include symptoms of mass effect from epidural hematoma related to dural sinus trauma or lower cranial never deficits.

In patients with midfacial trauma, injuries to the palate, maxilla, & mandible should be assessed at imaging, as lack of appropriate repair can result in malocclusion. Depending on the degree, orbital floor involvement in patients with a ZMC fx will likely require surgical reduction. Orbital wall fxs will be treated if there is entrapment of the extraocular muscles, impingement upon the orbital apex or middle cranial fossa, or to prevent globe malposition that is resulting in diplopia or enophthalmos. Traumatic telecanthus & damage to the lacrimal drainage pathway are complications of NOE fxs that require surgical intervention.

Selected References

1. Fraioli RE et al: Facial fractures: beyond Le Fort. Otolaryngol Clin North Am. 41(1):51-76, vi, 2008
2. Samii M et al: Skull base trauma: diagnosis and management. Neurol Res. 24(2):147-56, 2002

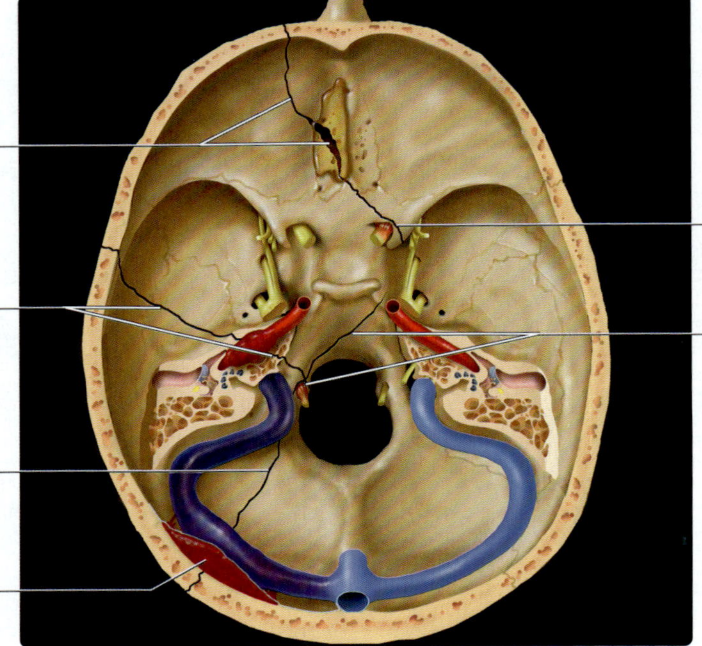

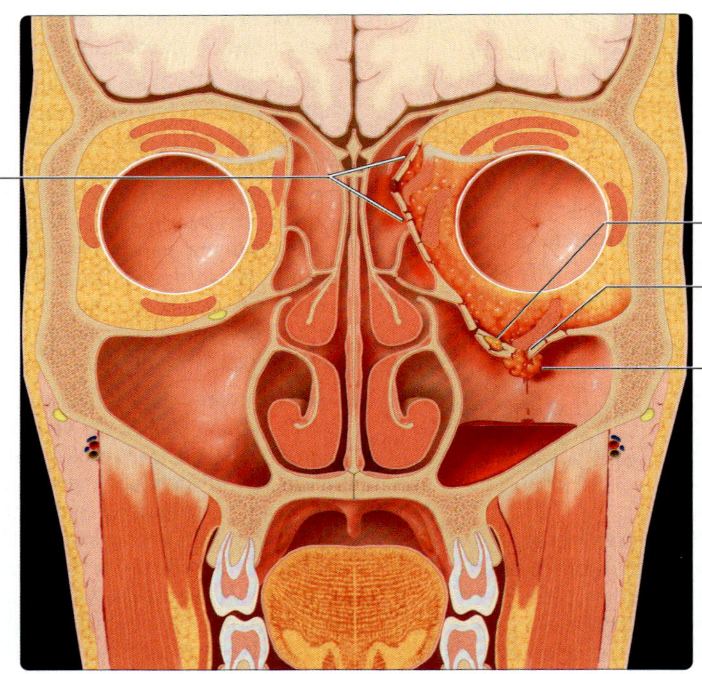

(Top) *Graphic of endocranial view of the skull base shows multiple fractures with expected complications. An anterior skull base fracture crosses the cribriform plate & extends into the optic canal. A fracture through the right middle fossa extends through the petrous apex involving the petrous carotid canal. An oblique clival fracture extends into the hypoglossal canal. A posterior fossa occipital fracture damages the transverse sinus & causes an extraaxial hemorrhage.* **(Bottom)** *Coronal graphic illustrates a medial & inferior blowout fracture on the left. The medial blowout fracture displaces the lamina papyracea medially into the ethmoid sinus. An inferior blowout fracture of the floor of the orbit (maxillary sinus roof) with infraorbital nerve injury is depicted. Herniation of the inferior rectus muscle & orbital fat into the maxillary sinus may occur with variably sized floor fractures. A blow to the anterior orbit/globe, such as from a baseball, may cause either both or one of these fractures.*

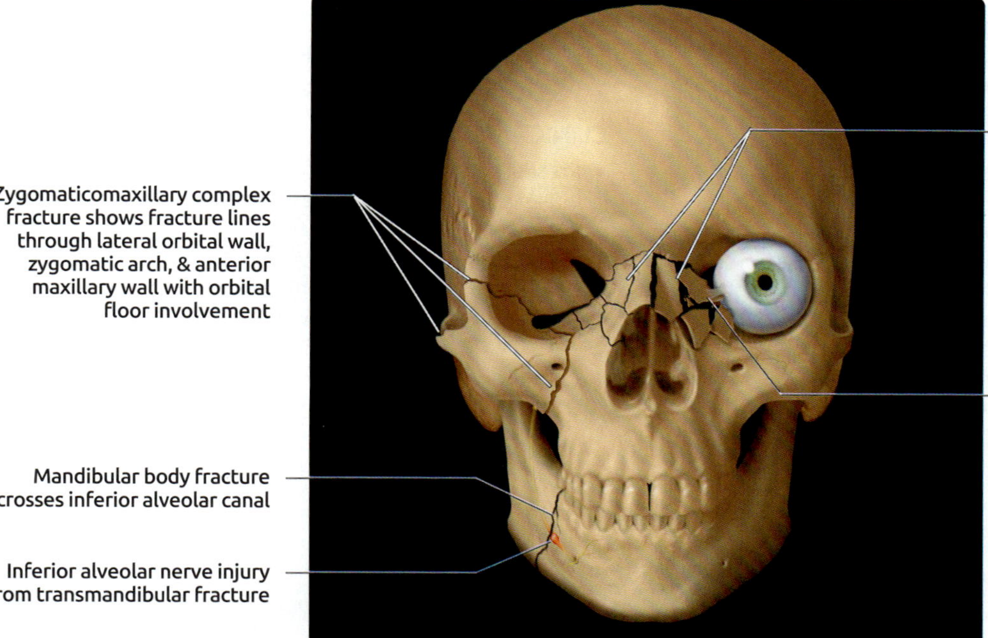

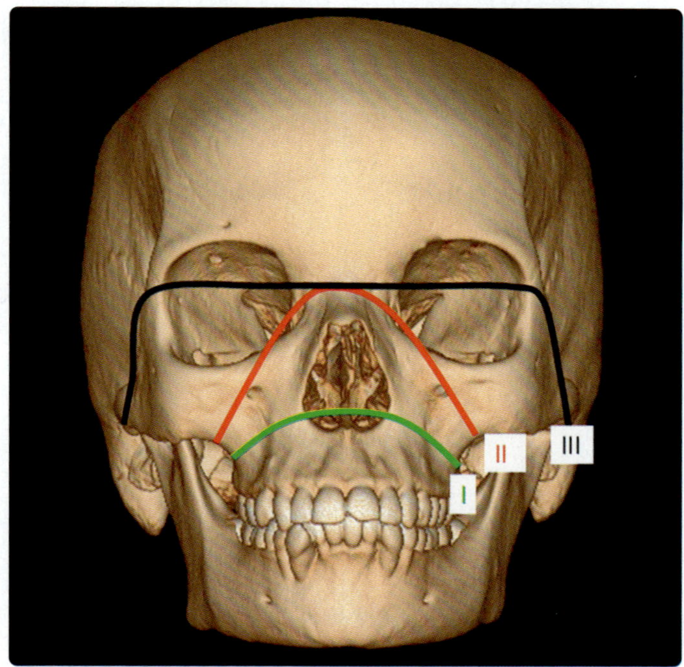

(Top) *Frontal graphic demonstrates fractures of the midface.* **(Bottom)** *Coronal graphic shows lines defining the 3 types of Le Fort fractures. Le Fort I (green) involves the nasal aperture & essentially separates the maxilla & palate from the remaining midface. Le Fort II (red) traverses the inferior orbital rim & is also known as the pyramidal fracture due to its configuration. The Le Fort III (black), or craniofacial separation, extends through the zygomatic arches. A common feature of all 3 Le Fort fracture types is involvement of the pterygoid plates (not shown).*

Temporal Bone Fractures

KEY FACTS

IMAGING

- Bone algorithm MDCT with coronal reconstructions, CTA/MRA for suspected vascular injury
  - Dedicated brain imaging critical to evaluate for intracranial injuries (present in up to 90%)
- **Longitudinal fractures**: Vertical plane parallels long axis of petrous ridge (PR)
  - EAC, middle ear (ME)/ossicular involvement common
    - Otic capsule (OC) involvement rare
- **Transverse fractures**: Perpendicular to PR long axis
  - OC involvement, facial nerve (CNVII) injury very common; EAC/ME involvement rare
- **Oblique fractures**: Mixed features, typically horizontal and parallel to PR long axis
- **OC-violating vs. OC-sparing** classification best predicts complications, such as hearing loss, CNVII injury, CSF leak
- **Ossicular injuries: Dislocations** > > fractures, incus most commonly involved
- **CNVII injuries**: Most commonly at **geniculate ganglion**; symptoms often resolve spontaneously
- All varieties: Assess for tegmen fracture (CSF leak), carotid canal injury, extension to central skull base

TOP DIFFERENTIAL DIAGNOSES

- Pseudofractures: Sutures, fissures, canaliculi, aqueducts

CLINICAL ISSUES

- Presentation: Depends on fracture location
  - Hearing loss: **Conductive** (ossicle injury, blood/fluid) or **sensorineural** (transotic fracture); audiogram typically obtained at ≥ 6 weeks to differentiate
  - Peripheral facial nerve paralysis
    - Electroneuronography and electromyography after 3 days to determine nerve integrity; explore if concern over transection
  - CSF leak (tegmen fracture) or perilymphatic fistula: typically resolve spontaneously

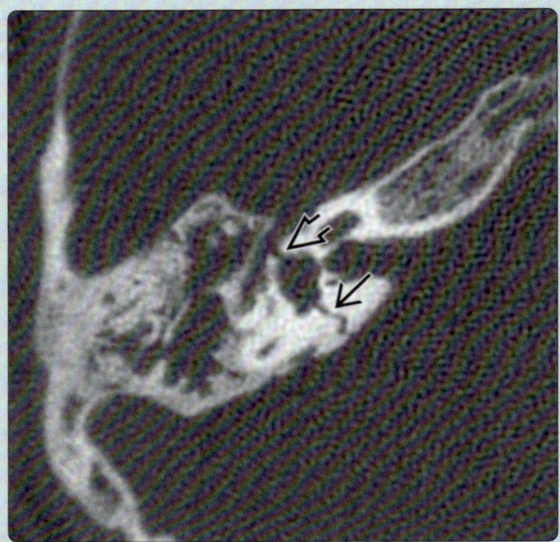

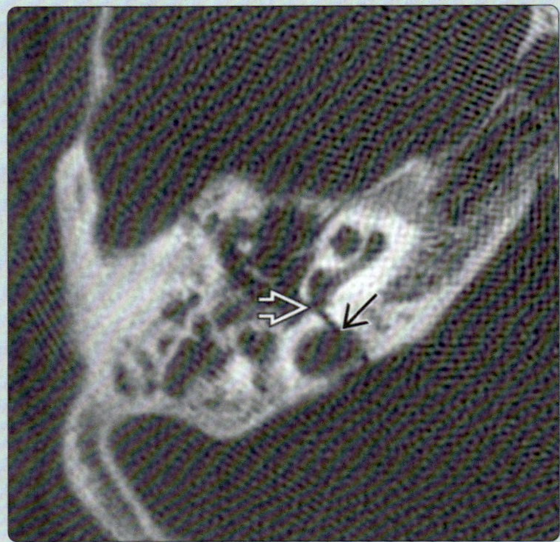

(Left) *Axial bone CT in a 14 year old following severe head injury shows a medial transverse, otic capsule-violating fracture → traversing the vestibule with extension into the medial aspect of the tympanic facial nerve canal ⇨.* **(Right)** *Axial bone CT more inferiorly in the same patient shows typical inferior extension of the fracture across the jugular foramen → into the round window niche ➡.*

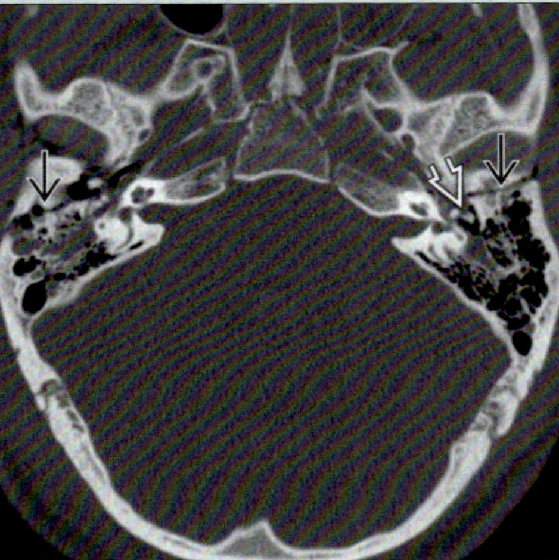

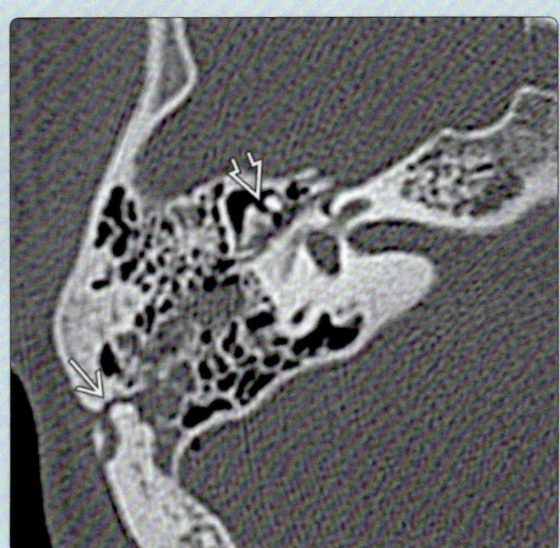

(Left) *Axial bone CT shows bilateral otic capsule-sparing fractures →. In addition, on the left is a malleoincudal dislocation ➡.* **(Right)** *Axial bone CT in a patient with head trauma shows the posterior aspect of a longitudinal temporal bone fracture ➡ and subtle medial subluxation of the malleus head ➡, seen as the "ice cream" sliding off of the "cone."*

KEY FACTS

TERMINOLOGY

- Injury to ossicles; dislocation or subluxation > > fracture

IMAGING

- **Malalignment or dislocation** of ossicle articulations
- **Incudostapedial** > incudomalleolar > complete incus dislocation > stapediovestibular disruption > malleus dislocation
- **Incudostapedial dislocation**
  - Incus lenticular process off stapes head
- **Incudomalleolar dislocation/disruption**
  - Axial CT: Ice cream falling off of cone appearance
  - Sagittal CT: Disruption of molar tooth
  - Coronal CT: Broken heart sign = malleus/incus seen adjacent to each other with dislocation cleft in between
- **Incus dislocation**
  - Disrupted incudomalleolar & incudostapedial joints → incus dissociating from malleus & stapes
- **Stapes dislocation/stapediovestibular disruption**
  - Suspect if transverse fracture through oval window
  - Actual disruption difficult to see, < 1-mm images may identify stapes fragments or footplate malalignment
- **Malleus dislocation**
  - Rare traumatic ossicle finding

TOP DIFFERENTIAL DIAGNOSES

- Congenital ossicular anomalies and fixation
- Ossicular prosthesis
- Chronic otomastoiditis with ossicular erosions
- Congenital or acquired cholesteatoma with ossicular erosions

CLINICAL ISSUES

- Posttraumatic **conductive hearing loss**
- Treatment options
  - Ossicular reconstruction with repositioning or interpositioning of various materials
    - PORP, TORP, incus interposition

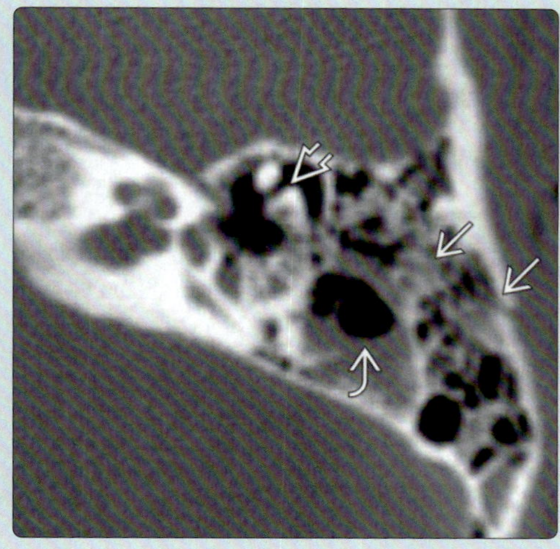

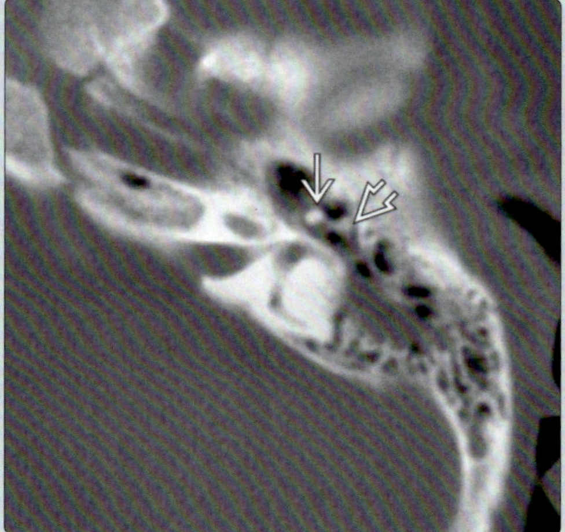

(Left) *Axial bone CT in a 7 year old who fell 8 feet shows a longitudinal, otic capsule-sparing temporal bone fracture ➡, mild widening of the incudomalleolar joint ➡, and blood in the antrum ➡.* **(Right)** *Axial bone CT in a 12 year old involved in an all-terrain vehicle accident demonstrates medial dislocation of the malleus head ➡ relative to the incus body ➡, resulting in the ice cream falling off of the cone appearance, typical of incudomalleolar dislocation.*

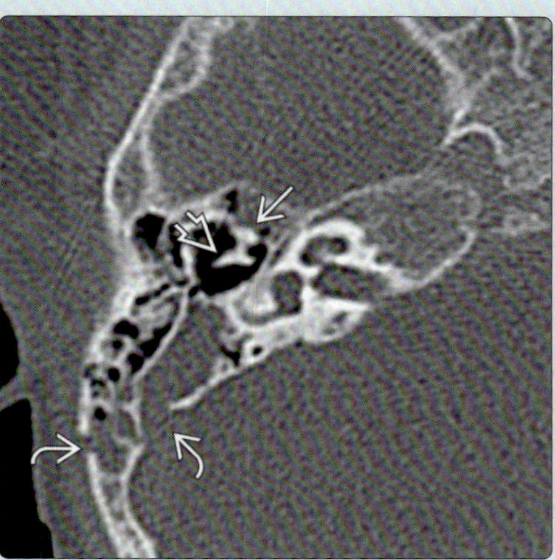

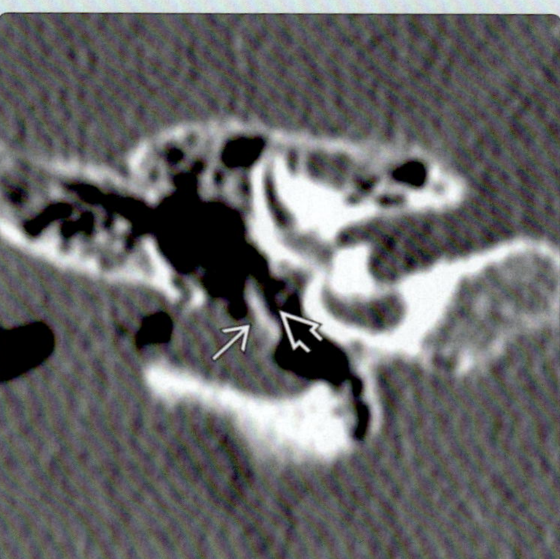

(Left) *Axial bone CT in an 18 month old after a TV fell on his head shows malposition and malrotation of the malleus head ➡ and the incus body ➡ as well as a diastatic mastoid fracture ➡.* **(Right)** *Coronal reformat bone CT in the same child also shows inferior position of the incus long process ➡ relative to the stapes head ➡, consistent with incus dislocation secondary to incudomalleolar and incudostapedial joint disruption.*

Skull Base Trauma

KEY FACTS

TERMINOLOGY

- Traumatic injury of bony anterior, middle, or posterior cranial fossa

IMAGING

- Noncorticated, noninterdigitating lucency + pneumocephalus or intraorbital emphysema
- Location
  - Anterior fossa: Frontal bone-sinus, cribriform plate
  - Middle fossa: Greater sphenoid wing, sphenoid sinus, clivus
  - Posterior fossa: Petrous temporal bone, occiput
- Protocol advice
  - Bone CT: Skull + facial bones + cervical spine
  - NECT: Brain + neck soft tissues
  - CTA or MRA/MRV: Suspected neurovascular injury
  - MR brain: Suspected cerebral injury

TOP DIFFERENTIAL DIAGNOSES

- Pseudofractures
  - Sutures and fissures
  - Canals and foramina
  - Emissary veins and venous sinuses

PATHOLOGY

- Associated abnormalities
  - Intracranial contusion, hematoma
  - Pneumocephalus
  - Neurovascular injury
  - CSF fistula/leak
  - Cranial nerve deficits

CLINICAL ISSUES

- Results from high-velocity impact: Motor or ATV vehicle accident, gunshot/missile
- Management triaged according to degree/severity of intracranial injury

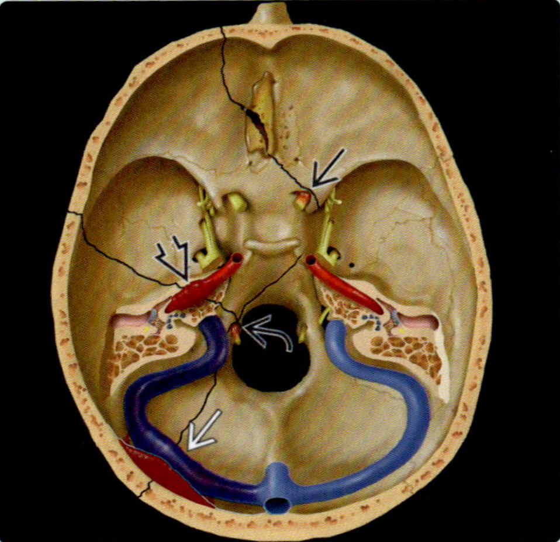

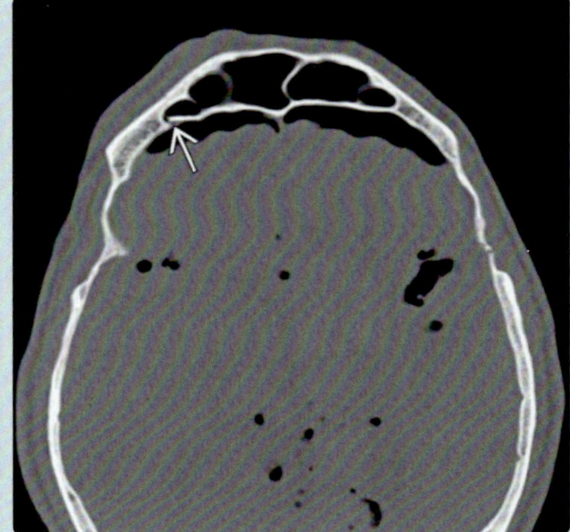

(Left) *Endocranial view of skull base (SB) fractures shows an anterior SB fracture crossing the cribriform plate and optic canal ➡. The middle fossa fracture injures the horizontal petrous internal carotid artery ➡. The posterior fossa fracture injures the hypoglossal nerve ➡ and transverse sinus ➡.* **(Right)** *Axial bone CT shows a fracture of the right frontal sinus posterior wall ➡. This fracture accounts for the source of pneumocephalus and places the patient at risk for meningitis.*

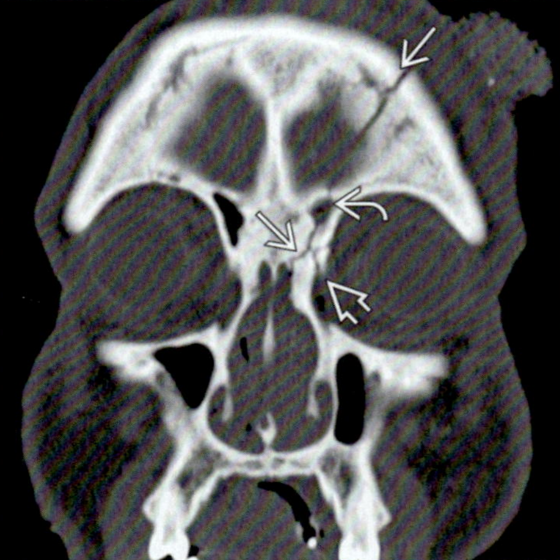

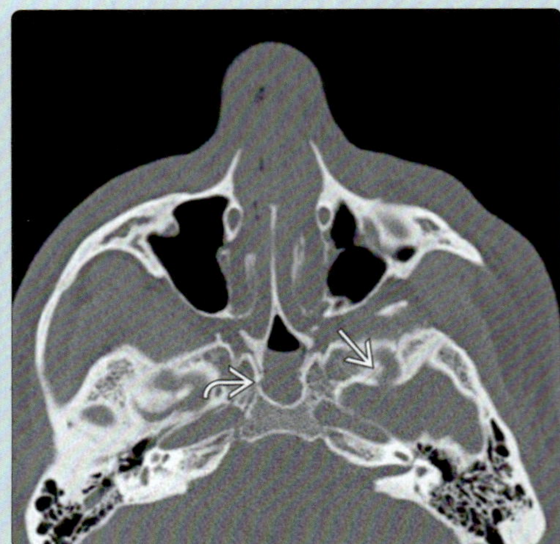

(Left) *Coronal bone CT shows an anterior skull base/type III frontobasal fracture with a large fracture ➡ extending through the left frontal bone to the nasoorbitoethmoid complex. The fracture traverses the left frontal sinus ➡ and terminates in the region of the left lacrimal sac ➡.* **(Right)** *Axial bone CT shows middle cranial fossa fractures through the left greater wing of the sphenoid bone ➡ and lateral wall of the right sphenoid sinus ➡. Fractures of the middle cranial fossa often involve vascular canals or neural foramina.*

Orbital Foreign Body

KEY FACTS

TERMINOLOGY

- Foreign material introduced into orbit via trauma

IMAGING

- CT is sensitive and safe modality for detecting foreign body (FB)
  - Density and shape indicate nature of object
  - **Metal** density > 1,000-2,000 HU, attenuation artifact
    - Firearms, workplace materials
  - **Glass** denser than bone, wide variation
    - Pane shards or safety glass fragments
  - **Wood** typically low density, similar to air when dry
    - Pencils with dense stylus core, tree branches
  - **Miscellaneous** objects of any origin
    - Plastic or sponge very low density, similar to air
    - Sand or gravel dense granular material
- Consider MR for possible FB if CT negative
  - Contraindicated if unknown ferromagneticity
  - Inflammation or granulation suggests organic material

TOP DIFFERENTIAL DIAGNOSES

- Ophthalmic surgical device
- Phthisis bulbi
- Dystrophic calcification

PATHOLOGY

- Most FB occur with high-velocity or projectile injury
  - Hammering, occupational, assault, MVA
  - May occur after apparently trivial trauma

CLINICAL ISSUES

- Organic FB more likely to incite cellulitis and abscess
- All puncture wounds require exploration
- Surgical decision depends on type and location of FB

DIAGNOSTIC CHECKLIST

- CT is study of choice and should be performed 1st
- Occult FB discoveries are surprisingly common
- Assess for globe rupture and optic nerve injury

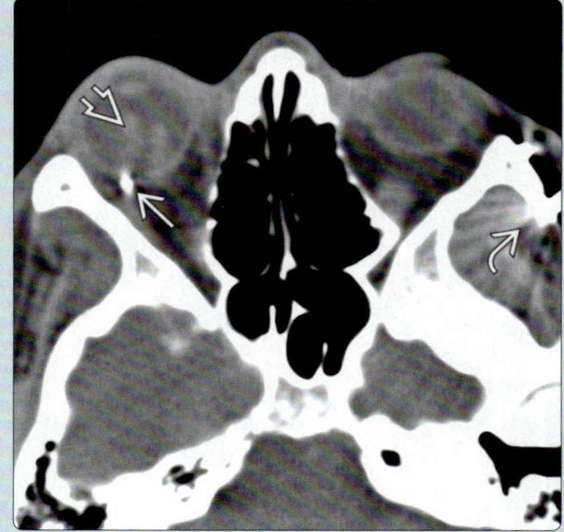

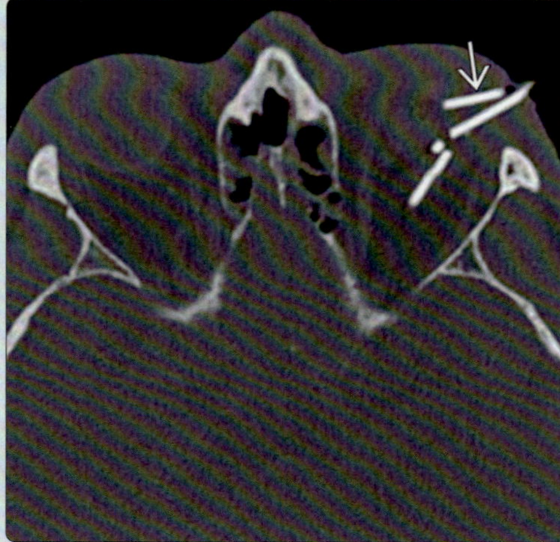

(Left) *Axial NECT in a patient who sustained a shotgun injury to the face shows shrapnel ➡ in the sclera posteriorly. The globe was ruptured, and there is intraocular hemorrhage ➡. Additional foreign body artifact is noted on the left ➡.* **(Right)** *Axial bone CT shows multiple well-defined hyperdense shards of glass penetrating the left orbit and perforating globe ➡. The patient had fallen face first onto a drinking glass while intoxicated.*

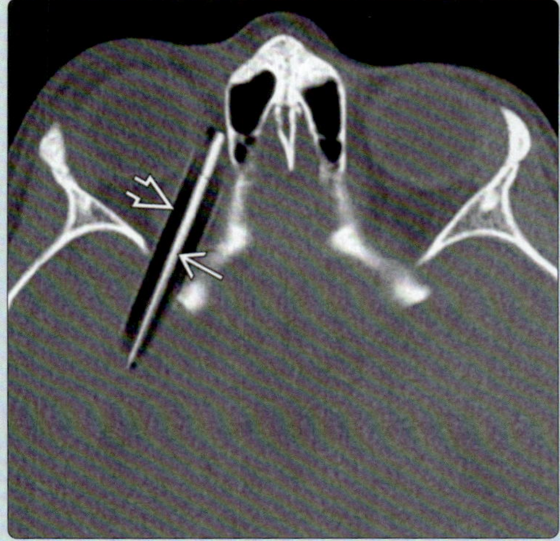

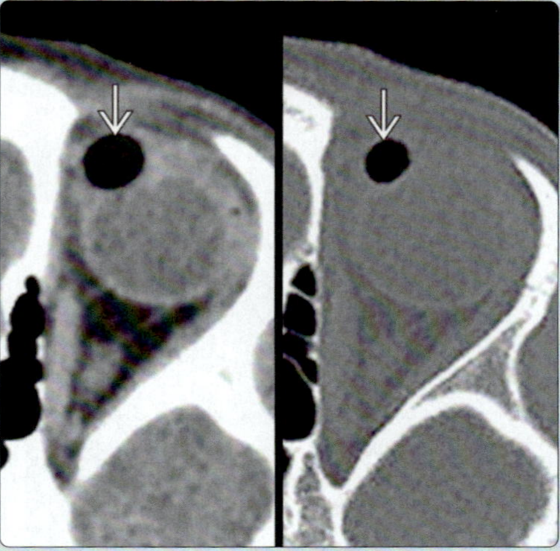

(Left) *Axial bone CT shows a piece of a broken pencil within the right orbit. The center dense core represents the pencil stylus ("lead") ➡. The outer casing of wood is low density ➡.* **(Right)** *Axial CT demonstrates a foreign body with very low density ➡ displayed at 2 different grayscale levels. Variable grayscale display is useful when assessing the nature of a foreign body, demonstrating in this case that the object is comprised of polystyrene foam, rather than air or a lipoid mass.*

KEY FACTS

TERMINOLOGY

- Traumatic deformity of orbital floor or medial wall resulting from impact of blunt object larger than orbital aperture

IMAGING

- High-resolution axial bone CT with coronal & sagittal reconstructions is modality of choice
- 2 broad categories of blowout fractures
  - Open door: Large, displaced, frequently comminuted
  - Trapdoor: Linear, hinged, minimally displaced
- Associated findings
  - Herniation of orbital contents through bony defect
  - Involvement of infraorbital canal
  - Orbital soft tissue injury
  - May occur in combination with other facial fractures (nasal, transfacial, zygomaticomaxillary complex)

TOP DIFFERENTIAL DIAGNOSES

- Dehiscent lamina papyracea
- Orbital decompression surgery
- Nasoorbitalethmoidal fracture

CLINICAL ISSUES

- Most common symptoms
  - Diplopia: Typically related to entrapment
  - Enophthalmos: Due to prolapse of orbital contents into sinuses
  - Hypesthesia of cheek and upper gum: Due to infraorbital nerve injury
- Treatment: Orbital floor reconstruction typically performed with alloplast (titanium mesh, porous polyethylene)

DIAGNOSTIC CHECKLIST

- Entrapment is clinical, not radiographic, diagnosis
  - Note abnormal position & morphology of extraocular muscles
- In children, minimally displaced but highly symptomatic trapdoor fractures are common

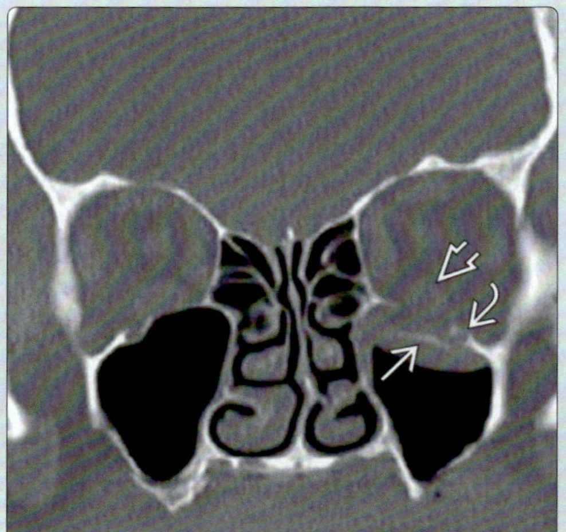

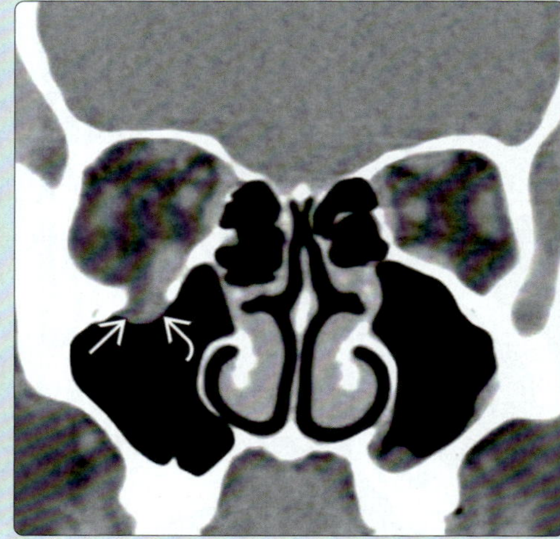

(Left) *Coronal bone CT demonstrates a mildly depressed left orbital floor orbital blowout fracture (OBF) ➡ just medial to the infraorbital canal ➡. The inferior rectus muscle ➡ is grossly normal in position and configuration.* **(Right)** *Coronal NECT reveals a chronic right orbital floor OBF with herniation of a small volume of fat ➡ and a portion of the inferior rectus muscle ➡ through the fracture defect. The muscle also demonstrates an abnormal vertical orientation.*

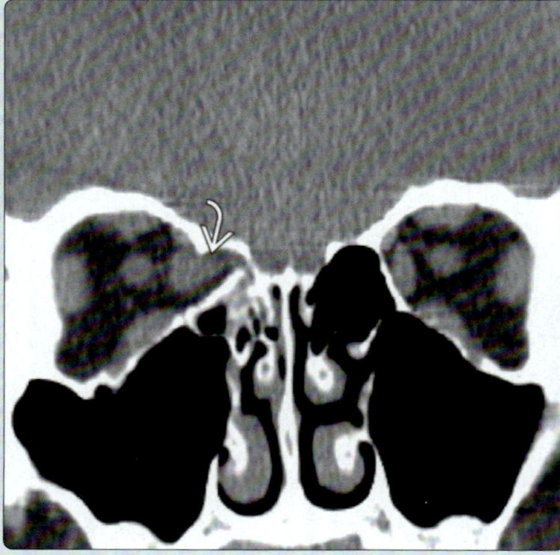

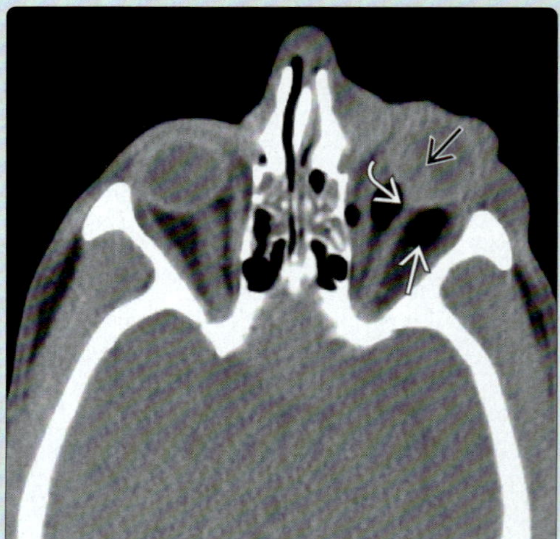

(Left) *Coronal soft tissue NECT shows deformity of the right medial rectus muscle entering the osseous defect of a lamina papyracea fracture ➡.* **(Right)** *Axial NECT shows retrobulbar orbital emphysema ➡ with associated proptosis and tenting of the optic nerve insertion ➡. There is also an intraocular hemorrhage ➡.*

KEY FACTS

TERMINOLOGY

- Fractures disrupting **pterygomaxillary junction**, disjoining portions of face (maxilla) from skull

IMAGING

- Best diagnostic clue: Pterygoid process and pterygoid plate fractures in patients with clinically mobile facial skeleton
- **Le Fort I**
  - Pyriform rim + medial & lateral walls of maxillary sinus or alveolus + nasal septum
- **Le Fort II**
  - Medial orbital wall, including frontomaxillary suture + nasofrontal junction; inferior orbital wall, including zygomaticomaxillary suture + inferior rim
- **Le Fort III**
  - Medial orbital wall, including frontomaxillary suture + nasofrontal junction; lateral orbital wall, including zygomaticofrontal suture + zygomaticosphenoid suture + zygomatic arch

TOP DIFFERENTIAL DIAGNOSES

- Zygomaticomaxillary complex fracture
- Nasoorbitalethmoidal fracture
- Complex facial fracture
- Pterygoid plate avulsion

PATHOLOGY

- **Type I: "Floating palate"**
  - Inferior portions of medial & lateral maxillary buttresses
- **Type II: "Pyramidal fracture"**
  - Superior portion of medial maxillary buttress + inferior portion of lateral maxillary buttress
- **Type III: "Craniofacial dissociation"**
  - Superior portions of lateral and medial maxillary buttresses + upper transverse maxillary buttress

DIAGNOSTIC CHECKLIST

- Involvement of pterygoid processes/plates is common feature and sine qua non of Le Fort fractures

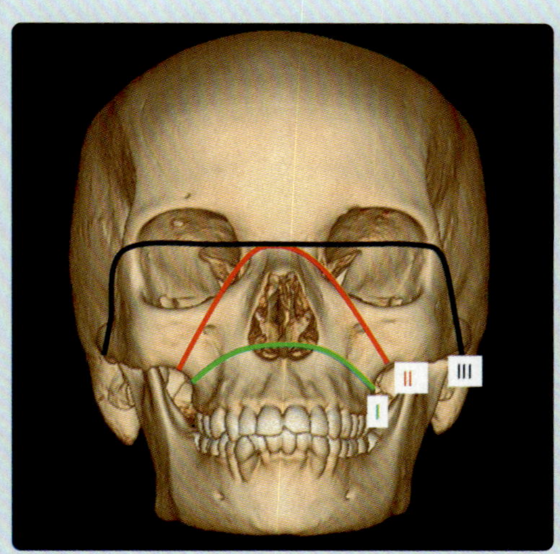

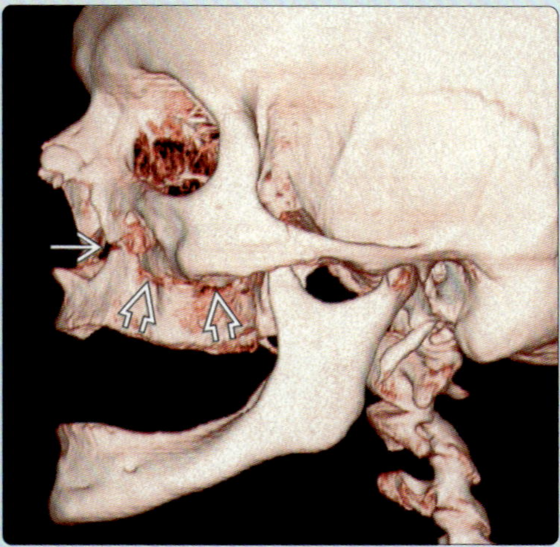

(Left) *Frontal graphic demonstrates the 3 types of Le Fort fractures: Le Fort I (green) involves the nasal aperture and piriform rim, Le Fort II (red) traverses the inferior and medial orbital walls, and Le Fort III (black) extends through the zygomatic arches and lateral and medial orbital walls.* **(Right)** *3D CT reformation shows a horizontal Le Fort I fracture ➡ separating the maxillary alveolus from the midface. Note the involvement of the nasal aperture ➡. The inferior orbital rim and zygomatic arch are intact.*

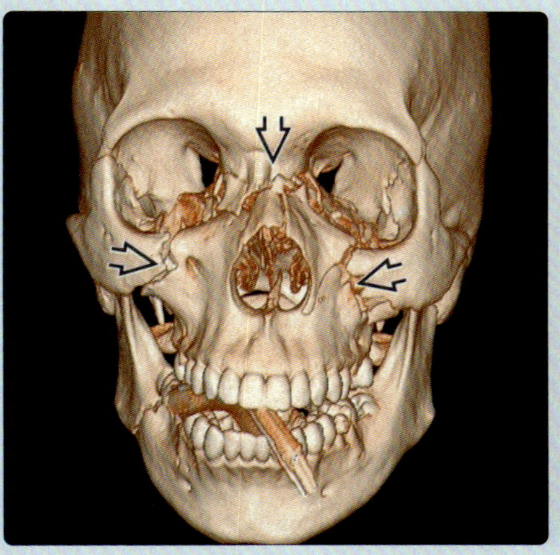

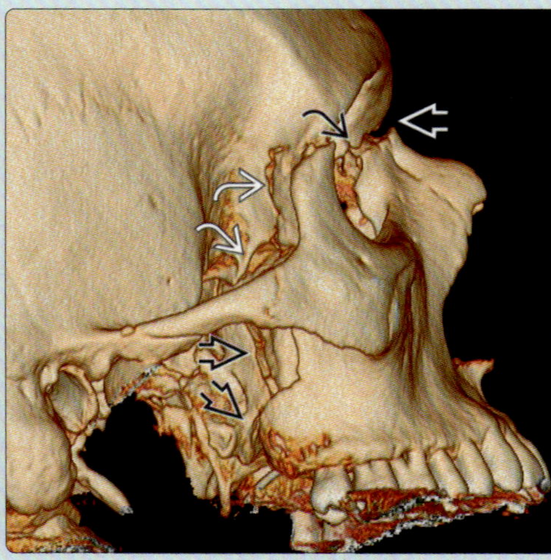

(Left) *AP 3D CT reformation shows a Le Fort II fracture ⇨ with subtle clockwise rotation of the midface and an asymmetric bite. Note the bilateral inferior orbital rim involvement with sparing of the nasal aperture.* **(Right)** *Lateral bone CT 3D reformation shows a right Le Fort III fracture with nasofrontal diastasis ➡, medial ⇨ and lateral ➡ orbital wall fractures, and pterygoid plate fractures ⇨. The inferior orbital rim is spared.*

Zygomaticomaxillary Complex Fracture

KEY FACTS

TERMINOLOGY

- ZMC definition: Fracture complex with fracture lines involving zygomatic arch, lateral orbital wall, anterior & lateral walls of maxillary sinus, & orbital floor
  - Previously called **trimalar** or **tripod** fracture; ZMC fracture terminology most accurate as fracture involves **lateral orbital wall** along zygomaticosphenoid suture

IMAGING

- Fracture lines through or near sutures of zygoma
  - Involves zygomatic arch, lateral orbital wall, anterior & lateral walls of maxillary sinus, & orbital floor
- Modality of choice: Thin-slice axial bone algorithm CT
  - Reformatted to coronal & sagittal planes
  - 3D reformatted images helpful for revealing degree of fracture displacement & angulation

TOP DIFFERENTIAL DIAGNOSES

- Complex midfacial fracture
- Transfacial (Le Fort) fractures
- Zygomatic arch fracture

PATHOLOGY

- Mechanism of injury: Direct malar eminence trauma
- Classification systems not often used to plan treatment since advent of miniplates & microplates

CLINICAL ISSUES

- Teenage to young adult males most commonly affected
- Signs & symptoms
  - Loss of cheek projection with increased facial width
  - Impaired sensation or anesthesia of cheek/upper lip
    - **Inferior orbital nerve** injury
  - Trismus: Depressed zygomatic arch impinges on temporalis muscle or coronoid process of mandible
- Surgical treatment issues
  - Observation for isolated, nondisplaced fracture
  - Gillies approach for minimally displaced fracture

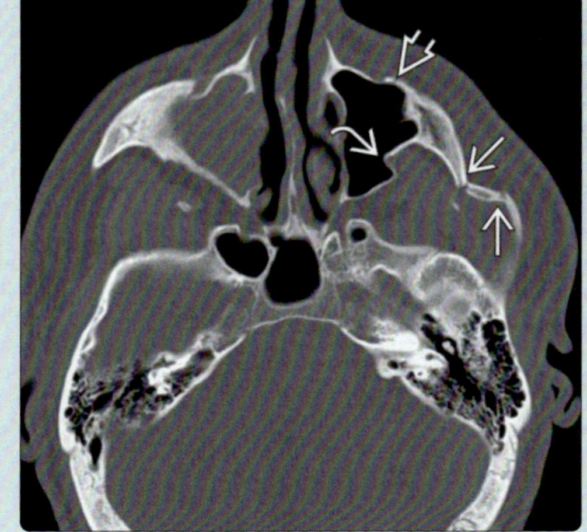

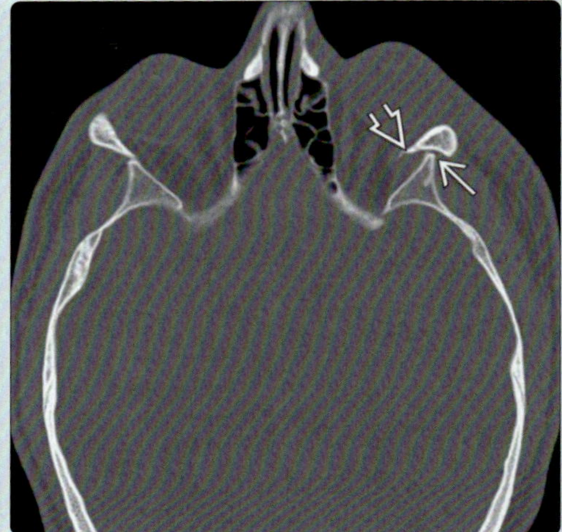

(Left) *Axial bone CT shows the typical fracture patterns of a zygomaticomaxillary complex (ZMC) fracture. There is a comminuted, depressed fracture of the left zygomatic arch → and a fracture of the lateral maxillary sinus wall that is buckled →. The anterior wall fracture is subtle →.* **(Right)** *Axial bone CT through the orbits in the same patient shows a displaced lateral orbital wall fracture →. The bone fragment protrudes into the extraconal fat near the lateral rectus muscle →.*

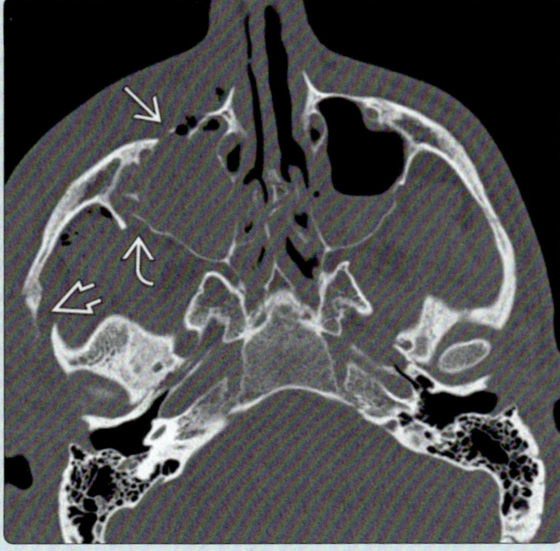

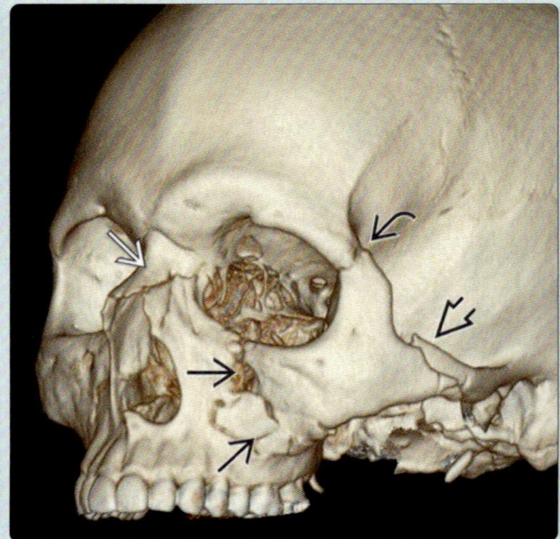

(Left) *Axial bone CT shows a right ZMC fracture. There is premaxillary soft tissue swelling. Fractures of the anterior → and lateral → right maxillary sinus walls are noted, in addition to a right zygomatic arch fracture →.* **(Right)** *3D reformation demonstrates the classic features of a ZMC fracture. Fractures involve the walls of the left maxillary sinus →, the left zygomatic arch →, and the lateral orbital wall →. This patient also sustained trauma to the nasal dorsum →.*

KEY FACTS

TERMINOLOGY

- Synonyms: Facial smash injury, panfacial fracture
- No widely accepted definition
  - Severely comminuted fractures involving multiple facial bones
  - Does not follow pattern described for traditional transfacial (Le Fort) fracture

IMAGING

- Thin-section axial bone CT with multiplanar reconstruction is modality of choice
  - 3D CT reformatted images improve appreciation of disrupted facial architecture for surgical planning
- Fractures may involve frontal, nasoethmoid, midfacial, or craniofacial regions
  - May also involve mandible
- CTA may be necessary to exclude carotid artery injury
- MR helpful for assessing associated intracranial & orbital injuries

TOP DIFFERENTIAL DIAGNOSES

- Transfacial (Le Fort) fracture
- Zygomaticomaxillary complex fracture
- Nasoorbitalethmoidal fracture

PATHOLOGY

- High association with intracranial injuries

CLINICAL ISSUES

- Soft tissue injuries & loss of bone structure may lead to malocclusion, "dish" face deformity, & enophthalmos
- Treatment often delayed because of other life-threatening injuries
  - Often require acute airway management
- Reconstruction often performed in multiple stages
- Preoperative CT, virtual surgical planning, intraoperative navigation, & 3D reconstructions aid in planning & execution of complex craniofacial fracture reconstruction

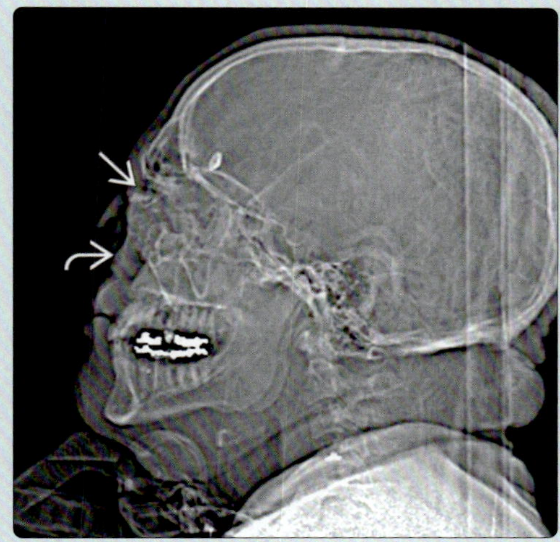

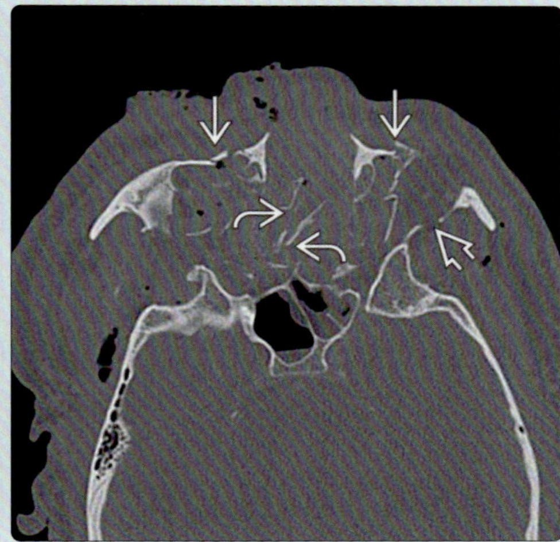

(Left) *Lateral CT scout image in a patient status post high-force blunt facial trauma demonstrates flattening of facial projection involving the nasal dorsum ➡ & midface ➡, referred to as "dish" face deformity.* **(Right)** *Axial bone CT in the same patient demonstrates extensive injuries to the facial soft tissues & underlying facial skeleton. Lacerations with soft tissue emphysema are noted. Severely comminuted fractures involve the maxillae ➡, orbital walls ➡, & nasal septum ➡. The entire face is depressed.*

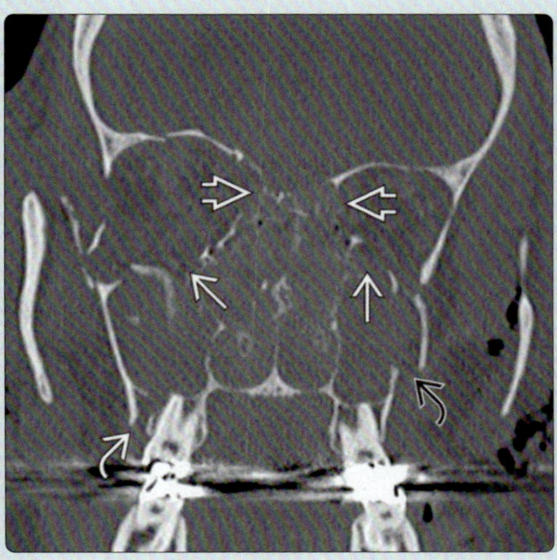

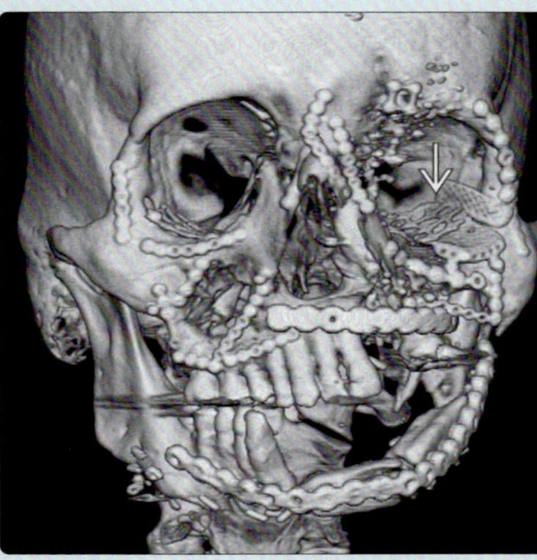

(Left) *Coronal bone CT demonstrates extensive fractures of the midface, involving the medial orbital walls ➡, orbital floors ➡, right maxillary alveolus ➡, & left lateral maxillary sinus ➡. These fractures do not conform to the classic Le Fort fracture pattern.* **(Right)** *Anteroposterior 3D reformation in a patient after reconstruction of panfacial injuries shows numerous malleable screw plates bridging fractures & mesh along the left orbital floor ➡.*

KEY FACTS

TERMINOLOGY

- **Central upper midface fracture** complex involving confluence of medial and upper maxillary buttresses and their posterior extensions
  - Disruption of medial canthal regions, ethmoids, and medial orbital walls

IMAGING

- Bone CT: Nasal bone fracture in combination with fractures of medial orbital wall and frontal process of maxilla

TOP DIFFERENTIAL DIAGNOSES

- Complex midfacial fracture
- Nasal bone fracture
- Medial orbital blowout fracture

PATHOLOGY

- Force transmitted through nasal bones and involves ethmoid sinuses and medial orbits
- May involve frontal recess resulting in impaired frontal sinus drainage
- May involve cribriform plate → CSF leak, meningoencephalocele, intracranial infection
- Markowitz-Manson classification
  - Type I: Medial canthal insertion on large fracture fragment
  - Type II: Canthal tendon attached to small bone fragment
  - Type III: Complete avulsion of medial canthal tendon

CLINICAL ISSUES

- Symptoms and signs
  - Loss of nasal projection in profile
  - Increased distance between inner corners of eyes (traumatic telecanthus)
  - Evaluate for CSF leak, epistaxis, lacrimal apparatus injury
- Nasoorbitalethmoidal fractures can be among most difficult facial fracture patterns to accurately repair

(Left) *Axial bone CT shows markedly comminuted fractures involving the nasoorbitalethmoidal (NOE) complex. Multiple small fracture fragments are noted in the medial canthal regions ➡, and there is a degree of telecanthus. Soft tissue swelling, emphysema, and a lateral orbital fracture ➡ are noted.* **(Right)** *Axial bone CT in the same patient (inferiorly) shows that the fractures involve both nasolacrimal ducts ➡. In such a patient, epiphora would be an expected complication of the injury.*

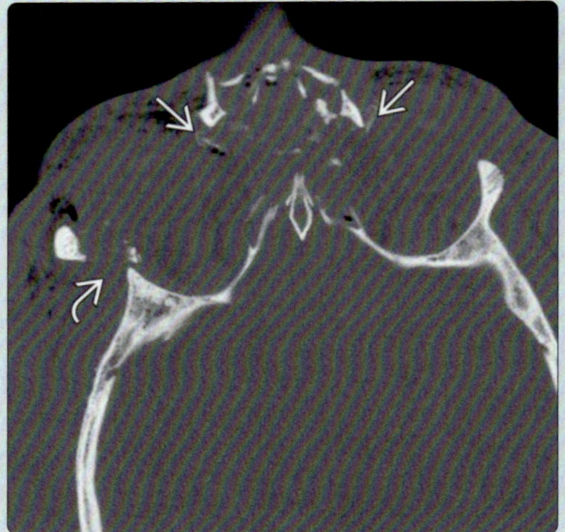

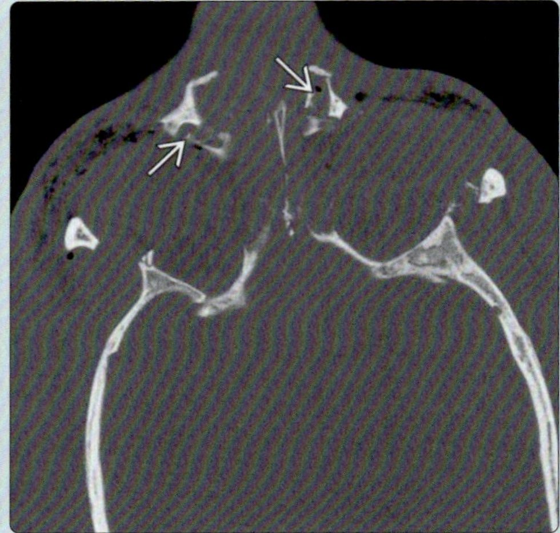

(Left) *Axial bone CT demonstrates comminuted fractures involving the NOE complex with retropulsion of the nasal bridge ➡ and fracture of the left lamina papyracea ➡.* **(Right)** *Anterior 3D reconstructed bone CT in a 20 year old demonstrates highly comminuted fractures involving the NOE ➡, orbit ➡, and maxilla ➡.*

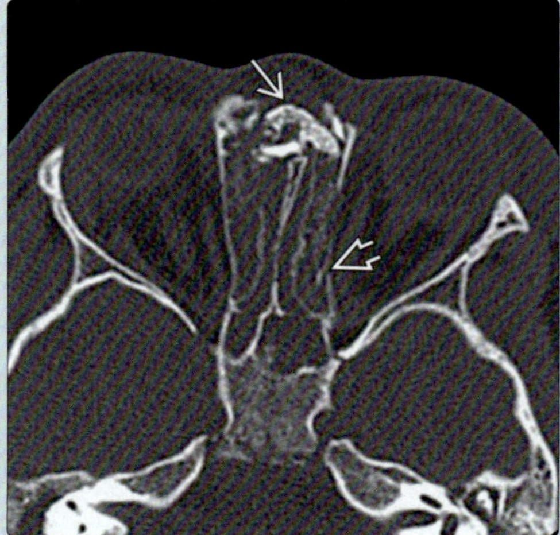

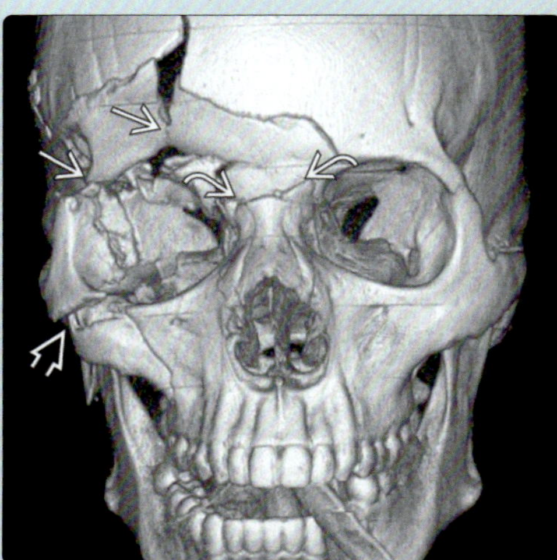

KEY FACTS

IMAGING

- Mandible simulates bony ring: **2 breaks** common (50%)
  - Parasymphyseal fracture often associated with contralateral angle/body or subcondylar fracture
  - Bilateral subcondylar fractures often result from direct impact to symphysis
- CT has largely replaced plain film evaluation of facial trauma
  - Thin-slice axial bone algorithm CT with coronal reformation & 3D reconstruction
- Bone CT appearance
  - **Radiolucent**, **noncorticated lines** with variable diastasis, angulation, & comminution
  - Fracture tends to follow along axis of teeth
  - In condylar neck fracture, condylar head **pulled medially** by lateral pterygoid muscle
  - Empty temporomandibular joint sign when temporomandibular joint dislocated

TOP DIFFERENTIAL DIAGNOSES

- **Pseudofractures**: Nutrient canal, inferior alveolar nerve canal, mental foramen

PATHOLOGY

- Causes of mandibular fracture
  - Motor vehicle accidents: 40%
  - Assault: 40%
  - Fall: 10%
  - Sports-related injury: 5%
- 15% have ≥ 1 other facial bone fracture

CLINICAL ISSUES

- 2nd most commonly fractured facial bone
- Goals of treatment
  - Restoration of normal occlusion & complete bony union
- Wound infection is potential complication of fracture to tooth-bearing portion of mandible, facial equivalent of open fracture

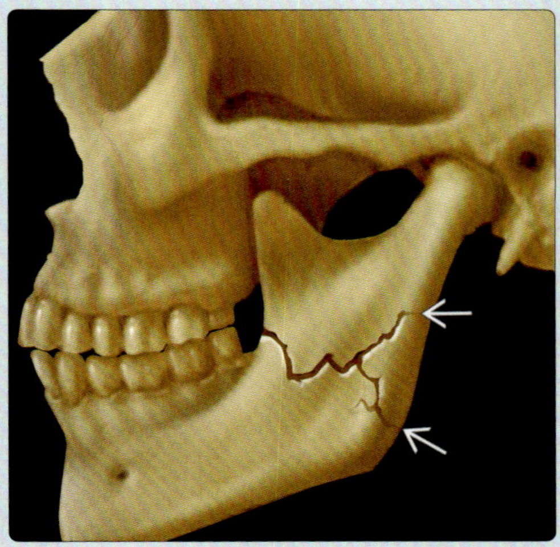

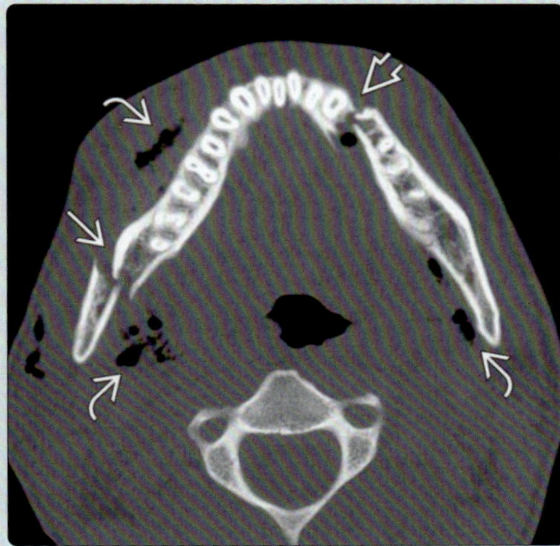

(Left) *Sagittal graphic shows a complex mandibular ramus fracture obliquely crossing the posterior margin of the mandible ➡. Inferior alveolar nerve may be injured in such a fracture, resulting in a numb chin.* **(Right)** *Axial bone CT shows displaced mandibular fractures of the right angle ➡ and left parasymphysis ➡. A fracture through the teeth is considered open, requiring antibiotics. Two fractures are often present as the mandible is essentially a fixed ring of bone. Extensive lacerations resulted in associated soft tissue emphysema ➡.*

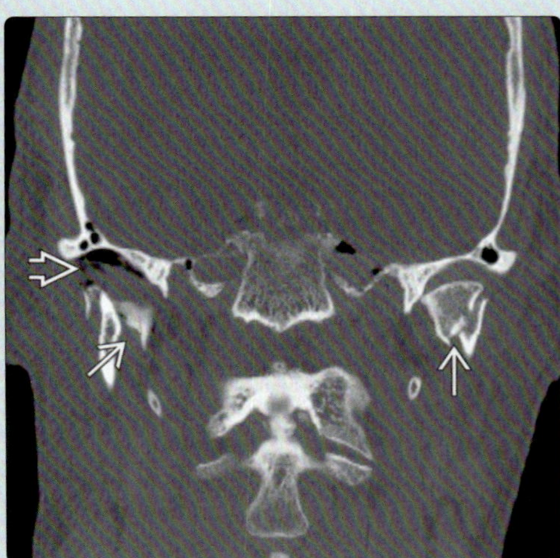

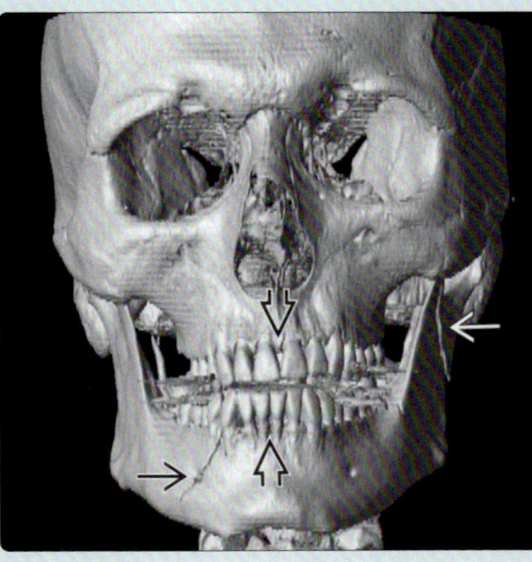

(Left) *Coronal bone CT demonstrates bilateral mandibular condyle fractures ➡ with severe displacement of fracture fragments on the right. Trauma to the right temporomandibular joint was significant, and air is noted in the joint ➡.* **(Right)** *3D reformation shows obliquely oriented fractures through the right mental foramen ➡ and left mandibular ramus ➡. There is associated malocclusion ➡. 3D reformatted images are often helpful for surgical repair of facial fractures.*

SECTION 6

Temporal Bone and CPA-IAC

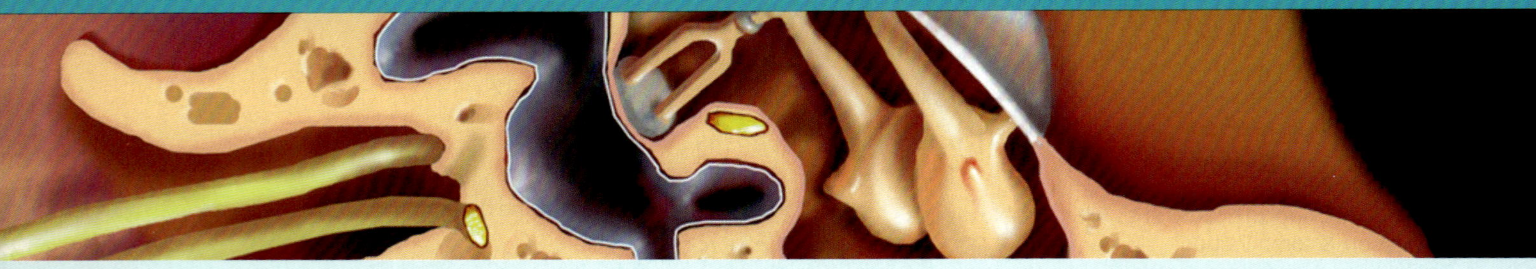

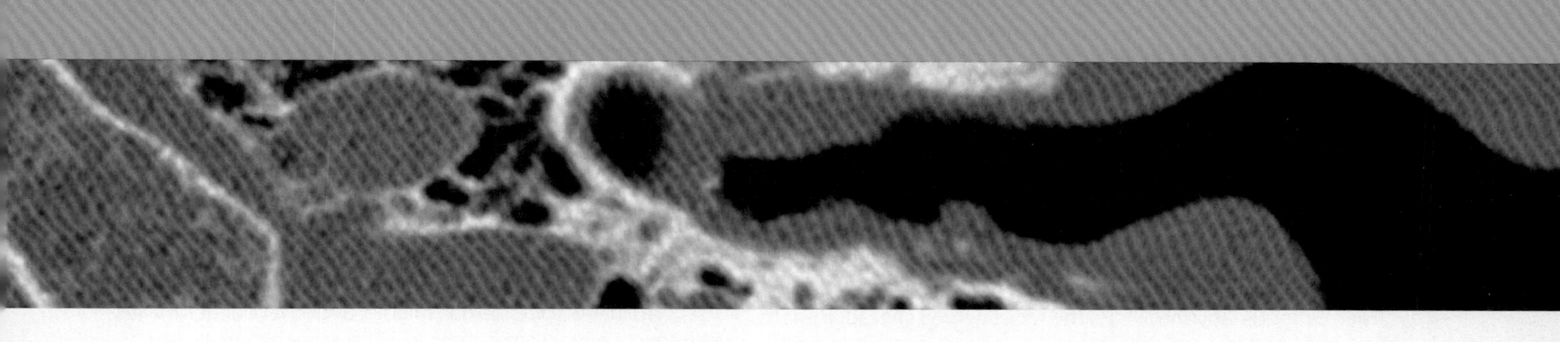

Petrous Apex

Intratemporal Facial Nerve

Temporal Bone, No Specific Anatomic Location

CPA-IAC

Summary Thoughts: Temporal Bone

The temporal bone (T-bone) is one of the most complex and intriguing areas of the head and neck. Understanding normal anatomy is key to accurate T-bone image interpretation. Incorporating the otologic findings of a middle ear mass also helps the clinician to arrive at a correct preoperative diagnosis. If the clinical question is conductive hearing loss (CHL), an abnormality on CT is almost always present and should be extensively searched for, especially in children.

Cholesteatoma is a very common clinical concern in most otolaryngology practices. The following questions should be addressed in a patient with a cholesteatoma: (1) Is the tegmen tympani intact? (2) Is there potential for a fistula into the membranous labyrinth? (3) Is the facial nerve canal adjacent to or eroded by the cholesteatoma? (4) Is there tissue in the sinus tympani? (5) What is the relationship of the mass to the ossicles? Where is the location of the sigmoid sinus? How contracted is the mastoid cavity?

Imaging Techniques & Indications

CT is the primary imaging tool for evaluating the fine bony detail of the T-bone. Current multislice CT scanners allow thin slices (≤ 1 mm) and provide excellent multiplanar reformatted images, which have become the mainstay for diagnosis of T-bone disease. Current protocols include direct axial and reformatted coronal views, vestibular oblique or short-axis views (Pöschl plane), and cochlear oblique or long-axis views (Stenver plane). A window width of 4,000 HU is ideal.

CT is the imaging study of choice when the clinical question is CHL, external auditory canal (EAC) atresia/stenosis, or chronic otitis media with cholesteatoma.

MR is best for evaluation of inner ear pathology, particularly sensorineural hearing loss (SNHL). High-resolution 3D MR cisternographic sequences provide an excellent screening examination for SNHL. These thin-section (≤ 1-mm) T2-weighted MR sequences (SPACE, FIESTA, etc.) in the axial and coronal planes can help identify mass lesions of the internal auditory canal (IAC), particularly a vestibular schwannoma. Sagittal oblique planes are excellent for evaluation of congenital SNHL to identify the 4 nerves within the IAC.

The gold standard for imaging patients with acquired SNHL is enhanced thin-section (≤ 3-mm) axial and coronal images through the T-bone with fat-saturated, postcontrast images. Precontrast T1-weighted images are helpful to evaluate for T1-hyperintense lesions, such as hemorrhage or lipoma. Nonecho planar diffusion-weighted imaging can be useful to detect cholesteatoma (down to 2-3 mm), which can sometimes avoid 2nd-look procedures for cholesteatoma.

When the clinical question is SNHL, a petrous apex lesion, or possible IAC or cerebellopontine angle (CPA) lesion, MR is the imaging study of choice. MR and CT imaging provide **complimentary** information to evaluate lesions of the petrous apex and jugular foramen and other intratemporal tumors.

Embryology

The otocyst buds from the neuroectoderm, migrates to the location of the inner ear, and becomes the membranous labyrinth. The EAC forms from the 1st branchial groove or cleft. The middle ear (tympanic) cavity forms from the 1st branchial (pharyngeal) pouch. The tympanic membrane (TM) forms where the EAC (1st branchial cleft) and middle ear (1st branchial pouch) meet. The middle ear cavity and the eustachian tube form from the same 1st branchial pouch. The middle ear cavity envelops the ossicles.

The **ossicles** form primarily from the 1st and 2nd branchial arches, separately from the inner ear. Epitympanic and mesotympanic components of the ossicles arise from the 1st and 2nd branchial arches, respectively. The medial portion of the bilaminar footplate comes from the otocyst. The endolymphatic system forms from the otocyst. The perilymphatic space and otic capsule form from surrounding mesenchyme.

In nonsyndromic aural atresia, the inner ear is spared, as it forms from migration of the otocyst, which is independent from the 1st and 2nd branchial groove-pouch-arch interaction. A combination of external, middle, and inner ear anomalies suggests a syndromic etiology or teratogenic insult.

Consider the following questions when evaluating a patient with **EAC atresia**: (1) Is the EAC atresia plate thick, thin, or part membranous in nature? (2) How small is the middle ear cavity? (3) What is the status of the ossicles (or ossicular mass), especially the stapes? (4) Is the facial nerve canal anomalous in its course or dehiscent? (5) What is the status of the oval and round windows? (6) Is there a congenital cholesteatoma? (7) Are the inner ear structures normal?

Imaging Anatomy

The T-bone is located in the middle cranial fossa posterolateral floor. Its boundaries include the sphenoid bone anteriorly, occipital bone posteriorly and medially, and parietal bone superiorly and laterally.

There are **5 bony parts** of the adult T-bone: Squamous, mastoid, petrous, tympanic, and styloid portions. The squamous portion forms the lateral wall of the middle cranial fossa. The mastoid process represents the postnatal development of the posteroinferior mastoid. The petrous portion of the T-bone contains the middle and inner ear, IAC, and petrous apex. The tympanic segment is a U-shaped bone that forms most of the bony external ear. The styloid portion forms the styloid process after birth.

The **petrous portion** of the T-bone includes 2 important structures anteriorly. The tegmen tympani (Latin for "roof of the cavity") serves as the roof of the tympanic cavity. The arcuate eminence is the bony prominence over the superior semicircular canal (SCC) and serves as an important surgical landmark along the middle cranial fossa floor.

There are 5 major anatomic components of the T-bone: EAC, middle ear-mastoid (ME-M), inner ear, petrous apex, and facial nerve. These anatomic components help define the various differential diagnosis lists of the T-bone.

The **EAC** is made up of the tympanic bone medially and fibrocartilage laterally. The medial border of the EAC is formed by the TM, which attaches to the scutum superiorly and the tympanic annulus inferiorly. The nodal drainage of the EAC and the adjacent scalp is to the parotid lymph nodes.

The **middle ear** includes the epitympanum, mesotympanum, and hypotympanum. The **epitympanum** (attic) is defined superiorly by the tegmen tympani, which forms the roof. The inferior margin is defined by a line between the scutum and the tympanic segment of the facial nerve. The tegmen tympani is the bony roof between the epitympanum and the middle cranial fossa dura. **Prussak space** represents the lateral epitympanic recess and is a classic location for primary acquired (pars flaccida) **cholesteatoma**. The malleus head and the incus short process are present in the epitympanum.

The **mesotympanum** is between the epitympanum above and the hypotympanum below. It is defined superiorly by a line between the scutum and tympanic segment of the facial nerve and inferiorly by a line between the tympanic annulus and the base of the cochlear promontory. The remainder of the ossicles (manubrium of the malleus, lenticular process of the incus, and stapes) is located in the mesotympanum. The 2 muscles of the middle ear, the tensor tympani and stapedius, are also in the mesotympanum and can dampen sound. The posterior wall of the mesotympanum has 3 important structures: Facial nerve recess, pyramidal process or eminence, and sinus tympani. The **facial nerve recess** contains the mastoid facial nerve and may be dehiscent or have a bony covering. The **pyramidal eminence** contains the belly and tendon of the stapedius muscle. The **sinus tympani** is a clinical blind spot during a standard mastoid surgical approach to the T-bone, where cholesteatomas may hide. The medial wall contains the lateral SCC, the tympanic segment of the facial nerve, and the oval and round windows. The **hypotympanum** is a shallow trough on the floor of the middle ear cavity.

The **mastoid** sinus contains 3 important anatomic structures. The **mastoid antrum** (Latin for "cave") is the large, central mastoid air cell. The **aditus ad antrum** (Latin for "entrance to the cave") connects the epitympanum to the mastoid antrum. **Körner septum** is part of the petrosquamosal suture running posterolaterally through the mastoid air cells. This septum functions as an important surgical landmark within the mastoid air cells and also serves as a barrier to the extension of infection from the lateral mastoid air cells to the medial mastoid air cells. The mastoid T-bone continues to develop after birth. As the mastoid eminence protects the facial nerve, this nerve is relatively unprotected until the eminence is formed. This is why the facial nerve is vulnerable to birth trauma and surgical trauma in young children.

The **inner ear** contains the **membranous labyrinth**, which is housed in the bony labyrinth (otic capsule). The membranous labyrinth consists of the fluid spaces within the bony labyrinth, including the fluid and soft tissues of the vestibule, SCCs and cochlea, the endolymphatic duct and sac, and cochlear duct. The vestibule houses the largest part of the membranous labyrinth, consisting of the utricle and saccule. The utricle is the more cephalad portion, and the saccule is the more caudal portion of the vestibule. The vestibule is separated laterally from the middle ear by the oval window niche. The SCCs project off the superior, posterior, and lateral aspects of the vestibule. The lateral (or horizontal) SCC is at risk for fistula formation from a cholesteatoma as it projects into the epitympanum. The endolymphatic duct and sac contain endolymph, whereas the cochlear duct contains perilymph.

The **bony labyrinth** (otic capsule) forms the cochlea, vestibule, SCCs, and vestibular and cochlear aqueducts. The **cochlea** has ~ 2.5 turns. The entire cochlea encircles a central bony axis, the **modiolus**. The modiolus houses the spiral ganglia, cell bodies of the cochlear nerve. The 3 spiral chambers of the cochlea are the scala tympani (posterior chamber), scala vestibuli (anterior chamber), and scala media (contains organ of Corti = hearing apparatus).

The **SCCs** project off the superior, lateral, and posterior aspects of the vestibule. The superior SCC projects cephalad. The bony ridge over the superior SCC in the roof of the petrous pyramid is the arcuate eminence, an important (though unreliable) surgical landmark. The lateral (or horizontal) SCC projects into the middle ear. The tympanic segment of the facial nerve is on the undersurface of the lateral SCC, a consistent surgical landmark. The posterior SCC projects posteriorly along the petrous ridge. The crus communis is the common origin of the superior and posterior SCCs, out of which travels the vestibular aqueduct.

The **petrous apex** is anteromedial to the inner ear and lateral to the petrooccipital fissure. It is pneumatized in ~ 33% of people. The abducens nerve (CNVI) passes along the medial surface of the petrous apex and through Dorello canal. The trigeminal nerve (CNV) passes through the porus trigeminus into Meckel cave on the medial surface of the petrous apex. In petrous apicitis, CNV and CNVI are commonly affected.

The petrous **internal carotid artery** (ICA) includes the vertical and horizontal segments within the petrous temporal bone. The vertical segment rises to the genu beneath the cochlea. The horizontal segment projects anteromedially to turn cephalad as the cavernous segment.

The **intratemporal facial nerve (CNVII)** is composed of the IAC and labyrinthine, tympanic, and mastoid segments. The IAC segment is located anterosuperiorly within the IAC. The labyrinthine segment extends from the IAC fundus to the geniculate ganglion. The geniculate ganglion is also known as the anterior genu, and the greater superficial petrosal nerve (GSPN) originates here. The tympanic segment leaves the geniculate ganglion and passes under the lateral SCC. The posterior genu is where the tympanic segment bends inferiorly to become the mastoid segment. The mastoid segment passes inferiorly to the stylomastoid foramen. It 1st gives off the motor nerve to the stapedius muscle, then the chorda tympani nerve. The facial nerve then exits the skull base through the stylomastoid foramen.

The motor root of CNVII innervates the muscles of facial expression, stapedius, platysma, and posterior belly of the digastric muscles. The sensory-parasympathetic root (nervus intermedius) contains special sensory visceral afferent fibers that convey taste to the anterior 2/3 of the tongue; the parasympathetic portion provides general visceral efferent secretomotor fibers to lacrimal (via GSPN), and submandibular and sublingual glands (via the chorda tympani).

CNVII has 4 major functions that help localize a lesion along its course. Lacrimation is via the GSPN. The stapedius nerve provides the stapedius reflex, which creates sound dampening. Taste to the anterior 2/3 of the tongue is via the chorda tympani nerve to the lingual nerve to the oral tongue. Motor branches supply muscles of facial expression.

The 2 muscles of the temporal bone, the **tensor tympani** and **stapedius** muscles, function to dampen sound. When dysfunctional, a patient may present with hyperacusis. The tensor tympani is innervated by a trigeminal nerve (CNV3) branch. It is located in the anteromedial wall of the mesotympanum. The tensor tympani muscle tendon goes through the semicanal, turns laterally at the cochleariform process to attach to the manubrium of the malleus. The stapedius muscle is innervated by CNVII and is located in the pyramidal process/eminence. The stapedius tendon attaches to the capitulum (head) of the stapes.

There are 3 ossicles: **Malleus**, **incus**, and **stapes**. The malleus is the most anterior ossicle and is composed of the umbo,

Differential Diagnosis: Location

External auditory canal	Inner ear
External auditory canal atresia/stenosis	Superior semicircular canal dehiscence
Cholesteatoma	Labyrinthitis & labyrinthine ossificans
Squamous cell carcinoma	Large endolymphatic sac anomaly
Exostoses (surfer's ear)	Fenestral & cochlear otosclerosis
Osteoma	Intralabyrinthine schwannoma
Medial canal fibrosis	Endolymphatic sac tumor
Keratosis obturans	Intralabyrinthine hemorrhage
Necrotizing otitis externa	Labyrinthine, cochlear-vestibular malformations
Middle ear-mastoid	**Petrous apex**
Acquired cholesteatoma	Trapped fluid
Congenital cholesteatoma	Cholesterol granuloma
Cholesterol granuloma	Congenital cholesteatoma
Acute coalescent mastoiditis	Cephalocele or arachnoid cyst
Chronic otitis media ± tympanosclerosis	Apical petrositis
Dehiscent jugular bulb	Mucocele
Aberrant internal carotid artery	**Intratemporal facial nerve**
Glomus tympanicum paraganglioma	Herpetic or varicella facial neuritis (Bell palsy or Ramsay Hunt)
Glomus jugulare paraganglioma	Facial nerve venous malformation ("hemangioma")
Meningioma	Facial nerve schwannoma
Rhabdomyosarcoma	Perineural parotid malignancy

manubrium, and head. The incus is located posteriorly and is composed of the short process, body, long process, and lenticular process. The stapes is located medially and is composed of the head, crura, and footplate.

Approaches to Imaging Issues of the Temporal Bone

When faced with a T-bone study, use a systematic approach through the 5 major functional components (EAC, ME-M, inner ear, petrous apex, and facial nerve). Evaluate and report on the location of the ICA, status of the ossicles, location of CNVII and integrity of the facial nerve canal, presence of the oval window, and integrity of the fissula ante fenestram (anterior margin of the oval window). If a lesion of the T-bone is found, its location as well as clinical findings help refine the differential diagnosis list.

CHL is caused by a disruption of the conductive chain, which may be due to diseases of the EAC, TM, ossicles, or oval window. Typical lesions causing CHL include acquired cholesteatoma, chronic otitis media, EAC atresia/stenosis, fenestral otosclerosis, and cholesterol granuloma. Less common etiologies include oval window atresia, congenital cholesteatoma, ossicular fixation, and medial canal fibrosis.

SNHL involves the cochlea, modiolus, or cochlear nerve. These lesions may occur in the T-bone, IAC, CPA, or brainstem. Inner ear abnormalities in congenital SNHL may provide clues to a specific syndromic etiology. Findings help direct genetic testing and affect patient management. The most common lesion to present with acquired, unilateral SNHL is vestibular schwannoma (~ 90% of lesions). Other much less common etiologies include meningioma, otosclerosis, facial nerve schwannoma, metastases, and labyrinthitis.

Whenever the T-bone is imaged, the entire facial nerve canal should be visualized and inspected. If a lesion of CNVII is found, it should be precisely localized to 1 of the CNVII segments: Cisternal segment (brainstem to porus acusticus), IAC (canalicular) segment, labyrinthine segment, tympanic segment, mastoid segment, or parotid segment.

Some lesions of the T-bone may result in **facial nerve paralysis**, including Bell palsy, T-bone fractures, cholesteatoma, schwannoma, venous malformation, glomus jugulare paraganglioma, meningioma, metastases, middle ear rhabdomyosarcoma, and Langerhans histiocytosis.

Clinical Implications

When a middle ear lesion is present, correlation with **otoscopic findings** provides critical clues to precise diagnosis. If a ruptured or deeply retracted TM is present, a cholesteatoma may be seen through the defect. Most retrotympanic lesions have a distinctive hue and location. When the clinician sees a **white** middle ear lesion behind an intact TM, diagnoses to consider include a congenital cholesteatoma or schwannoma. If there is a **red** hue, the list includes a paraganglioma or aberrant ICA. If there is a **blue** hue, cholesterol granuloma, hemotympanum, or a dehiscent jugular bulb should be considered.

Peripheral facial nerve paralysis is defined as unilateral facial nerve injury with involvement of the entire face, including the forehead. This type of CNVII injury includes loss of the 4 facial nerve functions: Lacrimation (parasympathetic), stapedius reflex (sound dampening), taste to the anterior 2/3 of the tongue, and facial expression. Injury to CNVII at any point through the T-bone results in peripheral facial nerve paralysis.

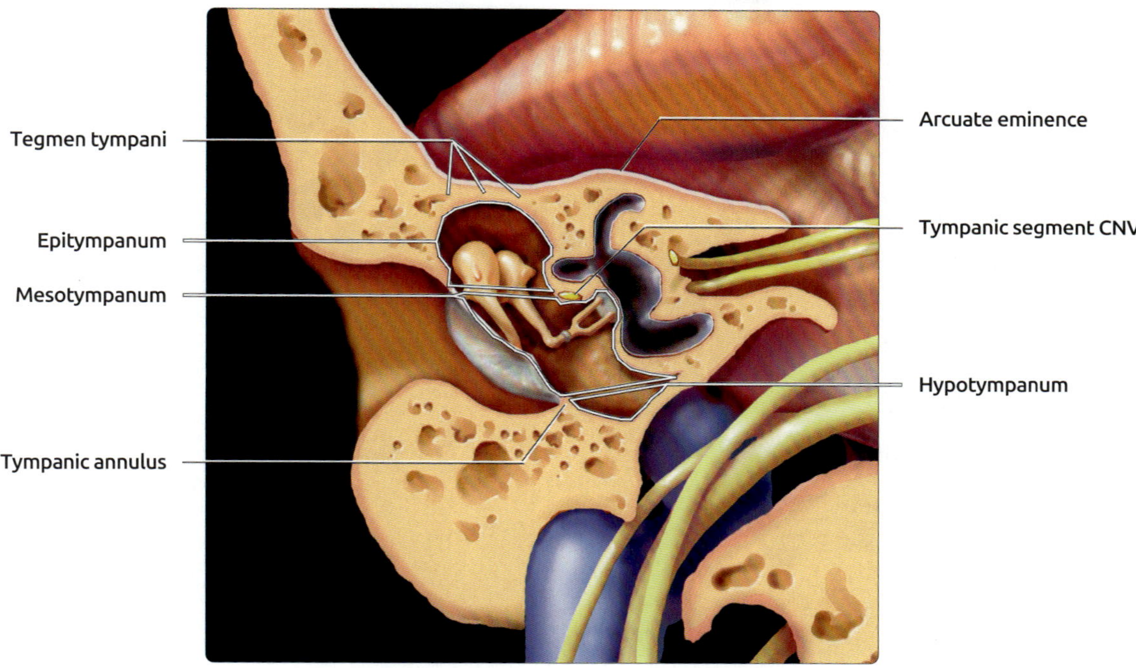

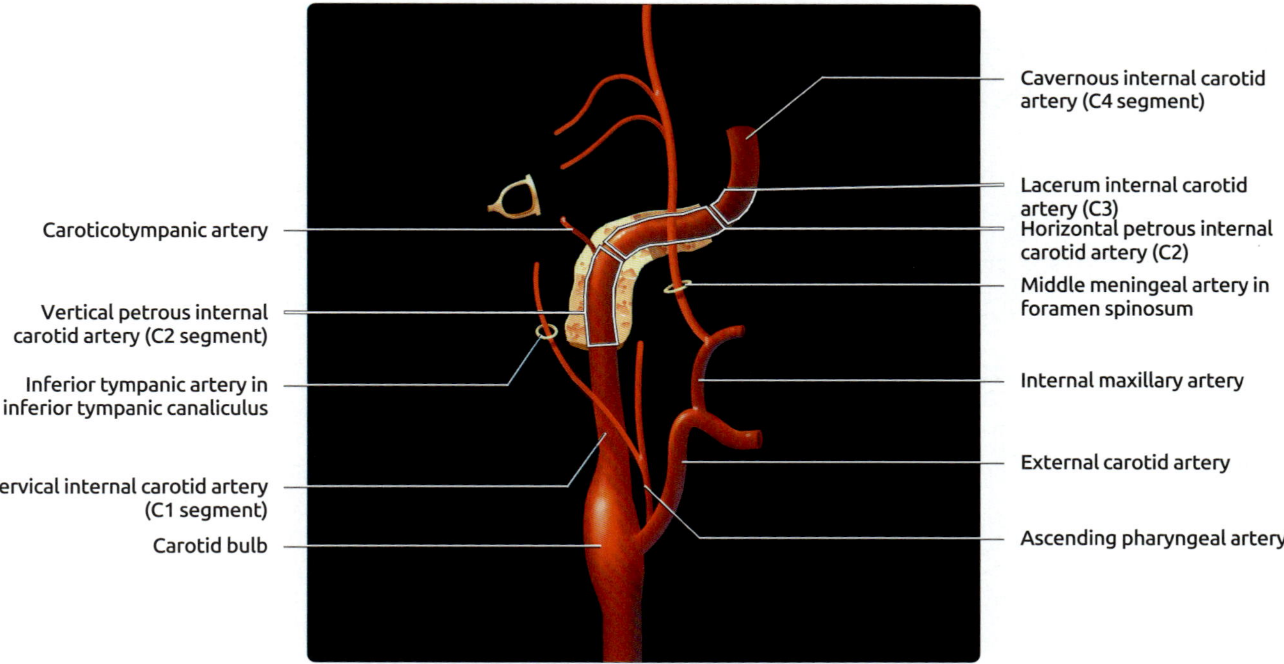

(Top) *Coronal magnified graphic shows the middle ear. The middle ear is divided into 3 portions: Epitympanum, mesotympanum, and hypotympanum. The epitympanum is defined as the middle ear cavity above a line drawn from the tip of the scutum to the tympanic segment of CNVII. The epitympanic roof is called the tegmen tympani. The mesotympanum extends from this line inferiorly to a line connecting the tympanic annulus to the base of the cochlear promontory.* **(Bottom)** *Sagittal graphic shows the petrous internal carotid artery (ICA). The cervical ICA enters the carotid canal of the skull base to become the vertical petrous ICA (C2 subsegment ICA). It then turns anteromedially to become the horizontal petrous ICA (C2 subsegment ICA). The segment of the intracranial ICA just above the foramen lacerum is called the lacerum segment (C3 ICA segment). Note that the inferior tympanic artery rises through the inferior tympanic canaliculus, and the middle meningeal artery arises off the internal maxillary artery passing through the foramen spinosum.*

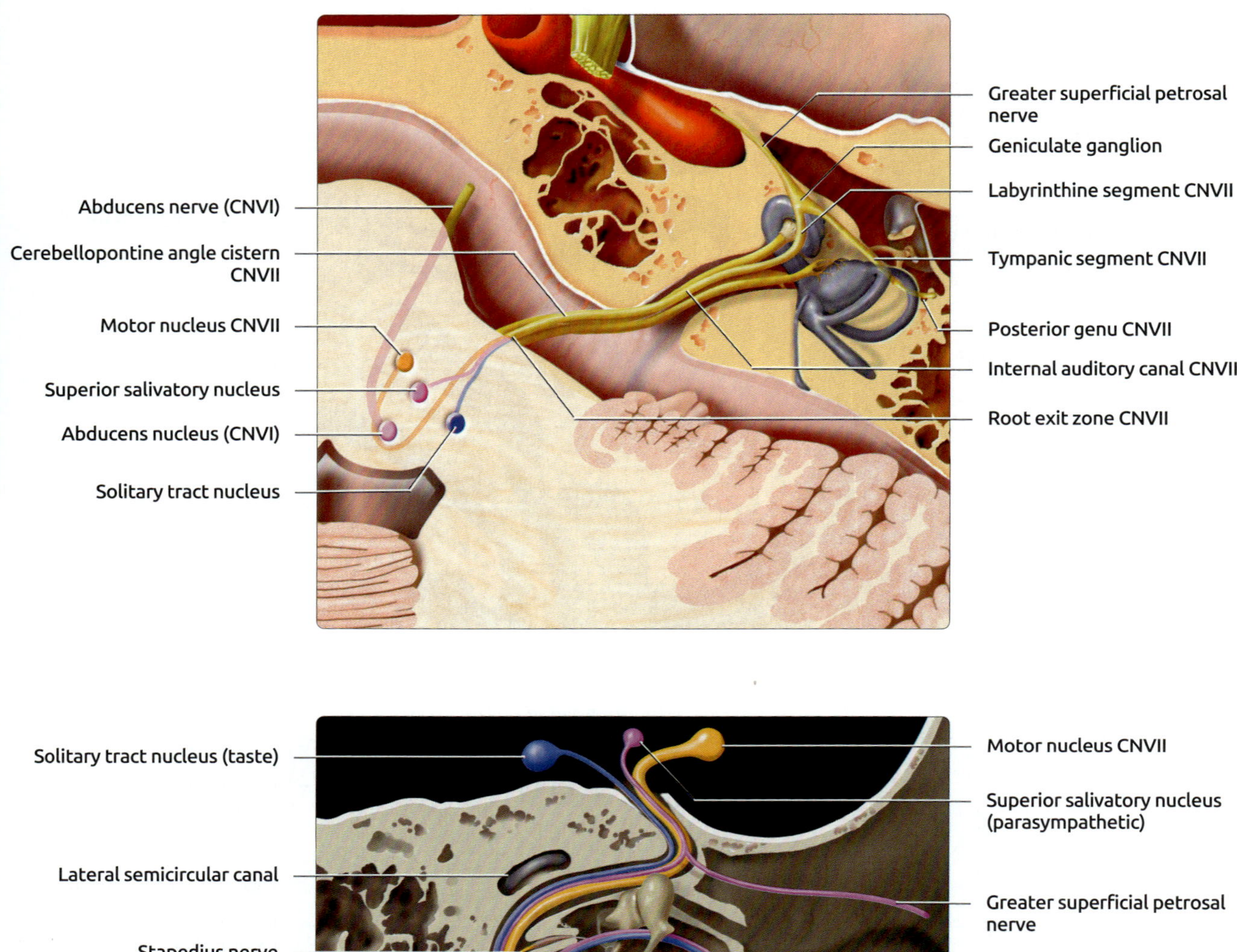

(Top) *Axial graphic shows the facial nerve from the brainstem nuclei to the posterior genu in the temporal bone (T-bone). The motor nucleus sends out fibers, which encircle the CNVI nucleus before reaching the root exit zone at the pontomedullary junction. Superior salivatory nucleus sends parasympathetic secretomotor fibers to the lacrimal, submandibular, and sublingual glands. The solitary tract nucleus receives the anterior 2/3 of tongue taste information, via the chorda tympani nerve, to the lingual nerve, to the oral tongue.* **(Bottom)** *Sagittal graphic depicts CNVII within the T-bone [motor fibers pass through the T-bone, giving off the stapedius nerve to the stapedius muscle, then exit via the stylomastoid foramen to the extracranial CNVII (entirely motor)]. Parasympathetic fibers from the superior salivatory nucleus reach the lacrimal gland via the greater superficial petrosal nerve and the submandibular-sublingual glands via the chorda tympanic nerve. The anterior 2/3 of tongue taste fibers come via the chorda tympani nerve, the cell bodies of which create the geniculate ganglion.*

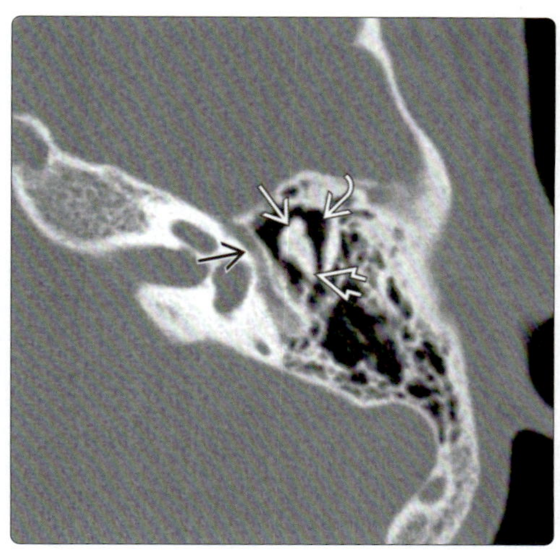

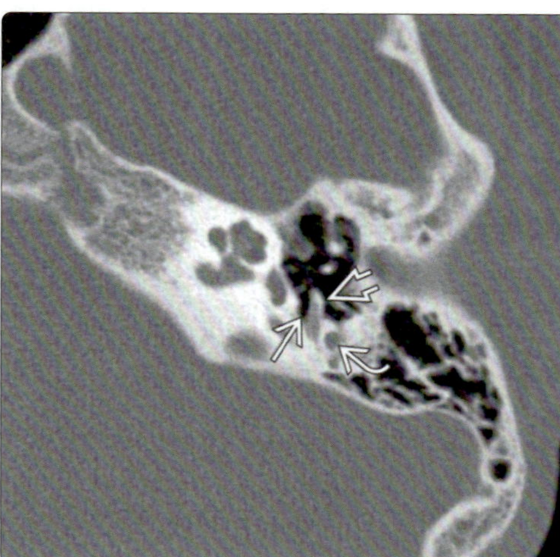

(Left) *Axial T-bone CT through the epitympanum shows the malleus head ➡ anterior to the incus short process ➡. The Prussak space is the lateral epitympanic recess ➡ and is a typical location for acquired cholesteatoma. Tympanic segment CNVII is well seen ➡.* **(Right)** *Axial T-bone CT through the mesotympanum shows the posterior wall sinus tympani ➡ and pyramidal eminence ➡, which contains the stapedius muscle and mastoid CNVII ➡. The most anterior ossicle is the malleus. The posterior ossicle is the incus.*

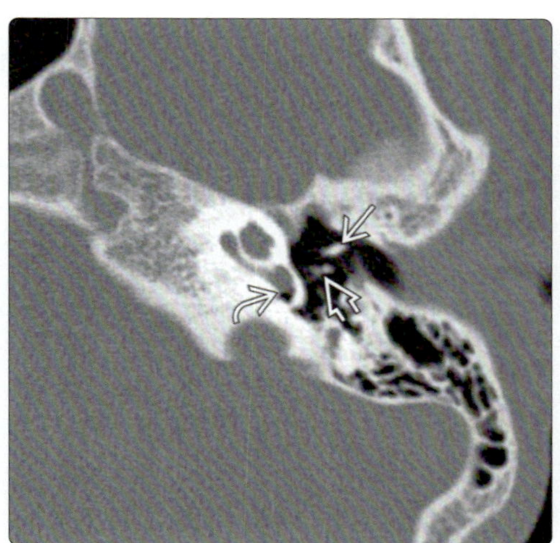

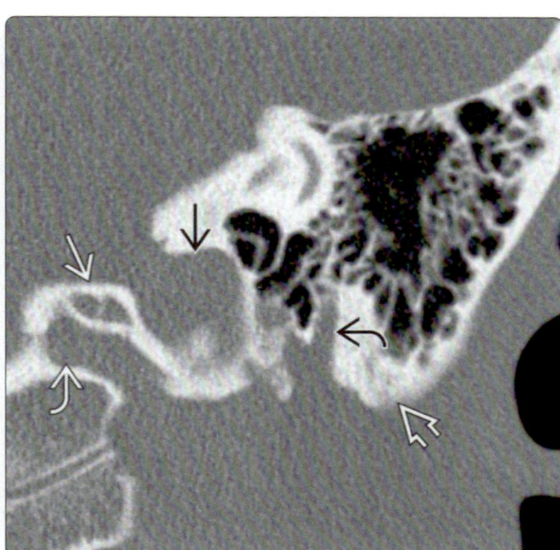

(Left) *Axial T-bone CT through the low mesotympanum shows the normal manubrium of malleus ➡ and the incudostapedial articulation ➡. Basal turn of the cochlea ends at the round window ➡.* **(Right)** *Coronal T-bone CT through the posterior mastoid region shows the mastoid segment of CNVII ➡, which then exits at the stylomastoid foramen. The mastoid tip ➡ helps protect this portion of CNVII. The jugular foramen ➡ and the hypoglossal canal ➡ are separated by the jugular tubercle ➡.*

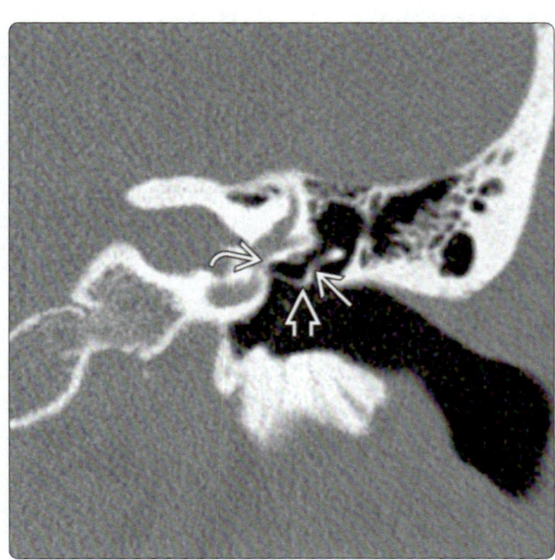

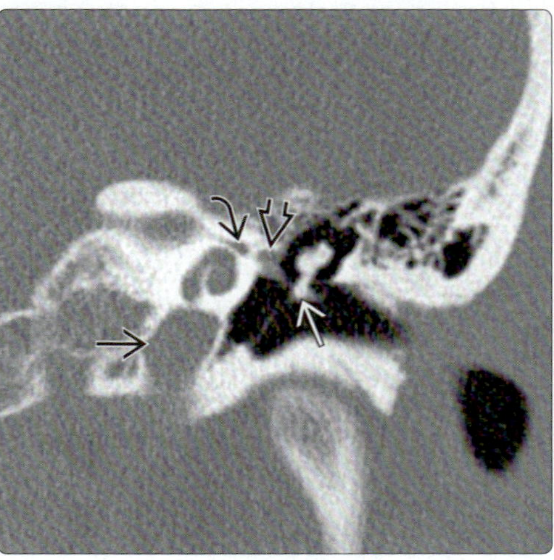

(Left) *Coronal T-bone CT through the semicircular canals demonstrates the long process ➡ and the lenticular process ➡ of the incus. Notice the normal absence of bone evident in the oval window niche ➡. The oval window and stapes are best visualized in the coronal plane.* **(Right)** *Coronal T-bone CT through the anterior middle ear shows the malleus ➡, labyrinthine ➡, and tympanic ➡ facial nerve segments. Notice the horizontal petrous ICA ➡ below the cochlea.*

Foramen Tympanicum

KEY FACTS

TERMINOLOGY

- Synonyms: Foramen of Huschke; tympanic bone dehiscence
- Definition: Developmental ossification defect in anteroinferior aspect of bony external auditory canal (EAC)
  - Should be considered normal EAC variant

IMAGING

- Axial temporal bone CT: ~ 4- to 6-mm bony dehiscence in medial, anteroinferior aspect of bony EAC
- Axial diameter: Variable; 2-8 mm (mean: ~ 4 mm)

TOP DIFFERENTIAL DIAGNOSES

- 1st branchial cleft cyst
- EAC cholesteatoma
- EAC squamous cell carcinoma

PATHOLOGY

- Foramen tympanicum is formed in tympanic plate of temporal bone before 1 year of age
  - Usually closes before 5 years of age
  - Persistence seen on bone CT after 5 years of age in ~ 5% of patients
- Pathology associated with foramen tympanicum
  - **Spontaneous herniation of TMJ soft tissues** into EAC
  - Parotid gland and synovial TMJ fistulas into EAC
  - Foramen tympanicum may facilitate ear injury during TMJ arthroscopy

CLINICAL ISSUES

- **Asymptomatic** normal variant found incidentally during temporal bone CT
- Otorrhea with otalgia possible if dehiscence is large
  - Physical examination reveals polypoid lesion in anteroinferior bony EAC
  - If patient opens mouth, polypoid lesion disappears
- Gustatory otorrhea (occurs with eating)
  - Sialo-aural fistula from parotid gland through foramen tympanicum to EAC

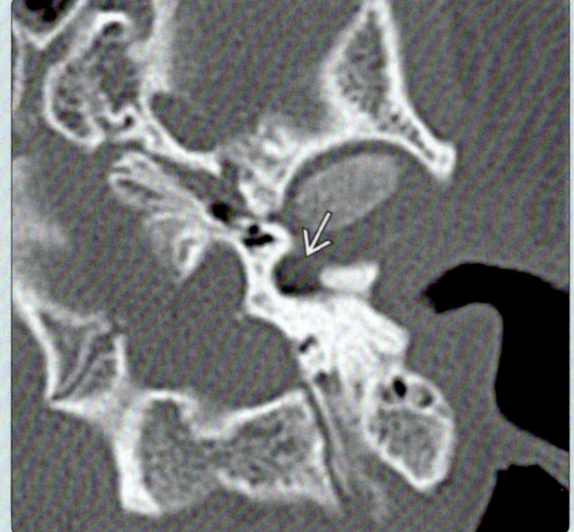

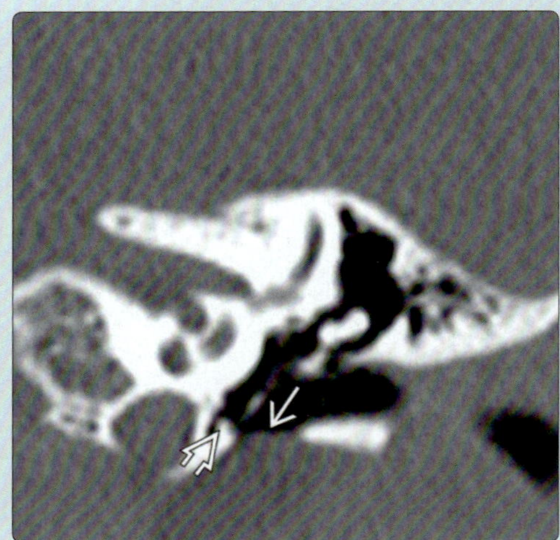

(Left) *Axial temporal bone CT of the left ear shows the appearance of incidental foramen tympanicum ➡ in a 3 year old. Notice the anteroinferior tympanic bone dehiscence that normally closes by 5 years of age.* **(Right)** *Coronal temporal bone CT in the same patient demonstrates the well-defined areas of incomplete ossification in the anterior medial aspect of the osseous external auditory canal (EAC) ➡. Note the proximal relationship of the foramen tympanicum to the tympanic annulus ➡.*

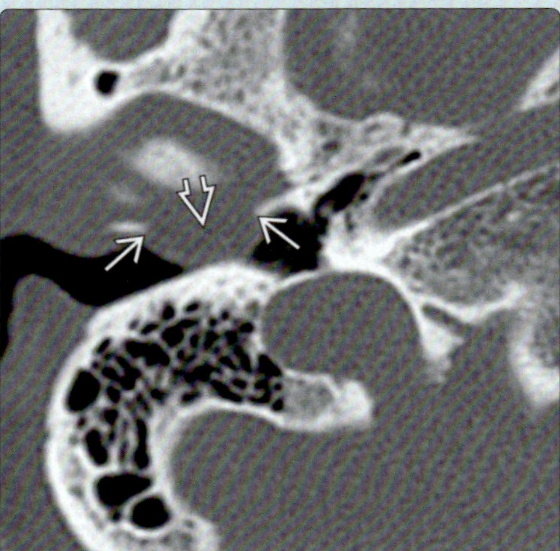

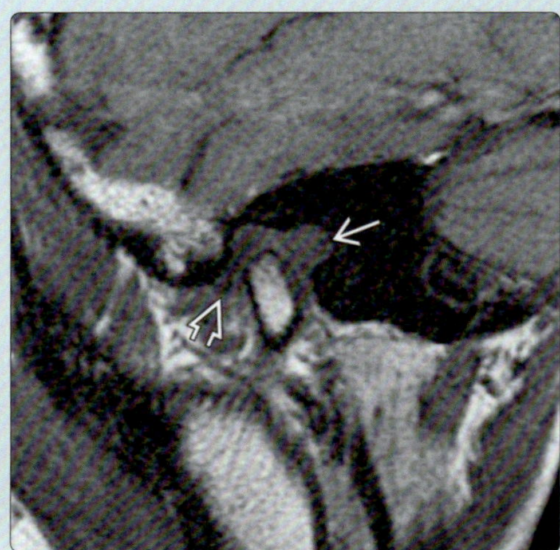

(Left) *Axial bone CT through the EAC reveals a large (14-mm) foramen tympanicum in the anteroinferior bony EAC ➡. The posterior TMJ soft tissues have prolapsed through a dehiscence ➡ into the EAC lumen.* **(Right)** *Sagittal T1 MR in the closed mouth position shows posterior TMJ soft tissues filling the lumen of the EAC ➡. The meniscus ➡ is in normal position. With the mouth open (not shown), soft tissue in the EAC diminishes considerably, suggesting it is the joint capsule that has prolapsed into the EAC.*

KEY FACTS

TERMINOLOGY

- Congenital external and middle ear malformation (CEMEM)

IMAGING

- Auricle: Anotia or microtia
- **EAC stenosis**: Narrow EAC, tympanic plate (TP) hypoplasia
    - Normal or thickened tympanic membrane (TM)
    - Small middle ear cavity
    - Subtle ossicular anomaly
- **EAC (aural) atresia**: Absent EAC, TP, and TM; moderate or severe CEMEM + middle ear findings
- **Moderate CEMEM** middle ear findings
    - Small middle ear cavity ± low tegmen tympani
    - Fusion, malformation, and rotation of malleus and incus
    - Mastoid CNVII more anterolateral than normal
- **Severe CEMEM** middle ear findings
    - Tiny or absent middle ear cavity, low tegmen tympani
    - Ossicles absent or rudimentary
    - Oval window atresia (35%) ± aberrant CNVII
    - Aberrant facial nerve canal course
    - Erosive opacity with scalloped edges in CEMEM suggests congenital cholesteatoma

TOP DIFFERENTIAL DIAGNOSES

- Acquired EAC stenosis (surfer's ear)
- EAC osteoma
- Tympanosclerosis

CLINICAL ISSUES

- Conductive hearing loss = most common symptom
- Severity of microtia approximates severity of CEMEM
- Treatment options
    - Atresiaplasty when ossicles (especially + stapes), middle and inner ear, facial nerve, and mastoid are favorable
    - **Imaging critical to determine surgical candidacy**
        - Jahrsdoerfer scale; ≥ 7 points predicts better hearing
    - Osseointegrated bone conduction solutions provide excellent hearing outcomes

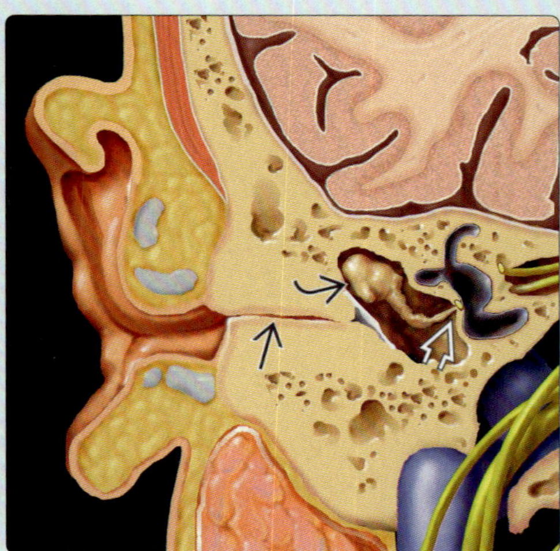

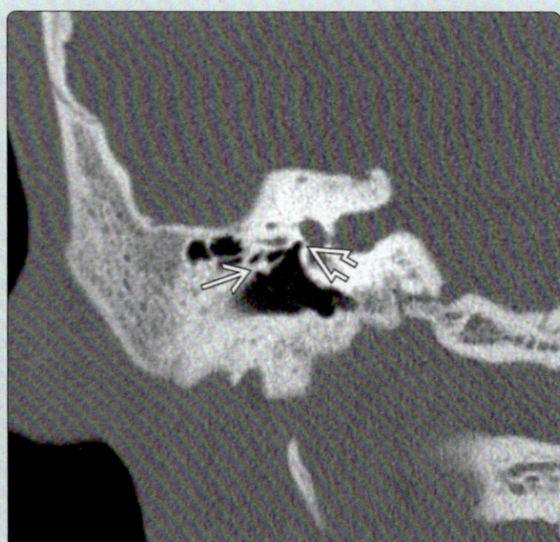

(Left) *Coronal graphic of the right ear shows deformed auricle with absent external auditory canal ➡. Ossicular fusion mass ➡ and rotation with oval window atresia ➡ are also present.* **(Right)** *Coronal bone CT in this patient with congenital external ear malformation shows the ossicular fusion mass ➡ ankylosed to the lateral wall (atretic plate) of the middle ear cavity. Oval window atresia is present, diagnosed by observing the narrowed oval window niche and thin bone covering the oval window itself ➡.*

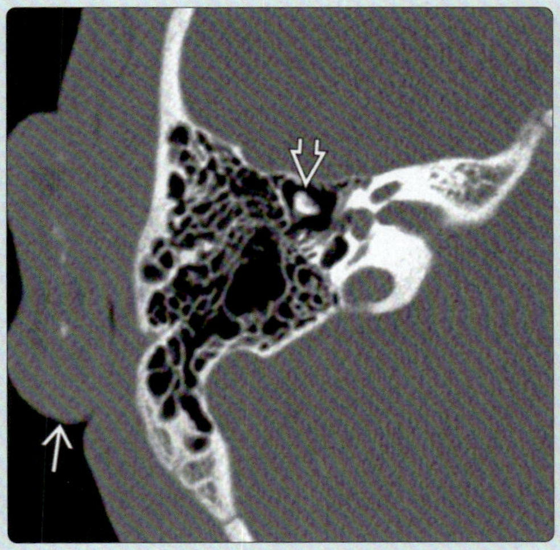

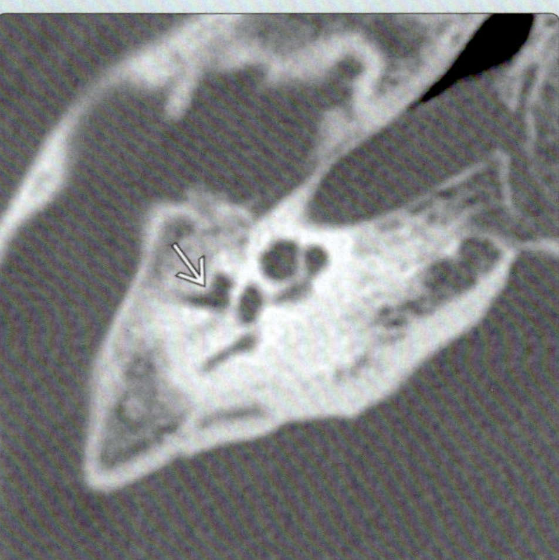

(Left) *Axial T-bone CT reveals a lumpy, featureless pinna ➡, normal mastoid complex, small middle ear cavity, and dysmorphic malleus head ➡. Inner ear structures and IAC are normal. This patient would likely be a candidate for atresiaplasty.* **(Right)** *Axial bone CT in a patient with severe microtia reveals a normal-appearing inner ear with a very small middle ear cavity ➡ and no ossicles. The absence of ossicles combined with near absence of the middle ear cavity makes surgical correction inadvisable.*

Necrotizing External Otitis

KEY FACTS

TERMINOLOGY

- Necrotizing external otitis (NEO); "malignant" otitis externa or skull base osteomyelitis
- NEO definition: Severe **invasive infection** of external auditory canal (EAC), adjacent soft tissues, and skull base

IMAGING

- Swollen EAC soft tissues with **bony erosion** (bone CT) and adjacent cellulitis or abscess
- MR findings
  - Low T1 signal in bony marrow: Osteomyelitis
  - Tissues of EAC and auricle diffusely enhance
- T1WI C+ MR findings
  - **Phlegmon**: Heterogeneously enhancing tissue
  - **Abscesses**: Rim-enhancing fluid collections
- Nuclear medicine findings
  - Bone and gallium scans often done together
  - If both positive with gallium scan showing larger activity area, high correlation with NEO

TOP DIFFERENTIAL DIAGNOSES

- EAC squamous cell carcinoma
- EAC cholesteatoma
- Postinflammatory medial canal fibrosis
- EAC keratosis obturans

PATHOLOGY

- Diabetic vasculopathy and immune dysfunction
- **Pseudomonas aeruginosa**: 98% NEO infections

CLINICAL ISSUES

- Presentation: Severe otalgia and otorrhea
  - "Silent" disease if **diabetic microangiopathy**
- 95% of adults with NEO have **diabetes**
  - Predisposition equal for types I and II
- Treatment
  - Glucose control, granulation biopsy and debridement
  - Topical and systemic antibiotic therapy
  - Surgical drainage of any abscess

(Left) *Axial bone CT shows external auditory canal (EAC) opacification with focal anterior wall ➡ and floor of middle ear ➡ erosion in this diabetic patient with painful otorrhea and early necrotizing external otitis.* **(Right)** *Coronal bone CT in the same patient demonstrates anterior EAC wall bony destruction ➡ accompanied by complete opacification of the EAC. The middle ear is also opacified. In this case, the Pseudomonas infection involved both the EAC and the middle ear cavity.*

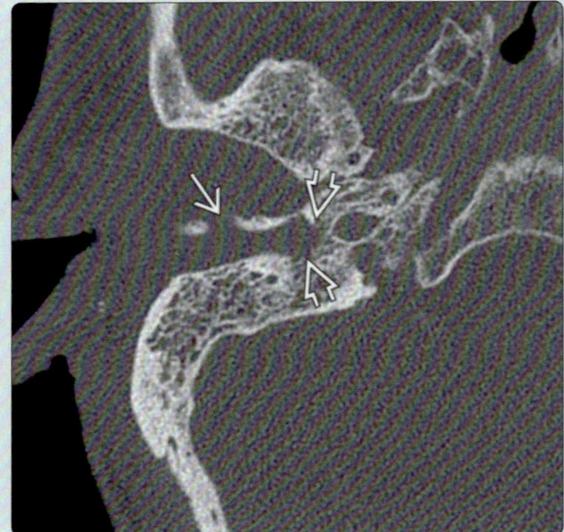

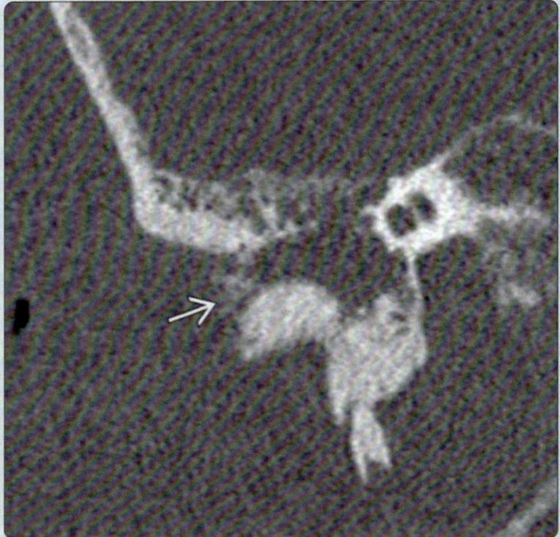

(Left) *Axial bone CT reveals EAC opacification associated with multiple areas of erosive bony change ➡. The mandibular condyle is also eroded ➡, indicating that the infection has spread to involve the TMJ.* **(Right)** *Axial T2WI FS MR in the same patient shows abnormal high signal in the masticator ➡, parapharyngeal ➡, and prevertebral ➡ spaces secondary to spread of the EAC infection into the subjacent spaces of the suprahyoid neck. Sigmoid sinus high signal is from thrombosis ➡.*

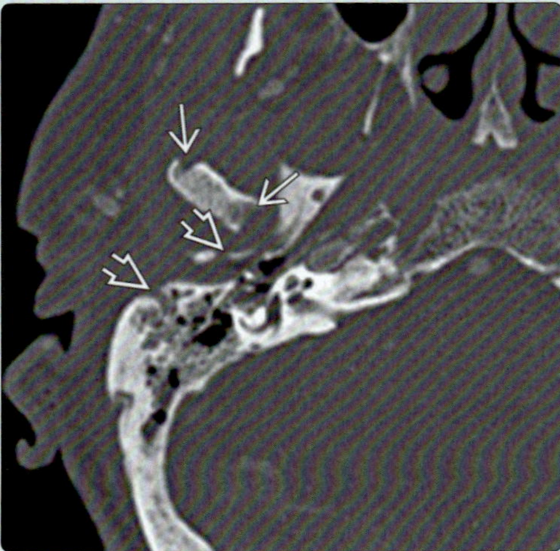

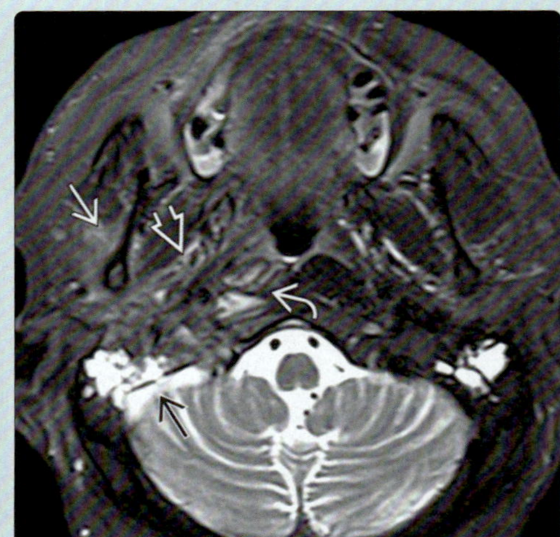

KEY FACTS

TERMINOLOGY

- Keratosis obturans (KO): Abnormal accumulation & obstruction of bony external auditory canal (EAC) from desquamated keratin without erosive bony changes

IMAGING

- Temporal bone CT findings
  - Benign-appearing **luminal** soft tissue lesion partially or completely filling EAC
  - May diffusely enlarge EAC and cause bony remodeling
  - **No** bony erosive change (cf. EAC cholesteatoma)
  - Bilateral (50%)
  - Middle ear spared unless KO neglected

TOP DIFFERENTIAL DIAGNOSES

- Benign EAC debris
- EAC cholesteatoma
- Necrotizing external otitis
- EAC squamous cell carcinoma

PATHOLOGY

- Benign keratin "plug" filling EAC without focal bony erosion

CLINICAL ISSUES

- Clinical presentation
  - Acute **severe otalgia**
  - Conductive hearing loss
- KO treatment
  - Excision of keratin "plug"
  - Removal of reaccumulated debris often required

DIAGNOSTIC CHECKLIST

- "KO" & "EAC cholesteatoma" terms often confused
  - KO: EAC luminal lesion **without** bony erosions
    - If large, may involve middle ear through damaged tympanic membrane
  - EAC cholesteatoma: Subepithelial lesion with EAC erosions ± bony flecks (50%)
    - If large, may involve mastoid air cells

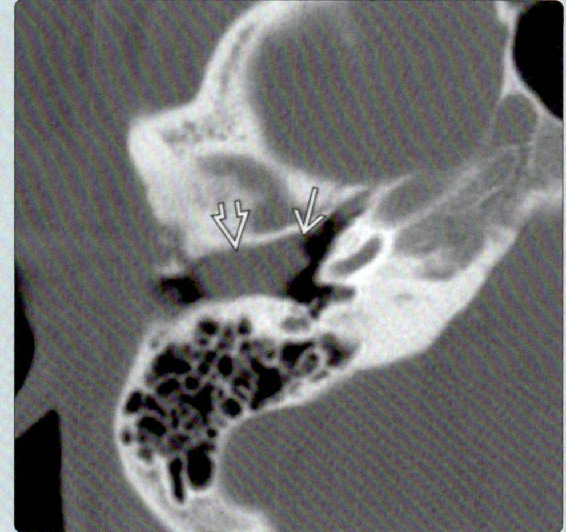

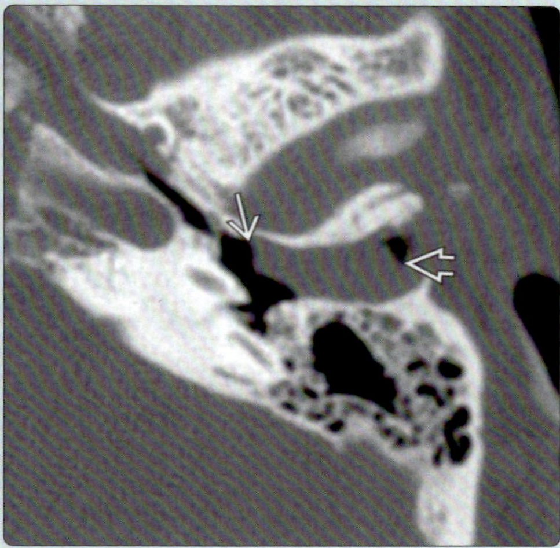

(Left) *Axial bone CT in this patient with otoscopic evidence of EAC obstruction shows a soft tissue "plug" ➡ in the EAC extending laterally from the tympanic membrane ➡. Note absence of underlying bony changes.* **(Right)** *Axial bone CT in a patient with conductive hearing loss demonstrates a benign-appearing soft tissue lesion in the left EAC extending from the tympanic membrane ➡ to the lateral bony EAC margin ➡. The middle ear and underlying EAC bone are not involved.*

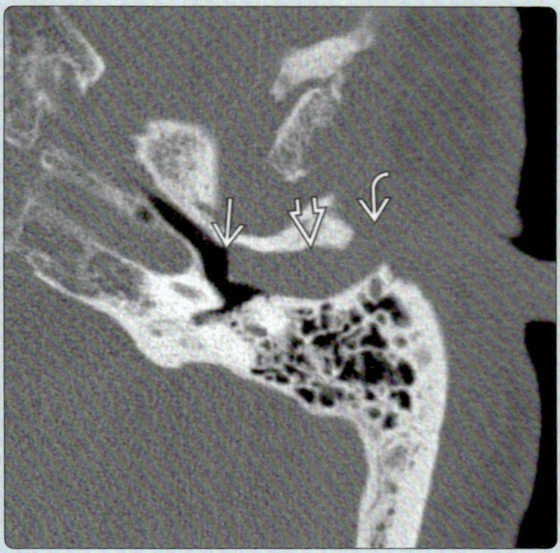

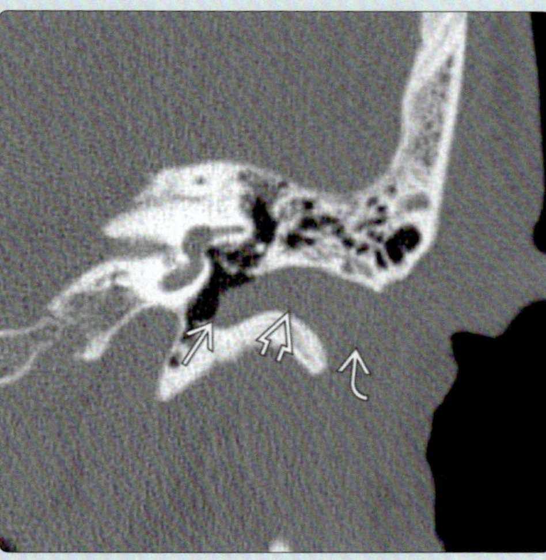

(Left) *Axial bone CT of the left ear shows the EAC is filled with soft tissue ➡. This bland-appearing lesion extends from the tympanic membrane ➡ laterally into the cartilaginous EAC ➡.* **(Right)** *Coronal bone CT in the same patient reveals benign-appearing soft tissue within the EAC ➡ extending from the tympanic membrane ➡ laterally into the cartilaginous EAC ➡. There is slight flaring of the lateral bony EAC but no other bony change is apparent.*

Medial Canal Fibrosis

KEY FACTS

TERMINOLOGY

- Medial canal fibrosis (MCF)
  - Discrete clinicopathological disease characterized by formation of fibrous tissue in medial aspect of bony external auditory canal (EAC)

IMAGING

- **Early-stage MCF**
  - Thickened tympanic membrane (TM) with edematous, thickened medial EAC
- **Late stage MCF**
  - Thick "crescent" fibrosis overlying lateral TM surface
  - TM **cannot** be resolved as separate from MCF fibrous mass; loss of TM landmarks
  - No underlying bony changes present

TOP DIFFERENTIAL DIAGNOSES

- Benign EAC debris; EAC keratosis obturans
- EAC cholesteatoma; EAC exostoses (surfer's ear)
- EAC squamous cell carcinoma
- Necrotizing external otitis

PATHOLOGY

- MCF is final common pathophysiologic pathway for multiple mechanisms of injury to EAC; possible autoimmune/inflammatory
  - Chronic otitis externa: Most common etiology
  - Secondary to surgical procedure or trauma
  - Suppurative otitis media
  - Radiotherapy to EAC

CLINICAL ISSUES

- Common presentation
  - Middle-aged woman with bilateral otorrhea, conductive hearing loss (CHL), history of chronic otitis
- Treatment options
  - Early: Topical steroids
  - Late phase: Surgery corrects CHL; recurrence frequent

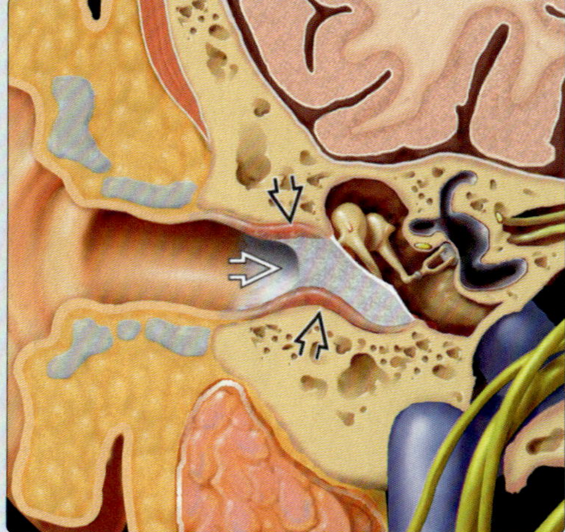

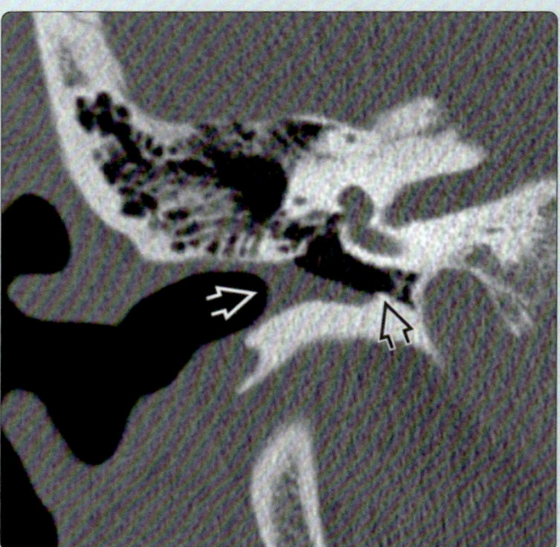

(Left) *Coronal graphic of the right ear shows medial canal fibrosis (MCF) as a thick fibrous crescent ➡ overlying the tympanic membrane (TM) and filling the medial external auditory canal (EAC). Inflammatory changes ➡ of medial EAC walls are also depicted.* **(Right)** *Coronal T-bone CT reveals a band of soft tissue ➡ filling the medial EAC and abutting the TM. The middle ear is unaffected by MCF. The inferior insertion of the TM is marked by the tympanic annulus ➡.*

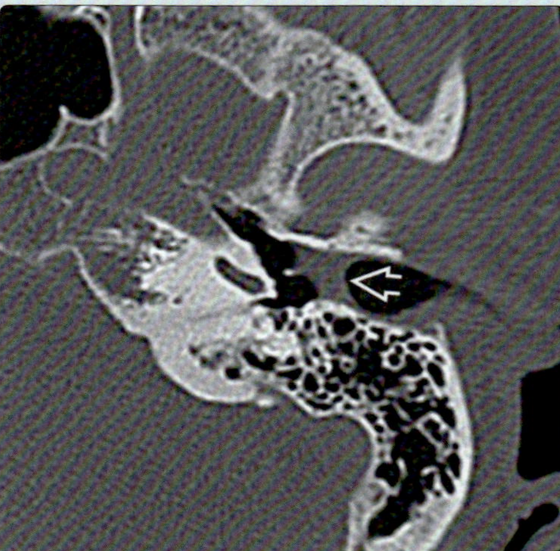

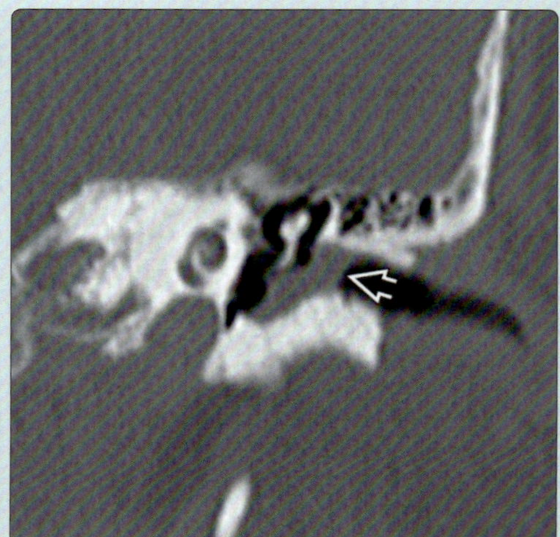

(Left) *Axial bone CT of the left ear demonstrates the characteristic appearance of mature MCF as a crescentic area of soft tissue thickening ➡ on the outer surface of the TM extending laterally into the EAC.* **(Right)** *Coronal bone CT in the same patient reveals the fibrous rind ➡ on the outer surface of the TM. Notice that the middle ear is spared, as is typical for MCF.*

KEY FACTS

TERMINOLOGY

- External auditory canal cholesteatoma (EACC)
- EACC: EAC erosive lesion composed of exfoliated keratin within stratified squamous epithelium

IMAGING

- **Unilateral** scalloping soft tissue bony EAC mass
- **Bone fragments** within soft tissue mass (50%)
- May extend locally into subjacent bony structures
- Tympanic membrane intact; middle ear spared

TOP DIFFERENTIAL DIAGNOSES

- Medial canal fibrosis of EAC
- Necrotizing external otitis
- Squamous cell carcinoma of EAC
- Keratosis obturans of EAC

PATHOLOGY

- Spontaneous: Abnormal migration of EAC ectoderm
- Secondary: Postoperative or posttraumatic
- Congenital: Ectodermal rest within EAC wall (rare)
  - May be associated with congenital ear malformation

CLINICAL ISSUES

- Presentation: Primary symptoms: Otorrhea, otalgia, conductive hearing loss if obstructive
- Demographics
  - Older population: 40-75 years old
- Natural history: Relentless increase in size & erosion of EAC bony wall
  - May show less aggressive behavior in pediatric patients
- Treatment options: Surgical excision for larger lesions with bony invasion
- Must rule out malignancy, especially in older patients

DIAGNOSTIC CHECKLIST

- Focal, unilateral EAC mass + EAC bony scalloping ± bony flecks = EACC

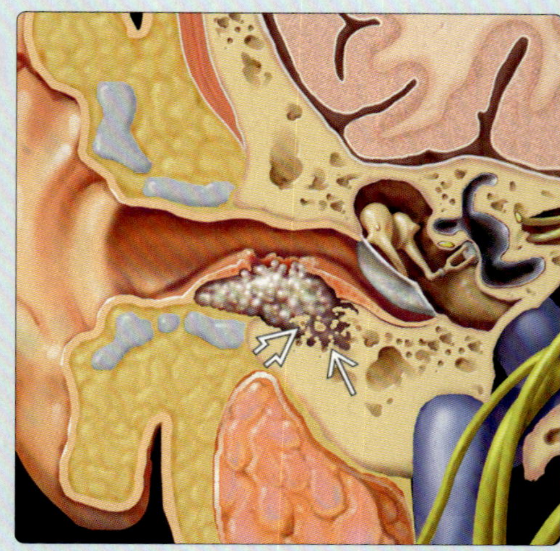

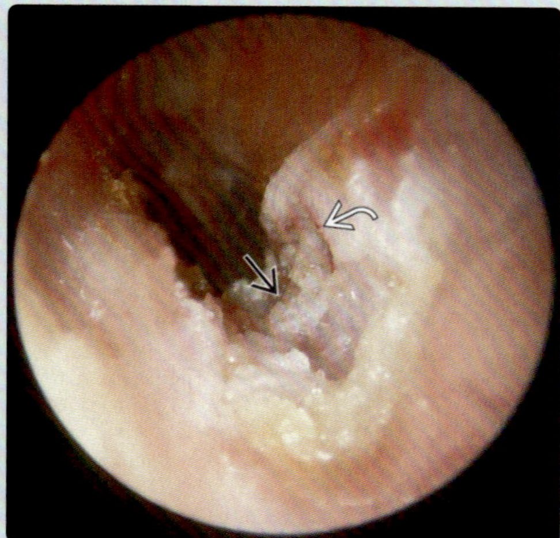

(Left) *Coronal graphic shows an external auditory canal cholesteatoma (EACC) as an erosive, scalloping subepithelial mass in the inferior bony EAC. Note bone erosion ➡ with bony flecks ⮕ within the cholesteatoma matrix.* **(Right)** *Otoscopic view of a left EACC demonstrates heaped-up squamous debris ⇨ that is seen with marked epithelial irregularities ➡.*

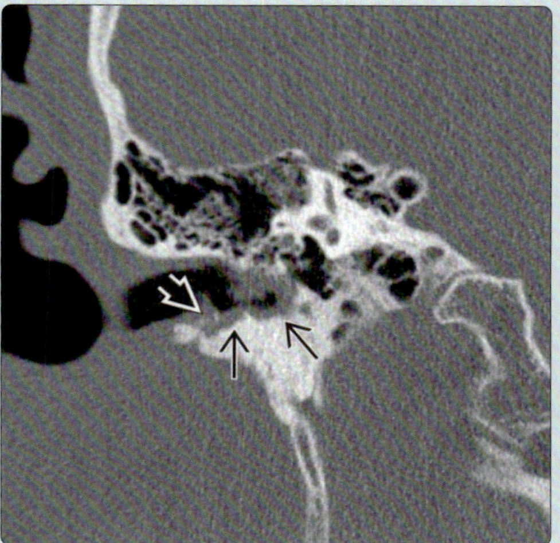

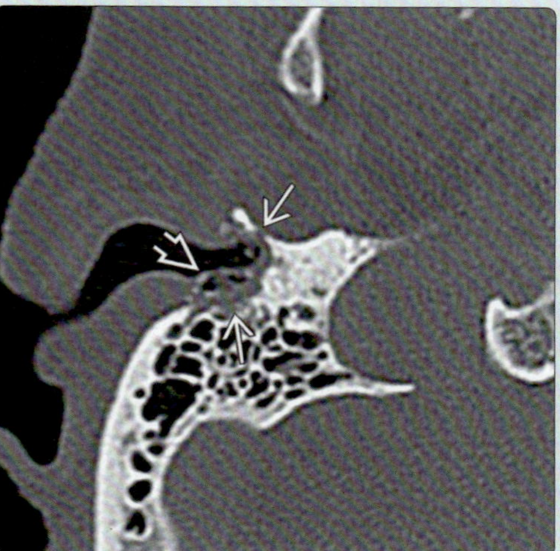

(Left) *Coronal bone CT reveals an EACC as a soft tissue mass along the inferior bony canal with underlying osseous erosion ⇨ and bony flecks within the cholesteatoma matrix ➡.* **(Right)** *An elderly woman presented with otorrhea, otalgia, and a heaped-up submucosal lesion in the EAC area. Axial bone CT shows an erosive lesion of the bony EAC ➡ affecting the anterior, posterior, and inferior walls. Note multifocal bony flecks ➡ within the soft tissue component of the lesion.*

EAC Osteoma

KEY FACTS

TERMINOLOGY

- Osteoma: Rare, benign, focal, pedunculated, bony overgrowth of osseous external auditory canal (EAC) with normal overlying squamous epithelium

IMAGING

- Most common site: Bony-cartilaginous EAC junction
- Bone CT: Benign-appearing, focal, **pedunculated**, bony overgrowth of osseous EAC
  - Cerumen entrapment, squamous debris accumulation, or **secondary canal cholesteatoma** possible with large, lateral lesions

TOP DIFFERENTIAL DIAGNOSES

- EAC exostoses (surfer's ear)
- EAC cholesteatoma
- Medial canal fibrosis
- Necrotizing external otitis
- Benign EAC debris

PATHOLOGY

- Irregularly oriented **lamellated bone** with surrounding discrete, fibrovascular channels
- Osteoma found in other temporal bone sites
  - Ossicles, mastoid, internal auditory canal

CLINICAL ISSUES

- Asymptomatic, usually incidental finding
- Treatment
  - Permanent cure with adequate surgical excision via canalplasty; often accomplished via transcanal approach

DIAGNOSTIC CHECKLIST

- Differentiate from EAC exostoses
  - EAC osteoma: Narrow-based, single lesion, lateral EAC, **unilateral**
  - EAC exostosis: Broad-based, circumferential, multilobular, medial EAC, history of cold water exposure, **bilateral**

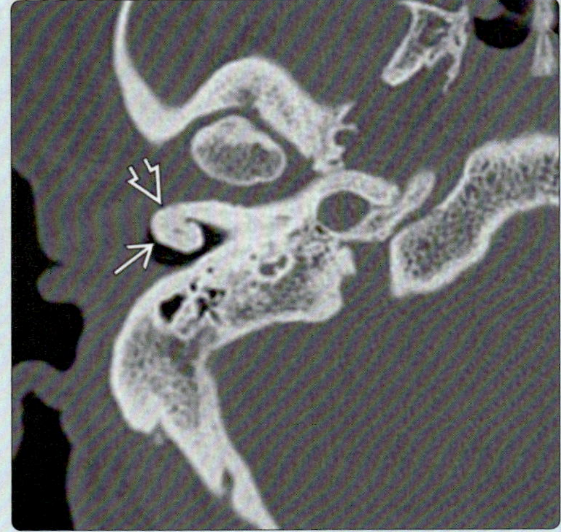
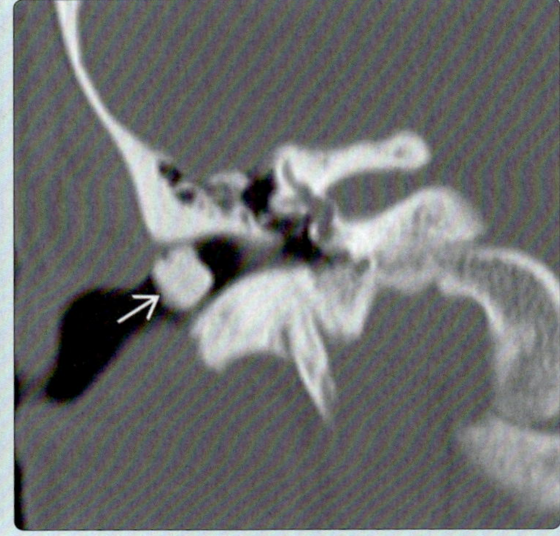

(Left) *Axial bone CT shows an osteoma ➡ pedunculating from the anterolateral aspect ➡ of the bony external auditory canal (EAC) in this patient who presents with hard submucosal mass in the mid EAC.* **(Right)** *Coronal bone CT in the same patient shows the osteoma ➡ almost completely plugging the EAC. There is still sufficient room for wax and squamous debris to exit the medial EAC.*

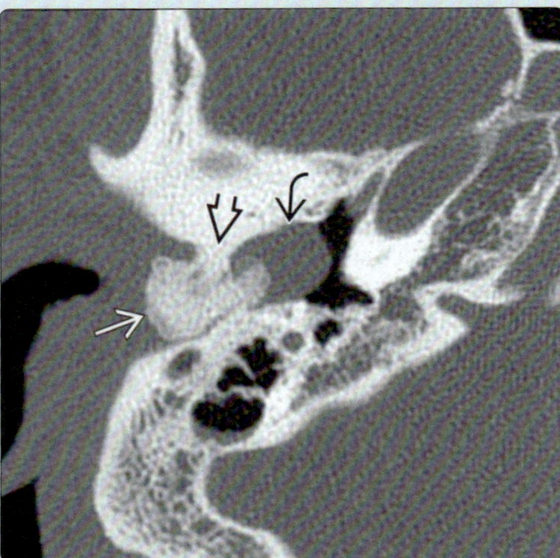
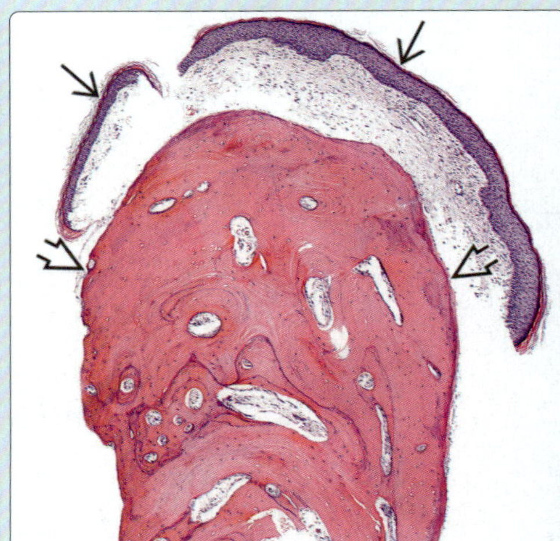

(Left) *Axial bone CT shows a pedunculated osteoma ➡ arising from the anterior EAC bony wall ➡. Clinical exam shows occlusion of the EAC. Note the secondary canal cholesteatoma ➡ within the medial EAC. The middle ear space is aerated.* **(Right)** *H&E micrograph reveals surface squamous epithelium ➡ is uninvolved by the osteoma ➡. There is well-formed, mature compact bone within the osteoma. This osteoma expanded from the adjacent bony EAC cortex, creating an obstructing subepithelial mass. (From DP: H&N 2e.)*

KEY FACTS

TERMINOLOGY

- Definition: Benign overgrowth of bony external auditory canal (EAC) in response to chronic cold water exposure

IMAGING

- Temporal bone CT
  - **Bilateral** lesions in almost all cases
  - Broad-based or more focal circumferential bony overgrowth of osseous EAC
  - Variable EAC stenosis results

TOP DIFFERENTIAL DIAGNOSES

- EAC osteoma
- EAC cholesteatoma
- EAC medial canal fibrosis
- Necrotizing external otitis

CLINICAL ISSUES

- Most common symptoms
  - Conductive hearing loss, chronic otitis externa, otorrhea, tinnitus, otalgia
- Patient profile
  - 20-50 years old, male predominance
  - 70% prevalence in surfers
    - Increased incidence with increased time of exposure
- Treatment options
  - Often require no treatment
  - May require surgical excision via canalplasty if conductive hearing loss or chronic otitis externa are present
  - Avoid intraoperative facial nerve injury in posterior-inferior EAC

DIAGNOSTIC CHECKLIST

- Image interpretation pearls
  - Most common differential diagnosis: EAC osteoma
  - EAC osteoma: Unilateral, focal, in lateral bony EAC
  - EAC exostoses: Bilateral mid bony EAC circumferential, multilobular narrowing

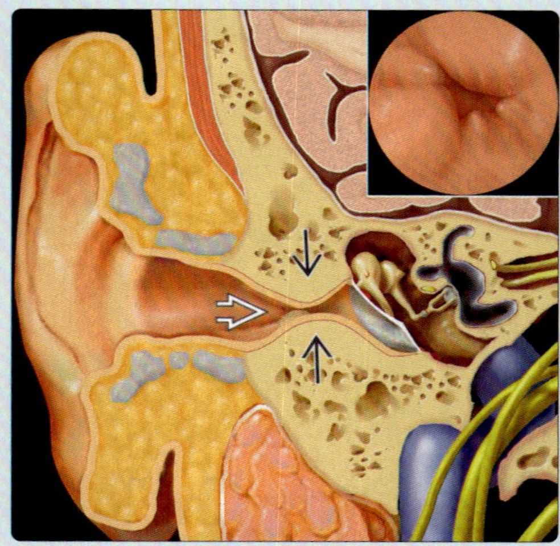

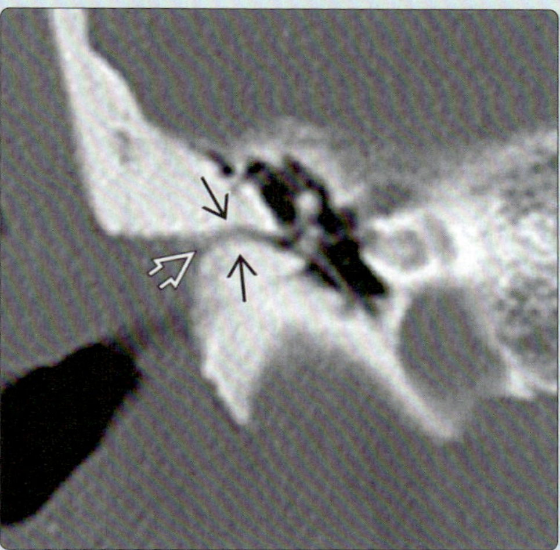

(Left) *Coronal graphic shows benign-appearing bony overgrowth of the right EAC ➾ in a case of external auditory canal (EAC) exostoses. Insert shows otoscopic view of circumferential subepithelial EAC narrowing ➡.* **(Right)** *Coronal bone CT of the right temporal bone shows severe EAC stenosis ➡ secondary to circumferential exostoses ➾ that developed bilaterally as a result of chronic cold water exposure (often from surfing).*

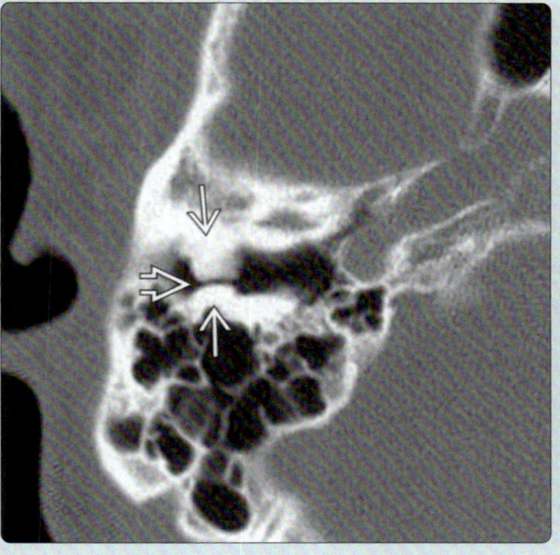

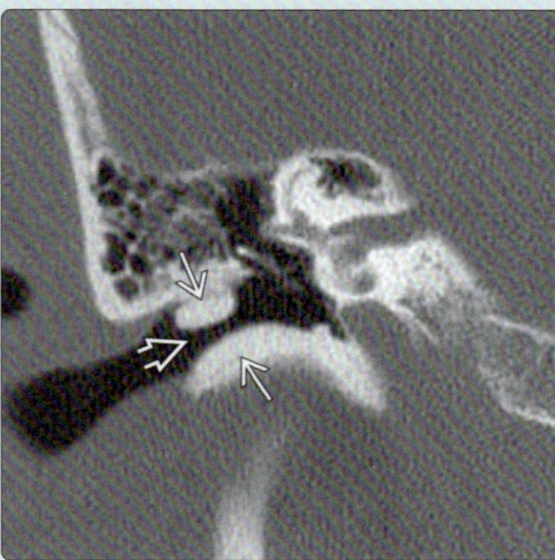

(Left) *Axial bone CT reveals bilateral EAC exostoses ➡ with moderate EAC luminal stenosis ➡. (Courtesy C. Schatz, MD.)* **(Right)** *Coronal temporal bone CT in the same patient shows EAC exostoses ➡ with moderate EAC luminal stenosis ➡. The bilaterality (not shown) and circumferential bony involvement differentiate this lesion from unilateral, focal EAC osteoma.*

EAC Skin Squamous Cell Carcinoma

KEY FACTS

TERMINOLOGY

- Squamous cell carcinoma (SCCa) of external ear with spread to external auditory canal (EAC); T-bone carcinoma

IMAGING

- Imaging done to assess soft tissue extent, bone or parotid invasion, intracranial extension, CNVII perineural spread
- T-bone CT best predicts osseous invasion
  - Bone destruction or soft tissue invasion indicates aggressive malignancy
  - Soft tissue window will show parotid nodes
- Enhanced MR superior for intracranial, parotid, and perineural spread

TOP DIFFERENTIAL DIAGNOSES

- Benign EAC debris
- EAC cholesteatoma
- Necrotizing external otitis
- Osteoradionecrosis

PATHOLOGY

- Disease of elderly (median age: 65 years)
- ↑ incidence in patients with otological diseases

CLINICAL ISSUES

- Clinical presentation: Pain, otorrhea, facial paresis
  - Patients with **known SCCa of auricle**; previously treated
  - SCCa spreads to EAC late
    - EAC SCCa 1st destroys bony canal then invades surrounding anatomic structures
  - Imaging done to assess extent of regional invasion
    - Imaging also done to assess for intraparotid, pre- & postauricular nodal metastases
- **5-year survival** for early stage (T1/T2) = 70%; advanced stage (T3) = 40%
- Treatment options
  - With early stage (T1-T2) tumors, en bloc resection via lateral temporal bone resection often curative
  - T3-T4 tumors: Surgery and radiation ± chemotherapy

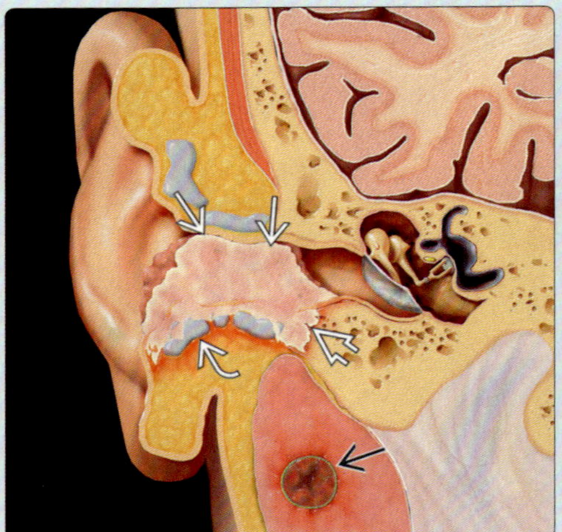

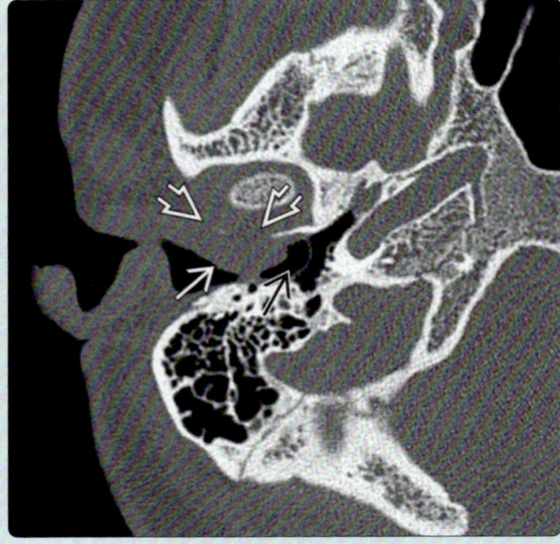

(Left) *Coronal graphic illustrates large external auditory canal (EAC) squamous cell carcinoma (SCCa) presenting as a mass ➡ filling the canal. Note the aggressive features with infiltration of the auricle & its cartilages ➡, invasion of the T-bone ➡, & metastatic intraparotid node ➡.* **(Right)** *Axial T-bone CT reveals SCCa of right EAC with prominent soft tissue mass ➡ filling the EAC. Osseous invasion through posterior wall of TMJ condylar fossa ➡ is present. Distal EAC at the tympanic membrane ➡ is clear of tumor.*

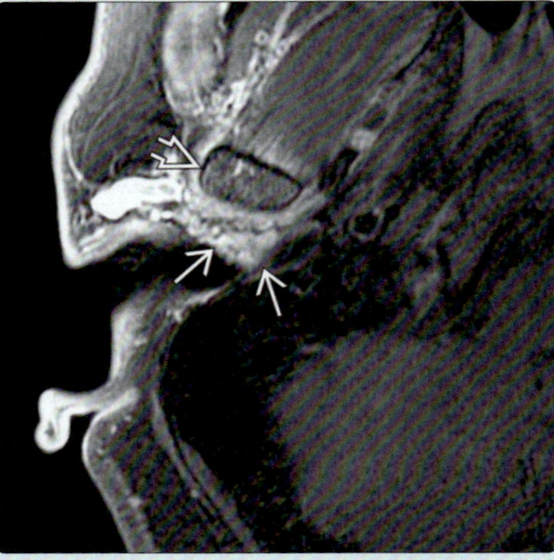

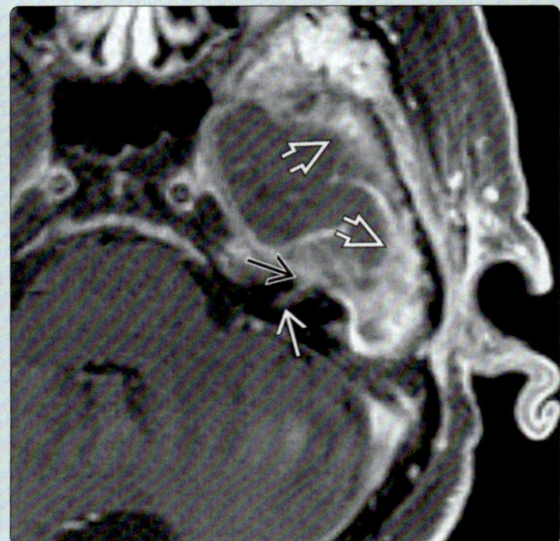

(Left) *Axial T1WI C+ MR shows a solidly enhancing EAC SCCa ➡ filling the canal and invading anteriorly into the TMJ. Note the soft tissue tumor around the right condylar head ➡.* **(Right)** *Axial T1WI C+ FS MR shows more advanced EAC SCCa with gross transdural ➡ extension into the left middle cranial fossa. Marked thickening and enhancement along CNVII at the geniculate ganglion ➡ and in the internal auditory canal ➡ represents a perineural tumor.*

Congenital Middle Ear Cholesteatoma

KEY FACTS

TERMINOLOGY

- Congenital middle ear cholesteatoma (CMEC)
- Definition: Cholesteatoma in middle ear behind intact tympanic membrane (TM) in patient with no history of surgery, otitis media, or otorrhea

IMAGING

- Temporal bone CT findings
  - Small: Well-circumscribed soft tissue middle ear mass medial to ossicles
  - Large: Erodes ossicles, middle ear wall, lateral semicircular canal, or tegmen tympani
  - Long process of incus & stapes superstructure most commonly destroyed ossicles
  - If aditus ad antrum occluded, mastoid air cells opacify with retained secretions
  - Mastoid pneumatization usually normal
- MR findings
  - T1WI C+: Rim-enhancing middle ear mass
  - Non-echo-planar DWI sequences recommended, especially if surveillance needed
    - Minimize susceptibility artifacts
    - ↑ sensitivity for detection of smaller lesions (2 mm)
    - CMEC **hyperintense**; due to high keratin content

TOP DIFFERENTIAL DIAGNOSES

- Pars tensa- or flaccida-acquired cholesteatoma
- Glomus tympanicum paraganglioma
- Facial nerve schwannoma of tympanic segment
- Middle ear cholesterol granuloma

CLINICAL ISSUES

- Younger patient (< 20 years old)
- **Often incidentally found**, pearly, avascular middle ear mass behind **intact TM**
- Unilateral conductive hearing loss (30%)
- Complete surgical extirpation = treatment of choice
  - Tympanoplasty, ± ossiculoplasty, ± mastoidectomy

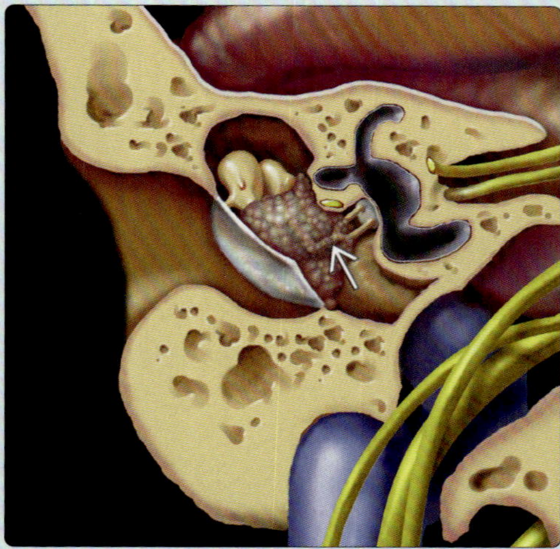

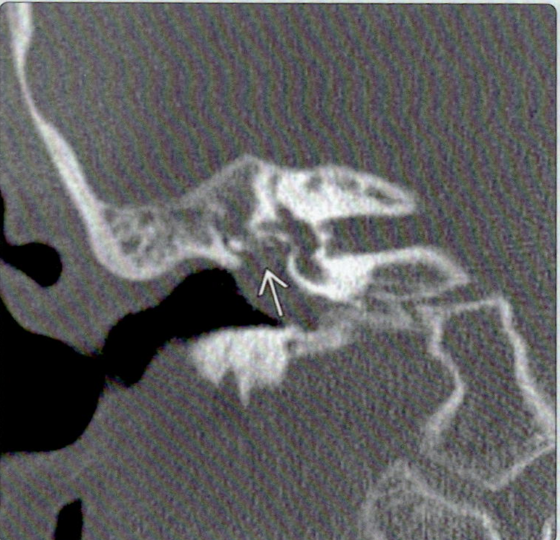

(Left) *Coronal graphic shows congenital middle ear cholesteatoma (CMEC). Notice that the lesion surrounds and is medial to the ossicles ➡. The tympanic membrane is intact.* **(Right)** *Coronal temporal bone CT of the right ear demonstrates a large congenital cholesteatoma filling the middle ear cavity with subtle long process of incus and stapes hub erosion ➡ and deossification. The tympanic membrane bulges laterally but is intact by otoscopic examination.*

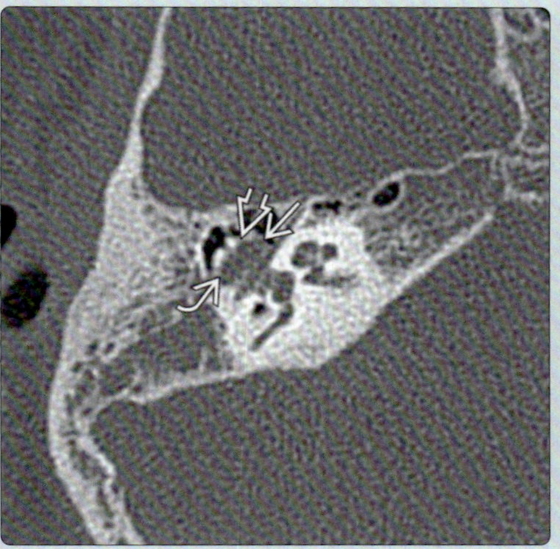

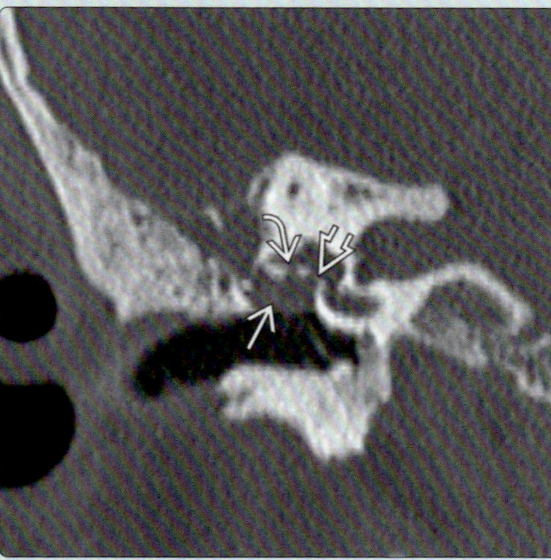

(Left) *Axial bone CT of the right ear reveals a medial epitympanic congenital cholesteatoma ➡ eroding the medial head of the malleus ➡ and short process of the incus ➡. Aditus ad antrum block causes mastoid effusion.* **(Right)** *Coronal bone CT in the same patient shows CMEC eroding the long process of the incus ➡ and filling the oval window niche ➡. The tympanic segment of CNVII canal enlargement ➡ is secondary to cholesteatoma focal invasion.*

Congenital Mastoid Cholesteatoma

KEY FACTS

TERMINOLOGY

- Definition: Cholesteatoma in mastoid secondary to epithelial rest

IMAGING

- Bone CT findings
  - Expansile soft tissue mass
  - Smooth erosion of mastoid bone
- MR findings
  - T1 low, T2 high
  - T1WI C+ nonenhancing; bows sigmoid sinus
  - **DWI hyperintensity** (restricted diffusion)
- Mastoid locations
  - Anywhere in mastoid area
  - Medial mastoid ± internal auditory canal ± petrous apex

TOP DIFFERENTIAL DIAGNOSES

- Large pars flaccida-acquired cholesteatoma
- Mastoid cholesterol granuloma
- Temporal bone fibrous dysplasia
- Temporal bone Langerhans cell histiocytosis

PATHOLOGY

- Microscopic: Stratified squamous epithelium with progressive exfoliation of keratinous material

CLINICAL ISSUES

- Presentations
  - Older patient group (20-40 years)
    - Compared to middle ear cholesteatoma
  - Retroauricular swelling and pain; ± headache
  - May be **incidentally found** on head MR
- Treatment
  - Surgical removal is treatment of choice
  - Sigmoid sinus preservation important

DIAGNOSTIC CHECKLIST

- DWI **restricted diffusion** confirms congenital mastoid cholesteatoma diagnosis

(Left) *Axial bone CT shows a multilobular congenital cholesteatoma involving the lateral clivus ➡ and the medial mastoid ➡. The expansile bony margins are suggestive of this diagnosis.* **(Right)** *Axial T2WI MR in the same patient reveals a giant temporal bone congenital mastoid cholesteatoma as a high-signal, sharply marginated mass ➡.*

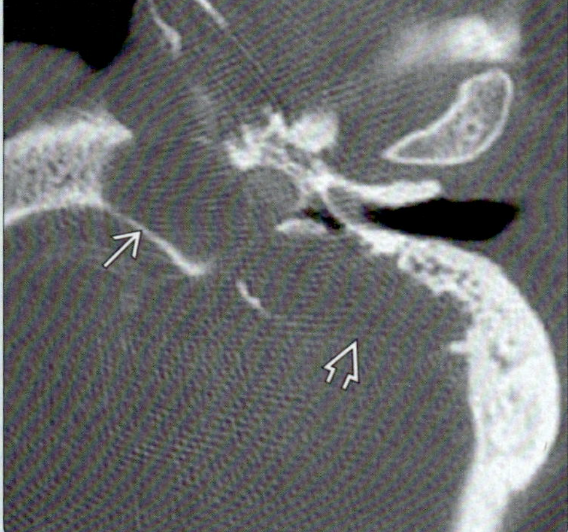

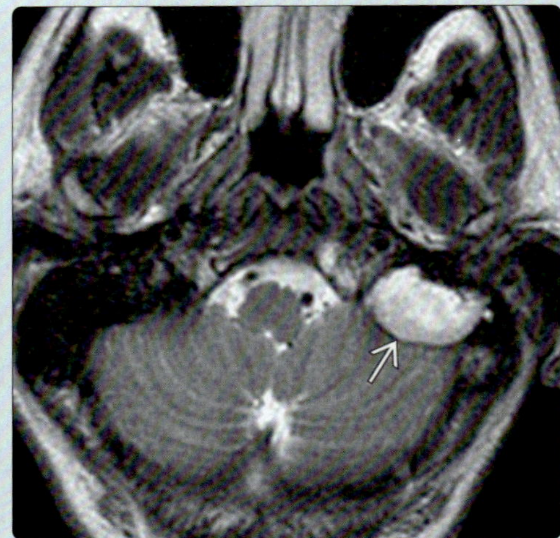

(Left) *Axial T1WI C+ MR in the same patient shows both the lateral clival ➡ and mastoid ➡ components of a large temporal bone congenital cholesteatoma. As in this case, nonenhancement would be expected.* **(Right)** *Axial DWI MR in the same patient shows high signal ➡ in the location of the giant temporal bone congenital cholesteatoma. Restricted diffusion within the lesion is highly suggestive of the diagnosis of cholesteatoma.*

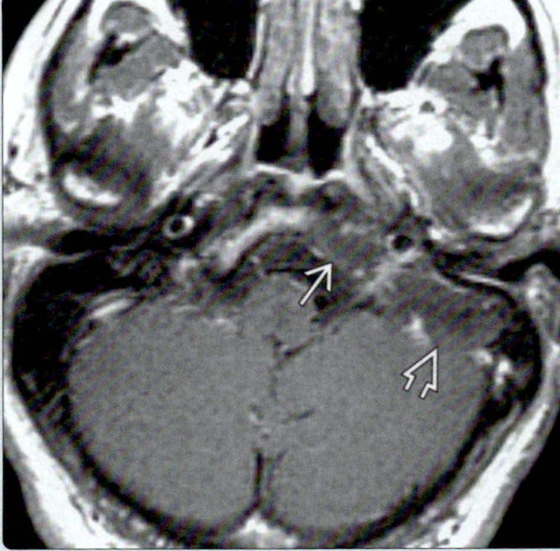

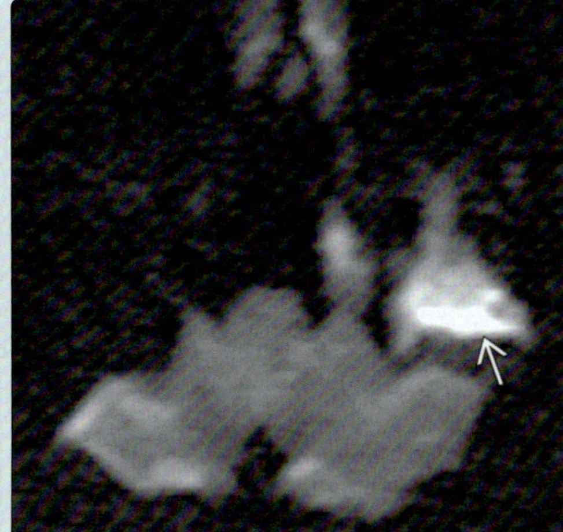

KEY FACTS

TERMINOLOGY

- Major anomaly: Anomaly of middle and external ear
- Minor anomaly: Isolated middle ear (ME) anomaly
- Ossicular fixation: Congenital ankylosis; rigid bar or fibrous band connects ossicle to wall of ME
- Ossicular malformation: Anomaly in shape, size, &/or orientation of ossicle
- Columellar stapes: 1 central, broad stapedial crus

IMAGING

- High-resolution bone CT critical to diagnosis (< 1 mm)
- **Malleus**: Normal or malformed; bony or fibrous fixation to lateral, superior, anterior epitympanum
- **Incus**: Normal or malformed; agenesis is rare
  - Deficient segment of incus is uncommon
  - Bony or fibrous fixation to attic; incus-malleus fusion
- **Stapes**: Normal or malformed; fixation of superstructure to promontory, pyramidal process, or CNVII canal
- **Ossicular joints**: Fusion or discontinuity
- **Oval window & CNVII canal**: Normal, stenotic, or atretic oval window; normal or anomalous ± dehiscent CNVII
- **Tegmen tympani**: Normal or low, abutting ossicles

TOP DIFFERENTIAL DIAGNOSES

- Tympanosclerosis involving ossicles
- Congenital external and ME malformation
- Calcified stabilizing ligaments
- Ossicular fixation, posttraumatic
- Ossicular prosthesis

PATHOLOGY

- Exact etiology unknown in most cases
- Isolated or syndromic; sporadic or familial

CLINICAL ISSUES

- Nonprogressive 40-60 dB conductive hearing loss
- Treatment: Surgery; maintain continuity of native ossicles when possible, ossicular reconstruction when necessary
- Imaging critical to determine surgical candidacy

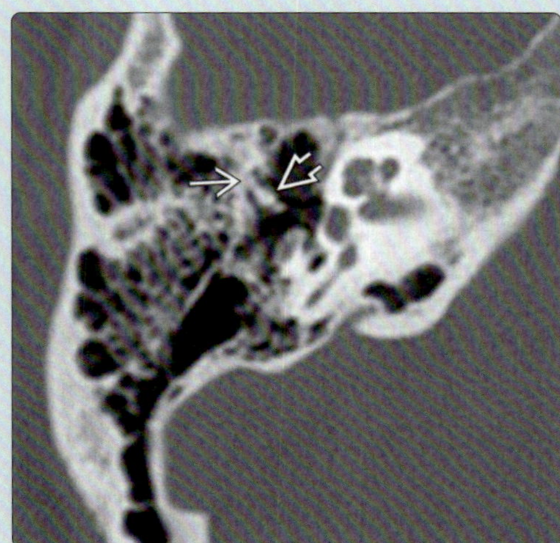

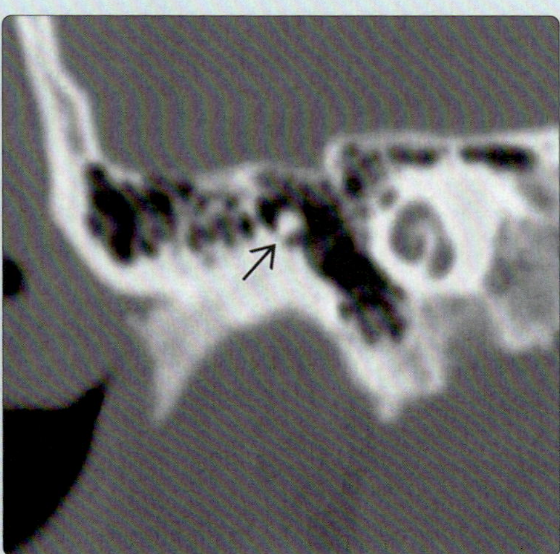

(Left) *Axial bone CT shows a bony bar ➡ between the malleus head ➡ and lateral epitympanic wall. Notice that there is no evidence of prior infection or trauma. The mastoid air cells are normally developed, and no inflammatory debris is present.* **(Right)** *Coronal bone CT in the same patient shows a bony bar ➡ between the malleus head and lateral epitympanic wall. The external auditory canal is normal (not shown), and there is no evidence of previous infection.*

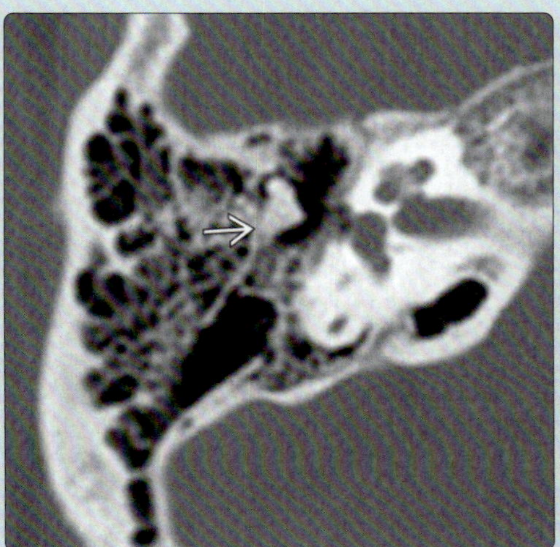

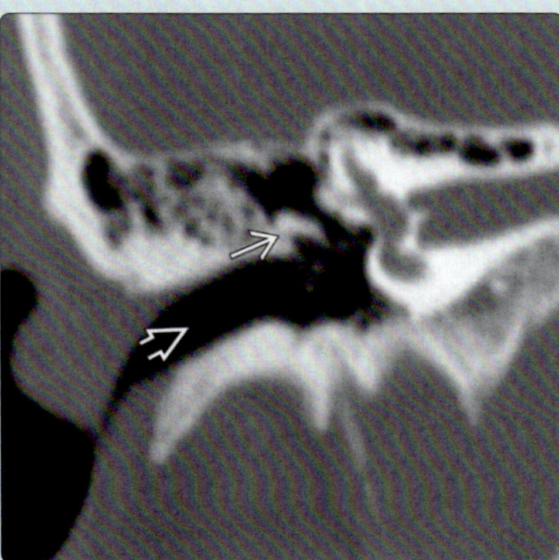

(Left) *Axial bone CT in this patient with conductive hearing loss reveals bony ankylosis of the lateral margin of the short process of the incus ➡ to the lateral epitympanic wall.* **(Right)** *Coronal bone CT in the same patient demonstrates the bony attachment of the short process of the incus ➡ to the lateral epitympanic wall. Notice the normal external auditory canal ➡ and absence of inflammatory changes.*

KEY FACTS

TERMINOLOGY

- Oval window atresia (OWA): Absent space between lateral semicircular canal above and cochlear promontory below associated with anomalous stapes and malpositioned CNVII

IMAGING

- **Imperative in congenital conductive hearing loss**: Evaluate for OWA, middle and inner ear malformations
- Temporal bone CT findings
  - Normal OW replaced by ossific "web" or plate
  - **Inferomedially positioned** tympanic segment **CNVII**
    - May completely overlie OW
    - May reside on superior or inferior OW margin
- Key surgical finding on CT = facial nerve location prevents safe surgical correction
- Best imaging tool: Multiplanar temporal bone CT
  - OW niche best seen in coronal plane
  - CNVII location relative to OW best seen in coronal plane
  - Stapes crura best seen in axial plane
- Bony plate over OW + inferomedially displaced tympanic CNVII = OWA
  - If both findings present, no differential diagnosis present

TOP DIFFERENTIAL DIAGNOSES

- Tympanosclerosis
- Fenestral otosclerosis or congenital stapes fixation
- Congenital external ear malformation

PATHOLOGY

- Best hypothesis for OW etiology: Primitive stapes fails to fuse with primitive vestibule during 7th week of gestation

CLINICAL ISSUES

- Clinical presentation
  - Nonprogressive conductive hearing deficit from birth
  - No history of otomastoiditis; normal EAC and TM
- Best treatment: Osseointegrated bone conduction devices
  - **Facial nerve ectopia** into OW niche in OWA is **surgical contraindication**, no need for exploration

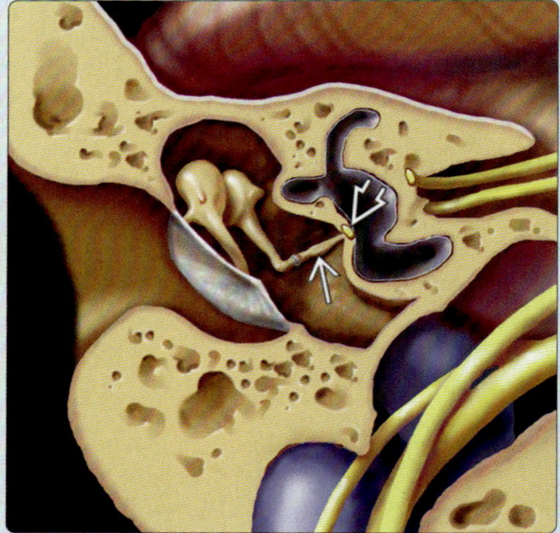

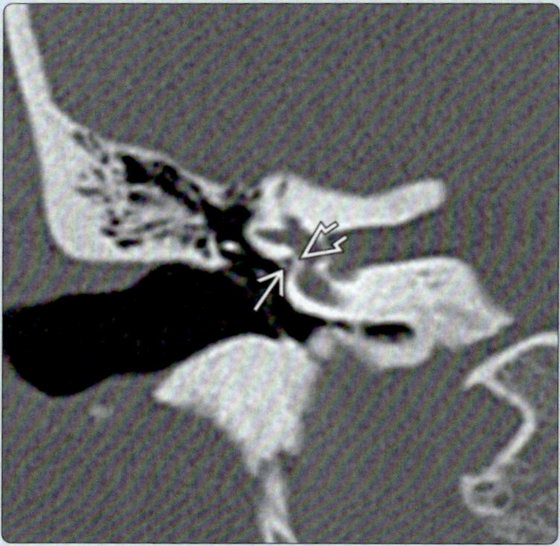

(Left) *Coronal graphic illustrates features of oval window atresia, including malformation of the stapes crura and footplate ➡ and tympanic segment of the facial nerve in an abnormal location ➡.* **(Right)** *Coronal bone CT through the IAC demonstrates that the oval window is absent with bone density ➡ in its expected location. The tympanic segment of the facial nerve is not in its expected location inferior to the horizontal semicircular canal but instead overlies the atretic window ➡. The stapes is not seen.*

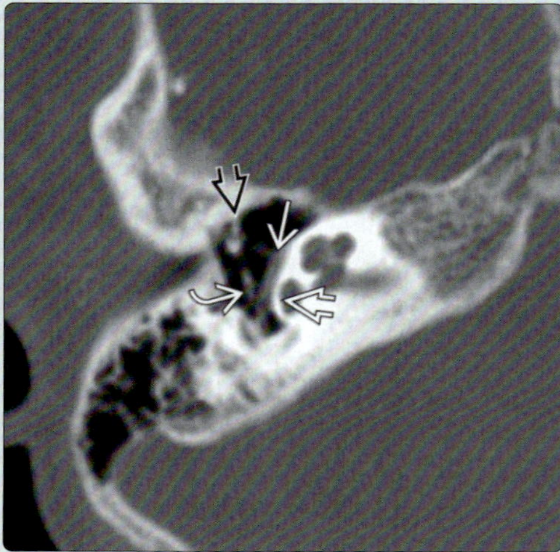

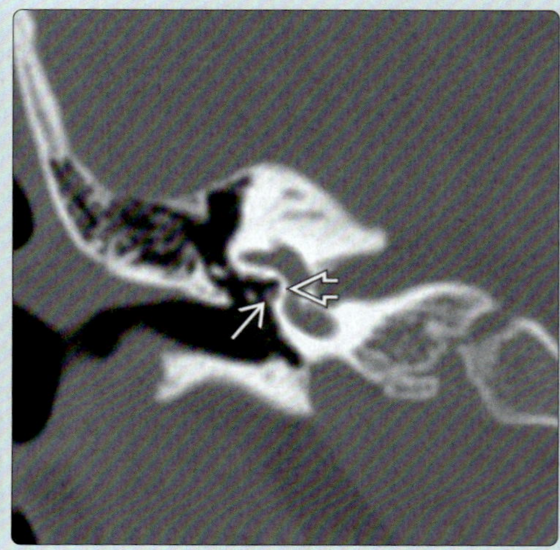

(Left) *Axial bone CT in an adolescent patient with conductive hearing loss shows deformed ossicles with angulation of the incus ➡ and anterior malleolar ligament calcification ➡. The oval window is bone covered ➡ with the tympanic segment of CNVII traversing its margin ➡.* **(Right)** *Coronal bone CT in the same patient reveals the bony plate within the oval window ➡. Notice that the tympanic segment is present along the inferior margin of the oval window niche ➡.*

Aberrant Internal Carotid Artery

KEY FACTS

TERMINOLOGY

- Aberrant internal carotid artery (AbICA): Congenital vascular anomaly resulting from failure of formation of extracranial ICA with arterial collateral pathway

IMAGING

- Appearance of AbICA on thin-section (< 1-mm) temporal bone CT is diagnostic
  - AbICA appears as **tubular lesion** crossing middle ear from posterior to anterior
  - **Enlarged inferior tympanic canaliculus** important observation
  - AbICA narrows as reenters horizontal petrous ICA
- Caution: AbICA mimics glomus tympanicum paraganglioma

TOP DIFFERENTIAL DIAGNOSES

- Other vascular middle ear lesions
  - Glomus tympanicum paraganglioma
  - Dehiscent jugular bulb
  - Lateralized internal carotid artery

PATHOLOGY

- Best explanation: "Alternative blood flow" theory
  - Persistence of pharyngeal artery system means **C1 portion of ICA is absent**
  - Mature arterial collateral system compensates for absent C1 and vertical petrous ICA segments
  - Ascending pharyngeal artery → inferior tympanic artery → caroticotympanic artery → posterolateral aspect of horizontal petrous ICA
- 30% of AbICA have **persistent stapedial artery**

CLINICAL ISSUES

- Typically asymptomatic and discovered at time of routine physical exam, during middle ear surgery, or as incidental imaging finding
- Associated symptoms
  - Pulsatile tinnitus, conductive hearing loss
- No treatment is best treatment

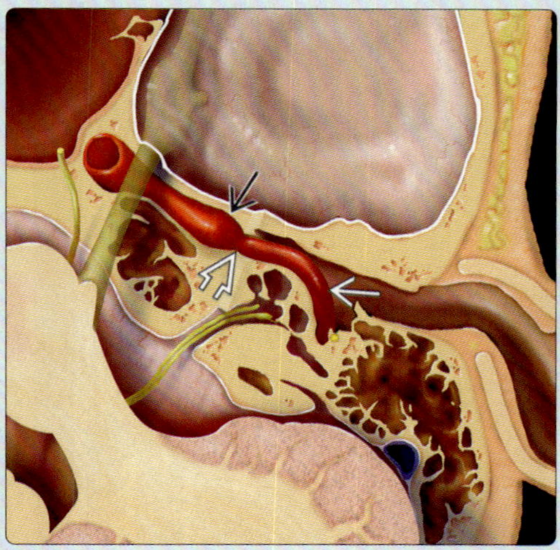

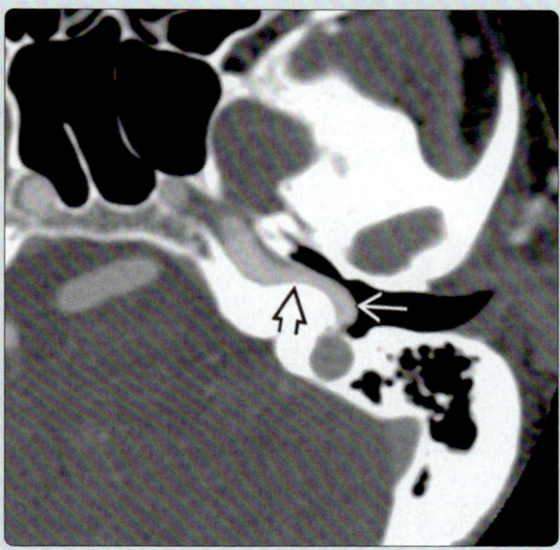

(Left) *Axial graphic of the left temporal bone illustrates classic aberrant internal carotid artery (AbICA) ➡ rising along the posterior cochlear promontory, crossing along the medial middle ear wall, & rejoining the horizontal petrous ICA ⇨. At the point of reconnection to the horizontal petrous ICA, stenosis ➡ is often present.* **(Right)** *Axial CTA through the middle ear shows the looping aberrant internal carotid ➡ on the low cochlear promontory. Note the caliber change ⇨ as the AbICA rejoins the normal horizontal segment of the ICA.*

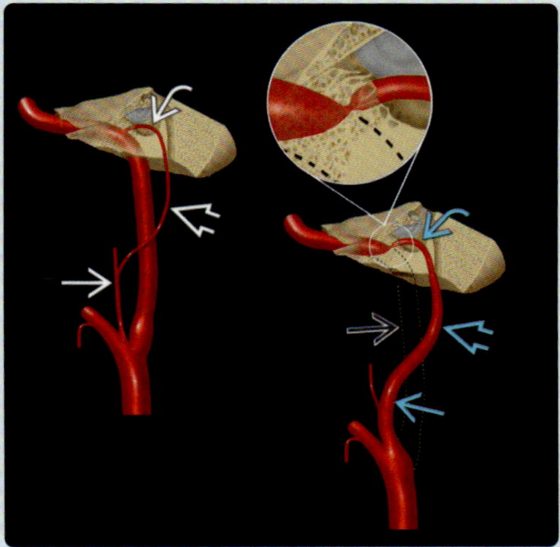

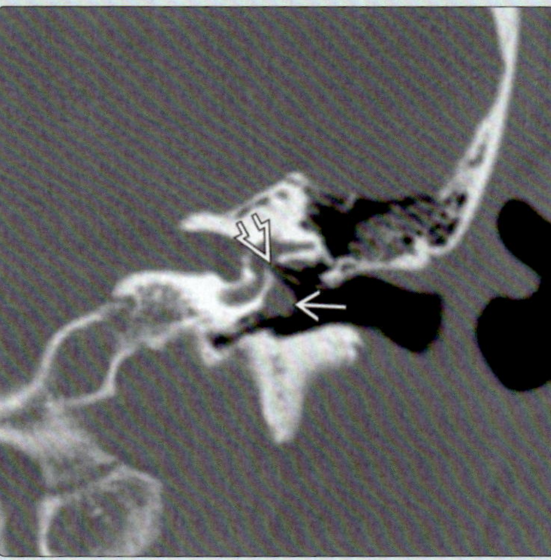

(Left) *Lateral graphic of the ICA (left) shows normal ascending pharyngeal ➡, inferior tympanic ➡, caroticotympanic ➡ arteries sequence and size. Lateral graphic (right) shows failure of cervical ICA to develop ⇨ with ascending pharyngeal ⇨, inferior tympanic ⇨, caroticotympanic ⇨ arteries as collateral arterial channel resulting in an AbICA.* **(Right)** *Coronal left bone CT at oval window ➡ shows the AbICA ➡ as a "mass" on the cochlear promontory resembling a glomus tympanicum paraganglioma. Beware!*

Persistent Stapedial Artery

KEY FACTS

TERMINOLOGY

- Persistent stapedial artery (PSA): Rare congenital vascular anomaly in which embryological stapedial artery persists

IMAGING

- Temporal bone **CT findings**
  - **Enlargement** of **anterior tympanic segment** of facial nerve canal
  - **Absent foramen spinosum**
    - Posterolateral from foramen ovale on axial bone CT

TOP DIFFERENTIAL DIAGNOSES

- Facial nerve venous malformation ("hemangioma")
- Facial nerve schwannoma
- Perineural parotid malignancy in CNVII canal

PATHOLOGY

- Primitive 2nd aortic arch gives rise to hyoid artery
- Hyoid artery gives rise to stapedial artery
- Stapedial artery divides into dorsal (**middle meningeal artery**) & ventral divisions (to maxilla & mandible)
- PSA courses from infracochlear ICA through stapedial obturator foramen
- PSA **enlarges tympanic** CNVII **canal** on its way to middle cranial fossa
- **PSA becomes middle meningeal artery**

CLINICAL ISSUES

- **Asymptomatic**; no treatment required
- Needs to be correctly identified as incidental congenital vascular anomaly on temporal bone CT
- If PSA found during stapes surgery, it is often most safe to abort surgery
- Frequently **bilateral**

DIAGNOSTIC CHECKLIST

- If **aberrant ICA** discovered, look for associated **PSA**
- Large anterior tympanic CNVII + absent foramen spinosum = persistent stapedial artery

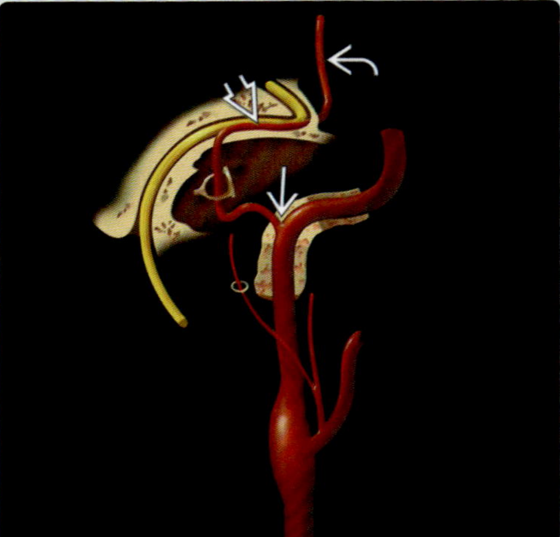

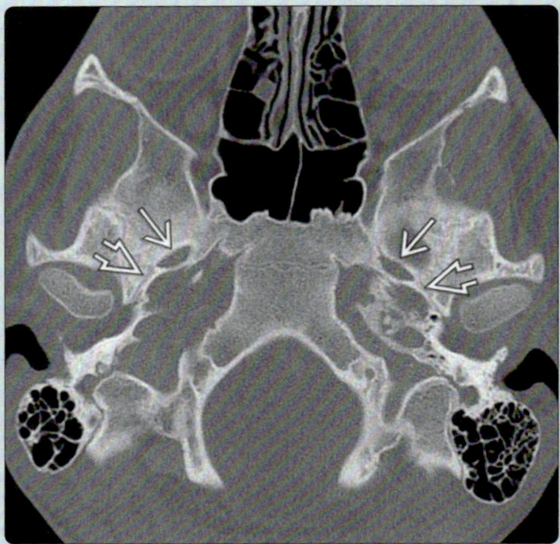

(Left) *Lateral graphic shows the persistent stapedial artery (PSA) arising from the vertical segment of the petrous ICA ➡, passing through the stapes, and traveling along the tympanic segment of the facial nerve ➡ to become the middle meningeal artery ➡.* **(Right)** *Axial temporal bone CT in a patient with bilateral PSAs shows the bilateral absence of the foramen spinosum ➡ in the central skull base just posterolateral to the foramen ovale ➡. The middle meningeal artery is fed by the PSA when present, not the internal maxillary artery.*

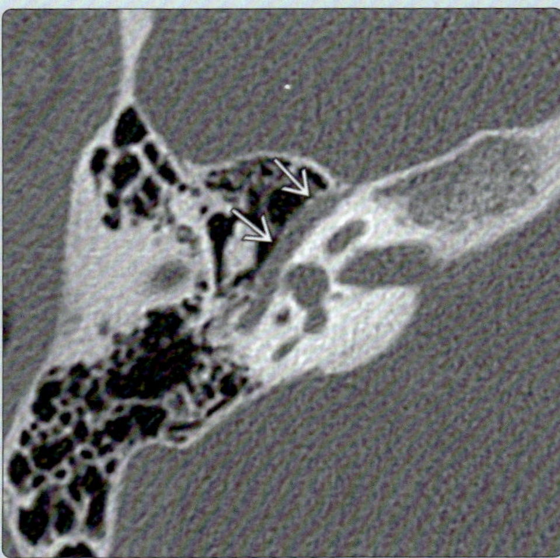

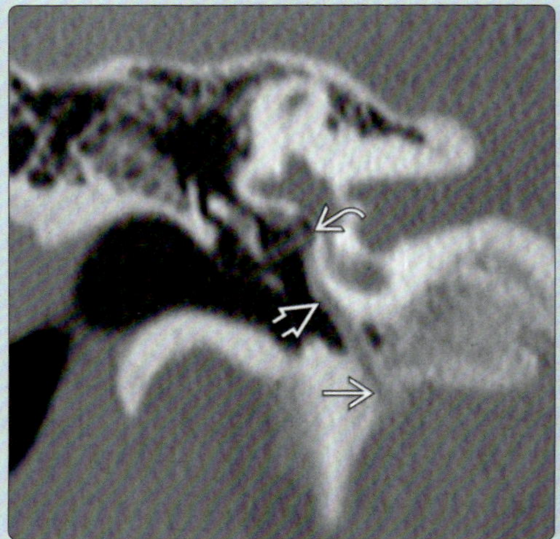

(Left) *Axial right temporal bone CT reveals an enlarged tympanic segment ➡ of the intratemporal facial nerve to the PSA.* **(Right)** *Coronal bone CT of the right ear in the same patient demonstrates the PSA arising from its takeoff origin from the genu of the petrous internal carotid artery ➡, ascending on the cochlear promontory ➡, and passing through the crura of the stapes ➡ on its way to join the tympanic segment of the facial nerve canal. (Courtesy K. Funk, MD.)*

KEY FACTS

TERMINOLOGY

- Acute coalescent otomastoiditis (ACOM): Acute middle ear-mastoid infection with progressive bony resorption due to intramastoid empyema ± osteomyelitis

IMAGING

- Bone CT findings: Mastoid cortex ± trabecula erosions (coalescent otomastoiditis)
- CECT or enhanced MR findings of **ACOM complications**
  - **Subperiosteal abscess**: Periauricular fluid collection
  - **Bezold abscess**: Walled-off pus in and around sternocleidomastoid muscle
  - **Middle cranial fossa abscess** (epidural or temporal lobe abscess)
  - **Posterior fossa abscess** (epidural or cerebellar abscess)
  - **Thrombosed sigmoid sinus** ± **internal jugular vein**

TOP DIFFERENTIAL DIAGNOSES

- Acquired cholesteatoma; apical petrositis
- Temporal bone Langerhans histiocytosis; temporal bone rhabdomyosarcoma/metastasis

PATHOLOGY

- Common pathophysiology
  - Granulation tissue or cholesteatoma blocks aditus ad antrum and prevents mastoid air cell drainage
- Less common pathophysiology
  - Mastoid cortex remains intact with septic thrombophlebitis of **emissary veins** seeding periosteum

CLINICAL ISSUES

- Symptoms: Otalgia, fever, otorrhea, ± postauricular swelling
- IV antibiotics, wide myringotomy, ± tube placement
- Drainage of focal pus ± canal wall up mastoidectomy, removal of cholesteatoma
- Drainage of extratemporal abscess (intra- or extracranial) as indicated

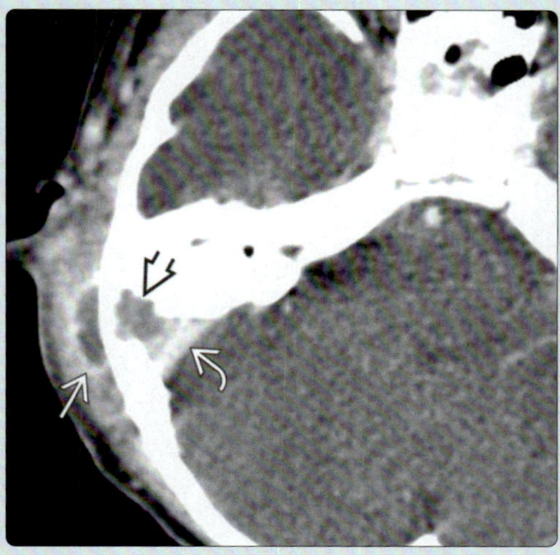

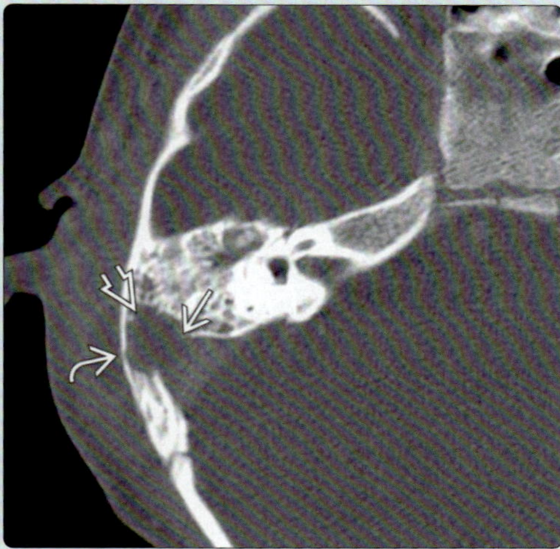

(Left) *Axial CECT in a patient with a postauricular tender mass, headache, and fever reveals a postauricular abscess ➡ and coalescent otomastoiditis ⇨, resulting in epidural extension of infection with a nonthrombosed sigmoid sinus ➡.* **(Right)** *Axial bone CT of the same patient shows loss of mastoid trabecula ➡ and a dehiscent sigmoid plate ➡ that is diagnostic of coalescent otomastoiditis. Subtle erosion of the lateral mastoid cortex ➡ indicates continuity of mastoid infection with the postauricular abscess.*

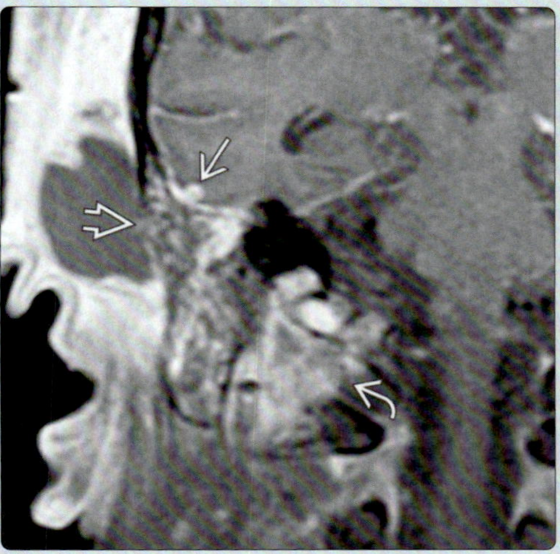

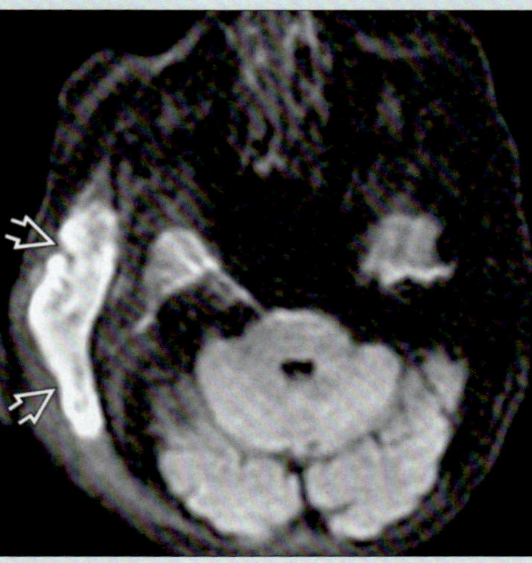

(Left) *Coronal T1WI C+ FS MR reveals mastoid enhancement with a large periauricular abscess. The lateral mastoid is focally dehiscent ➡ with thick and enhancing proximal meninges ➡. The subjacent skull base enhances ➡, indicating extensive associated osteomyelitis.* **(Right)** *Axial DWI MR of the same patient reveals restricted diffusion within an extensive periauricular abscess ➡. (Courtesy N. Fischbein, MD.)*

KEY FACTS

TERMINOLOGY

- Synonyms: Noncholesteatomatous ossicular erosion; postinflammatory ossicular erosion
- Definition: Erosive changes involving ossicles in absence of cholesteatoma in patient with history of chronic otomastoiditis (COM)

IMAGING

- Axial bone CT
  - Absence of part of posterior line of normal "2 parallel lines" of ossicles
  - Incudostapedial joint (ISJ) may be replaced by fibrous tissue
  - ISJ appears widened on axial CT
  - Erosion of "cone" (incus body/short process) also occurs
  - Associated findings of chronic otitis media
    - Underpneumatization of mastoid air cells
    - Inflammatory debris in middle ear and mastoid
- Coronal bone CT
  - Long process of incus most commonly absent
  - Vertical segment of **"right angle" at ISJ missing**
  - Tympanic membrane retraction often present

TOP DIFFERENTIAL DIAGNOSES

- Mild congenital external ear malformation, acquired cholesteatoma + ossicular erosion, congenital middle ear cholesteatoma + ossicle erosion, postoperative ossicular loss, posttraumatic ossicular dislocation

PATHOLOGY

- COM initially causes periostitis and osteitis
- Subsequent osteoclasia and decalcification creates bone loss

CLINICAL ISSUES

- Clinical presentation: Chronic otitis media history
  - Postinflammatory conductive hearing loss
- Primary treatment: Surgical repair of ossicles
  - Tympanomastoidectomy with ossicular reconstruction

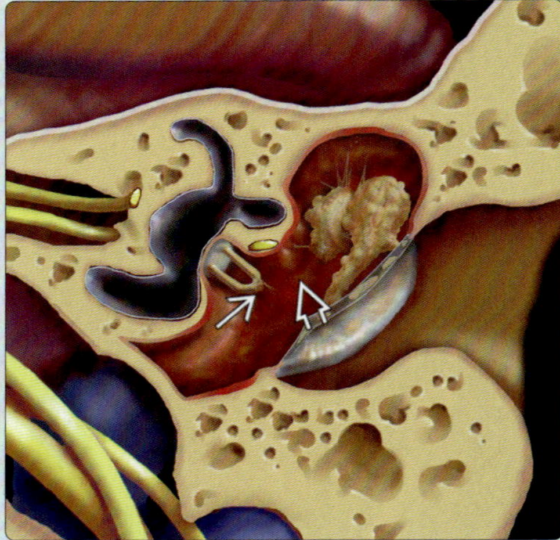

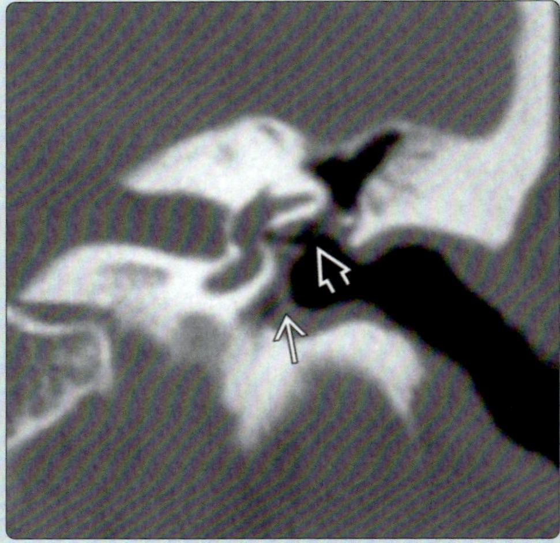

(Left) *Coronal graphic of the left ear shows postinflammatory ossicular erosion of the incus long process ➡ and stapes hub ➡. Note the changes of tympanosclerosis of tympanic membrane and remaining ossicles.* **(Right)** *Coronal bone CT reveals retraction of a thickened tympanic membrane ➡ with demineralization of the long process of incus ➡. Stranding soft tissue in the middle ear is associated inflammatory debris.*

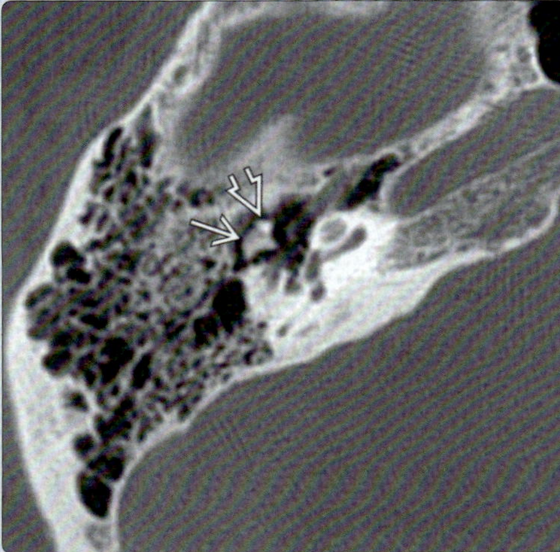

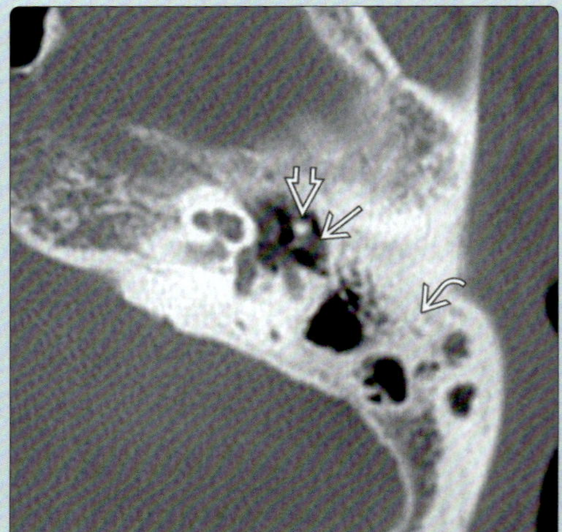

(Left) *Axial bone CT shows a normal short process of the right incus ➡ and head of malleus ➡. Notice the well-pneumatized mastoid.* **(Right)** *Axial bone CT of the left ear in a patient with history of chronic otitis media demonstrates deossification of the left short process of the incus ➡. The head of the malleus ➡ is normal in density and size. The mastoid is underpneumatized ➡ from otomastoiditis during mastoid formation.*

KEY FACTS

TERMINOLOGY

- Definition: Calcific, bony, or fibrous middle ear foci secondary to **suppurative** chronic otomastoiditis (COM)

IMAGING

- Bone CT: Common locations of tympanosclerotic **calcification**
  - Tympanic membrane
  - Ossicle surface
  - Stapes footplate
  - Muscle tendons
  - Ossicle ligaments
- Focal tympanosclerotic **ossifications**
  - May be seen anywhere in middle ear or mastoid
- Chronic otomastoiditis findings associated

TOP DIFFERENTIAL DIAGNOSES

- Chronic otitis media
- COM with ossicular erosions
- COM with ossicular fixation
- Fenestral otosclerosis
- Ossicular prosthesis

PATHOLOGY

- Etiology: Healing response to repeated inflammatory events in middle ear-mastoid
- True tympanosclerosis: Diffuse hyalinization & deposition of calcium & phosphate crystals
- New bone formation (osteoneogenesis)

CLINICAL ISSUES

- Clinical presentation
  - **Conductive hearing loss** out of proportion to inflammatory debris + **history of COM**
- Treatment options
  - Atticotomy ± mastoidectomy, mobilization of ossicles
  - Ossiculoplasty with insertion of prosthesis or homograft device

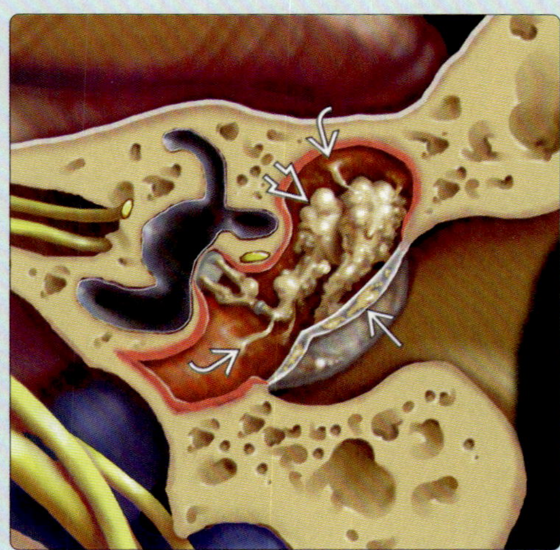

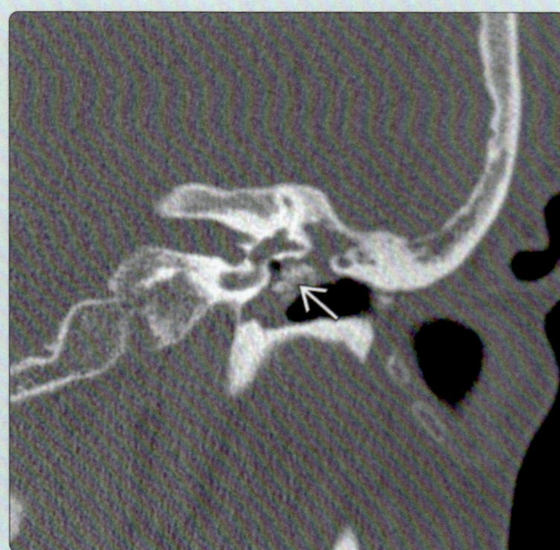

(Left) *Coronal graphic shows severe tympanosclerosis in the setting of chronic otomastoiditis. Postinflammatory calcification can be seen in the tympanic membrane ➡, ossicles ➡, and ossicle ligament ➡.* **(Right)** *Coronal bone CT reveals the ossicles as a fuzzy ball ➡. This appearance is due to tympanosclerotic calcific foci deposited on the surface of the middle ear ossicles.*

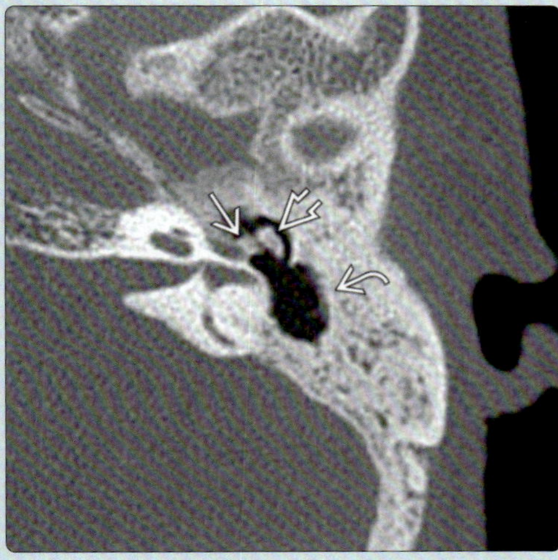

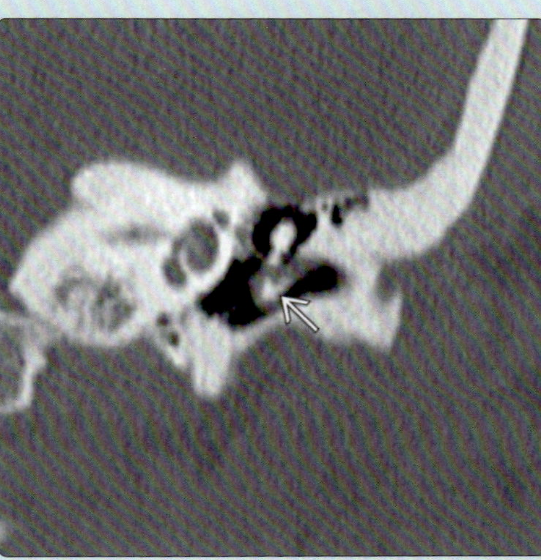

(Left) *Axial bone CT shows a focal area of ossific tympanosclerosis ➡ just medial to the ossicles in the medial wall of the epitympanum. Also note that the malleus-incus articulation is fused ➡ and the mastoid contains an antral cavity ➡ only.* **(Right)** *Coronal bone CT reveals thickening of the tympanic membrane with a linear focus of calcification ➡ along its surface. Tympanosclerotic calcifications can affect ligaments, tendons, ossicles, or the tympanic membrane, as in this case.*

Pars Flaccida Cholesteatoma

KEY FACTS

TERMINOLOGY

- "Attic" or "Prussak space" cholesteatoma

IMAGING

- T-bone CT: Smaller pars flaccida cholesteatoma (PFC)
  - Soft tissue in Prussak space + scutum & ossicle erosions
- T-bone CT: Larger PFC
  - Look for **lateral semicircular canal, CNVII canal, & tegmen tympani ± mastoideum dehiscence**
  - Exclude sinus tympani extension
    - Associated with high postoperative recurrence rate
- T-bone MR: Complementary; higher sensitivity & specificity
  - Nonecho-planar DWI superior to conventional EPI DWI
  - May obviate need for 2nd-look revision surgery if hearing outcomes from primary surgery acceptable

TOP DIFFERENTIAL DIAGNOSES

- Acquired pars tensa cholesteatoma
- Congenital middle ear cholesteatoma
- Middle ear cholesterol granuloma
- Glomus tympanicum paraganglioma

PATHOLOGY

- Starts at pars flaccida of tympanic membrane
- Microscopically consists of exfoliated keratin within stratified squamous epithelium

CLINICAL ISSUES

- Most common type (**80%** of all acquired cholesteatoma)
- Patient with chronic middle ear inflammatory disease, conductive hearing loss, & tympanic membrane (TM) abnormality
  - TM retraction: PFC may **not** be visible; CT helps make diagnosis based on ossicle or bone loss
  - TM perforation: PFC visible; diagnosis known
- Treatment options
  - Tympanomastoidectomy with ossiculoplasty, often performed at-2nd stage surgery; residual disease often in sinus tympani, facial recess

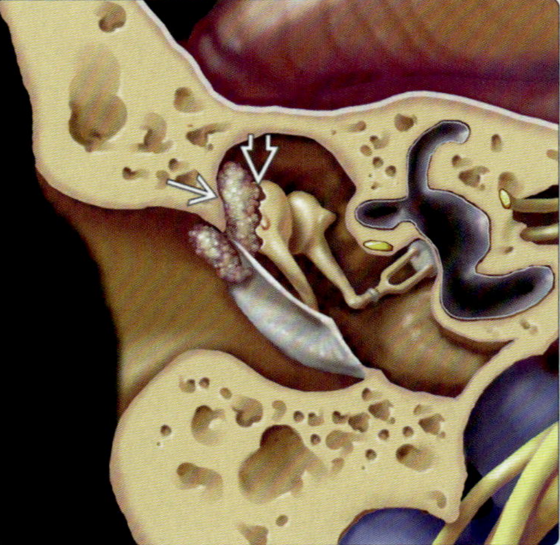
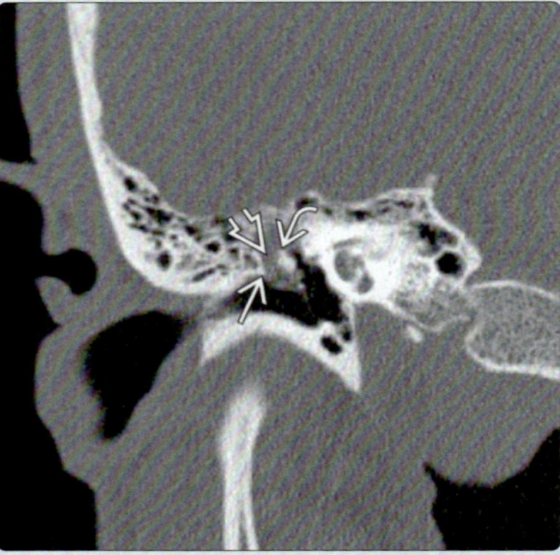

(Left) *Coronal graphic shows small cholesteatoma originating at the pars flaccida portion of the tympanic membrane with filling of the Prussak space ➡. Slight erosion ➡ with medial displacement of the head of malleus is present.* **(Right)** *Coronal bone CT reveals a small pars flaccida cholesteatoma filling the Prussak space ➡ with blunting of the scutum ➡. The head of the malleus is mildly eroded and medially displaced ➡.*

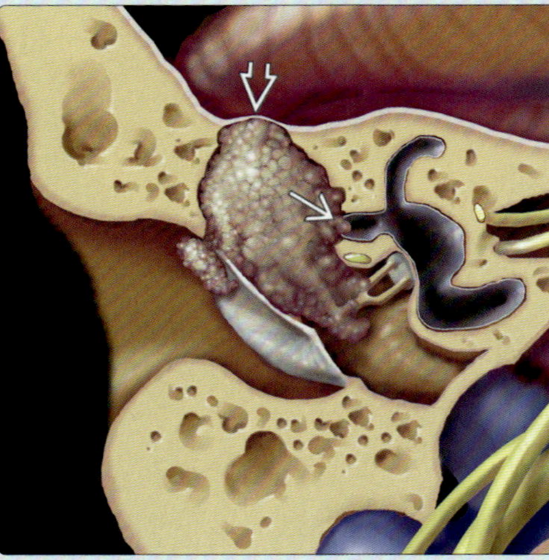
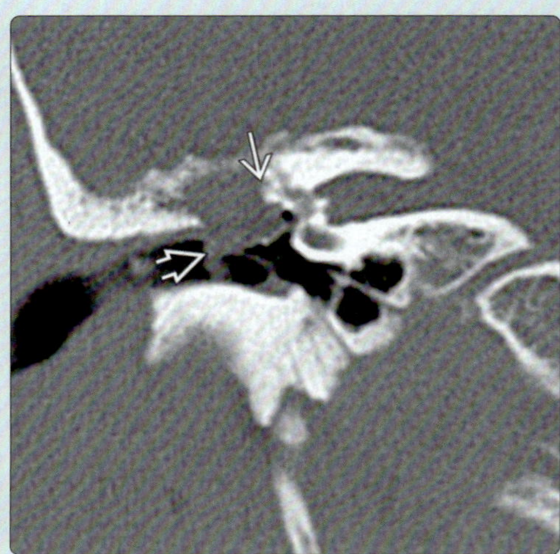

(Left) *Coronal graphic shows a large pars flaccida cholesteatoma. Complications include erosion of ossicles, dehiscence of the lateral semicircular canal ➡, and scalloping of the tegmen tympani ➡.* **(Right)** *Coronal bone CT shows a large pars flaccida cholesteatoma as a soft tissue mass within the right middle ear and mastoid cavity. There is fistulation with the lateral semicircular canal ➡. Cholesteatoma is also visible protruding through the tympanic membrane perforation into the external auditory canal ➡.*

KEY FACTS

TERMINOLOGY

- Definition: Focal accumulation of exfoliated keratin within stratified squamous epithelium at site of perforation or retraction pocket at pars tensa tympanic membrane (TM)

IMAGING

- Axial and coronal temporal bone CT is study of choice
  - Erosive mass in **posterior mesotympanum**
  - Usually found **medial** to ossicles; may involve sinus tympani, facial recess, and aditus ad antrum ± mastoid
  - Ossicular erosion common along medial incus long process, stapes superstructure, + malleus manubrium
- MR adjunctive; answers issues raised by bone CT
  - **Nonecho-planar DWI** superior to conventional echo-planar DWI; may obviate need for 2nd-look surgery

TOP DIFFERENTIAL DIAGNOSES

- Middle ear congenital cholesteatoma
- Pars flaccida-acquired cholesteatoma
- Middle ear cholesterol granuloma

PATHOLOGY

- Migrated/implanted epithelium through TM perforation → nidus of stratified squamous epithelium with keratin squames in middle ear → cholesteatoma

CLINICAL ISSUES

- **10-20%** of all middle ear cholesteatoma
- Clinical presentation
  - History of chronic otitis media ± TM perforation
  - Otoscopy: Retraction pocket, perforation, mucopurulent otorrhea, or visible cholesteatoma at pars tensa
- Treatment options: Tympanomastoidectomy, preferably canal wall up, with ossiculoplasty
  - Residual disease often seen in sinus tympani or facial recess
    - Otoendoscope may be helpful adjunct to see around corners

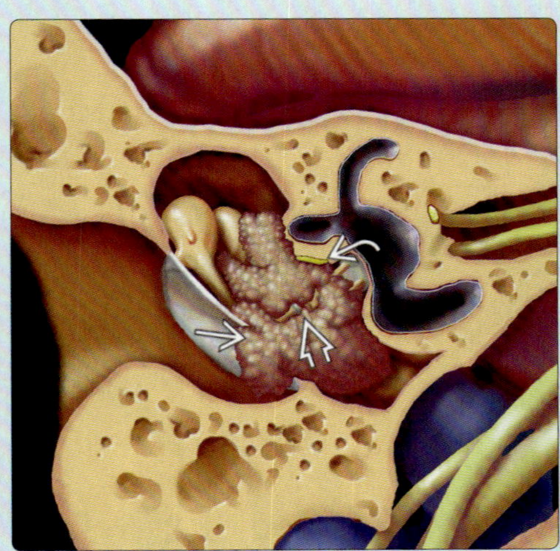

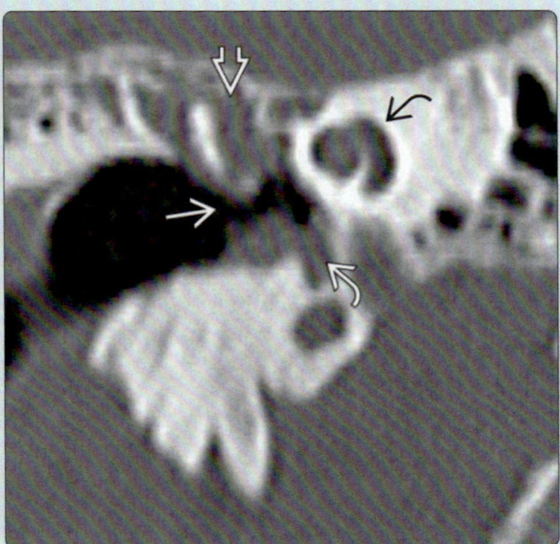

(Left) *Coronal graphic of pars tensa cholesteatoma (PTC) shows the cholesteatoma extending laterally through an inferior tympanic membrane (TM) rupture ➡. The middle ear PTC erodes ossicles ➡, invades and flattens the tympanic CNVII canal ➡, and is primarily medial to the ossicles.* **(Right)** *Coronal bone CT at the level of the cochlea ➡ demonstrates a pars tensa TM perforation ➡. The most anterior aspect of the PTC is seen above ➡ and below ➡ the perforation in the middle ear cavity.*

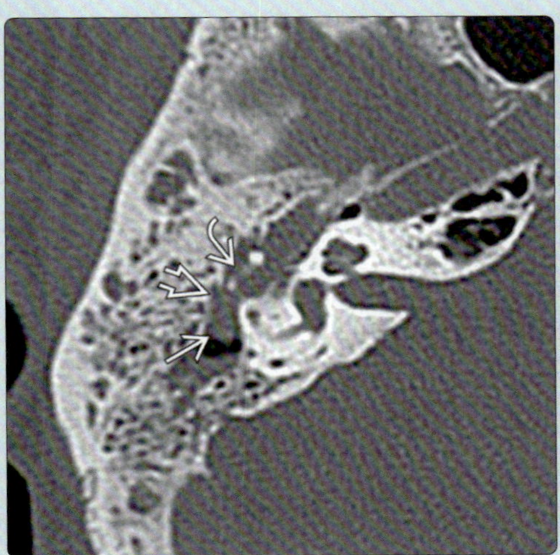

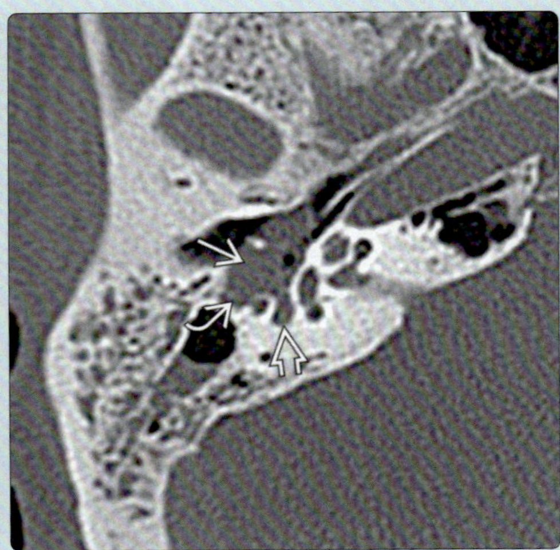

(Left) *Axial bone CT in the same patient reveals the PTC eroding the short process of the incus ➡ and extending through the aditus ad antrum ➡ into the mastoid antrum ➡.* **(Right)** *Axial bone CT at the level of the oval window reveals erosion of the incus and hub of the stapes ➡ with invasion of the facial nerve recess ➡ and sinus tympani ➡. Sinus tympani involvement must be reported, as this area is blind to the surgeon and may serve as nidus for recurrence if unnoticed.*

KEY FACTS

TERMINOLOGY

- Synonyms: Automastoidectomy; "shell" or "rind" cholesteatoma
- Rare variant of acquired cholesteatoma
- Definition: Residual cholesteatoma "rind" left behind after acquired middle ear-mastoid cholesteatoma extrudes central matrix through dehiscent **EAC bony wall**

IMAGING

- Temporal bone CT findings
  - Mastoidectomy cavity with residual soft tissue "rind" along cavity wall **without** history of mastoidectomy
  - Large lesion can fistulize any area of inner ear
  - Focal dehiscence of posterior or superior EAC wall
- CT findings suggest mastoidectomy but none has occurred: **Automastoidectomy**
- With mural cholesteatoma, check for ossicle destruction, inner ear or CNVII canal dehiscence, EAC wall erosion

TOP DIFFERENTIAL DIAGNOSES

- Coalescent mastoiditis
- Mastoidectomy
- Keratosis obturans with automastoidectomy

PATHOLOGY

- "Rind" of tissue found along wall of cavity
- Only "lining" of cholesteatoma seen by pathologist
- Microscopic features: Aggressive keratinizing stratified squamous epithelium

CLINICAL ISSUES

- Older patient with chronically draining ear
  - May report material "falling out of ear"
- Long history of chronic otitis media **without** mastoidectomy
- Surgery depends on lesion size and extent
  - Excision of tissue lining of cavity key
  - Tympanomastoidectomy with ossicular reconstruction

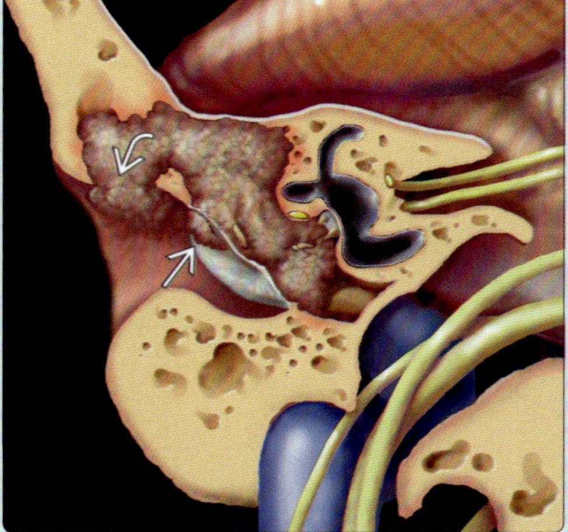

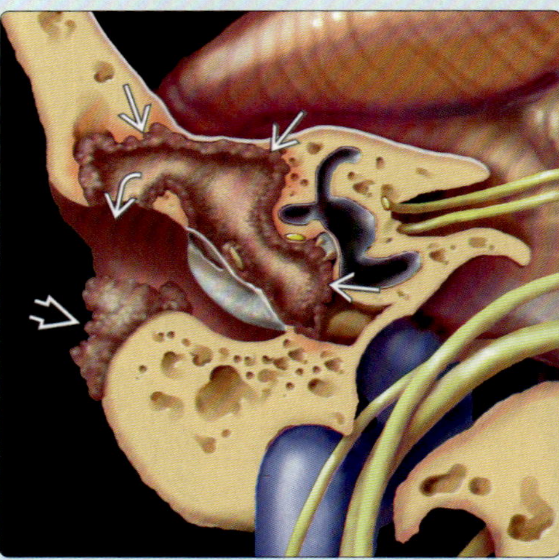

(Left) *Coronal graphic shows a large cholesteatoma beginning at a pars flaccida perforation ➡. The lesion has eroded the middle ear walls, ossicles, mastoid cavity, and external auditory canal (EAC) bony walls ➡.* **(Right)** *Coronal graphic reveals that the large cholesteatoma in the previous drawing has evacuated its central material through the EAC dehiscence ➡ into the external ear canal ➡. A mural cholesteatoma is left behind as a cholesteatoma "rind" along the walls of the middle ear and mastoid ➡.*

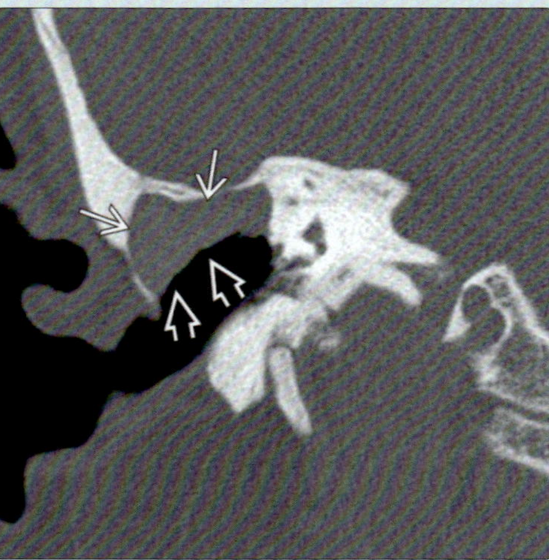

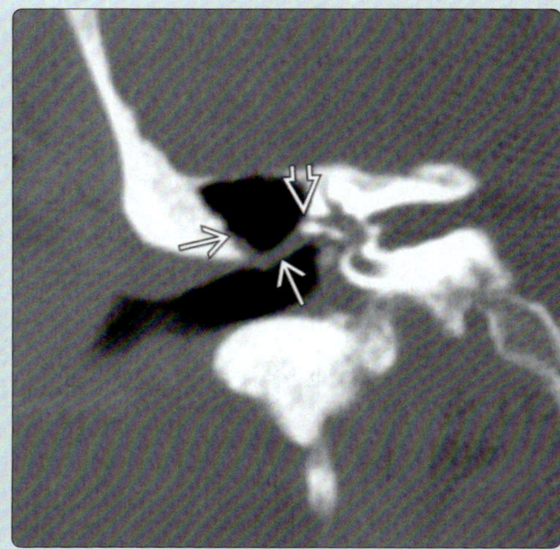

(Left) *Coronal temporal bone CT demonstrates a partially extruded mural cholesteatoma ➡ in an enlarged mastoid cavity with a broad EAC posterosuperior wall dehiscence ➡.* **(Right)** *Coronal temporal bone CT shows a thin-walled mural cholesteatoma ➡ in a "hollowed out" mastoid cavity. Lateral semicircular canal fistula ➡ is present. The thickness of the mural cholesteatoma "rind" is dependent on the amount of the lesion that has been extruded.*

KEY FACTS

TERMINOLOGY

- Cholesterol granuloma (CG): Recurrent hemorrhage into middle ear (ME) cavity causes inflammatory mass of granulation tissue

IMAGING

- Bone CT: Smoothly **expansile mass** of ME ± mastoid air cells
- MR: **High T1** and T2 signal in ME

TOP DIFFERENTIAL DIAGNOSES

- Dehiscent jugular bulb
- Aberrant internal carotid artery
- Chronic otitis media + hemorrhage
- Pars flaccida-acquired cholesteatoma
- Paraganglioma
  - Glomus tympanicum paraganglioma
  - Glomus jugulare paraganglioma
- Encephalocele of ME
- Traumatic hemotympanum

CLINICAL ISSUES

- Clinical presentation
  - Symptoms: Conductive hearing loss
  - Otoscopy: Nonpulsating bluish discoloration of tympanic membrane = "blue" eardrum
  - Symptoms arise years after initial otitis media
- Treatment options
  - Initial surgery: Resection of wall and contents
  - Intractable disease: Mastoidectomy + ventilation tube
- Natural history
  - Most ME CGs grow over decades
- Recurrence rates for ME CG are much lower than for petrous apex CG

DIAGNOSTIC CHECKLIST

- "Blue" tympanic membrane + **expansile** bone changes (on bone CT) + **high T1** (on MR) = CG of ME

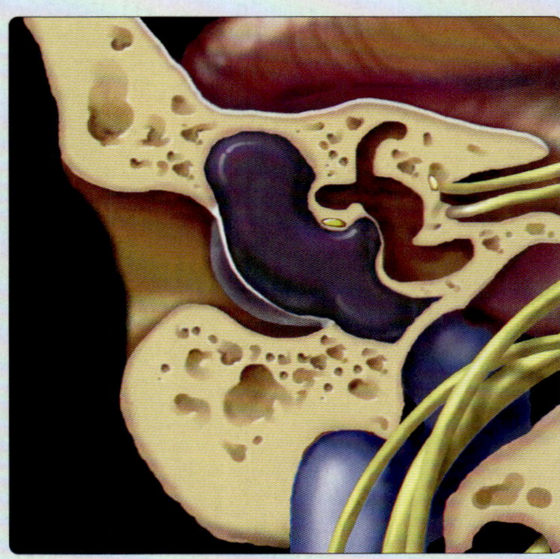

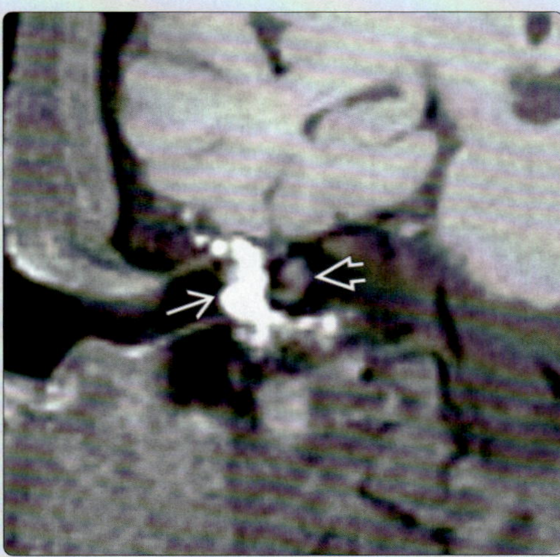

(Left) *Coronal graphic depicts a large middle ear cholesterol granuloma. The entire middle ear is filled with dark brown ("chocolate") fluid with the ossicles no longer present. Otoscopy reveals a "blue-black" eardrum.* **(Right)** *Coronal T1WI MR demonstrates a retrotympanic high-signal cholesterol granuloma ➡ that causes the tympanic membrane to bulge into the external auditory canal. Notice the signal of the cochlea medially ⇨. The cholesterol granuloma fills the entire middle ear cavity.*

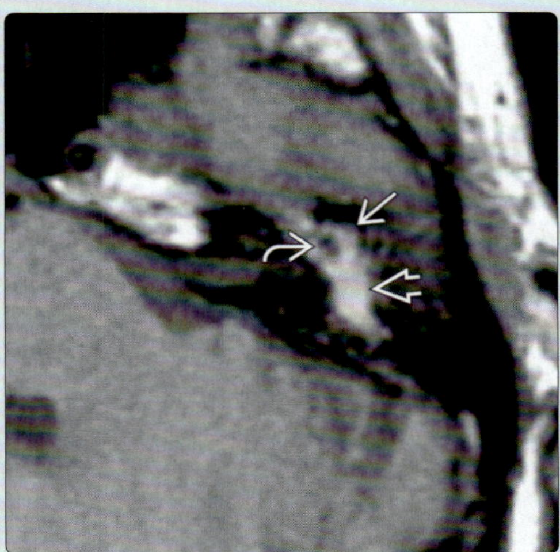

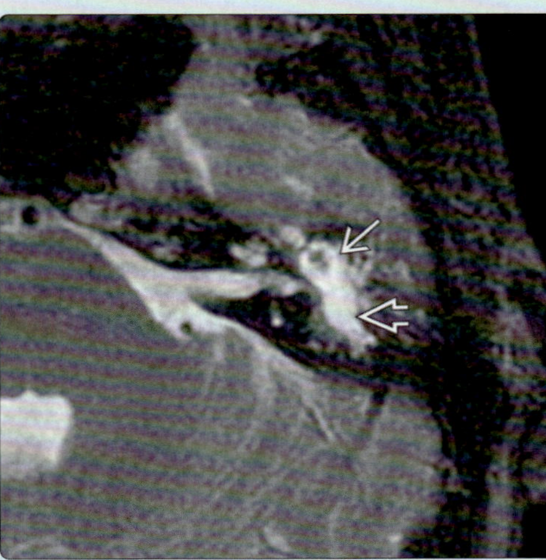

(Left) *Axial T1WI MR in a patient with a "blue-black" retrotympanic lesion shows a high-signal cholesterol granuloma filling the middle ear ➡ and mastoid antrum ⇨. Note the low-signal head of the malleus and short process of incus ➡ visible within the lesion.* **(Right)** *Axial T2WI fat-saturated MR in the same patient reveals hyperintense cholesterol granuloma in the epitympanum ➡ and mastoid antrum ⇨. Early-phase disease preserves the ossicles and shows no evidence of bony scalloping.*

Glomus Tympanicum Paraganglioma

KEY FACTS

TERMINOLOGY

- Abbreviation: Glomus tympanicum paraganglioma (GTP)
- Benign tumor arising from glomus bodies situated on **cochlear promontory**

IMAGING

- Best imaging study: Bone CT without contrast
- CT: Mass with flat base on cochlear promontory
- MR: Enhancing mass with flat base on cochlear promontory
- Floor of middle ear cavity is typically **intact** (if dehiscent, consider glomus jugulare paraganglioma)
- Evaluate integrity of bone on jugular bulb, carotid canal

TOP DIFFERENTIAL DIAGNOSES

- Glomus jugulare paraganglioma
- Aberrant internal carotid artery (AbICA)
- Dehiscent jugular bulb
- Congenital cholesteatoma, middle ear
- Facial nerve schwannoma, tympanic segment

PATHOLOGY

- Arises from glomus (Latin for ball) bodies (paraganglia) found along inferior tympanic nerve (Jacobson nerve) on cochlear promontory
- GTP is most common tumor of middle ear

CLINICAL ISSUES

- Clinical presentation
  - Often seen in middle age: 40-60 years, M:F = 1:3
  - Pulsatile tinnitus + vascular retrotympanic mass
- Treatment options
  - Surgical resection; approach depends on extent of GTP; transcanal, postauricular
  - Preoperative embolization and control of great vessels not typically necessary
- GTP may be clinically indistinguishable from glomus jugulare paraganglioma or AbICA
  - Imaging differentiates GTP from glomus jugulare paraganglioma, AbICA, and dehiscent jugular bulb

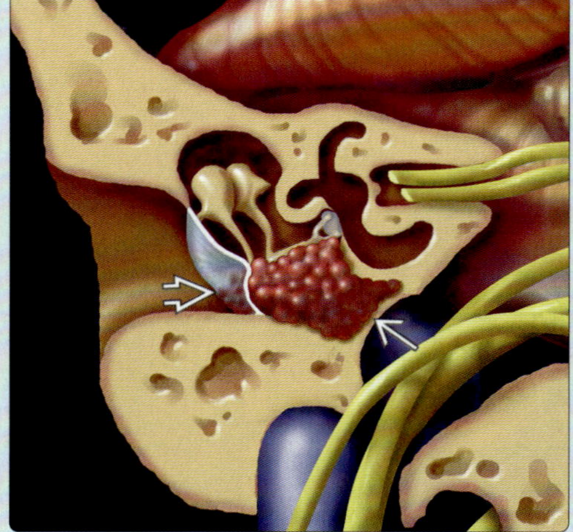

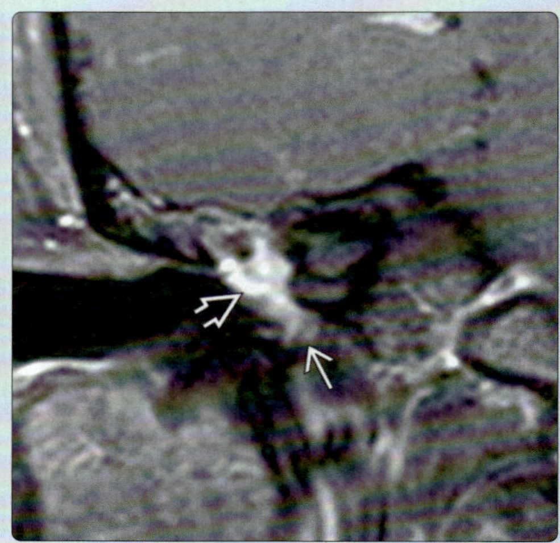

(Left) *Coronal graphic shows a vascular glomus tympanicum paraganglioma (GTP) over the cochlear promontory and filling the inferior middle ear cavity. The bony floor of the middle ear cavity is intact →. Otoscopy reveals this tumor as a reddish, pulsatile mass behind the lower tympanic membrane ⇒.* **(Right)** *Coronal T1 C+ FS MR demonstrates a large GTP filling the middle ear cavity ⇒. The floor is intact →, separating the tumor from the jugular bulb below.*

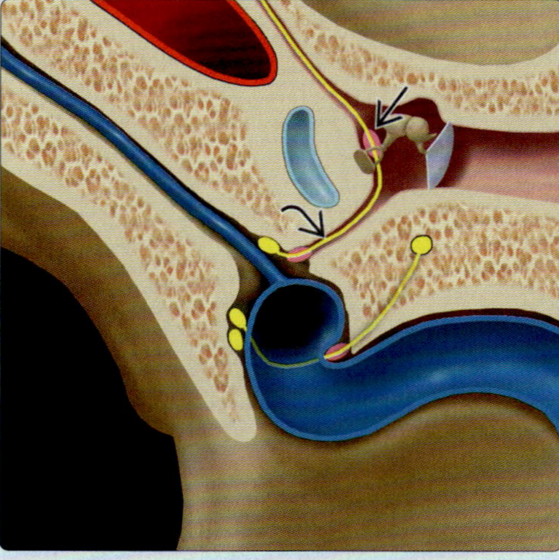

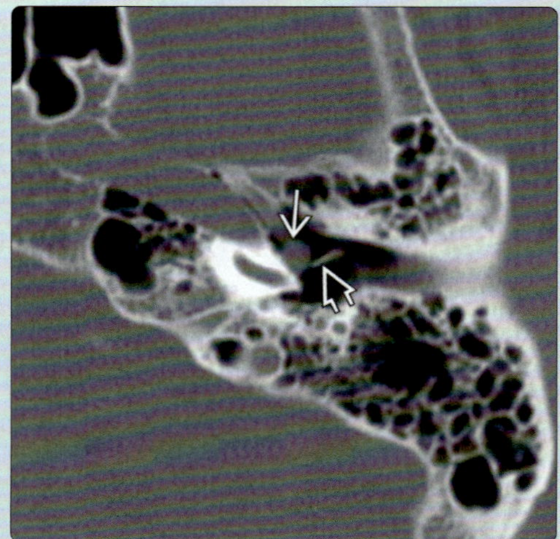

(Left) *Axial graphic shows glomus bodies → along the course of the inferior tympanic nerve (branch of Jacobson nerve ↷) on the cochlear promontory. Glomus tympanicum tumors arise from this normal cellular collection.* **(Right)** *Axial bone CT reveals an ovoid glomus tympanicum tumor on the low cochlear promontory → abutting the manubrium of the malleus ⇒. The patient's history of conductive hearing loss is secondary to the restricted motion of the inferior malleus-tympanic membrane by the tumor.*

KEY FACTS

TERMINOLOGY

- Synonym: Intratympanic or intraosseous meningioma
- Definition: Meningioma involving middle ear (ME) or inner ear of temporal bone

IMAGING

- Morphology: Dural-based globular or en plaque mass
  - Extension via tegmen, internal carotid artery, or jugular foramen
- Bone CT findings
  - **Permeative-sclerotic** or **hyperostotic** changes
  - May underestimate extent of tumor
  - Intratumoral **calcification** common
  - **Ossicles intact** without destruction typically
- MR findings
  - Avidly enhancing mass involving temporal bone
  - If **dural tail** present, helps make diagnosis
- 3 principal sites of origin + specific vector of spread
  - Tegmen tympani tumor grows inferiorly into ME
  - Jugular foramen tumor grows centrifugally into ME if superolateral spread present
  - Internal auditory canal (IAC) tumor grows into inner ear
- Imaging protocol suggestion
  - Thin T1 C+ FS IAC MR best shows tumor extent
  - Especially with extensive intraosseous component

CLINICAL ISSUES

- Hearing loss patterns
  - Conductive: Tegmen tympani meningioma affecting ME
  - Sensorineural: IAC meningioma
  - Mixed: Jugular foramen meningioma
- Otoscopy: Vascular retrotympanic mass if extends to ME
- Treatment: Surgical removal to extent possible; subtotal resection may be necessary with diffuse disease

DIAGNOSTIC CHECKLIST

- Permeative-sclerotic CT findings + dural tail on MR
- Identify site of origin, vector of spread, and extent

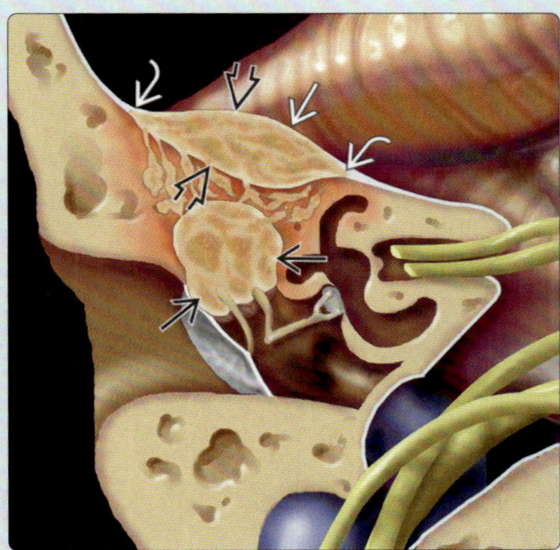

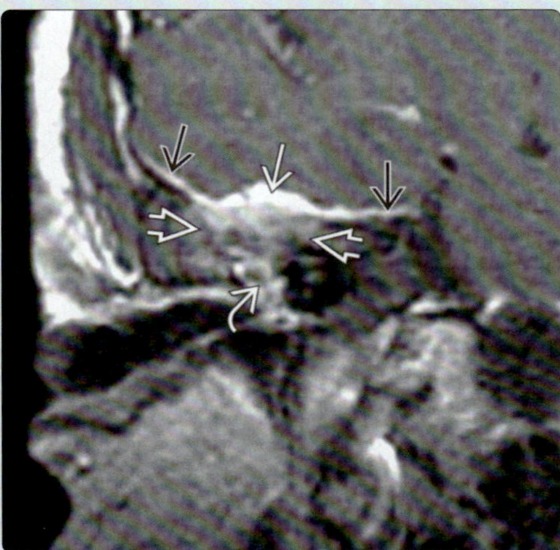

(Left) *Coronal graphic of tegmen tympani meningioma reveals en plaque dural origin of the tumor ➡ with spread through the tegmen ⇨ thickened by hyperostosis into the superior middle ear cavity. The ossicles have been engulfed by the tumor ⇨. Dural tails are visible along the tumor margins ➡.* **(Right)** *Coronal T1 C+ FS MR shows en plaque meningioma arising along the middle cranial fossa floor ➡. Note the enhancing dural tails ⇨. Transosseous tegmen tumor ➡ spreads into the middle ear cavity and engulfs the ossicles ➡.*

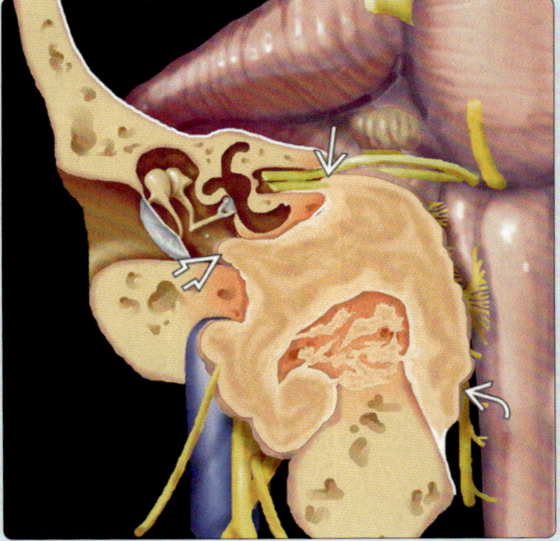

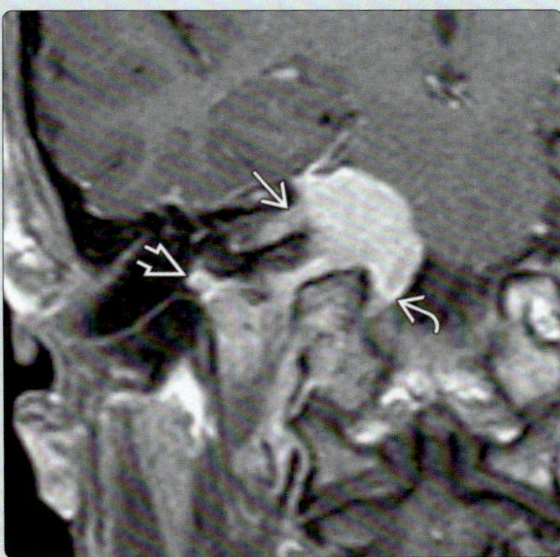

(Left) *Coronal graphic of a jugular foramen meningioma depicts the centrifugal spread pattern reaching the IAC ➡, middle ear ➡, and basal cistern ➡. When a jugular foramen meningioma reaches the middle ear, it can mimic glomus jugulare paraganglioma.* **(Right)** *T1 C+ FS MR reveals an extensive jugular foramen meningioma that spreads to the IAC ➡, middle ear ➡, and basal cistern ➡. Centrifugal spread pattern, dural-based morphology, and absence of flow voids suggest a diagnosis of meningioma.*

Middle Ear Schwannoma

KEY FACTS

TERMINOLOGY

- **Primary schwannoma**: Primary to middle ear (ME) cavity
  - Tympanic segment CNVII > > tympanic branch nerve (CNIX branch), chorda tympani nerve (CNVII branch)
- **Secondary schwannoma**: Arises outside ME
  - Jugular foramen schwannoma involves ME
  - Translabyrinthine CNVIII schwannoma
  - Primary inner ear schwannoma → ME

IMAGING

- Bone CT findings
  - **CNVII schwannoma**: Well-marginated mass emanating from CNVII canal
  - **Transotic intralabyrinthine schwannoma** (spread from inner ear with ME protrusion): Labyrinth erosions with mass protruding into ME via round or oval window
  - **ME schwannoma** (from chorda tympani or Jacobson nerve): Focal mass filling ME without involving CNVII canal
- T1 C+ MR findings
  - CNVII schwannoma: Enhancing mass contiguous with tympanic or mastoid CNVII
  - Transotic intralabyrinthine schwannoma: Enhancing mass contiguous with IAC & inner ear spaces
  - ME schwannoma: Mass primary to ME cavity
  - **Intramural cysts** may be visible when large

TOP DIFFERENTIAL DIAGNOSES

- Congenital ME cholesteatoma
- Glomus tympanicum paraganglioma
- Pars flaccida, acquired cholesteatoma
- Middle ear adenoma

CLINICAL ISSUES

- Presentation: Conductive hearing loss, facial paresis
- Otoscopy: Fleshy-white mass behind intact TM
- Imaging depends on erosion of surrounding structures
- Treatment: Surgical removal; approach depends on location

(Left) *Axial temporal bone CT of the left ear reveals the middle ear component of the schwannoma pushing the ossicles laterally. The mastoid air cells are opacified as a result of the aditus ad antrum block created by the schwannoma.* **(Right)** *Axial T1WI C+ MR shows a transotic schwannoma extending from the cerebellopontine angle through the inner ear and into the middle ear cavity. The original clinical diagnosis in this case was congenital cholesteatoma of the middle ear.*

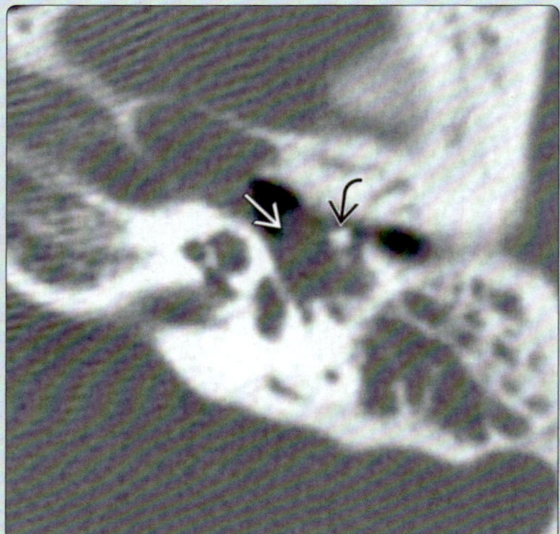

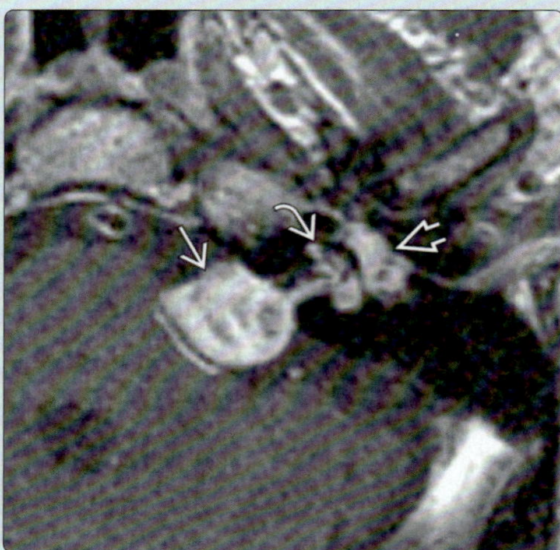

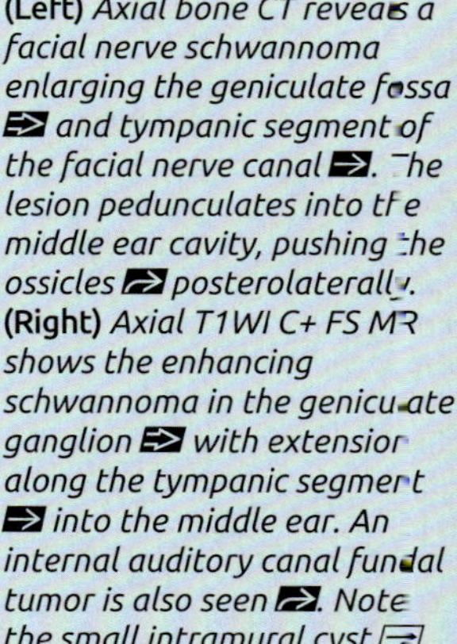

(Left) *Axial bone CT reveals a facial nerve schwannoma enlarging the geniculate fossa and tympanic segment of the facial nerve canal. The lesion pedunculates into the middle ear cavity, pushing the ossicles posterolaterally.* **(Right)** *Axial T1WI C+ FS MR shows the enhancing schwannoma in the geniculate ganglion with extension along the tympanic segment into the middle ear. An internal auditory canal fundal tumor is also seen. Note the small intramural cyst.*

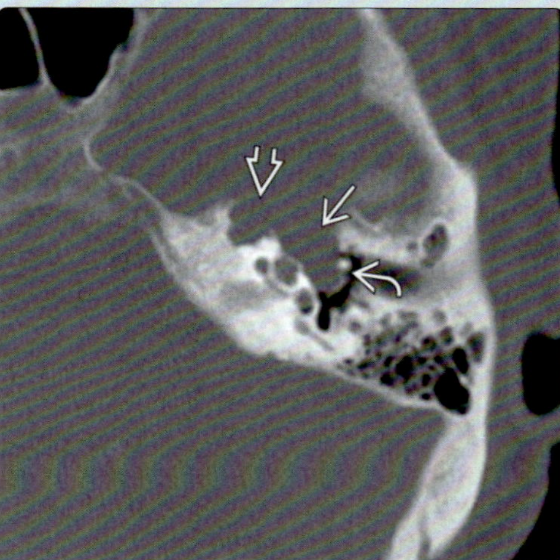

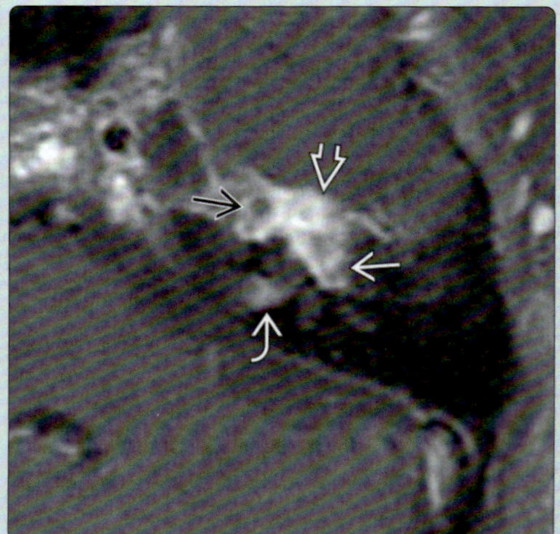

KEY FACTS

TERMINOLOGY

- Middle ear adenoma (MEA)
  - Very rare, benign tumor of mixed exocrine & neuroendocrine origin

IMAGING

- Soft tissue mass in middle ear
- Temporal bone CT findings
  - Middle ear mass behind intact tympanic membrane (TM)
  - Indistinguishable on bone CT from glomus tympanicum & pedunculated middle ear schwannoma
  - Well-pneumatized mastoid (no history of chronic otitis media)
  - May show areas of **local bone invasion**
- MR findings
  - If large adenoma present, T1 C+ MR may be helpful in defining lesion extent
  - MEA **enhances** like glomus tympanicum & pedunculated CNVII schwannoma
  - Enhancement excludes middle ear congenital cholesteatoma

TOP DIFFERENTIAL DIAGNOSES

- Glomus tympanicum paraganglioma
- Pedunculated facial nerve schwannoma
- Middle ear congenital cholesteatoma

CLINICAL ISSUES

- Otoscopy appearance
  - Tan-pink soft tissue mass behind intact TM
- Principal symptoms
  - Tinnitus and conductive hearing loss
  - "Ear fullness"
- Mean age at presentation: 45 years
- Natural history of tumor
  - If aggressive type, facial nerve injury possible
- Treatment options
  - Complete surgical excision is treatment of choice

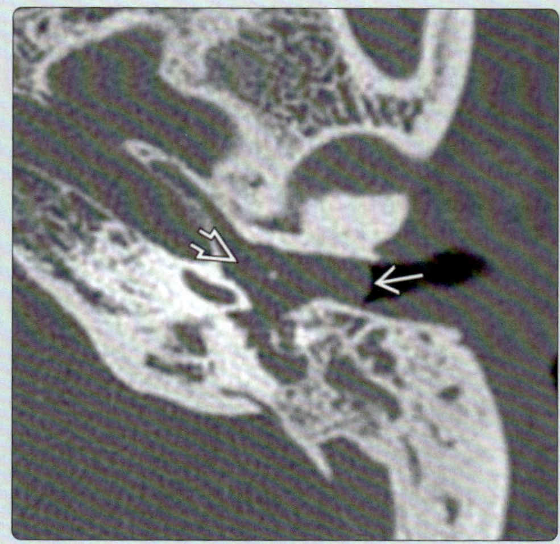

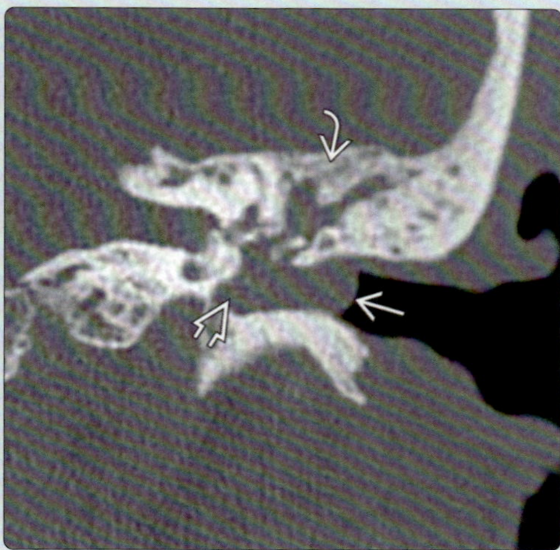

(Left) *Axial bone CT through the middle ear shows a soft tissue mass filling the middle ear ➡ with polypoid extension into the external auditory canal (EAC) ➡. Mastoid opacification is present due to obstruction at the aditus ad antrum (not shown).* **(Right)** *Coronal bone CT reveals a mass filling the middle ear ➡ and extending into the EAC ➡. Permeative changes are seen in the middle ear walls ➡ but not to the EAC. Pathology showed the lesion to be middle ear adenoma.*

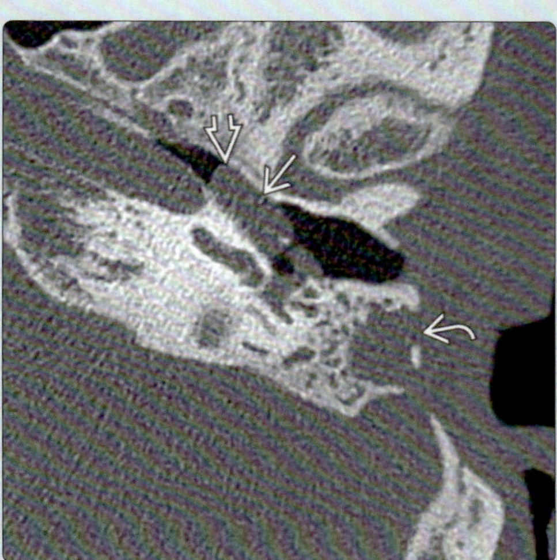

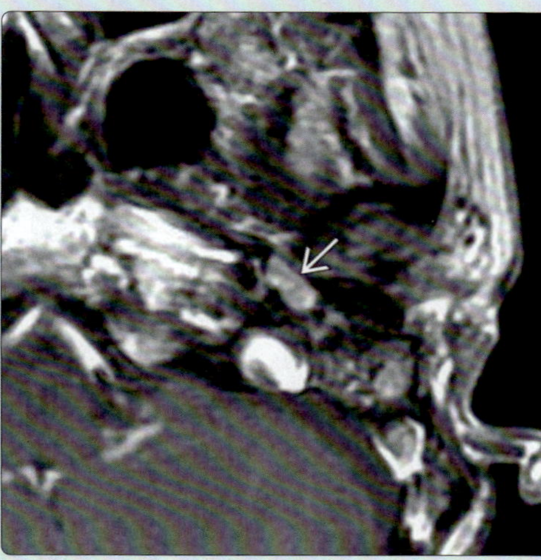

(Left) *Axial bone CT through the low mesotympanum reveals a noninvasive middle ear adenoma ➡ extending into the entrance of the bony eustachian tube ➡. Postmastoidectomy changes are also present ➡.* **(Right)** *Axial T1 C+ MR shows a well-circumscribed, enhancing lesion ➡ within the middle ear cavity. The lesion enhancement makes middle ear adenoma a possible diagnosis. Without otoscopy, one must also consider glomus tympanicum paraganglioma and middle ear schwannoma.*

KEY FACTS

TERMINOLOGY

- **Rhabdomyosarcoma (RMS): Rare pediatric destructive T-bone lesion**
  - Arises from embryonic skeletal muscle precursor cells or pluripotential mesenchymal cells

IMAGING

- Middle ear-mastoid or petrous apex destructive mass with variable contrast enhancement
  - Middle ear RMS often with associated external auditory canal extension (aural polyp)
  - Petrous apex RMS may be primary or spread from parameningeal RMS
  - Skull base and cranial nerve involvement common
- Both CT and MR recommended to stage skull base destruction and middle ear and intracranial extension
- T1 C+ FS MR best to detect intracranial extension via tegmen, mastoid roof, ± skull base foramina
- T2 MR helpful to differentiate obstructed mastoid secretions (more hyperintense than RMS)

TOP DIFFERENTIAL DIAGNOSES

- Acquired cholesteatoma
- Langerhans cell histiocytosis of T-bone
- Acute otomastoiditis with coalescence
- Metastatic neuroblastoma
- Cholesterol granuloma of middle ear

CLINICAL ISSUES

- Clinical presentation
  - Child (< 6 years old) with chronic otitis media
  - Other symptoms: Otorrhea, hearing loss, facial paresis, ear pain, external auditory canal polyp
- Most common soft tissue sarcoma in children
- Up to 40% of RMSs in children occurs in H&N
  - 7% of H&N RMSs occur in T-bone
- Surgery for biopsy, debulking; adjuvant chemoXRT

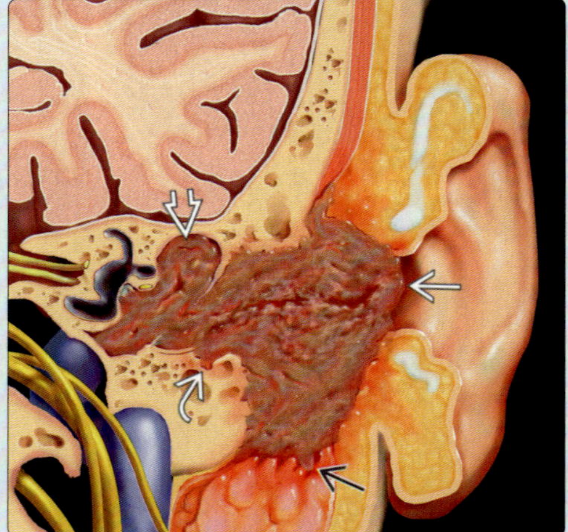

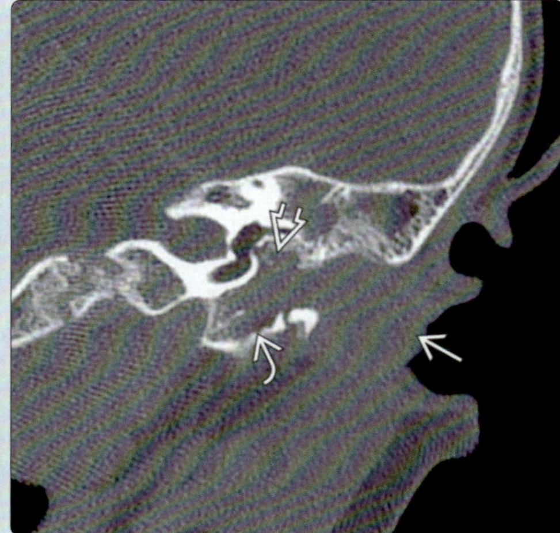

(Left) *Coronal graphic of temporal bone rhabdomyosarcoma (RMS) shows a mass filling the middle ear ➡, spreading laterally to fill the EAC, and appearing clinically as an EAC polyp ➡. Note invasion of the bony medial floor of the EAC ➡ and subjacent parotid ➡.* **(Right)** *Coronal bone CT in a 2-year-old child with an EAC polyp and bleeding shows rapidly growing RMS of left EAC ➡, middle ear cavity ➡, and mastoid air cells. This tumor causes osseous erosion of the floor of the hypotympanum ➡.*

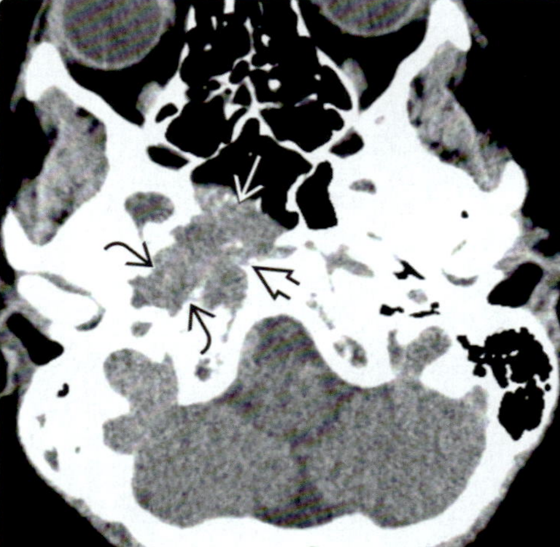

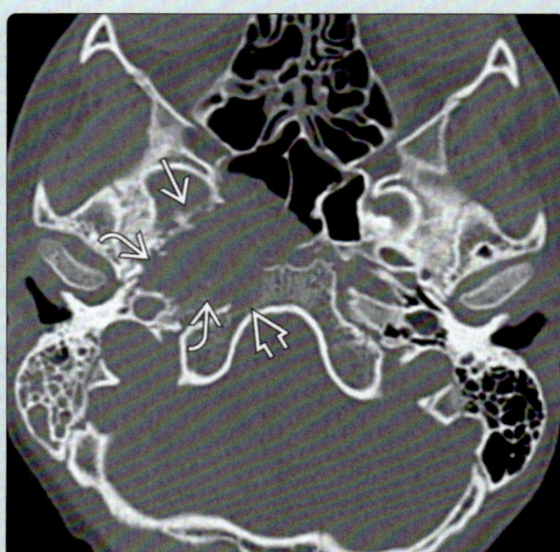

(Left) *Axial NECT of the skull base of an 11-year-old boy with nasopharyngeal RMS shows superior extension of the mass into the sphenoid sinus ➡, adjacent skull base/clivus ➡, and inferior aspect of the petrous apex ➡.* **(Right)** *Axial bone CT in the same patient clearly defines erosion of the petrous apex ➡, clivus ➡, and middle cranial fossa floor ➡. This is a characteristic pattern of spread in parameningeal RMS.*

KEY FACTS

TERMINOLOGY

- Definition: Protrusion of cranial contents into middle ear (ME) or mastoid through dehiscence of tegmen
- Synonyms: Temporal lobe meningocele, encephalocele, or meningoencephalocele; defined by content

IMAGING

- CT: **Tegmen tympani** (ME roof) or **mastoideum** (mastoid roof) dehiscence
  - Tegmen defect does not necessarily result in cephalocele
  - Evaluate for concurrent superior canal dehiscence
- MR: Temporal lobe herniation ± CSF into ME or mastoid

TOP DIFFERENTIAL DIAGNOSES

- Large cholesteatoma with tegmen dehiscence
- ME cholesterol granuloma
- Temporal bone bone arachnoid granulation

PATHOLOGY

- Temporal bone cephalocele has multiple etiologies
  - Congenital
  - Acquired
    - Traumatic: Postsurgical or posttrauma/fracture
    - Nontraumatic: Cholesteatoma induced
    - Related to **idiopathic intracranial hypertension**
      - Obese, middle-aged women
    - Spontaneous: Predisposition with thin tegmen

CLINICAL ISSUES

- Clinical presentation
  - 85% conductive hearing loss with middle ear fluid
  - PE tubes result in persistent **clear otorrhea**
- Treatment options
  - Surgery: Multilayer closer with middle fossa ± transmastoid approaches ± lumbar drain
  - Threat of **meningitis** catalyzes this action
  - Treat idiopathic intracranial hypertension if present

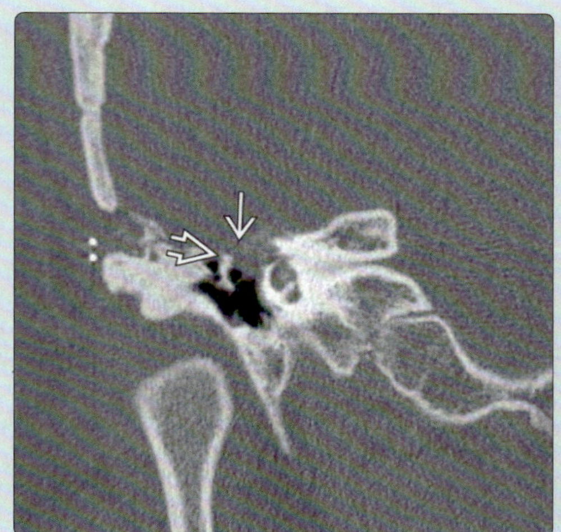

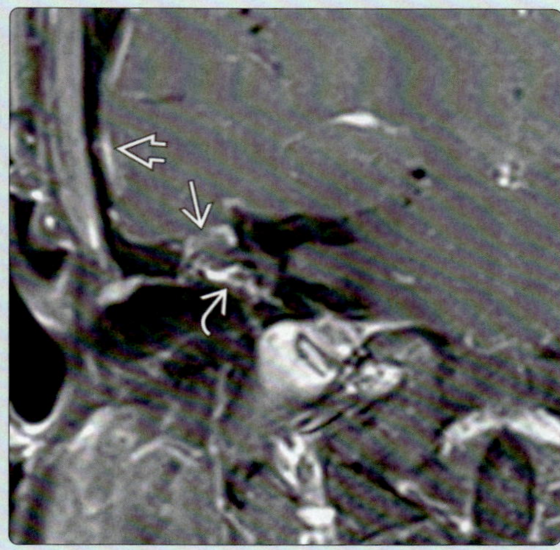

(Left) *Coronal bone CT in a patient with a history of severe temporal bone trauma and conductive hearing loss reveals complete absence of the tegmen tympani ➡ with cephalocele surrounding the head of the malleus ➡.* **(Right)** *Coronal T1WI C+ FS MR in a patient with "fluid" behind an intact tympanic membrane shows a spontaneous tegmen tympani area cephalocele ➡. Enhancing tissue in the middle ear ➡ and dural enhancement ➡ is seen. At surgery, CSF leakage accompanied the cephalocele.*

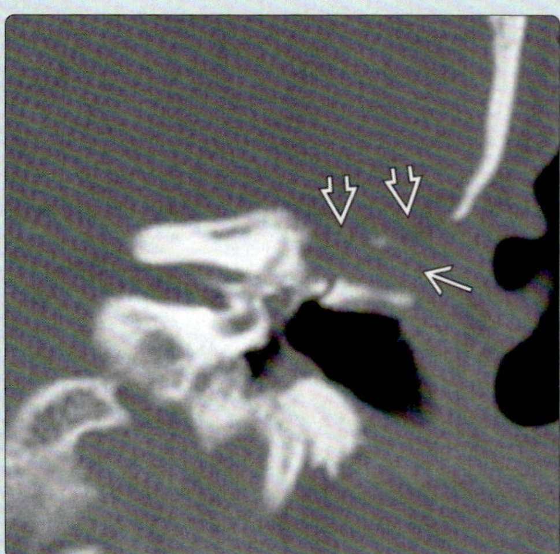

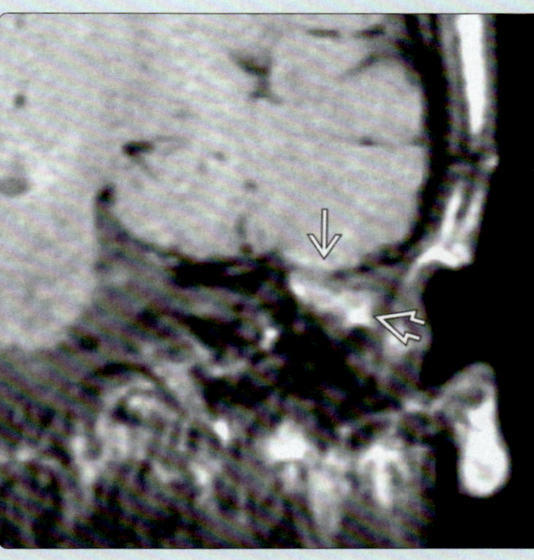

(Left) *Coronal bone CT in a patient with CSF leakage following mastoidectomy demonstrates a broad tegmen dehiscence ➡ accompanied by opacification ➡ of the epitympanum and lateral mastoid air cells below the area of dehiscence. The possibility of cephalocele was raised by this coronal CT appearance.* **(Right)** *Coronal FLAIR MR in the same patient reveals a hammock-like encephalocele of the temporal lobe through the tegmen post surgical defect ➡. High-signal surgical fat packing is visible below the encephalocele ➡.*

Ossicular Prosthesis

KEY FACTS

TERMINOLOGY

- Ossicular replacement prosthesis (ORP)
  - Partial (PORP = to stapes), total (TORP = to footplate)
- **Ossiculoplasty**: Surgical reconstruction of malfunctioned ossicular chain to improve or to maintain residual conductive hearing function
- Common ORP types
  - Stapes prosthesis
  - Incus interposition graft
  - PORP, TORP

IMAGING

- Temporal bone CT = best imaging tool
  - All or part of ossicular chain, replaced by tissue graft (autograft, homograft, autolograft) or allograft
  - CT may over- or underestimate (< 1 mm) size of metallic ORP due to metallic artifacts
  - CT may underestimate fluoroplastic portion of ORP if surrounded by soft tissue
  - Allow some leeway when commenting on medial-lateral position of ORP
- **Prosthesis malfunction** findings on CT
  - Displacement, dislocation, protrusion, extrusion
  - Stapes prostheses should be just within vestibule, TORPs should not (ends at footplate)
  - Abnormal soft tissue-embedded ORP
  - Recurrent/progressive primary disease
    - Cholesteatoma, otosclerosis, tympanosclerosis
- Prosthetic MR safety
  - Most modern ossicular replacement prostheses are tested safe or conditional at 1.5T or 3T
  - Check specific product against known MR safety record

TOP DIFFERENTIAL DIAGNOSES

- Chronic otitis media with tympanosclerosis
- Posttraumatic incus dislocation
- Foreign body in middle ear
- Semiimplantable direct drive hearing device

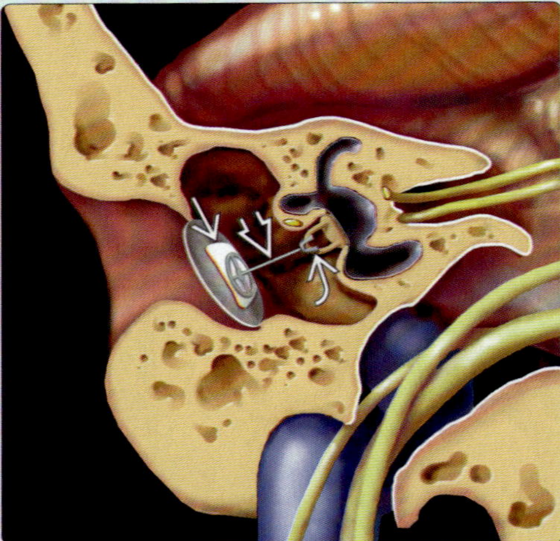
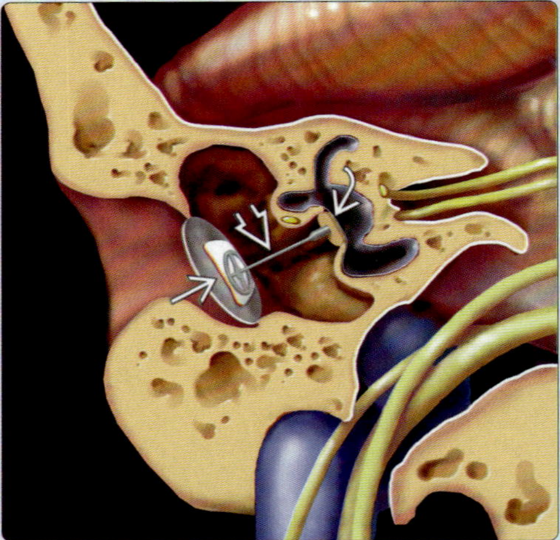

(Left) *Coronal graphic shows a titanium PORP ➡ connecting the tympanic membrane (TM) to the capitulum of stapes ➡. A cartilage graft ➡ is often placed between the TM and head of prosthesis to reduce incidence of implant extrusion. Prostheses connecting any part of ossicular chain to capitulum are called PORP.* **(Right)** *Coronal graphic shows a TORP ➡ connecting the TM to the footplate ➡ at the oval window. A TORP is used when the stapes is absent. Intervening cartilage cap ➡ is between TM and prosthesis head.*

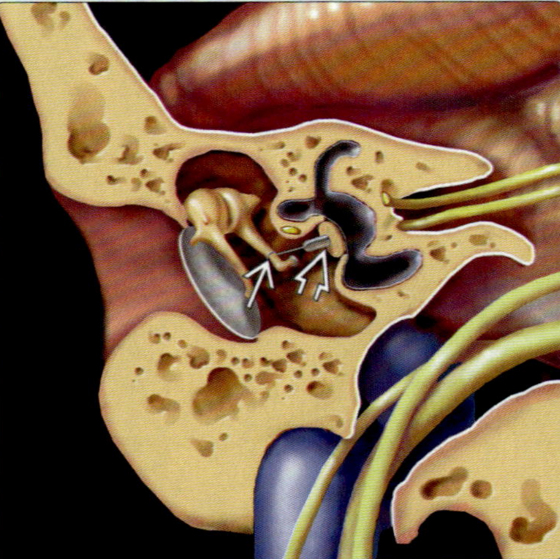
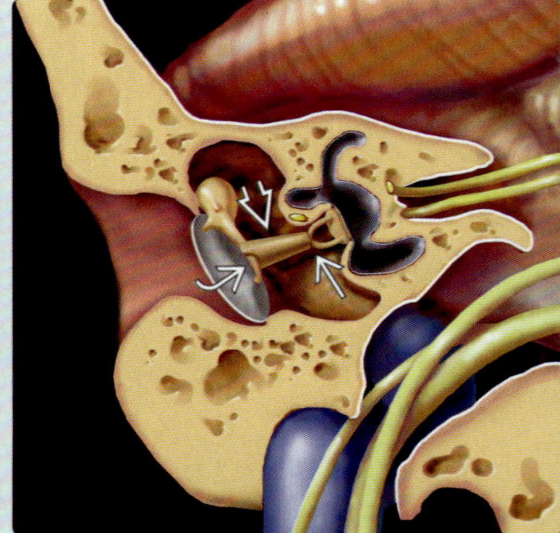

(Left) *Coronal graphic shows a stapes prosthesis. The incus end ➡ is crimped to the incus long process. Piston base ➡ is placed through the footplate (fixed by otosclerosis) via stapedotomy.* **(Right)** *Coronal graphic reveals an example of an incus interposition graft where the incus ➡ is sculpted and rotated to connect the handle of malleus to the capitulum of stapes. A groove ➡ is created in the remaining long process of the incus to anchor it to the manubrium. A hole ➡ is drilled in the incus body to accommodate the stapes capitulum.*

Petromastoid Canal

KEY FACTS

TERMINOLOGY

- Petromastoid canal (PMC) definition: **Normal temporal bone osseous canal** that passes through arch of superior semicircular canal conveying subarcuate artery to otic capsule
- Synonyms: Subarcuate canal or canaliculus

IMAGING

- Osseous canal passing **beneath superior semicircular canal**
  - Infant: Globoid to tubular + CSF in subarachnoid space
    - Best seen on axial high-resolution T2 MR
  - Adult: Linear with sclerotic margins on CT; unseen on MR

TOP DIFFERENTIAL DIAGNOSES

- Large vestibular aqueduct (IP-II)
- Prominent cochlear aqueduct
- Temporal bone fracture involving inner ear

PATHOLOGY

- Maximum size of PMC occurs at week 21 of embryonic development
  - Then ↓ in size to form subarcuate fossa & PMC
- Contains subarcuate artery & vein
- PMC in child < 2 years of age
  - **Dural-lined subarachnoid space** connected to cerebellopontine angle cistern
- PMC in child > 2 years of age
  - Involutes with disappearance of dura, subarachnoid space, & CSF

DIAGNOSTIC CHECKLIST

- **PMC may be mistaken for pathology**
  - In infant: Inner ear or petrous apex anomaly
  - In adult: Temporal bone fracture
- PMC = potential route of spread of infection

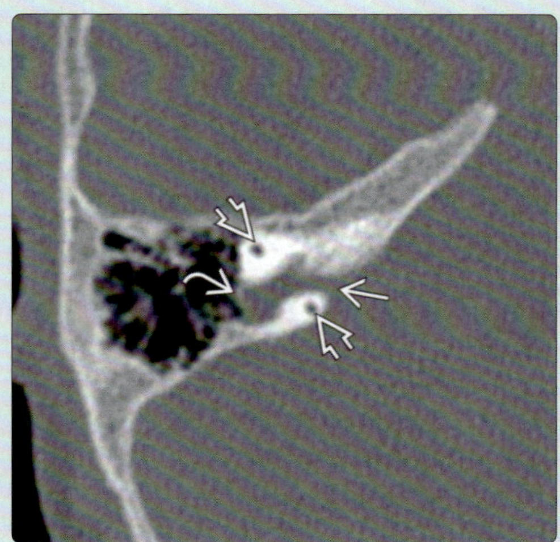

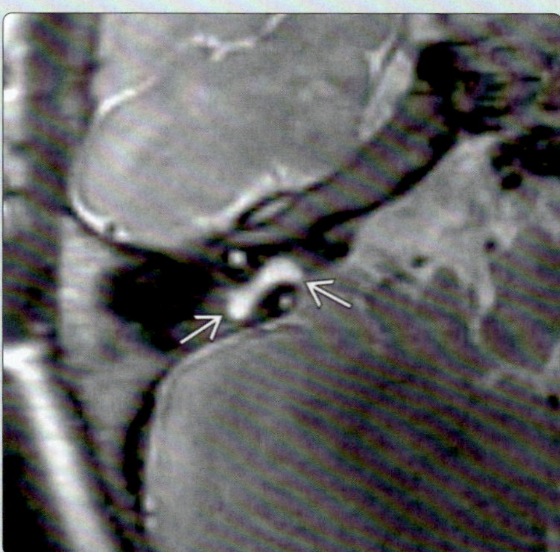

(Left) *Axial bone CT in a 9 month old shows a prominent petromastoid canal (PMC) extending from the medial petrous ridge ➡, beneath the superior semicircular canal ➡, to the medial mastoid antrum wall ➡. Note the thin bony wall at its medial margin.* **(Right)** *Axial T2 MR in the same infant shows the conspicuous high-signal PMC ➡. Early in life (< 2 years of age), this developing structure is a dural-lined subarachnoid space filled with high-signal CSF that may be confused with pathology.*

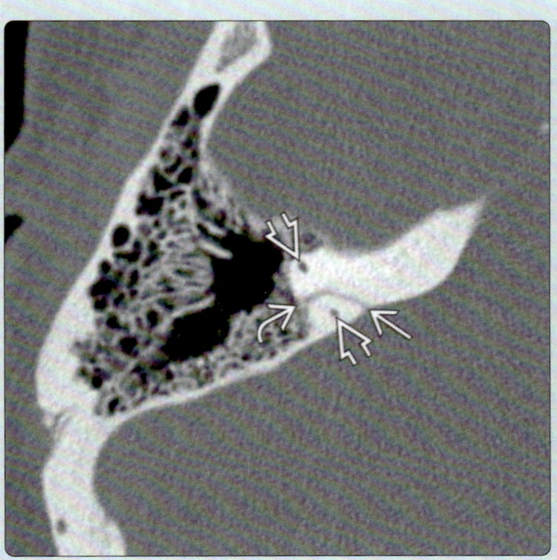

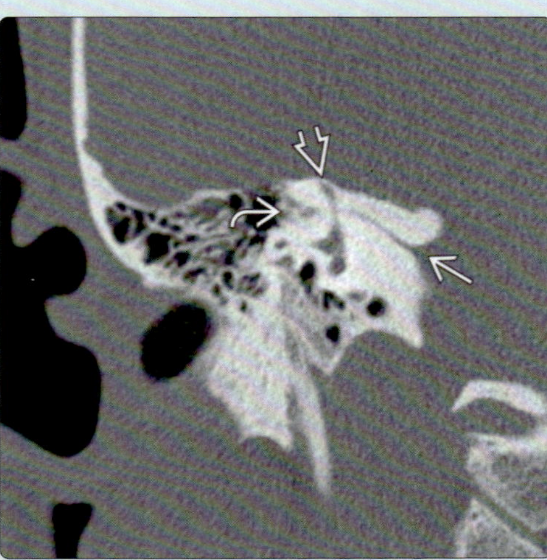

(Left) *Axial temporal bone CT of an adult right ear shows a normal, linear, arching PMC passing from the medial petrous ridge ➡ under the superior semicircular canal ➡ to the lateral wall of the mastoid antrum ➡.* **(Right)** *Coronal CT in the same adult shows a normal curvilinear PMC passing from the subarcuate fossa of medial petrous ridge ➡ beneath the superior semicircular canal ➡ to the medial wall of the mastoid antrum ➡. PMC may be mistaken for a fracture.*

KEY FACTS

TERMINOLOGY

- Synonyms for cochlear cleft
  - Localized pericochlear hypoattenuating foci
  - Cochlear capsule space
- Cochlear cleft definition
  - Developmental curvilinear lucency attributed to **nonosseous otic capsule space** adjacent to cochlea in children seen on temporal bone CT

IMAGING

- Bone CT (< 1-mm thick images)
  - Bilateral > unilateral
  - C-shaped, thin, sharply defined lucency in otic capsule
  - Adjacent to middle & apical portions of first 2 cochlear turns
  - Adjacent lateral > medial aspect of cochlea
  - May extend to apical turn on axial images
  - Anterior to oval window
  - Does not extend to oval window
- Parallel to cochlea on coronal images
  - Lucency curved in shape of cochlear promontory

TOP DIFFERENTIAL DIAGNOSES

- Fenestral otosclerosis
- Cochlear otosclerosis
- Temporal bone osteogenesis imperfecta
- Postirradiated temporal bone

CLINICAL ISSUES

- Clinical presentation
  - **Incidental finding** in child
- Becomes less conspicuous & disappears with age
  - Medial lucency disappears 1st
- Age vs. incidence of cochlear cleft
  - **< 4 years**: Present in **~ 60%**
  - 4-7 years: Present in ~ 45%
  - 7-10 years: Present in ~ 25%
  - 10-19 years: Present in ~ 20%

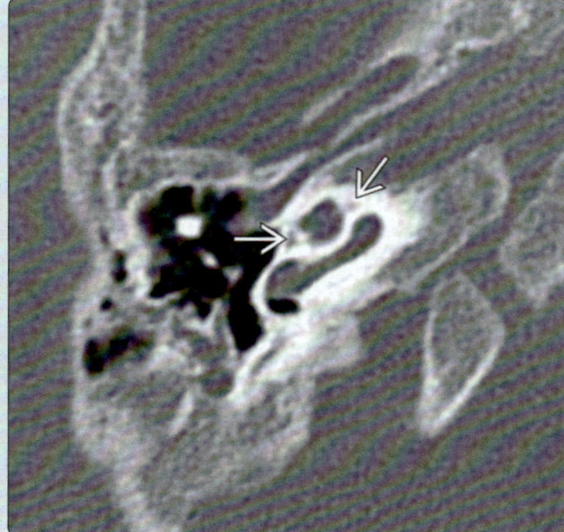

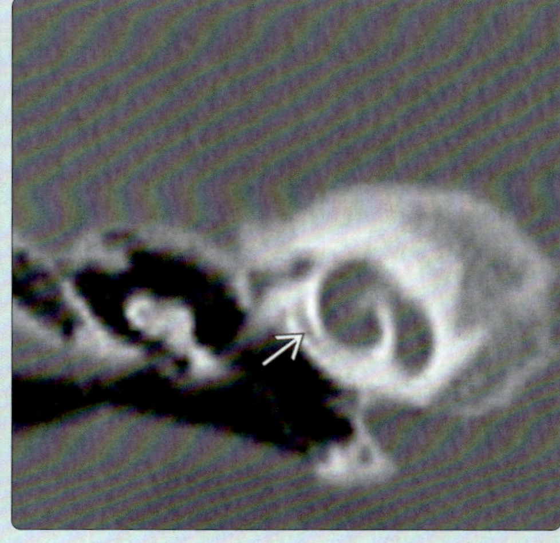

(Left) *Normal temporal bone CT in a 2-month-old girl with sensorineural hearing loss demonstrates well-defined curvilinear lucency ➡ within the otic capsule bone parallel to the cochlear turns. The lucency is more pronounced laterally than medially. These findings are characteristic of developmental cochlear cleft.* **(Right)** *Right ear coronal reformatted bone CT reveals the curvilinear lucency ➡ within the otic capsule bone parallel to the cochlea, just deep to the surface of the cochlear promontory.*

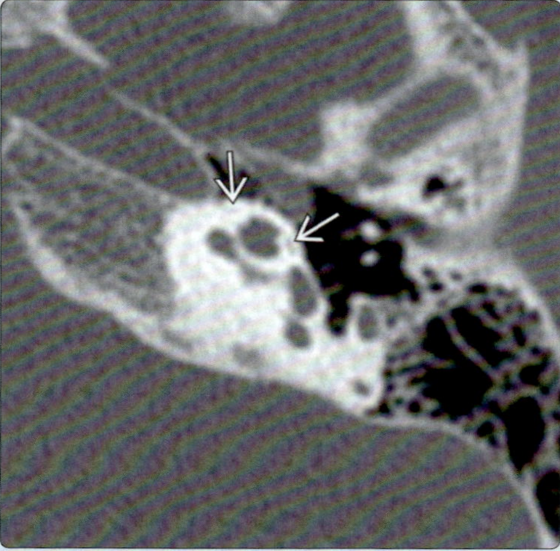

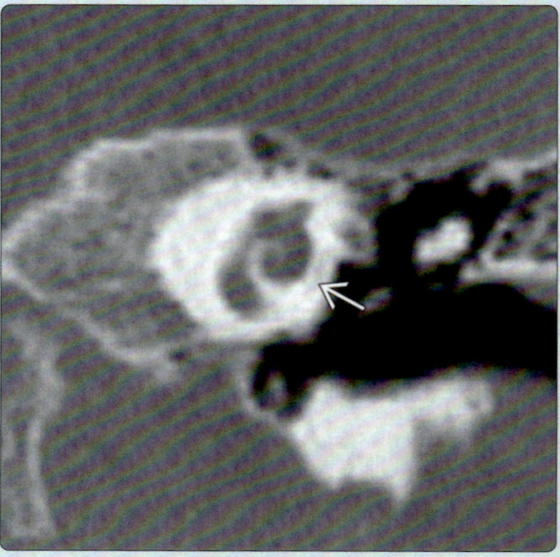

(Left) *Axial bone CT in a 3-year-old boy with sensorineural hearing loss and a normal CT exam shows an evolving cochlear cleft. At this stage, a linear lucency ➡ is present medial & lateral to the apical portions of the first 2 cochlear turns.* **(Right)** *Coronal CT reformation in the same patient shows a faint cochlear cleft lucent line ➡ lateral to the cochlea deep to the cochlear promontory surface.*

KEY FACTS

TERMINOLOGY

- Synonym: Complete labyrinthine aplasia
  - Michel aplasia/anomaly (old synonym)

IMAGING

- Bilateral or unilateral anomaly
- Temporal bone CT findings
  - Otic capsule bone: Aplasia/hypoplasia
  - Absent cochlea, vestibule, semicircular canals, & vestibular aqueduct
  - Cochlear promontory: Absent/flattened
  - Ossicles: Normal or malformed stapes
  - Tegmen tympani: Normal, low, or defective
  - Facial nerve canal: Aberrant course
  - Petrous apex: Hypoplasia
  - Internal auditory canal: Aplasia/hypoplasia
  - Carotid canal: Normal or absent
- MR: Absent vestibular & cochlear nerves

TOP DIFFERENTIAL DIAGNOSES

- Cochlear aplasia
- Common cavity
- Labyrinthine ossification, obliterative type

PATHOLOGY

- Genetic mutation (e.g., *HOXA1*), thalidomide exposure, or unknown etiology
- **Arrested otic placode development** before 3rd week of gestation

CLINICAL ISSUES

- Extremely rare anomaly
- Congenital sensorineural hearing loss
- Horizontal gaze palsy or abnormal teeth suggest underlying syndrome

DIAGNOSTIC CHECKLIST

- Often asymmetric: Contralateral common cavity, inner ear hypoplasia, or cochlear IP-I anomaly

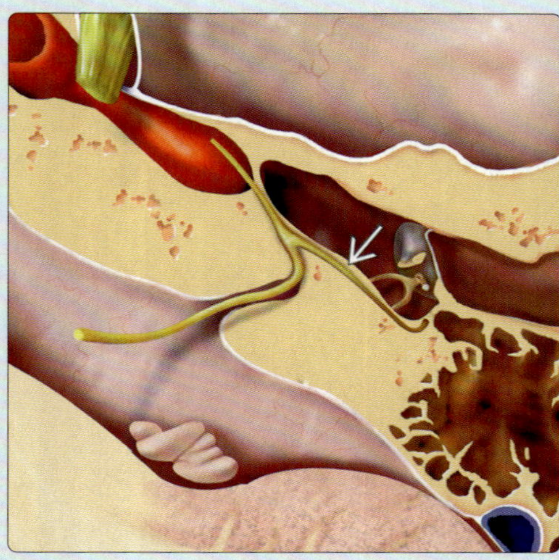

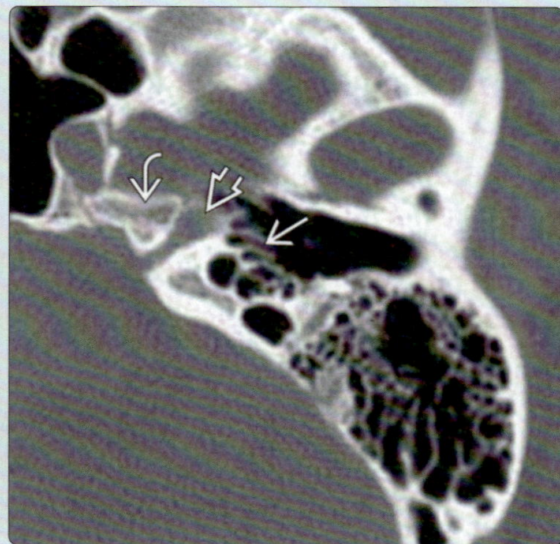

(Left) *Axial graphic depicts labyrinthine aplasia. Note the complete absence of all inner ear structures with the exception of a small IAC with only CNVII. The lateral wall of the inner ear (promontory) is flattened ➡.* **(Right)** *Axial bone CT in 21-year-old woman with SNHL shows severe hypoplasia of otic capsule bone with air cells in expected location of the promontory ➡. Inner ear structures are absent. CNVII canal is present with a broadened anterior genu ➡. Note petrous apex is hypoplastic ➡, narrow in width.*

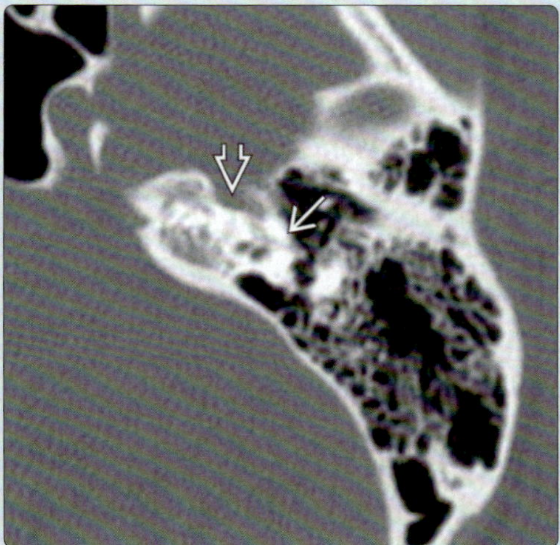

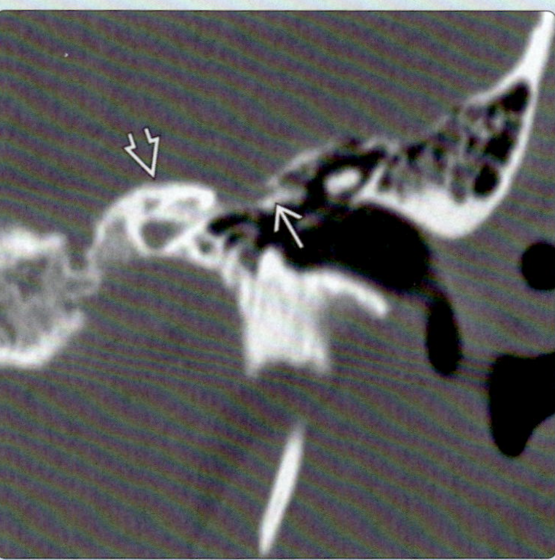

(Left) *Axial bone CT, in the same patient at a more cephalad level, shows hypoplastic otic capsule bone ➡. The anterior genu and proximal tympanic segment of the anomalous CNVII canal are visible ➡.* **(Right)** *Coronal bone CT in the same patient reveals complete absence of inner ear structures and severe hypoplasia of the otic capsule bone ➡ and petrous apex ➡. Note normal middle ear and ossicles despite complete inner ear aplasia.*

KEY FACTS

TERMINOLOGY

- Common cavity (CC) is cystic space representing **undifferentiated cochlea & vestibule**

IMAGING

- **Cochlea, vestibule, & horizontal semicircular canal (SCC)**: CC, variable size
- Posterior & superior SCC: Usually absent or malformed
- IAC: Variable size, anomalous course, deficient fundus
  - Small CC: Stenotic IAC; large CC: Widened IAC
- CNVIII: Small or absent components
- Facial nerve canal: Anomalous course
- Vestibular aqueduct: Not dilated, may be absent
- Ossicles: Normal or anomalous stapes & stenotic oval window

TOP DIFFERENTIAL DIAGNOSES

- Cochlear aplasia
- Cystic cochleovestibular anomaly

PATHOLOGY

- Unknown or genetic mutation
- *HOXA1* mutations: Bosley-Salih-Alorainy syndrome

CLINICAL ISSUES

- Congenital sensorineural hearing loss (SNHL)
- Rare: < 1% of all congenital inner ear malformations
- Bilateral profound SNHL: Cochlear implantation can be successful in CC; often need lateral wall electrode
- Potential risk of recurrent meningitis for large CC & large IAC with associated perilymph fistula

DIAGNOSTIC CHECKLIST

- **Common cavity** if **cochlea, vestibule, & horizontal SCC form single cavity** without differentiation
- Consider cystic cochleovestibular anomaly if differentiated into separate but featureless cochlea & vestibule
- If IAC enters anterior CC, can be difficult to distinguish from cochlear aplasia + globular vestibule & horizontal SCC

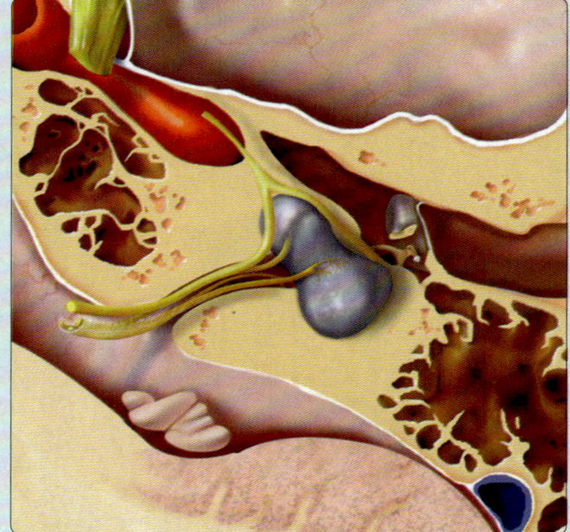

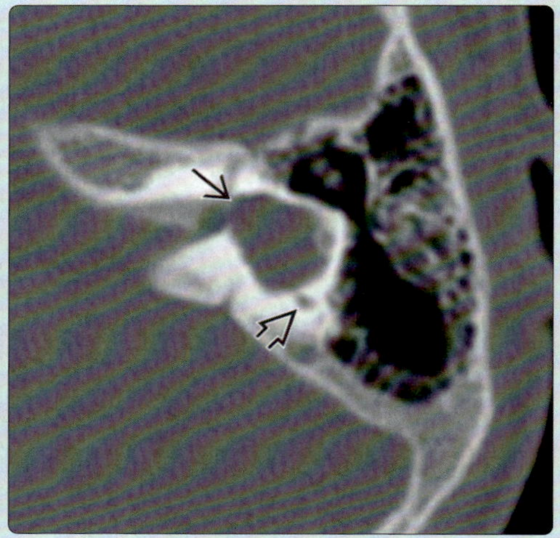

(Left) *Axial graphic shows features of a common cavity malformation. Note that the cochlea and vestibule are melded into 1 common cyst. Semicircular canals (SCCs) are not distinct from the cystic vestibular component.* **(Right)** *Axial bone CT shows the internal auditory canal entering the anterior aspect of the common cavity malformation ⇒ where the cochlea is fused with the vestibule. (Middle ear & mastoids formed later, during the 2nd trimester, & were normal.) A tiny portion of the posterior SCC is present ⇒.*

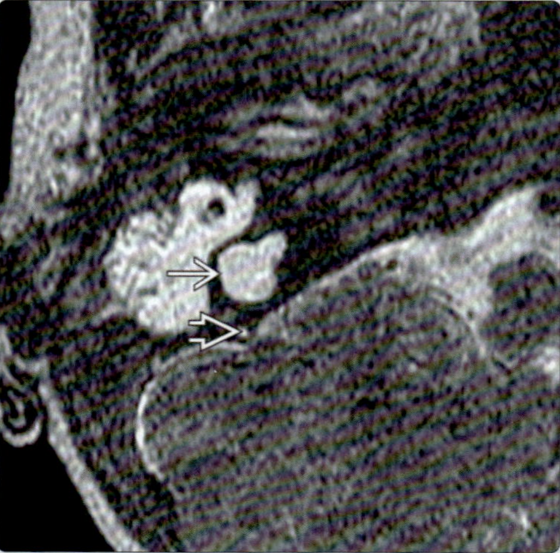

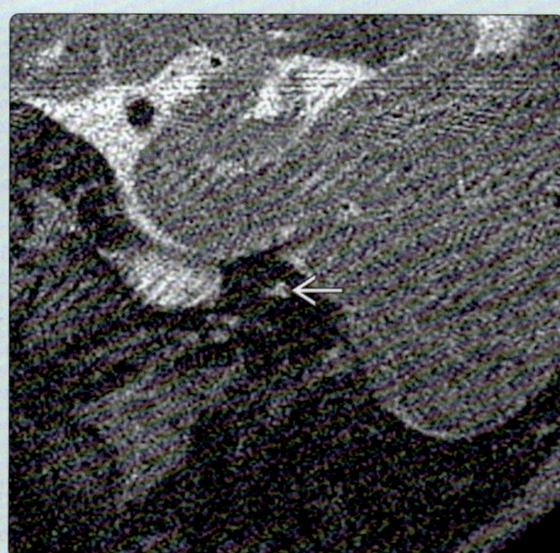

(Left) *Axial 3D FIESTA image in an 18-month-old child with bilateral congenital sensorineural hearing loss demonstrates a common cavity anomaly with a cystic structure representing the vestibule, rudimentary cochlear bud, and horizontal semicircular canal ⇒. There is a small posterior SCC ⇒.* **(Right)** *Oblique 2D FIESTA MR in the same patient shows a small internal auditory meatus containing only a single, posteriorly located vestibular nerve ⇒. No facial nerve is present.*

Cystic Cochleovestibular Malformation (IP-I)

KEY FACTS

TERMINOLOGY

- Cochlear incomplete partition type I: **Dilated vestibule** and **horizontal semicircular canal** (SCC)

IMAGING

- Cochlea: Absent internal septation & modiolus (incomplete partition type I, IP-I)
- Vestibule & SCC: Dilated vestibule & horizontal SCC form single cavity, wide communication with cochlea
- CNVII canal: Normal or mildly obtuse anterior genu angle; normal or dehiscent tympanic segment
- Internal auditory canal: Small or dilated, defective fundus
- CNVIII: Nerves hypoplastic or absent
- Vestibular aqueduct: Usually normal
- Oval window: Normal or stenotic + stapedial anomaly

TOP DIFFERENTIAL DIAGNOSES

- **Cochlear aplasia**
    - Absent cochlea; vestibule & SCC normal, dilated, or hypoplastic
- **Common cavity**
    - Cystic cochlea & vestibule form ovoid or rounded common cavity

CLINICAL ISSUES

- Presentation
    - Congenital sensorineural hearing loss
    - Isolated symptom or with syndromic features (cardiac, spine anomalies, etc.)
- Cystic cochleovestibular malformation (CCVM) accounts for < 2% of all congenital labyrinthine lesions

DIAGNOSTIC CHECKLIST

- CCVM (IP-I)
    - **Figure 8 cochlea & vestibule lacking internal architecture**
    - Risk of CSF leak & meningitis from translabyrinthine fistula

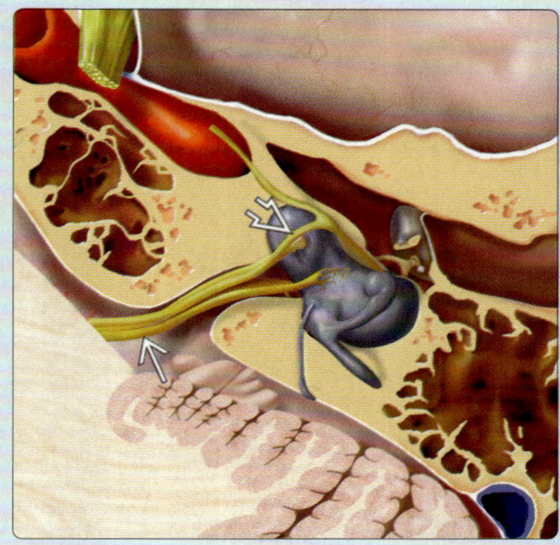

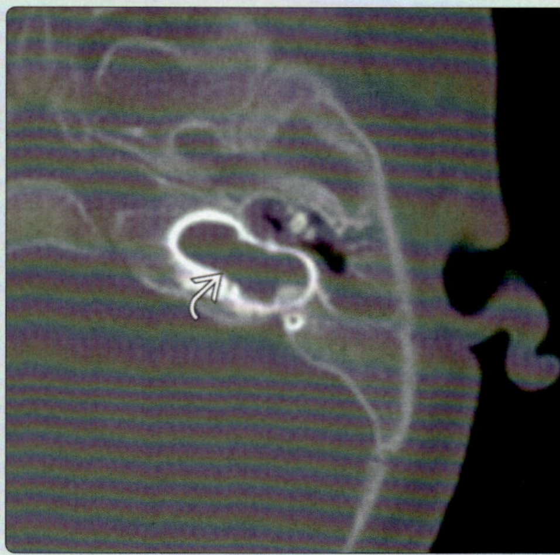

(Left) *Figure 8 morphology of featureless cochlea & vestibule is shown. Cochlear interscalar septum & modiolus are absent. CNVIII components are hypoplastic ➡. IAC is narrow & shortened. CNVII labyrinthine segment has lost its anteriorly curving shape & appears straightened ➡ as it ends at the geniculate ganglion.* **(Right)** *Axial bone CT in a 6-month-old girl with unilateral sensorineural hearing loss (SNHL) & multiple congenital anomalies shows typical figure 8 morphology of cystic cochleovestibular malformation (CCVM) ➡.*

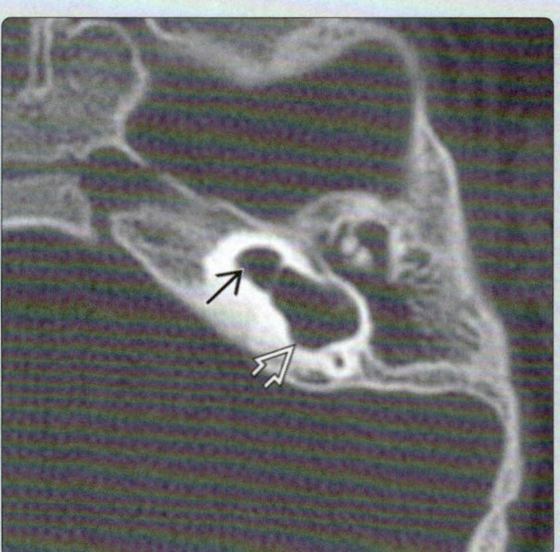

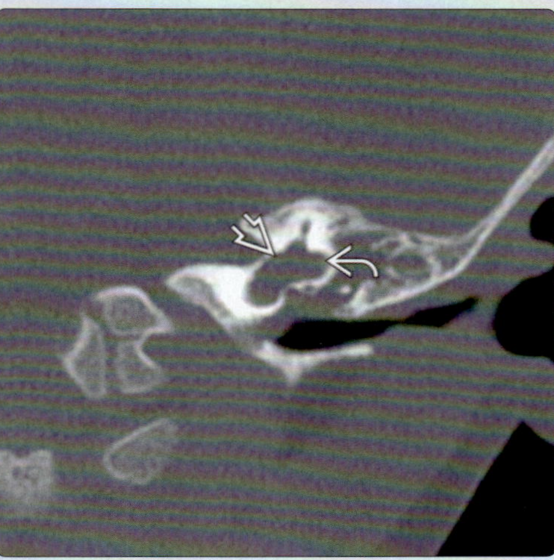

(Left) *CT in an 18-month-old boy with congenital SNHL and CCVM shows a cochlea that lacks internal architecture ➡, also termed incomplete partition type I malformation. The vestibule and horizontal semicircular canal (SCC) form a single globular cavity ➡. The middle ear space and mastoid air cells are opacified. This patient had a contralateral common cavity anomaly.* **(Right)** *Coronal bone CT in the same patient demonstrates the globular vestibule ➡ and horizontal SCC ➡.*

KEY FACTS

TERMINOLOGY

- IP-I spectrum of anomalies: **Mild** (cochlea lacks modiolus and interscalar septum) to **severe** [cystic cochleovestibular malformation (CCVM)]
- Cochlear incomplete partition type I (IP-I): Milder form of IP-I; cochlea has some external structure, variable anomaly vestibule & semicircular canal (SCC)
- CCVM: Least differentiated manifestation of IP-I involving cochlea, vestibule, & SCC

IMAGING

- IP-I has absent interscalar septum & modiolus
- Spectrum of IP-I severity
  - Amorphous sac, wide communication between cochlea & vestibule; figure 8 morphology (CCVM)
  - Some external structure, dilated vestibule, & horizontal SCC (most common)
  - External indentations suggesting cochlear turns, ± normal vestibule (rare)
- Cochlear nerve canal & IAC: Normal, wide (most common), or narrow; absent macula cribrosa
- Cochlear nerve: Usually hypoplastic or absent
- Vestibule & horizontal SCC: Usually dilated
- Vestibular aqueduct: Usually normal

TOP DIFFERENTIAL DIAGNOSES

- **Cochlear hypoplasia**: Small cochlea, < 2 turns
- **Cochlear incomplete partition type II (IP-II)**
  - Defective septation between middle & apical cochlear turns, normal basal turn
  - Large vestibular aqueduct/endolymphatic sac
- **Common cavity malformation**
  - Single cystic structure = cochlea + vestibule

CLINICAL ISSUES

- When profound bilateral SHNL: Cochlear implantation variably successful, lateral wall electrode usually preferred
  - Risk of CSF gusher, pack opening to prevent leak

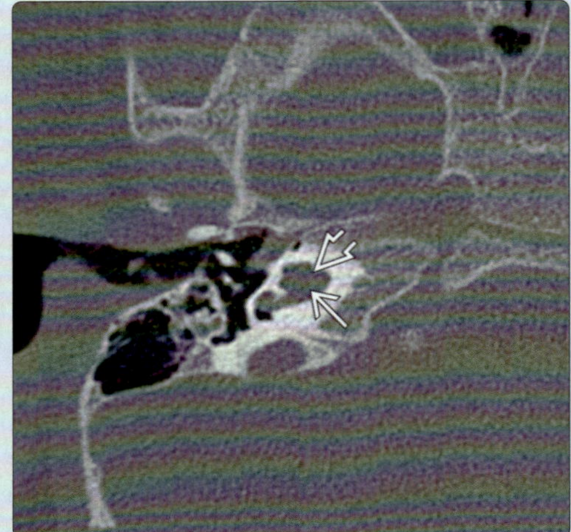

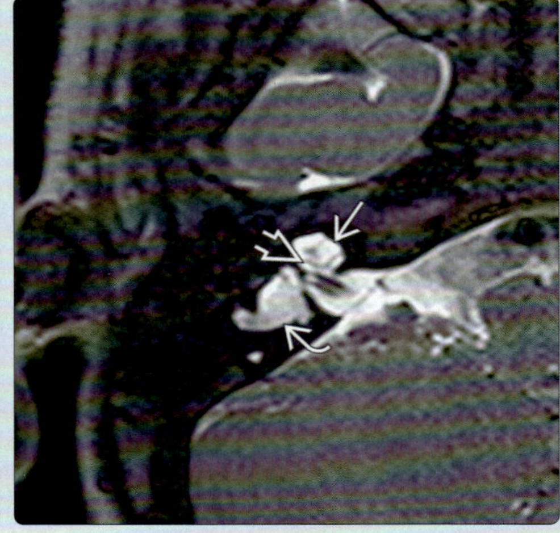

(Left) *Axial bone CT in a 9-month-old girl with right SNHL shows complete absence of the cochlear modiolus ➡ & interscalar septum ➡. The anomaly affects the entire cochlea. In this relatively mild & uncommon manifestation of IP-I, there is some external "shape" to cochlea.* **(Right)** *Axial T2 MR in a 1-year-old boy with SNHL shows a large, amorphous cochlea ➡. The modiolus & osseous interscalar septum are absent. Curvilinear internal hypointensity presumably represents the spiral lamina ➡. The vestibule ➡ & lateral SCC are dilated.*

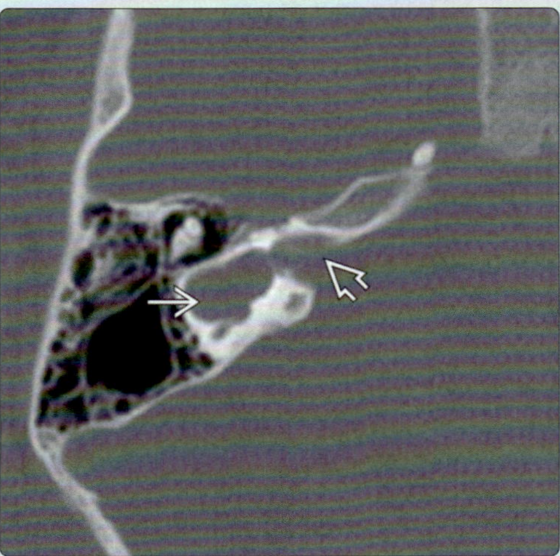

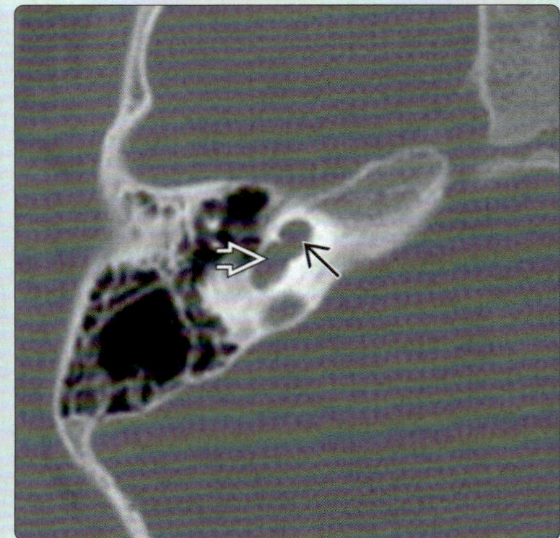

(Left) *Axial bone CT in a 4-year-old boy with right SNHL shows dilatation of the vestibule & horizontal SCC ➡. The vestibular aqueduct is not enlarged. The internal auditory meatus is widened ➡.* **(Right)** *Axial bone CT in the same patient shows cystic cochlea that lacks internal structure ➡. Note wide communication between the cochlea and vestibule ➡. This is the more common form of IP-I, with a cystic cochlea and dilatation of the vestibule and horizontal SCC, also referred to as CCVM.*

KEY FACTS

TERMINOLOGY

- IP-II: Incomplete partition due to deficient interscalar septum (ISS) between middle & apical cochlear turns
- Mondini anomaly (historic terminology): IP-II + large vestibular aqueduct (LVA)

IMAGING

- Cochlea
  - Absent ISS between plump middle & apical turns
  - Do not mistake osseous spiral lamina for ISS on MR
  - Smooth external contour between middle & apical turns posterolaterally (baseball cap cochlea)
  - Asymmetric scalar chambers
  - Deficient or absent modiolus
- Vestibular aqueduct/endolymphatic sac
  - Typically large (most cases) or borderline large & flared; rarely normal
- Vestibule: Normal or large
- SCC: Normal or mildly plump anterior limb lateral SCC

TOP DIFFERENTIAL DIAGNOSES

- Cochlear IP-I
- Cochlear hypoplasia
- CHARGE syndrome
- X-linked stapes gusher (DFNX2)

PATHOLOGY

- *SLC26A4* mutation (PDS gene, chromosome 7) most common
- Syndromic deafness: Pendred syndrome
- Nonsyndromic deafness: DFNB4
- ~ 20% of temporal bones with LVA have IP-II anomaly

CLINICAL ISSUES

- Bilateral or unilateral, severe or profound SNHL
- SNHL precipitated by minor trauma
- Fluctuating, progressive SNHL (or mixed hearing loss)
- Avoid contact sports & try to prevent head trauma
- Severe-profound bilateral SNHL: **Cochlear implantation**

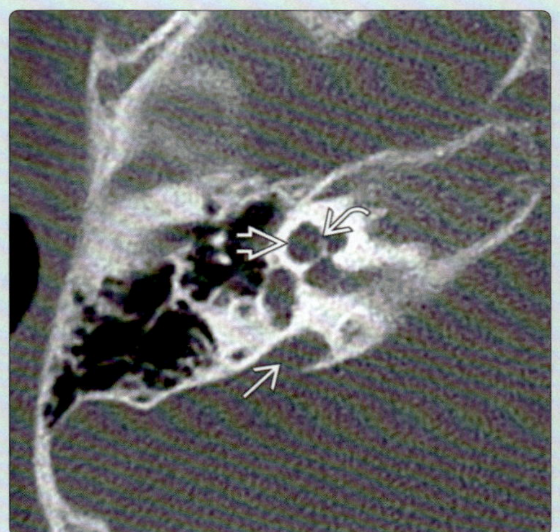

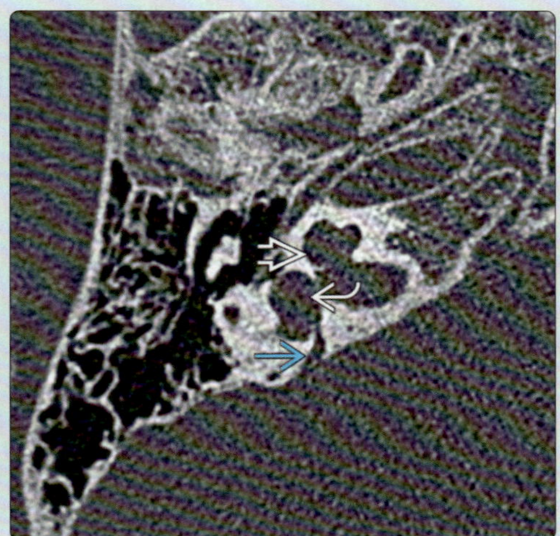

(Left) *Axial bone CT in 4-year-old girl with mixed hearing loss shows large vestibular aqueduct (LVA) ➡ & IP-II cochlear anomaly with smooth contour laterally & deficiency of interscalar septum (ISS) between apical & middle turns ➡; modiolus is malformed ➡.* **(Right)** *Axial bone CT in 2-year-old boy with sensorineural hearing loss (SNHL) shows mild LVA ➡ with absence of ISS between plump apical & middle cochlear turns ➡ & absence of modiolus. Cochlea resembles a baseball cap. Vestibule is mildly enlarged ➡.*

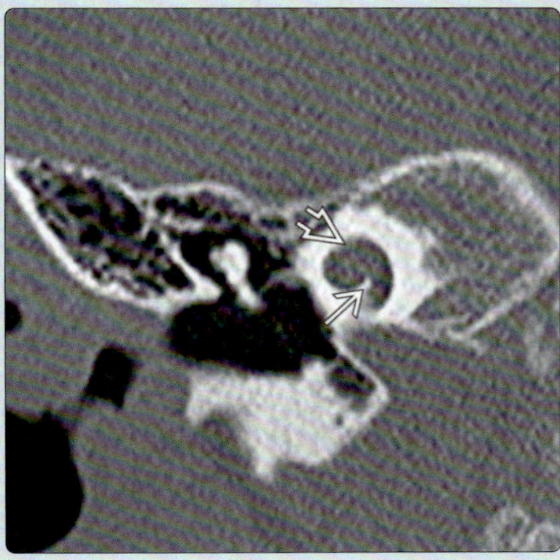

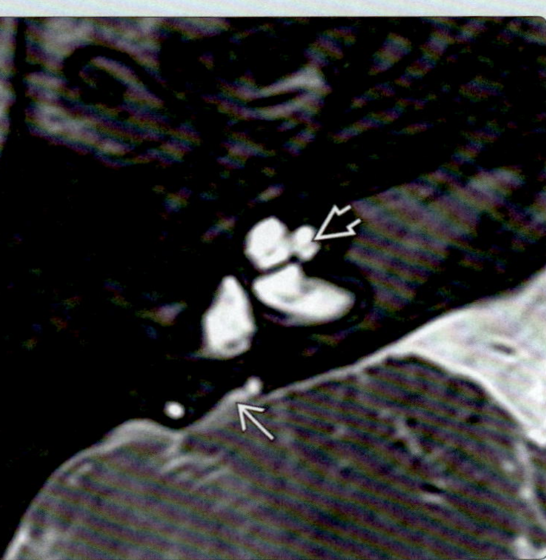

(Left) *Coronal reformatted bone CT in the same patient shows the tapered ISS between the basal and middle cochlear turns ➡. The ISS between the apical and middle turns ➡ is absent.* **(Right)** *Axial T2 SPACE MR in the same patient shows the mildly enlarged endolymphatic sac ➡. Notice again the baseball cap configuration of the cochlea with absence of the ISS between the apical and middle cochlear turns. The osseous spiral lamina ➡ is faintly seen within the middle cochlear turn and should not be mistaken for the ISS.*

Large Vestibular Aqueduct (IP-II)

KEY FACTS

TERMINOLOGY

- Large vestibular aqueduct (LVA) includes enlarged endolymphatic sac and duct
- IP-II: Incomplete partition type II between middle and apical cochlear turns often seen with LVA
- IP-II + LVA: Mondini anomaly (historic terminology)

IMAGING

- Axial CT: **LVA ≥ 1.0 mm at midpoint** &/or ≥ 2.0 mm at operculum; short-axis CT reformat: LVA ≥ 1.2 mm at midpoint, ≥ 1.3 mm at operculum; LVA > posterior SCC
- MR (high-res T2): **Enlarged endolymphatic sac and duct**
- Cochlea: **Abnormal in ~ 75% of LVA cases**
  - Absent septation between middle and apical turns
  - Deficient modiolus, asymmetric scalar chambers
- Vestibule and semicircular canal: Normal or mildly enlarged

TOP DIFFERENTIAL DIAGNOSES

- Cystic cochleovestibular malformation (IP-I)
- Cochlear hypoplasia
- CHARGE syndrome (funnel-shaped LVA)
- Branchiootorenal syndrome (funnel-shaped LVA)

PATHOLOGY

- *SLC26A4* mutations
  - Autosomal recessive, ~ 5-10% of prelingual hearing loss
  - Syndromic deafness + goiter: **Pendred syndrome**
  - Nonsyndromic deafness: DFNB4
  - ~ 50% of LVA patients have *SLC26A4* mutations

CLINICAL ISSUES

- Most common imaging abnormality in pediatric sensorineural hearing loss (SNHL); often **bilateral**
- Congenital cause of acquired SNHL or mixed hearing loss
- **Progressive/fluctuating SNHL**
- Avoid contact sports and try to prevent head trauma
- **Cochlear implantation** for profound bilateral SNHL; may encounter perilymph gusher

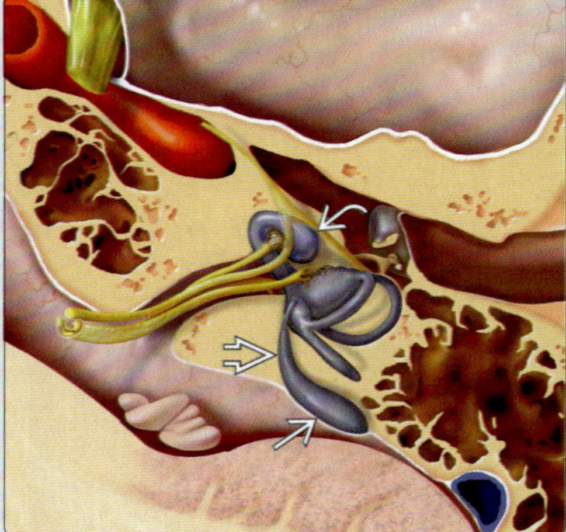

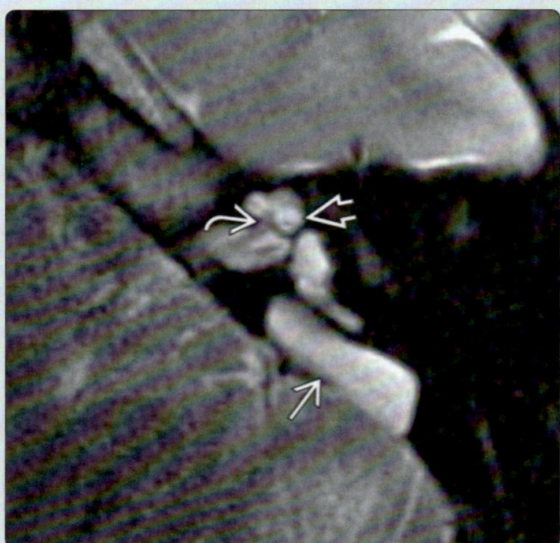

(Left) *In the left inner ear in the large vestibular aqueduct (IP-II), note the large endolymphatic sac epidural ➡ and intraosseous ➡ components. The cochlea is malformed with absent septation between middle and apical turns, which appear bulbous ➡.* **(Right)** *Axial T2WI MR shows a magnified view of the left inner ear in a patient with a large vestibular aqueduct (IP-II). Notice the high-signal, fluid-filled large endolymphatic sac ➡, asymmetrically large scala vestibuli ➡, and modiolar deficiency ➡.*

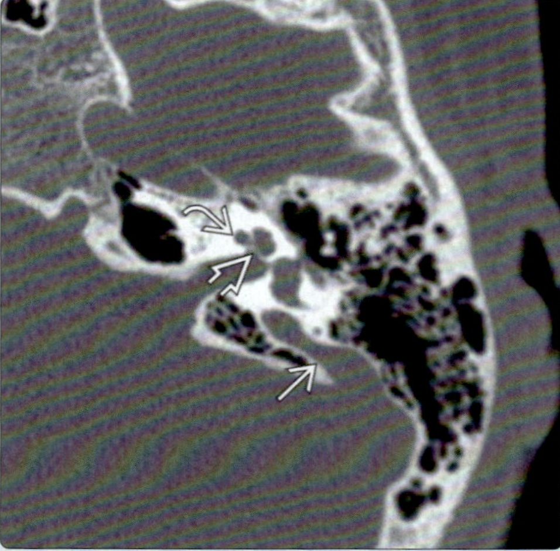

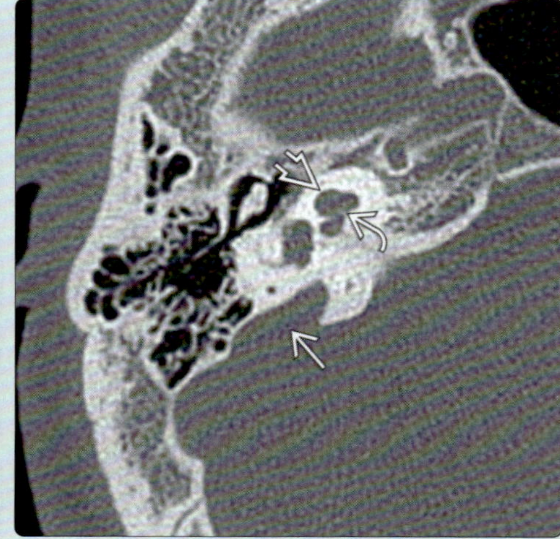

(Left) *Axial left bone CT in a 15-year-old boy with sensorineural hearing loss shows a large vestibular aqueduct ➡. Interscalar septum is present between apical and middle cochlear turns, but modiolus is narrow ➡, and scalar chambers are asymmetric (posterior > anterior) ➡.* **(Right)** *Axial temporal bone CT in a patient with Pendred syndrome shows a large vestibular aqueduct ➡ and absent septation between the middle and apical cochlear turns ➡ with absence of the modiolus ➡.*

KEY FACTS

TERMINOLOGY

- Definition: Absent cochlea; vestibule, semicircular canals (SCC), & internal auditory canal (IAC) present in some form

IMAGING

- Cochlea: **Absent** bilaterally or unilaterally
- Cochlear nerve canal & cochlear nerve: **Absent**
- Cochlear promontory: Hypoplastic, **flattened**
- Vestibule & SCC: Often malformed, globular, & dilated or hypoplastic
- Vestibular aqueduct: **Normal**
- Facial nerve canal: **Anomalous**, obtuse angle anterior genu
- IAC: **Hypoplastic**
- Middle ear: Normal size
- Ossicles: Normal or malformed stapes
- Oval window: Normal or stenotic/atretic

TOP DIFFERENTIAL DIAGNOSES

- Labyrinthine aplasia
    - **Cochlea, vestibule, & SCC absent**
- Common cavity deformity
    - **Dilated cochlea & vestibule form common cavity**
- Cystic cochleovestibular anomaly
    - **Cochlea & vestibule are cystic with no internal architecture**
- Labyrinthine ossificans
    - **Acquired sensorineural hearing loss (SNHL)**, usually postmeningitic

PATHOLOGY

- Absent cochlea, remainder of inner ear usually abnormal

CLINICAL ISSUES

- Extremely rare, congenital SNHL, usually bilateral

DIAGNOSTIC CHECKLIST

- Cochlear aplasia if no cochlea is seen on CT or T2 MR but rest of membranous labyrinth is present
- Distinguish from obliterative cochlear ossification

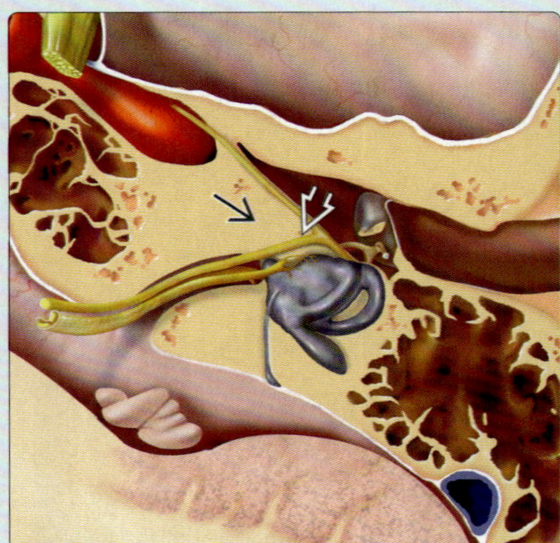

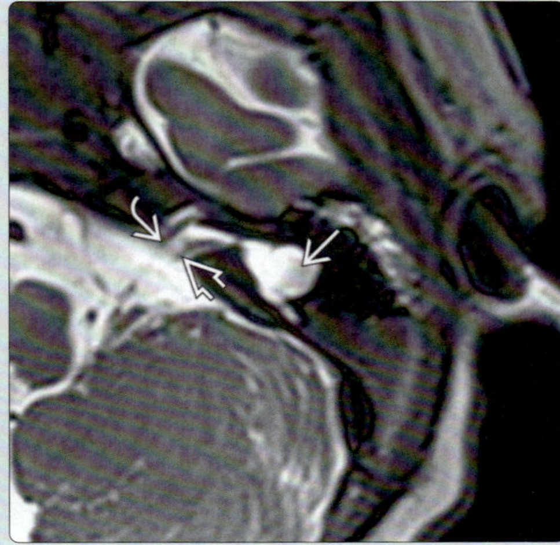

(Left) *Axial graphic shows findings of cochlear aplasia, including a small internal auditory canal (IAC) with absence of the cochlear nerve, absent cochlea ➔, vestibular & semicircular canal (SCC) malformation, & flattening of CNVII anterior genu ➔.* **(Right)** *Axial T2 SPACE in a 4-month-old girl with congenital SNHL reveals cochlear aplasia. There is globular vestibule-horizontal SCC anomaly ➔. A short, narrow internal auditory meatus contains vestibular ➔ & facial ➔ nerves. No cochlear nerve was seen.*

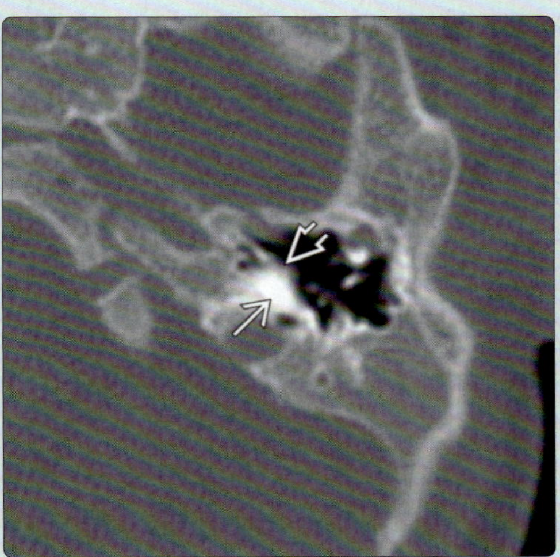

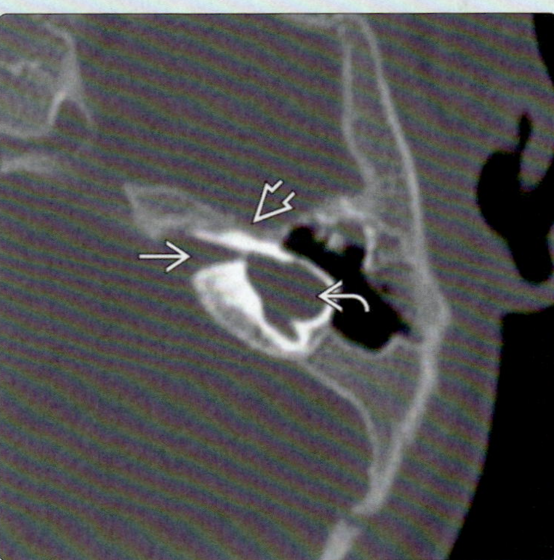

(Left) *Axial bone CT in the same patient demonstrates absence of the cochlea ➔ and mild flattening of the cochlear promontory ➔.* **(Right)** *Axial bone CT in the same patient shows a globular, malformed vestibule-horizontal SCC ➔. A shortened, narrowed IAC is seen ➔. An obtuse anterior genu of the facial nerve canal is partially visualized ➔ with an anomalous course of the facial nerve canal.*

Cochlear Hypoplasia

KEY FACTS

TERMINOLOGY

- Small, underdeveloped cochlea, usually < 2 turns

IMAGING

- Cochlea (variable severity)
  - **Primitive single turn or bud-like**
  - Small, cystic, no modiolus or interscalar septum
  - Small, + internal architecture, short modiolus
- Cochlear nerve canal: Absent, narrow, normal, wide
- Cochlear nerve: **Often absent or hypoplastic; best seen with high-resolution T2, sagittal cut**
- Facial nerve canal: Aberrant course ± dehiscence
- Internal auditory canal: Normal or narrow/anomalous
- Vestibule: Normal, dilated, or hypoplastic
- Vestibular aqueduct: Normal or large

TOP DIFFERENTIAL DIAGNOSES

- **Cochlear incomplete partition**
  - Cochlea size is normal to large; absent interscalar septum & modiolus
- **Cochlear incomplete partition**
  - Deficient modiolus, absent interscalar septum between plump apical & middle turns, large vestibular aqueduct
- **Branchiootorenal syndrome**
  - Hypoplastic offset middle & apical turns, ± funnel-shaped large vestibular aqueduct
- **CHARGE syndrome**
  - Small/absent semicircular canal (SCC), variable cochlear hypoplasia, ± funnel-shaped large vestibular aqueduct

CLINICAL ISSUES

- Congenital sensorineural hearing loss

DIAGNOSTIC CHECKLIST

- Consider CHARGE syndrome: Cochlear hypoplasia, cochlear nerve canal stenosis, small vestibule, & small/aplastic SCC
- Consider branchiootorenal syndrome: Tapered basal turn, hypoplastic, offset middle & apical turns

(Left) *Axial bone CT in a 2 1/2-year-old boy with bilateral profound congenital sensorineural hearing loss shows a small bud-like structure, consistent with cochlear hypoplasia ➔, that is isolated from the internal auditory canal (IAC). The round window is absent.* **(Right)** *Coronal CT reconstruction in the same patient shows the small bud-like hypoplastic cochlea ➔ with no internal architecture.*

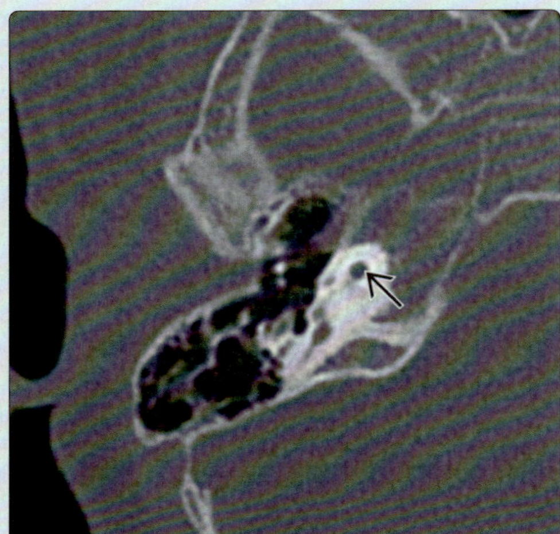

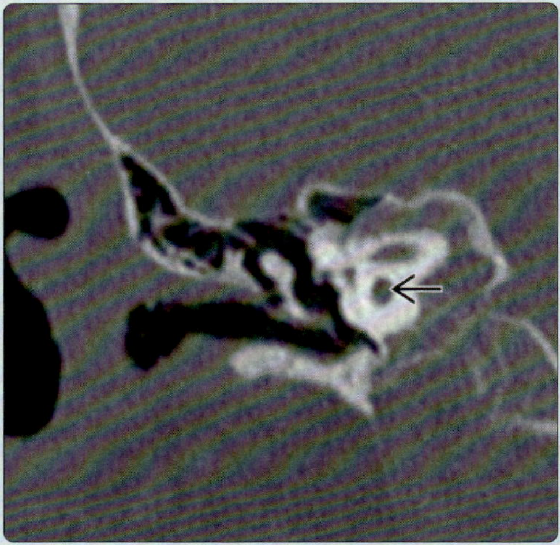

(Left) *3D T2 SPACE MR in an infant boy with bilateral profound sensorineural hearing loss shows a single, rounded cochlear turn ➔ without a modiolus.* **(Right)** *A more cephalad image in the same infant reveals the superior aspect of the single cochlear turn ➔. The IAC and inferior vestibular nerve ➔ appear normal. The cochlear nerve is not identified, and the cochlear nerve canal is absent ➔.*

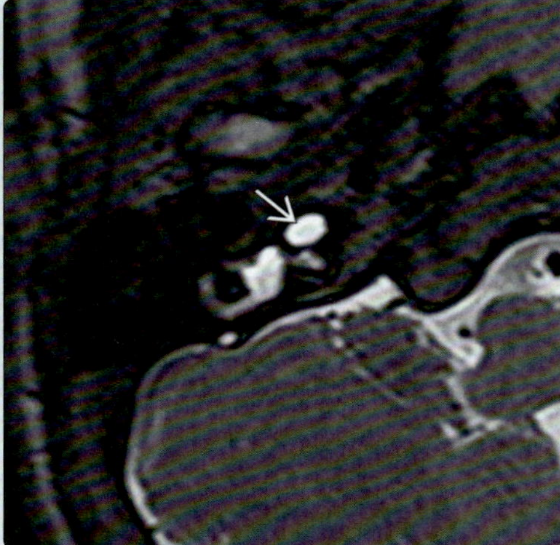

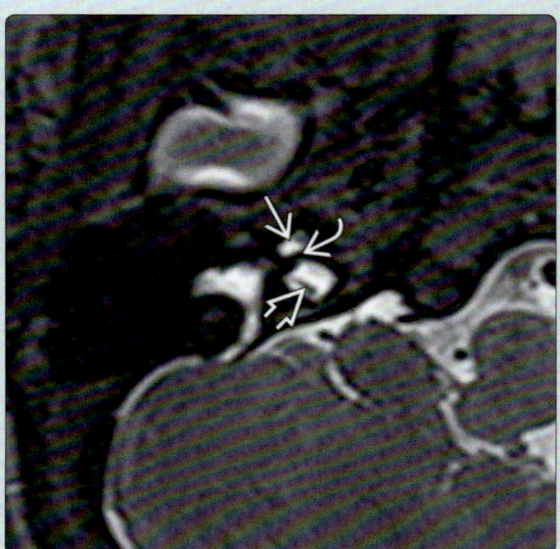

KEY FACTS

TERMINOLOGY

- Stenosis or atresia of cochlear nerve canal (CNC)
- Cochlear nerve deficiency (CND): Cochlear nerve (CN) hypoplasia/aplasia

IMAGING

- CNC extends from internal auditory canal (IAC) fundus to modiolus
  - Diameter measured at narrowest point
  - **CNC stenosis**: **< 1.7 mm**
- Cochlea (spectrum of findings)
  - Normal
  - Normal modiolus + mildly stenotic CNC
  - Thickened modiolus + stenotic/atretic CNC
  - Cochlear anomaly + stenotic/atretic CNC
- IAC: Normal, small, absent or "duplicated" (separate CNVII canal)
- CND: **CN smaller** than normal CNVII (hypoplasia) **or absent** (aplasia)

TOP DIFFERENTIAL DIAGNOSES

- CHARGE syndrome
- Cochlear aplasia or hypoplasia

PATHOLOGY

- Unclear whether CN fails to form or forms initially then degenerates

CLINICAL ISSUES

- Presents with congenital sensorineural hearing loss
- ~ 70% incidence of CN aplasia in pediatric unilateral neural sensorineural hearing loss
- CND used to be contraindication to cochlear implantation; however, patients can benefit; outcomes less predictable

DIAGNOSTIC CHECKLIST

- Most cases of CND have normal cochlea ± modiolar thickening ± CNC stenosis or atresia
- Assess CNs on axial & **oblique sagittal** 3D T2 SPACE/FIESTA MR sequences: **4 nerves** should be present in IAC

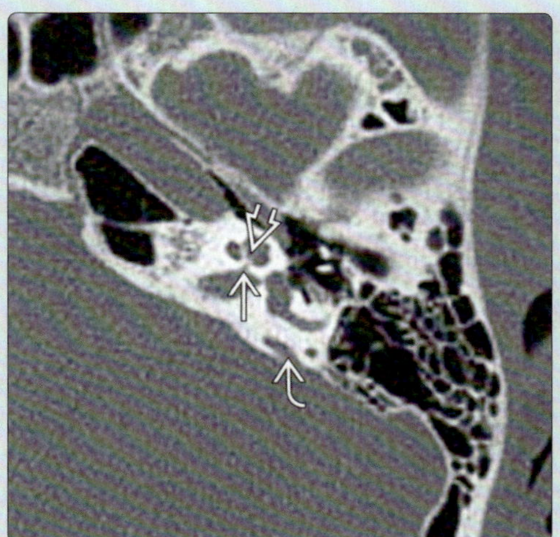

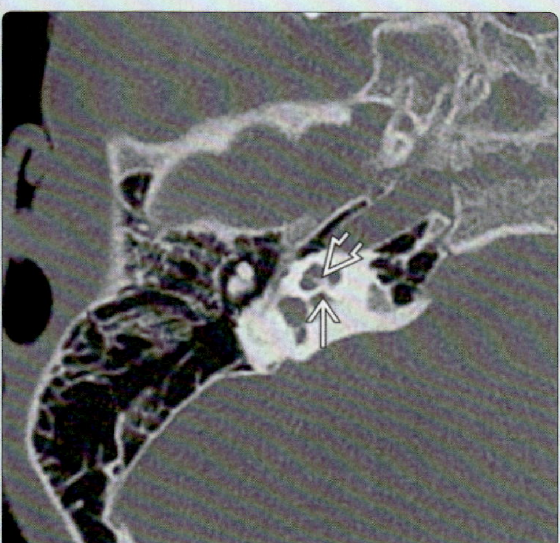

(Left) *Axial bone CT in an 11-year-old girl with profound bilateral sensorineural hearing loss (SNHL) is shown. There is severe stenosis of the cochlear nerve canal (CNC) ➔. The modiolus ➔ and scalar chambers appear asymmetric. This patient also has a mildly enlarged vestibular aqueduct ➔.* **(Right)** *Axial bone CT in a 4-year-old girl with profound right SNHL is shown. There is absence of the CNC ➔ and marked thickening of the modiolus ➔.*

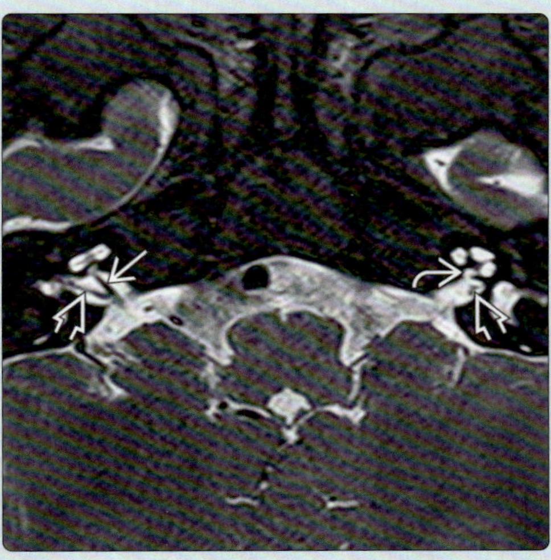

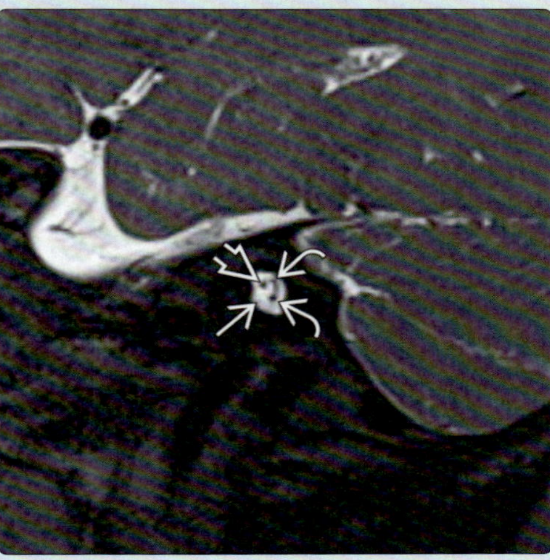

(Left) *Axial T2 SPACE MR shows a 1-year-old boy with profound left SNHL. A normal right CN ➔ and normal vestibular nerves ➔ are seen. The left CN is absent, and the left CNC is mildly stenotic ➔.* **(Right)** *Sagittal oblique T2 SPACE MR shows a 1-year-old boy with profound left SNHL. Absence of the left CN ➔ and a normal facial nerve ➔ and vestibular nerves ➔ are visible.*

KEY FACTS

TERMINOLOGY

- Definition: Hypoplasia/aplasia of 1 or multiple semicircular canals (SCCs) ± hypoplastic vestibule

IMAGING

- Hypoplastic vestibule + hypoplasia/aplasia of horizontal or all SCCs in **CHARGE syndrome**
  - Oval window stenosis/atresia & anomalous CNVII
  - Cochlea: Variable malformation; thickened modiolus, flattened apical ± middle turns or single turn/hypoplasia
  - Cochlear nerve canal: Stenosis/atresia
  - Vestibular aqueduct: Dilated, funnel-shaped
- Hypoplasia of single SCC + normal (or large) vestibule
  - Posterior SCC (PSCC) + normal or flattened cochlear apical turn: Waardenburg & Alagille syndromes
  - PSCC + hypoplastic, offset middle & apical cochlear turns: Branchiootorenal (BOR) syndrome
  - Horizontal SCC (HSCC): Oval window stenosis/atresia & anomalous ± dehiscent tympanic segment CNVII

TOP DIFFERENTIAL DIAGNOSES

- **Down syndrome**
  - Small or absent HSCC bone island; globular SCC-vestibule (anlage) anomaly
  - Cochlear nerve canal stenosis, internal auditory canal stenosis, left vertebral artery, variably present
- **Labyrinthine ossificans**: Prior meningitis or surgery

DIAGNOSTIC CHECKLIST

- **CHARGE** is diagnosed if **vestibular hypoplasia & horizontal SCC or multiple SCCs**
- Axial & coronal temporal bone to assess oval window & CNVII tympanic segment
- Consider **BOR** for hypoplastic, offset middle & apical turns cochlea; look for PSCC anomaly
- Consider Waardenburg syndrome for PSCC anomaly & Hirschsprung disease
- Consider Alagille syndrome for PSCC anomaly, pulmonary stenosis, & cholestatic liver disease

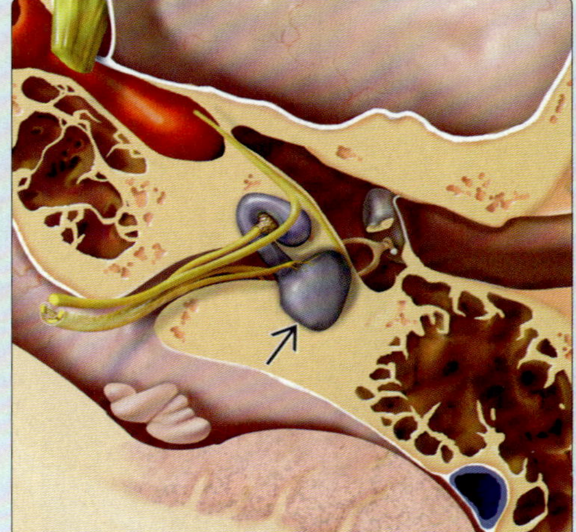

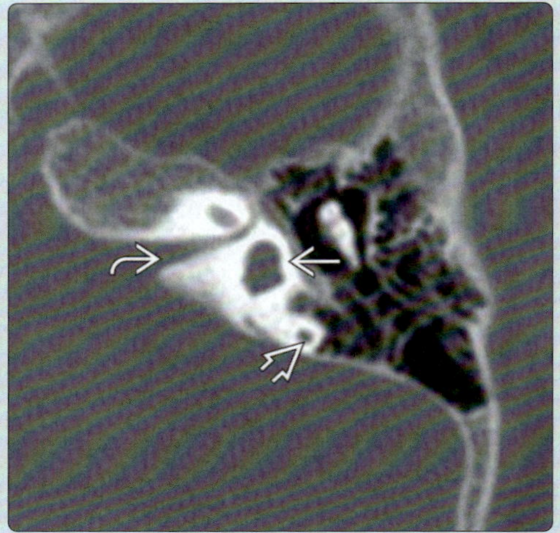

(Left) *Axial graphic depicts severe, syndromic type of semicircular canal (SCC) anomaly with complete absence of all SCCs, cochlear malformation, and dysmorphic small vestibule ⇨.* **(Right)** *Axial bone CT in a 12-month-old boy with profound sensorineural hearing loss shows complete absence of the horizontal SCC ➡ at the level of the vestibule. A normal posterior SCC is seen ➡. The internal auditory canal is narrow ➡.*

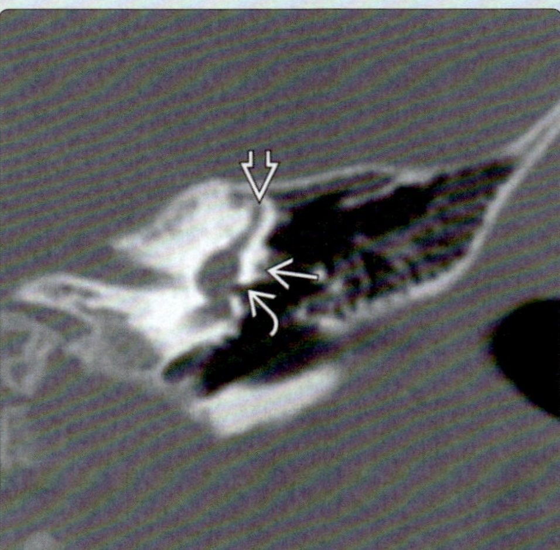

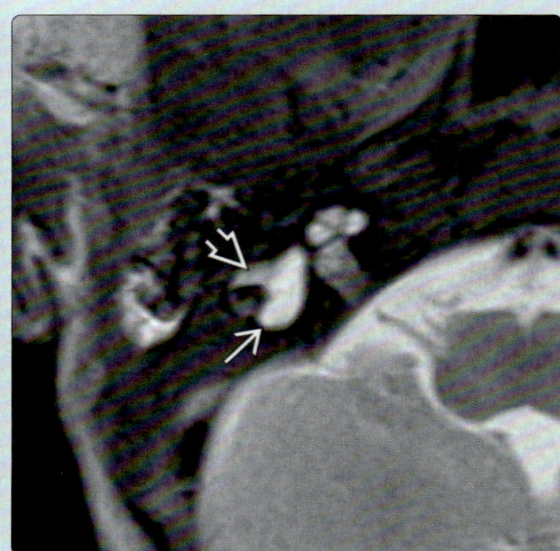

(Left) *Coronal bone CT demonstrates the facial nerve canal ➡, absence of the horizontal SCC, and a normal superior SCC ➡. There is mild stenosis of the oval window ➡.* **(Right)** *Axial T2WI MR in a 1-day-old girl with Waardenburg syndrome shows a rudimentary posterior SCC bud along the posterior aspect of the vestibule ➡. A normal horizontal SCC is seen ➡.*

KEY FACTS

TERMINOLOGY

- Dilatation of semicircular canal (SCC) & globular vestibule
- Bone island between vestibule & affected SCC is small or absent (persistent SCC anlage anomaly)

IMAGING

- Most frequently seen SCC & vestibular anomaly
- Usually affects lateral SCC (LSCC): Last to develop
- Isolated finding or with other temporal bone anomalies
- SCC: Widened lumen of 1 limb or entire SCC; small or absent bone island
- Vestibule: Normal or large, less commonly small
- Cochlea: Normal or malformed

TOP DIFFERENTIAL DIAGNOSES

- **Large vestibular aqueduct (LVA)**
  - LVA, ± IP-II anomaly, ± globular vestibule/LSCC
- **Apert syndrome**
  - Craniosynostosis, polysyndactyly, LSCC anlage anomaly
- **Trisomy 21**
  - Vestibule normal or small; small LSCC bone island or persistent SCC anlage anomaly
- **22q11.2 deletion syndrome**
  - Vestibule normal, large or small; small LSCC bone island or persistent SCC anlage anomaly

CLINICAL ISSUES

- Mild form may be asymptomatic
- Vestibular symptoms: Normal or imbalance, vertigo
- Caloric testing: Absent or decreased caloric responses
- Hearing: Normal, sensorineural, mixed, or conductive hearing loss (ossicular or inner ear origin)

DIAGNOSTIC CHECKLIST

- LSCC + external & middle ear malformation
  - Syndromic or chromosomal/genetic anomaly
  - Craniofacial anomaly (most)
  - Toxic exposure

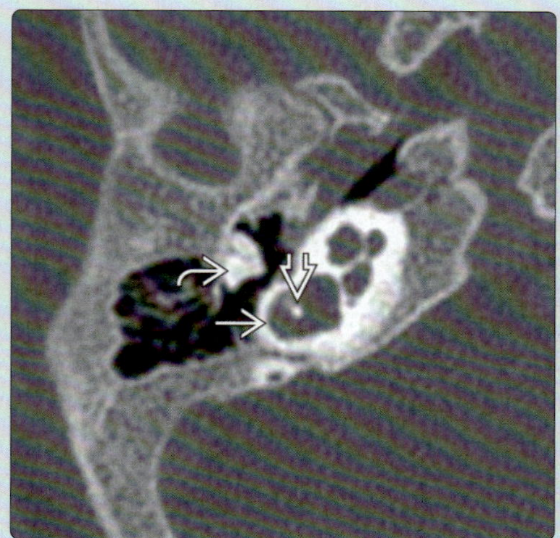

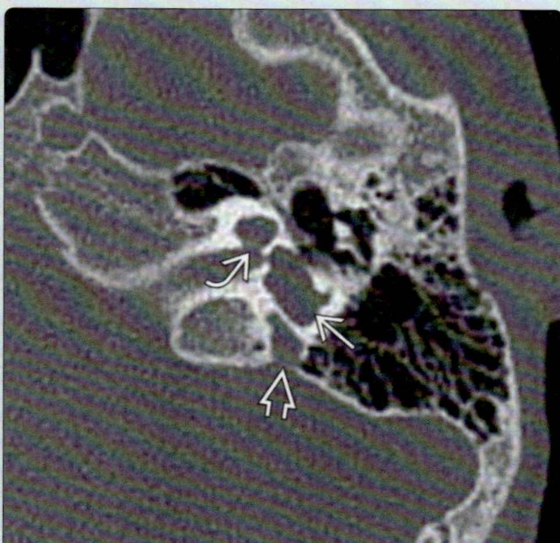

(Left) *Axial bone CT in a 9-month-old boy with oculoauriculovertebral spectrum shows dilated lateral semicircular canal (LSCC) ➡ & a small bone island ➡ between the LSCC & globular vestibule. Malformed ossicles are fixed to the lateral wall of the attic ➡.* **(Right)** *Axial bone CT in 7-year-old girl with severe SNHL & in utero exposure to maternal drugs shows dilatation of posterior SCC ➡ & vestibule & funnel-shaped, large, vestibular aqueduct ➡. Cochlear modiolus ➡ & cochlear septation are deficient.*

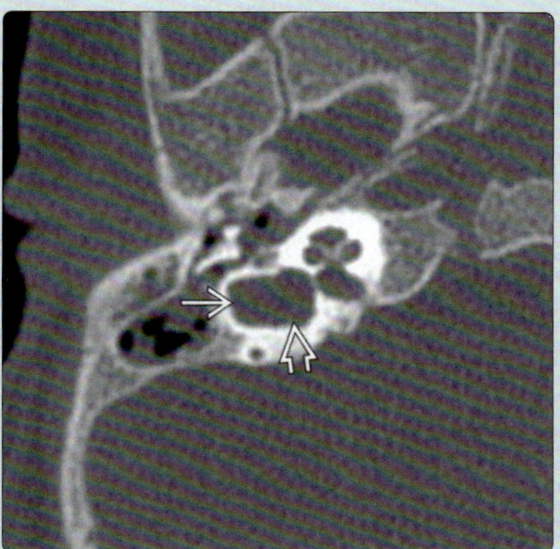

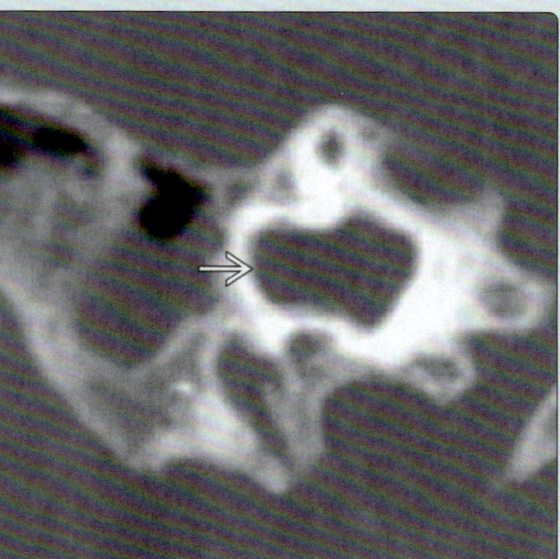

(Left) *Axial bone CT in a 10-month-old girl with profound SNHL demonstrates a large, globular LSCC ➡ that communicates with a dilated vestibule ➡, forming a single cavity.* **(Right)** *Coronal CT reconstruction reveals massive dilatation of the LSCC ➡ in this patient with persistent anlage anomaly. Oval window atresia was also noted on a more anterior image (not shown).*

Labyrinthitis

KEY FACTS

TERMINOLOGY

- Definition: Subacute inflammatory or infectious disease of fluid-filled spaces of inner ear

IMAGING

- **MR findings**
  - T1 C+ FS: Faint to moderate **enhancement within inner ear fluid**
  - T2: Normal high fluid signal preserved
  - T1: Normal to mildly increased signal; if hemorrhage, increased inner ear signal
- **T-bone CT findings**
  - Normal in acute/subacute labyrinthitis
  - **Labyrinthine ossificans** possible if suppurative labyrinthitis
    - Subacute to chronic imaging finding

TOP DIFFERENTIAL DIAGNOSES

- Labyrinthine ossificans; intralabyrinthine schwannoma
- Intralabyrinthine hemorrhage

PATHOLOGY

- Labyrinthitis classification
  - Viral labyrinthitis: Unilateral most commonly
  - Bacterial labyrinthitis: Meningogenic (bilateral) > > tympanogenic (unilateral)
  - Posttraumatic/postsurgical: Unilateral
  - Autoimmune: Related to systemic disease (bilateral)

CLINICAL ISSUES

- Viral vs. vascular: Sudden onset unilateral sensorineural hearing loss (SNHL) + vertigo
  - Treatment: High-dose steroids, oral &/or intratympanic
- Bacterial: Child with bacterial meningitis → bilateral, progressive SNHL; labyrinthitis ossificans (LO) may develop
  - Evaluate for LO with serial imaging
  - If severe profound SNHL develops, cochlear implantation as soon as medically feasible

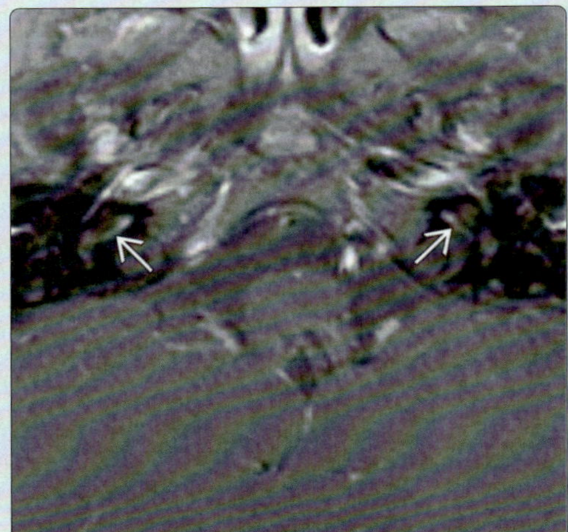

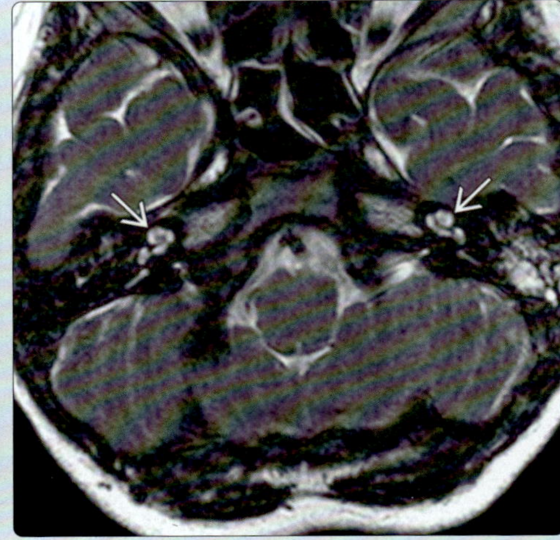

(Left) *Axial T1WI C+ FS MR in a 1-year-old boy with a prior history of meningitis and sensorineural hearing loss demonstrates abnormal bilateral enhancement of the basal turn of the cochlea ➡ consistent with meningogenic labyrinthitis.* **(Right)** *Axial T2WI FSE MR in a patient with bilateral labyrinthitis shows normal, hyperintense fluid within the cochlea bilaterally ➡. Normal to slightly decreased fluid signal helps distinguish labyrinthitis from labyrinthine mass(es).*

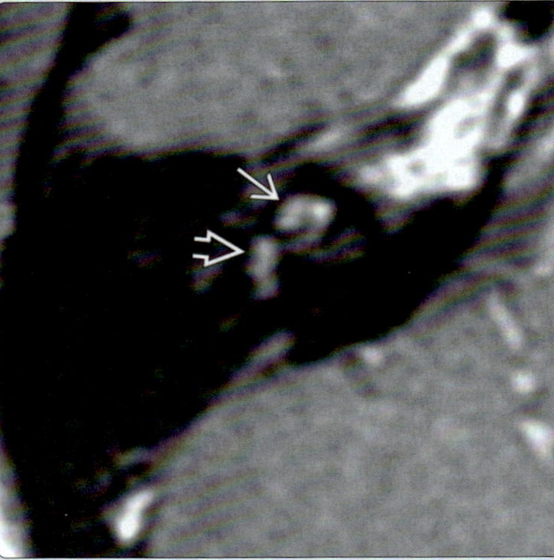

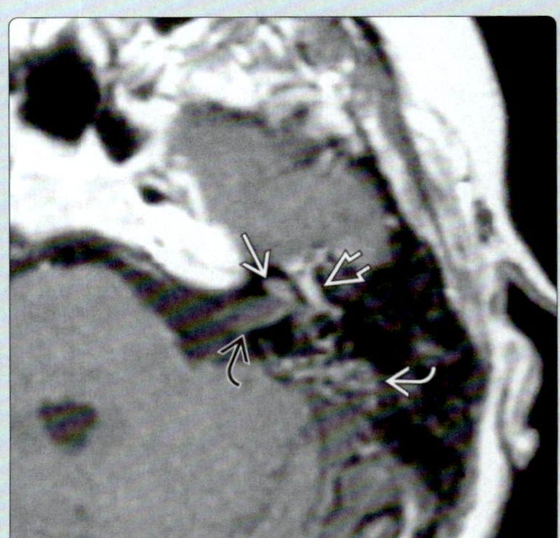

(Left) *Axial T1WI C+ MR in a case of labyrinthitis shows pathologic enhancement of the cochlear turns ➡ and vestibule ➡ in a patient with an acute onset of vertigo and hearing loss.* **(Right)** *Axial T1WI C+ MR reveals enhancement of the cochlea ➡ & internal auditory canal ⇨ in a patient with bacterial otomastoiditis ➡ presenting with otalgia, CNVII palsy, and hearing loss. Tympanic CNVII is also thickened & enhancing ➡ in this example of tympanogenic labyrinthitis. (Courtesy C. Schatz, MD.)*

KEY FACTS

TERMINOLOGY

- Definition: Sexually transmitted disease caused by bacterium spirochete *Treponema pallidum* affecting inner ear

IMAGING

- Temporal bone CT
  - **Moth-eaten permeative demineralization** of temporal bone (syphilitic osteitis)
  - Inner ear, middle ear mastoid, ossicles may all be involved
- T1 C+ MR findings
  - **Enhancement** of **CNVII & CNVIII** in IAC
    - **Membranous labyrinth** may also enhance (syphilitic labyrinthitis-meningitis)

TOP DIFFERENTIAL DIAGNOSES

- Cochlear otosclerosis
- Temporal bone osteogenesis imperfecta
- Temporal bone Paget disease
- Temporal bone fibrous dysplasia
- Postirradiated temporal bone

PATHOLOGY

- **Osteitis**: Inflammatory resorptive osteitis
- **Labyrinthitis**: Obliterative endarteritis

CLINICAL ISSUES

- Diagnosis: Otologic symptoms + positive serology
- Hearing loss (80%) & vertigo; uni- or bilateral facial nerve paralysis
  - Often acute & fluctuating
  - Simulates Ménière disease
- Treatment: Antibiotics (penicillin) & corticosteroids

DIAGNOSTIC CHECKLIST

- Consider: If HIV patient with hearing loss & permeative inner demineralization, test for positive syphilis serology before diagnosing otosyphilis

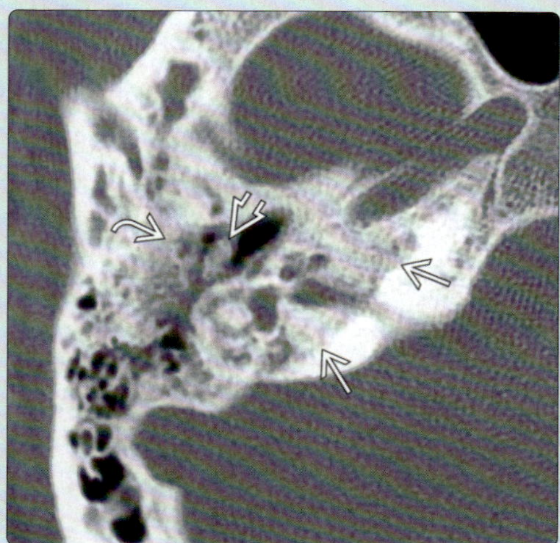

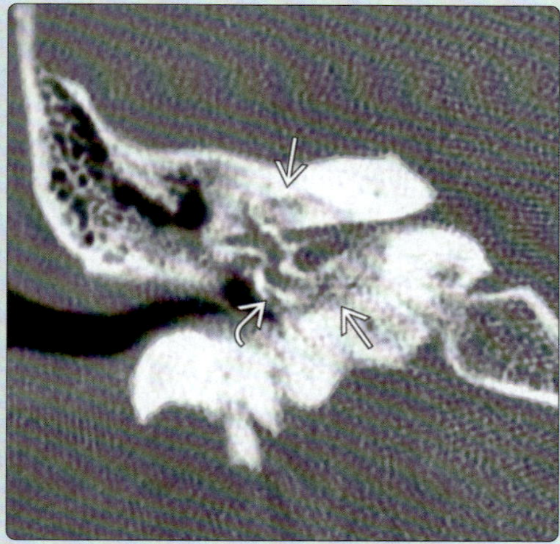

(Left) *Axial temporal bone CT shows typical findings of advanced middle and inner ear otosyphilis. There are extensive moth-eaten permeative bony changes of the inner ear ➡, middle ear mastoid ➡, and ossicles ➡. (Courtesy M. Sandlin, MD.)* **(Right)** *Coronal temporal bone CT in the same patient demonstrates permeative demineralization of the otic capsule ➡ with otosclerosis-like plaque on cochlear promontory ➡. These findings are secondary to inflammatory resorptive osteitis.*

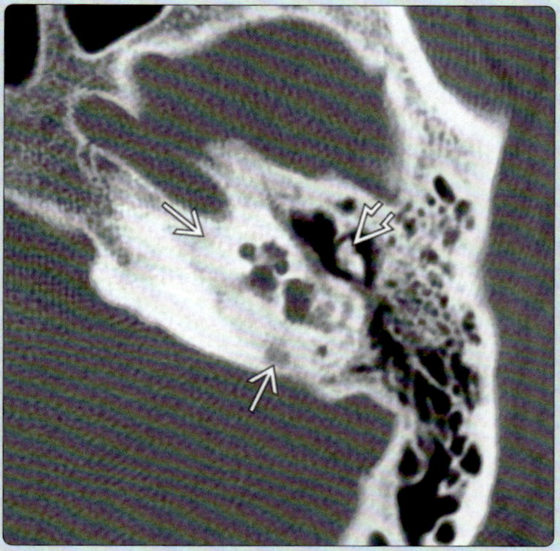

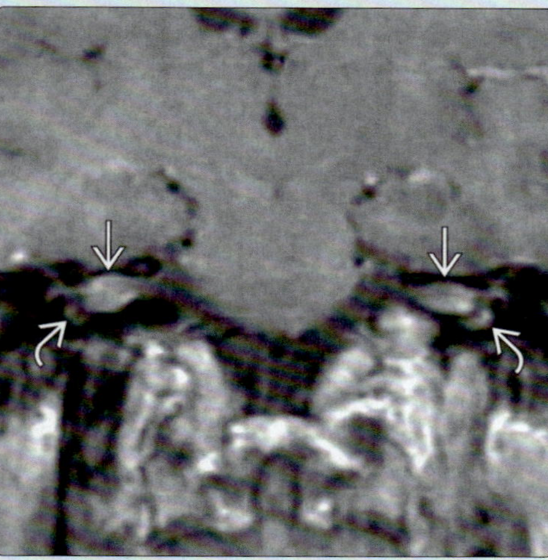

(Left) *Axial temporal bone CT shows similar but less severe changes of otosyphilis of the otic capsule ➡ and ossicles ➡ with the remainder of the middle ear osseous structures and mastoid being normal. CT findings of the radiated temporal bone may mimic this appearance. (Courtesy M. Sandlin, MD.)* **(Right)** *Coronal T1 C+ MR reveals pathologic leptomeningeal enhancement in the internal auditory canals ➡ and membranous labyrinths ➡. This is the labyrinthitis-meningitis form of otosyphilis.*

KEY FACTS

TERMINOLOGY

- **Membranous labyrinth ossification**: Healing response to inner ear infection, inflammation, trauma, or surgery

IMAGING

- Varies with severity
  - Mild: "Enlarged" modiolus; subtle inner ear new bone
  - Severe: All inner ear fluid replaced by bone
- Temporal bone CT: **High-density** bone deposition within membranous labyrinth
- T2 MR: **Low-intensity** foci within high-signal fluid of membranous labyrinth; loss of fluid signal

TOP DIFFERENTIAL DIAGNOSES

- Labyrinthine aplasia
- Cochlear aplasia
- Intravestibular lipoma
- Cochlear otosclerosis
- Labyrinthine schwannoma

PATHOLOGY

- **Fibrous stage**: Fibroblast proliferation
- **Ossific stage**: Osteoblasts forming abnormal bony trabeculae within membranous labyrinthine spaces

CLINICAL ISSUES

- Most common: Bilateral sensorineural hearing loss (SNHL) in child weeks to months after acute meningitis episode
  - When hearing loss is sequelae from meningitis, imaging is critical to evaluate for labyrinthine ossificans (LO)
- Less common: Unilateral SNHL with previous surgery, trauma, mastoid/middle ear infection
- Cochlear implantation for severe-profound SNHL with LO
  - Early implantation during fibrous stage is preferable
- Bilateral cochlear LO is serious detriment to cochlear implantation
  - May require split-electrode array or cochlear drill out
- Precochlear implant evaluation of temporal bone in children: Look for LO and inner ear congenital anomalies

(Left) *Axial bone CT in a 2-year-old boy with bilateral sensorineural hearing loss 7 months after an episode of bacterial meningitis shows subtle ossification at the midportion of the basal turn of the left cochlea ➔ with sparing of the middle and apical turns.* **(Right)** *Axial bone CT in the same patient demonstrates subtotal ossification of the anterior and midportion of the lateral semicircular canal ➔. The posterior and superior semicircular canals were also involved (not shown).*

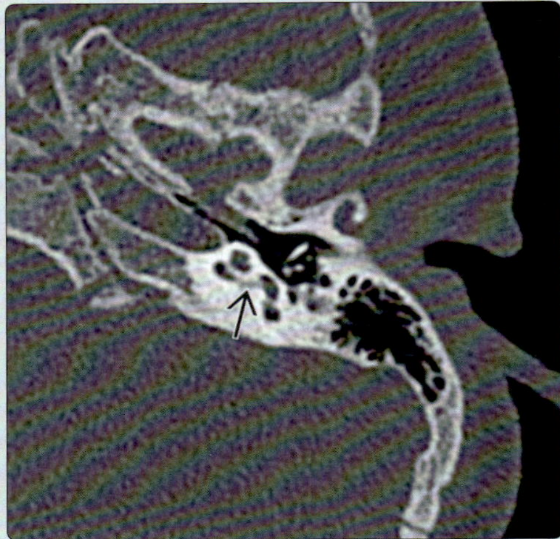

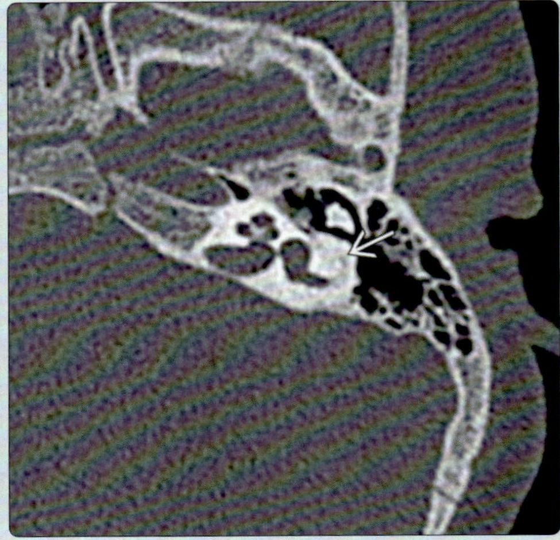

(Left) *Axial thin section T2WI MR in a 2 year old with bacterial meningitis 3 weeks prior shows diffuse, bilateral decrease in normal hyperintense inner ear fluid involving the cochlea ➔, vestibule ➔, and visualized portions of semicircular canals ➔. These findings are consistent with early fibroosseous replacement of normal inner ear fluid.* **(Right)** *Axial T1WI C+ FS MR in the same patient shows bilateral abnormal inner ear enhancement in the cochlea ➔, vestibule ➔, and lateral semicircular canal ➔.*

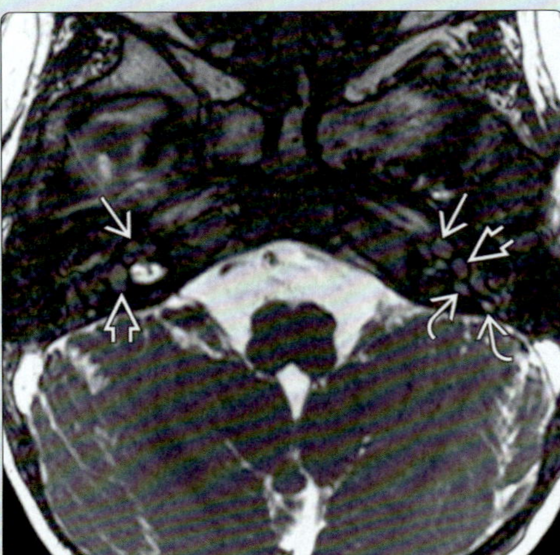

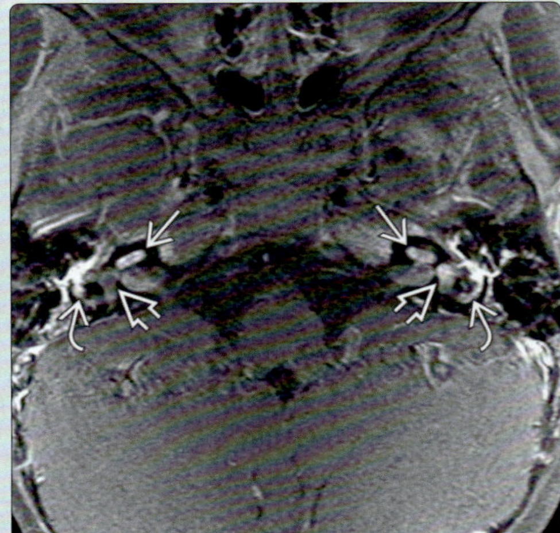

KEY FACTS

TERMINOLOGY

- Synonym: **Otospongiosis**
- Fenestral otosclerosis (FOto), cochlear otosclerosis (COto)
- Pathologic appearance of lytic spongy bone foci in bony labyrinth of unknown cause
  - Starts perifenestral (FOto), progresses to surround cochlea (FOto + COto)
- **Fissula ante fenestram**: Cleft of fibrocartilaginous tissue between inner & middle ears just anterior to oval window

IMAGING

- Best diagnostic clue: Temporal bone CT shows **lytic (otospongiotic) foci** involving bony labyrinth
- FOto: Starts at anterior margin of oval window (fissula ante fenestram)
- COto: Affects pericochlear bony labyrinth, "far advanced"
  - Halo sign with pericochlear lucency
- Postoperative imaging: Tip of stapes prosthesis should pass through oval window, slightly engage vestibule

TOP DIFFERENTIAL DIAGNOSES

- Chronic otitis media with tympanosclerosis
- Temporal bone Paget disease
- Temporal bone fibrous dysplasia
- Temporal bone osteoradionecrosis
- Temporal bone osteogenesis imperfecta

PATHOLOGY

- Enchondral layer of bony labyrinth displays spongy, vascular, decalcified, irregular bone formation

CLINICAL ISSUES

- Uni- or bilateral progressive conductive (FOto) or mixed (FOto + COto) hearing loss in young adult
- Treatment options
  - **Stapedectomy** with stapes prosthesis
  - **Cochlear implantation** with severe-profound sensorineural hearing loss in COto
  - **Fluoride** treatment if COto present, controversial

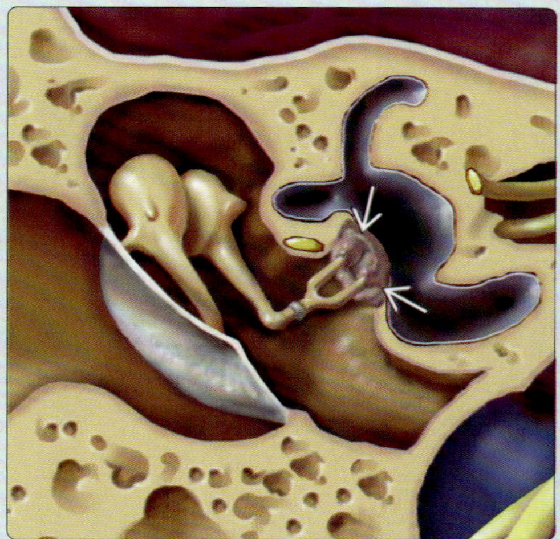

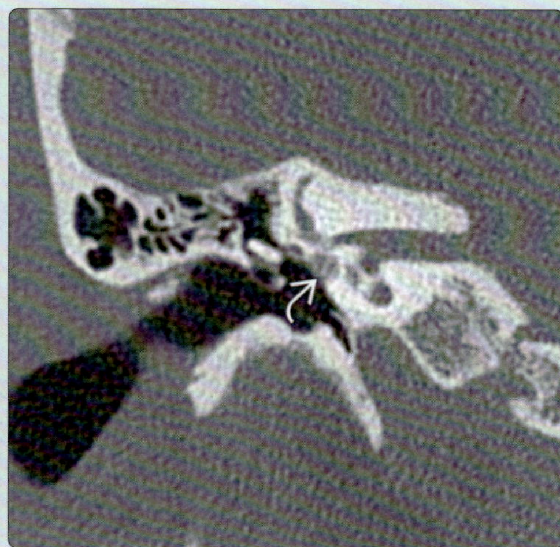

(Left) *Coronal graphic illustrates findings of fenestral otosclerosis with a "donut" otospongiotic plaque ➡ surrounding the stapes footplate in the oval window. The crisp margins of the oval window are obscured by plaque.* **(Right)** *Coronal right temporal bone CT shows a lytic focus anterior to the oval window ➡, the typical appearance and location of an otospongiotic plaque of fenestral otosclerosis.*

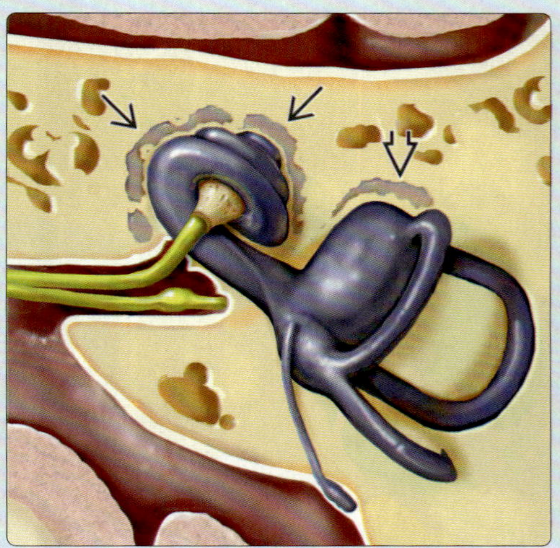

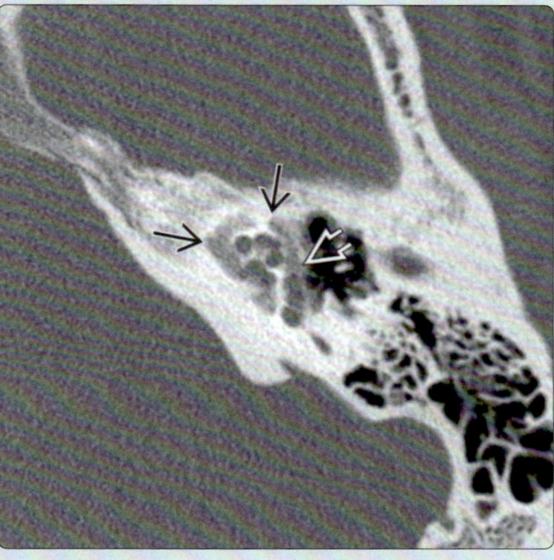

(Left) *Axial graphic demonstrates a classic example of cochlear otosclerosis. Note otospongiotic plaques in a halo around the cochlea ➡ with concurrent fenestral otosclerosis ➡.* **(Right)** *Axial left temporal bone CT shows cochlear otosclerosis as osteolytic foci surrounding the cochlea ➡. This is the halo sign. Concurrent fenestral otosclerosis is noted as bony lucency along cochlear promontory extending from fissula ante fenestram ➡.*

KEY FACTS

TERMINOLOGY

- Osteogenesis imperfecta (OI): Inherited connective disorder characterized by bone fragility and fractures

IMAGING

- Skull: ± undermineralized, **wormian bones**, fractures
- Bones: Fractures ± osteopenia, ± deformity
- Ossicles: Tendency to fracture, deformity, stapes fixation
- Inner ear: Normal or **progressive otic capsule demineralization** (OI type I)
  - Early: Band-like pericochlear lucency
  - Late: Lucent otic capsule bone (CT), enhances on MR
- ± jugular vein stenosis and large mastoid emissary veins

TOP DIFFERENTIAL DIAGNOSES

- **Otosclerosis**: Demineralized otic capsule, similar to OI
- **Nonaccidental injury**: Unexplained fractures
- **Paget disease**: Involves entire petrous bone, asymmetric
- **Cochlear cleft**: Faint pericochlear lucency < 4 years

PATHOLOGY

- Most OI is **autosomal dominant** (AD); *COL1A1* or *COL1A2* mutations (95%) → **defective collagen**
- **OI type I** (AD): **Mild ± later onset; fractures**, ± minimal deformity, **blue sclerae**, **hearing loss (HL)**
- **OI type II** [AD, autosomal recessive (AR)]: **Perinatal lethality**; osteopenia, severe deformity, multiple fractures
- **OI type III** (AD, AR): Progressive deformity, short stature, dentinogenesis imperfecta, ± blue sclerae
- **OI type IV** (AD): Mild/moderate deformity and fracture, mild blue sclerae, dentinogenesis imperfecta, HL

CLINICAL ISSUES

- Most common heritable connective tissue disorder
- **Multiple fractures from minimal trauma** ± osteopenia, deformity, short stature, blue sclerae
- HL in ~ 60%: Conductive, SNHL, or mixed ± vertigo
- Often presents with conductive HL due to stapes fixation; treat with stapes surgery or hearing aid

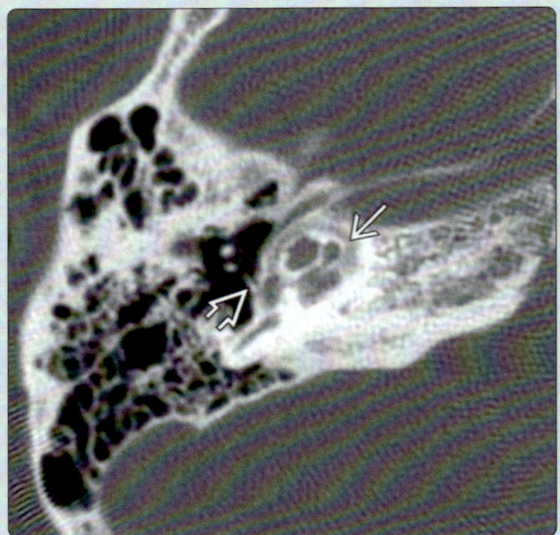

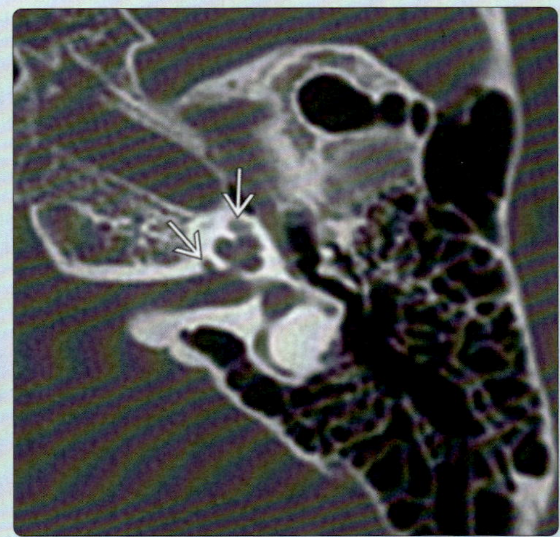

(Left) *Axial right T-bone CT shows extensive otic capsule bony demineralization ➡ of the inner ear in a patient with osteogenesis imperfecta (OI). The posterior crus of the stapes is also thickened ➡.* **(Right)** *Axial T-bone CT of a case of OI demonstrates focal otic capsule lucencies adjacent to the cochlea and internal auditory canal ➡. OI is indistinguishable from cochlear otosclerosis on T-bone CT. Regions of demineralization may be multifocal as in this case or band-like.*

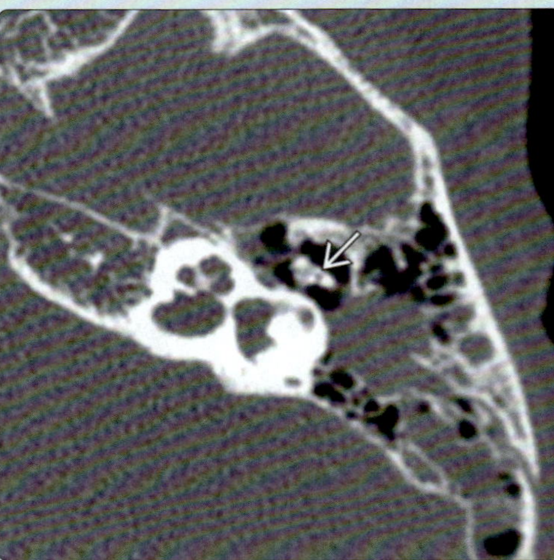

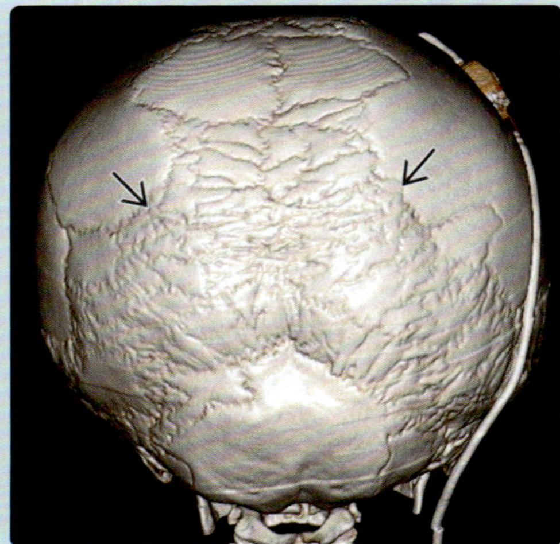

(Left) *Axial bone CT in a 13-year-old boy with OI who fell and hit his head on the ground shows a fracture of the short process of the incus ➡. In addition, there were tympanic plate and mastoid fractures.* **(Right)** *Posterior 3D skull reformation shows innumerable intrasutural, or wormian, bones ➡ in a child with OI. Basilar impression and craniocervical junction stenosis result in hydrocephalus in this patient, requiring shunting. Bony demineralization and multiple old fracture deformities can often also be seen in OI.*

KEY FACTS

TERMINOLOGY

- Intralabyrinthine schwannoma (ILS): Benign tumor arising from Schwann cells within membranous labyrinth

IMAGING

- These tumors can be subtle and easily overlooked
- T1 C+ MR: Focal enhancing mass in membranous labyrinth
- High-resolution T2 MR: Filling defect within perilymph
- Focal intralabyrinthine mass named by location
  - **Intracochlear**: Schwannoma within cochlea
  - **Intravestibular**: Within vestibule of inner ear
  - **Vestibulocochlear**: Involves both vestibule and cochlea
  - **Transmodiolar**: Crosses modiolus from cochlea to fundus of internal auditory canal (IAC)
  - **Transmacular**: Crosses from vestibule into fundus of IAC
  - **Transotic**: Involves inner ear, fundus of IAC to middle ear
- Use focused T1 C+ with high-resolution T2 imaging of cerebellopontine angle (CPA)-IAC to make diagnosis of ILS
  - T2 artifact can mimic tumor; compare with T1 C+

TOP DIFFERENTIAL DIAGNOSES

- Labyrinthitis
- Labyrinthine ossificans
- Intralabyrinthine hemorrhage
- Facial nerve schwannoma with inner ear dehiscence

CLINICAL ISSUES

- Tumor location-specific symptoms
  - When in vestibule: Tinnitus, episodic vertigo with nausea and vomiting, sensorineural hearing loss
  - When in cochlea: Slowly progressive sensorineural hearing loss, ± vestibular symptoms
- Conservative management vs. surgical resection
  - Conservative: Follow for 2-5 years to assess for growth
    - If no such growth, continue conservative mgmt
  - Removal if disabling symptoms (intractable vertigo)
    - Labyrinthectomy or IT gentamicin injections
  - Surgery or radiation if transmodiolar, transmacular or transotic, and documented growth into CPA-IAC

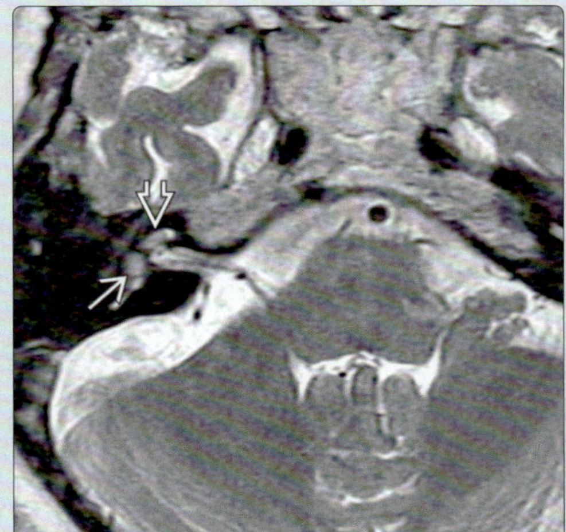

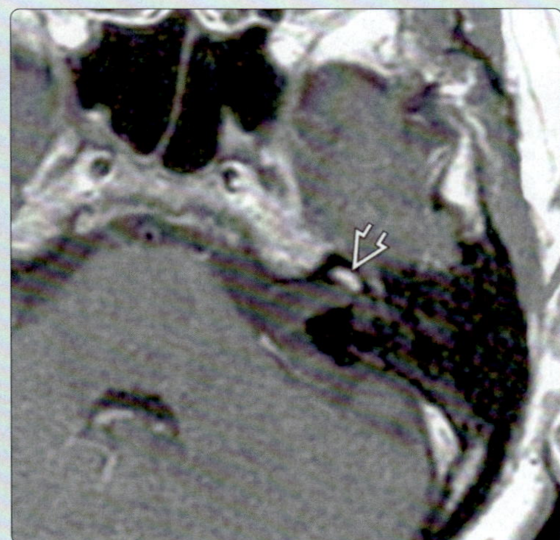

(Left) *Axial T2WI MR shows a classic example of an intralabyrinthine schwannoma (ILS). This is a vestibulocochlear type as it involves both the vestibule ➡ and cochlea ➡. Note soft tissue intensity replacing the normal perilymphatic tissue of the membranous labyrinth.* **(Right)** *Axial T1WI C+ MR shows an intracochlear schwannoma as focal enhancement of the cochlea ➡. It is important to review precontrast T1WI and T2WI to exclude intralabyrinthine hemorrhage and labyrinthitis, which may mimic this tumor.*

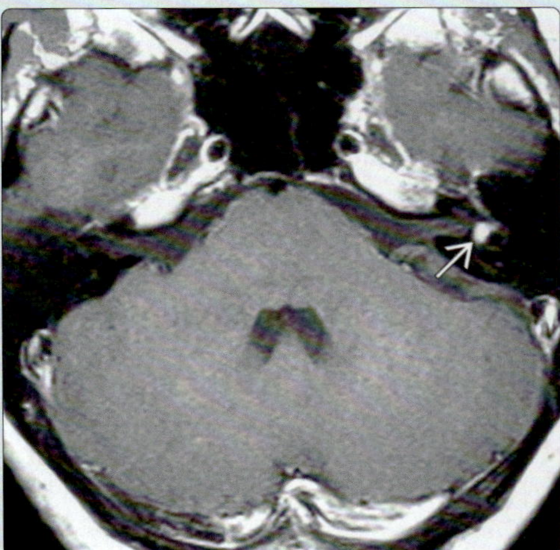

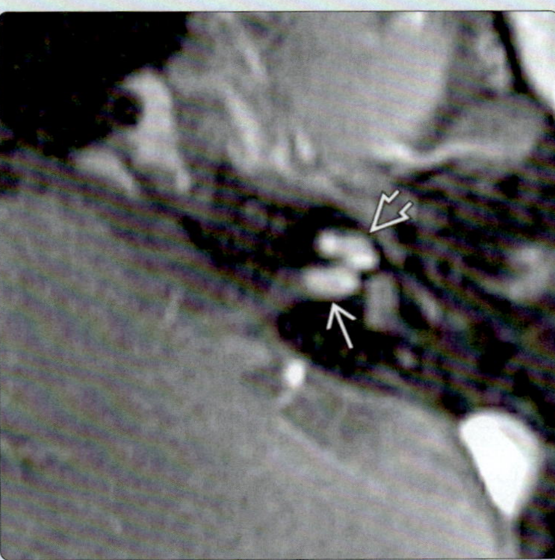

(Left) *Axial T1WI C+ MR shows intense enhancement of this intravestibular schwannoma ➡. When these tumors are small, they may be treated conservatively unless the patient has intractable vertigo or the tumor shows signs of interval transmacular growth into the internal auditory canal.* **(Right)** *Axial T1WI C+ MR shows enhancement of the distal internal auditory canal fundus ➡ and cochlea ➡ in this transmodiolar type of ILS. This tumor needs careful imaging follow-up and treatment if it continues to grow toward the brainstem.*

KEY FACTS

TERMINOLOGY

- Endolymphatic sac tumor (ELST)
- Papillary cystadenomatous tumor of ELS
  - Originates from epithelium of ELS

IMAGING

- CT findings
  - **Permeative-destructive** retrolabyrinthine mass
  - Central spiculated tumor **Ca^{++}** (100%)
  - Thin, **calcified rim** at posterior tumor margin
- MR findings
  - T1-hyperintense foci in 80%
  - Inhomogeneous T2 signal
  - Heterogeneous enhancement
  - Intralabyrinthine hemorrhage often seen with sudden hearing loss
- Angiographic findings
  - Tumors < 3 cm supplied by ECA branches
  - Tumors > 3 cm also recruit ICA branches

TOP DIFFERENTIAL DIAGNOSES

- Petrous apex cholesterol granuloma
- Glomus jugulare paraganglioma
- Petrous apex meningioma
- T-bone metastasis

PATHOLOGY

- Sporadic occurrence more common than von Hippel-Lindau disease (VHL)-associated ELST
  - **15% of VHL patients** develop **ELST**, 30% **bilateral**
- VHL
  - Cerebellar & spinal cord hemangioblastoma, renal cell carcinoma, pheochromocytoma
  - Kidney & pancreas cysts

CLINICAL ISSUES

- Sensorineural hearing loss is most common symptom
- Treatment: Complete surgical resection
- If sporadic ELST, check patient & family for VHL

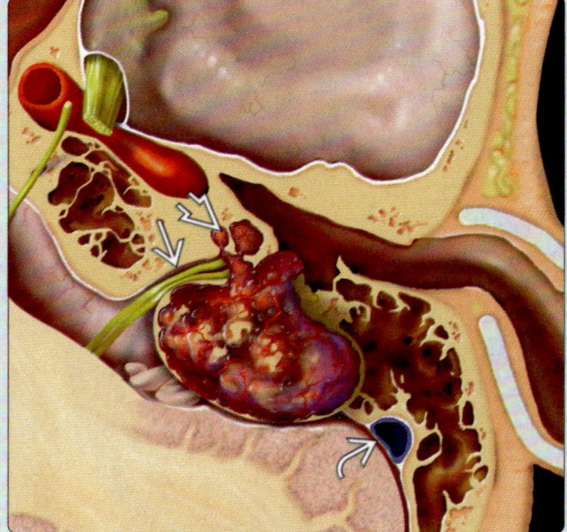

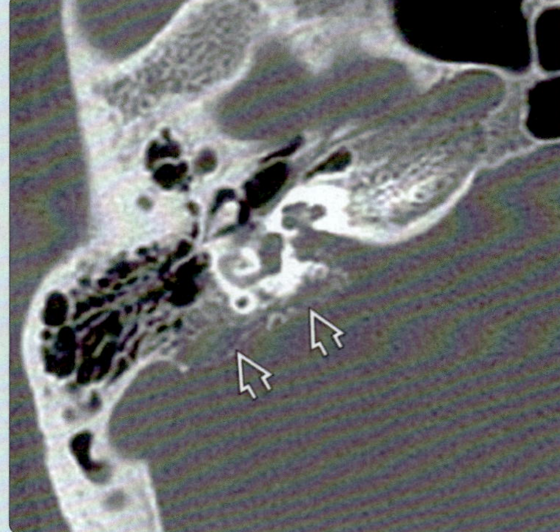

(Left) *Axial graphic of the T-bone illustrates the typical appearance of an endolymphatic sac tumor (ELST). Important features include its vascular nature, tendency to fistulize in inner ear ➡, & bone fragments within the tumor matrix. Note the classic retrolabyrinthine location between the IAC ➡ & sigmoid sinus ➡.* **(Right)** *Axial bone CT shows imaging features of ELST, including tumor centered in posterior T-bone in an area of fovea of the endolymphatic sac, spiculated tumor matrix Ca^{++} ➡, & permeative bone changes.*

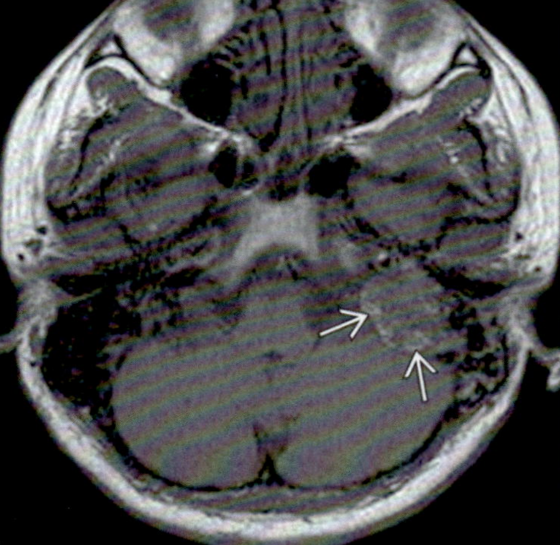

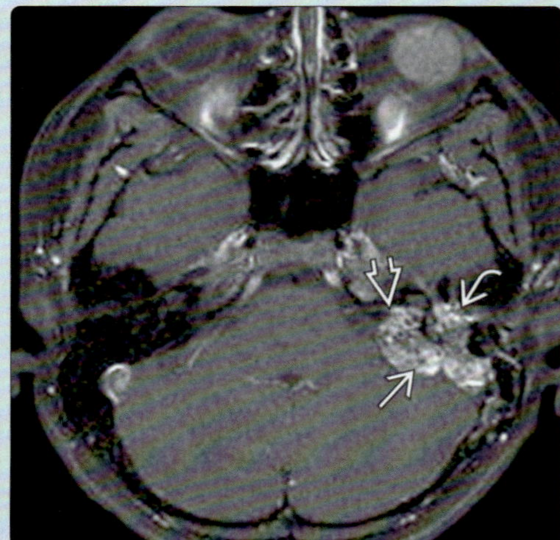

(Left) *Axial T1WI MR shows an expansile, lobular mass centered in the left T-bone with areas of ↑ T1 signal, which are common in ELST and are typically peripheral in location ➡.* **(Right)** *Axial T1WI C+ FS MR in the same patient reveals the typical intense, heterogeneous contrast enhancement ➡ expected in ELST. This tumor has also grown into the left IAC ➡, middle ear ➡, & mastoid. Note diffuse abnormal signal in the left globe indicating retinal angioma with detachment that is seen in von Hippel-Lindau disease.*

Intralabyrinthine Hemorrhage

KEY FACTS

TERMINOLOGY

- Blood within normally fluid-filled spaces of labyrinth

IMAGING

- T1 MR: **High signal** within normally fluid-filled space of labyrinth
- T2 MR: Variable depending on age of hemorrhage
- T1 C+: High signal, not to be confused with enhancement
- T1 FS: High inner ear signal remains on fat-saturated images
  - Not if intralabyrinthine lipoma present

TOP DIFFERENTIAL DIAGNOSES

- Labyrinthitis
- Vestibular schwannoma
- Intralabyrinthine schwannoma
- Congenital intralabyrinthine lipoma

PATHOLOGY

- Shortened T1 relaxation time caused by intra-/extracellular methemoglobin

CLINICAL ISSUES

- Presentation: Acute onset of unilateral sensorineural hearing loss
- History: Anticoagulant therapy, sickle cell disease, or trauma
- Prognosis: Variable return of hearing
- Treatment: Aimed at underlying condition

DIAGNOSTIC CHECKLIST

- Always evaluate unenhanced T1 MR and evaluate for evidence of intralabyrinthine high signal
- Differentiate from intralabyrinthine lipoma with fat-saturated images

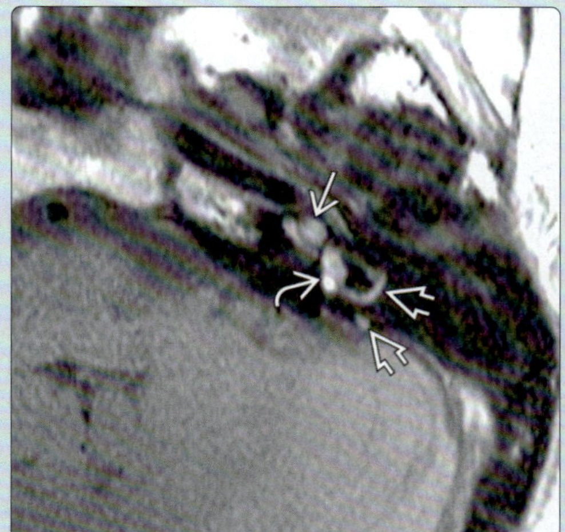
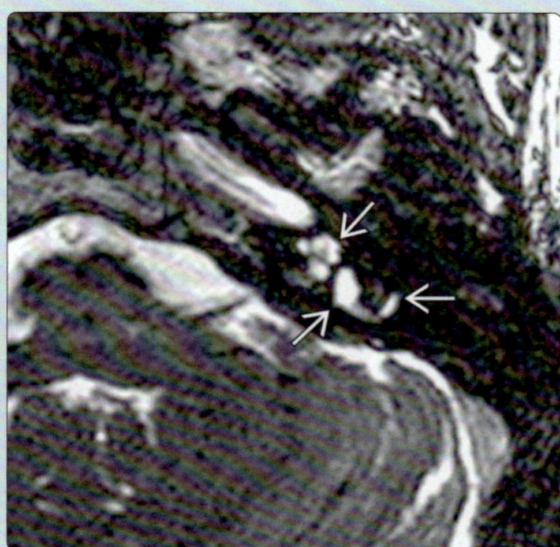

(Left) *Axial T1 MR without contrast shows the classic findings of intralabyrinthine hemorrhage (ILH) with hyperintense blood (methemoglobin) within the membranous labyrinth of the cochlea ➡, vestibule ➡, and semicircular canals ➡.* **(Right)** *Axial T2 MR in the same patient reveals corresponding high T2 signal within the inner ear ➡. T2 signal is variable in ILH, depending on the age of the blood. When T2 signal is decreased, the diffuse involvement of the labyrinth can distinguish ILH from intralabyrinthine masses.*

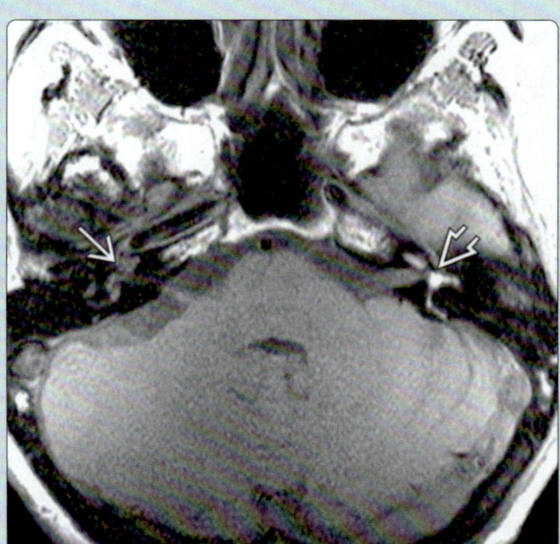
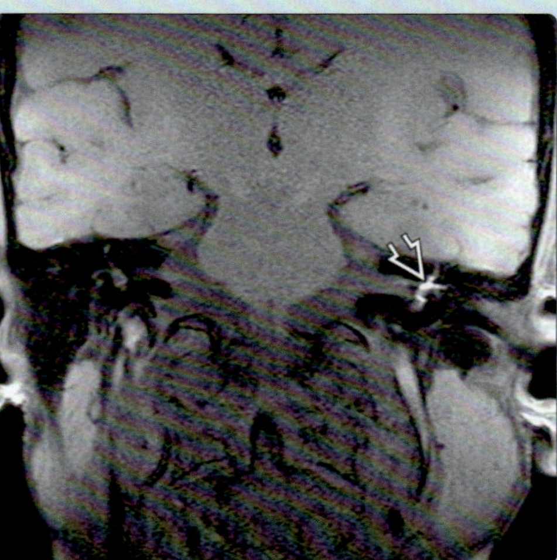

(Left) *Axial T1 MR without contrast at the level of the internal auditory canals shows hyperintense signal in the left inner ear membranous labyrinth ➡, representing ILH. Compare to normal fluid signal on the right ➡.* **(Right)** *Coronal T1 FS MR in the same patient demonstrates that the high signal in the left inner ear ➡ is not fat, as it persists despite fat-saturation sequence. Findings exclude the possibility of intralabyrinthine lipoma and confirm the diagnosis of ILH.*

KEY FACTS

TERMINOLOGY

- Definition: Extreme thinning or absence of otic capsule and bony roof over superior semicircular canal (SSCC)

IMAGING

- Thinning of **tegmen tympani and mastoideum** often associated; evaluate for bilateral semicircular canal dehiscence (SCCD)
- Transverse oblique T-bone CT reformats
  - In-plane view of SSCC dehiscent roof
- Axial T-bone CT
  - In rare **posterior** SCCD, provides in-plane view of SCCD

PATHOLOGY

- Unknown; developmentally thinned ± acquired component
  - Evaluate for structural cause of dehiscence
    - Venous anomaly (superior petrosal sinus) or arachnoid granulation
- Bony opening overlying SSCC creates **3rd mobile window** into inner ear
- 3rd window allows SSCC to respond to sound & pressure changes in membranous labyrinth

CLINICAL ISSUES

- Presenting signs and symptoms: "Great otologic mimicker" capable of causing most otologic symptoms
  - Sound ± pressure-induced vestibular symptoms ± eye movements
  - Chronic disequilibrium may be debilitating
  - Oscillopsia (oscillating vision)
  - Autophony, also hearing body noises (eye and neck movements, footsteps)
- **Tullio phenomenon**
  - Vertigo ± nystagmus related to sound
- **Treatment issues**
  - Middle fossa vs. transmastoid approaches both viable
  - Treat by plugging vs. resurfacing

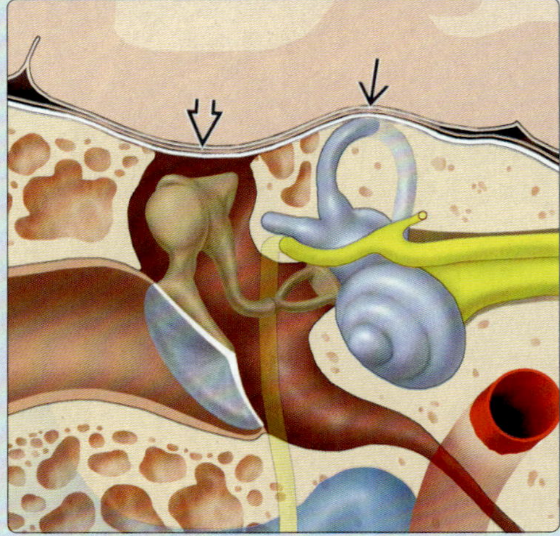

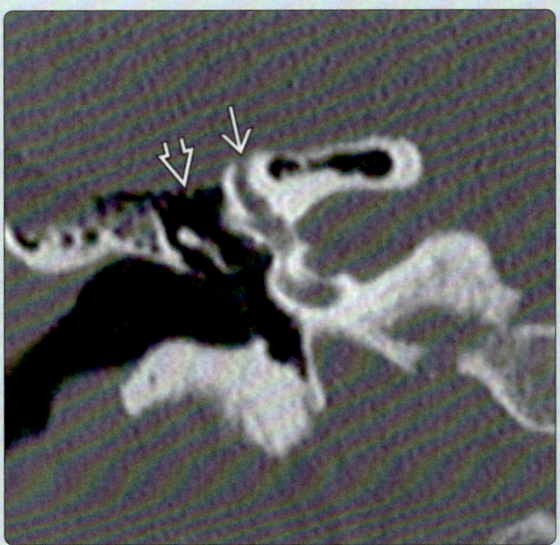

(Left) *Coronal graphic illustrates the principal findings of superior semicircular canal dehiscence, including absence of bone overlying the superior semicircular canal ⇨ and associated thinning of the tegmen tympani ⇨.* **(Right)** *Coronal T-bone CT shows no bone covering the roof of the superior semicircular canal ➡, representing superior semicircular canal dehiscence. Note thinning of the tegmen tympani and mastoideum ➡, a common associated finding on T-bone CT.*

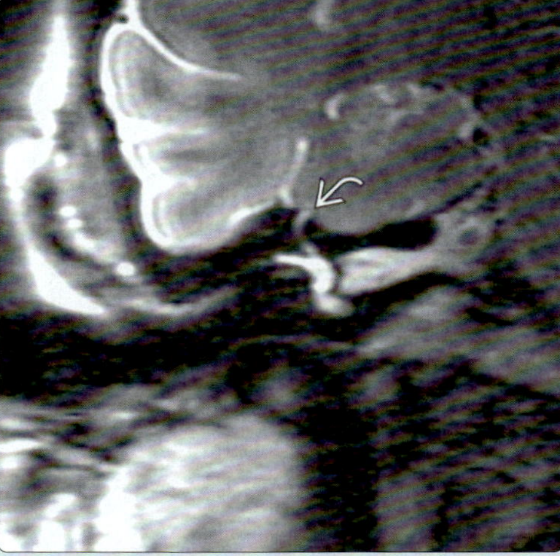

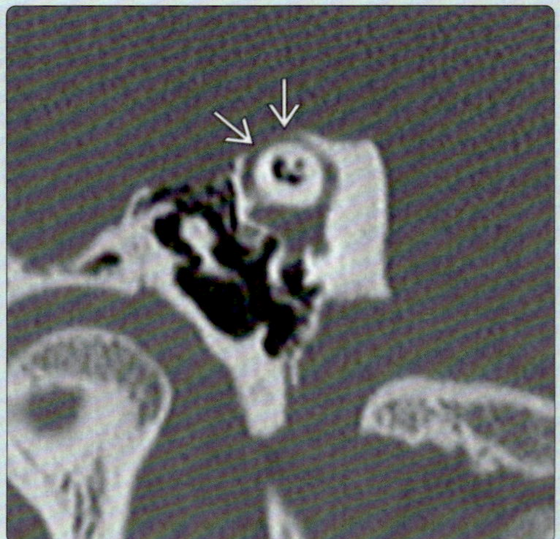

(Left) *Coronal T2WI MR reveals the absence of cortical bone covering the superior semicircular canal ➡, which is diagnostic of superior semicircular canal dehiscence. Coronal bone CT is the preferred imaging modality in this diagnosis.* **(Right)** *Transverse oblique T-bone CT formation clearly demonstrates an in-plane view of the superior semicircular canal showing the entire extent of superior semicircular canal dehiscence ➡ in a single image. Although not critical for diagnosis, it is very helpful in measuring the extent.*

KEY FACTS

TERMINOLOGY

- Cochlear implant (CI): Multicomponent electronic device that directly stimulates spiral ganglion neurons

IMAGING

- Preop evaluation: CT or MR depending on clinician preference (in congenital hearing loss, MR helpful to evaluate presence of cochlear nerve)
- Postop CI evaluation: T-bone CT; plain film imaging or fluoroscopy can be used during surgery
- Electrode tip should be in basal turn or 2nd turn of cochlea
  - No wire in cochlea signifies malpositioning
- Wire fracture or kinking may be demonstrated in malfunctioning CI; this imaging finding should be interpreted with caution in normally functioning device

CLINICAL ISSUES

- Torque experienced by CI in 1.5T MR is sufficient to cause implant movement; see protocols for head wrapping
- MR-compatible implants with self-aligning magnets are available; still create artifactual shadow with brain imaging

DIAGNOSTIC CHECKLIST

- Key **absolute contraindications** to CI placement
  - Cochlear aplasia
- Key **relative contraindications** to CI placement
  - Labyrinthine ossificans; would require drill out or split electrode array
  - Malformed cochlea (common cavity, cystic cochleovestibular anomaly); lateral wall electrodes typically best
  - Cochlear nerve aplasia/hypoplasia (may still get some auditory signals via crossover nerve fibers; hearing outcome less predictable)
- Key imaging findings that may complicate surgery
  - Contracted mastoid; aberrant facial nerve; otosclerosis with round window obliteration; otomastoiditis or otitis media; inner ear abnormalities; cochlear ossification

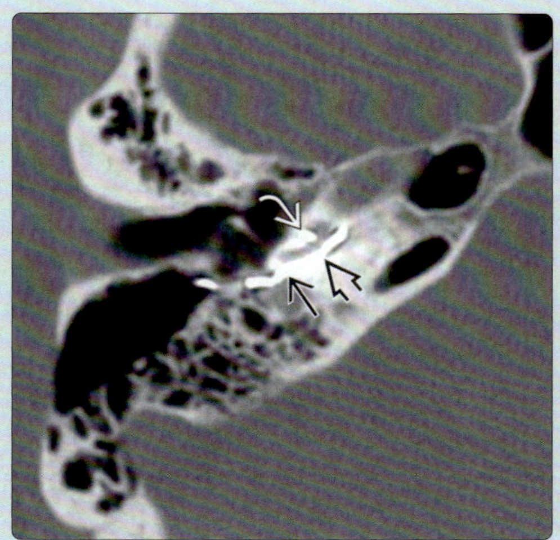

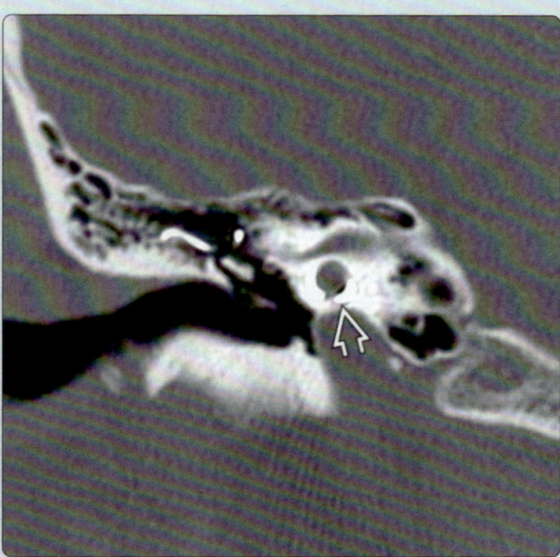

(Left) *Axial right T-bone CT shows the normal appearance and location of a cochlear implant. The wire enters the round window ➡ and traverses the basal turn of the cochlea ➡ to reach the cochlear 2nd turn ➡.* **(Right)** *Coronal T-bone CT in the same patient demonstrates normal positioning of the cochlear implant wire in the basal turn of the cochlea ➡.*

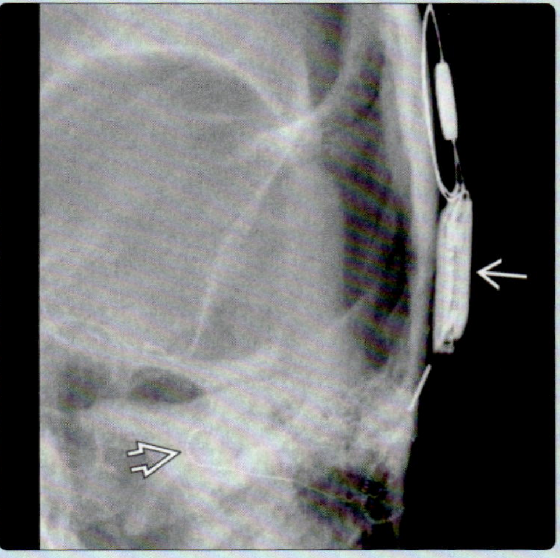

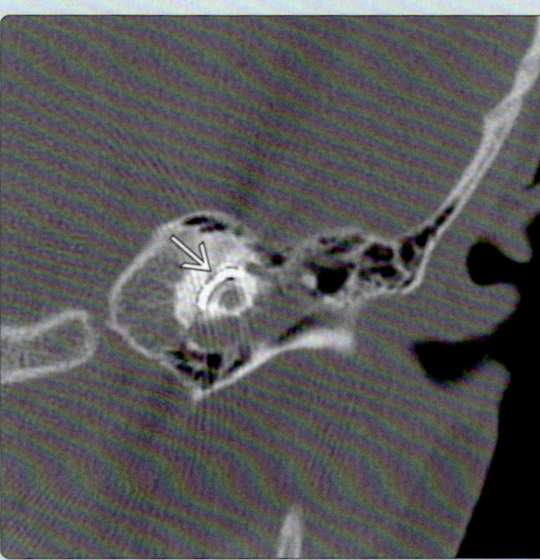

(Left) *AP plain film skull x-ray performed after left cochlear implantation shows the internal receiver-stimulator adjacent to the skull ➡. The electrode should assume a cochlear-shaped conformation ➡ as it curls through the basal and mid turn. Clinicians can use the x-ray to look for tip fold-over, depth of insertion, and for a grossly misplaced electrode.* **(Right)** *Coronal left T-bone CT shows a normally positioned cochlear implant electrode wire in the basal turn of the cochlea ➡.*

KEY FACTS

TERMINOLOGY

- Petrous apex (PA) asymmetric marrow: Asymmetric pneumatization of PA with nonpneumatized marrow space in opposite PA simulating mass lesion
- Synonym: PA pseudolesion

IMAGING

- Temporal bone CT findings
  - Normal PA marrow space
  - Normal air cells visible in contralateral PA
  - **No expansile changes** present
- MR findings
  - Nonpneumatized PA contains normal fatty marrow, hyperintense on T1WI
  - Mimics cholesterol granuloma
  - **Fat-saturated sequences** confirm fatty nature of lesion

TOP DIFFERENTIAL DIAGNOSES

- PA cholesterol granuloma
- PA trapped fluid
- PA congenital cholesteatoma
- Apical petrositis

PATHOLOGY

- Congenital normal variant in PA pneumatization-marrow space spectrum
- Embryology/anatomy
  - **33%** have pneumatized petrous apices
  - 5% are asymmetrically pneumatized

CLINICAL ISSUES

- Clinical presentation
  - **Asymptomatic** by definition
- Patient undergoing brain MR for unrelated symptoms
  - Incidental MR finding
- Requires no treatment or follow-up
- If mentioned in radiology report, important to understand incidental nature

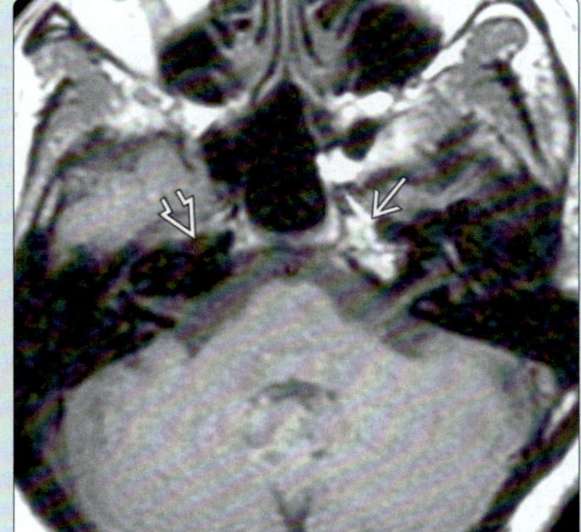

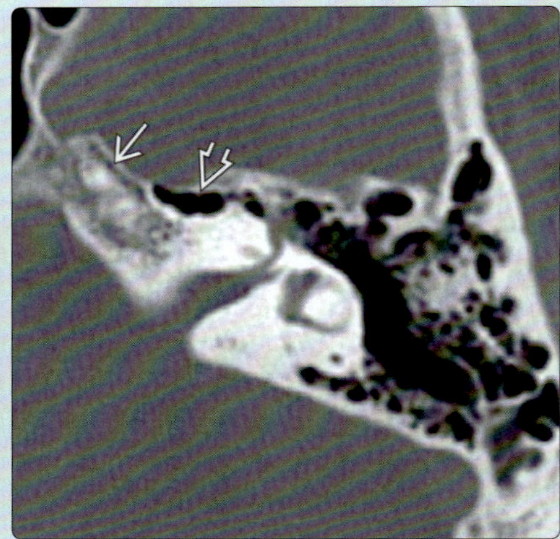

(Left) *Axial T1WI MR demonstrates an irregularly shaped high-signal fatty marrow focus ➡ in the left petrous apex. The right petrous apex is low signal ➡ due to air in petrous apex air cells. Fatty marrow must not be mistaken for cholesterol granuloma.* **(Right)** *Axial bone CT in the same patient reveals only minimal petrous apex pneumatization ➡. The remainder of the petrous apex is marrow space ➡. There is no evidence for any expansile change in this area.*

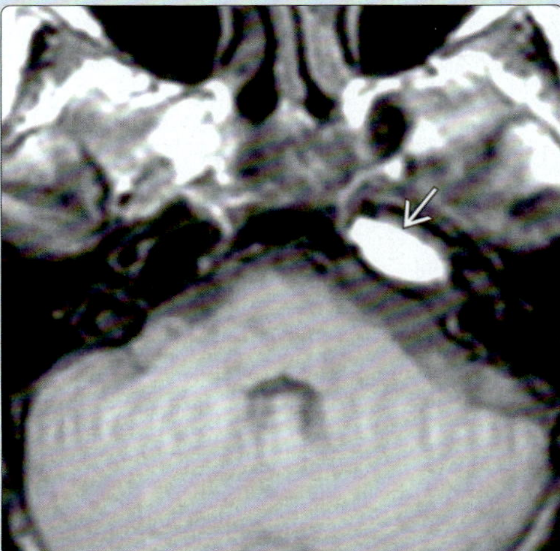

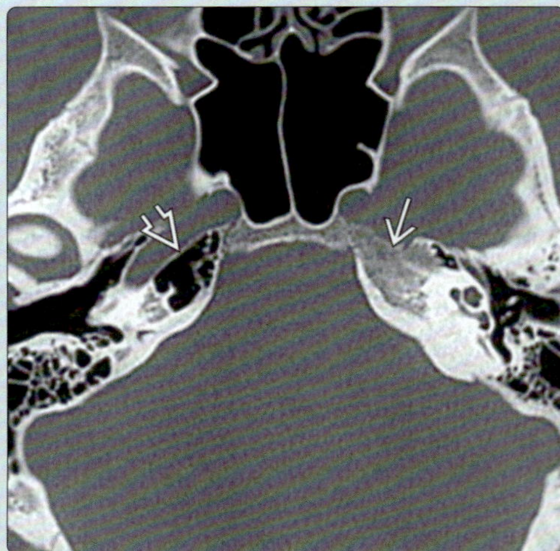

(Left) *Axial T1WI MR shows a conspicuous bright lesion in the left petrous apex ➡ suspicious for cholesterol granuloma. Bone CT was ordered to further define the nature of this finding.* **(Right)** *Axial bone CT in the same patient demonstrates asymmetric marrow in the left petrous apex ➡. Notice that the opposite petrous apex is pneumatized ➡. Asymmetric fatty marrow spaces may appear quite conspicuous on T1WI MR. Review of fat-saturated MR sequences sorts this finding into the normal category.*

Petrous Apex Cephalocele

KEY FACTS

TERMINOLOGY

- Synonyms: Petrous apex (PA) arachnoid cyst
- Definition: Congenital or acquired herniation of posterolateral wall of Meckel cave (MC) into PA

IMAGING

- Bone CT findings
  - Unilateral or bilateral expansile PA lesions
  - Enlarges porus trigeminus PA notch
- MR findings
  - CSF intensity ovoid PA lesion on all sequences
  - Directly communicates with MC
  - Appears to "spill out" of patulous MC

TOP DIFFERENTIAL DIAGNOSES

- PA cholesterol granuloma
- PA congenital cholesteatoma
- PA mucocele

CLINICAL ISSUES

- Common clinical presentation
  - Most commonly **incidental asymptomatic** MR finding
- Rare clinical presentation
  - Symptomatic lesion (CSF otorrhea, trigeminal neuralgia, meningitis); lesion breaks into temporal bone air cells
  - Headache from idiopathic intracranial hypertension
    - If see empty sella, consider enlarged optic nerve CSF spaces associated with PA cephalocele (PAC)
- **No treatment** in most cases
- Surgical treatment
  - If lesion communicates with PA air cells ± CSF otorrhea
    - If CSF is actively leaking, patient at risk for meningitis

DIAGNOSTIC CHECKLIST

- PAC = "leave alone" lesion of PA
- PAC requires **no further work-up** or surgical intervention in most cases

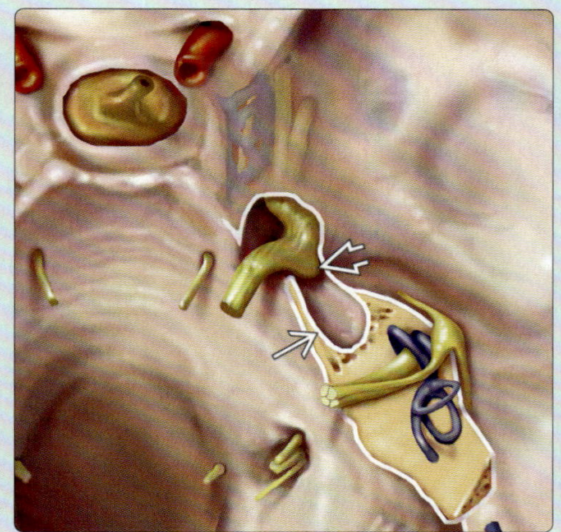

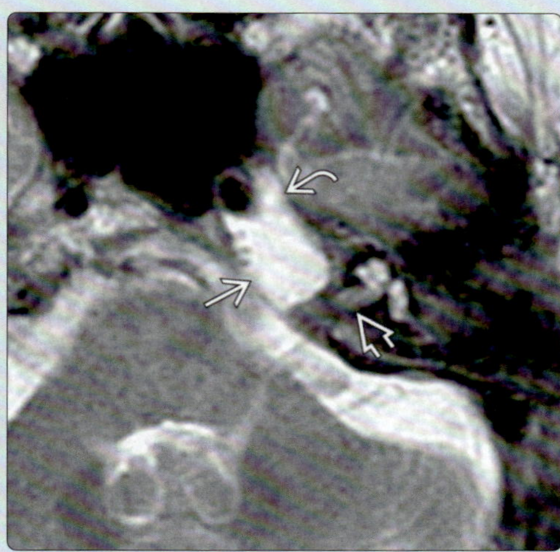

(Left) *Axial graphic illustrates the herniation of a cephalocele from the Meckel cave into the petrous apex (PA) ➡. A portion of the trigeminal ganglion is depicted protruding into the cephalocele ⇨.* **(Right)** *Axial T2WI MR shows a cephalocele ➡ protruding into the left PA just anteromedial to the internal auditory canal ⇨. Notice the connection of the lesion to the Meckel cave ↩.*

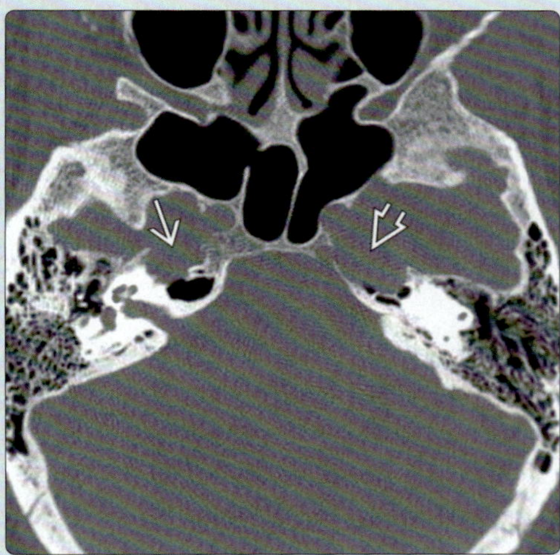

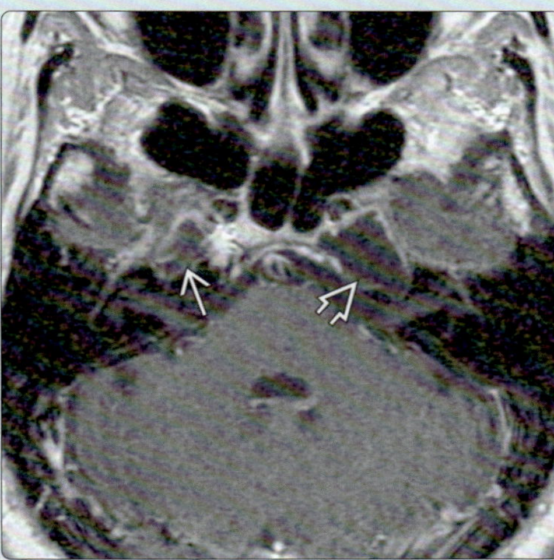

(Left) *Axial bone CT demonstrates a right ➡ and left ⇨ PA ovoid with scalloping lesions projecting into the PA air cells from the posterolateral Meckel cave area. Bilateral PA cephaloceles (PACs) were suspected, and MR was ordered for confirmation.* **(Right)** *Axial T1WI C+ MR in the same patient reveals bilateral, left ⇨ larger than right ➡, fluid intensity PACs that arise from the inferior aspect of the Meckel cave.*

Congenital Petrous Apex Cholesteatoma

KEY FACTS

TERMINOLOGY

- Petrous apex (PA) cholesteatoma or epidermoid: PA focus of cholesteatoma due to **epithelial rest** of embryonal origin

IMAGING

- May simultaneously involve adjacent areas
  - Horizontal petrous internal carotid artery (ICA) canal
  - Inner ear structures (otic capsule)
  - Internal auditory canal
  - Meckel cave
  - Medial mastoid air cells
  - Facial nerve canal (labyrinthine and anterior tympanic segments)
- Bone CT: **Expansile** mass with **smooth, lobular bone remodeling**
  - Shows smooth, expansile, lobulated lesion of PA
- MR: Expansile PA lesion with low T1, high T2 signal but **without** enhancement
  - **Restricted diffusion** (high signal on DWI)

TOP DIFFERENTIAL DIAGNOSES

- PA arachnoid cyst
- PA trapped fluid or mucocele
- PA cholesterol granuloma
- Petrous ICA aneurysm

PATHOLOGY

- **Aberrant PA epithelial rest** of **exfoliated keratin** within stratified squamous epithelium
  - Growth from **progressive desquamation of epithelium**

CLINICAL ISSUES

- Clinical profile: 40-year-old adult with unilateral sensorineural hearing loss
- Surgical treatment: Removal via transpetrous or middle fossa approach
- May get infected, spreads intracranially (meningitis)
- High rate of recurrence; requires serial MR imaging

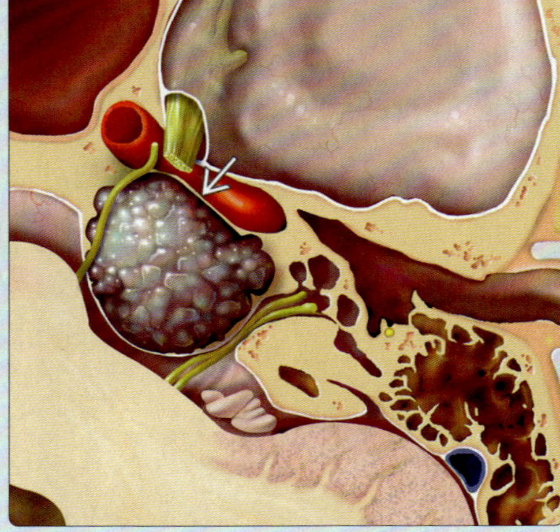
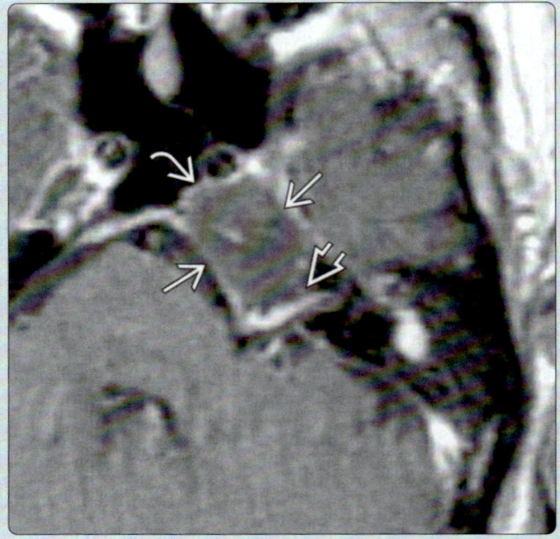

(Left) *Axial graphic depicts typical petrous apex (PA) congenital cholesteatoma or epidermoid. Notice the benign expansile nature of the PA bone as it responds to the growing cholesteatoma. The horizontal petrous internal carotid artery (ICA) posterior wall is thinned ➡ by cholesteatoma growth.* **(Right)** *Axial T1WI C+ MR reveals a large PA cholesteatoma ➡ with minimal rim enhancement. The lesion is impinging on the internal auditory canal ➡ and sphenoid sinus ➡.*

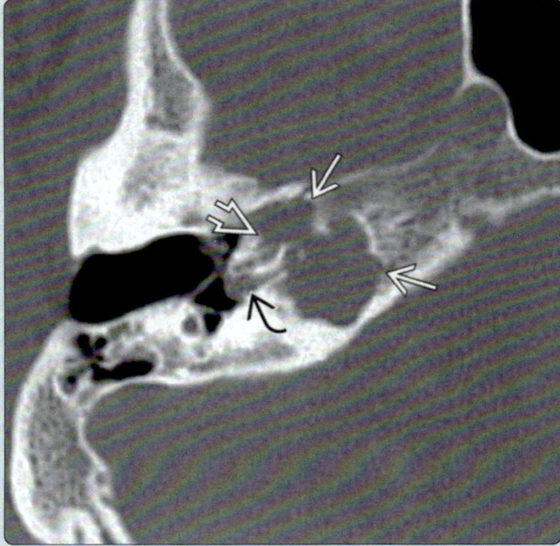
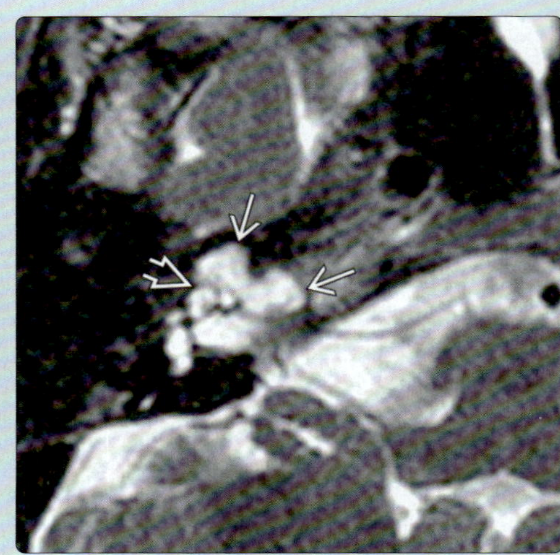

(Left) *Axial bone CT in the right ear shows an expansile, smoothly marginated cholesteatoma remodeling the PA ➡ and eroding the bony labyrinth around the cochlea ➡. The cholesteatoma can also be seen emerging from the round window niche ➡.* **(Right)** *Axial T2WI MR in the same patient shows the hyperintense congenital cholesteatoma eroding the PA ➡ and the bone of the cochlea ➡. PA congenital cholesteatoma often involves more than just the PA. In this case, the inner ear is affected.*

KEY FACTS

TERMINOLOGY

- Definition: Sterile residual fluid collection in petrous apex (PA) air cells, sometimes resulting from remote otomastoiditis
- a.k.a. PA effusion

IMAGING

- Variable T1, high T2 signal in PA on MR with bone CT showing opacified PA air cells **without** trabecular loss or expansion
- Temporal bone CT findings
  - Opacified PA air cells; middle ear-mastoid clear
  - **No expansile component** to lesion
  - **No PA cortical or trabecular erosions**
- MR findings
  - T1 intermediate to high signal most common
  - High T2 signal in normal-appearing PA

TOP DIFFERENTIAL DIAGNOSES

- PA cholesterol granuloma
- PA congenital cholesteatoma
- Apical petrositis

PATHOLOGY

- Pathophysiology
  - May also follow remote otomastoiditis
  - May occur as normal developmental variant
- Sterile PA air cell fluid

CLINICAL ISSUES

- Principal presenting symptom: **None**
- **Incidental finding** on brain MR for unrelated symptoms
- Bone CT shows typical trapped fluid findings, no bone remodeling or breakdown
- Treatment: **None**: This is considered "no touch" lesion

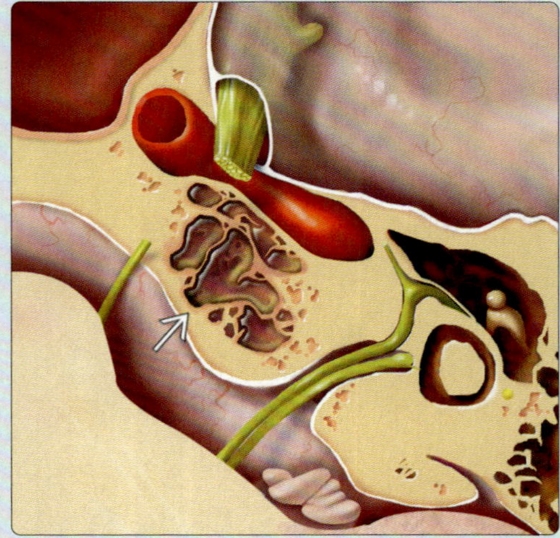

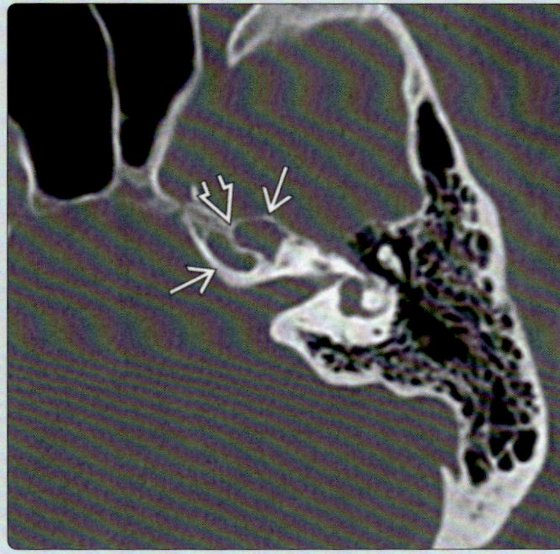

(Left) *Axial graphic of the left temporal bone demonstrates fluid-filled petrous apex air cells ➡. Notice that trapped fluid in the petrous apex has no associated expansion or trabecular breakdown.* **(Right)** *Axial bone CT demonstrates a typical example of petrous apex trapped fluid as a group of nonexpansile opacified petrous apex air cells ➡ with preservation of the trabecula ➡ and cortical margins. Also notice the absence of fluid opacification of the middle ear and mastoid air cells.*

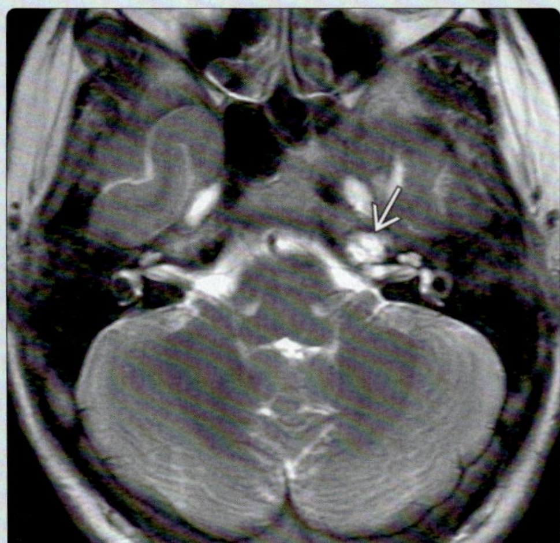

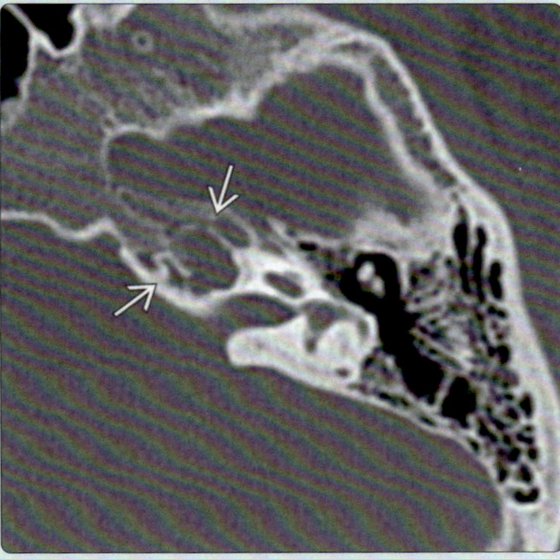

(Left) *Axial T2WI MR shows a conspicuous area of high signal in the left petrous apex ➡ on brain MR performed for loss of consciousness. The radiologist queried the diagnosis of cholesterol granuloma in the radiologic report and suggested temporal bone CT for further evaluation.* **(Right)** *Axial bone CT in the same patient shows opacified air cells in the left petrous apex ➡ without evidence for expansion or trabecular loss. The diagnosis of trapped fluid was made with no follow-up recommended.*

Petrous Apex Mucocele

KEY FACTS

TERMINOLOGY

- Mucus-containing, expanded petrous apex (PA) air cells(s) lined by secretory epithelium resulting from chronic ostial obstruction

IMAGING

- Requires pneumatized PA
- CT: Fluid-filled, **expanded PA air cell(s)**
- MR: Nonenhancing, T1 low, T2 high signal; DWI with no restricted diffusion

TOP DIFFERENTIAL DIAGNOSES

- PA trapped fluid
- PA cholesterol granuloma
- PA congenital cholesteatoma
- PA cephalocele

PATHOLOGY

- Results from **obstruction to PA air cell drainage**
- Obstruction from middle ear-mastoid infection, trauma, previous surgery
- Secretion of mucus into obstructed air cells
- Air cell expansion from pressure remodeling of wall

CLINICAL ISSUES

- Often incidental and asymptomatic
- Headache or rare cranial neuropathy from compression
- Treatment issues: Controversial if patient asymptomatic
  - Consider follow-up CT to see if mucocele increases in size
  - Surgical obliteration if enlarges

DIAGNOSTIC CHECKLIST

- When bone CT shows **expansile PA lesion**
  - Consider **mucocele** if T1 is low, T2 is high, DWI shows no restricted diffusion
  - Consider **cholesterol granuloma if T1 signal** is **high**
  - Consider **congenital cholesteatoma if DWI** shows **restricted diffusion**

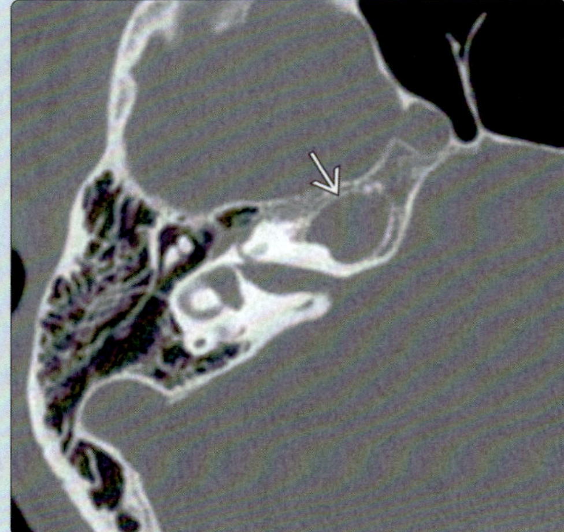

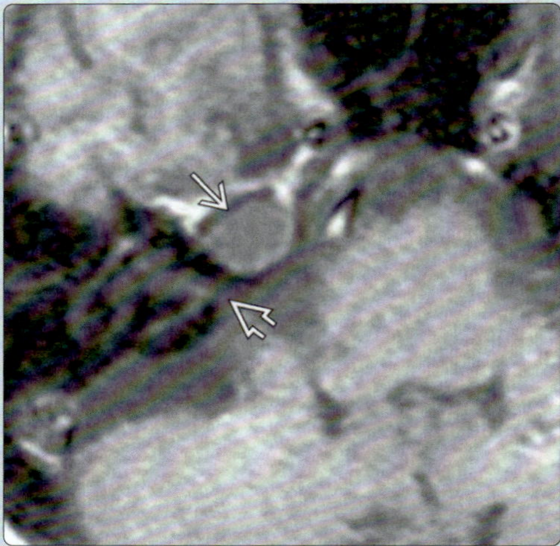

(Left) *Axial bone CT shows an expansile right petrous apex (PA) lesion ➡ with loss of the normal air cell trabeculations. The differential diagnosis is congenital cholesteatoma, cholesterol granuloma, and mucocele.* **(Right)** *Axial T1WI MR in the same patient demonstrates an expansile PA mucocele ➡ with minimally higher signal than CSF. Note low-signal CSF of the internal auditory canal ➡ just posterolateral to the lesion. Low signal on T1WI MR excludes cholesterol granuloma.*

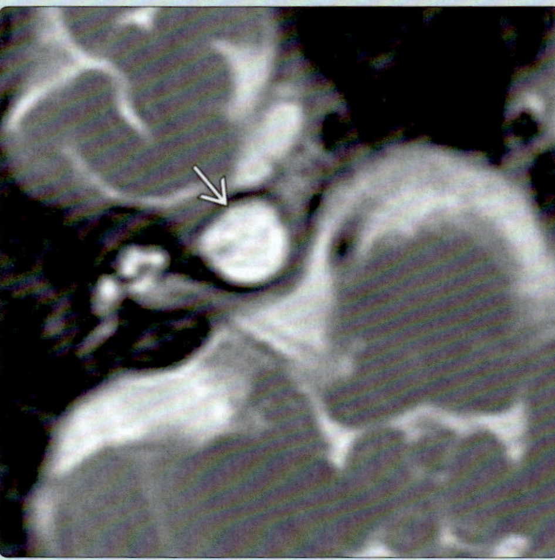

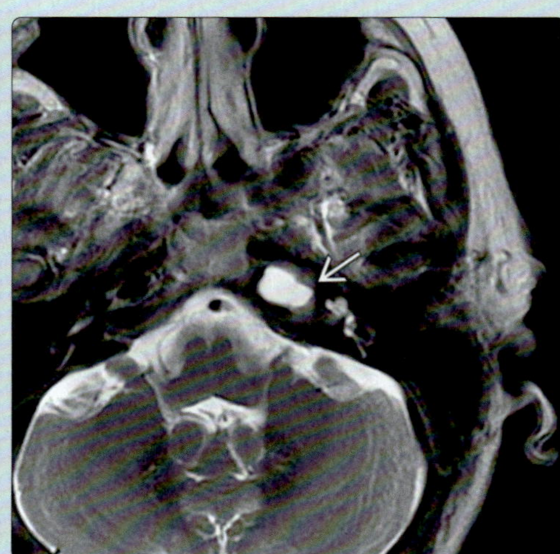

(Left) *Axial T2WI MR demonstrates the PA mucocele is uniformly hyperintense ➡. DWI (not shown) had no restricted diffusion. An expansile PA lesion with low T1, high T2, and no restricted diffusion is highly suggestive of a mucocele.* **(Right)** *Axial T2WI MR in demonstrates bright T2 signal in an expanded PA mucocele ➡. T1 signal was low (not a cholesterol granuloma), and there was no restricted diffusion (not a congenital cholesteatoma).*

KEY FACTS

TERMINOLOGY

- Petrous apex (PA) cholesterol granuloma: **Expansile** PA lesion resulting from foreign-body giant cell reaction to deposition of cholesterol crystals in apical air cells with fibrosis and vascular proliferation
- a.k.a. cholesterol cyst, "chocolate" cyst

IMAGING

- Temporal bone CT findings
  - **Sharply marginated**, **expansile** PA lesion
  - Trabecular breakdown with cortical thinning of PA expected; pneumatized PA air cells **required**
  - Larger lesions will have areas of **focal bony wall dehiscence**
- Temporal bone MR findings
  - **High T1 internal signal**
  - High T2 internal signal
  - **Peripheral low-signal hemosiderin ring** (T2)
  - No internal enhancement

TOP DIFFERENTIAL DIAGNOSES

- PA asymmetric marrow
- PA trapped fluid
- PA congenital cholesteatoma
- PA internal carotid artery aneurysm
- PA mucocele
- Apical petrositis

PATHOLOGY

- Obstruction-vacuum pathogenesis (classic hypothesis)
- Exposed bone marrow pathogenesis (recent alternative hypothesis)

CLINICAL ISSUES

- May be incidental, asymptomatic lesion
- Most common symptoms: Headache, dizziness
  - Facial pain/weakness, diplopia, or hearing loss
- Multiple approaches for drainage: Infracochlear allows dependent drainage; endoscopic transsphenoidal

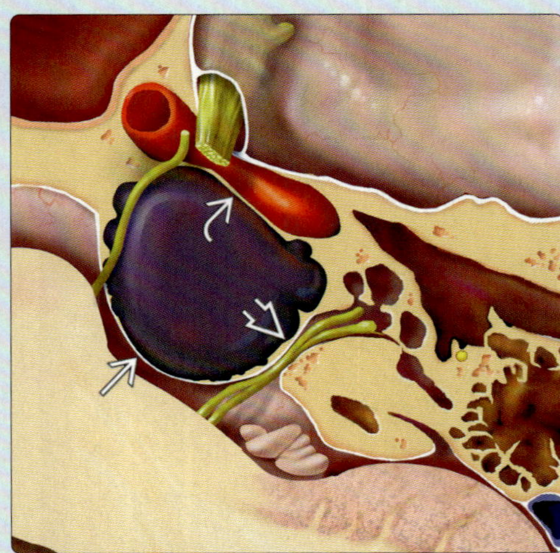

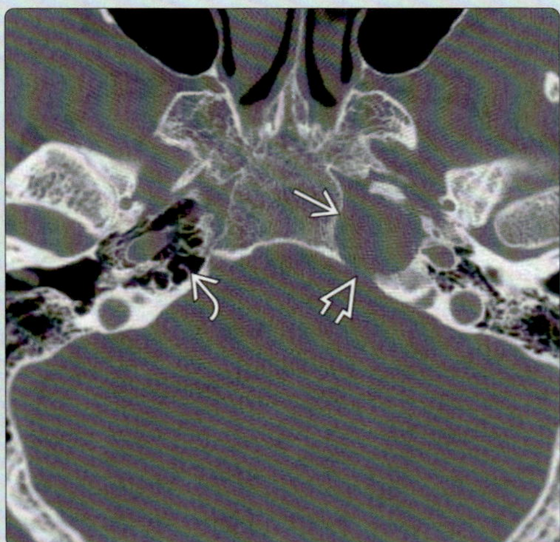

(Left) *Axial graphic shows a cholesterol granuloma (CG) of the petrous apex (PA). The lesion is expansile with air cell trabecular loss and "eggshell" medial cortex ➡. The lesion compresses the internal auditory canal ➡ and thins the posterior wall of the horizontal petrous internal carotid artery canal ➡.* **(Right)** *Axial bone CT reveals an expansile CG in the left PA ➡ with marginal bone dehiscence present ➡. The right PA is well pneumatized ➡. PA-CG most commonly occurs in a pneumatized PA.*

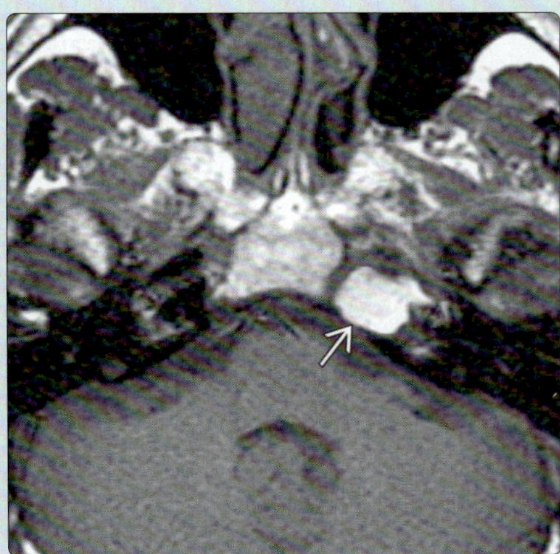

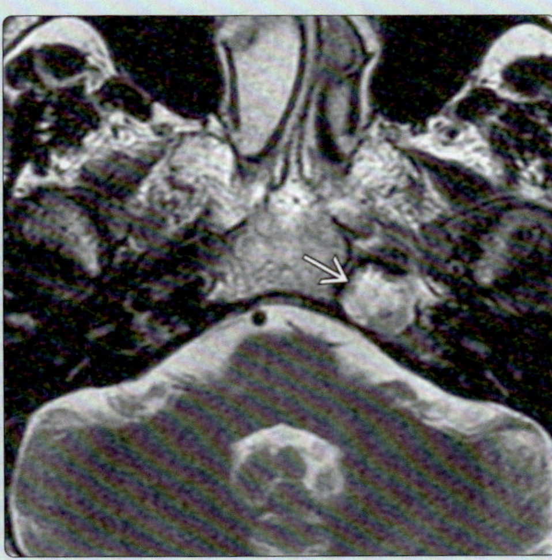

(Left) *Axial T1WI unenhanced MR in the same patient shows characteristic high signal ➡ of PA-CG. If no fat saturation is applied to the enhanced sequences through this lesion, it will appear to enhance when in fact it does not.* **(Right)** *Axial T2WI MR in the same patient demonstrates the lesion has inhomogeneous high signal ➡. CG contains "old blood." The T1 signal is therefore high (methemoglobin) and T2 signal inhomogeneous (methemoglobin and hemosiderin).*

Apical Petrositis

KEY FACTS

TERMINOLOGY

- Definition: Extension of middle ear-mastoid (ME-M) infection into pneumatized petrous apex (PA) with resulting **suppurative apical petrositis**

IMAGING

- Bone CT: **Trabecular breakdown ± cortical erosions** in opacified PA air cells
- Enhanced T1 findings: Early disease
  - **Rim-enhancing fluid-filled PA**
  - Adjacent **meningeal thickening**
- Enhanced T1 findings: Advanced disease
  - Thickened, C+ Meckel cave, & cavernous sinus
  - Skull base osteomyelitis (enhancing clival marrow)
  - Enhancing cranial nerves, especially CNV, CNVI
  - Petrous ± cavernous internal carotid artery spasm
  - Epidural or brain abscess, meningitis

TOP DIFFERENTIAL DIAGNOSES

- PA trapped fluid
- PA metastasis
- PA cholesterol granuloma
- PA congenital cholesteatoma
- Petrooccipital fissure chondrosarcoma

PATHOLOGY

- Pathophysiology: Suppurative ME-M infection spreads via air cells or venous channels to PA

CLINICAL ISSUES

- Complete clinical syndrome = **Gradenigo syndrome**
  - Acute otomastoiditis with **otorrhea**, deep facial or **retroorbital pain** (CNV), & **abducens nerve palsy** (CNVI)
- Treatment: Antibiotics (IV) alone are usually sufficient
  - If severe symptoms at presentation, surgical intervention with mastoidectomy ± petrous apicotomy

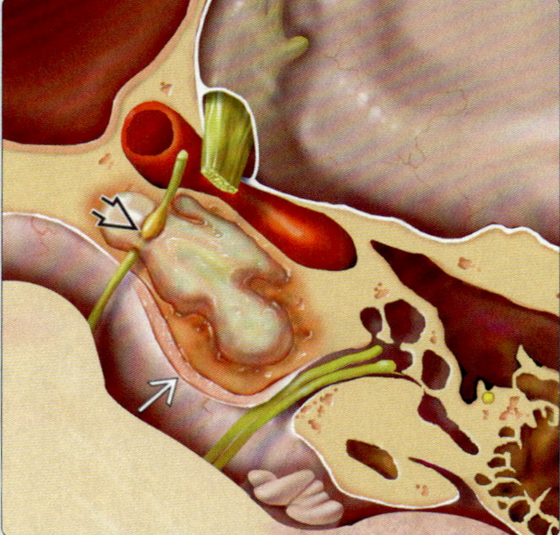

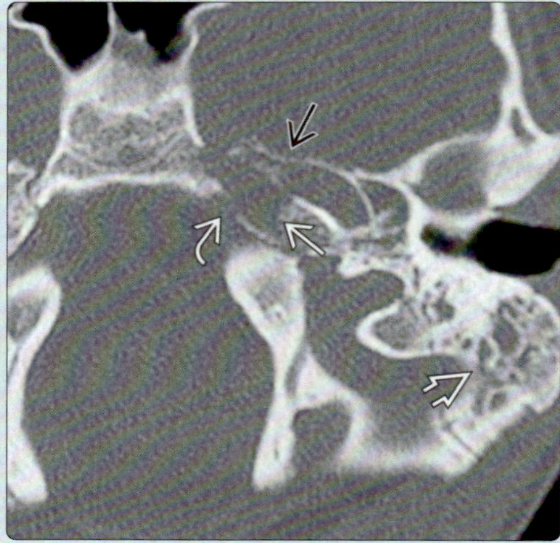

(Left) *Axial graphic of the left petrous apex (PA) shows "confluent apical petrositis" with PA abscess formation. Pus surrounds the 6th cranial nerve* ➡ *and associated inflammation thickens adjacent meninges* ➡. **(Right)** *Axial temporal bone CT in a young patient with petrous apicitis demonstrates left PA opacification and trabecular destruction* ➡ *as well as cortical disruption* ➡. *Note accompanying mastoid opacification* ➡. *Cortical irregularity of petrous carotid canal raises suspicion of spread into canal* ➡.

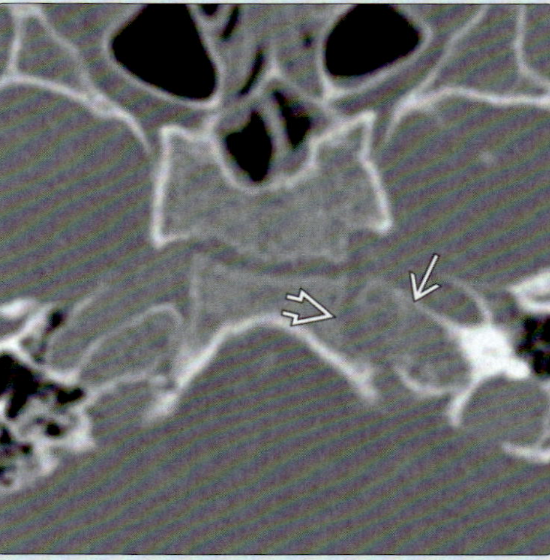

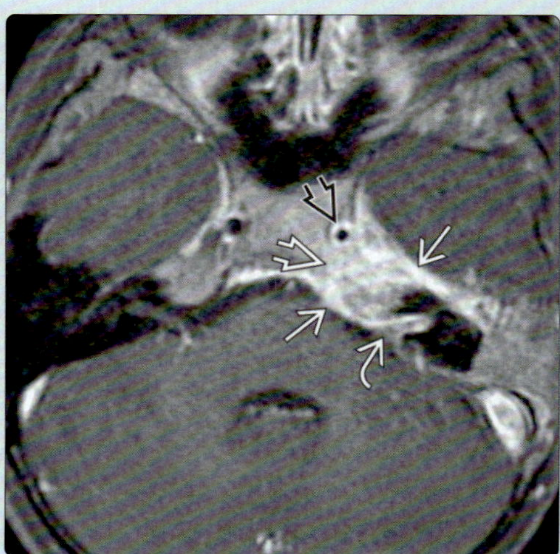

(Left) *Axial bone CT in a child with full-blown Gradenigo syndrome (retroorbital pain, abducens nerve palsy, and otorrhea) reveals infection of the left PA cortical bone* ➡ *with infection crossing the petrooccipital fissure to involve the bone of the lateral clivus* ➡. **(Right)** *Axial T1WI C+ FS MR in the same patient shows infection of the PA with adjacent involvement of the clivus* ➡, *dura* ➡, *and internal auditory canal* ➡. *Note the spasm of cavernous internal carotid artery* ➡ *secondary to adjacent infectious process.*

Petrous Apex Internal Carotid Artery Aneurysm

KEY FACTS

TERMINOLOGY

- Rare congenital or acquired aneurysm of petrous internal carotid artery (ICA)

IMAGING

- Rarity makes errors in imaging diagnosis common
- Complex expansile mass of petrous ICA canal with internal flow on CTA, MRA, or angiography
  - Size: Variable; 1-5 cm
  - Shape: Focal ovoid to fusiform
- Bone CT findings
  - **Ovoid** or **fusiform** enlargement of petrous ICA canal
  - **Curvilinear calcifications** in aneurysm wall
- CTA: **Aneurysmal dilation** of petrous ICA is **diagnostic**
- MR findings
  - T1: **Complex signal mass**
  - High signal: Intraluminal clot, slow flow
  - Low signal: Wall calcification, high flow

TOP DIFFERENTIAL DIAGNOSES

- Petrous apex cholesterol granuloma
- Aberrant ICA
- Dehiscent jugular bulb

PATHOLOGY

- **Congenital aneurysm** (true aneurysm)
  - Forms at congenital weakness at origin of obliterated embryologic vessel (caroticotympanic)
- **Acquired aneurysm** (false or pseudoaneurysm)
  - Posttraumatic, postinfectious, postradiation

CLINICAL ISSUES

- Sensorineural hearing loss, Horner syndrome, pulsatile tinnitus, stroke
- Gradual enlargement; progressive risk of rupture
- **Endovascular therapy**
  - Obliteration of ICA or stent placement

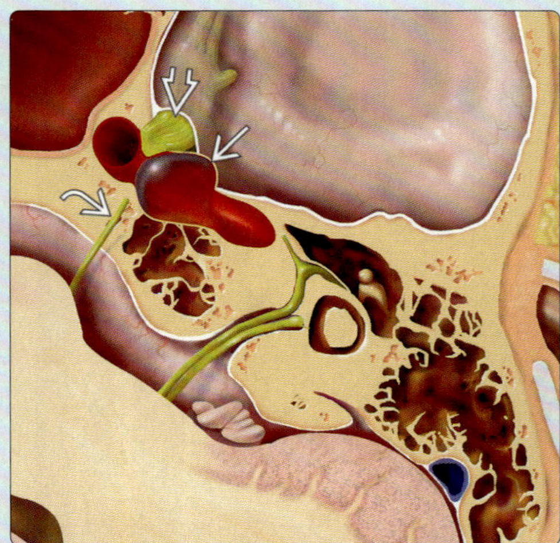

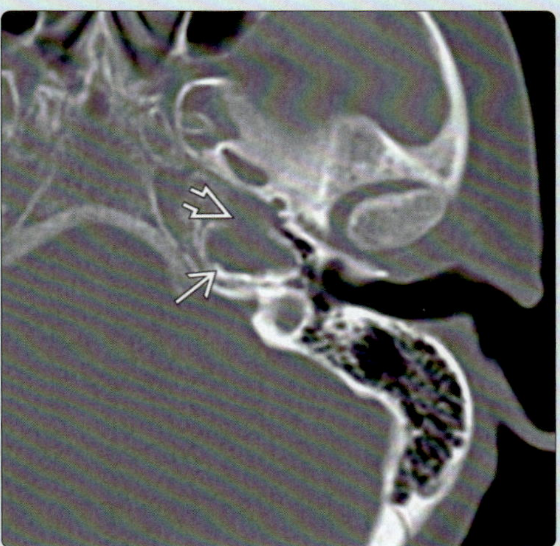

(Left) *Axial graphic through the left temporal bone shows focal aneurysmal dilation ➡ of the horizontal petrous internal carotid artery (ICA). Note the proximity to the trigeminal nerve ➡ and the abducens nerve ➡ to the petrous ICA aneurysm.* **(Right)** *Axial bone CT in a patient presenting with recurrent transient ischemic attacks shows an expansile ovoid lesion ➡ in the left petrous apex (PA). Note the anterior wall dehiscence ➡ where the aneurysm connects to the horizontal petrous ICA.*

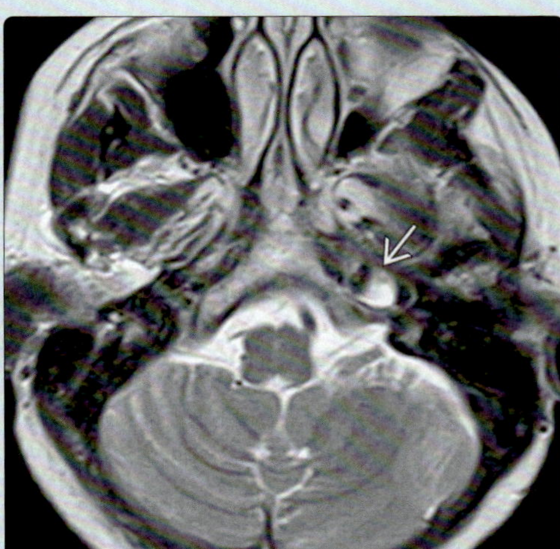

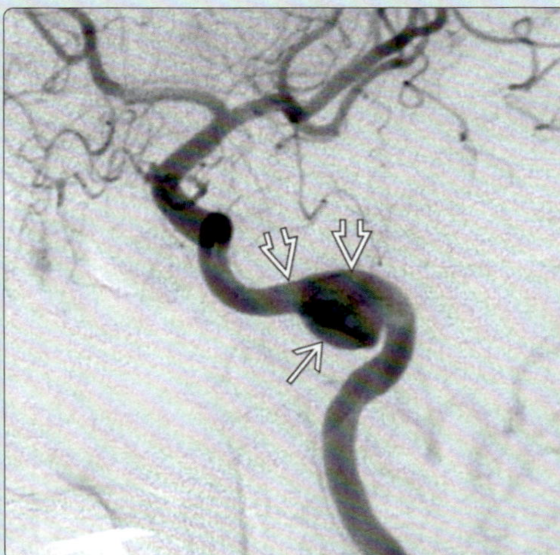

(Left) *Axial T2WI MR in the same patient demonstrates a complex signal ovoid mass ➡ in the PA. Without CTA or MRA, it might be possible to mistake this petrous ICA aneurysm for a cholesterol granuloma.* **(Right)** *Oblique left ICA angiogram in the same patient reveals the PA aneurysm ➡ projecting off the undersurface of the horizontal petrous ICA ➡.*

Intratemporal Facial Nerve Enhancement

KEY FACTS

TERMINOLOGY

- Definition: Normal contrast enhancement on T1 C+ MR along course of intratemporal facial nerve (CNVII) without abnormal bony changes on bone CT

IMAGING

- T1 C+ MR enhancement along CNVII
  - Mastoid > geniculate ganglion > tympanic segments
- Bone CT: Normal CNVII canal

TOP DIFFERENTIAL DIAGNOSES

- Bell palsy
- Perineural parotid tumor of intratemporal CNVII
- Facial nerve schwannoma within temporal bone

PATHOLOGY

- Lush **circumneutral arteriovenous plexus** surrounds CNVII within temporal bone
  - Labyrinthine segment is **least** well vascularized

CLINICAL ISSUES

- Clinical presentation: **Asymptomatic** by definition
- Treatment options
  - None; do not mistake for Bell palsy
- Imaging recommendations
  - Bone CT used when MR shows asymmetric contrast enhancement to rule out underlying bony changes
  - If CNVII bony canal is enlarged, consider CNVII schwannoma or perineural tumor

DIAGNOSTIC CHECKLIST

- Asymmetric contrast enhancement along canalicular (internal auditory canal), labyrinthine segment, or extracranial (parotid) CNVII segments **not** normal
- Higher field strength (3T) ± IR-FSPGR MR sequences makes normal CNVII contrast enhancement more conspicuous
- If fundal vestibular schwannoma present, labyrinthine segment of CNVII may enhance normally
  - Arteriovenous plexus congestion is likely cause

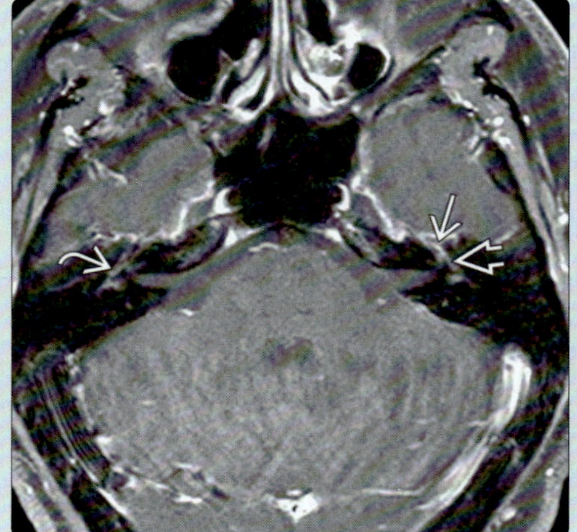

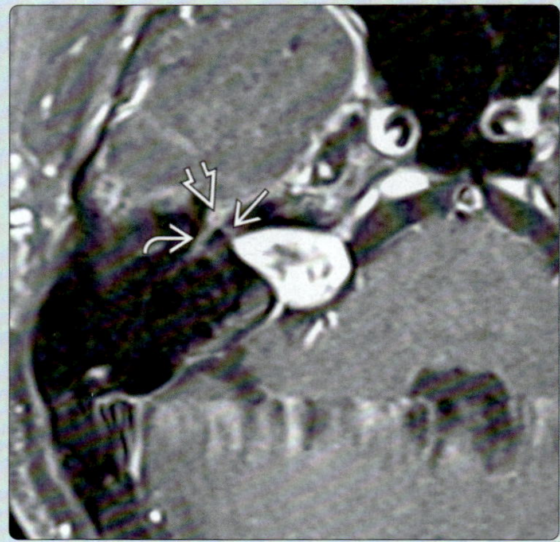

(Left) *Axial T1WI C+ FS MR through the internal auditory canals reveals a normal geniculate ganglion ➡ and anterior tympanic segment CNVII ➡ enhancement on the left. On the right, normal anterior tympanic segment enhancement ➡ is visible.* **(Right)** *Axial T1WI C+ FS MR in a patient with right vestibular schwannoma demonstrates increased enhancement of the labyrinthine ➡ CNVII, geniculate ganglion ➡, and anterior tympanic segment ➡ CNVII.*

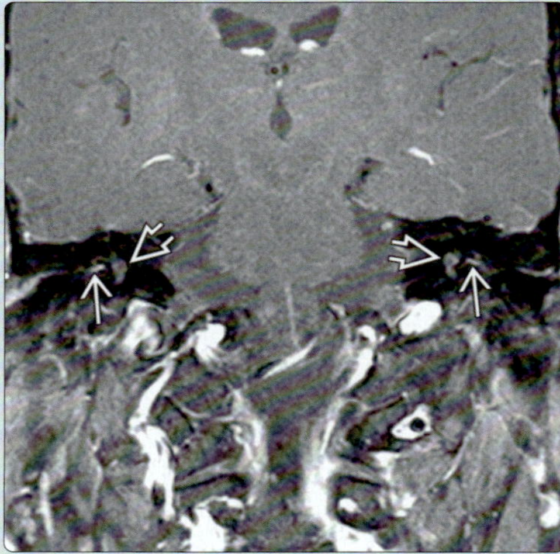

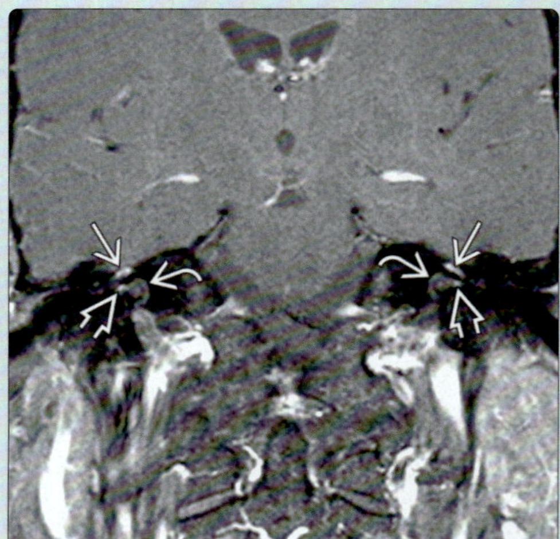

(Left) *Coronal T1WI C+ FS MR at the level of the vestibules ➡ reveals normal enhancement of the midtympanic segment of the facial nerves ➡.* **(Right)** *Coronal T1WI C+ FS MR in the same patient shows the normal geniculate ganglion enhancement ➡ just superior to the cochleas ➡. Note that the tensor tympani muscles ➡ both also enhance. With 3T imaging, more normal enhancement of structures within the temporal bone is seen.*

Middle Ear Prolapsing Facial Nerve

KEY FACTS

TERMINOLOGY

- Definition: Midtympanic facial nerve (CNVII) segment protrudes through bony dehiscence
  - **CNVII dehiscence** refers only to segmental absence of bony covering of CNVII
  - **Prolapsing CNVII**: CNVII protrudes through dehiscence in tympanic CNVII canal

IMAGING

- **Incidental finding** on temporal bone CT
  - Tubular soft tissue extends from midtympanic CNVII into oval window niche
- Coronal bone CT
  - Soft tissue mass in oval widow niche
  - Along undersurface of lateral semicircular canal
  - Contiguous with midtympanic segment of CNVII
- Axial bone CT
  - Hammock-like CNVII spanning middle ear cavity under lateral semicircular canal

TOP DIFFERENTIAL DIAGNOSES

- Intratemporal facial nerve schwannoma
- Oval window atresia
- Congenital cholesteatoma in facial nerve canal
- Persistent stapedial artery

CLINICAL ISSUES

- Clinical presentation
  - Most commonly **asymptomatic**
  - Rarely conductive hearing loss present from impingement on stapes
- Treatment option
  - None; do not mistake for small CNVII schwannoma
- Warning to clinician: Prolapsed CNVII in peril during stapedectomy
  - Most conservative decision is to avoid surgery or abort if found intraoperatively
  - If prolapse is mild, occasionally CNVII can be gently retracted, but this is high risk

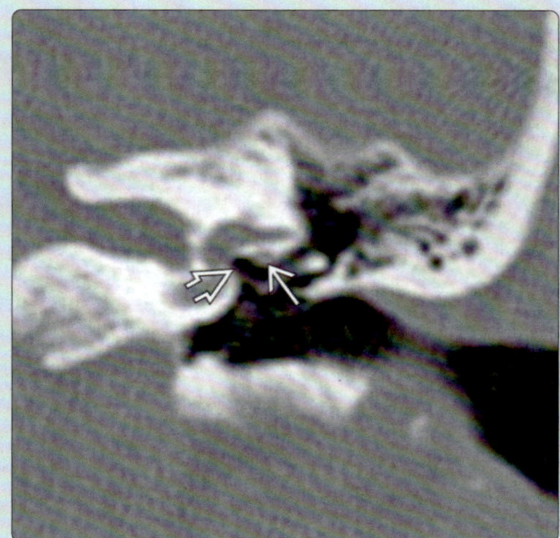

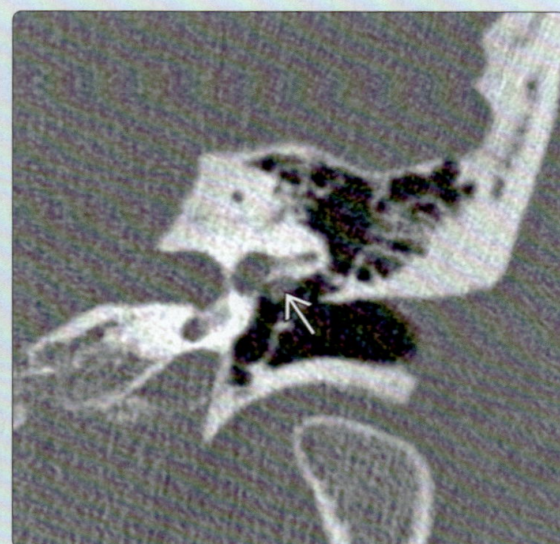

(Left) *Coronal left ear temporal bone CT shows the normal tympanic segment of the facial nerve in cross section ➔ along the undersurface of the lateral semicircular canal. Note subtle bone covering and relationship to the oval window niche ➔.* **(Right)** *Coronal left ear temporal bone CT reveals a focal mass projecting from the midtympanic facial nerve ➔. The lesion is a prolapsed facial nerve, not a facial nerve schwannoma. Facial nerve prolapse can create significant surgical difficulties during stapedectomy.*

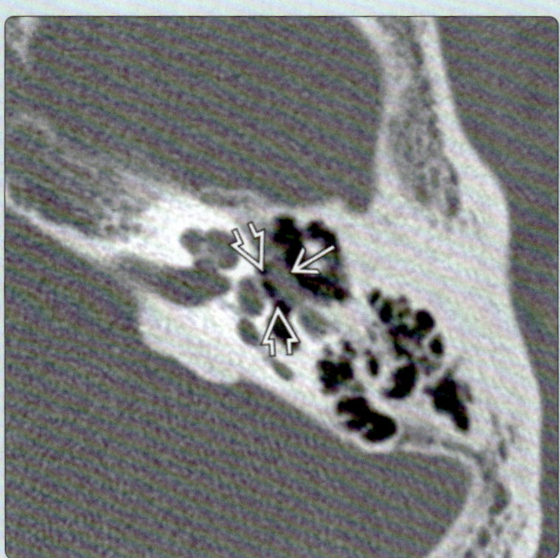

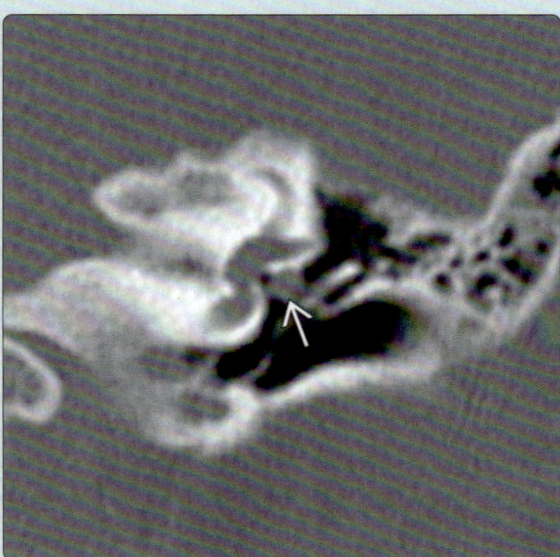

(Left) *Axial bone CT in the same patient demonstrates the hammock-like protruding tympanic segment of CNVII ➔ strung across middle ear cavity. Notice that CNVII touches the crura ➔ of the stapes, explaining the conductive hearing loss presentation.* **(Right)** *Coronal left ear temporal bone CT shows a round soft tissue mass ➔ projecting off the midtympanic segment of CNVII. Enhanced MR can differentiate protrusion of CNVII (no enhancement) vs. facial nerve schwannoma (enhancement).*

Bell Palsy

KEY FACTS

TERMINOLOGY

- Bell palsy (BP): Herpetic peripheral facial nerve paralysis secondary to herpes simplex virus; rapid onset, all ipsilateral facial nerve branches involved, no other etiology

IMAGING

- Imaging note: For typical BP, **routine imaging is not recommended**
- If **atypical BP**, search with imaging for underlying lesion
- T1WI C+ fat-saturated MR: Fundal tuft and labyrinthine segment CNVII show intense asymmetric enhancement
  - Entire intratemporal CNVII may enhance

TOP DIFFERENTIAL DIAGNOSES

- Normal physiologic enhancement of intratemporal CNVII
- Ramsay Hunt syndrome
- Facial nerve schwannoma
- Facial nerve venous malformation (hemangioma)
- Perineural tumor from parotid

PATHOLOGY

- Etiology-pathogenesis (current hypothesis)
  - Latent **herpes simplex** infection of geniculate ganglion with reactivation causing neural edema and constriction at labyrinthine segment and distal nerve fiber degeneration

CLINICAL ISSUES

- Classic clinical presentation
  - Acute-onset peripheral CNVII paralysis (36-hr onset)
- Medical therapy for BP
  - High dose oral steroids (prednisone), then taper; begin within 3 days of symptoms for best outcome
  - Steroids + antiviral agents may provide additional benefit
- Surgical therapy for BP has been proven effective but is still controversial
  - Profound denervation (> 90% out on ENoG and with no EMG response) treated with facial nerve decompression at labyrinthine segment via middle fossa craniotomy

(Left) *Axial T1WI C+ FS MR shows classic findings of Bell palsy with the internal auditory canal (IAC) fundal tuft sign ➡, labyrinthine ➡, and tympanic ➡ facial nerve segment enhancement.* **(Right)** *Axial T1WI C+ FS MR in the same patient again shows the IAC fundal tuft sign ➡ and tympanic segment of the facial nerve enhancement ➡. Remember that the geniculate ganglion and posterior genu/upper mastoid segment of the facial nerve may normally enhance.*

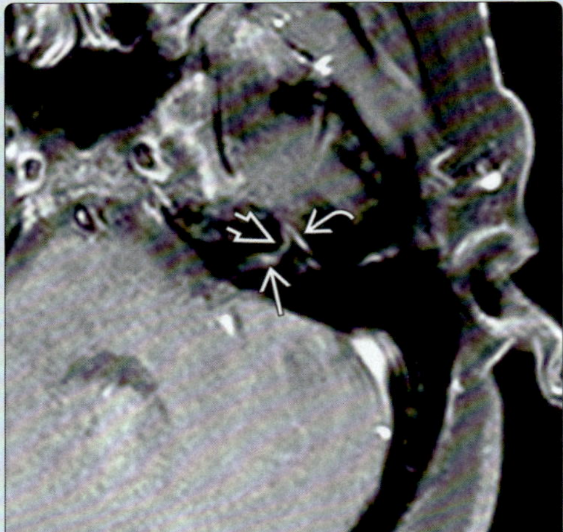

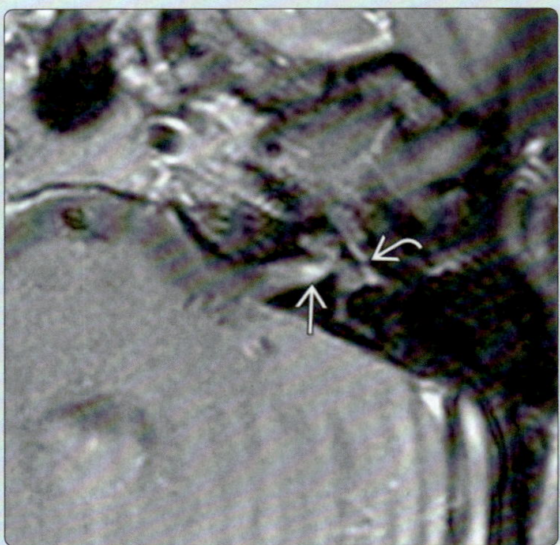

(Left) *Axial T1WI C+ FS MR in the same patient through the stylomastoid foramen demonstrates an enhancing, slightly enlarged facial nerve ➡. Swelling of the facial nerve is possible outside the bony facial nerve canal within the temporal bone.* **(Right)** *Coronal T1WI C+ FS MR in the same patient reveals avid enhancement in the mastoid ➡, stylomastoid ➡, and extracranial facial nerve ➡ in this patient with typical Bell palsy.*

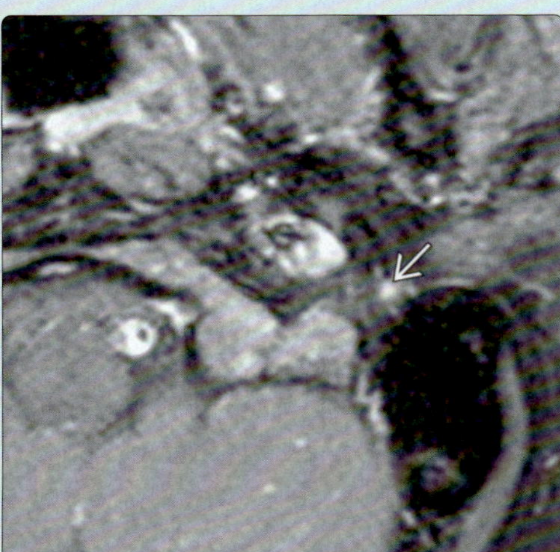

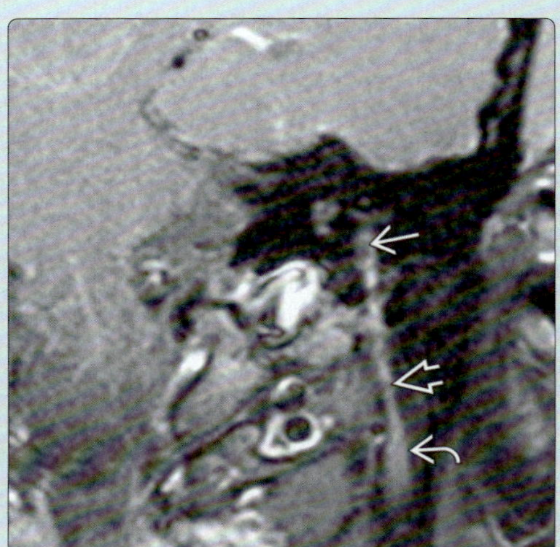

KEY FACTS

TERMINOLOGY

- Facial nerve venous malformation (FNVM)
- Older terms: Facial nerve hemangioma/ossifying hemangioma
- Definition: Benign developmental lesion near intratemporal CNVII in geniculate fossa area

IMAGING

- Bone CT
  - **Honeycomb high-density matrix** lesion (50%)
  - Most commonly located in geniculate fossa
- T1 C+ FS MR
  - Enhancing geniculate ganglion area lesion
  - Usually with irregular margins

TOP DIFFERENTIAL DIAGNOSES

- Normal intratemporal facial nerve enhancement
- Intratemporal facial nerve schwannoma
- Bell palsy
- Perineural parotid malignancy on intratemporal CNVII
- Congenital cholesteatoma within intratemporal CNVII canal

PATHOLOGY

- **Immunohistochemical markers** critical to correct venous malformation (hemangioma) diagnosis
  - Endothelial lining of vascular channels stain negatively for hemangioma-associated markers (**GLUT1 and LeY**)
  - **Podoplanin** staining utilizing D2-40 antibody **negativity** excludes lymphatic malformation

CLINICAL ISSUES

- Intratemporal FNVM produces **peripheral CNVII paralysis** early in its natural history; + SNHL if cochlea involved
  - Caveat: May be described as "**atypical Bell palsy**"
- Treatment: Surgical resection with graft if needed when facial nerve function is poor
  - Final CNVII function depends on duration of preoperative CNVII deficit
  - Smaller lesion are extraneural, larger lesion invade CNVII

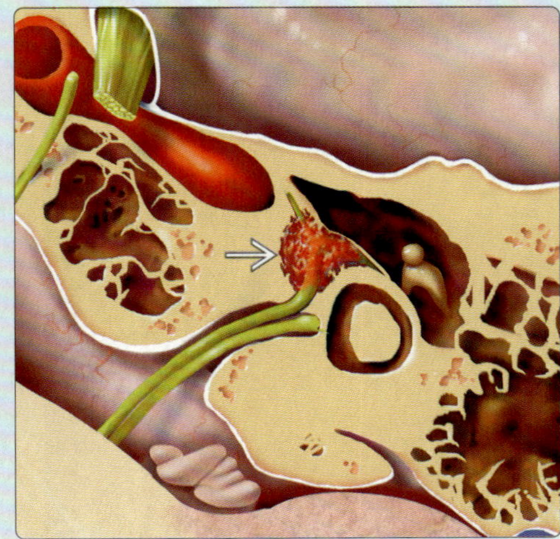

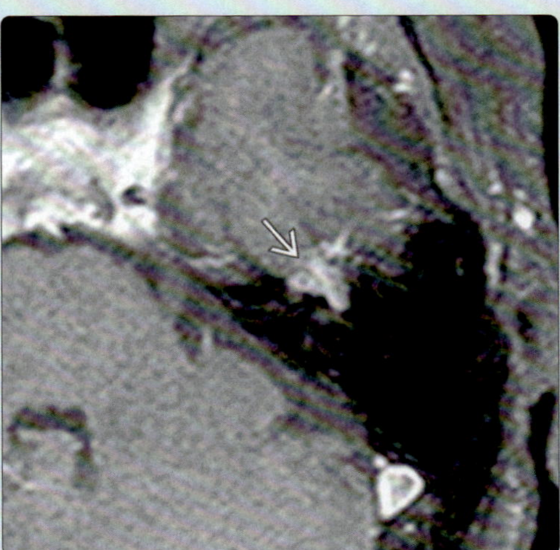

(Left) *Axial graphic illustrates a classic example of a medium-sized facial nerve venous malformation (FNVM) centered in the geniculate fossa ➡ of the temporal bone. Notice the honeycomb bone within the lesion matrix.* **(Right)** *Axial T1 C+ MR with fat saturation in a patient with a left atypical Bell palsy reveals a classic left geniculate fossa enhancing FNVM ➡. Punctate areas of high density on bone CT (not shown) confirmed this imaging impression.*

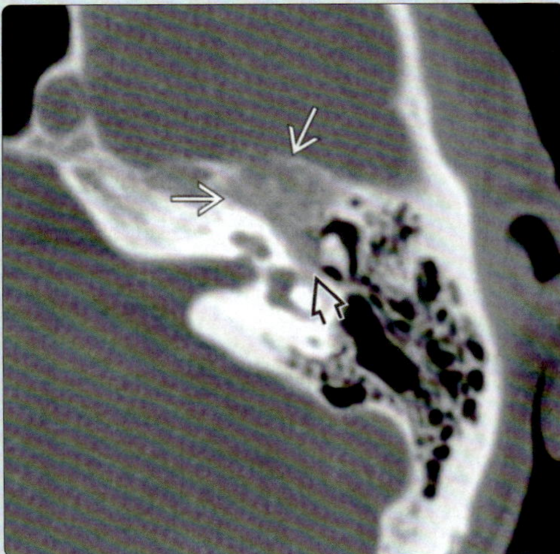

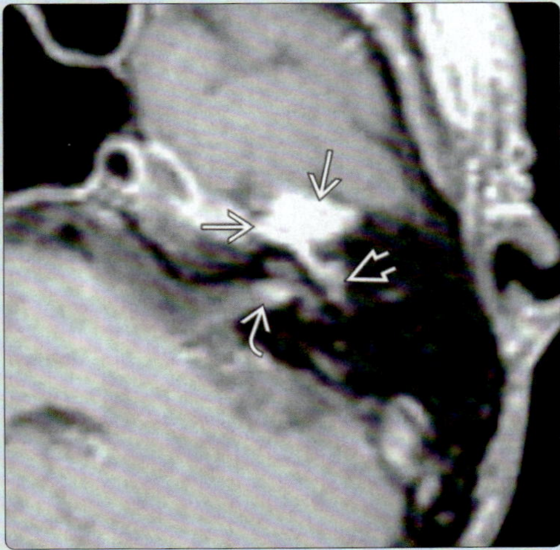

(Left) *Axial bone CT demonstrates the honeycombing appearance of FNVM centered in the geniculate fossa ➡. Note extension of the lesion along the proximal tympanic CNVII segment ➡.* **(Right)** *Axial T1 C+ MR in the same patient shows a poorly marginated, avidly enhancing lesion in the geniculate fossa ➡. Note extension along the tympanic segment of CNVII ➡ and into the fundus of the internal auditory canal (IAC) ➡. IAC extension occurred via the labyrinthine segment of CNVII (not shown).*

KEY FACTS

TERMINOLOGY

- Facial nerve schwannoma (FNS): Rare benign tumor of Schwann cells that invests intratemporal facial nerve (CNVII)

IMAGING

- Temporal bone CT: Tubular mass spanning multiple intratemporal CNVII segments with smooth enlargement of bony CNVII canal
    - **> 90%** of FNS span ≥ 3 intratemporal CNVII segments
- T1 C+ MR: Homogeneously enhancing tubular mass ± intramural cysts
- Temporal bone CT appearance dictated by specific location
    - **Geniculate fossa FNS**: Ovoid smooth enlargement of geniculate fossa with projections into labyrinthine ± anterior tympanic segments of CNVII
    - **Tympanic segment FNS**: Pedunculated FNS emanates from tympanic CNVII into middle ear
        - May displace ossicles laterally
    - **Mastoid segment FNS**: Either tubular with sharp margins or globular with irregular margins (breaks into mastoid air cells); can prolapse to external auditory canal
    - **Greater superficial petrosal nerve (GSPN) schwannoma**: Enlargement of GSPN canal

TOP DIFFERENTIAL DIAGNOSES

- Normal intratemporal FN enhancement
- Bell palsy (herpetic facial paralysis)
- Intratemporal FN venous malformation
- Intratemporal CNVII perineural malignancy

CLINICAL ISSUES

- Symptoms: Hearing loss (70%), CNVII paresis (50%)
- Treatment options
    - Conservative: Observation until facial function worsens > House-Brackmann 3-4/6
    - Surgery: Complete tumor removal with FN graft is goal
    - Radiotherapy: Viable option to control tumor growth

(Left) *Axial graphic shows a tubular facial nerve schwannoma (FNS) involving the labyrinthine ➡ segment, geniculate ganglion ➡, and anterior tympanic segment ➡ of the intratemporal FN.* **(Right)** *Axial T1WI FS enhanced MR through left IAC shows an enhancing FNS involving the fundal ➡, labyrinthine ➡, and geniculate ganglion ➡ portions of the FN.*

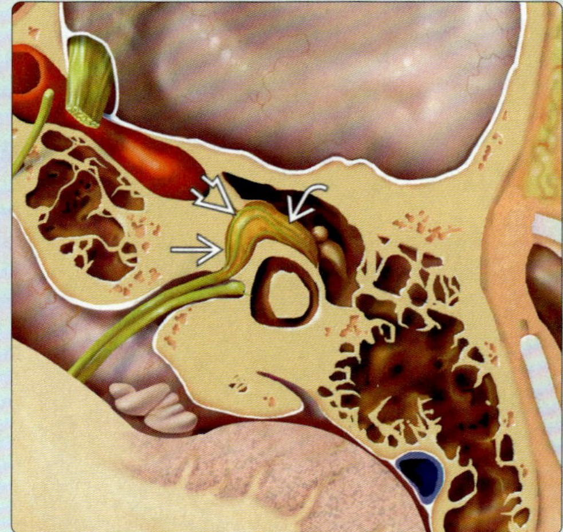

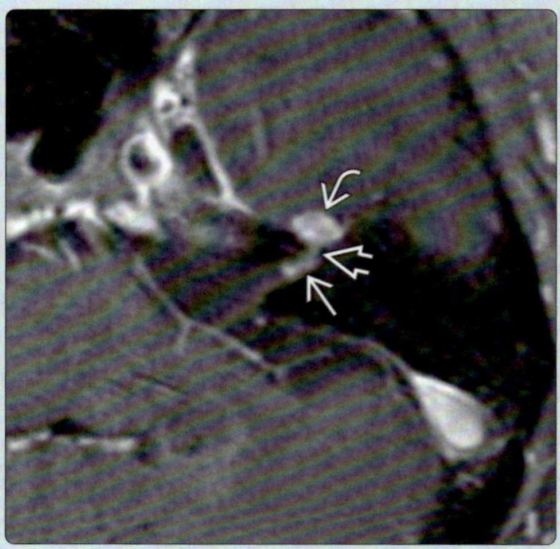

(Left) *Axial bone CT in a patient with CNVII paresis shows tubular enlargement of the distal labyrinthine segment ➡, geniculate fossa ➡, and anterior tympanic segment ➡ of the CNVII canal. Involvement of multiple segments of the FN, as in this case, is highly suggestive of FNS.* **(Right)** *Coronal bone CT in the same patient reveals the FNS involving the midtympanic segment ➡ of the FN. Notice that the FN bony canal "opens" into the middle ear mass ➡.*

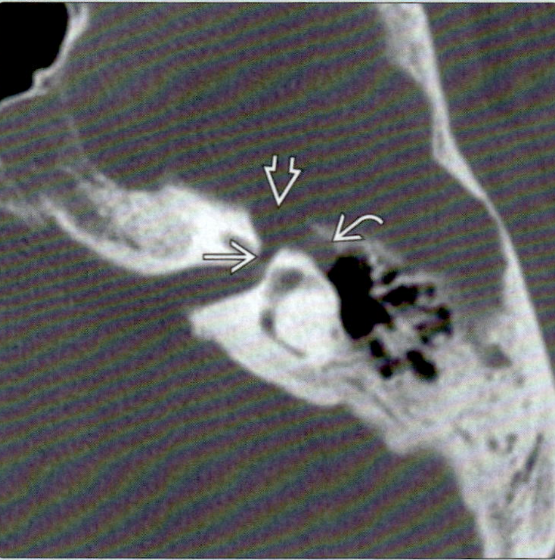

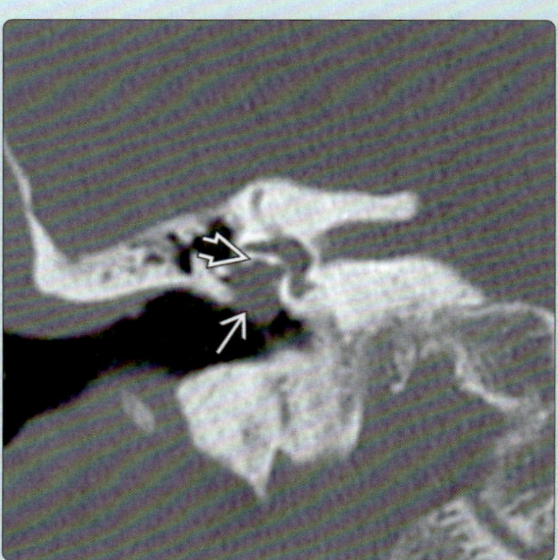

KEY FACTS

TERMINOLOGY

- Perineural tumor (PNT) on CNVII in T-bone: Local extension of malignant tumor along intratemporal CNVII

IMAGING

- Best clue: Poorly circumscribed, enhancing, tubular lesion extending from intraparotid tumor through stylomastoid foramen (SMF) to involve at least mastoid CNVII segment
  - **Contiguous spread** or **skip lesions** along CNVII
  - Image entire CNVII from end organ to brain stem
- T-bone CT findings
  - Intratemporal CNVII PNT may be difficult to detect
  - Mastoid CNVII canal may be slightly enlarged
  - Adjacent air cell opacification
- MR findings
  - Loss of SMF fat best seen on axial T1 MR
  - Axial images best delineate tympanic, geniculate ganglion, & labyrinthine CNVII PNT
  - Coronal & sagittal images through T-bone best show PNT extending through SMF into mastoid CNVII segment

TOP DIFFERENTIAL DIAGNOSES

- Bell palsy
- T-bone CNVII venous malformation ("hemangioma")
- T-bone CNVII schwannoma
- Transmodiolar cochlear nerve schwannoma
- Ramsay Hunt syndrome

CLINICAL ISSUES

- Clinical presentation
  - Asymptomatic (60%) but with imaging findings
  - "All that palsies is not Bell": Gradual, progressive, segmental CNVII paralysis typify PNT
- Treatment options
  - Surgery combined with postoperative radiation therapy
    - Obtain clear margins on nerve, graft if possible
  - 1° radiation therapy for surgically unresectable tumors

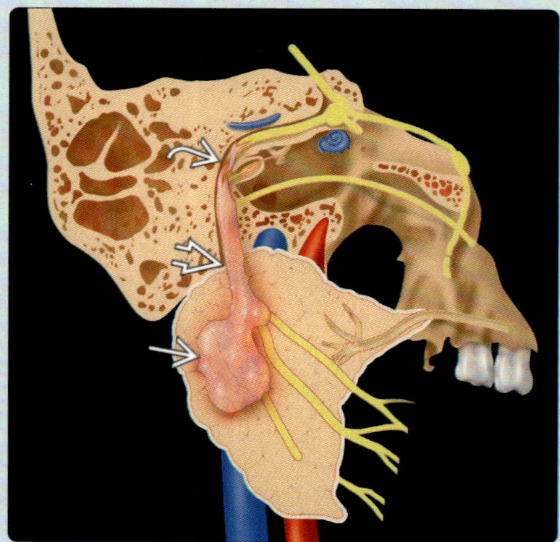

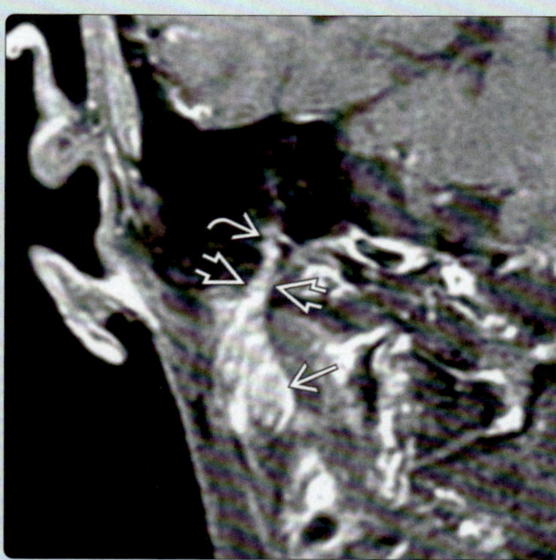

(Left) *Sagittal graphic depicts an intraparotid neoplasm ➡ spreading along CNVII through the stylomastoid foramen ⇨. Note that it travels superiorly on the mastoid segment of CNVII to the posterior genu ↪.* **(Right)** *Coronal T1 C+ FS MR shows parotid adenoid cystic carcinoma ➡ spreading along proximal extracranial CNVII through the stylomastoid foramen ⇨ then up the mastoid segment of CNVII ↪.*

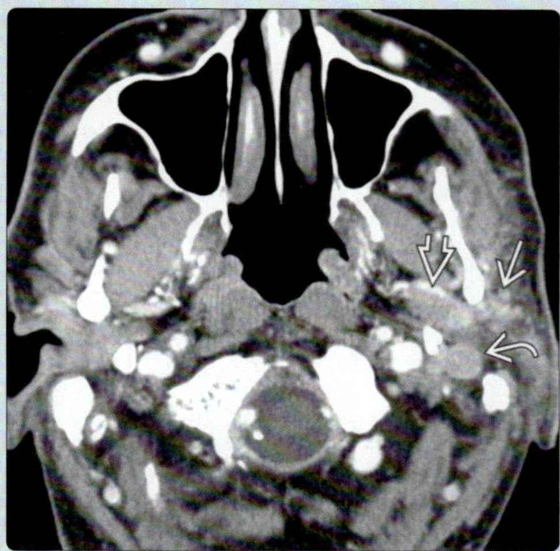

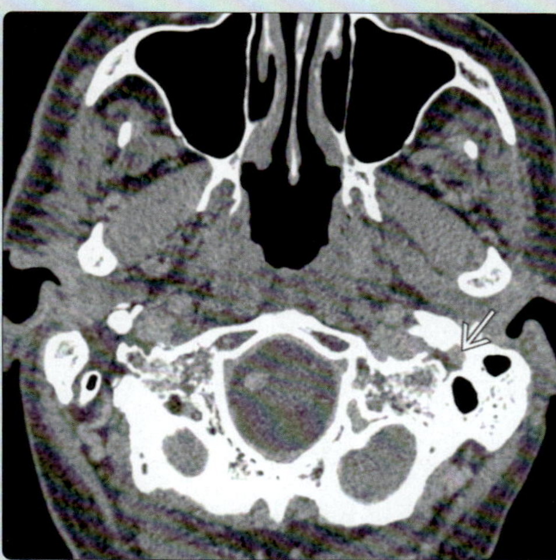

(Left) *Axial CECT shows infiltrating parotid adenoid cystic carcinoma ➡ with perineural spread along the auriculotemporal nerve ⇨. Perineural spread along intraparotid CNVII is seen as a round lesion ↪ in the fat just below the stylomastoid foramen.* **(Right)** *Axial CECT demonstrates an enlarged facial nerve from a perineural tumor ➡ in the left stylomastoid foramen in this patient with primary parotid adenoid cystic carcinoma.*

Temporal Bone CSF Leak

KEY FACTS

TERMINOLOGY

- CSF leak into middle ear (ME) cavity
- Leak of CSF either from congenital or acquired tegmen or inner ear (IE) defect

IMAGING

- Axial bone CT (≤ 1 mm) + coronal reformats
  - Coronal best shows tegmen defect
- Bone CT findings
  - Opacified ME-mastoid air cells
  - Tegmen defect: Isolated or with **cephalocele**
  - Possible associated findings: **Fracture**, **arachnoid granulation** or osseous dural defect, **postsurgical findings**, **IE anomaly, superior semicircular canal dehiscence**
- MR findings if suspect cephalocele
  - T2 coronal: Meningocele (fluid-filled sac) or encephalocele (brain)
  - Extends through tegmen defect into ME
- Imaging recommendations
  - CT: Include all paranasal sinuses & both temporal bones

TOP DIFFERENTIAL DIAGNOSES

- Rhinorrhea without CSF leak
  - Cribriform plate, ethmoid roof, sphenoid sinus walls intact on HRCT; **β2**-transferrin negative
- Otorrhea without CSF leak

CLINICAL ISSUES

- Watery fluid leaking from nose or external auditory canal, often seen after PE tube placement
- Fluid positive for **β2-transferrin** = CSF protein
- **Obesity** with **increased intracranial hypertension** increasing in frequency
  - Spinal tap pressures unreliable while actively leaking
- Treatment: Posttraumatic leak: Bed rest, lumbar drain
  - Middle fossa ± transmastoid approach ± lumbar drain
    - Requires multilayer closure

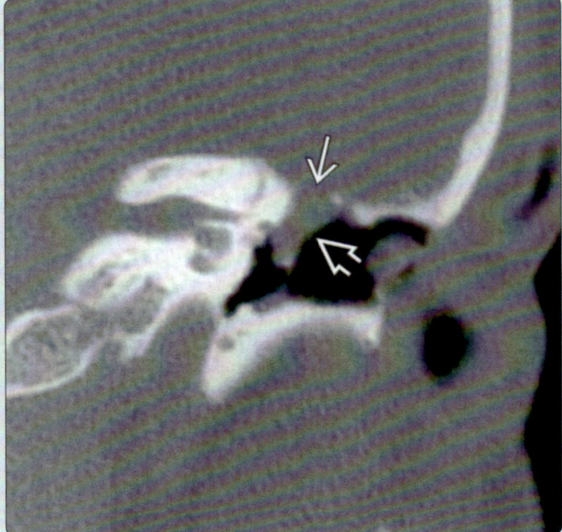

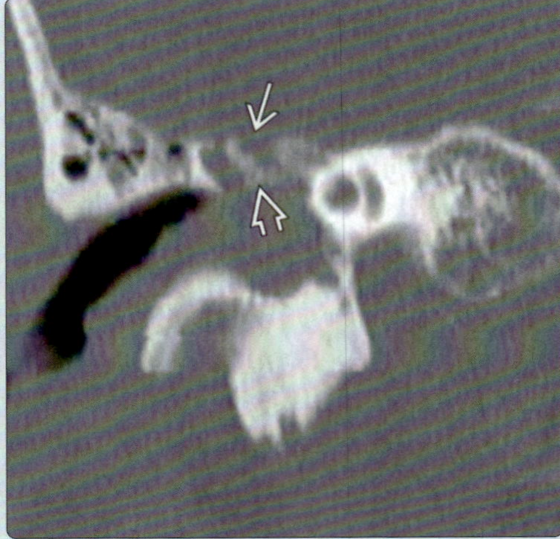

(Left) *Coronal left ear bone CT in patient with CSF leak shows tegmen tympani dehiscence ➡ & cephalocele projecting into the middle ear behind the tympanic membrane ➡. High-resolution coronal T2 MR would determine type of cephalocele.* **(Right)** *Coronal bone CT, right ear, reveals a comminuted posttraumatic tegmen fracture ➡ with bone fragments ➡ in the epitympanum. Some CSF leaks resolve spontaneously, but a defect this large will likely need surgery. MR can best characterize soft tissue/fluid filling the middle ear.*

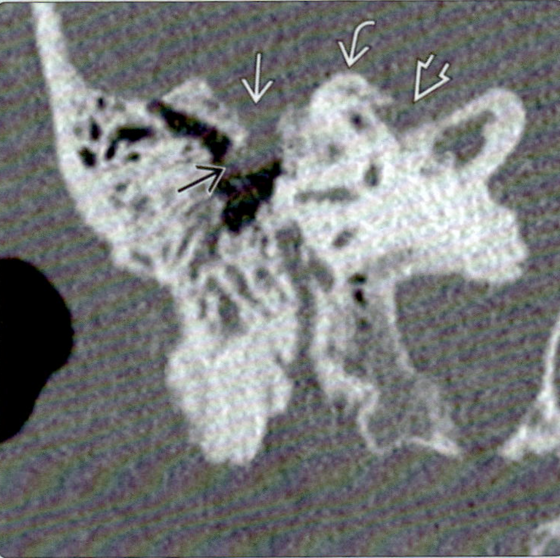

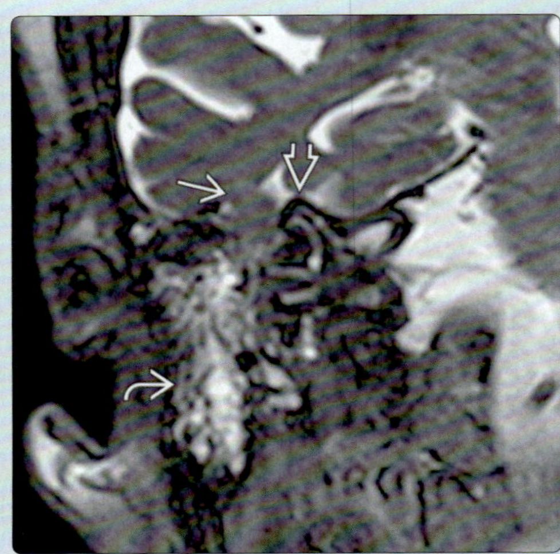

(Left) *Coronal right ear bone CT in an 80 year old with spontaneous CSF leak ➡ shows 2 areas of dehiscence on either side of the arcuate eminence ➡: Lateral tegmen roof dehiscence ➡ & medial petrous apex roof dehiscence ➡.* **(Right)** *Coronal T2WI FS MR in the same patient reveals that tegmen dehiscence lateral to the arcuate eminence ➡ is accompanied by an encephalocele involving a inferior temporal gyrus ➡. Note CSF ➡ high signal in mastoid air cells.*

KEY FACTS

TERMINOLOGY

- Definition: **Nonvenous sinus-related** (aberrant) pseudopodial **pia-arachnoid projection** into tegmen tympani or posterior wall of temporal bone

IMAGING

- Bone CT findings
  - Ovoid/tubular scalloping erosion in temporal bone wall
- MR findings
  - T1 C+: Nonenhancing low signal
  - T2: Homogeneous high signal
- Locations
  - Lateral 1/3 of posterior temporal bone wall
    - Between posterior semicircular canal and anterior margin of sigmoid sinus
  - Tegmen tympani and mastoideum: Hard to see on CT/MR
- Size variation of posterior wall arachnoid granulations (AG)
  - Few millimeters to 2-3 centimeters (**giant AG**)

TOP DIFFERENTIAL DIAGNOSES

- Endolymphatic sac tumor
- Large vestibular aqueduct (incomplete partition type II)
- Skull base dural arteriovenous fistula

PATHOLOGY

- **Temporal bone AG** = form of **aberrant AG**
  - Aberrant AG = AG that penetrates dura but **fails to reach venous sinus**
  - CSF pulsations suspected to enlarge AG causing arachnoid pouch to bulge into temporal bone
    - Idiopathic intracranial hypertension may accelerate

CLINICAL ISSUES

- **Incidental asymptomatic** finding
  - Rarely CSF leak associated ± meningitis
- Posterior wall AG **prevalence ↑ with age**
- On bone CT, posterior wall AG seen in **2.5%** of patients
- Treatment: None, unless CSF leak associated

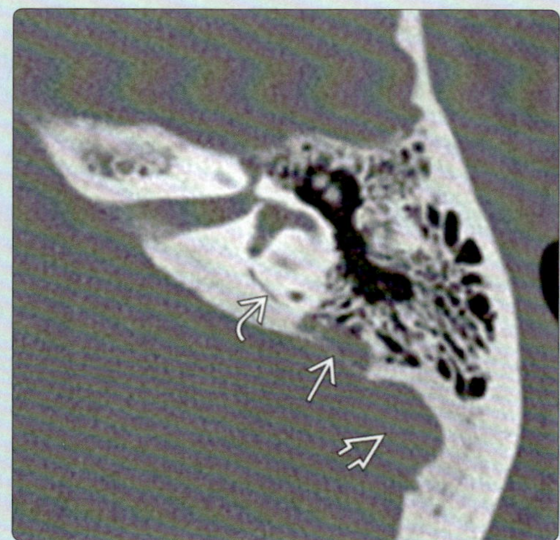

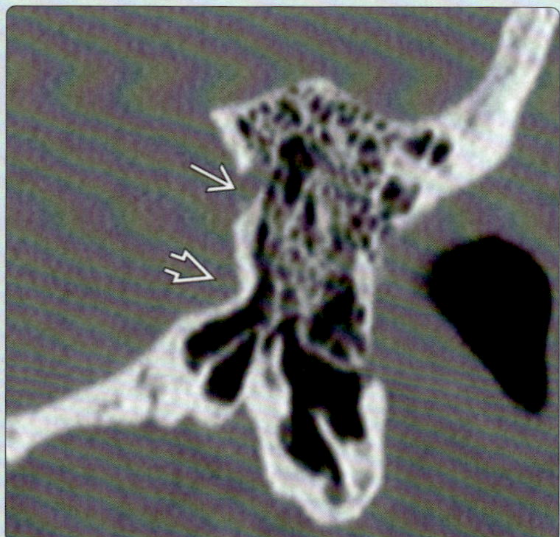

(Left) *Axial bone CT of the left ear in a patient with right ear symptoms shows a medium-sized incidental arachnoid granulation (AG) in the medial mastoid wall ➡ projecting into the mastoid air cells. Note the proximity of the sigmoid sinus ➡ and bony vestibular aqueduct ➡.* **(Right)** *Short-axis oblique bone CT of the left temporal bone reveals a small AG ➡ in the medial mastoid wall. Note that the lesion is on the superior margin of the sigmoid sinus ➡.*

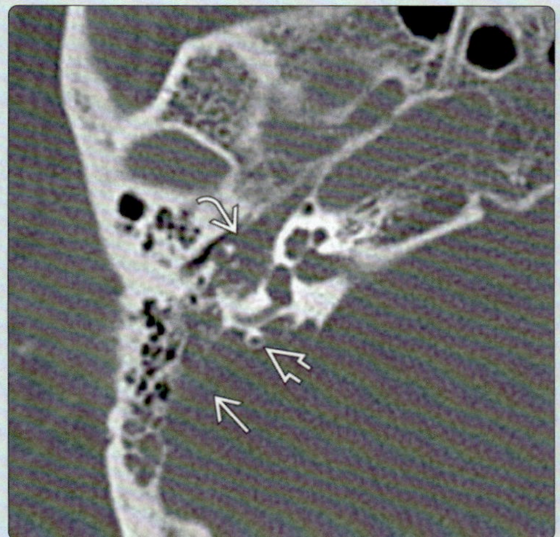

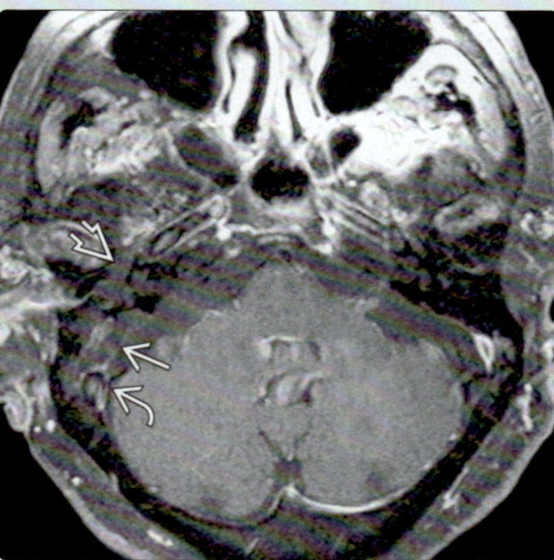

(Left) *Axial bone CT of the right temporal bone in a patient with clinically obvious CSF leak demonstrates a giant AG eroding the medial mastoid wall ➡. The posterior semicircular ➡ canal appears to float in the AG. The middle ear is full of fluid (CSF) ➡.* **(Right)** *Axial T1WI C+ FS MR in the same patient reveals the giant AG ➡ as a lobular fluid signal structure with subtle rim enhancement. The middle ear fluid is low signal ➡. Note the proximity of the sigmoid sinus ➡ to the giant AG.*

Temporal Bone Fibrous Dysplasia

KEY FACTS

TERMINOLOGY

- Fibrous dysplasia (FD) definition: Congenital disorder with **defect in osteoblastic differentiation & maturation** resulting in progressive replacement of normal cancellous bone by mixture of **fibrous tissue** & **immature woven bone**

IMAGING

- Bone CT shows **expansile ground-glass** bony matrix
  - Expansile lesion centered in medullary space with variable attenuation
  - **Pagetoid (mixed) pattern (50%)**: Mixed radiopacity & radiolucency
  - **Sclerotic FD (25%)**: Ground-glass density
  - **Cystic FD (25%)**: Centrally lucent lesions with thinned but sclerotic borders
- T1 MR: Expansile lesion with ↓ signal
- T2 MR: ↓ signal in ossified ± fibrous areas
- T1 C+ FS MR: Diffuse, rim, or no enhancement possible

TOP DIFFERENTIAL DIAGNOSES

- Temporal bone Paget disease
- Skull base giant cell tumor
- Temporal bone meningioma
- Temporal bone metastasis

PATHOLOGY

- Benign **tumor-like lesion** of bone with local arrest of normal structural/architectural development
  - Contains fibrous tissue (spindle cell stroma) with intramural woven bone trabeculae

CLINICAL ISSUES

- Clinical setting: Often asymptomatic lesion when small
  - Young affected (< 30 years old); can be monostotic or polyostotic
  - Polyostotic seen in McCune-Albright syndrome
- History: Most show growth cessation by age 25-30
- Aggressive surgery not recommended in most cases

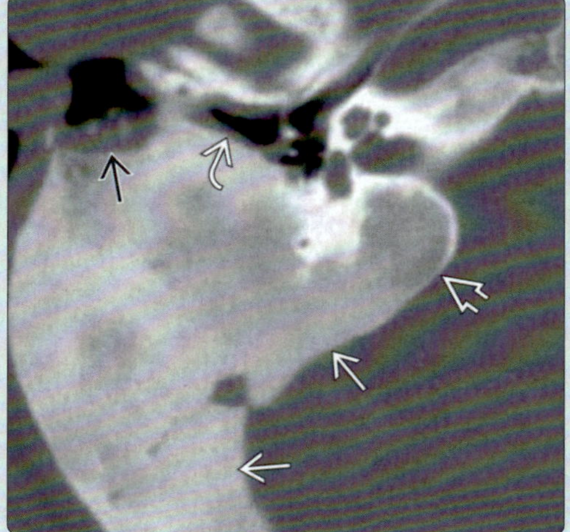

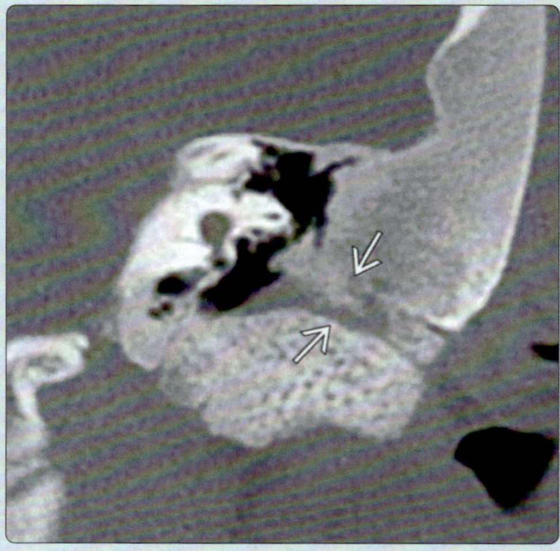

(Left) *Axial bone CT reveals the common sclerotic variety of fibrous dysplasia (FD) involving the mastoid ➡ and inner ear ➡ and encroaching on the posterior middle ear. FD expansion causes external auditory canal (EAC) stenosis ➡. Anterolaterally, note previous biopsy site ⇨.* **(Right)** *Coronal bone CT shows sclerotic FD that has expanded to occlude the EAC ➡. Clinically significant conductive hearing loss can be expected. Otoscopy revealed findings similar to congenital EAC malformation.*

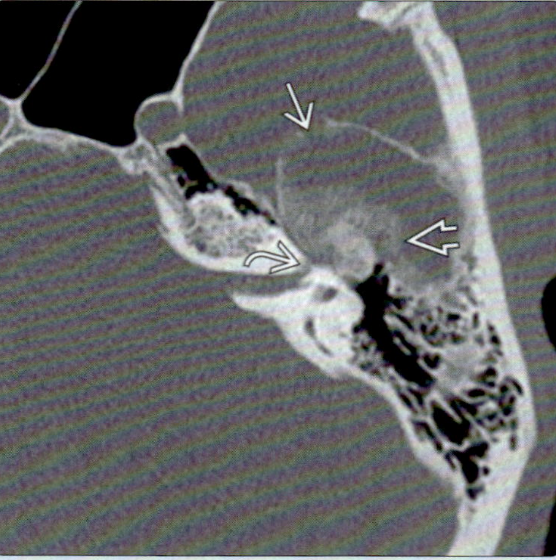

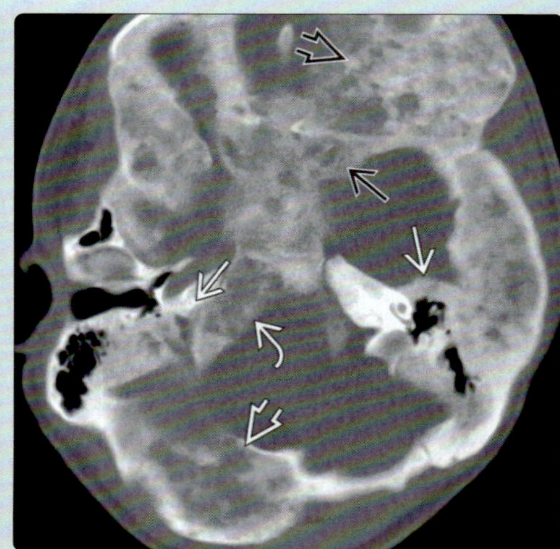

(Left) *Axial left temporal bone CT reveals aggressive-appearing anterior left temporal bone foci of cystic FD ➡. Subtle ground-glass component ➡ is visible within the lesion. Note the labyrinthine segment of the facial nerve canal is visible ➡, but the lesion involves the geniculate fossa.* **(Right)** *Axial bone CT shows polyostotic FD affecting both temporal bones ➡. Multiple other foci are apparent, including the right occipital bone ➡, clivus ➡, sphenoid bone ⇨, and frontal bone ⇨.*

Temporal Bone Paget Disease

KEY FACTS

TERMINOLOGY

- Paget disease (PD) definition: Bone dysplasia characterized by **excessive remodeling** of bone resulting from alternating waves of osteoclastic & osteoblastic activity

IMAGING

- Location of involvement of PD
  - Calvarium > cranial base > temporal bone
- Bone CT
  - Calvarium & cranial base: Diffuse thickening with mixed-density bone
  - Temporal bone: Sclerotic & erosive bone change affecting all areas
    - Includes otic capsule when advanced
  - External auditory canal: Tortuosity & stenosis
  - Middle ear: Middle ear cavity constriction; ossicles & ligaments with pagetoid changes
  - Inner ear/otic capsule: Otic capsule demineralization (peripheral to central) involves all 3 layers
  - Internal auditory canal (IAC): Enlarging bone narrows IAC & compresses CNVII & CNVIII
- MR: Diminished T1 signal of enlarged bones
  - T1 C+ FS: Avid enhancement

TOP DIFFERENTIAL DIAGNOSES

- Temporal bone fibrous dysplasia
- Temporal bone osteoradionecrosis
- Otosclerosis

CLINICAL ISSUES

- Clinical presentation
  - Progressive bilateral mixed hearing loss → deafness
  - Conductive hearing loss: Ossicles & ligaments affected
  - Sensorineural hearing loss: Otic capsule erosions; IAC compression
- Age at presentation
  - > 40 years
  - Compare to < 30 years for fibrous dysplasia

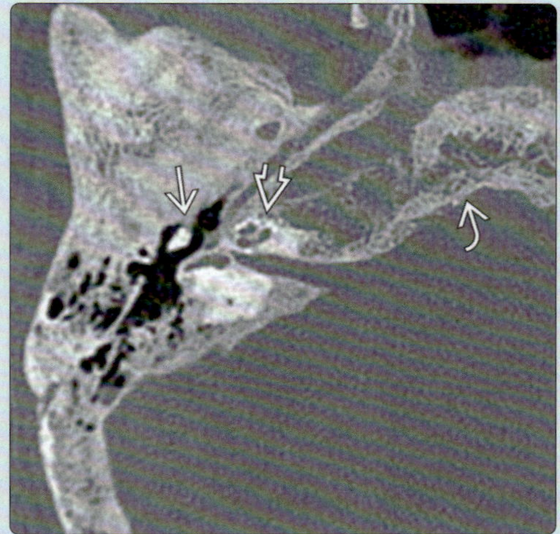

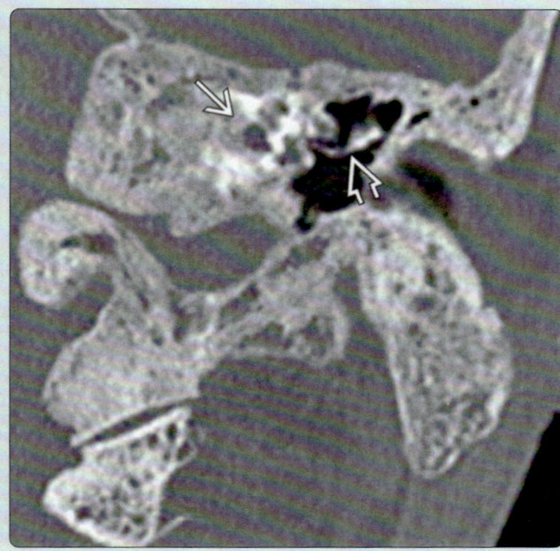

(Left) *Axial right ear temporal bone CT shows Paget disease causing diffusely thickened bones of the clivus ➡, petrous apex, and bones around the middle and inner ear. Notice the thickened ligament ➡ connected to the malleus and the erosion of the otic capsule ➡.* **(Right)** *Coronal bone CT in the opposite ear in the same patient reveals diffuse bony enlargement of all bones of the skull base and temporal bone. Erosive changes ➡ of the otic capsule and thickening of the ossicles ➡ are evident.*

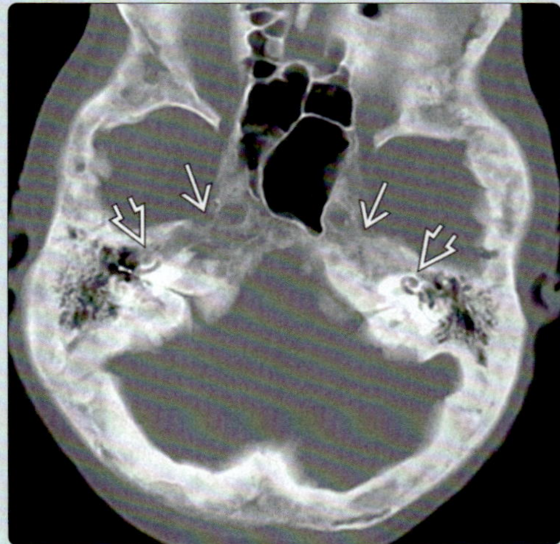

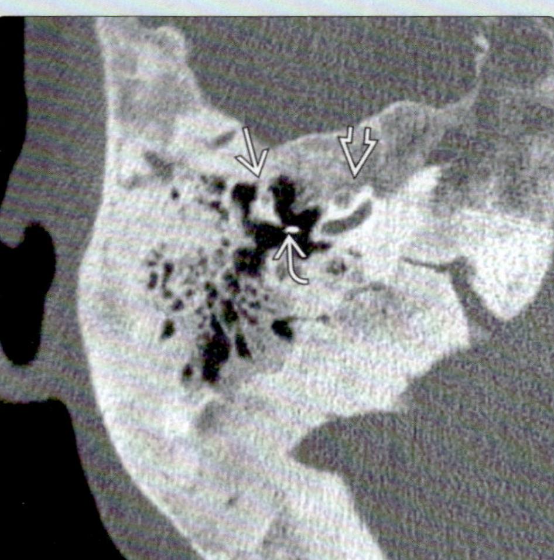

(Left) *Axial bone CT shows diffuse enlarged bones of the skull base with a cotton wool pattern appearance. The petrous apices ➡ are enlarged but demineralized, which indicates that earlier, more active disease is present. The anteromedial otic capsules are eroded ➡.* **(Right)** *Axial bone CT of the right ear in a patient with hearing loss shows malleal ligament ossification ➡ as well as subacute erosive phase of Paget disease affecting the otic capsule ➡. Stapedectomy with stapes prosthesis ➡ had been performed.*

Temporal Bone Langerhans Cell Histiocytosis

KEY FACTS

TERMINOLOGY

- Synonyms: Histiocytosis X
- Old classification: Eosinophilic granuloma, Hand-Schüller-Christian disease, Abt-Letterer-Siwe disease
- Proliferative disorder of Langerhans-type histiocytes, which form granulomas in T-bone & surrounding soft tissues

IMAGING

- Well-defined **lytic lesions** of T-bone with associated enhancing soft tissue masses
  - **Squamous & mastoid bones** > petrous apex
- Both enhanced CT & MR often performed in complex cases
  - Bone CT best for evaluating osseous structures
  - Contrast-enhanced MR best for soft tissue evaluation

TOP DIFFERENTIAL DIAGNOSES

- Coalescent otomastoiditis
- T-Bone rhabdomyosarcoma
- T-Bone metastasis

PATHOLOGY

- Histiocyte proliferation & infiltration; poorly understood
- **New classification system based on risk factors**
  - Multifocal involvement, young age, multiorgan dysfunction, disease relapse

CLINICAL ISSUES

- Otologic symptoms in **25%** of T-bone cases
  - **Conductive hearing loss** ± **otorrhea**
- Presents in **1st decade** of life
- Other symptoms: Otalgia, vertigo, otitis media ± externa, periauricular soft tissue swelling, CNVII palsy, sensorineural hearing loss, aural polyp
- Treatment options
  - Depends on symptoms, location, extent
  - Observation (solitary lesions may spontaneously regress)
  - Surgical curettage or mastoidectomy for localized mastoid-middle ear disease
  - Systemic disease: Chemoradiation therapy

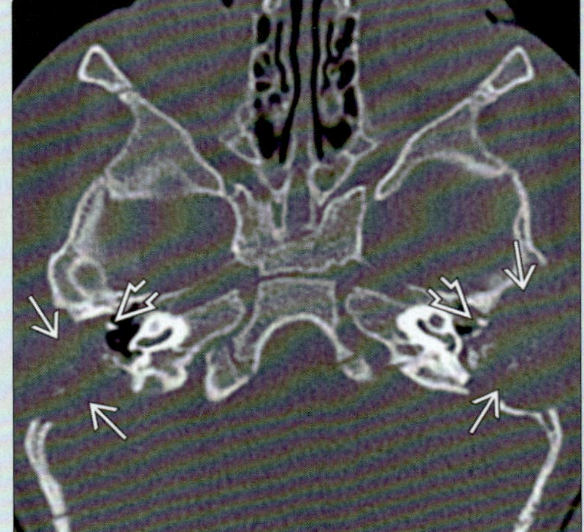

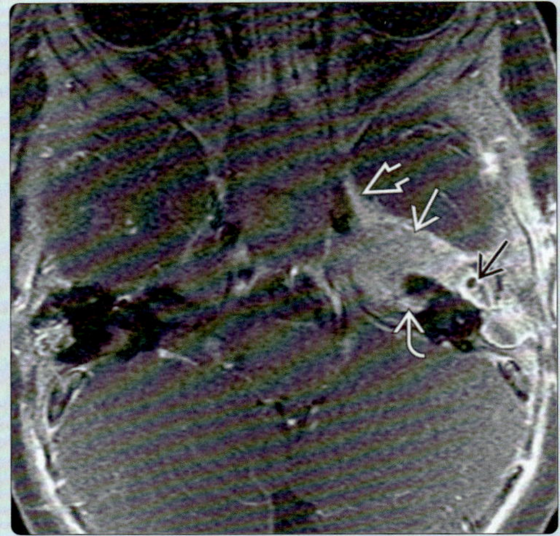

(Left) *Axial bone CT in a 2-year-old girl with bilateral otorrhea shows well-defined destructive lesions of Langerhans cell histiocytosis (LCH) involving bilateral mastoid & left squamous temporal bones ➡, opacified middle ear cavities, & near-complete ossicular destruction ➡. The lesions lack typical aggressive periosteal reaction of metastatic neuroblastoma.* **(Right)** *Axial T1 C+ FS MR shows enhancing LCH extending into the left middle cranial fossa ➡, cavernous sinus ➡, & IAC ➡. Ossicles are encased ➡ by tumor.*

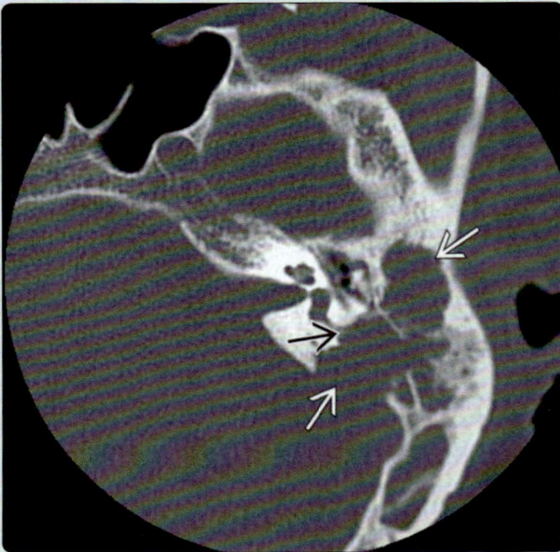

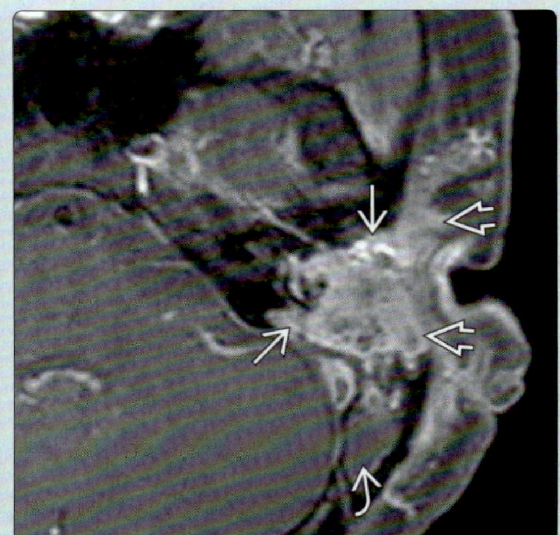

(Left) *Axial bone CT demonstrates sharply punched-out lytic destruction of the left T-bone due to LCH ➡, including involvement of the otic capsule ➡ (which is uncommonly eroded by most processes).* **(Right)** *Axial T1 C+ FS MR shows extensive enhancement within the left T-bone ➡ due to involvement by LCH with extension into the adjacent extracranial soft tissues ➡. Trapped mastoid fluid is noted posteriorly ➡.*

KEY FACTS

TERMINOLOGY

- Hematogenous spread from distant primary neoplasm
- Bony metastatic disease to petrous apex [(PA), most common site] or mastoid/middle ear

IMAGING

- Bone CT
  - Focal **lytic** or **permeative**, rarely **blastic** lesion
  - Commonly other bone metastases are present
  - Subtle appearance in pneumatized portions of T-bone
  - Enhances significantly in most cases
  - CT differentiates benign lesions (fibrous dysplasia, osteoma)
- MR
  - T1: Lesion hypointense to normal fatty marrow
  - T1 C+ FS: Delineates tumor vs. normal fatty marrow

TOP DIFFERENTIAL DIAGNOSES

- Apical petrositis
- Cholesterol granuloma of PA
- Langerhans cell histiocytosis of T-bone
- Plasmacytoma of T-bone

CLINICAL ISSUES

- Often asymptomatic
  - Hearing loss if any symptoms
  - Cranial nerve (CN) palsy (CNVIII > CNVII > CNV or CNVI)
- Breast > lung > renal > prostate cancer origin
- Neuroblastoma and leukemia most common in children
- Often requires systemic (chemo-) therapy; palliative radiation for individual lesions

DIAGNOSTIC CHECKLIST

- Remember background PA marrow/pneumatization is commonly asymmetric
- Isolated T-bone lesion is less likely to be metastasis
- Look for dura, dural venous sinus, and brain invasion
- Include whole-body imaging to eval for other mets

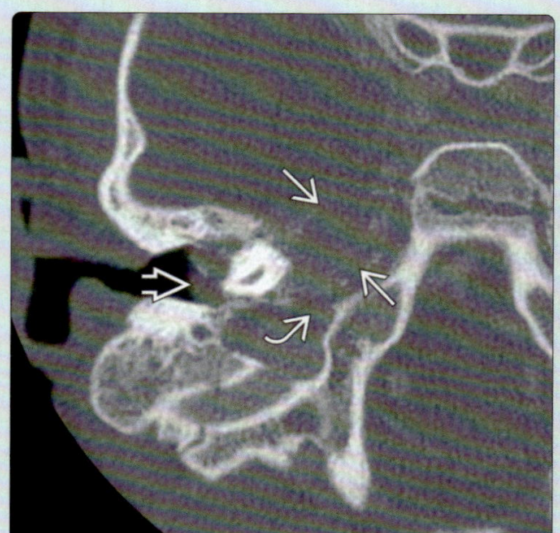

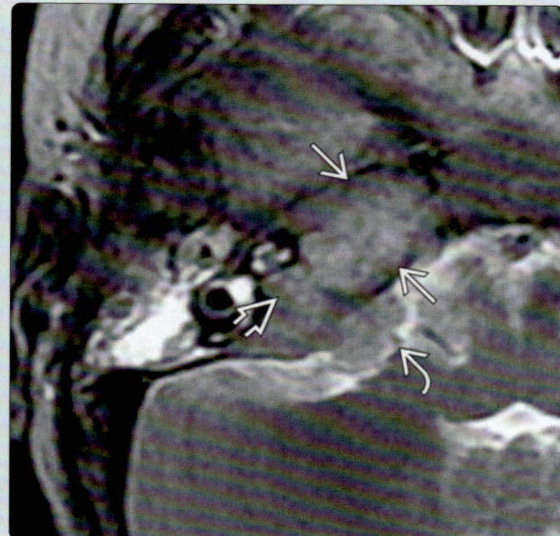

(Left) *T-bone CT in an infant with right CNVII palsy shows permeative, lytic petrous apex destruction ➡ with sparing of the dense otic capsule bone. The neuroblastoma extends into the middle ear cavity ➡ and erodes the anterior wall of the jugular foramen ➡.* **(Right)** *Axial T2WI FS MR in the same patient shows a hypointense petrous apex mass ➡ consistent with cellular tumor. It extends into the right IAC ➡ and CPA ➡. Biopsy revealed neuroblastoma. Subsequent imaging revealed an adrenal primary.*

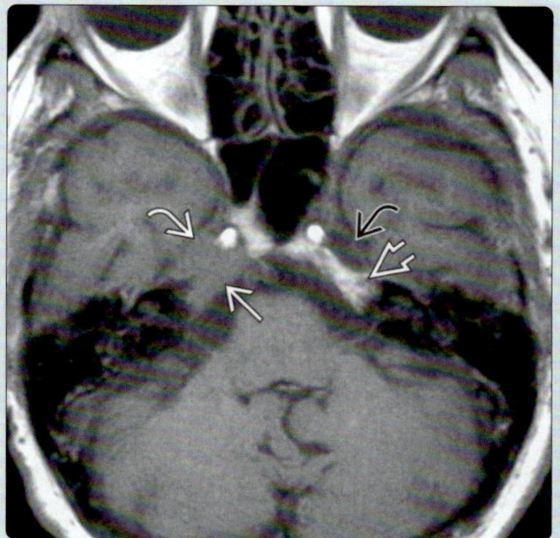

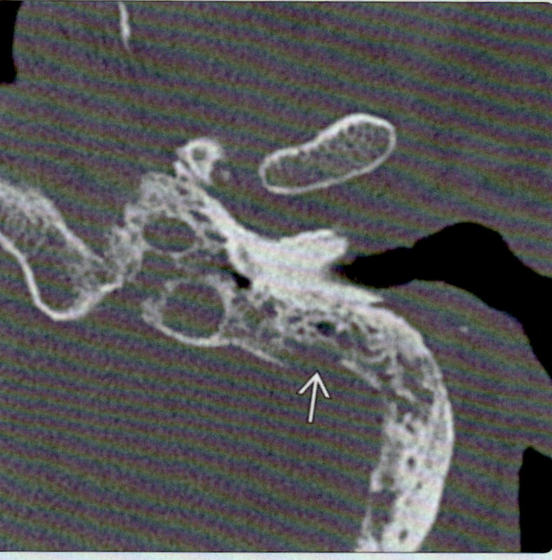

(Left) *Axial T1WI MR shows the typical appearance of right petrous apex metastasis replacing fatty marrow ➡ with expansion into the right Meckel cave ➡ in this patient with right facial numbness. On the left, note the normal marrow signal in the petrous apex ➡ and CSF Meckel cave ➡.* **(Right)** *Osseous mastoid bone metastasis, with cortical destruction of the inner cortex/sigmoid plate ➡, puts the sigmoid sinus at risk for invasion/thrombosis. Smaller metastases are easily missed, secondary to aerated/varied appearance of the T-bone.*

KEY FACTS

TERMINOLOGY

- Radiation therapy (RT)-induced injury to temporal bone

IMAGING

- Bone CT findings
  - **Moth-eaten destruction** of temporal bone and adjacent skull base ± **sequestrum**
- T2 MR findings
  - High-signal mucosal injury of external auditory canal (EAC), middle ear cavity, mastoid
  - High signal of adjacent brain → radiation necrosis
  - Meningitis, abscess, dural sinus thrombosis

TOP DIFFERENTIAL DIAGNOSES

- Malignant external otitis
- Coalescent mastoiditis
- Aggressive cholesteatoma
- EAC carcinoma
- Paget disease

PATHOLOGY

- **Avascular bone necrosis** from **obliterative endarteritis**
- Susceptible to infection, which accelerates ORN

CLINICAL ISSUES

- Presentation: Otalgia, otorrhea, hearing loss after RT
- Occurs few months to many years post RT (> 60 Gy)
  - Most common in setting of regional RT for parotid, EAC, or nasopharynx carcinoma
- Treatment options
  - Conservative management: 1st-line option
  - Surgical management and adjuvant therapy as indicated; may require subtotal petrosectomy
  - Pentoxifylline, vitamin E, and clodronate (PENTOCLO) for prevention and treatment

DIAGNOSTIC CHECKLIST

- CT for bone changes, extent of involvement; MR for complications

(Left) *Axial bone CT reveals abnormal soft tissue ➡ filling the left external auditory canal (EAC) and mastoid air cells with obvious destruction of the posterior EAC wall and mastoid septations ➡. Note mixed sclerotic and lytic ➡ bone. These findings represent the classic appearance of temporal bone osteoradionecrosis.* **(Right)** *Axial bone CT shows radiation-induced necrosis of the bony EAC ➡ and confluent destruction of mastoid air cells. Note "floating" bony sequestrum ➡, all indicating severe osteoradionecrosis.*

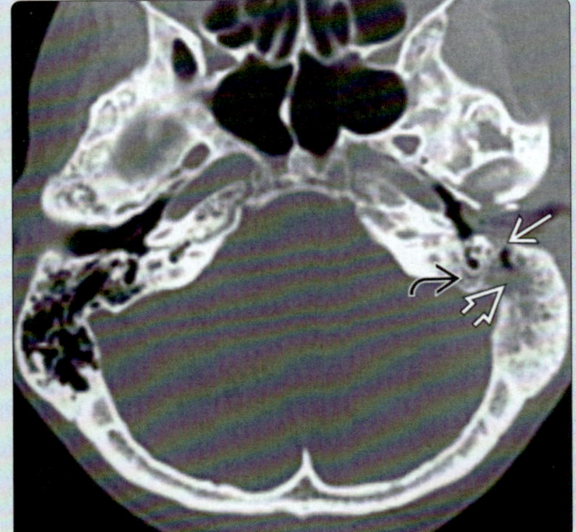

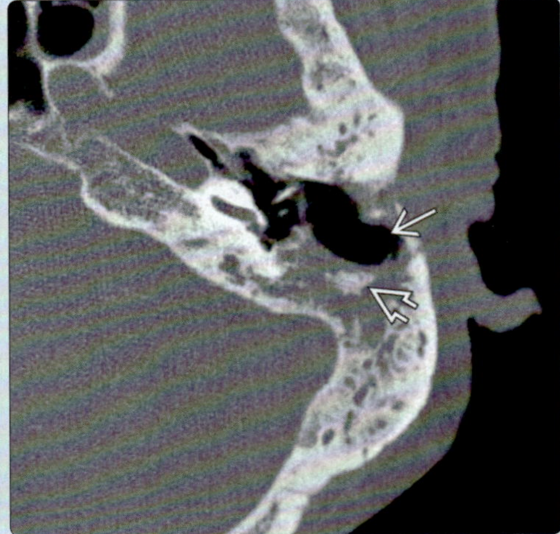

(Left) *Axial bone CT shows diffuse opacification of the middle ear and mastoid in association with permeative-destructive bony changes in this previously radiated patient. Focal bone necrosis is seen in the petrous bone ➡ and lateral mastoid cortex ➡.* **(Right)** *Axial T1 C+ FS MR in a previously radiated patient reveals nonspecific enhancing tissue in the middle ear ➡, mastoid ➡, and petrous apex ➡. Although radiation changes can be suggested by MR, osteoradionecrosis of bone is a diagnosis best made by temporal bone CT.*

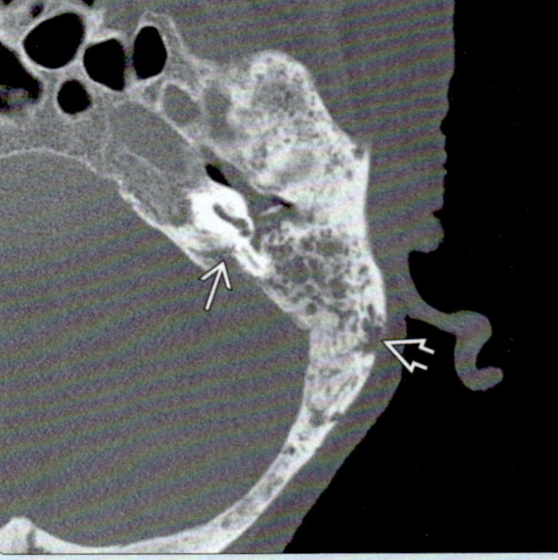

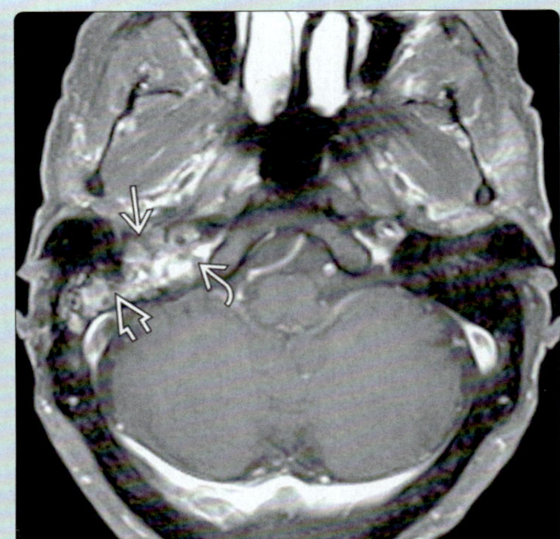

TERMINOLOGY

Abbreviations

- Osteoradionecrosis (ORN)

Synonyms

- Radiation osteitis, radiation necrosis, irradiation osteomyelitis, avascular bone necrosis

Definitions

- Radiation-induced injury to temporal bone
  - Localized (more common): Limited to external auditory canal (EAC)
  - Diffuse: Involves mastoid septations and middle ear cavity (MEC), possibly skull base

IMAGING

General Features

- Best diagnostic clue
  - Bone CT shows moth-eaten demineralization and destruction of temporal bone ± sequestrum

CT Findings

- CECT
  - Mucosal involvement may enhance
  - Contrast not needed to make diagnosis
- Bone CT
  - Diffuse mucosal thickening in EAC, MEC, and mastoid
  - **Permeative bone destruction** ± **sequestrum**

MR Findings

- T2WI
  - Nonspecific high signal in EAC, MEC, and mastoid
  - High-signal adjacent brain indicates **cerebral radiation necrosis**
- T1WI C+
  - Variable enhancement in osteitic bone
  - Mucosal injury will enhance

Imaging Recommendations

- Best imaging tool
  - Temporal bone CT
- Protocol advice
  - Thin-section axial and coronal bone CT
  - MR for complications
    - Cerebral radiation injury
    - Meningitis or abscess
    - Dural sinus thrombosis

DIFFERENTIAL DIAGNOSIS

Necrotizing External Otitis

- Immunocompromised, often diabetic patient; no radiation history
- EAC soft tissue and bone infection

Coalescent Mastoiditis

- Disruption of mastoid septa in acute/chronic otomastoiditis

Aggressive Cholesteatoma

- Cholesteatoma seen at otoscopy; no radiation history
- CT: Otic capsule invasion late finding

Paget Disease

- Bilateral sensorineural hearing loss
- Entire cranial base usually involved

EAC Carcinoma

- Skin lesion of EAC
- No prior radiation therapy (RT)

PATHOLOGY

General Features

- Etiology
  - Radiation dose > 60 Gy
  - **Avascular bone necrosis** from obliterative endarteritis
  - Susceptible to infection, which accelerates ORN
- Temporal bone at higher risk for ORN
  - Poorly vascularized bone
  - Thin protective overlying soft tissue
  - Exposure to respiratory pathogens via eustachian tube

Gross Pathologic & Surgical Features

- **Dead bone** and **soft tissue fibrosis**

CLINICAL ISSUES

Presentation

- Most common signs/symptoms
  - Purulent, foul-smelling otorrhea with spicules of exposed bone
  - Hearing loss
- Intracranial complications
  - Meningitis, abscess, sinus thrombosis, CSF leak

Natural History & Prognosis

- Occurs few months to many years post RT
  - More commonly in setting of parotid, EAC, or nasopharynx cancer
- Mastoid air cell destruction: Poor prognostic indicator

Treatment

- Conservative: Initial management for most patients
  - Local debridement of EAC
  - Antibiotics; otic prep (may need systemic treatment)
  - Pentoxifylline, vitamin E, and clodronate (PENTOCLO)
- Surgical: If conservative management fails
  - **Resect all necrotic tissue** ± repair with vascularized flap
  - Adjuvant PENTOCLO ± hyperbaric oxygen

DIAGNOSTIC CHECKLIST

Image Interpretation Pearls

- CT for bone changes; MR for soft tissue complications

SELECTED REFERENCES

1. Glicksman JT et al: Pentoxifylline-tocopherol-clodronate combination: a novel treatment for osteoradionecrosis of the temporal bone. Head Neck. 37(12):E191-3, 2015
2. Kammeijer Q et al: Treatment outcomes of temporal bone osteoradionecrosis. Otolaryngol Head Neck Surg. 152(4):718-23, 2015
3. Ahmed S et al: CT findings in temporal bone osteoradionecrosis. J Comput Assist Tomogr. 38(5):662-6, 2014

Terminology

The contents of the cerebellopontine angle (CPA) and internal auditory canal (IAC) cisterns include the facial nerve (CNVII), the vestibulocochlear nerve (CNVIII), and the anterior inferior cerebellar artery (AICA) loop. The bony IAC, its fundal crests (vertical and horizontal), and its opening in the porus acusticus are also included as part of this discussion.

Embryology

The temporal bone forms as 3 distinct embryological events: (1) The external and middle ear, (2) the inner ear, and (3) the IAC. The practical implications of these 3 related, but distinct, embryological events are that the presence or absence of the IAC is independent of the development of the inner, middle, or external ear.

The IAC develops in response to formation and migration of the facial and vestibulocochlear nerves through this area. IAC size depends on the number of migrating nerve bundles. The fewer the nerve bundles, the smaller the IAC. If the IAC is very small and only 1 nerve is seen, it is usually the facial nerve.

Imaging Anatomy of Cochlea-IAC-CPA

The cochlear nerve portion of the vestibulocochlear nerve begins in the modiolus of the cochlea where the bipolar **spiral ganglia** are found. Distally projecting axons reach the organ of Corti within the scala media. Proximally projecting axons coalesce to form the cochlear nerve itself within the fundus of the IAC.

CNVIII in the IAC and CPA cisterns is made up of vestibular (balance) and cochlear (hearing) components. The cochlear nerve is located in the anteroinferior quadrant of the IAC. In the region of the porus acusticus, the cochlear nerve joins the superior and inferior vestibular nerve bundles to become the vestibulocochlear nerve in the CPA cistern.

The vestibulocochlear nerve crosses the CPA cistern as the posterior nerve bundle (CNVII is the anterior nerve bundle) to enter the brainstem at the junction of the medulla and pons. The entering cochlear nerve fibers pierce the brainstem and bifurcate to form synapses with both the **dorsal** and the **ventral cochlear nuclei**. These 2 nuclei are found on the lateral surface of the inferior cerebellar peduncle. Their location can be accurately determined by looking at high-resolution T2 axial images and identifying the contour of the inferior cerebellar peduncle. The entering vestibular nerve fibers divide into 4 branches to form synapses with the superior, inferior, medial, and lateral nuclei. The vestibular nuclei are clustered in the inferior cerebellar peduncle just anteromedial to the cochlear nuclei.

Remembering the normal orientation of nerves within the IAC cistern is assisted by the mnemonic "7-Up, Coke down." CNVII is found in the anterosuperior quadrant, whereas the cochlear nerve is confined to the anteroinferior quadrant. Given this information, it is simple to remember that the superior vestibular nerve (SVN) is posterosuperior, while the inferior vestibular nerve (IVN) is posteroinferior.

Other normal structures to be aware of in the IAC include the **horizontal or transverse crest** (crista falciformis) and the **vertical crest** ("Bill bar"). The horizontal crest is a medially projecting horizontal bony shelf in the IAC fundus that separates the CNVII and SVN above from the cochlear nerve and IVN below. The vertical crest is found between CNVII and the SVN along the superior fundal bony wall. The horizontal crest is easily seen on both bone CT and high-resolution MR. The vertical crest is more readily seen on bone CT.

Openings from the IAC fundus into the inner ear are numerous. The largest is the anteroinferior **cochlear nerve canal**, which conveys the cochlear nerve from the modiolus to the IAC fundus. Anterosuperiorly, the **meatal foramen** opens into the labyrinthine segment of CNVII. The **macula cribrosa** is the multiply perforated bone that separates the vestibule of the inner ear from the IAC fundus.

Other nonneural normal anatomy of interest in the CPA cistern includes the AICA loop, flocculus, and choroid plexus. The **AICA** arises from the basilar artery, courses superolaterally into the CPA cistern, and then travels into the IAC cistern. Within the IAC, the AICA feeds the internal auditory artery of the cochlea. The AICA loop in the IAC or CPA cisterns may mimic a cranial nerve bundle on high-resolution T2WI MR. AICA vascular territory includes the cochlea, flocculus of the cerebellum, and anterolateral pons in the area of cranial nerve nuclei for CNV, CNVII, and CNVIII. The **flocculus** is a lobule of the cerebellum that projects into the posterolateral CPA cistern, and **can sometimes be mistaken for a CPA mass**. The 4th ventricle **choroid plexus** typically passes through the foramen of Luschka in the CPA cistern.

Imaging Techniques & Indications

The principal clinical indication requiring clinicians to examine the CPA-IAC is **sensorineural hearing loss (SNHL)**. Three principal parameters must be satisfied when completing the MR study in SNHL: (1) Use contrast-enhanced T1 fat-saturated thin-section sequences through the CPA-IAC to identify enhancing lesions in this location, (2) utilize high-resolution T2-weighted sequences to answer presurgical questions when a mass lesion is found, and (3) screen the brain for intraaxial causes, such as multiple sclerosis.

The gold standard for imaging patients with acquired SNHL is enhanced thin-section (≤ 3 mm) axial and coronal fat-saturated MR through the CPA-IAC. With these enhanced sequences, it is highly unlikely that a lesion causing SNHL will be missed. Be sure to obtain an axial or coronal precontrast T1 sequence and use fat saturation when contrast is applied to avoid the rare but troublesome mistake of calling a CPA-IAC lipoma a vestibular schwannoma. In the absence of fat saturation, the inherent high signal of lipoma will appear to enhance, leading to the misdiagnosis of vestibular schwannoma.

High-resolution T2-weighted thin-section (≤ 1 mm) MR sequences (CISS, FIESTA, T2 space) in the axial and coronal planes can be used as a screening exam without contrast to identify patients with mass lesions in the CPA-IAC area or for serial imaging for patients with known vestibular schwannomas. However, these sequences are currently more commonly used as supplements when a vestibular schwannoma is found on the enhanced T1 sequences to answer specific surgically relevant questions: What size is the fundal cap? What is the nerve of origin? Does the lesion enter the cochlear foramen?

Whenever MR is ordered for SNHL, remember to include whole-brain FLAIR, GRE, and DWI sequences. FLAIR will identify the rare multiple sclerosis patient presenting with SNHL as well as other intraaxial causes. GRE will demonstrate micro- or macrohemorrhage within a vestibular schwannoma and may help with aneurysm diagnosis when blooming of

CPA Mass Differential Diagnosis

Pseudolesions	Vascular
Asymmetric cerebellar flocculus	Aneurysm (vertebrobasilar, posterior and anterior inferior cerebellar artery)
Asymmetric choroid plexus	Arteriovenous malformation
High jugular bulb	**Benign tumor**
Jugular bulb diverticulum	Choroid plexus papilloma
Marrow foci around internal auditory canal	Facial nerve schwannoma
Congenital	Hemangioblastoma, cerebellum
Arachnoid cyst	Internal auditory canal hemangioma (venous malformation)
Epidermoid cyst	Meningioma
Lipoma	Vestibular schwannoma
Neurofibromatosis type 2	**Malignant tumor**
Infectious	Brainstem glioma, pedunculated
Cysticercosis	Ependymoma, pedunculated
Meningitis	Melanotic schwannoma
Inflammatory	Metastases, systemic or subarachnoid spread ("drop")
Idiopathic intracranial pseudotumor	
Sarcoidosis	

blood products or calcium in an aneurysm wall is seen. When **DWI** shows restricted diffusion in a CPA mass, the diagnosis of **epidermoid** is easily made.

Approaches to Imaging Issues of CPA-IAC

Approach to Sensorineural Hearing Loss in Adult

Asymmetric SNHL in an otherwise healthy adult is evaluated with an enhanced thin-section fat-saturated T1WI MR of the CPA-IAC area, with high-resolution T2WI sequences providing help in surgical planning if a lesion is identified. Despite audiometric and brainstem-evoked response testing, positive MR studies for lesions causing the SNHL are infrequent (< 5% even in highly screened patient groups). **Vestibular schwannoma** is by far the most common cause of asymmetric SNHL (~ 90% of lesions found with MR). It is important for the clinician to become familiar with the wide range of appearances of vestibular schwannoma, including intramural cystic change, micro- and macroscopic hemorrhage, and associated arachnoid cyst.

Meningioma, epidermoid cyst, and CPA aneurysm are responsible for ~ 8% of lesions found in adult patients with asymmetric SNHL. A long list of rare lesions, including facial nerve, labyrinthine and jugular foramen schwannomas, IAC hemangioma, CPA metastases, labyrinthitis, sarcoidosis, lipoma, and superficial siderosis, make up < 2% of lesions causing unilateral SNHL in an adult that are found by MR.

Approach to Sensorineural Hearing Loss in Child

When a child presents with unilateral or bilateral SNHL, the emphasis in the imaging work-up veers away from the typical adult tumor causes. Instead, congenital inner ear or CPA-IAC lesions are sought as the cause of the hearing loss. Complications of suppurative labyrinthitis (labyrinthine ossificans) are also included in the differential diagnosis.

When the child's presentation is bilateral profound SNHL, imaging is usually obtained as part of the work-up for possible **cochlear implantation**. High-resolution T2 MR imaging is obtained in the axial and **oblique sagittal** planes to look for inner ear anomalies and labyrinthine ossificans as well as the presence or absence and size of a cochlear nerve in the IAC. If complex congenital inner ear disease is found, bone CT is often obtained to further define the inner ear fluid spaces and look for an absent cochlear nerve canal.

In reviewing the MR and CT in a child with SNHL, it is important to accurately describe any inner ear congenital anomaly, if present. If there is a history of meningitis, labyrinthine ossificans may be present. Look for bony encroachment on the fluid spaces of the inner ear. In particular, make sure the basal turn of the cochlea is open because occlusion by bony plaque may thwart successful cochlear implantation. Check the T2 oblique sagittal MR images for the presence of a normal cochlear nerve. If absent, cochlear implantation results may be negatively affected. Finally, look carefully at the IAC and CPA for signs of epidermoid cyst (restricted diffusion on DWI), lipoma (high signal on T1 precontrast sequences), and neurofibromatosis type 2 (bilateral CPA-IAC vestibular or facial schwannoma).

Selected References

1. Giesemann AM et al: The vestibulocochlear nerve: aplasia and hypoplasia in combination with inner ear malformations. Eur Radiol. 22(3):519-24, 2012
2. Burmeister HP et al: Identification of the nervus intermedius using 3T MR imaging. AJNR Am J Neuroradiol. 32(3):460-4, 2011
3. Sheth S et al: Appearance of normal cranial nerves on steady-state free precession MR images. Radiographics. 29(4):1045-55, 2009
4. Trimble K et al: Computed tomography and/or magnetic resonance imaging before pediatric cochlear implantation? Developing an investigative strategy. Otol Neurotol. 28(3):317-24, 2007
5. Rabinov JD et al: Virtual cisternoscopy: 3D MRI models of the cerebellopontine angle for lesions related to the cranial nerves. Skull Base. 14(2):93-9; discussion 99, 2004
6. Daniels RL et al: Causes of unilateral sensorineural hearing loss screened by high-resolution fast spin echo magnetic resonance imaging: review of 1,070 consecutive cases. Am J Otol. 21(2):173-80, 2000
7. Schmalbrock P et al: Assessment of internal auditory canal tumors: a comparison of contrast-enhanced T1-weighted and steady-state T2-weighted gradient-echo MR imaging. AJNR Am J Neuroradiol. 20(7):1207-13, 1999

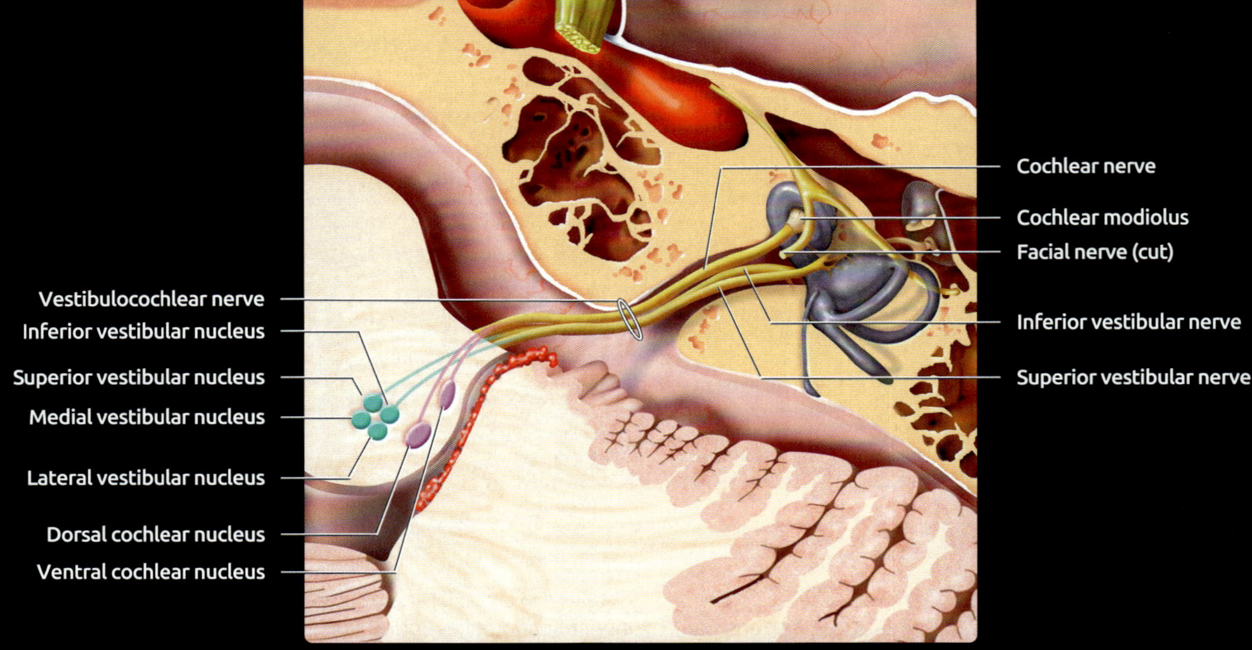

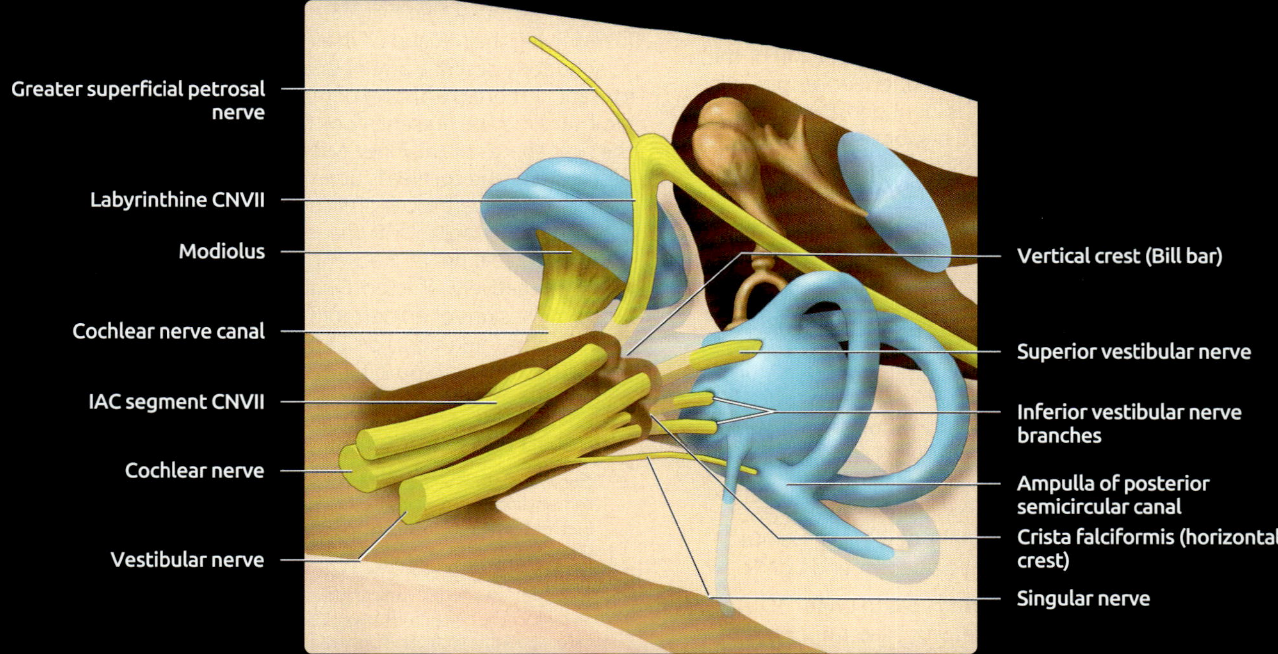

(Top) *Axial graphic depicts the vestibulocochlear nerve (CNVIII). The cochlear component of CNVIII begins in bipolar cell bodies within the spiral ganglion in the modiolus. Central fibers run in the cochlear nerve to the dorsal and ventral cochlear nuclei on the lateral margin of the inferior cerebellar peduncle. Inferior and superior vestibular nerves begin in cell bodies in the vestibular ganglion; from there, they course centrally to 4 vestibular nuclei.* **(Bottom)** *Graphic shows the normal facial nerve and vestibulocochlear nerve in the internal auditory canal (IAC) and temporal bone. Notice that by the mid IAC, there are 4 main nerves present, including the facial, cochlear, superior vestibular, and inferior vestibular nerves. The singular nerve branches off the inferior vestibular nerve midway through the IAC on its way to the ampulla of the posterior semicircular canal. Multiple inferior vestibular nerve branches pierce the macular cribrosa, as does the superior vestibular nerve, on their way to the vestibule.*

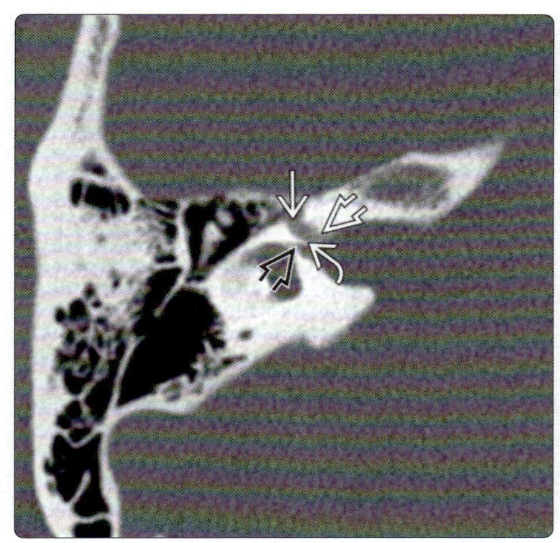

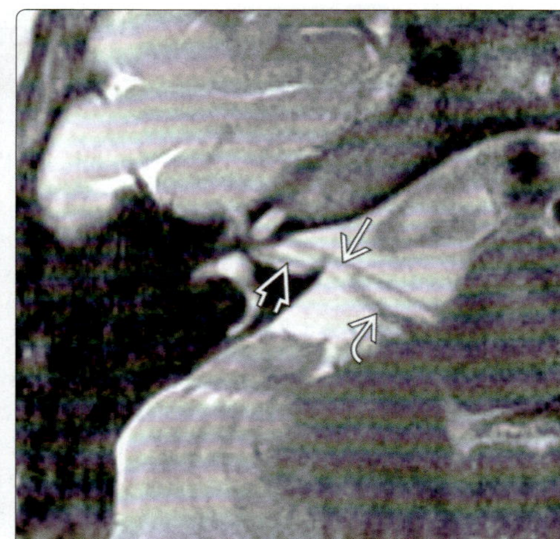

(Left) *Axial bone CT through the superior IAC reveals the labyrinthine segment of CNVII ➡, the meatal foramen ➡, the vertical crest ➡, and the superior vestibular nerve ➡ connecting the IAC to the vestibule through the macula cribrosa.* **(Right)** *Axial T2WI MR through the superior IAC shows the anterosuperior CNVII ➡, the superior vestibular nerve ➡, and the vestibulocochlear nerve ➡.*

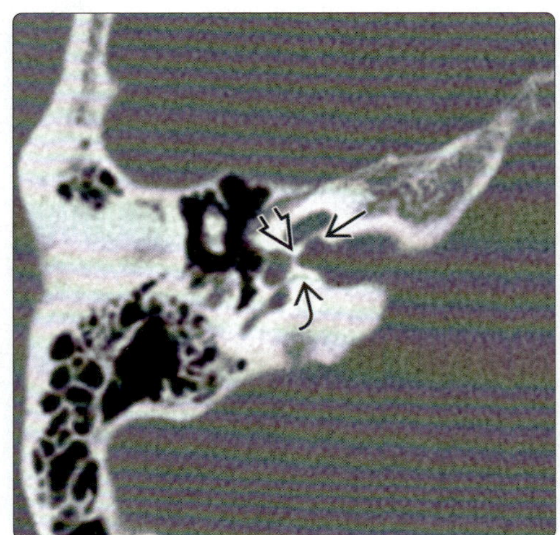

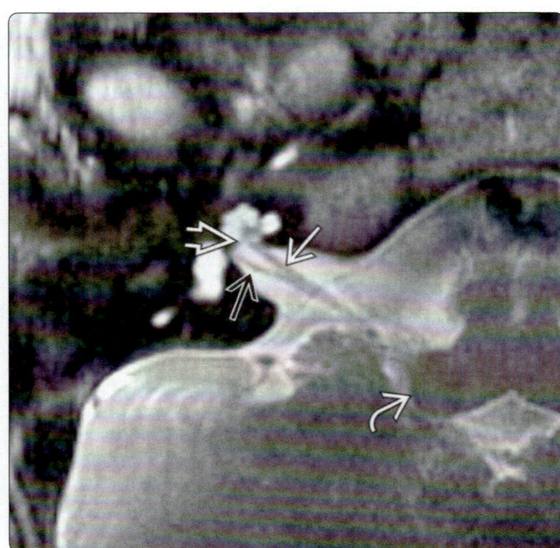

(Left) *Axial bone CT through the mid IAC shows the cochlear nerve canal ➡, inferior vestibular nerve leaving the fundus ➡, and singular nerve canal containing the posterior branch of the inferior vestibular nerve ➡.* **(Right)** *Axial T2WI MR through the inferior IAC reveals the cochlear nerve ➡ projecting into the cochlear nerve canal ➡. Dorsal and ventral cochlear nuclei are not seen but are known to reside in the lateral inferior cerebellar peduncle margin ➡. Note the inferior vestibular nerve ➡.*

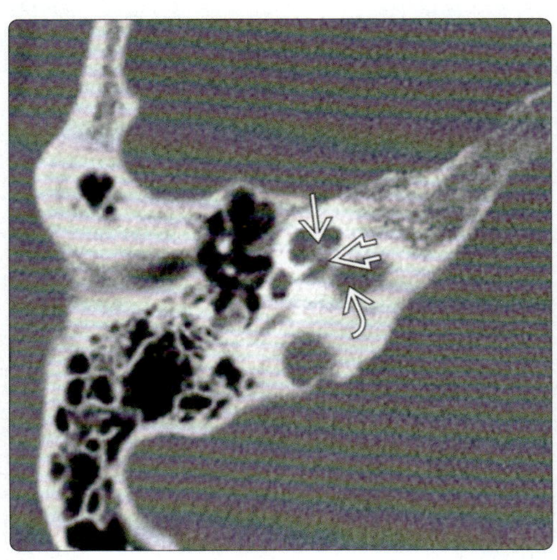

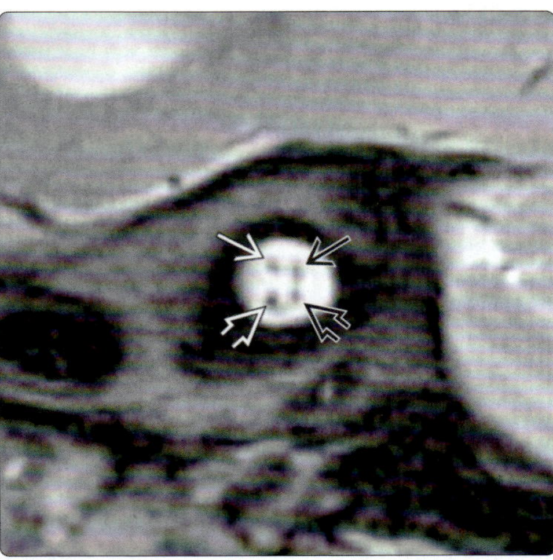

(Left) *Axial bone CT through the inferior IAC demonstrates the cochlear modiolus as a high-density structure at the cochlear base ➡. The cochlear nerve canal ➡ and the fundus of the IAC ➡ are also labeled.* **(Right)** *Oblique sagittal T2WI MR shows the 4 nerve bundles of the mid IAC cistern. CNVII is anterosuperior ➡, the cochlear nerve is anteroinferior ➡, and the superior ➡ and inferior ➡ vestibular nerves are posterosuperior and posteroinferior, respectively.*

CPA-IAC Epidermoid Cyst

KEY FACTS

TERMINOLOGY

- Definition: Congenital inclusion of ectodermal epithelial elements during neural tube closure

IMAGING

- Cerebellopontine angle (CPA) cisternal **insinuating** mass with high signal on DWI MR
    - 90% intradural, 10% extradural
    - Margins usually scalloped or irregular
    - Cauliflower-like margins with "fronds" possible
- T1 and T2: Isointense or slightly hyperintense to CSF
- DWI: **Restricted diffusion** makes diagnosis

TOP DIFFERENTIAL DIAGNOSES

- Arachnoid cyst in CPA
- Cystic neoplasm in CPA
    - Cystic vestibular schwannoma; cystic meningioma
    - Infratentorial ependymoma; pilocytic astrocytoma
- Neurenteric cyst
- Neurocysticercosis, CPA

PATHOLOGY

- Surgical appearance: Pearly white CPA cistern mass
- Cyst wall: Squamous epithelium with fibrous capsule

CLINICAL ISSUES

- Clinical presentation
    - Principal presenting symptom: Dizziness and headache
        - Sensorineural hearing loss also common
    - If extends to lateral pons: Trigeminal neuralgia
    - Rarer symptoms: Facial palsy, seizure
- Treatment: Complete surgical removal is goal; high risk to involved cranial nerves during resection
    - If adherent to neural structures, complete removal may not be possible; if recurs, takes many years to grow
    - DWI MR key to diagnosing recurrence on surveillance imaging

(Left) *Axial graphic shows a large CPA epidermoid cyst within a typical bed of pearls appearance. Note that the V →, VII →, and VIII → cranial nerves along with the anterior inferior cerebellar artery loop → are characteristically engulfed by this insinuating mass.* **(Right)** *Axial CECT shows a large CPA epidermoid cyst →. Note that this nonenhancing low-density lesion appears to invade the left cerebellar hemisphere →. Minimal rim enhancement is visible along the posterior margin of the cyst →.*

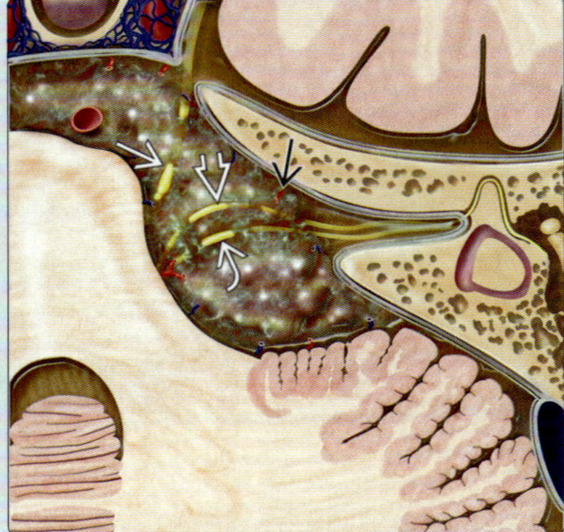

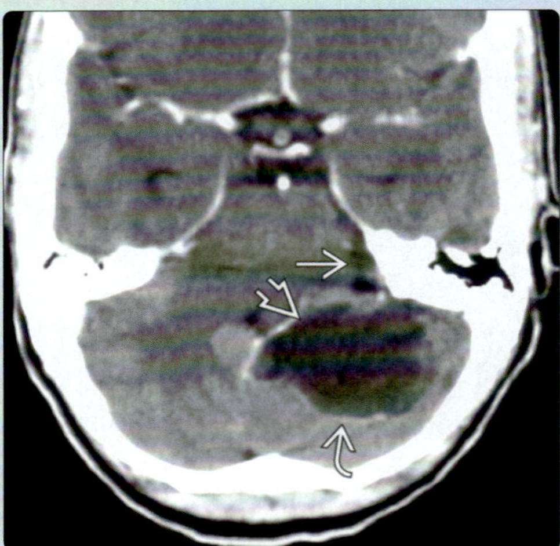

(Left) *Axial FLAIR MR of the same patient shows "incomplete" or partial nulling of the signal of this large epidermoid cyst. Associated high signal → along the deep margins of the lesion is most likely due to gliosis of the cerebellar hemisphere.* **(Right)** *Axial DWI MR in the same patient reveals the expected high signal → from epidermoid cyst diffusion restriction. DWI sequence allows straightforward differentiation of this epidermoid cyst from an arachnoid cyst.*

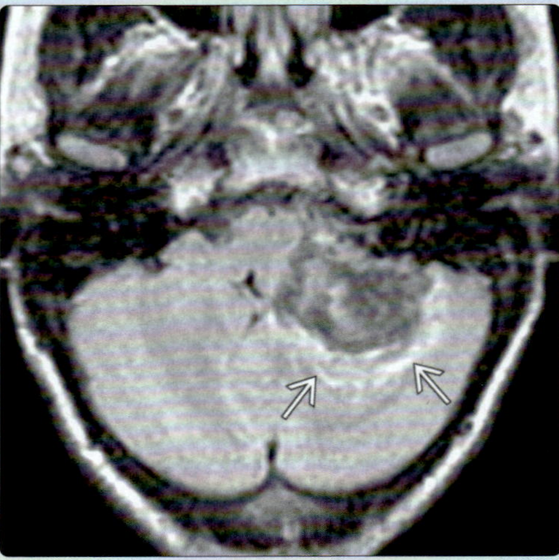

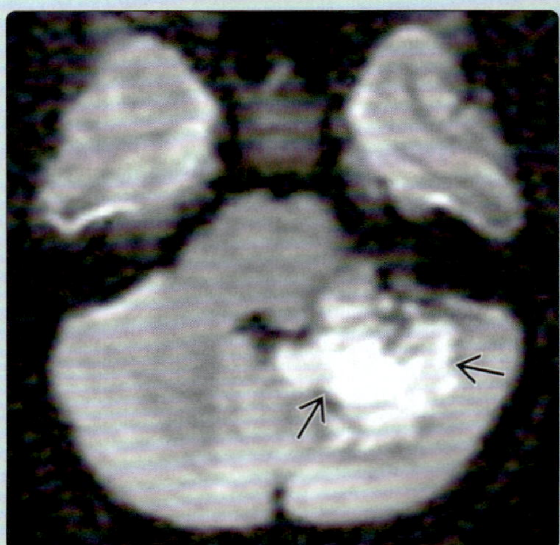

KEY FACTS

TERMINOLOGY

- Arachnoid cyst (AC) definition: Developmental arachnoid duplication anomaly creating CSF-filled sac

IMAGING

- Sharply demarcated ovoid extraaxial cisternal cyst with imperceptible walls with CSF density (CT) or intensity (MR)
- AC signal parallels (is isointense) CSF on **all** MR sequences
- Complete fluid attenuation on FLAIR MR
- **No** diffusion restriction on DWI MR imaging

TOP DIFFERENTIAL DIAGNOSES

- Epidermoid cyst in cerebellopontine angle (CPA)
- Cystic vestibular schwannoma
- Neurenteric cyst
- Cystic meningioma in CPA
- Cystic infratentorial ependymoma
- Cerebellar pilocytic astrocytoma

CLINICAL ISSUES

- Clinical presentation
  - Small AC: Asymptomatic, incidental finding (MR)
  - Large AC: Mostly asymptomatic
    - Symptoms may arise from direct compression ± ↑ intracranial pressure
- Natural history
  - Vast majority of ACs **do not** enlarge over time
- Treatment options
  - Often found incidentally; most cases require **no** treatment
  - Treatment is highly selective process when patient's symptoms are clearly referable to anatomic location of AC

DIAGNOSTIC CHECKLIST

- Differentiate AC from epidermoid cyst
- AC: No restriction on DWI = best clue

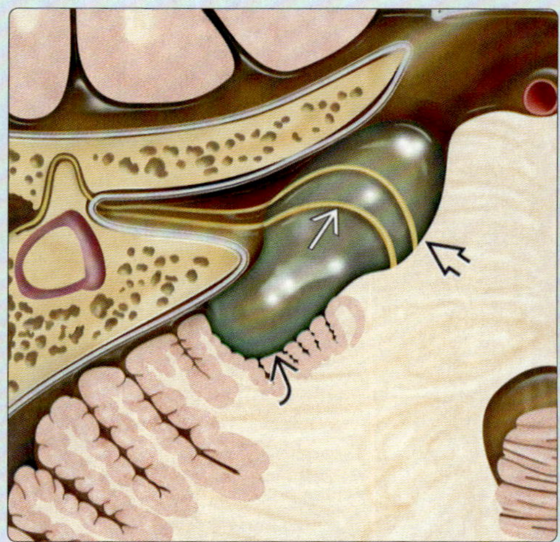

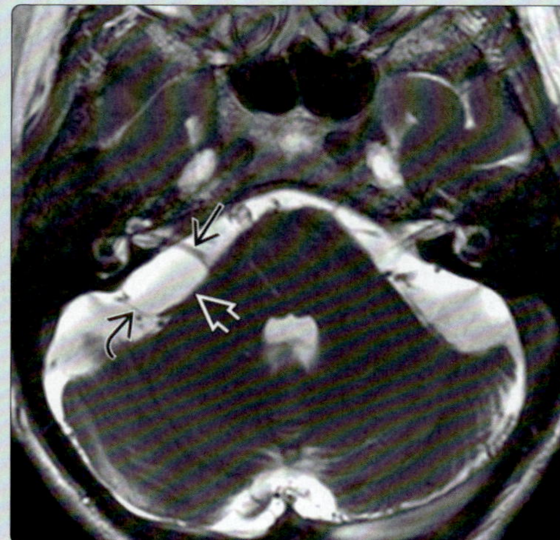

(Left) *Axial graphic of an arachnoid cyst in the cerebellopontine angle (CPA) shows a thin, translucent wall. Notice the cyst bowing the VII and VIII cranial nerves anteriorly ➡ and effacing of the brainstem ⇨ and cerebellum ⇨.* **(Right)** *Axial T2WI MR reveals a right CPA arachnoid cyst causing bowing of the facial and vestibulocochlear nerves anteriorly ⇨, small bridging veins posteriorly ⇨, and flattening of the lateral margin of the brachium pontis ➡.*

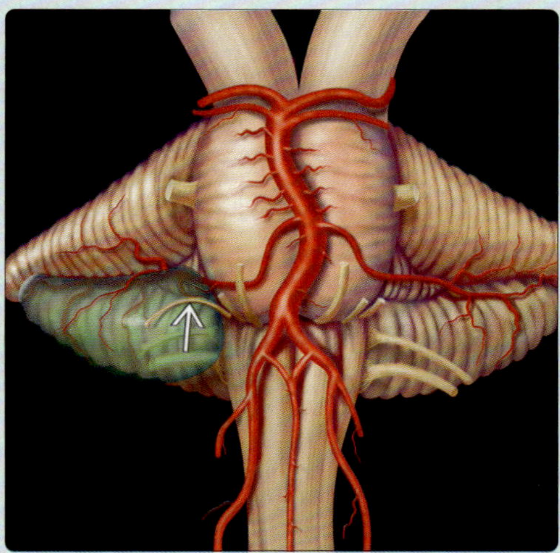

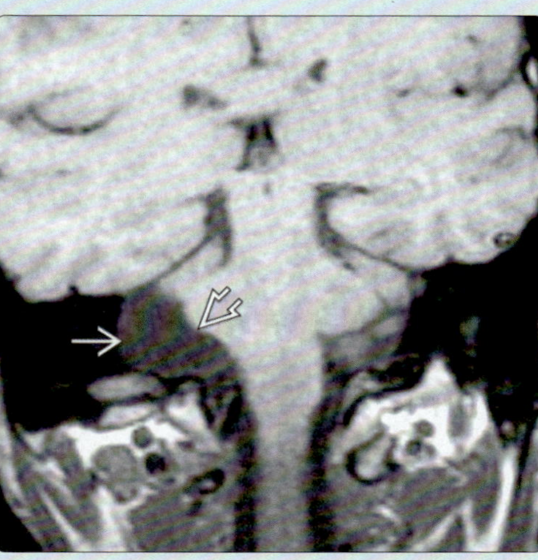

(Left) *Coronal graphic of a CPA arachnoid cyst depicts a typical translucent cyst wall. CNVII and CNVIII are pushed by the cyst ➡ without being engulfed by it. In an epidermoid cyst, cranial nerves are usually engulfed.* **(Right)** *Coronal T1WI MR demonstrates a small CSF intensity CPA arachnoid cyst ➡ with subtle mass effect on the adjacent brainstem ➡. Complete fluid attenuation on FLAIR MR helps differentiate this lesion from an epidermoid cyst, which is the primary imaging differential diagnosis.*

Lipoma in CPA-IAC

KEY FACTS

TERMINOLOGY

- Lipoma in CPA-IAC: Nonneoplastic mass of adipose tissue in CPA-IAC area

IMAGING

- Focal benign-appearing CPA-IAC mass, which follows fat density (CT) and intensity (MR)
- Concurrent intralabyrinthine deposit may be seen in association with CPA-IAC lipoma
- MR: Hyperintense CPA mass (parallels subcutaneous and marrow fat intensity)
  - Becomes **hypointense** with **fat saturation**
  - Caveat: Fat-saturated MR sequences avoid mistaking lipoma for "enhancing CPA mass"

TOP DIFFERENTIAL DIAGNOSES

- Hemorrhagic vestibular schwannoma
- Aneurysm in CPA-IAC
- Neurenteric cyst
- Ruptured dermoid cyst

PATHOLOGY

- Aberrant differentiation of embryonic meninx primitiva (meningeal precursor tissue)
- Lipoma composed of mature lipocytes (fat cells)

CLINICAL ISSUES

- Most common presentation: Adult presenting with unilateral sensorineural hearing loss
  - CNVIII compression: Tinnitus (40%), vertigo (45%)
  - Compression of CNV root entry zone: Trigeminal neuralgia (15%)
  - Compression of CNVII root exit zone: Hemifacial spasm, facial nerve weakness (10%)
  - Incidentally seen on brain CT or MR completed for unrelated reasons (33%)
- Treatment: **No treatment** is most often best treatment
  - If surgery required (cranial neuropathy), subtotal resection (debulking) only recommended

(Left) *Axial graphic shows a CPA lipoma ➔ abutting the lateral pons. Notice that the facial nerve ➔, vestibulocochlear nerve ➔, and anterior inferior cerebellar artery (AICA) loop ➔ all pass through the lipoma on their way to the IAC.* **(Right)** *Axial T1WI MR shows a right CPA lipoma ➔ adherent to the lateral pontine pial surface. Note the 2nd smaller lipoma ➔ along the lateral margin of the IAC. A portion of the AICA loop ➔ passes through the anterolateral lipoma.*

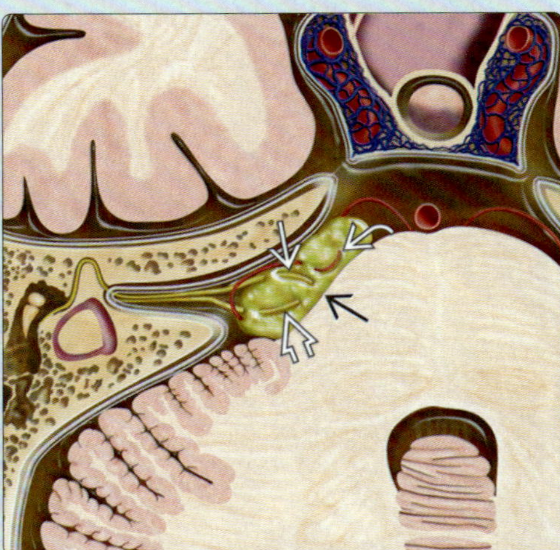

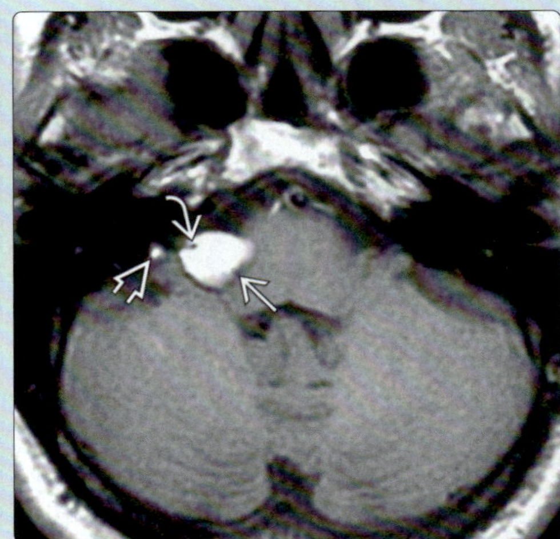

(Left) *Axial T1WI MR reveals a hyperintense CPA lipoma ➔ abutting the lateral pons. Note the 2nd ➔ focus of hyperintensity representing a small intravestibular lipoma. Such intralabyrinthine lipomas are very rare and may exist with or without CPA lipoma.* **(Right)** *Axial T1WI C+ FS MR in the same patient shows both lesions have disappeared. Fat-saturation MR sequences are key to confirming the diagnosis of lipoma and to avoid mistaking a lipoma for an enhancing CPA mass.*

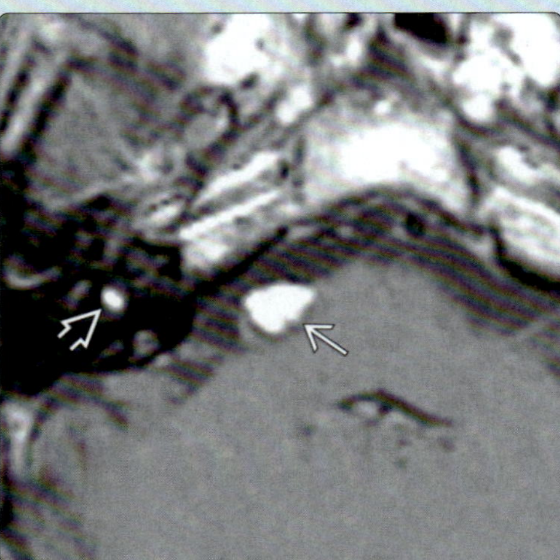

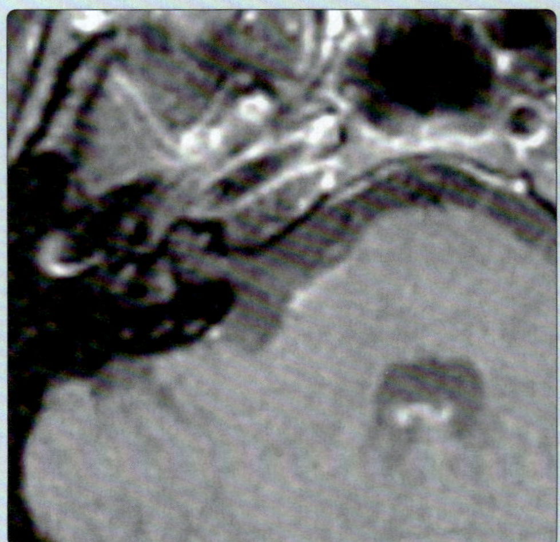

KEY FACTS

TERMINOLOGY

- IAC-VM: Benign developmental lesion associated with CNVII in IAC
  - May extend to geniculate ganglion
- IAC "hemangioma" is misnomer for IAC-VM

IMAGING

- Temporal bone CT findings
  - **Stippled ossifications** in lesion matrix
- Enhanced T1 MR findings
  - Enhancing IAC mass (< 10 mm) in fundus
  - Focal intralesional low-signal foci possible
  - If extends along labyrinthine CNVII to geniculate ganglion, creates **dumbbell** appearance
- IAC enhancing mass + CNVII paralysis ± punctate ossifications = IAC VM (hemangioma)

TOP DIFFERENTIAL DIAGNOSES

- Vestibular schwannoma
- Meningioma of IAC-CPA
- Facial nerve schwannoma of IAC-CPA
- Metastases of IAC-CPA

PATHOLOGY

- Etiology
  - Benign congenital VM arising in close approximation to CNVII in IAC
  - "Malformation" is term used for **errors of vascular morphogenesis** that develop in utero and persist postnatally
- Microscopic features
  - Immunohistochemical markers critical to VM diagnosis
  - Vascular channel endothelium **stain negatively** for hemangioma-associated markers (**GLUT1 & LeY** antigen)

CLINICAL ISSUES

- Presentation: Hearing loss associated with **CNVII paralysis**
- Treatment: Nerve-sparing surgical resection

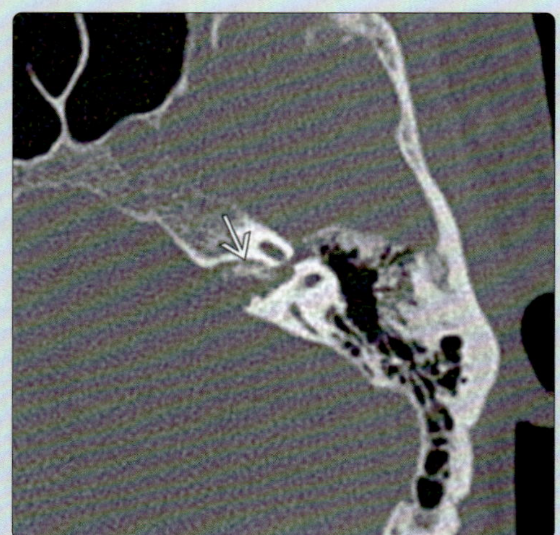

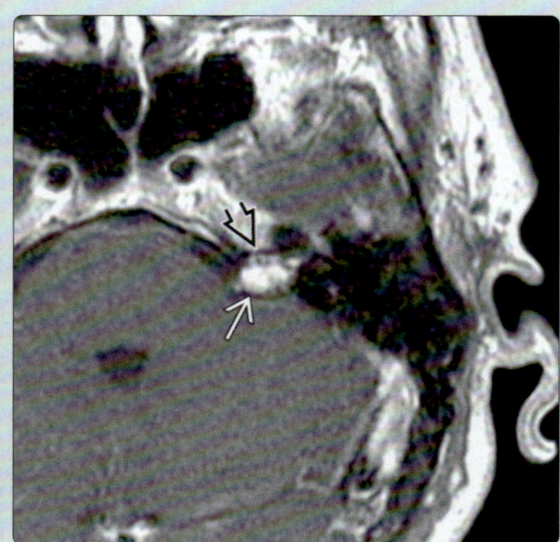

(Left) *Axial bone CT shows typical CT stippled ossifications ➡ in the matrix of an IAC-VM ("hemangioma"). When found, ossifications help differentiate IAC-VM from IAC acoustic schwannoma.* **(Right)** *Axial T1WI C+ MR in the same patient demonstrates an enhancing IAC-VM ➡. The low-signal foci ⇨ along the anterior margin of the lesion are secondary to intratumoral ossifications.*

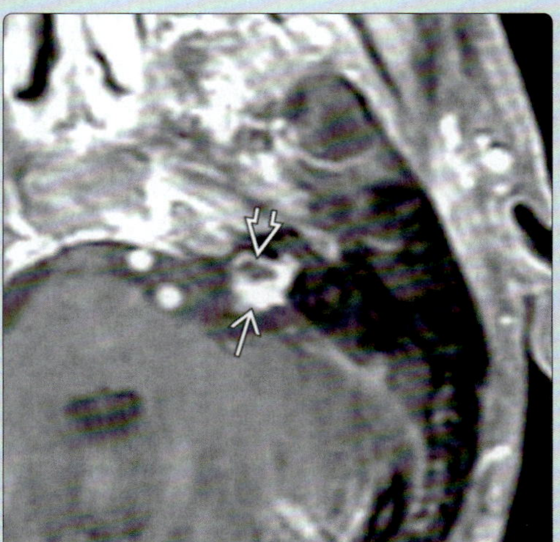

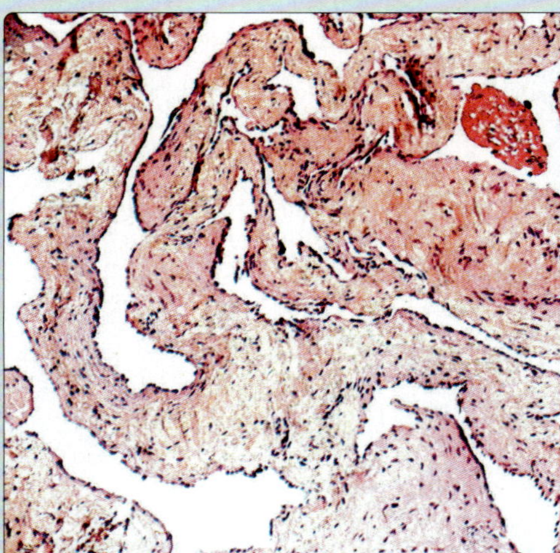

(Left) *Axial T1WI C+ FS MR reveals an enhancing IAC-VM ➡ with an area of low signal along the anterior margin of the lesion ➡ secondary to intratumoral ossification.* **(Right)** *Micropathology shows dilated vascular spaces with collagenous walls lined by a single layer of endothelium. The endothelial lining stains are negative for GLUT1 and LeY antigens. These antigens are considered hemangioma-associated markers.*

KEY FACTS

TERMINOLOGY

- Definition: Acute or chronic infectious infiltrate of pia, arachnoid, and CSF in vicinity of T-bone, internal auditory canal (IAC), and cerebellopontine angle (CPA)

IMAGING

- CT shows underlying lesion causing meningitis ± CSF leak
  - Congenital: Inner ear lesions, cephalocele, patent petromastoid canal
  - Acquired: Coalescent mastoiditis or apical petrositis
  - Acquired: Tegmen or posterior wall arachnoid granulations
  - Acquired: T-bone fractures of tegmen or inner ear
- MR may show meningitis
  - Meningeal exudate + brain surface C+
    - Thickened meninges: Local or diffuse
  - Hyperintensity in posterior fossa sulci ± cisterns

TOP DIFFERENTIAL DIAGNOSES

- Meningeal metastases
- Neurosarcoidosis, CPA-IAC
- Increased FLAIR signal in CSF from acute stroke, subarachnoid hemorrhage, or artifact

PATHOLOGY

- Meningitis focused along deep surfaces of T-bone or in floor of middle cranial fossa is secondary to T-bone disease until proven otherwise
- Complications: Cerebritis, abscess, empyema, ventriculitis
- Cerebrovascular complications: Venous sinus or arterial thrombosis

CLINICAL ISSUES

- Meningitis = clinical/laboratory, **not imaging**, diagnosis
- Imaging used to identify underlying lesions
- Treatment: Address underlying cause, often requires IV antibiotic

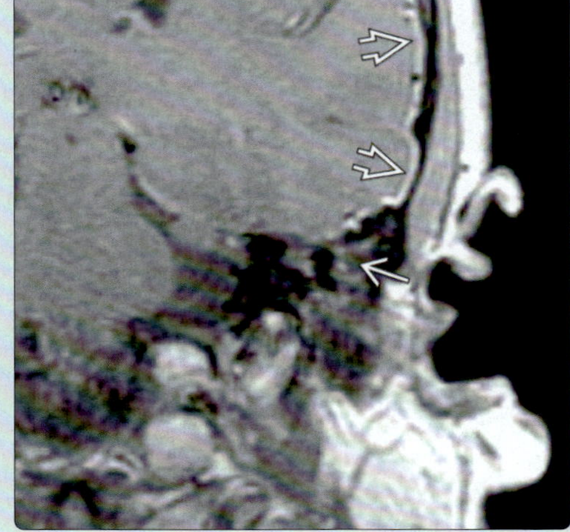

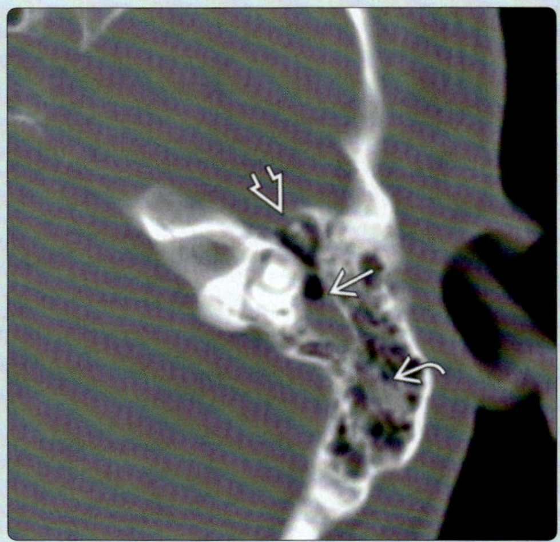

(Left) *Coronal T1WI C+ MR shows enhancing mastoid tissue ➡ along with meningeal enhancement (meningitis) ➡ in this patient with severe headache and recurrent otomastoiditis.* **(Right)** *Axial bone CT through the left T-bone in the same patient demonstrates an air-fluid level in mastoid ➡ with thinning of the anterior epitympanic recess wall ➡. Notice the partial opacification of the mastoid air cells ➡. In this case, bacterial otomastoiditis spread locally to cause the meningitis.*

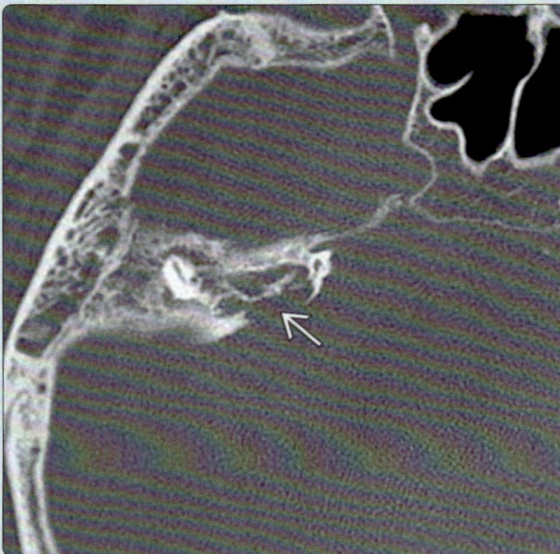

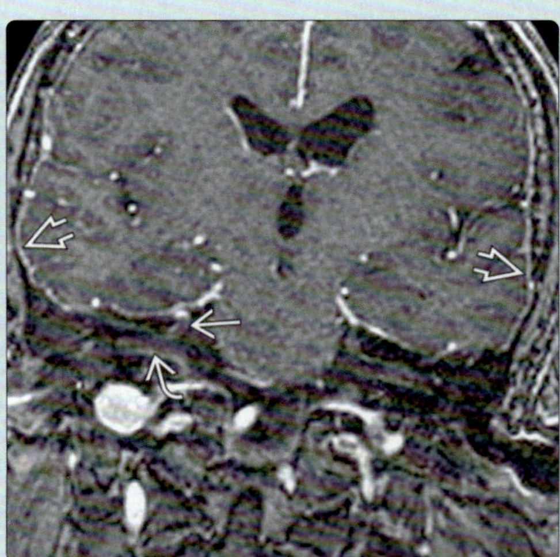

(Left) *Axial bone CT of the right T-bone in this patient with CSF-proven meningitis reveals an arachnoid granulation ➡ in the location of the subarcuate canaliculus. CSF otorrhea was present.* **(Right)** *Coronal T1WI C+ FS MR in the same patient after antibiotic treatment shows the arachnoid granulation as a focal fluid collection ➡ just above the right internal auditory canal ➡. Notice the diffuse leptomeningeal enhancement ➡ sometimes seen in the setting of meningitis.*

KEY FACTS

TERMINOLOGY

- Varicella-zoster virus infection involving sensory fibers of CNVII & CNVIII & portion of **external ear** supplied by auriculotemporal nerve

IMAGING

- Imaging Dx: Pathologic enhancement on T1 C+ MR of CNVII ± CNVIII in IAC fundus along with all or part of membranous labyrinth
- Enhanced MR findings by location
  - External ear: Enhancing external ear vesicles & associated inflammation
  - Intratemporal CNVII: Entire intratemporal CNVII enhancement typical
  - Membranous labyrinth: Fluid spaces of cochlea, vestibule, & semicircular canals may all be variably affected
  - IAC: Linear to fusiform enhancement in IAC fundus (CNVII & CNVIII)
  - Brainstem: Facial nucleus in brainstem enhances infrequently in Ramsay Hunt syndrome (RHS)

TOP DIFFERENTIAL DIAGNOSES

- Bell palsy
- Meningitis
- Neurosarcoidosis in cerebellopontine angle-IAC

CLINICAL ISSUES

- Clinical presentation
  - CNVII palsy & sensorineural hearing loss associated with external ear vesicular rash
  - Fever, vertigo, nausea, & vomiting; deep, burning pain in ear
  - Electroneuronography and electromyography can be predictive of severity
- Treatment options: Corticosteroids ± acyclovir
  - Surgical decompression of CNVII labyrinthine segment for complete paralysis is controversial in RHS

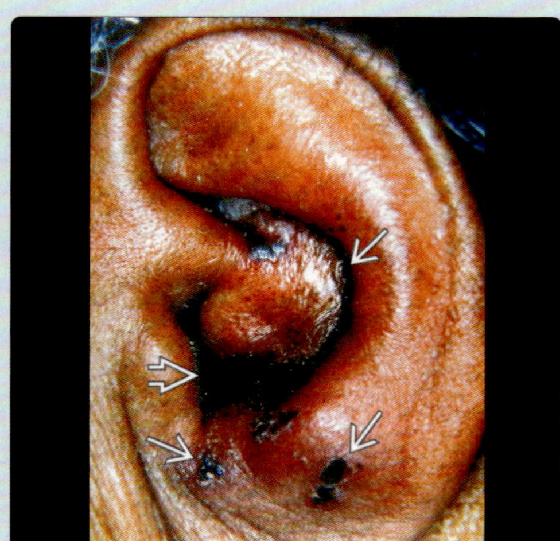

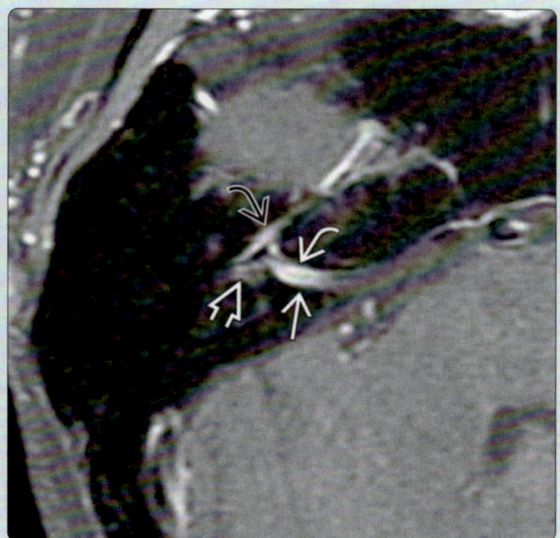

(Left) *Clinical photograph of the external ear demonstrates a hemorrhagic vesicular rash affecting the auricle ➡ and external auditory canal ➡. This often painful rash, along with facial and vestibulocochlear neuropathy, makes the clinical diagnosis of Ramsay Hunt syndrome (RHS) obvious.* **(Right)** *Axial T1WI C+ FS MR in a RHS patient shows linear enhancement of CNVII in the IAC fundus ➡ extending into the labyrinthine and tympanic segments ➡. The superior vestibular nerve also enhances in the IAC fundus ➡ and on into the vestibule ➡.*

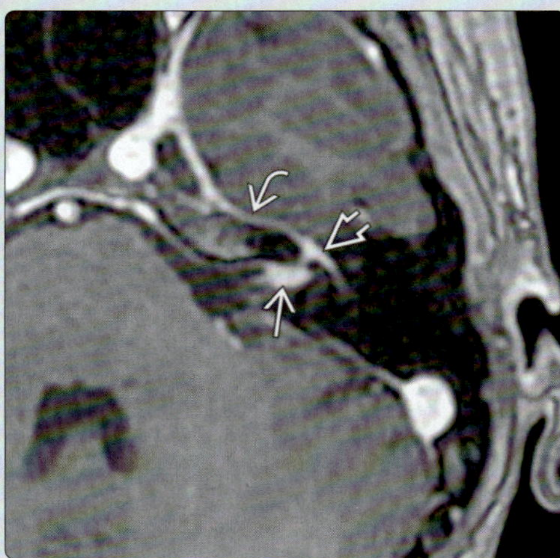

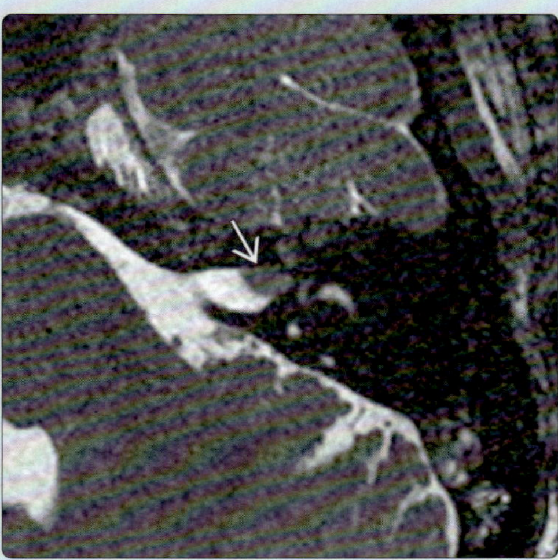

(Left) *Axial SPGR C+ reveals enhancement of the left IAC fundus ➡ as well as enhancement of the labyrinthine segment, geniculate ganglion, and anterior tympanic segment of CNVII ➡. In addition, the greater superficial petrosal nerve branch of CNVII ➡ enhances along the anterior margin of the petrous apex.* **(Right)** *Magnified axial T2WI FS MR in the same patient shows the thickened, inflamed CNVII and CNVIII as brain intensity material ➡ in the fundus of the IAC.*

KEY FACTS

TERMINOLOGY

- Vestibular schwannoma (VS): Benign tumor from Schwann cells surrounding vestibular nerves of CNVIII at glial-Schwann cell junction

IMAGING

- T1WI fat-saturated enhanced MR = gold standard
  - Focal, enhancing mass of CPA-IAC cistern centered on porus acusticus
  - **Small VS**: Ovoid enhancing intracanalicular mass
  - **Large VS**: Ice cream on cone shape in CPA and IAC
  - 15% with intramural cysts (low-signal foci)
  - 0.5% with associated arachnoid cyst/trapped CSF
- High-resolution T2 space, CISS, or FIESTA: Filling defect in hyperintense cerebrospinal fluid of CPA-IAC cistern
  - Effective for screening protocols, active surveillance
- FLAIR: ↑ cochlear signal from ↑ protein
- T2* GRE: Microhemorrhages ↓ signal foci (common)
  - Characteristic VS finding when present
  - Not seen in meningioma

TOP DIFFERENTIAL DIAGNOSES

- Meningioma in CPA-IAC
- Epidermoid cyst in CPA
- Aneurysm in CPA
- Facial nerve schwannoma in CPA-IAC
- Metastases in CPA-IAC

CLINICAL ISSUES

- Demographics and symptoms
  - Adults with **unilateral sensorineural hearing loss**
- Surgical approaches
  - Translabyrinthine resection if no hearing or large tumor
  - Middle cranial fossa approach for IAC VS
  - Retrosigmoid approach for medial location + hearing
- Fractionated or stereotactic radiotherapy with documented tumor growth; smaller tumors, older patients
- Active surveillance for smaller tumors, older patients

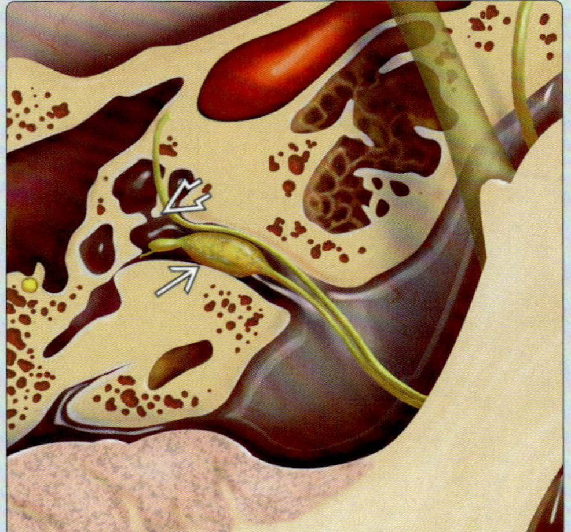

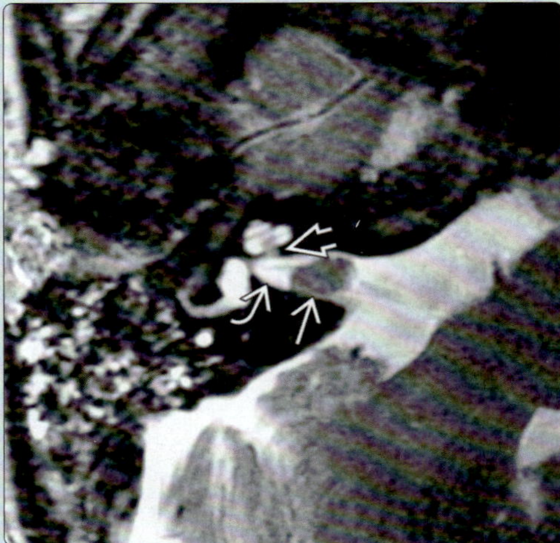

(Left) *Axial graphic shows small intracanalicular vestibular schwannoma ➡ arising from the superior vestibular nerve. Notice that the cochlear nerve canal is uninvolved ➡.* **(Right)** *Axial T2WI MR reveals a small intracanalicular vestibular schwannoma ➡ visualized as a soft tissue intensity mass surrounded by high-intensity CSF. The cochlear nerve canal ➡ is not involved, and an 8-mm fundal cap ➡ is present.*

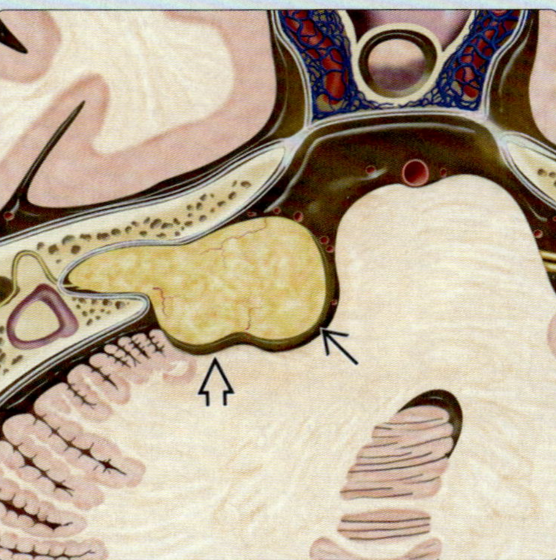

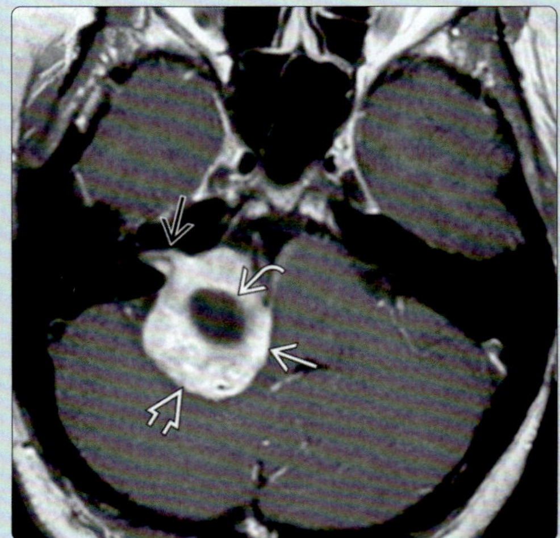

(Left) *Axial graphic of a large vestibular schwannoma reveals the typical ice cream on cone CPA-IAC morphology. Mass effect on the middle cerebellar peduncle ➡ and cerebellar hemisphere ➡ is evident.* **(Right)** *Axial T1WI C+ MR demonstrates a large CPA-IAC vestibular schwannoma compressing the middle cerebellar peduncle ➡ and cerebellar hemisphere ➡. Enhancement within the IAC ➡ and the large intramural cyst ➡ makes the imaging diagnosis certain.*

KEY FACTS

TERMINOLOGY

- **PHACES**: Association of craniofacial hemangioma and 1 or more features listed in PHACES acronym
  - **P**osterior fossa malformations
  - **H**emangioma
  - **A**rterial lesions
  - **C**ardiac abnormalities/aortic coarctation
  - **E**ye abnormalities
  - **S**ternal defects or supraumbilical raphe

IMAGING

- **Proliferating regional or midline cervicofacial hemangioma**: Lobulated or plaque-like, prominent vascularity
- Unilateral cerebellar hypoplasia and prominent retrocerebellar CSF space
- Widened IAC ± hemangioma ± persistent stapedial artery
- Hypoplasia, aplasia, aberrancy, ectasia, tortuosity, and stenoocclusive changes of major cerebral arteries

TOP DIFFERENTIAL DIAGNOSES

- Sturge-Weber syndrome
- Marfan syndrome
- Schwannoma

PATHOLOGY

- Suspected genetic defect with possible environmental factors

CLINICAL ISSUES

- Hemangioma appears at birth or in neonate
- Gender: 80-90% female
- Cutaneous manifestations in beard-like distribution
  - Large regional or midline craniofacial hemangioma
    - 20% of patients have PHACES
- Treatment
  - Propranolol accelerates involution; cardiology will often monitor for safety
  - Neurosurgical revascularization

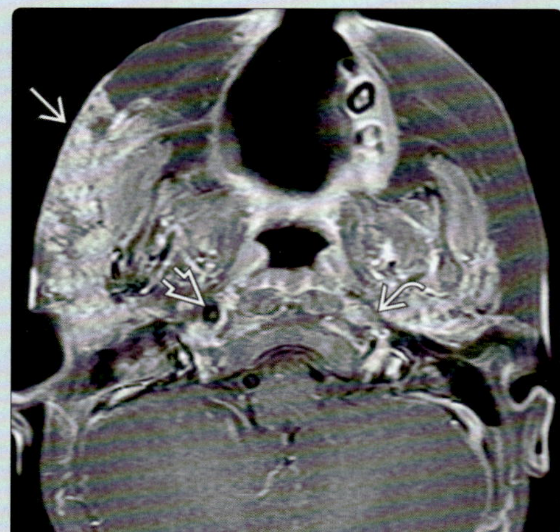

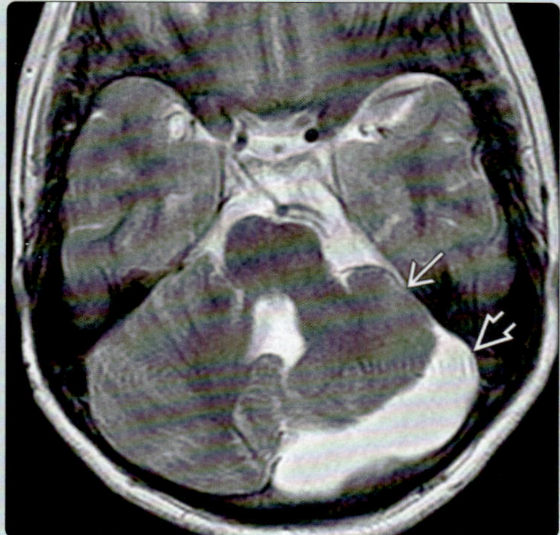

(Left) *Axial T1WI C+ FS MR shows an enhancing right facial hemangioma ➡ with cutaneous and subcutaneous involvement. A normal right internal auditory canal (ICA) flow void is seen ➡. There is no left ICA flow void as a result of ICA atresia ➡.* **(Right)** *Axial T2WI MR in the same patient reveals cerebellar hypoplasia and cerebellar cortical malformation ➡ with a prominent retrocerebellar CSF space ➡. The ventral aspect of the pons is flattened and small.*

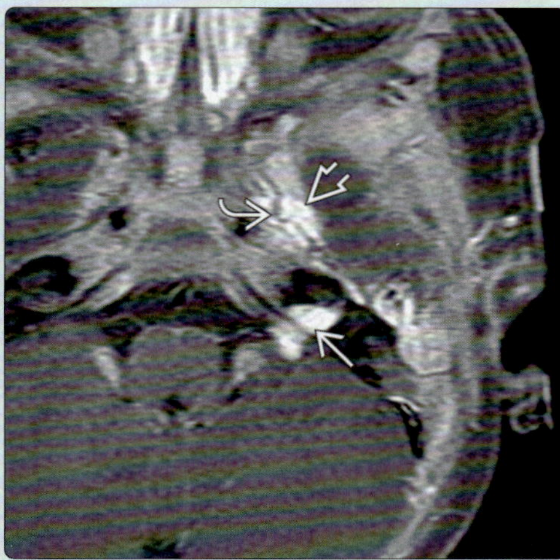

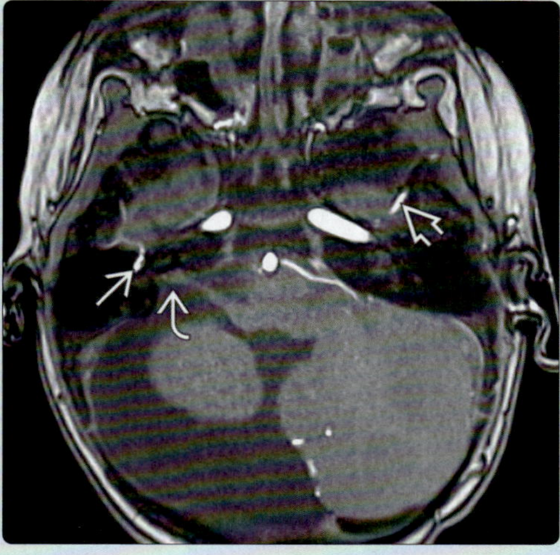

(Left) *Three-week-old boy with left facial palsy shows avidly enhancing masses within the left IAC ➡ and cavernous sinus ➡ with a prominent flow void within the left cavernous sinus mass ➡. The IAC mass mimics a schwannoma. These hemangiomas involuted after the 1st year of life.* **(Right)** *Axial MRA of infant girl with PHACES and right cerebellar hypoplasia is shown. There is a right persistent stapedial artery ➡. Note the normal left middle meningeal artery ➡. Right porus acusticus of the IAC ➡ is widened.*

KEY FACTS

TERMINOLOGY

- Definition: Benign, unencapsulated neoplasm arising from meningothelial arachnoid cells of CPA-IAC dura

IMAGING

- 10% occur in posterior fossa
- When in CPA, asymmetric to IAC porus acusticus
- NECT: 25% calcified; 2 types seen
  - Homogeneous, sand-like (psammomatous)
  - Focal sunburst, globular, or rim pattern
- Bone CT: Hyperostotic or permeative-sclerotic bone changes possible (en plaque type)
- T2WI MR: Pial blood vessels seen as surface flow voids between tumor and brain
  - High-signal crescent from CSF ("CSF cleft")
- T1WI C+ MR: Enhancing dural-based mass with dural tails centered along posterior petrous wall
  - When IAC tail present, usually dural reaction, not tumor

TOP DIFFERENTIAL DIAGNOSES

- Vestibular schwannoma
- Epidermoid cyst, CPA-IAC
- Dural metastases, CPA-IAC
- Sarcoidosis, CPA-IAC
- Idiopathic inflammatory pseudotumor

CLINICAL ISSUES

- 2nd most common CPA tumor
- Slow-growing tumor, displacing adjacent structures
- Often found as incidental brain MR finding
- < 10% symptomatic
- Treatment
  - Follow with imaging if smaller size and older patient
  - Surgical removal if medically safe; cranial nerve morbidity often less than vestibular schwannoma of similar size and location
  - Stereotactic radiation to arrest growth

(Left) *Axial graphic at the level of the IAC shows a large CPA meningioma causing mass effect on the brainstem-cerebellum. Notice the broad dural base creating the shape of a mushroom cap. Dural tails ➡ are present in ~ 60% of cases, typically representing reactive rather than neoplastic change. CSF-vascular cleft is also visible ➡.* **(Right)** *Coronal CT through the IAC shows a focal area of meningioma-associated hyperostosis ➡ that may suggest osteoma of the IAC. Isolated intracanalicular meningioma is a rare lesion.*

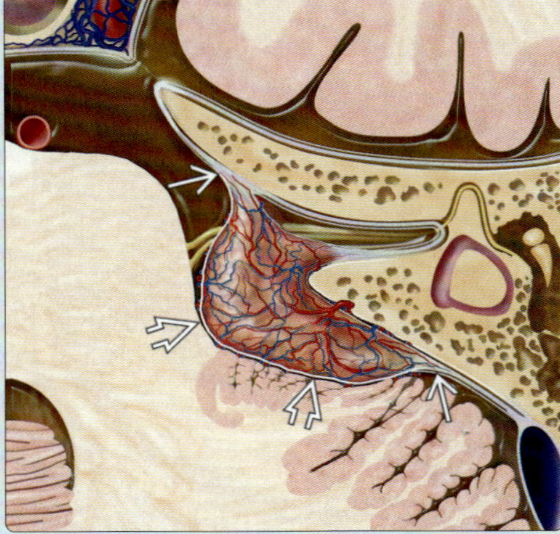

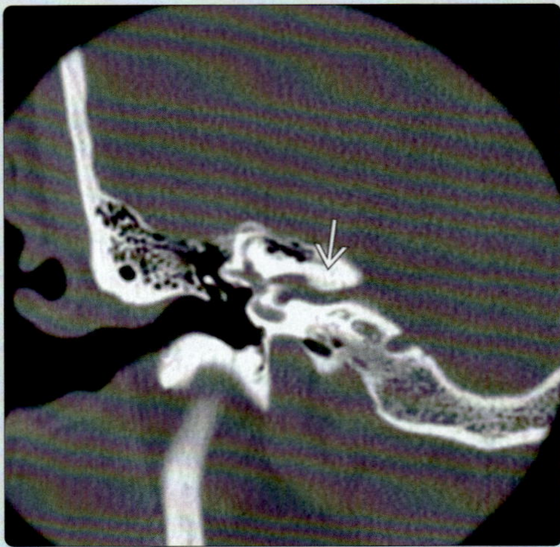

(Left) *Axial T1WI C+ FS MR through the IAC shows a meningioma overlying the porus acusticus. Note the dural tail ➡ extending along the temporal bone posterior wall. A dot of enhancement in the IAC fundus ➡ suggests that the low-signal area in the IAC is a nonenhancing meningioma.* **(Right)** *Axial T2WI FS MR in the same patient reveals a high-velocity flow void ➡ representing a dural artery feeder penetrating the meningioma core. Low signal in the IAC ➡ is a intracanalicular meningioma.*

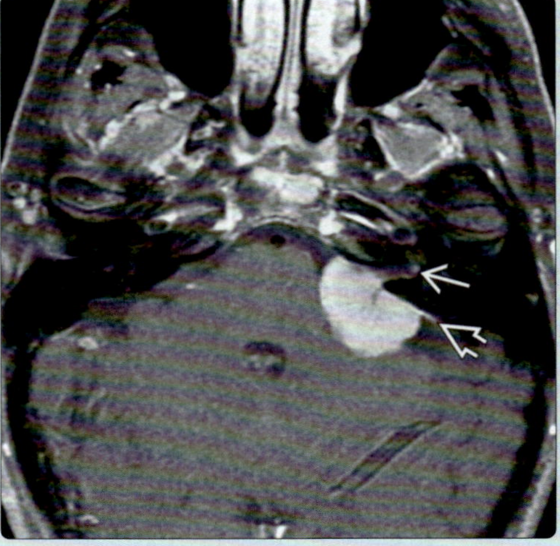

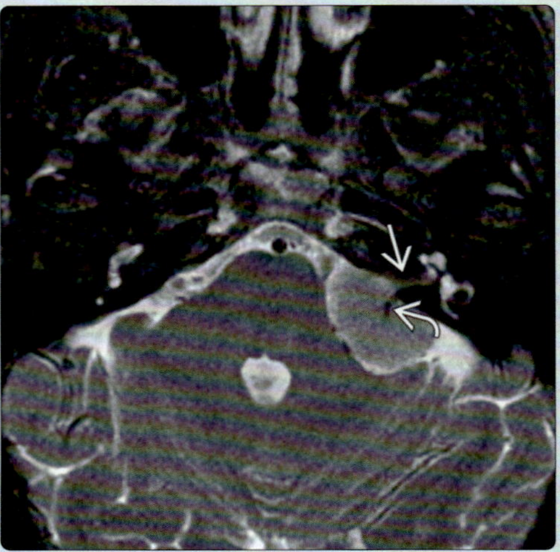

KEY FACTS

TERMINOLOGY

- Abbreviation: Facial nerve schwannoma (FNS)
- FNS definition: Rare benign tumor of Schwann cells that surrounds CNVII in CPA-IAC ± labyrinthine CNVII

IMAGING

- Temporal bone CT findings
  - ↑ size of labyrinthine CNVII canal ± geniculate fossa
- MR findings
  - T1 C+: CPA-IAC-labyrinthine CNVII canal C+ mass

TOP DIFFERENTIAL DIAGNOSES

- Bell palsy (herpetic facial paralysis)
- Vestibular schwannoma
- CPA-IAC meningioma
- Neurofibromatosis type 2

PATHOLOGY

- Tumor of Schwann cells lining CNVII
- Neurofibromatosis type 2
  - **Bilateral** CPA-IAC schwannomas
  - May be of **vestibular nerve** or **FN** origin

CLINICAL ISSUES

- Clinical presentation
  - Sensorineural hearing loss (SNHL)
  - FN paralysis
  - SNHL and FN paralysis similar in frequency
- Treatment options
  - Conservative management: Active surveillance until CNVII paralysis at HB 3-4/6 present
  - Surgical management: Used when CNVII paralysis + other symptoms evolving
    - Debulking also effective but high risk of FN weakness
  - Stereotactic radiotherapy
    - Used for poor surgical candidates
    - Recent use in small- to medium-sized FNS with CNVII function and hearing relatively preserved

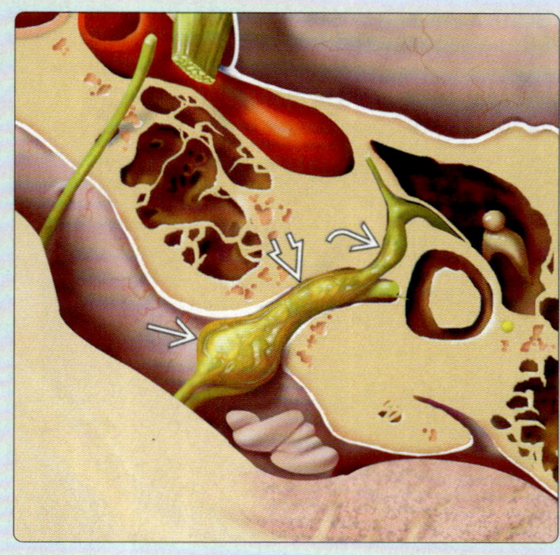

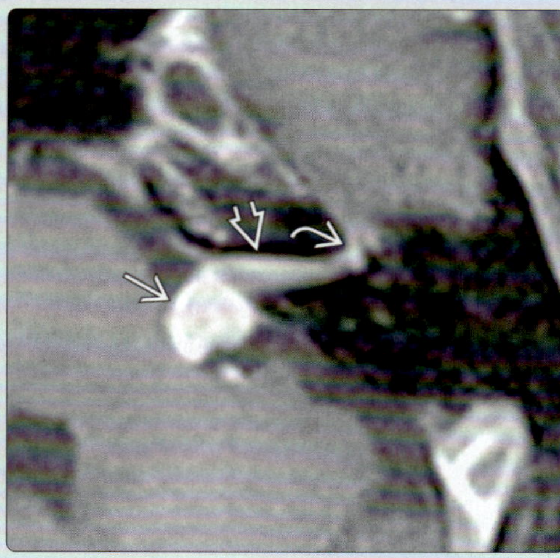

(Left) *Axial graphic of a larger facial nerve schwannoma (FNS) shows CPA ("ice cream") and IAC ("cone") components that mimic vestibular schwannoma. The labyrinthine segment of FN involvement makes the diagnosis.* **(Right)** *Axial T1WI C+ FS MR in a patient with unilateral sensorineural hearing loss shows FNS with CPA and IAC components. Note the labyrinthine segment FN tail, which differentiates FNS from vestibular schwannoma.*

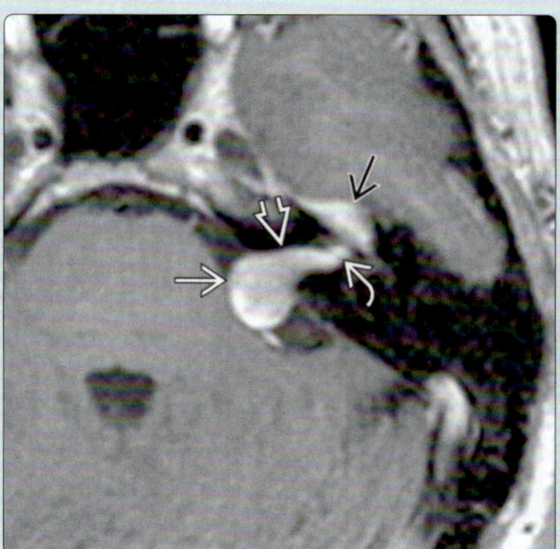

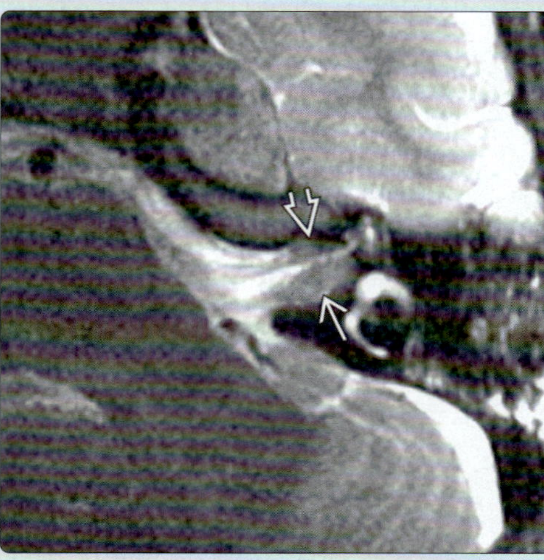

(Left) *Axial T1WI C+ MR in a patient with facial paresis reveals a C+ FNS that involves the CPA, IAC, labyrinthine segment, and geniculate ganglion of CNVII. When the FNS is confined to IAC only, it exactly mimics vestibular schwannoma.* **(Right)** *Axial thin-section magnified T2WI MR of left IAC fundus in a patient with neurofibromatosis type 2 (NF2) shows the superior vestibular nerve and FN schwannomas. A caveat is that in NF2, not all IAC lesions are vestibular schwannoma.*

CPA-IAC Metastases

KEY FACTS

TERMINOLOGY

- Definition: CPA-IAC metastases refers to systemic or CNS neoplasia affecting area of CPA-IAC

IMAGING

- 4 major sites: Leptomeningeal (pia-arachnoid), dura, flocculus, and choroid plexus
- T1WI C+ MR
  - **Leptomeningeal metastases**: Diffuse thickening and enhancement of cranial nerves in IAC
  - **Dural metastases**: Thickened enhancing dura; may be diffuse or focal
  - **Floccular metastases**: Enhancing floccular mass extends into CPA cistern
  - **Choroid plexus metastases**: Enhancing nodular lesion along normal course of choroid plexus
  - Focal, enhancing brain metastases may be present
- FLAIR MR
  - Parenchymal brain metastases usually high signal

TOP DIFFERENTIAL DIAGNOSES

- Bilateral vestibular schwannoma (NF2)
- Sarcoidosis
- Meningitis
- Ramsay Hunt syndrome

CLINICAL ISSUES

- Rapidly progressive unilateral or bilateral facial nerve paralysis and sensorineural hearing loss
- Patient with past history of treated malignancy
- Treatment: Radiotherapy as indicated

DIAGNOSTIC CHECKLIST

- If trying to diagnose bilateral "vestibular schwannoma" in adult as NF2, consider CPA metastases
- Rapidly progressive CNVII and CNVIII palsies + CPA mass suggests metastatic focus
  - Vestibular schwannoma rarely causes CNVII palsy
- Whole-body imaging may be required to find primary lesion

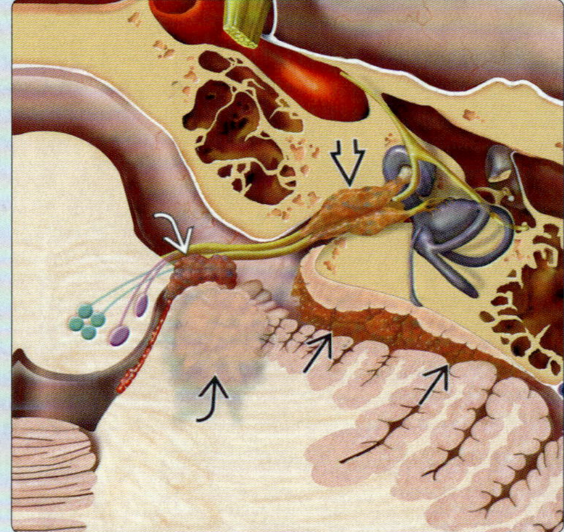

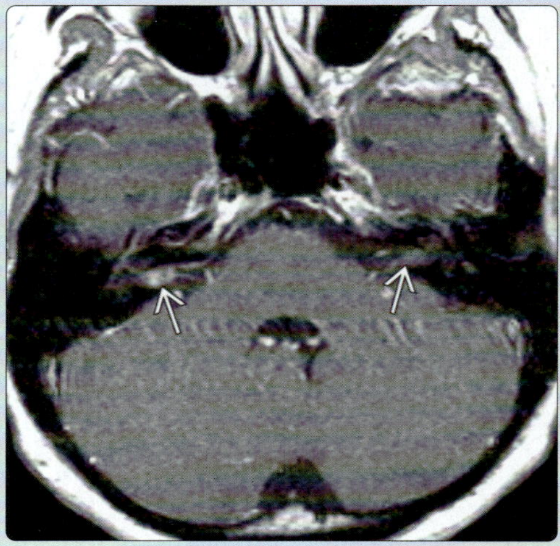

(Left) *Axial graphic depicts the 4 major types of CPA-IAC area metastases. Along the posterolateral margin of the IAC, thickened dural metastases ⇨ are visible. Within the IAC, metastatic leptomeningeal (pia-arachnoid) ⇨ involvement is present. Choroid plexus ➡ and floccular ⇨ metastases are also depicted.* **(Right)** *Axial T1WI C+ MR shows bilateral leptomeningeal breast carcinoma metastases ➡ within the IACs. The left-sided disease is more subtle than the right.*

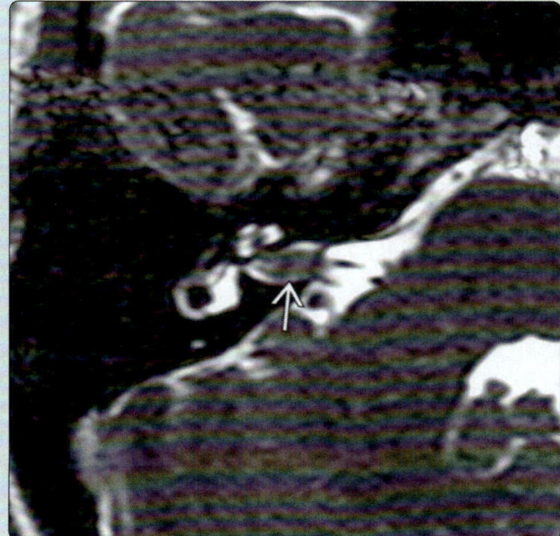

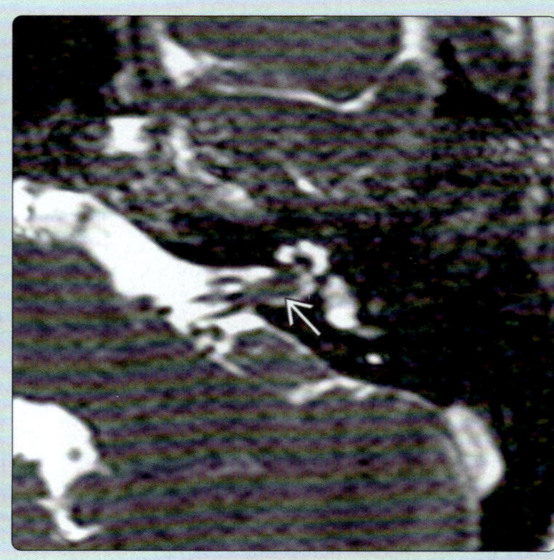

(Left) *Axial T2WI MR demonstrates right IAC leptomeningeal metastatic foci as thickening of the branches of CNVII and CNVIII ➡ within the IAC.* **(Right)** *Axial T2WI MR reveals left IAC metastatic disease as subtle thickening of the branches of CNVII and CNVIII ➡ within the IAC. In an adult patient with suspected bilateral vestibular schwannoma, consider metastatic disease rather than neurofibromatosis type 2.*

KEY FACTS

TERMINOLOGY

- Definition: Vascular loop compressing trigeminal nerve (CNV) at its root entry zone (REZ) or preganglionic segment (PGS)

IMAGING

- High-resolution MR: Serpiginous asymmetric signal void (vessel) in CPA CNV REZ or PGS
  - CNV PGS atrophy: Severe, prolonged compression; compressing vessel will bow PGS
- Offending vessels: **Superior cerebellar artery** (55%) > AICA (10%) > basal artery (5%) > variant vein (5%) > other

TOP DIFFERENTIAL DIAGNOSES

- Aneurysm in CPA-IAC
- Arteriovenous malformation in CPA
- Developmental venous anomaly in posterior fossa

PATHOLOGY

- CNV REZ or PGS experiences "irritation" from vessel

CLINICAL ISSUES

- Trigeminal neuralgia symptoms
  - Lancinating pain following V2 ± V3 distributions
  - May occur spontaneously or in response to "trigger" from tactile stimulation
- Treatment: Begin with conservative drug therapy; microvascular decompression or focused radiotherapy (~ 70% long-term success rate)

DIAGNOSTIC CHECKLIST

- 1st look for multiple sclerosis or DVA with draining vein along PGS
  - Also check for cisternal mass: Schwannoma, meningioma, epidermoid
- Next, follow CNV distally into cavernous sinus & face
  - Exclude perineural tumor, malignancies of face
- Lastly, view high-resolution thin-section MR for causal vessel
  - Causal vessel will bow PGS or deform REZ

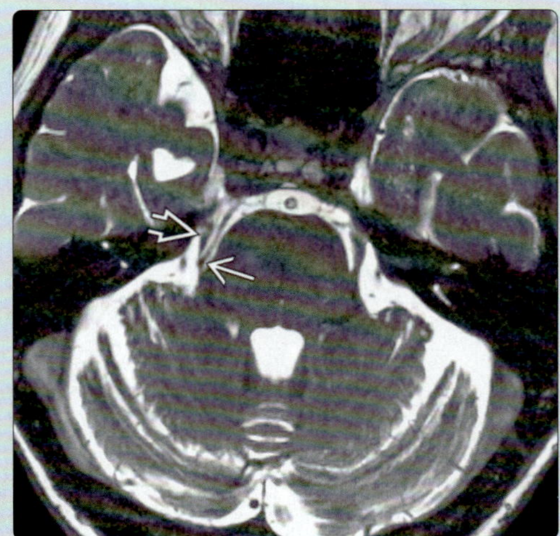

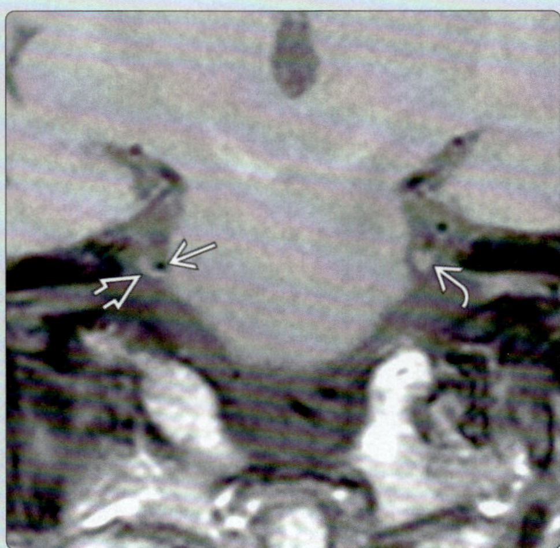

(Left) *Axial T2WI MR in this patient with right trigeminal neuralgia (TN) shows the low-signal superior cerebellar artery ➡ impinging on the root entry zone of the preganglionic segment ➡ of the trigeminal nerve.* **(Right)** *Coronal T1WI MR in the same patient reveals the superior cerebellar artery ➡ compressing and deforming the right proximal preganglionic segment of CNV ➡. Notice the larger, normal left preganglionic CNV ➡ that indicates atrophy is a feature of the affected right side.*

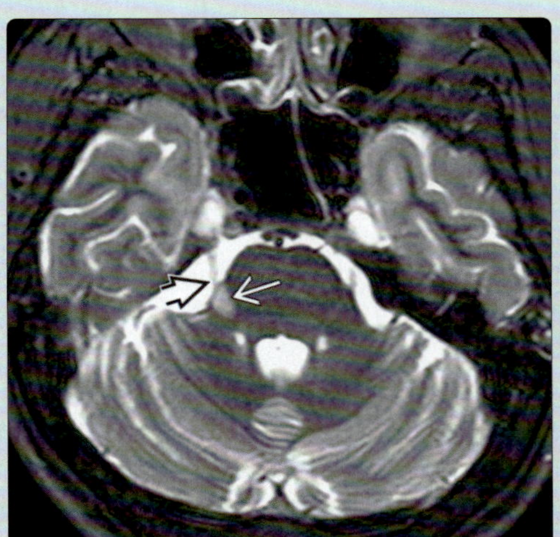

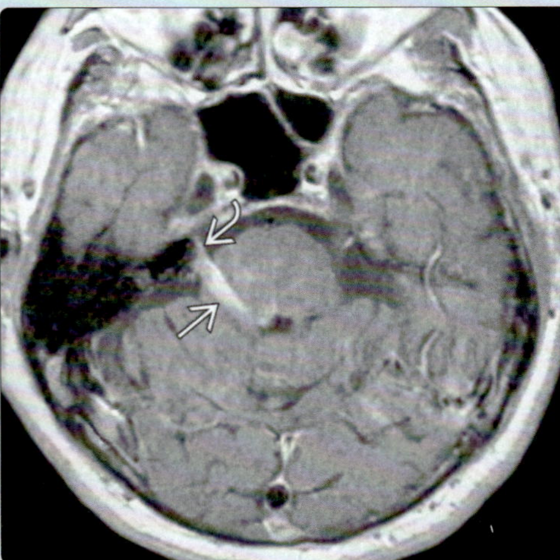

(Left) *Axial T2WI FS MR in a patient with right TN reveals a multiple sclerosis lesion ➡ involving the lateral pons at the root entry zone of the trigeminal nerve ➡. Rarely, cisternal masses or MS may present with TN.* **(Right)** *Axial T1WI C+ MR in a patient with right TN shows a developmental venous anomaly of the cerebellum draining through the lateral pons ➡ and root entry zone ➡ of CNV. Less than 5% of patients with TN have a venous explanation for their symptoms.*

Hemifacial Spasm

KEY FACTS

TERMINOLOGY

- Definition: Vascular loop compressing facial nerve at its root exit zone within cerebellopontine angle (CPA) cistern causing hemifacial spasm

IMAGING

- High-resolution T2WI MR or source MRA images show serpentine asymmetric signal void (vessel) in medial CPA
  - AICA (50%) > PICA (30%) > VA (15%) > vein (5%)

TOP DIFFERENTIAL DIAGNOSES

- Aneurysm, CPA-internal auditory canal
- Arteriovenous malformation, CPA
- Developmental venous anomaly, posterior fossa

PATHOLOGY

- CNVII bundle experiences "irritation" from vessel
- Rare, nonvascular causes of hemifacial spasms (HFS)
  - Multiple sclerosis
  - Cisternal masses
    - Epidermoid, meningioma, schwannoma
  - Temporal bone and parotid lesions
    - Perineural CNVII malignancy

CLINICAL ISSUES

- Clinical presentation
  - Unilateral involuntary facial spasms (HFS)
  - HFS begins with orbicularis oculi spasms
  - Tonic-clonic bursts become constant over time
- Microvascular decompression is highly effective

DIAGNOSTIC CHECKLIST

- Positive MR findings present in ~ 50% HFS patients
- 1st look for cisternal mass lesions, multiple sclerosis
- Then follow CNVII distally into temporal bone and parotid
  - Exclude CNVII venous malformation, parotid malignancy
- Determine if MRA source images or high-resolution T2WI images identify causal vessel

(Left) *Axial MRA source image in a patient with right hemifacial spasm shows a tortuous right vertebral artery ➡ and associated PICA ➡ pushing on the root exit zone of the facial nerve. The facial nerve is visible in the cerebellopontine angle (CPA) cistern ➡.* **(Right)** *Axial CISS MR through the CPA cisterns in a patient with a right hemifacial spasm demonstrates a PICA loop ➡ pushing the cisternal CNVII and CNVII posteriorly, causing them to drape over the posterior margin of the porus acusticus ➡.*

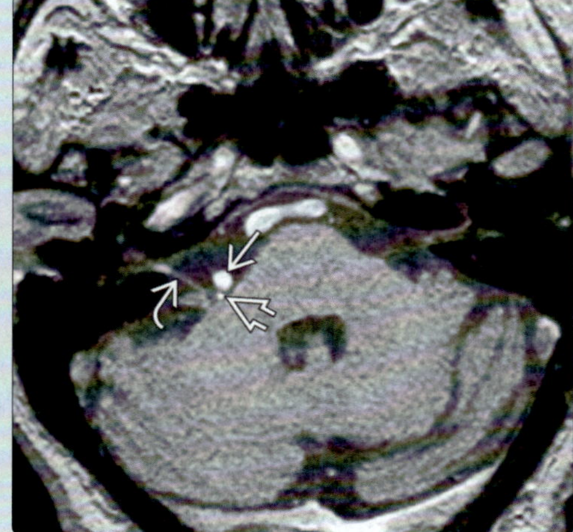

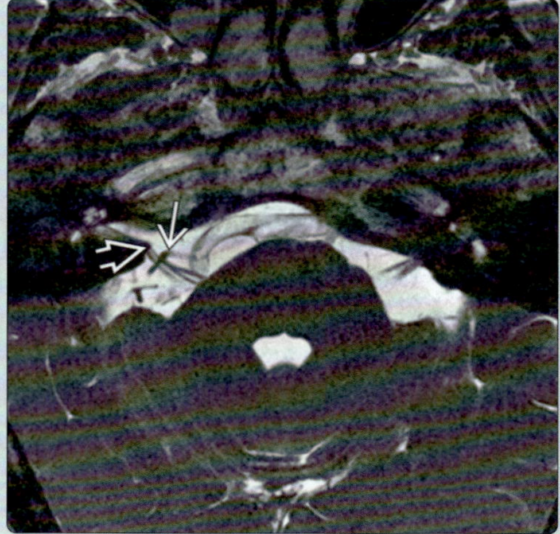

(Left) *Axial CISS MR in a patient with left hemifacial spasm reveals the left vertebral artery ➡ looping into the CPA cistern where it impinges on the proximal facial nerve ➡ at the root exit zone.* **(Right)** *Axial T2WI MR reveals a dolichoectatic vertebral artery ➡ impinging on the root exit zone ➡ of the facial nerve in the medial CPA cistern in this patient with hemifacial spasm. Approximately 50% of patients with hemifacial spasm have positive MR findings, typically on thin-section T2 or MRA sequences.*

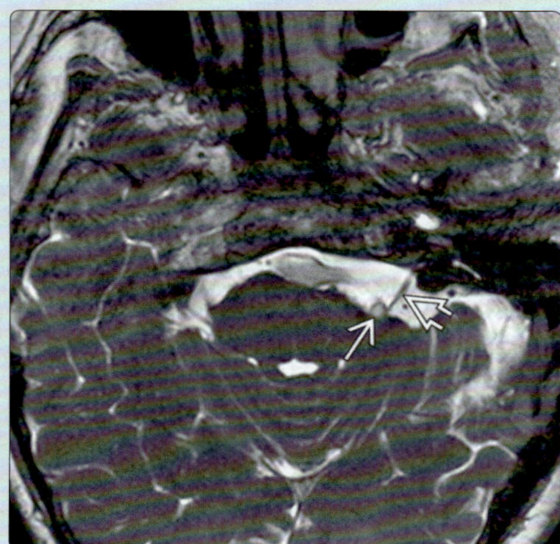

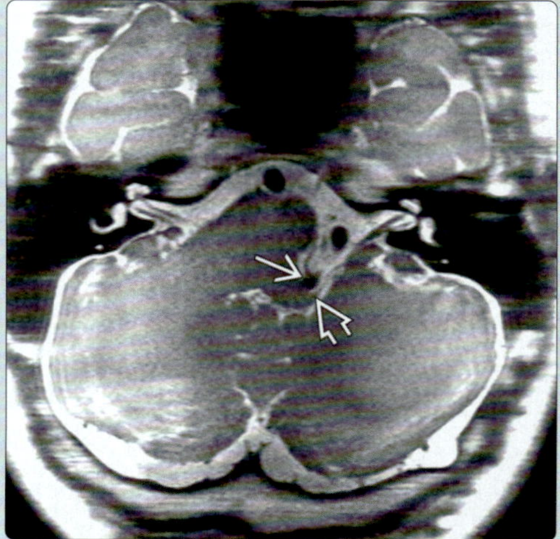

CPA-IAC Aneurysm

KEY FACTS

TERMINOLOGY

- Focal ballooning or fusiform dilatation of posterior inferior cerebellar artery (PICA), vertebral artery (VA), or anterior inferior cerebellar artery (AICA) in CPA-IAC cistern

IMAGING

- CPA aneurysm incidence: PICA > VA > AICA
  - 10% all intracranial aneurysms are vertebrobasilar
- CPA-IAC aneurysm: Mass with **calcified rim** (CT) or layered **complex signal** in wall (MR)
- CECT of partially thrombosed aneurysm
  - Complex mass with central or eccentric enhancing lumen, nonenhancing mural thrombus
  - Often has **calcified rim**
- CTA: Shows neck and originating artery (PICA, VA, AICA)
- MR findings
  - MR complex signal from Ca^{++}, clot, flow
  - T1: **Subacute luminal clot** is **hyperintense** secondary to **methemoglobin T1 shortening**
  - T2: Signal varies from hypointense flow void to **complex mixed-signal** appearance
- Angiogram: Visible lumen may be smaller than overall aneurysm if clot is present
  - May **underestimate** aneurysm size

TOP DIFFERENTIAL DIAGNOSES

- Vertebrobasilar dolichoectasia
- Dural arteriovenous fistula + venous varix
- Arteriovenous malformation

CLINICAL ISSUES

- Clinical presentation
  - Sensorineural hearing loss (70%)
  - Headache from subarachnoid hemorrhage (50%)
  - Hemifacial spasm or facial nerve palsy
- Treatment options
  - Surgical clipping
  - Endovascular coiling depending on configuration

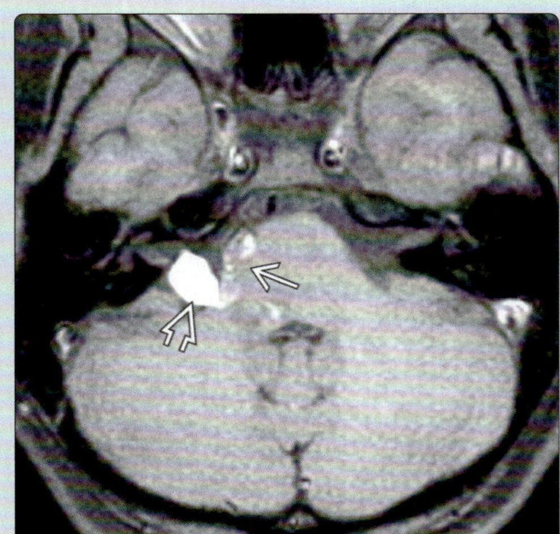

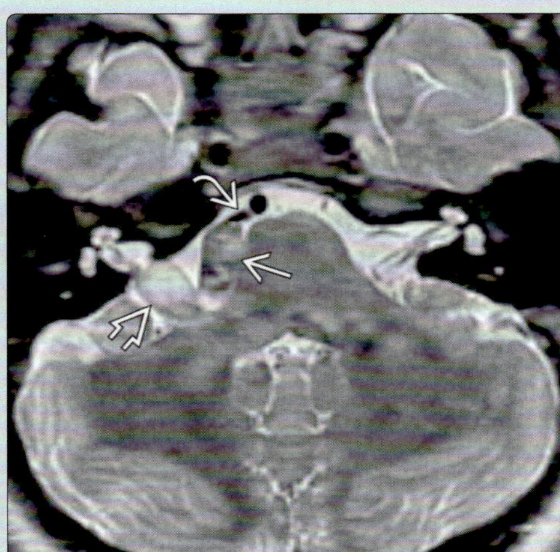

(Left) *Axial T1WI MR shows a tubular hyperintense mass extending laterally from the basilar artery into the CPA cistern. The more medial portion of the mass shows complex signal from flow and subacute clot ➡, while the more lateral component is completely thrombosed and filled with high-signal subacute clot ➡.* **(Right)** *Axial T2WI MR in the same patient reveals the patent PICA-AICA complex takeoff from the basilar artery ➡ with areas of partial ➡ and complete thrombosis ➡ of the aneurysm.*

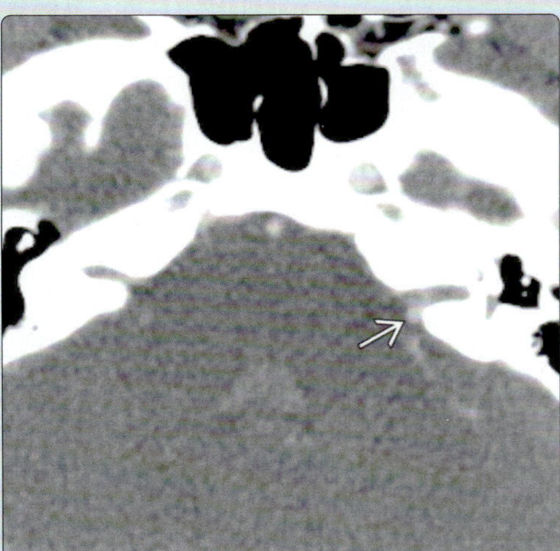

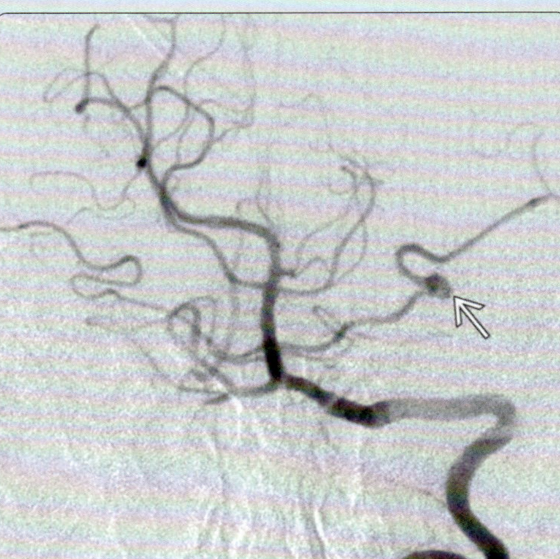

(Left) *Axial CTA through the IAC demonstrates a focal area of enhancement on the posterior margin of the porus acusticus ➡.* **(Right)** *Anteroposterior left vertebral angiogram in the same patient demonstrates the AICA aneurysm ➡ looping into the vicinity of the internal auditory canal. AICA aneurysm in the CPA-IAC is the rarest of the aneurysms affecting the CPA-IAC area.*

INDEX

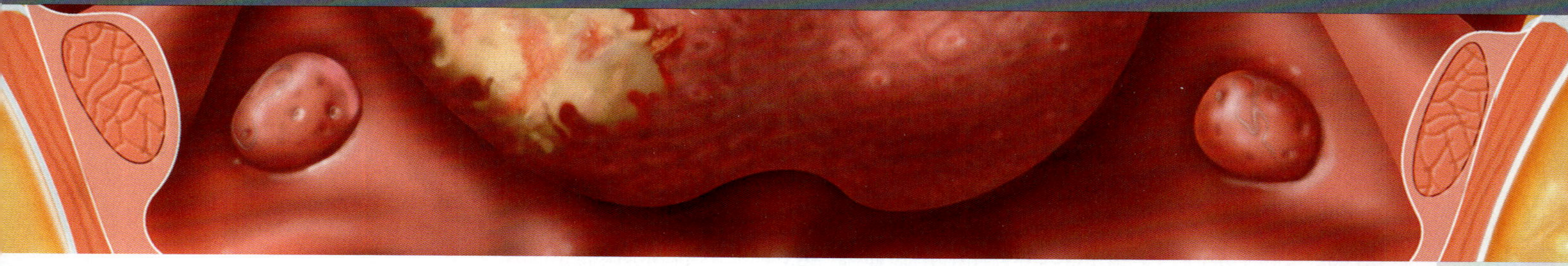

A

INDEX

B

C

INDEX

INDEX

INDEX

INDEX

D

INDEX

E

F

G

H

I

INDEX

J

INDEX

K

L

INDEX

M

INDEX

INDEX

N

INDEX

P

INDEX

INDEX

INDEX

R

S

INDEX

INDEX

INDEX

INDEX

T

INDEX

INDEX

INDEX

U

V

W

X

Z